BSAVA Manual of Canine and Feline Anaesthesia and Analgesia
third edition

Editors:

Tanya Duke-Novakovski
BVetMed MSc DVA DipACVAA DipECVAA
Department of Small Animal Clinical Sciences,
Western College of Veterinary Medicine,
University of Saskatchewan, Saskatoon, SK S7N 5B4, Canada

Marieke de Vries
CertVA DipECVAA DVM MRCVS
Davies Veterinary Specialists,
Manor Farm Business Park, Higham Gobion, Hertfordshire SG5 3HR, UK

Chris Seymour
MA VetMB DVA DipECVAA PGCert(MedEd) FHEA MRCVS
Royal Veterinary College, University of London,
Hawkshead Lane, North Mymms, Hatfield, Hertfordshire AL9 7TA, UK

Published by:

British Small Animal Veterinary Association
Woodrow House, 1 Telford Way,
Waterwells Business Park, Quedgeley,
Gloucester GL2 2AB

A Company Limited by Guarantee in England
Registered Company No. 2837793
Registered as a Charity

First edition 1999 · Second edition 2007 · Third edition 2016
Reprinted 2017, 2018, 2019, 2020, 2021, 2022
Copyright © 2022 BSAVA

T0340735

Figures 16.1, 18.4, 19.6, 22.10 and 24.6 were drawn by S.J. Elmhurst BA Hons (www.livingart.org.uk) and are printed with her permission.

A catalogue record for this book is available from the British Library.

ISBN 978 1 905319 61 9

The publishers, editors and contributors cannot take responsibility for information provided on dosages and methods of application of drugs mentioned or referred to in this publication. Details of this kind must be verified in each case by individual users from up to date literature published by the manufacturers or suppliers of those drugs. Veterinary surgeons are reminded that in each case they must follow all appropriate national legislation and regulations (for example, in the United Kingdom, the prescribing cascade) from time to time in force.

Printed in the UK by Cambrian Printers Ltd., Pontllanfraith NP12 2YA
Printed on ECF paper made from sustainable forests

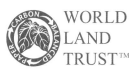

www.carbonbalancedpaper.com
CBP006075

Carbon Balancing is delivered by World Land Trust, an international conservation charity, who protects the world's most biologically important and threatened habitats acre by acre. Their Carbon Balanced Programme offsets emissions through the purchase and preservation of high conservation value forests.

17840PUBS22

Titles in the BSAVA Manuals series

For further information on these and all BSAVA publications, please visit our website: **www.bsava.com**

Contents

Contributors

Hatim I.K. Alibhai
BVSc MVM PhD DipECVAA FHEA
Royal Veterinary College, University of London,
Hawkshead Lane, North Mymms,
Hatfield, Hertfordshire AL9 7TA, UK

Adam Auckburally
BVSc CertVA DipECVAA FHEA MRCVS
School of Veterinary Medicine,
University of Glasgow,
Bearsden Road, Glasgow G61 1QH, UK

Kieran Borgeat
BSc BVSc MVetMed CertVC DipACVIM DipECVIM-CA (Cardiology)
MRCVS
Highcroft Veterinary Referrals,
615 Wells Road, Bristol BS14 9BE, UK

Jacqueline C. Brearley
MA VetMB PhD DVA DipECVAA MRCA MRCVS
Department of Veterinary Medicine,
University of Cambridge,
Madingley Road, Cambridge CB3 OES, UK

Andrew Claude
DVM DipACVAA
College of Veterinary Medicine,
Mississippi State University, MS 39762, USA

Marieke de Vries
CertVA DipECVAA DVM MRCVS
Davies Veterinary Specialists,
Manor Farm Business Park, Higham Gobion,
Hertfordshire SG5 3HR, UK

Tanya Duke-Novakovski
BVetMed MSc DVA DipACVAA DipECVAA
Department of Small Animal Clinical Sciences,
Western College of Veterinary Medicine,
University of Saskatchewan,
Saskatoon, SK S7N 5B4, Canada

Christine M. Egger
DVM MVSc CVA CVH DipACVAA
College of Veterinary Medicine,
University of Tennessee,
Knoxville, TN 37996, USA

Derek Flaherty
BVMS DVA DipECVAA MRCA FHEA MRCVS
School of Veterinary Medicine,
University of Glasgow,
Bearsden Road, Glasgow G61 1QH, UK

Tamara Grubb
DVM PhD DipACVAA
College of Veterinary Medicine,
Washington State University,
Pullman, WA 99164, USA

Matthew Gurney
BVSc CertVA DipECVAA MRCVS
Northwest Surgeons,
Delamere House, Ashville Point,
Sutton Weaver, Cheshire WA7 3FW, UK

Richard Hammond
BVetMed BSc(Hons) MMedSci(MedEd) PhD DVA DipECVAA FHEA
MRCVS
School of Veterinary Sciences,
University of Bristol,
Langford House, Langford,
North Somerset BS40 5DU, UK

Lynne Hughes
MVB DipECVAA DVA FCARCSI MRCVS
School of Veterinary Medicine, Veterinary Sciences
Centre, University College Dublin,
Belfield, Dublin 4, Ireland

Colette Jolliffe
BVetMed CertVA DipECVAA MRCVS
Animal Health Trust, Lanwades Park,
Kentford, Suffolk CB8 7UU, UK

Ronald S. Jones OBE
MVSc Dr Med Vet DVSc DVA DipECVAA DipACVAA CBiol FSB FLS
FRSA FRCA FRCVS
School of Veterinary Science, University of Liverpool,
Leahurst Campus, Chester High Road,
Neston, Cheshire CH64 7TE, UK

Sabine B.R. Kästner
Prof Dr med vet MVet Sci, DipECVAA
Tierärztliche Hochschule Hannover, Klinik für Kleintiere,
Bünteweg 9, D-30559 Hannover

Carolyn L. Kerr
DVM DVSc PhD DipACVAA
Department of Clinical Studies,
Ontario Veterinary College, University of Guelph,
Guelph, Ontario, Canada

Mary P. Klinck
BSc DVM DipACVB
Faculté de Médecine Vétérinaire, Université de Montréal,
Saint Hyacinthe, Québec, Canada

Elizabeth A. Leece
BVSc CVA DipECVAA MRCVS
Dick White Referrals,
Veterinary Specialist Centre, Station Farm,
London Road, Six Mile Bottom,
Cambridgeshire CB8 0UH, UK

Samantha Lindley
BVSc MRCVS
School of Veterinary Medicine,
University of Glasgow,
Bearsden Road, Glasgow G61 1QH, UK

Robert E. Meyer
DVM DipACVAA
College of Veterinary Medicine,
Mississippi State University,
MS 39762, USA

Lisa Milella
BVSc DipEVDC
53 Parvis Road, Byfleet, Surrey KT14 7AA, UK

Martina Mosing
DipECVAA PD
Division of Anaesthesiology,
Equine Department Vetsuisse-Faculty,
University of Zürich Winterthurerstr. 258 c,
8057 Zürich, Switzerland

Pamela J. Murison
BVMS PhD DipECVAA DVA FHEA MRCVS
Royal (Dick) School of Veterinary Studies,
University of Edinburgh,
Easter Bush, Midlothian EH25 9RG, UK

Joanna C. Murrell
BVSc(Hons) PhD DipECVAA MRCVS
School of Veterinary Sciences, University of Bristol,
Langford House, Langford,
North Somerset BS40 5DU, UK

Daniel S.J. Pang
BVSc PhD DipECVAA DipACVAA MRCVS
Department of Veterinary Clinical and
Diagnostic Sciences, Faculty of Veterinary Medicine,
University of Calgary, 3280 Hospital Dr NW,
Calgary, Alberta T2N 4Z6, Canada

Peter J. Pascoe
BVSc DVA DipACVAA DipECVAA
Department of Surgical and Radiological Sciences,
School of Veterinary Medicine, University of California,
Davis, CA 95616, USA

Ludovic Pelligand
Dr med vet Cert VA DipECVAA DipECVPT FHEA PhD MRCVS
Royal Veterinary College, University of London,
Hawkshead Lane, North Mymms,
Hatfield, Hertfordshire AL9 7TA, UK

Lysa P. Posner
DVM DipACVAA
College of Veterinary Medicine,
North Carolina State University,
1060 William Moore Drive,
Raleigh, NC 27607, USA

Clara F. Rigotti
DVM PhD MRCVS
School of Veterinary Science, University of Liverpool,
Leahurst Campus, Chester High Road,
Neston, Cheshire CH64 7TE, UK

Eva Rioja Garcia
DVM DVSc PhD DipACVAA MRCVS
School of Veterinary Science,
University of Liverpool,
Leahurst Campus, Chester High Road,
Neston, Cheshire CH64 7TE, UK

Rebecca Robinson
BVSc MVetMed DipECVAA MRCVS
Animal Health Trust,
Lanwades Park, Kentford,
Suffolk CB8 7UU, UK

Sandra Sanchis Mora
DVM MVetMed MRCVS
Royal Veterinary College, University of London,
Hawkshead Lane, North Mymms,
Hatfield, Hertfordshire AL9 7TA, UK

Stijn Schauvliege
DVM PhD DipECVAA
Department of Surgery and Anaesthesiology of
Domestic Animals, Faculty of Veterinary Medicine,
Ghent University, Salisburylaan 133,
B-9820 Merelbeke, Belgium

Ian Self
BSc BVSc PGCert Vet Ed FHEA CertVA DipECVAA MRCVS
School of Veterinary Medicine and Science,
University of Nottingham,
College Road, Sutton Bonington,
Loughborough, Leicestershire LE12 5RD, UK

Chris Seymour
MA VetMB DVA DipECVAA PGCert(MedEd) FHEA MRCVS
Royal Veterinary College, University of London,
Hawkshead Lane, North Mymms, Hatfield,
Hertfordshire AL9 7TA, UK

Julie A. Smith
DVM DipACVAA
MedVet Medical and Cancer Centers for Pets,
300 E. Wilson Bridge Road,
Worthington, OH 43085, USA

Eric Troncy
DV MSc PhD DUn
Faculté de Médecine Vétérinaire,
Université de Montréal, Saint Hyacinthe,
Québec, Canada

Kata O. Veres-Nyéki
Dr Med Vet DipECVAA PhD MRCVS
Royal Veterinary College, University of London,
Hawkshead Lane,
North Mymms, Hatfield,
Hertfordshire AL9 7TA, UK

Foreword

I am pleased to have the opportunity to write the 'Foreword' for this third edition of the *BSAVA Manual of Canine and Feline Anaesthesia and Analgesia*. Anaesthetic drugs have not changed greatly since the last edition nine years ago but the manner in which they are used has done so, and equipment and monitoring devices are always evolving. This new edition reflects the continuing need for sophisticated and supportive techniques of anaesthesia and analgesia necessitated by the advances in veterinary diagnosis and surgery. Owners of pets expect that their animal can receive the same treatments as they themselves may receive; no longer is 'too old' or 'too sick' considered a reason not to treat.

The majority of the chapters have been extensively updated by the original or by new authors, most of whom are experienced Diplomates of the relevant American or European Colleges. Some new chapters have been added. For example, there are now five chapters on analgesia; assessment of pain is awarded a full chapter, as is the treatment of chronic pain. This reflects the continuing emphasis placed on providing perioperative pain relief for our patients. There is a new chapter on providing cardiovascular support during anaesthesia, and in addition the chapter on cardiovascular disease provides a comprehensive account of such conditions in animals, including diagnosis and effects. Other chapters on anaesthesia for 'special' conditions cover the majority of situations likely to be met in small animal general or referral practice. A chapter on anaesthesia for MRI is a very useful addition, as this procedure involves a number of special problems. The final chapter is about complications, accidents and emergencies, but if the words of wisdom earlier in the book are heeded, hopefully the need for this last chapter will be very rare.

The first BSAVA book on small animal anaesthesia, published in 1979, was a very slim handbook which provided a simple guide for those working in general practice. The book 'metamorphosed' through various editions to this *Manual of Canine and Feline Anaesthesia and Analgesia*, with each new version expanding the depth of the subject. The final result is now a comprehensive textbook for all small animal veterinary surgeons wishing to advance their knowledge in veterinary anaesthesia.

I thank the Editors, their authors and the BSAVA team assisting them from behind the scenes for all their work and congratulate them on the final outcome.

K.W. Clarke
MA VetMB DVetMed DVA DipECVAA FRCVS
Honorary Professor of Veterinary Anaesthesia,
Royal Veterinary College, London, UK

Preface

The provision of safe anaesthesia and optimal analgesia is an ethical obligation for all practitioners in the veterinary field. There is an increasing awareness not only among veterinary surgeons (veterinarians) but also the general public that veterinary anaesthesia is – indeed literally – a vital discipline within the veterinary profession.

Nine years have passed since the last edition of this manual was published. Although the basic principles may not have changed much, veterinary anaesthesia and analgesia is a speciality that continues to progress. This new manual provides in-depth and up-to-date coverage of all aspects of canine and feline anaesthesia and analgesia. Not only have new anaesthetic and analgesic drugs appeared over the last decade, but also old techniques have been refined and new ones developed. Compared with the last edition, chapters have been updated with the latest available knowledge and, where possible, with evidence-based information. Detailed illustrations have been included in several chapters to visually enhance understanding of the text. A new chapter is specifically dedicated to anaesthesia of patients undergoing magnetic resonance imaging; a topic worthy of inclusion considering the increased use of this diagnostic imaging technique in veterinary practice.

Although there is still much scope for improvement, fortunately both recognition and treatment of acute and chronic pain in our patients have undergone tremendous development during the last 10 years and clear evidence exists that the use of multimodal analgesic protocols should be advocated. To emphasize this development, five chapters are specifically dedicated to the pathophysiology of pain, pain recognition and scoring, and to various analgesic agents, local anaesthetic and adjuvant analgesic techniques.

This manual is by no means meant to be the 'Holy Grail' of veterinary anaesthetic and analgesic wisdom. A thorough understanding of all aspects of perioperative medicine and familiarity with anaesthetic drugs and protocols is as important to provide safe anaesthesia as the use of the latest, state of the art techniques. However, it is time to step back from applying fixed anaesthetic protocols, and to regard each of our patients as unique individuals for which an individual protocol should be considered. Our aim is for this manual to be used as a reference and guide, to provide extra knowledge behind the rationales for drug choices and techniques, and to support a logical approach to the development of anaesthetic protocols.

We would like to express our gratitude to all those authors involved in writing this manual; their combined knowledge and expertise will hopefully make this manual a worthwhile aid in ensuring the provision of optimal anaesthesia and analgesia in our much loved patients. We are also very grateful to all of those at the BSAVA involved in the successful completion of this the third edition of the *BSAVA Manual of Canine and Feline Anaesthesia and Analgesia*.

Tanya Duke-Novakovski
Marieke de Vries
Chris Seymour
April 2016

Chapter 1

The practice of veterinary anaesthesia and analgesia: legal and ethical aspects

Ronald S. Jones

The most fundamental consideration in the practice of veterinary medicine and surgery is the health and welfare of the animals that are entrusted to our care. The prevention of pain and suffering is paramount. Although there have been dramatic developments in pain assessment and treatment in animals over the past 25 years, there is still considerable scope for improvement. Pain is a subjective experience that is dependent both on the mental and physical state of the patient and its environment. In animals, the perception of pain has to be inferred because they lack the ability to communicate verbally with humans. There are, however, no anatomical or physiological reasons to assume that animals do not perceive pain in a similar manner to humans. There are certain differences in the manifestation of, and responses to, pain, but these can be attributed to species variation. This is a basic aspect of pain in animal species; for example, different behavioural reactions are observed in the cat and horse in response to a given painful stimulus.

Aims of anaesthesia and analgesia

In general, the aims of anaesthesia and analgesia are to:

- Prevent awareness of, and response to, pain
- Provide restraint and immobility of the animal and relaxation of skeletal muscles when this is required for a particular procedure
- Achieve both of the above without jeopardizing the life and safety of the animal before, during and after anaesthesia.

Until relatively recently, it was thought that a single drug could achieve all of these aims, and occasionally this is still true. However, the trend in modern anaesthesia is to use several drugs with selective and complementary actions. The term *balanced anaesthesia* refers to the use of smaller doses of a combination of drugs to achieve the various components of anaesthesia, thus reducing the disadvantages associated with using large doses of any one drug. Balanced anaesthesia also offers a multidimensional approach to pain control; not only does it help to block autonomic responses to surgery and provide analgesia postoperatively, but it may also pre-empt postoperative hypersensitivity to pain.

Choice of anaesthetic technique

The choice of anaesthetic technique is influenced by a wide range of factors, including:

- **Facilities.** If facilities are poor and likely to prejudice the outcome of anaesthesia, they should not be used. For example, a well–administered intravenous technique may be much safer than an inhalational agent delivered with inferior equipment
- **Skill and experience of the anaesthetist and surgeon.** These are extremely important and particularly evident when working as a team
- **Facilities for postoperative recovery and care.** These are important considerations when deciding whether the animal is to be hospitalized or returned to its owner following anaesthesia (see legal aspects below). It is imperative to ensure that adequate postoperative analgesia is provided
- **Temperament of the animal.** In animals of good temperament, only minimal sedative pre-anaesthetic medication may be required before the intravenous induction of anaesthesia. Competent and sympathetic assistance in restraint can be invaluable. Some cats may be so unruly that crush cages or inhalation anaesthetic induction chambers are needed. Aggressive dogs and cats may require heavy sedation, which can influence the subsequent doses of drugs for both induction and maintenance of anaesthesia
- **Species and breed of animal.** Some breeds respond adversely to intravenous agents, and some Boxers are sensitive to acepromazine (see Chapter 2)
- **Age of the animal.** Doses of anaesthetic agents may need to be reduced in both young and elderly animals. In very young kittens and puppies, inhalational agents are generally the drugs of choice for induction and maintenance of anaesthesia. Smaller size and impaired thermoregulatory mechanisms predispose to hypothermia (see Chapter 30)
- **Health status of the animal.** Physical status is often classified according to the categories of the American Society of Anesthesiologists (ASA) (see Chapter 2). Endotoxaemia is one of the most important disease conditions as it is often accompanied by cardiac problems often accompanied by haemodynamic instability. Great caution is needed in the administration of precalculated doses of intravenous anaesthetic

drugs to such animals, which may require much lower doses than healthy animals. In addition, sick animals may have a longer circulation time, which should be taken into consideration in order to avoid anaesthetic overdose. Problems with fluid balance should be corrected and, for example, diabetic animals stabilized before the induction of anaesthesia. It is important to ensure that animals are in optimal health before anaesthesia for non-urgent procedures, even if this means deferring anaesthesia for some days

- **Site and nature of the procedure.** Endotracheal intubation is mandatory for oral, dental and pharyngeal surgery. Special care must be taken during these procedures to prevent the accumulation of blood, fluid and other detritus in the pharynx, which may be inhaled after removal of the endotracheal tube. The use of an endoscope within the respiratory tract presents difficulties because of competition for the airway, and anaesthetic techniques need to be adapted to deal with this problem
- **Use of neuromuscular blocking agents.** Intermittent positive pressure ventilation (IPPV) is essential when these drugs are used as part of an anaesthetic technique, e.g. for ocular, abdominal, thoracic and some orthopaedic procedures
- **Anaesthesia for Caesarean section.** This requires special techniques as multiple lives are involved (see Chapter 26)
- **Examination under anaesthesia.** Although such procedures often require only short periods of anaesthesia, the same high level of care is required. The adage that 'there may be minor procedures but never minor anaesthetics' certainly applies
- **Proposed duration of surgery.** Short procedures can often be performed with a single dose of an intravenous drug. If required, anaesthesia may be extended for short periods with incremental doses. However, even under these circumstances, equipment must be readily available to carry out endotracheal intubation, administer oxygen and provide IPPV if necessary. In situations where the procedure is likely to be prolonged, it is important to ensure that either proper inhalation anaesthetic techniques or total intravenous anaesthesia (TIVA), is used.

Legislation

Veterinary Surgeons Act 1966

In the UK, the practice of veterinary medicine and surgery is governed by the Veterinary Surgeons Act 1966. Under the provisions of that Act, no person may practise unless they are registered with the Royal College of Veterinary Surgeons (RCVS). There are certain minor exceptions under Schedule 3, which relate to certain procedures that may be performed by veterinary nurses or by trained lay personnel. None of these exemptions apply to the induction and maintenance of anaesthesia in animals.

Protection of Animals (Anaesthetics) Act 1964

The Protection of Animals (Anaesthetics) Act 1964 governs anaesthesia of animals in the UK. It basically states that the performance of any operation, with or without the use of instruments and involving interference with the sensitive tissues or bone structures of an animal, shall constitute an offence unless an anaesthetic is administered to prevent any pain to the animal during the operation. Some exceptions to this general rule are included in the Act. They include:

- Castration of farm animals up to certain ages (anaesthesia is always required for the castration of dogs and cats)
- Amputation of the dewclaws of a dog before its eyes are open
- Any minor operation performed by a veterinary surgeon which by reason of its quickness or painlessness is customarily performed without the use of an anaesthetic
- Any minor operation (whether performed by a veterinary surgeon or some other person) which is not customarily performed by a veterinary surgeon. Other procedures not covered in the previous sentence are listed in the Act but apply mainly to farm animals.

Misuse of Drugs Act 1971

In the UK, the Misuse of Drugs Act 1971 and its various regulations, including the regulations in 2001, govern the use of several drugs that are administered to cats and dogs to provide anaesthesia and analgesia. The regulations impose legal obligations on all veterinary surgeons (as well as doctors, dentists, pharmacists and nurses) prescribing, supplying and administering these drugs, which relate mainly to the potential for harm to, and abuse by, humans.

- Schedule 1 Controlled Drugs (such as cannabis and LSD) have no veterinary use and veterinary surgeons have no authority to prescribe them.
- Schedule 2 Controlled Drugs include morphine, fentanyl, methadone and ketamine. A record of their purchase and supply must be kept in a Controlled Drugs Register (see below). A handwritten requisition is required by a supplier/wholesaler before delivery is permitted. When writing treatment orders for a Schedule 2 Controlled Drug (e.g. on inpatient kennel sheets), it is a legal requirement to specify both the dose in mg/kg and the volume in millilitres.
- Schedule 3 Controlled Drugs include buprenorphine and barbiturates. These drugs require a written requisition to the supplier/wholesaler but their purchase and use do not have to be recorded in the Controlled Drugs Register.
- Schedule 4 Controlled Drugs include benzodiazepines and are exempt from most controls.
- Schedule 5 Controlled Drugs include preparations of certain Controlled Drugs (such as codeine and morphine) which are exempt from full control when present in medicinal products of low strength.

Controlled Drugs must be kept in a locked safe/cabinet that can be opened only by an authorized person or with their consent. The cabinet should preferably be made of steel, with suitable hinges, and fixed to a wall or floor with anchor bolts (which should not be accessible from outside the cabinet). Ideally, the safe/cabinet should be within a cupboard or in some other position to avoid easy detection by intruders. In addition, the room containing the cabinet should be lockable. A locked motor vehicle is *not* classed as a as a locked receptacle. It makes good sense to store all Schedule 3 drugs (with Schedule 2 drugs) in the Controlled Drugs cabinet.

The Controlled Drugs Register must:

- Be either a computerized system or a bound book, which does not include any form of loose-leaf register or card index
- Be separated into sections for each class of drug
- Have a separate page for each strength and form of a particular drug, which must be specified at the top of each page
- Have the entries in chronological order and made on the day of the transaction or, if this is not reasonably practicable, the next day
- Have the entries written in ink or in a computerized form in which every entry is capable of being audited
- Have no cancellations, obliterations or alterations
- Be kept on the premises to which it relates and be available for inspection at any time. A separate register must be kept for each premises
- Not be used for any other purpose
- Be kept for a minimum of **2 years** after the date of the last entry.

Further information is available on the websites of the BSAVA (www.bsava.com/Resources/BSAVAMedicinesGuide/ControlledDrugs.aspx) and the Veterinary Medicines Directorate (www.vmd.defra.gov.uk/pdf/vmgn/VMGNote20.pdf).

Controlled Drugs in Schedules 1 and 2 may be destroyed only in the presence of a person authorized by the Secretary of State, e.g. a police officer or Home Office inspector. Such an authorized person is required to be present for the destruction of all out-of-date stock items in Schedule 1 or 2. Details of the drug being destroyed must be entered in the Controlled Drugs Register, including the drug name, form, strength and quantity, as well as the date of destruction and signature of the person in whose presence the drug was destroyed.

Although the legislation may differ in detail from country to country (and between states and provinces within certain countries), similar laws apply to the secure storage and record keeping of this group of drugs.

Animals (Scientific Procedures) Act 1986

The Animals (Scientific Procedures) Act 1986 governs the use and care of experimental animals for research purposes. It is specific about the use of analgesic and anaesthetic agents. Similar legislation exists in the European Union and there is federal legislation in the USA. The Canadian Council on Animal Care issues welfare guidelines for animals used for research in Canada, including guidelines on anaesthetic and analgesic use.

Animal Welfare Act 2006

The Animal Welfare Act 2006 is an all-embracing Act relating to animal welfare. It sets out the duties of owners and keepers of animals and, in addition, covers mutilations of animals.

Duty of care

The principles of the duty of care, as defined in *Halsbury's Laws of England*, apply equally to veterinary surgeons as to medical practitioners, with one distinct difference, namely that the duty of care is to the client/animal owner when making a number of decisions relating to anaesthesia. These include:

- A duty of care when deciding whether anaesthesia may be performed with a reasonable degree of safety
- A duty of care in the selection of the most appropriate anaesthetic technique
- A duty of care in the administration of the anaesthetic
- A duty of care in fully consulting other veterinary surgeons dealing with the case and offering full and proper advice to the animal owner.

Negligence

Veterinary surgeons (veterinarians) must bring to their task a reasonable degree of skill and knowledge and must exercise a reasonable degree of care. Whether this has been done is a matter that must be determined by the facts pertaining to each individual case. It is clear, however, that failure to do so, which results in injury to (or death of) an animal, will give the owner the right to bring a legal action for damages. In general, a veterinary surgeon in general practice will be judged against the standard of the good, careful and competent general practitioner. This has been established in the English Courts and is known as the *Bolam Test*. It has been subsequently refined by application of the *Bolitho Test*, which would suggest that veterinary surgeons of specialist or consultant status will be judged against the standard of their peers.

There is also the important aspect of the responsibility of a veterinary surgeon for the negligence of any person assisting them with anaesthesia of an animal. In general practice, it is likely that a veterinary surgeon, as an employer, would be responsible for the negligence of an employee. It is likely that when assessing an action for negligence of a lay assistant, the Courts would take into account the assistant's level of training and qualifications. Hence, it is essential to ensure that any person asked to assist with anaesthesia is competent to carry out the tasks assigned to them.

While it is relatively rare for claims for negligence to be brought in relation to anaesthesia, there have been two relatively high-profile actions brought against veterinary surgeons in recent years. These involved dogs being returned to their owners before they were fully recovered from anaesthesia; both animals died. The Courts found the veterinary surgeons to be negligent in both cases.

There is often confusion between negligence and disgraceful professional conduct, which could lead to disciplinary action by the RCVS. Negligence *per se* does not necessarily amount to disgraceful professional conduct unless it is so gross and excessive that it is likely to bring the veterinary profession into disrepute. It is only then that a disciplinary action may ensue.

Consent

There is a distinct difference in law between the duty to obtain consent from an owner for a particular procedure to be carried out on an animal, and the duty to inform the owner of the material risks. While there is considerably more information and case law on the subject in human medicine than in the veterinary field, it is reasonable to assume that the Courts would follow a similar course of action. Failure to obtain consent may constitute a trespass, whereas failure to warn of material risks may give rise to an obligation to compensate for damages caused by that breach of duty. It could result in a claim for compensation in respect of a complication or adverse effect of the treatment even if the procedure was conducted properly. Consent is a state of mind – a decision by the animal owner (or occasionally by their agent). The competent adult owner, over 18 years of age, has a fundamental right under common law to give or withhold consent to examination, investigation or treatment of their animal. Consent may be *implied or express*:

- **Consent is implied** when an owner brings an animal to a veterinary surgeon for examination and there is physical contact between the veterinary surgeon and the animal. Implied consent does not necessarily imply that the material risks of any procedures have been explained or understood
- **Express consent** should be obtained for any procedure that carries a material risk. This, of course, applies to anaesthesia or sedation. While express consent may be obtained orally or in writing, it is always preferable to obtain written consent wherever possible. It is not acceptable for an owner to sign a blank piece of paper. It is essential that they have given their consent for a procedure and that there is evidence that the material risks have been explained to them, although it is a matter of judgement as to how much information is provided. It is important, but not always easy, to give the owner time to reflect on the information they have been given. In the exceptional situation that verbal consent is obtained, it is essential that a record of the advice offered, and that consent was given, be written in the case notes with a time and date. Written consent is not necessary to defend an action, although it provides evidence that consent was obtained.

It may occasionally be necessary to provide treatment and carry out a procedure without consent. This situation is rare, except for life-saving procedures where it is not possible to contact the animal owner. When this is done, a note should be made in the case notes to explain the absence of formal consent.

Adult owners have a right to refuse consent to a particular procedure with or without good reason. If the owner refuses consent for an anaesthetic or sedation procedure that is considered to be the most appropriate, then reasonable attempts should be made to persuade the owner that the technique carries the least risk of adverse sequelae. However, it is not acceptable to coerce owners into consenting to a specific technique. In certain situations it may be necessary to point out to owners that a failure to prevent suffering may breach animal welfare legislation. A copy of the specimen consent form recommended by the RCVS can be accessed via their website (www.rcvs.org.uk/home/).

A veterinary surgeon may administer a veterinary medicine outside the datasheet recommendations ('off-label'), a specially prepared medicine or an imported medicine under certain circumstances. The veterinary surgeon should explain fully what is involved and ideally obtain the owner's consent. If there are any concerns regarding this matter, veterinary surgeons are advised to consult their defence or insurance company. It is also necessary to inform the owner and obtain their informed consent when drugs or appliances are being used in a clinical trial.

When veterinary surgeons wish to carry out clinical trials on animals, they are strongly advised to seek an ethical review of their proposed project. While it is relatively easy for veterinary surgeons working in academic institutions to gain access to ethical committees, it is less straightforward for those in general practice, who are therefore strongly advised to seek advice from colleagues working in such institutions. Advice is available from the Association of Veterinary Anaesthetists Ethical Review Group.

Personnel

The role of the veterinary nurse or veterinary technician in anaesthesia has been a subject of considerable debate within the veterinary profession. It is well accepted that both the maintenance of anaesthetic equipment and preparation for anaesthesia can be delegated to these staff. They also play an important role in the restraint and management of animals during induction of anaesthesia. However, in the UK the induction and maintenance of anaesthesia is an act of veterinary surgery under the Veterinary Surgeons Act 1966. Veterinary nurses are often involved in the monitoring of anaesthesia, but the ultimate responsibility is that of the veterinary surgeon (see negligence above). Further guidance on delegation to veterinary nurses is available on the RCVS website (www.rcvs.org.uk/advice-and-guidance/code-of-professional-conduct-for-veterinary-nurses/supporting-guidance/delegation-to-veterinary-nurses/).

A similar situation applies in North America, although it appears that veterinary technicians are able to take more responsibility and in some states there is a specific additional qualification in veterinary anaesthesia available. In most states and provinces the law clearly states that the veterinary technician must be under the supervision of a veterinary surgeon, and most laws specify that the technician must be under *direct* supervision. This has come to be interpreted as that the veterinary surgeon must be on the premises if not in close proximity to the animal; this appears to be legal and acceptable. However, under this legislation, if problems do develop then the veterinary surgeon bears the ultimate responsibility.

Health and safety

Whilst all general aspects of health and safety in veterinary practice apply to anaesthesia, there are specific aspects relating to anaesthetic gases and vapours. Published studies have suggested that exposure to waste anaesthetic gases may have a large number of effects on human health. These include the risk of spontaneous abortion in pregnant women; the risk is greatest during the first trimester when the relative incidence is 1.5–2 times that in unexposed women. Exposure to nitrous oxide can result in bone marrow suppression with an alteration of DNA synthesis in bone marrow and mild megaloblastic anaemia. However, these changes are only temporary and are reversed within days. Most of the medical studies that provided these results were conducted in the 1970s when scavenging of waste anaesthetic gases was often not performed. Recent studies have not demonstrated any links with infertility or problems with unborn children among women working in operating theatres or anaesthetic practice; Burm (2003) provides further information on this topic. However, in order to reduce the risk in the working environment as much as possible, it is important that exposure to waste anaesthetic gases be kept to a minimum. This is achieved by the use of suitable scavenging equipment, preferably of the active type, and general ventilation of the workplace. If sidestream capnography is utilized (see Chapter 7), then it is important to scavenge gases from the monitor after analysis has taken place (Figure 1.1). Further details of scavenging systems can be found in Chapter 5. Maximum workplace exposure limits for the commonly available anaesthetic gases in the UK are given in Figure 1.2.

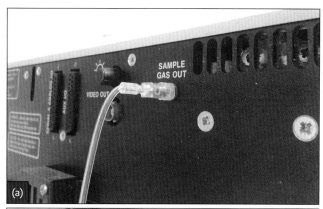

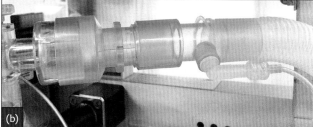

1.1 Scavenging from a capnograph. (a) Tubing attached to the exhaust port of the monitor. (b) The distal end of the tubing can be attached via an adaptor to the scavenging system.
(Courtesy of Marieke de Vries, Davies Veterinary Specialists, Higham Gobion, UK)

Agent	Concentration
Halothane	10 ppm
Isoflurane	50 ppm
Sevoflurane	20 ppm
Desflurane	None available to date
Nitrous oxide	100 ppm

1.2 Maximum allowed airborne concentrations of waste gases for inhalational anaesthetic agents commonly available in the UK. ppm = parts per million.

Environmental considerations

It is important that veterinary surgeons give due consideration to the effects of working practices on the environment. It has been suggested that waste anaesthetic gases may contribute to global warming (Sneyd *et al.*, 2010), hence it is essential that veterinary surgeons modify their practice to avoid the use of high fresh gas flows and to choose techniques that will reduce the environmental impact. In the future, it may become possible to capture the exhaled gases and recycle the agents. In addition, anaesthetic procedures also involve the use of a number of disposable equipment items, most of which are made from plastic. These contribute to landfill, if disposed of via this route, generate dioxins when incinerated and contain plasticizers, which can have effects on human health. Veterinary surgeons should be aware of these problems and take whatever steps are feasible to reduce the impact on the environment.

References and further reading

Allweiler SI and Kogan LR (2013) Inhalation anesthetics and the reproductive risk associated with occupational exposure among women working in veterinary anesthesia. *Veterinary Anaesthesia and Analgesia* **40**, 285–289

Burm AGL (2003) Occupational hazards of inhalational anaesthetics. *Best Practice and Research in Clinical Anaesthesiology* **17**, 147–161

Health and Safety Executive (2011) EH40/2005 Workplace exposure limits: containing the list of workplace exposure limits for use with the Control of Substances Hazardous to Health Regulations (as amended). (www.hse.gov.uk/pubns/books/eh40.htm)

Mads P, Andersen S, Nielsen OJ *et al.* (2012) Assessing the impact on global climate from general anaesthetic gases. *Anesthesia and Analgesia* **114**, 1081–1085

Nunn G (2008) Low-flow anaesthesia. *Continuing Education in Anaesthesia, Critical Care and Pain* **8**, 1–4

Ryan SM and Nielsen CJ (2010) Global warming potential of inhaled anesthetics: application to clinical use. *Anesthesia and Analgesia* **111**, 92–98

Sherman J, Lamers V and Eckelman M (2012) Life cycle greenhouse gas emissions of anesthetic drugs. *Anesthesia and Analgesia* **114**, 1086–1090

Sneyd JR, Montgomery H and Pencheon D (2010) The anaesthetist and the environment. *Anaesthesia* **65**, 435–437

Chapter 2

Pre-anaesthetic assessment and preparation

Lysa P. Posner

The benefits of evaluating veterinary patients before general anaesthesia are often underestimated and with recent advances in veterinary science, the veterinary surgeon (veterinarian) nowadays will routinely anaesthetize older and sicker patients. The recent Confidential Enquiry into Perioperative Small Animal Fatalities (CEPSAF) found an overall mortality of 0.17% (1.7/1000) for dogs and 0.24% (2.4/1000) for cats (Brodbelt *et al.*, 2008). By comparison, peri-anaesthetic mortality in humans has been reported to be 0.001% (1/100,000 patients). Thus, there is still room for mortality rates in veterinary medicine to be decreased. One approach to minimize morbidity and mortality is to identify at-risk patients and modify the anaesthetic plan accordingly.

Physical status

The American Society of Anesthesiologists (ASA) has developed a scale to rate physical status (Figure 2.1). This scale was originally developed for use in human patients but is commonly used in veterinary medicine. A patient is assigned a category status from 1 (healthy) to 5 (moribund). The letter 'E' following the number denotes 'emergency'. This scale has been shown to be predictive of anaesthetic morbidity and mortality in veterinary

patients (Hosgood and Scholl, 2002; Brodbelt *et al.*, 2008). Animals with an ASA score of 3 or higher are over 10 times more likely to suffer peri-anaesthetic complications compared with those in ASA categories 1 or 2. Accurately assigning an ASA score is a proven way to identify at-risk patients.

In order to assign an ASA status properly, a thorough pre-anaesthetic evaluation must be performed. It is important to be aware that while specific breed or species concerns (see below) are not directly linked to ASA status, they can influence the ASA status of a patient. For example, brachycephalic breeds such as bulldogs may suffer from brachycephalic airway syndrome, which could put them at greater risk for airway obstruction, and this would affect their ASA status.

Patient assessment

Veterinary patients are a heterogeneous group in terms of both physical stature and disease state. It is therefore important to assess each patient individually and tailor the anaesthetic plan to the patient.

History

For each patient, a complete history should be taken from the owner. This is an opportunity to not only gather useful information about the patient, but also to engage the owners and allow them to ask questions and raise any concerns. Some fractious animals will not tolerate handling for physical examination or diagnostic testing, and the history may be the only information available for the veterinary surgeon to consider before anaesthesia is induced. The history should include the following:

- Signalment
- Chief complaint/reason for sedation or general anaesthesia
- Complete medical history.

Signalment

Basic information should include species, breed, age, weight, sex and reproductive/neuter status. It is of note that the CEPSAF report found that cats have a higher risk of mortality than dogs, but it is unclear whether this is due to their size, anatomical or physiological characteristics, a

ASA scale	Physical description	Veterinary patient examples
1	Normal patient with no disease	Healthy patient scheduled for ovariohysterectomy or castration
2	Patient with mild systemic disease that does not limit normal function	Controlled diabetes mellitus, mild cardiac valve insufficiency
3	Patient with moderate systemic disease that limits normal function	Uncontrolled diabetes mellitus, symptomatic heart disease
4	Patient with severe systemic disease that is a constant threat to life	Sepsis, organ failure, heart failure
5	Patient that is moribund and not expected to live 24 hours without surgery	Shock, multiple organ failure, severe trauma
E	Describes patient as an emergency	Gastric dilatation–volvulus, respiratory distress

2.1 American Society of Anesthesiologists (ASA) physical status and classifications scale.

sensitive airway, or whether their veterinary care is different from that of dogs.

Knowledge of the breed characteristics and any associated medical conditions is also important as there are some specific risks associated with anaesthesia (see later). Age might influence whether further diagnostic tests are warranted, and influence the choice of drugs and the dosages used (see Chapter 30). Obesity is becoming a problem in companion animals and requires special consideration when planning anaesthesia (see Chapter 24).

Chief complaint/reason for sedation or general anaesthesia

This information should include the duration and severity of the presenting problem. Abnormal physical signs and any treatment received should be documented. Although consideration of the presenting problem alone will narrow the focus, it is imperative that the whole patient is assessed.

Complete medical history

This should include any other pertinent medical history, including nutrition, treatment with parasiticides, vaccination status and heartworm status. It is important to ask the owner directly about each individual organ system (Figure 2.2) as this might provide information about concurrent diseases that could affect the way anaesthesia is managed. Good-quality medical records kept within the practice can provide useful information. It is also useful to ask the owner about any previous anaesthetics performed at other practices and whether there were any adverse effects (e.g. prolonged sedation).

Physical examination

Ideally, every patient should have a complete physical examination within the week before anaesthesia and a further cursory examination on the day of the procedure. Patients presented for emergency anaesthesia should be evaluated as completely as possible. General assessment should include the following areas:

Parameter	Points of interest
Owner	Complete contact information, special considerations (e.g. consent, 'do not resuscitate' orders)
Medical history	Present and previous illness, surgery and anaesthetic history, current medications, vaccination status, heartworm status
Pre-anaesthetic preparedness	Fasted, clean, signed consent form
General	Attitude, activity, appetite, gain or loss of weight, water uptake/thirst
Integument	Pruritus, hair loss, wounds, infection
Cardiovascular system	Activity, stamina, cough, syncope
Respiratory system	Cough, sneeze, wheeze, dyspnoea, gagging, change of voice
Gastrointestinal system	Faeces, vomiting, regurgitation, endoparasites
Genitourinary system	Urination, reproductive status, neuter status, pregnancy, polyuria/polydipsia
Central nervous system	Mentation, balance, jumping, seizures, aggression

2.2 Guidelines for which areas to concentrate on when taking a patient history.

- Body condition score
- Hydration
- Cardiovascular system
- Respiratory system
- Gastrointestinal and urinary systems
- Integument
- Central nervous system (CNS).

Body condition score

Cats and dogs are generally given a body condition score from 1 (cachectic) to 9 (obese) (Freeman et al., 2011). Body condition can provide information about chronicity of a disease process and can serve to highlight potential problems during anaesthesia. In general, obese animals have diminished cardiovascular function and are at risk for hypoventilation, while cachectic animals are at risk of developing hypothermia and hypoglycaemia.

Hydration

All patients should have their hydration status evaluated. Laboratory results can be used alongside physical examination. It is important to estimate hydration status because dehydrated animals are likely to have decreased intravascular volume and electrolyte abnormalities. Whenever possible, rehydration and electrolyte stabilization should take place before anaesthesia (see Chapter 18).

Cardiovascular system

Cardiovascular system reserve is vital for the patient to cope with anaesthetic stresses. Heart rate, rhythm and any murmurs may affect the choice of drugs and course of anaesthesia. Any cardiovascular problems should be thoroughly investigated (e.g. by radiography, electrocardiography, echocardiography) and any problems stabilized (see Chapter 21).

Respiratory system

As with the cardiovascular system, the respiratory system should have enough reserves to enable the patient to tolerate anaesthesia. Patients with compromised pulmonary function are unable to tolerate heavy sedation without oxygen supplementation or support of ventilation. For details on respiratory system evaluation, see Chapter 22.

Gastrointestinal and urinary systems

Evaluation of the gastrointestinal and urinary systems is also important for patients requiring anaesthesia (see Chapters 24 and 25). The gastrointestinal system is often considered irrelevant in the pre-anaesthetic evaluation, but disease states affecting this system can have an effect on anaesthetized patients. Viscus dilatation, pancreatitis and abdominal cavity inflammation are painful conditions. Enlargement of abdominal organs can impede venous return and place pressure on the diaphragm, causing hypoventilation. Furthermore, protein loss (e.g. protein-losing enteropathy, nephropathy) can decrease oncotic pressure and lead to hypovolaemia and hypotension.

Integument

The skin should be evaluated for infection and characteristics such as turgor and thickness. Catheters and epidural or spinal needles should not be placed through infected skin as this increases the possibility of transferring infection to sites within the body. In addition, skin characteristics can point to other concurrent disease processes (e.g. thin, friable skin with Cushing's disease, ulcerated skin with autoimmune diseases). Some breeds tend to have thicker skin, which can make venous catheterization challenging.

Central nervous system

A basic neurological examination should be performed because anaesthetic drugs have their desired actions on the CNS and it is important to identify any problems before anaesthesia is induced. Patients with CNS depression are sensitive to many anaesthetic drugs and an exaggerated response may be observed with even low doses. Patients with neuromuscular disease can have weakened respiratory musculature leading to hypoventilation and hypoxaemia during anaesthesia (see Chapter 28).

Clinical diagnostic tests

Laboratory data can provide information that is useful in designing an appropriate anaesthetic plan. The choice of tests performed is based on the patient's age, the procedure planned, concurrent disease processes and cost. It is prudent to perform additional tests where results may alter the anaesthetic plan. As more information is obtained, the risk assessment associated with anaesthesia may change and the owners should be updated with this information before the animal is anaesthetized.

There is controversy regarding the percentage of outwardly healthy (ASA 1 and 2) patients that benefit from routine pre-anaesthetic haematology and biochemistry. Some reports indicate that <10% of patients have results that change their ASA status or the anaesthetic plan (Alef *et al.*, 2008); however, if testing is not performed, no abnormalities can be found. Some practices choose to perform basic bloodwork (see below) before anaesthesia unless the physical examination reveals any abnormalities for which further information is required. However, some practices perform basic haematology and biochemistry only for patients >7 years old.

Packed cell volume, total solids/total protein, blood glucose, blood urea nitrogen and creatinine

In young, healthy animals requiring elective procedures, if pre-anaesthetic bloodwork is undertaken, the recommended basic tests are for packed cell volume (PCV), total solids/total protein (TS/TP), blood glucose, blood urea nitrogen (BUN) and creatinine. These five tests can detect anaemia, hypo- and hyperproteinaemia, kidney disease and hypo- and hyperglycaemia. These tests require little blood or equipment and are relatively inexpensive. If any abnormalities are detected, further testing and/or evaluation can be undertaken.

Haematology, serum biochemistry and urinalysis

In older or infirm animals, haematology, serum biochemistry and urinalysis are more comprehensive and may be helpful in identifying some occult problems. These tests can be diagnostic for diseases such as diabetes mellitus (see Chapter 27) or indicate the need for further tests (e.g. bile acids to check liver function).

Tests for heartworm

The use of tests for heartworm depends on the geographical location or travel history of the patient. In endemic areas, heartworm status should be known before anaesthesia is induced, as heart failure and sudden death are possible with this disease.

Tests for thyroid function

Ideally, any animal showing physical evidence of thyroid dysfunction should be evaluated and stabilized before anaesthesia (see Chapter 27). Hypothyroidism in dogs is associated with obesity and a hypometabolic state. Hyperthyroid cats are generally underweight, have high metabolic demands and often have hypertrophic cardiomyopathy. Both of these thyroid conditions increase anaesthetic risk.

Coagulation profile

Animals at risk of increased bleeding based on breed (e.g. Dobermann), disease (e.g. thrombocytopenia) or procedure (e.g. liver biopsy) should be screened for the presence of coagulopathies. When possible, blood coagulation tests or specific factor determination should be performed in advance of the scheduled procedure. Knowledge of coagulation status allows for preparation in cases where excessive bleeding might occur, and alerts to the possible requirement for blood products (see Chapter 18).

Electrocardiography

Routine electrocardiographic screening is recommended for geriatric animals, patients with evidence of cardiac disease and patients with evidence of another disease that might cause arrhythmias (e.g. hyperkalaemia, splenomegaly, gastric dilatation–volvulus (GDV), post-traumatic myocarditis) (see Chapter 21). Veterinary surgeons who are uncomfortable evaluating electrocardiograms (ECGs) can make use of services providing remote evaluation of ECGs by a cardiologist.

Diagnostic imaging
Radiography

Radiography is useful to assess the size and shape of the internal organs (e.g. heart, liver, kidney) and can identify abnormal organ position (e.g. GDV), structures (e.g. tumour) or densities (e.g. air, fluid). Radiographs can be taken for routine screening (e.g. post-trauma or in geriatric patients) or to evaluate a particular problem (e.g. tumour metastasis, vomiting).

Echocardiography

An echocardiographic examination should be performed in patients with evidence of cardiac disease on physical examination, radiographic changes to the heart and/or an abnormal ECG. Echocardiography should also be performed if a disease is associated with changes in cardiac function (e.g. feline hyperthyroidism). This examination provides further information on anatomical or contractile changes. It is also useful for evaluating anaesthetic risk and to assess the ability of the cardiovascular system to cope with stress.

Computed tomography and magnetic resonance imaging

More specialized diagnostic imaging techniques can provide further information, but unfortunately they necessitate heavy sedation or general anaesthesia and therefore are not useful for pre-anaesthetic screening purposes. Specialized diagnostic imaging is described in Chapter 29.

Other considerations
Recent trauma

Traumatized patients can have multiple injuries that increase anaesthetic risk. Recently traumatized animals often require anaesthesia to repair obvious injuries (e.g. fractured limbs, ruptured urinary bladder). It should be borne in mind that traumatized patients often have more than one injury (see Chapters 18, 21, 23 and 28) and may have hidden injuries that are potentially life-threatening (e.g. pneumothorax). Traumatized patients should be evaluated for the presence of hypovolaemia, shock, bleeding, abdominal or thoracic injuries, cardiac abnormalities and neurological status. It is important to consider the whole patient in such cases, and some surgical repairs may need to be delayed until the patient is stabilized.

Breed considerations

Official Kennel Clubs list over 150 different breeds of dog and some of these breeds may require different anaesthetic management. Some breeds may have a predisposition to certain diseases that can affect the course of anaesthesia. Large dogs generally require lower dosages of drugs compared with toy breeds, and relative overdosage may be the cause of some misinformation regarding 'sensitivities' of certain large breeds to sedation and anaesthetic drugs. Below is a short list of breeds that have known risk factors associated with anaesthesia.

Dobermann: Abnormal plasma concentrations of von Willebrand factor occur in 73% of Dobermanns. Given this high prevalence, all Dobermanns should be screened before elective surgery. If a Dobermann is presented for emergency anaesthesia and the status is unknown, a buccal mucosal bleeding time (BMBT) test should be performed. A dog deficient in von Willebrand factor or with an abnormal BMBT may require additional treatment (e.g. desmopressin acetate, cryoprecipitate or fresh whole blood) to limit bleeding during surgery (see Chapter 18).

Miniature Schnauzer: Miniature Schnauzers, particularly females, are at risk of developing sick sinus syndrome. These dogs may appear normal on physical examination, but it is possible for occult disease to be unmasked by anaesthesia, and this can be fatal unless a pacemaker is available. It is therefore recommended that all Miniature Schnauzers have an ECG evaluated before any anaesthetic drugs are given. If sick sinus syndrome is detected, anaesthesia should be cancelled if possible and the heart disease fully evaluated (see Chapter 21).

Boxer: Certain familial lines of Boxers have been reported to be sensitive to the effects of acepromazine; they have an exaggerated response to the sedative and hypotensive effects of the drug and may faint as a result of hypotension. Bradycardia has been observed alongside hypotension, prompting the recommendation that an anticholinergic (e.g. glycopyrronium or atropine) be used in conjunction with acepromazine in Boxers, or that acepromazine be avoided altogether in this breed (see Chapter 17).

Brachycephalic breeds: The brachycephalic breeds (e.g. Bulldog, Pug) are thick-necked dogs that often have hypoplastic tracheas, elongated soft palates, everted laryngeal saccules and stenotic nares (see Chapter 22). A good physical examination of the respiratory system will indicate the severity of the condition. The cardiovascular system should also be examined for any abnormalities. Heavy sedation should be avoided unless the patient can be closely monitored with attention to oxygenation and ventilation. Brachycephalic airway syndrome has also been associated with gastrointestinal disease (Poncet *et al.*, 2005). In addition, Bulldogs and Shar Peis are at greater risk for congenital hiatal hernias, and some veterinary anaesthetists routinely administer proton pump inhibitors to dogs in this category (Lorinson and Bright, 1998; Guiot *et al.*, 2008).

Greyhounds and sighthounds: After the induction of anaesthesia with injectable drugs, recovery occurs through redistribution of the drug from the brain to the bloodstream and then to fat. Any drug in the circulation is removed through hepatic metabolism (see Chapter 14). Animals with low body fat stores, either through genetics or disease, tend to have higher concentrations of these drugs in the circulating blood, which in turn maintains the concentration of the drug in the brain. This can lead to prolonged recovery times. Sighthounds (e.g. Irish Wolfhound, Whippet) tend to have a low fat:body mass ratio. In addition to low body fat content, Greyhounds lack the cytochrome P450 microsomal enzyme needed for metabolism of barbiturates (Kukanich *et al.*, 2007). Thus, recovery from thiobarbiturates in this breed can be up to four times longer than in mixed-breed dogs. Although thiobarbiturates do not depress the cardiovascular system in Greyhounds and other sighthounds more than in other dogs, the prolonged recovery precludes the use of thiobarbiturates in these breeds. Alternatives for induction of anaesthesia include a ketamine/benzodiazepine combination, alfaxalone or propofol. Although Greyhounds metabolize propofol more slowly than other dogs, it is unlikely to significantly prolong anaesthesia (Zoran *et al.*, 1993).

*Multidrug resistance (*MDR1*) gene:* Some herding dogs (e.g. Australian Shepherds, collies) have a genetic mutation that affects their ability to transport certain drugs across cell membrames, such as parasiticides (e.g. ivermectin, milbemycin), antidiarrhoea drugs (e.g. loperamide) and anticancer agents (e.g. vincristine, doxorubicin) (Mealy, 2004). Currently, only acepromazine and butorphanol have been found to produce exaggerated effects in dogs with this mutation. These agents should therefore be cautiously used at a reduced dose. Definitive testing for the gene mutation is available. Further information is available on the Washington State University College of Veterinary Medicine website (www.vetmed.wsu.edu/deptsVCPL drugs.aspx).

Concurrent drug use

Many veterinary patients require anaesthesia while receiving medication for other disease processes. It is very important that these drugs are documented and a decision should be made to continue or discontinue them during the peri-anaesthetic period.

Antibiotics: Many animals will be concurrently receiving antibiotic therapy, but most antibiotics do not interfere or cause a problem with anaesthesia. However, the aminoglycoside antibiotics (e.g. gentamicin) can be nephrotoxic. Patients receiving aminoglycosides should be screened for renal disease, and good perfusion and hydration maintained during anaesthesia to limit renal damage. In addition, aminoglycosides can interfere with neuromuscular transmission and can potentiate neuromuscular block produced by peripherally acting neuromuscular blocking agents (e.g. atracurium) or disease (e.g. myasthenia gravis) (see Chapters 16 and 28). Occasionally, antibiotics given intravenously (e.g. sodium penicillin or co-amoxiclav) can result in vomiting, anaphylactic reactions and hypotension during anaesthesia, and patients should be monitored as appropriate.

Cardiac drugs: It is imperative that the veterinary surgeon understands the pharmacology of any cardiac drugs used and their potential effects during anaesthesia. In general, cardiac drugs should be continued during the peri-anaesthetic period and adverse effects should be anticipated (see Chapter 21 for further details).

Angiotensin-converting enzyme inhibitors: Angiotensin-converting enzyme (ACE) inhibitors (e.g. ramipril, enalapril, benazepril) are commonly used as vasodilators to prevent and treat heart failure (decrease afterload) and renal disease. These drugs interfere with the renin–angiotensin–aldosterone pathway by preventing the formation of angiotensin II. The diuretic effects coupled with vasodilation can result in clinically significant hypotension, particularly during anaesthesia. The cardiac benefits probably outweigh the risks of hypotension and if ACE inhibitors are continued on the day of anaesthesia, the patient should be closely monitored for hypotension.

Calcium sensitizers: Calcium sensitizers (e.g. pimobendan) are classed as inodilators because they exert both positive inotropic effects by increasing calcium binding, and vasodilator effects through the selective inhibition of phosphodiesterase III (PDE3). They are commonly used in dogs, and off-label in cats, to treat congestive heart failure. Although there are few documented interactions with anaesthetic drugs, there are reports that calcium sensitizers may increase the incidence of cardiac arrhythmias.

Cardiac glycosides: Cardiac glycosides (e.g. digoxin) are positive inotropes used to treat heart failure and atrial fibrillation. They increase cardiac contractility and output, and reduce heart rate. These drugs have a narrow therapeutic margin and overdose can result in ECG abnormalities and altered contractility. Patients treated with cardiac glycosides are more sensitive to hypomagnesaemia, hypokalaemia, hypovolaemia and hypoxaemia, and these conditions increase the incidence of ventricular arrhythmias. Patients receiving digoxin should not receive anticholinergic drugs.

Beta blockers: Beta blockers (e.g. propranolol, esmolol) are class II antiarrhythmic drugs. They mainly block beta-1 adrenoreceptors but can also block beta-2 adrenoceptors. These drugs are primarily used to treat tachyarrhythmias. Their use alongside anaesthetic drugs can result in bradycardia and decreased cardiac contractility. When prescribed for continued use (e.g. supraventricular tachycardia), the cardiac benefits generally outweigh the risks of decreased cardiac output; therefore, in such cases beta blockers should be administered on the day of anaesthesia and the patient carefully monitored.

Analgesics:
Opioids: Opioids (e.g. morphine, methadone, buprenorphine, hydromorphone, fentanyl) are drugs that bind to opioid receptors and provide analgesia. These drugs can also cause clinically significant sedation, bradycardia, second-degree atrioventricular block, respiratory depression and vomiting. Thus, it is helpful if the anaesthetic protocol is designed around the use of any opioids already being administered for pain, and these drugs should not cause problems if adverse effects are considered in the plan (see Chapter 10). The inclusion of a full mu opioid receptor agonist in the anaesthetic plan when butorphanol (a kappa agonist and mu antagonist) has already been administered can result in drug antagonism and unpredictable analgesic effects.

Tramadol: This drug is by classification a mu opioid receptor agonist, but exerts its analgesic effects mainly through the inhibition of noradrenaline (norepinephrine) and serotonin reuptake. Tramadol became popular in veterinary medicine because it was an unscheduled drug, had few side effects and could be administered orally. However, tramadol is now a Schedule 3 Controlled Drug, and the active metabolite responsible for much of its analgesic effect in humans is not formed in dogs. Although there are anecdotal reports of tramadol providing good analgesia, its analgesic effects in dogs and cats are now in question. Tramadol should be used with caution in patients receiving monoamine oxidase inhibitors (MAOIs; e.g. selegiline), tricyclic antidepressants (TCAs; e.g. amitriptyline) and selective serotonin reuptake inhibitors (SSRIs; e.g. fluoxetine), which also increase circulating serotonin concentrations. The increase in circulating serotonin levels can lead to 'serotonin syndrome', which can manifest as drowsiness, restlessness, altered mentation, muscle twitching, high body temperature, shivering, diarrhoea, unconsciousness and death.

Anti-inflammatory drugs:
Non-steroidal anti-inflammatory drugs: Non-steroidal anti-inflammatory drugs (NSAIDs; e.g. carprofen, meloxicam, coxibs) are frequently used to provide analgesia before or during anaesthesia. These drugs are potent analgesics and their mechanism of action is through interference with prostaglandin synthesis via the arachidonic acid pathway (see Chapter 10). These drugs can also inhibit other prostaglandins necessary for normal physiological functions, which can be detrimental. NSAIDs can interfere with gastric mucosal protection, renal blood flow and coagulation. Different NSAIDs have different adverse effects and safety profiles, particularly in different species, and therefore their indiscriminate use should be avoided. Dehydration, hypovolaemia and hypotension aggravate the adverse effects of NSAIDs and the potential risks and benefits need to be considered on a patient by patient basis.

Corticosteroids: Corticosteroids (e.g. prednisolone) bind to and activate the glucocorticoid receptor, which results in up-regulation of anti-inflammatory proteins and attenuation of pro-inflammatory proteins. Corticosteroids have powerful anti-inflammatory and immunomodulatory activity and are commonly used to prevent inflammation (to relieve itch and pain) and to suppress the immune system (e.g. allergies, cancer). They can also be administered to patients lacking normal physiological amounts of cortisol (hypoadrenocorticism, adrenal depletion; see Chapter 27). Corticosteroids are generally contraindicated in animals with systemic infections or gastrointestinal disease or in patients receiving NSAIDs.

N-methyl-D-aspartate receptor antagonists: N-methyl-D-aspartate (NMDA) receptor antagonists have analgesic properties and have been shown to interrupt central sensitization ('wind-up') (see Chapter 8).

Ketamine and amantadine: Ketamine can be used at subanaesthetic doses to treat refractory pain. To break wind-up pain, ketamine should be administered as an intravenous infusion for approximately 24 hours. Alternatively, amantadine (an oral NMDA receptor antagonist) should be administered for at least 2 weeks. When used in this way, these drugs should be compatible with other anaesthetics and are unlikely to produce unwanted behavioural or physiological adverse effects.

Behaviour-modifying drugs: The following drugs exert their effects through altering serotonin concentrations within the brain:

* Trazodone
* Fluoxetine
* Selegiline
* Clomipramine and amitryptyline.

Patients receiving these drugs should not be given pethidine (meperidine), tramadol or other drugs that can interfere with serotonin reuptake (e.g. SSRIs or TCAs), as this can lead to 'serotonin syndrome' (see above).

Trazodone: This drug is classified as an antidepressant, but is often used in veterinary medicine as a mild sedative, particularly postoperatively. The mechanism of action of trazodone is complex. The antidepressant effects are attributed to serotonin reuptake inhibition, while the sedative effect is likely to be the result of an alpha-adrenergic blocking action as well as modest histamine blockade (Jay *et al.*, 2013).

Fluoxetine: This drug is classified as an antidepressant of the SSRI class. It is widely used in veterinary medicine for behaviour modification in a variety of patients (e.g. separation anxiety, compulsive disorders).

Selegiline: This drug is used to treat dogs with canine cognitive disorder ('old dog dementia') and separation anxiety. Selegiline is a MAOI which results in increased levels of dopamine, as well as other monoamines such as serotonin.

Clomipramine and amitriptyline: These drugs are TCAs that prevent reuptake of serotonin and noradrenaline.

Incontinence drugs:
Phenylpropanolamine: This drug is a sympathomimetic that increases urethral sphincter tone due to increased noradrenaline release. The increase in noradrenaline may result in hypertension and/or tachycardia but generally does not appear to greatly modify the course of anaesthesia.

Ephedrine/pseudoephedrine: These drugs are sympathomimetics which increase urethral sphincter tone by increasing noradrenaline release (pseudoephedrine is an isomer of ephedrine). Clinical signs and cautions are the same as for phenylpropanolamine.

Anticonvulsants:
Phenobarbital: This barbiturate drug is commonly used to treat epilepsy. Like many other anaesthetic drugs, phenobarbital is a gamma-aminobutyric acid (GABA$_A$) receptor agonist. Patients treated with phenobarbital may have exaggerated CNS effects (synergy) to usual doses of anaesthetic drugs, and therefore doses should be adjusted. Phenobarbital should not be stopped in these patients.

Phenobarbital saturates liver enzyme systems for the first 7 days of administration, but following this period enzyme induction occurs and all exogenous drugs may have a shorter duration of action.

Chemotherapy drugs: There are many drugs used for cancer treatment in cats and dogs. Most of these drugs affect the bone marrow while others may be nephrotoxic, cardiotoxic or hepatotoxic. The reader should consult the relevant literature and examine the patient for changes in body systems that may affect the course of anaesthesia.

Nutraceuticals: Many owners administer a variety of 'natural' or 'complementary' therapies to their pets. Owners may assume that these products are benign, and may not report their use to the veterinary surgeon when asked if the animal is receiving any medication. However, many over-the-counter remedies and nutraceuticals have chemical properties that can react with anaesthetic drugs; for example, St John's wort has been linked to serotonin syndrome in people also taking TCAs or MAOIs. It is reasonable to assume that St John's wort might have similar interactions with tramadol. It is therefore prudent to ask the owner whether they are giving their animal any of these therapies and to research the potential interactions of any non-medically prescribed drug (Wong and Townley, 2011).

Concurrent disease states
Many patients requiring anaesthesia will have concurrent diseases. It is prudent to be familiar with the diseases and how they might affect the patient in the peri-anaesthetic period (see Chapters 19–28).

Preparation for anaesthesia
Fasting/water deprivation
Fasting is routinely recommended before general anaesthesia to decrease the amount of food and fluid in the stomach and decrease the risk of vomiting, regurgitation and aspiration in the peri-anaesthetic period. However, fasting can be deleterious in young or thin animals, or patients with a rapid metabolic rate, as they may become hypoglycaemic. Patients with increased fluid requirements (e.g. with fever, renal insufficiency, diabetes mellitus) can quickly become dehydrated during long periods of water deprivation. In healthy human patients, use of an abbreviated fasting period does not result in increased morbidity (Brady *et al.*, 2003). Furthermore, prolonged fasting in animals has been associated with an increased incidence of reflux and increased gastric acidity. On the basis of this information, it is probably prudent to have a moderate fasting period (6–8 hours for food and 2–4 hours for water) before administering pre-anaesthetic medication in reasonably healthy patients (Galatos and Raptopoulos, 1995).

Owner comprehension and permission
Before anaesthesia, the owner should understand both the anaesthetic and surgical risks. A frank discussion should take place about what to do in an emergency situation such as cardiac arrest and the wishes of the client for intervention (e.g. 'do not resuscitate' orders or open/closed chest resuscitation). The owner should also sign a consent form (see Chapter 1).

Cleanliness

Many veterinary surgeons recommend that all anaesthetic/surgical patients are recently bathed and are free from fleas and ticks. The patient's coat, the season, geographical location and the procedure to be performed should dictate whether this is necessary.

References and further reading

Alef M, Von Praun F and Oechtering G (2008) Is routine pre-anaesthetic haematological and biochemical screening justified in dogs? *Veterinary Anaesthesia and Analgesia* **35**, 132–140

Brady M, Kinn S and Stuart P (2003) Preoperative fasting for adults to prevent perioperative complications. *Cochrane Database of Systematic Reviews*, CD004423

Brodbelt DC, Blissitt KJ, Hammond RA *et al.* (2008) The risk of death: the confidential enquiry into perioperative small animal fatalities. *Veterinary Anaesthesia and Analgesia* **35**, 365–373

Freeman L, Becvarova I, Cave N *et al.* (2011) World Small Animal Veterinary Association (WSAVA) Nutritional Assessment Guidelines. *Journal of the South African Veterinary Association* **84**, 254–263

Galatos A and Raptopoulos D (1995) Gastro-oesophageal reflux during anaesthesia in the dog: the effect of preoperative fasting and premedication. *Veterinary Record* **137**, 479–483

Guiot LP, Lansdowne JL, Rouppert P *et al.* (2008) Hiatal hernia in the dog: a clinical report of four Chinese Shar Peis. *Journal of the American Animal Hospital Association* **44**, 335–341

Hosgood G and Scholl DT (2002) Evaluation of age and American Society of Anesthesiologists (ASA) physical status as risk factors for perianesthetic morbidity and mortality in the cat. *Journal of Veterinary Emergency and Critical Care* **12**, 9–15

Jay AR, Krotscheck U, Parsley E *et al.* (2013) Pharmacokinetics, bioavailability, and hemodynamic effects of trazodone after intravenous and oral administration of a single dose to dogs. *American Journal of Veterinary Research* **74**, 1450–1456

Kukanich B, Coetzee JF, Gehring R *et al.* (2007) Comparative disposition of pharmacologic markers for cytochrome P-450 mediated metabolism, glomerular filtration rate, and extracellular and total body fluid volume of Greyhound and Beagle dogs. *Journal of Veterinary Pharmacology and Therapeutics* **30**, 314–319

Lorinson D and Bright R (1998) Long-term outcome of medical and surgical treatment of hiatal hernias in dogs and cats: 27 cases (1978–1996). *Journal of the American Veterinary Medical Association* **213**, 381–384

Mealy KL (2004) Therapeutic implications of the MDR-1 gene. *Journal of Veterinary Pharmacology and Therapeutics* **27**, 257–264

Poncet CM, Dupre GP, Freiche VG *et al.* (2005) Prevalence of gastrointestinal tract lesions in 73 brachycephalic dogs with upper respiratory syndrome. *Journal of Small Animal Practice* **46**, 273–279

Wong A and Townley SA (2011) Herbal medicines and anaesthesia. *Continuing Education in Anaesthesia, Critical Care & Pain* **11**, 14–17

Zoran DL, Riedesel DH and Dyer DC (1993) Pharmacokinetics of propofol in mixed-breed dogs and greyhounds. *American Journal of Veterinary Research* **54**, 755–760

Chapter 3

General principles of perioperative care

Martina Mosing

Management of the perioperative period plays an important role in reducing anaesthetic-related mortality in cats and dogs. This chapter describes the scientific facts of perioperative risk revealed by one major study that investigated small animal anaesthetic fatalities (Brodbelt et al., 2007, 2008) and discusses the often underestimated importance of perioperative management of the small animal patient.

Anaesthetic risk

The Confidential Enquiry into Perioperative Small Animal Fatalities (CEPSAF) (Brodbelt et al., 2008) examined risk factors for peri-anaesthetic mortality and included data from sedation and anaesthetic records for over 98,000 dogs and 79,000 cats. The overall risk for anaesthesia- and sedation-related death in the first 48 hours following the procedure was 0.17% (1 of 601) in dogs and 0.24% (1 of 419) in cats. When the patients were categorized into those which were healthy (American Society of Anesthesiologists (ASA) physical status categories 1 and 2) and those which were debilitated (ASA physical status categories 3 and above), the risk was found to be 0.05% (1 of 1849) in healthy dogs and 0.11% (1 of 895) in healthy cats. Of the debilitated patients, 1.33% (1 of 75) of dogs and 1.4% (1 of 71) of cats died in the perioperative period. One of the most striking findings of this study was that 47% and 61% of canine and feline fatalities, respectively, occurred during the postoperative period, and most commonly within the first 3 hours of recovery.

Risk factors for perioperative mortality in cats and dogs include the presence of pre-existing pathology, being overweight (cats and dogs) or underweight (dogs), and the duration, complexity and urgency of the procedure. In dogs, specific risk factors include age (>12 years) and bodyweight (<5 kg). There is no apparent breed predisposition, although brachycephalic dogs tend to have a higher risk. Specific factors found to increase mortality in dogs include:

- Mask induction
- Use of volatile anaesthetic for both induction and maintenance of anaesthesia
- Use of intermittent positive pressure ventilation (IPPV) especially in sick dogs.

In cats, mortality increases in patients >12 years of age and in those with a bodyweight <2 kg. Specific factors found to influence mortality in cats include:

- Endotracheal intubation (increases mortality)
- Perioperative fluid therapy (increases mortality)
- Counting the pulse rate and/or using a pulse oximeter (decreases mortality)
- Sedation was associated with the same mortality as general anaesthesia.

The following sections describe how the findings of the CEPSAF study might influence the perioperative management of small animal patients, and how careful perioperative management can aid in reducing fatalities.

Procedure

Efficient time management is a crucial factor in reducing the duration of anaesthesia and its associated problems. Mismanagement and delays in preparation should be avoided, as they can increase the likelihood of prolonging anaesthetic time. Preoperative stabilization of emergency patients is vital to decrease mortality in this subset of patients. In an emergency situation any pre-existing health problems can easily be overlooked and this may lead to higher perioperative mortality. Recent guidelines from the American Animal Hospital Association (AAHA) recommend that fluid and electrolyte abnormalities be adequately corrected before anaesthesia (Davis et al., 2013).

Body condition score

Obesity is well recognized as a factor that increases anaesthetic risk in humans owing to its associated co-morbidities (e.g. type 2 diabetes mellitus, hypoventilation, cardiovascular disease, hypertension, osteoarthritis). Furthermore, in obese patients the closing volume (the volume at which the alveoli and small airways begin to collapse during expiration) exceeds functional residual capacity (FRC). This causes airway collapse and atelectasis, which leads to rapid development of hypoxaemia during periods of hypoventilation or apnoea during induction of anaesthesia. In obese dogs, a direct correlation has been demonstrated between poor arterial oxygenation and increased body fat during deep sedation, which might partially explain the higher mortality observed for obese animals (Mosing et al., 2013). Conversely, low bodyweight is also a risk factor for perioperative mortality. Underweight animals may have underlying co-morbidities such as chronic gastrointestinal or renal disease (see Chapters 24 and 25).

Bodyweight and size

The difficulty of using monitoring devices designed for larger patients may partially explain the higher mortality observed in cats and smaller dogs. The inability to adequately monitor a patient increases the likelihood of poor recognition of potentially life-threatening complications. Both non-invasive and invasive arterial blood pressure (ABP) measurement techniques can be challenging in dogs <5 kg and cats <2 kg because of unsuitable commercially available cuff sizes or reduced access to appropriate arteries. Furthermore, smaller animals are prone to hypothermia because of their high surface area:volume ratio. In addition, overestimation of their actual bodyweight is a frequent problem and may lead to accidental overdoses if an inappropriate volume of a drug is administered.

Age

In older animals, changes in physiology and altered drug pharmacokinetics and pharmacodynamics can lead to decreased compensatory reserve (see Chapter 30). Although the CEPSAF study indicated that age by itself is not a predictor of poor outcome, the effect of age is undoubtedly correlated with the presence of underlying disease.

Risk factors in dogs

Mask induction and mono-inhalational anaesthesia

The use of an inhalant as the sole agent for induction and maintenance of anaesthesia does not provide adequate analgesia and the relatively high concentrations needed for surgery cause profound cardiorespiratory depression and may even result in cardiac arrest. These risk factors emphasize the importance of providing adequate pre-anaesthetic medication and the application of a balanced anaesthetic protocol.

Intermittent positive pressure ventilation

The high mortality observed when IPPV is used is more difficult to explain, especially considering that, in anaesthetized humans, IPPV does not result in an increased risk. One possible cause may be the use of inadequate equipment or ventilation strategies that do not make use of recommended tidal volumes and respiratory rate settings to ensure normocapnia (see Chapter 6). The CEPSAF study did not distinguish between manually and mechanically applied IPPV; manual ventilation can potentially damage the lungs because excessive intrathoracic pressures and lung volumes are less easily recognized when using this method. In addition, the increased mean intrathoracic pressure associated with IPPV reduces venous return to the heart and may also have a detrimental effect on ABP, especially in hypovolaemic patients and/or those deeply anaesthetized patients.

Risk factors in cats

Endotracheal intubation

Mortality among cats is higher when they are intubated, even when health status and procedure are taken into account (Brodbelt et al., 2007). The feline larynx is very sensitive and delicate, and a gentle intubation technique should be applied to minimize risk. Various causes, such as irritation by the endotracheal tube (ETT) and manipulation during intubation, can result in breathing problems. The use of 1% lidocaine spray (Xylocaine 10mg Spray) should be avoided in cats as it contains preservatives that have been shown to cause (fatal) laryngeal oedema (Watson, 1992). Although occlusion of the ETT can cause problems in situ, the CEPSAF study demonstrated that the majority of deaths (>60%) occurred after extubation, indicating that laryngospasm, laryngeal oedema and/or post-traumatic swelling are all possible causes of death. These results also highlight the need for a sufficient depth of anaesthesia before intubation is attempted, which should be done gently and with as little force as possible.

Perioperative fluid therapy

Volume overload in the perioperative period is the most likely cause of feline perioperative mortality related to fluid therapy. The 2013 AAHA fluid therapy guidelines recommend fluid administration rates during anaesthesia of 5 ml/kg/h in dogs and 3 ml/kg/h in cats (Davis et al., 2013); these values are relatively lower than those previously reported. The lower value for cats is related to their lower circulating blood volume (55 ml/kg) compared to that of dogs (85 ml/kg). Veterinary practices often do not have infusion pumps and are more likely to apply gravity-fed infusion. The administration of intravenous fluids without using safety systems such as in-line burettes or rate-limiters can lead to unnoticed accidental fluid overload in cats. This should not discourage the veterinary surgeon (veterinarian) from using perioperative fluid therapy to treat either absolute or relative fluid deficits in cats; however, the volume administered should be carefully monitored and high intravenous infusion rates should be applied only with monitoring of the physiological response.

Monitoring peripheral pulse and/or use of a pulse oximeter

Anaesthetic risk in cats is reduced when either the peripheral pulse is assessed or a pulse oximeter is used; combining these techniques results in a greater reduction of risk. Monitoring the pulse quality and rate and arterial oxygenation will facilitate early detection of problems, which can be rapidly treated (see Chapter 31). The CEPSAF study did not evaluate the benefit of monitoring the electrocardiogram (ECG), measuring ABP and using capnography or spirometry because these techniques are, unfortunately, not commonly used in general practice. However, their use is highly recommended as they will help to detect problems earlier.

Sedation versus general anaesthesia

The perception that sedation carries less risk than general anaesthesia is incorrect. Generally, for cats with a high ASA physical status classification, sedation is often preferred over general anaesthesia. However, the absence of a patent and protected airway in a heavily sedated cat, combined with the often stressful situation for the patient and less than optimal monitoring, will be more problematic than a well managed general anaesthetic. Further discussion of this topic can be found in Chapters 13, 14 and 21.

Positioning the patient

It is important that the whole theatre team shares the responsibility for proper patient positioning throughout the perioperative period.

General principles

The animal should always be positioned on a soft, padded surface. The joints should be in natural positions as far as possible (Figure 3.1). Ideally, the head should be at the same level as the heart. Positioning the head above the heart (>30 degrees) will reduce cerebral perfusion pressure; when the head is lower than the heart, an increase in both intracranial and intraocular pressure will occur. Over-extension of the head can cause the ETT to exert pressure on laryngeal structures; excessive flexion of the head can kink the ETT and cause it to migrate towards the bronchi. The eyes should be protected against external pressure.

Cardiovascular and respiratory compromise

The use of general anaesthetic drugs interferes with the cardiovascular and respiratory systems and their homeostatic reflexes (see Chapters 17 and 22). During anaesthesia, the cardiovascular reflexes responsible for maintaining ABP during postural changes are blunted. Gravity can cause blood to pool in areas of the body below the level of the heart, thereby reducing venous return and consequently cardiac output. Thus, body position should be changed slowly and only when necessary; this is especially important in patients with cardiovascular instability. Placing the whole body in a head-down (Trendelenburg) or head-up (reverse Trendelenburg) position will increase or decrease venous return, respectively. After neuraxial (epidural or spinal) anaesthesia, sympathetic nerve fibres can become blocked where they leave the spinal cord, resulting in vasodilation in the areas innervated by these nerves. Blood will pool in the caudal extremities and viscera, which reduces venous return and consequently leads to hypotension. To facilitate venous return to the heart, the pelvic limbs should be placed slightly higher than heart level (see Figure 3.1).

Anaesthesia causes a reduction in FRC and an increase in atelectasis because of decreased respiratory muscle tone. In spontaneously breathing patients, chest and diaphragm movements can be compromised by unnatural positioning of the thoracic limbs (see Figure 3.1a). The work of breathing can also increase, eventually resulting in hypoventilation. The Trendelenburg position will cause abdominal organs to push against the diaphragm; this will further decrease FRC and increase atelectasis formation and intrapulmonary shunting of deoxygenated venous blood into the systemic arterial system. The reverse Trendelenburg position can reduce the pressure of abdominal organs on the diaphragm, but can compromise venous return and possibly also cerebral perfusion during periods of hypotension.

IPPV decreases atelectasis formation and removes the work of breathing. Its use should be considered with patients in all body positions that may hinder normal respiratory movement, although its effect on venous return should be taken into account.

Peripheral nerve injury

Peripheral nerve injury may be the result of compression, stretching or ischaemia. Although there are no published reports for small animals there is anecdotal evidence of facial, peroneal, ulnar and brachial plexus neuropathies. This emphasizes the necessity of careful body positioning and padding of areas where nerves run superficially. Neuropathies often take months to heal (see Chapter 31).

Eye injury and loss of vision

Corneal abrasions can occur as a result of direct trauma (fingers, equipment or drapes accidently touching the cornea), chemical injuries (antiseptic solutions), excessive drying (forced warm air blanket) and reduced tear production (anticholinergics, perioperative analgesics and inhalational anaesthetics). Animals with lagophthalmos are prone to direct trauma to the globe and special attention is needed when positioning the head of these patients. In dogs, corneal ulcers are more likely to develop with long and multiple anaesthetic periods. In brachycephalic dogs, the palpebral reflex returns later during recovery owing to a lower density of corneal sensory nerve fibres than in other breeds (Park *et al.*, 2013); decreased corneal innervation has also been described in Persian cats (Kafarnik *et al.*, 2008) making them prone to perioperative corneal ulcer development. Supportive care in the form of appropriate eye lubricants is a basic requirement in the perioperative period. Pressure must never be applied to the eyes, and proper padding and positioning of the patient to prevent eye injury is essential (see Chapter 19).

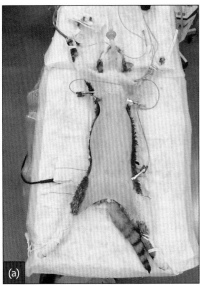

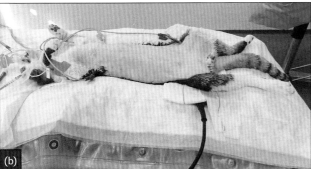

3.1 (a) Poor positioning of a cat for laparotomy. The limbs are over-extended and the tension on the thorax impairs thoracic movements. The pelvic limbs are pulled below the level of the heart. (b) The same cat after repositioning to a better position. Sandbags underneath the heating blanket are used to keep the cat in stable dorsal recumbency. The limbs are in a relaxed position and higher than the heart to avoid pooling of blood in the limbs.

Cats can be particularly prone to blindness as a complication of general anaesthesia. The use of a mouth gag to open the mouth widely for dental procedures or endoscopy has been linked to postoperative visual loss and central nervous system (CNS) deficits in this species (Stiles *et al.*, 2012). This is probably because overstretching both maxillary arteries (supplying the brain and retina), and the surrounding musculature, results in disruption of retinal and brain perfusion (Barton-Lamb *et al.*, 2013). Reduced perfusion of the brain during periods of hypotension and hypoxia of the visual cortex may also be contributing factors. Although recovery may take days, 70% of affected cats are likely to recover vision (Stiles *et al.*, 2012).

Body temperature and its regulation

General considerations

In mammals, body temperature is tightly regulated because metabolic function deteriorates during both hypo- and hyperthermia. All anaesthetic drugs depress the thermoregulatory centre and cause hypothermia. In humans, hypothermia (decrease in body temperature of 1–2°C) results in an increased incidence of postoperative wound infections, impaired coagulation, increased intraoperative blood loss and prolonged recovery and hospitalization. The CEPSAF study demonstrated that the majority of fatalities in cats and dogs occur during the postoperative period; intraoperative hypothermia can result in a prolonged recovery, with increased susceptibility to hypoventilation and aspiration.

In the conscious animal, heat is not uniformly distributed throughout the body. The core (trunk and head) temperature is kept stable by the central thermoregulatory control centre (variation <0.5°C), while the temperature in the rest of the body is variable (Figure 3.2). This temperature gradient is preserved by thermoregulatory vasoconstriction.

Thermoregulation during general anaesthesia

Inadvertent hypothermia is far more common during anaesthesia than hyperthermia. Hypothermia results from impairment of the central thermoregulatory control mechanisms by anaesthetic drugs and exposure of skin and open body cavities to low ambient temperatures. Inadvertent hypothermia in dogs and cats can be classified as slight (38.49–36.5°C), moderate (36.49–34.0°C) or severe (<34.0°C) (Redondo *et al.*, 2012ab). Studies have shown that >80% of dogs and 97% of cats were hypothermic (<38.5°C) at the end of an anaesthetic procedure when no active heating was applied during anaesthesia. Among these animals, 3% of dogs and 10% of cats were severely hypothermic (Redondo *et al.*, 2012ab).

If uncorrected, the decrease in body temperature during anaesthesia is dynamic and follows a defined pattern (Figure 3.3):

- Phase 1: initial rapid decrease in core temperature (first hour). This initial phase of hypothermia is induced by a centrally mediated decrease in temperature threshold, which causes increased peripheral blood flow to remove the 'excess heat'. Additionally, most general anaesthetics induce peripheral vasodilation, thus increasing redistribution of heat from the central to the peripheral compartment (Figure 3.3)
- Phase 2: slow linear reduction in core temperature (subsequent 2–3 hours). During the following hours of anaesthesia, a further decrease in body temperature results from heat loss exceeding heat production, associated with a significant reduction in metabolism and heat production from skeletal muscles. This phase is the main determinant for the severity of hypothermia
- Phase 3: after 3–4 hours of anaesthesia body temperature reaches a plateau phase during which heat production equals heat loss.

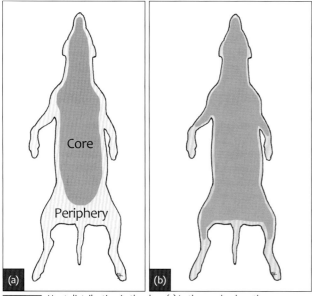

3.2 Heat distribution in the dog. (a) In the awake dog, the core compartment varies little in temperature. The peripheral compartment absorbs or releases heat to maintain normothermia. The temperature in the peripheral compartment can vary by up to 8°C. (b) Internal redistribution of body heat following induction of general anaesthesia (phase 1). Heat is redistributed into the peripheral compartment through vasodilation, leading to a drop in core temperature.

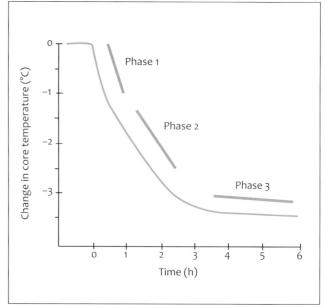

3.3 Typical curve for the development of hypothermia during general anaesthesia. The initial decrease (phase 1) results from a redistribution of body heat from the core to the periphery. This is followed by phase 2, in which a further decrease in temperature results from heat loss exceeding heat production. Finally, a plateau is reached where heat production equals heat loss (phase 3).

Causes of heat loss

The temperature of surface body layers is more suscep-tible to environmental factors than the core temperature. Heat is transferred from the animal to the environment in four ways:

- *Radiation* of infrared waves to the surroundings accounts for most heat loss in the anaesthetized patient
- Heat is continuously lost from blood flowing under the skin to air molecules moving over the skin surface via *convection*, which is the second most important cause of heat loss in anaesthetized patients. Surgical draping will prevent air movement around the patient, but clipping of hair increases air flow over the skin. Heat loss by convection is especially high in operating rooms equipped with laminar air flow
- Temperature differences between two adjacent surfaces (e.g. patient and operating table) results in transfer of heat via *conduction*. Use of foam pads, towels or other insulating material will easily prevent heat transfer
- *Evaporation* of water occurs mainly from the respiratory tract (dry medical gases), but only accounts for a small amount of total heat loss. However, evaporative heat losses from surgical sites and open body cavities can contribute markedly to total heat loss.

Perioperative complications and consequences of hypothermia

Hypothermia reduces the minimal alveolar concentration (MAC) of volatile agents and increases their solubility in tissues. Therefore, in hypothermic patients, less volatile drug is required compared with the requirement of normothermic patients undergoing similar procedures. The pharmacokinetics of many injectable drugs used dur-ing anaesthesia are altered by hypothermia. The effective duration of most non-depolarizing neuromuscular block-ing agents (NMBAs) is prolonged; in humans, the duration of action of vecuronium has been shown to double following a decrease in body temperature of 2–3°C. Temperature-dependent Hofmann degradation of atra-curium and cisatracurium is slower in hypothermic patients, thereby prolonging their action. Plasma concen-trations of propofol and fentanyl increase during hypo-thermia due to changes in redistribution and metabolism. In cats, a significant link between low body temperature and time from end of anaesthesia to extubation has been demonstrated (Steinbacher *et al.*, 2010).

Blood coagulation is also impaired due to a 'cold-induced' defect in platelet function and because the clotting factors and enzymes involved in the coagulation cascade have a reduced function. The changes in enzyme function that occur under clinical conditions often go undetected as all coagulation tests are carried out in the laboratory at 37°C, thus not reflecting the true picture *in vivo* in the hypothermic patient. In human anaesthesia, hypothermia is associated with a 20% increase in blood loss during surgery.

Hypothermia also reduces immune system function, which can result in substantial increases in the incidence of postoperative wound infections. Furthermore, hypothermia causes vasoconstriction, which reduces blood flow and oxygen delivery to the wound. In humans, hypothermia can delay wound healing and result in prolonged hospitalization even in patients without wound infections (Kurz *et al.*, 1996).

Postoperative shivering can increase oxygen consump-tion by up to 400% (in young children), and this may result in hypoxaemia when supplemental oxygen is no longer being provided. The residual respiratory depressant effects of anaesthetic agents can cause hypoventilation during the early postoperative period; in these circumstances, oxygen uptake may not be enough to meet demand. In one study, the incidence of postoperative shivering in cats was reported to be 33% and shivering stopped at body temper-atures between 36.5 and 38.1°C (Steinbacher *et al.*, 2010). People report shivering to be the worst aspect of the postanesthetic experience, and severe shivering may increase pain sensation through movement-induced shear-ing forces on the wound. It is difficult to predict if, and when, a patient is likely to shiver during recovery. In humans, postoperative shivering can be due not just to hypothermia but also to pain. Therefore, the patient should be warmed during anaesthesia and kept as normothermic as possible and adequate analgesia should be provided to treat pain before the animal recovers.

Thermoregulatory shivering does not occur at body temperatures below 35°C. Shivering can be treated by 'arti-ficially' reducing the shivering threshold with an alpha-2 adrenoceptor agonist (medetomidine 1 µg/kg i.v. or dex-medetomidine 0.5 µg/kg i.v.) or pethidine at a low dose (0.5–1.0 mg/kg i.m.).

Prevention of hypothermia
Prewarming

Physical warming of dogs and cats before induction of anaesthesia (for 30 minutes to 2 hours) significantly reduces the incidence of intraoperative hypothermia and postoperative shivering. Warming raises the peripheral temperature and reduces the initial drop in core body temperature observed during Phase 1, as redistribution of heat depends on the gradient between core and peripheral temperature: the higher the peripheral temperature at the beginning of anaesthesia, the less the redistribution of heat during the initial phase.

Clipping and surgical preparation

Clipping of the surgical field should be kept to a minimum because fur is a natural insulator against heat loss. Excessive scrubbing of the surgical field and the use of alcohol and other disinfectants should be avoided to mini-mize evaporative heat loss.

Environmental temperature

The operating room temperature will determine the extent of heat loss by radiation and convection from the skin, and by evaporation from surgical incisions. Room temper-atures below 26°C have been associated with significantly lower body temperatures in cats (Steinbacher *et al.*, 2010); however, a temperature of 26°C will be uncomfortably warm for personnel working in the operating room.

A substantial drop in body temperature can occur between administration of pre-anaesthetic medication and induction of anaesthesia (Redondo *et al.*, 2012ab). During this period, animals are often exposed to cold environ-ments and heat production will already be reduced by the drugs used. Excessive heat loss can be limited by provi-sion of a warm environment, by covering the patient with a blanket and avoidance of excessive air movement around the patient.

Warmed intravenous fluids

The temperature of intravenously administered fluids should not exceed the patient's body temperature; therefore, intravenous fluids cannot be used to warm the patient. In cats, the use of a sophisticated fluid warming device (providing a fluid temperature of 39°C when fluid entered the intravenous catheter at 10 ml/kg/h) resulted in body temperature being maintained at a temperature only 0.5°C higher than when fluids were administered at room temperature (Steinbacher et al., 2010). Prewarmed infusion fluid bags have no thermodynamic benefit (Soto et al., 2014). However, heat loss can become significant when large volumes of colder solutions are administered intravenously.

It is essential to use warmed fluids to flush body cavities and joints in order to reduce heat loss, although care must be taken to avoid lavaging with excessively warm fluids: the maximal temperature should be as for intravenous fluids (≤40°C).

Airway heating, humidification and low-flow anaesthesia

Only 10% of metabolically produced heat is lost via the respiratory tract, even when patients breathe dry, cool gas mixtures. Heat and moisture exchangers have not been shown to prevent hypothermia in anaesthetized dogs when used in a rebreathing system with an oxygen flow of 1.3 l/min (Hofmeister et al., 2011). It is not known whether such devices are more effective when used with a non-rebreathing system and/or with a higher fresh gas flow. Using low-flow or minimal-flow anaesthesia (fresh gas flow <200 ml/min or rebreathing fraction >75%) will conserve heat and moisture within the breathing system. In addition, the reaction of carbon dioxide with soda lime and other absorbents is exothermic and this will add heat to the gas in a rebreathing system (see Chapter 5).

Passive surface warming methods

Passive insulation reduces cutaneous heat loss by 30% (one layer) to 50% (three layers), and can be achieved with blankets, surgical drapes, metallic sheets or plastic blankets such as 'bubble wrap'. These materials reduce radiant, conductive and convective heat losses but do not attenuate the reduction in core temperature during the initial phase. Placing bandages around the limbs can reduce heat loss during Phase 2, after the redistribution of heat to the periphery. Metallic blankets can effectively reduce radiation heat loss due to their reflective properties (Figure 3.4).

Active surface warming methods

For most patients, some form of active warming will be required to prevent intraoperative hypothermia during procedures lasting more than 1 hour. Circulating warm water blankets are relatively ineffective when placed under the animal because the bodyweight reduces capillary blood flow in the areas in direct contact with the mattress and can prevent heat transfer to the central compartment. Furthermore, the combination of externally supplied heat and reduced local tissue perfusion can cause thermal injuries even when the temperature of the mattress does not exceed 40°C. It is advisable to use some form of insulation between the warming device and the patient, such as a towel, and even then caution should be exercised (Figure 3.5). A novel resistive heating system for small animals is the Hot Dog®: the blanket can be used over the body or placed around the animal, increasing the amount of body surface covered by the device (Figure 3.6).

Forced warm air (Figure 3.7) is by far the most commonly used and most effective intraoperative warming technique (Machon et al., 1999). This technique may be

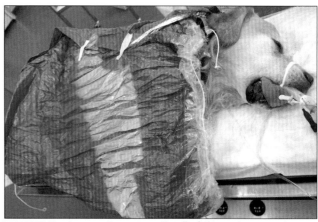

3.4 Passive warming system. Metallic foil is used to cover the patient, reducing radiant, conductive and convective heat losses.
(Courtesy of Rima Bektas, University of Zürich)

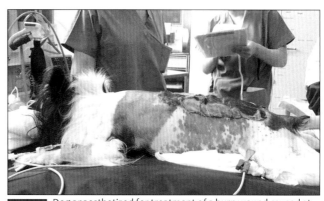

3.5 Dog anaesthetized for treatment of a burn wound caused at an earlier stage by an electrical heating mat placed beneath the dog during ovariohysterectomy in dorsal recumbency.
(Courtesy of Stephanie Picek, University of Zürich)

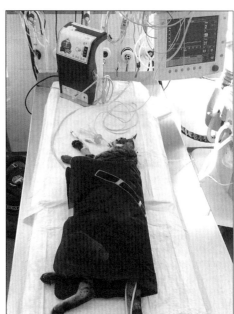

3.6 Cat under general anaesthesia. The blanket of an electrical heating system (Hot Dog® device) is wrapped around the patient to minimize heat loss.
(Courtesy of Charlotte Marly-Voquer, University of Zürich)

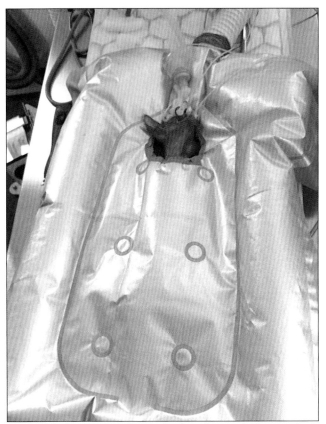

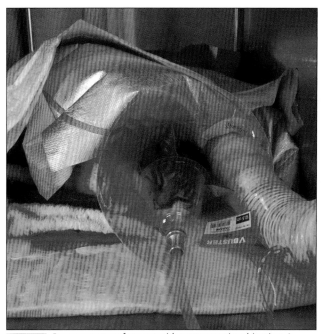

3.8 Recovery set-up for a cat with postoperative shivering. A forced warm air system and a heat lamp are used to rewarm the patient. Oxygen is being delivered via facemask to compensate for the increase in oxygen demand due to the shivering.

3.7 Active warming of a cat using forced warm air. The cover has been cut to allow surgical access and the edges of the cut are sealed with tape to avoid escape of the warm air.

more expensive than other methods, as the warm air blankets are disposable and should not be reused in a sterile setting. However, these blankets are very versatile, can be placed either underneath or on top of the patient and are available in several sizes and forms from different manufacturers (e.g. Bair Hugger, Cocoon).

Heat packs and plastic heat pads, home-made wheat bags, hot water bottles or water-filled gloves can be heated in a microwave and then used to provide active warming; all of these methods should be used with caution as they can cause thermal injuries and should never be placed in direct contact with the patient.

Rewarming the hypothermic patient

In order to rewarm a patient, the applied heat must be transferred from the periphery to the core. Skin surface warming is therefore far more effective at increasing core temperature when the patient is in a vasodilated state. It is easier to rewarm a patient during anaesthesia because the vasculature is dilated as a result of the anaesthetic drugs used. Rewarming during the postoperative period may take longer as vasoconstriction occurs during this period. Some anaesthetists prefer to wait until body temperature has reached 36.5°C before recovering their patients to avoid severe and moderate hypothermia in the recovery period (Redondo *et al.*, 2012ab). However, rewarming during anaesthesia will increase anaesthesia time and thus may increase the risk of mortality and total treatment costs. Therefore, hypothermic patients should still be diligently rewarmed postoperatively. As well as the active heating methods mentioned above, incubators designed for human infants, and heat lamps can also be used with care (Figure 3.8).

Recovery

Most fatalities occur during recovery suggesting greater vigilance is required during this period. The reasons for these fatalities are likely to be multifactorial, but the main contributing factors are lack of monitoring and observation.

Recovery area and criteria for monitoring

During recovery, developing complications may be missed as the patient is often left alone. Ideally, there should be a dedicated recovery area in the practice to facilitate close observation of the patient. The recovery facilities should reflect the number and type of cases that are normally seen. The area should be well ventilated to eliminate exhaled anaesthetic gases and equipped to provide oxygen via dedicated flowmeters and also the means to efficiently rewarm patients should be present. The necessary equipment for dealing with emergencies (see Chapter 31) should also be readily available such as an anaesthetic machine, breathing systems, ETTs and laryngoscope, suction apparatus, monitoring equipment, emergency drugs and, if possible, a defibrillator. It is also important to ensure that staff members are trained in good recovery techniques. Ideally, the following should be monitored postoperatively:

- Level of consciousness, activity and recovery of physiological reflexes
- Body temperature
- Oxygenation
- Ventilation and airway patency
- Circulation (heart or pulse rate, pulse quality, mucous membrane colour, capillary refill time)
- Postoperative analgesia.

Patients should only be left alone to recover if the following criteria are fulfilled:

- The animal is alert, can lift its head, is swallowing, and shows normal ocular reflexes. Jaw tone indicates good muscle strength
- No shivering is apparent and the body temperature is above the shivering threshold (>35°C)
- The mucous membranes are pink while the patient is breathing room air. If in doubt, a pulse oximeter should be used to check the oxygen saturation of haemoglobin, which should be >94%
- The animal is breathing freely and deeply without an ETT in place. No signs of upper airway obstruction are present
- Heart rate and ABP (if measured) are within 20% of pre-anaesthetic values; peripheral pulses are strong and regular
- Effective analgesia has been provided and is likely to last until the next assessment is due.

Complications during recovery

The most common complications occurring during the recovery period are:

- Upper airway obstruction
- Hypoxaemia
- Hypothermia and postoperative shivering
- Inadequately controlled pain
- 'Rough' recovery or emergence excitement
- Delayed recovery
- Bleeding from the surgical wound
- Hyperthermia
- Haemodynamic instability.

Upper airway obstruction

The patient should never be left unattended during early recovery, when the ETT is still in place. Extubation can be performed once the swallowing reflex has returned in dogs, and when there are clear palpebral reflexes or pro-voked ear twitches in cats. After extubation, the patient's neck and head should be extended and the tongue gently pulled forward to maintain a patent airway.

The most common causes of upper airway obstruction are loss of pharyngeal muscle tone, regurgitation, vomiting, laryngospasm and laryngeal oedema.

Loss of pharyngeal tone: The persistent effect of anaesthetic drugs, especially volatile anaesthetics, opioids, benzodiazepines and NMBAs, causes loss of pharyngeal muscle tone, which is a common cause of upper airway obstruction after extubation. The effort of breathing against a partially or completely obstructed larynx is characterized by snoring, flaring of the nostrils and a paradoxical breathing pattern. Extension of the neck and gentle withdrawal of the tongue often opens up the airway and this position should be maintained until the patient has adequately recovered. The effect of opioids and benzodiazepines can be antagonized if necessary (see Chapter 31). If residual neuromuscular block is a potential reason for the loss of pharyngeal tone, specific reversal agents can be administered (see Chapter 16). In rare cases the patient will need to be reintubated.

Brachycephalic dogs and cats often struggle to maintain a patent upper airway due to instability of the laryngeal cartilages, even when awake. Furthermore, the elongated fleshy soft palate, thickening of nasopharyngeal soft tissues, enlargement of the root of the tongue, everted pharyngeal tonsils and laryngeal ventricles characteristic of these breeds can, alone or in combination, cause airway obstruction during recovery. One way of overcoming this problem is to extubate later during recovery when all reflexes have sufficiently recovered, although this does increase the risk of regurgitation (see below). Placement of a supraglottic airway device (see Chapter 5) or a bandage roll in the mouth and pulling out the tongue may help to overcome lack of pharyngeal tone until the patient has recovered sufficiently (Figure 3.9).

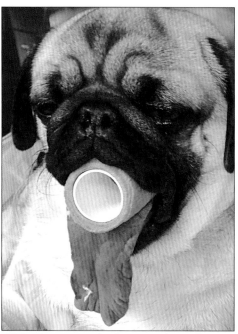

3.9 Pug recovering from anaesthesia after upper airway surgery. A bandage roll is placed in the mouth to keep the tongue pulled out and to maintain a patent airway.

Regurgitation or vomiting: Brachycephalic breeds are generally also prone to regurgitation. Unfortunately, while late extubation can be helpful in avoiding airway obstruction it can also cause regurgitation. Placing the patient in sternal recumbency with the head higher than the stomach for recovery can avoid aspiration in patients that have not already regurgitated. If regurgitation or vomiting occurs during recovery, it is important to remove all regurgitated material gently using suction (where possible) as soon as possible and to place the head below the trunk to allow material to drain.

Laryngospasm and laryngeal oedema: Laryngospasm, which can completely obstruct the laryngeal opening, requires immediate treatment. Spasm typically occurs immediately after extubation, often following dental procedures, difficult intubation, airway irrigation, and upper airway surgery. Cats are more prone to laryngospasm and/or laryngeal oedema than dogs and require close observation in the immediate post-extubation period. Details regarding treatment of laryngospasm and laryngeal oedema can be found in Chapter 31.

Hypoxaemia

During the postoperative period the residual effects of sedative and anaesthetic agents and opioids will often depress ventilation. Hypoventilation can also be caused by hypothermia or CNS disease (high intracranial pressure). The alveolar gas equation (see Chapter 7) demonstrates clearly that a high arterial (and therefore high alveolar) carbon dioxide tension decreases alveolar oxygen tension, which in turn decreases arterial oxygen tension, with consequent hypoxaemia. Hypoxaemia due to hypoventilation should be treated with supplemental oxygen to increase the inspired oxygen fraction (F_iO_2). Antagonizing the effect of benzodiazepines or opioids may also be indicated. In cases of severe hypoventilation it will be necessary to reintubate the patient and provide IPPV (see Chapter 31).

Diffusion hypoxaemia may occur if nitrous oxide and oxygen delivery are stopped at the same time and the animal is immediately disconnected from the breathing system. It can persist for up to 10 minutes with the patient breathing room air. To avoid this, nitrous oxide should be switched off earlier and the patient should breathe only oxygen and volatile anaesthetic agent for the last 5–10 minutes of the anaesthetic before being disconnected from the anaesthetic machine.

Diffusion impairment commonly occurs when there is underlying lung disease such as pneumonia, acute respiratory distress syndrome (ARDS) or airway disease. Ideally, the underlying disease will have been diagnosed before anaesthesia. Diffusion impairment in the postoperative period can be the result of interstitial and alveolar lung oedema caused by iatrogenic fluid overload. This can be further exacerbated by acute renal or congestive heart failure. Pulmonary oedema occurring after airway obstruction is the result of the high negative intrathoracic pressures generated by increased inspiratory efforts against a high resistance within the upper airway. These pressures increase the hydrostatic pressure gradient between the lung capillaries and alveoli, resulting in interstitial and alveolar oedema. Alveolar oedema can be diagnosed by auscultation and radiography, but interstitial lung oedema may be undetectable. Alveolar and interstitial lung oedema will both increase the diffusion distance and time for oxygen to reach the capillary blood and consequently can result in hypoxaemia.

A reduced ventilation (V_A)/perfusion (Q) ratio (see Chapter 22) is another common cause of hypoxaemia during the post-anaesthetic period. Low V_A/Q ratios indicate areas of high perfusion with low ventilation. Impaired ventilation of perfused alveoli results in an increased volume of deoxygenated blood entering the systemic arterial circulation (venous admixture). Hypoxaemia due to low V_A/Q mismatch areas can be treated by increasing F_iO_2 although this technique is ineffective in raising low arterial oxygen tensions caused by shunt. Complete intrapulmonary shunting represents blood flowing through atelectatic lung areas and is an extreme form of low V_A/Q mismatch where perfusion occurs in the absence of any ventilation. Atelectasis can rapidly develop in dependent areas of the lung and is a common problem during anaesthesia.

A reduced FRC will result in closure of small airways and absorption into the blood of all gases within the alveoli beyond the closed airways (absorption atelectasis); surfactant depletion also plays a role. Obese dogs are more prone to atelectasis formation and hypoxaemia because their FRC is already reduced (Mosing et al., 2013; see also earlier in this chapter). Atelectasis may persist for several days after anaesthesia, and can be a focus of infection and contribute to postoperative pulmonary complications.

Oxygen delivery systems in the postoperative period:
The choice of system used to deliver oxygen to the patient during recovery will depend on the patient's degree of hypoxaemia, stress level and cooperation, and the procedure that has been performed.

- *Flow-by technique*, in which an oxygen delivery system (tubing connected to an oxygen flowmeter or pressure regulator) is placed in front of the patient's nose. This technique is relatively ineffective as F_iO_2 will not exceed 0.4 even with high flows. The flow-by technique is easy to use and well tolerated, but will become ineffective the moment the patient moves its head away from the oxygen source.
- *Facemasks* are very efficient at increasing F_iO_2 even with low oxygen flows. The black diaphragm should be removed from the mask if there is no means of releasing pressure within the system. Patient acceptance of the facemask over the muzzle is well tolerated during early recovery (see Figure 3.8).
- *Elizabethan collars* with plastic wrap covering the lower two-thirds of the front aspect can be used in cats for a long period after anaesthesia.
- *Unilateral or bilateral nasal catheters* can be placed in the ventral nasal meatus, at the end of anaesthesia, before recovery. The distal tip of the catheter should reach the level of the medial canthus; this distance should be pre-measured and indicated on the catheter before placement. Oxygen flow rates of 100 ml/kg/min can produce an F_iO_2 >0.4 (Zimmerman et al., 2013). Bilateral nasal catheters can provide an F_iO_2 of approximately 0.6 (Dunphy et al., 2002). Nasal catheters should be used in combination with a bubble-through humidifier (see Chapter 5). They should not be used in brachycephalic animals, or in patients with head trauma (in which sneezing should be avoided) or other nasal pathology.
- *Oxygen cages or human paediatric incubators* can be used for recovery of small patients. However, this method does not allow the patient to be easily handled and results in oxygen wastage when the door is opened.

Hypothermia and postoperative shivering

These complications are covered earlier, in the section on perioperative complications and consequences of hypothermia.

Inadequately controlled postoperative pain

Pain assessment and treatment is discussed in Chapters 9–11. It is especially important to treat pain in the immediate postoperative period in order to facilitate a smooth recovery. Pain can also contribute to postoperative shivering. The analgesic plan should be re-evaluated in any patient with a dysphoric recovery and adapted if necessary.

Another common cause of sympathetic stimulus with resulting postoperative pain is a distended bladder. Manually expressing the bladder before recovery should be mandatory for every patient.

'Rough' recovery or emergence excitement

Animals often experience a transient state of confusion when emerging from general anaesthesia. This can be accompanied by vocalization, aggression, general excitement and escape behaviours. Emergence delirium is more likely when animals recover quickly from anaesthetics that are eliminated rapidly from the CNS, such as volatile anaesthetics. Once hypoxaemic delirium has been ruled out, intravenous administration of a low dose of a fast- and short-acting anaesthetic (alfaxalone or propofol) to calm the animal may be indicated. Thereafter, a rapidly acting sedative and/or analgesic drug can be administered to smooth the subsequent recovery (alpha-2 adrenoceptor agonist alone or in combination with an opioid). If excitation is moderate the intravenous administration of an alpha-2 adrenoceptor agonist with an onset time of 1–2 minutes (medetomidine or dexmedetomidine) might be sufficient. Acepromazine should only be used to sedate patients during recovery if adequate postoperative pain control is guaranteed, as it only causes sedation and exerts no analgesic effects. It is preferable to use acepromazine as part of the pre-anaesthetic medication if a rough recovery is expected. This is especially the case in dog breeds that may have an excitable temperament (e.g. Border Collie, Husky), as the onset of action of acepromazine is slow and therefore administration during emergence excitement may be too late to have an optimal effect.

Delayed recovery

Cats and dogs generally respond to external stimulation within an hour after the end of anaesthesia. Patients with a slow recovery should be examined for the presence of hypoxaemia, hypoventilation, hypovolaemia, hypoglycaemia, hypothermia, neurological disorders, drug interactions, or pre-existing problems such as endocrine, hepatic or renal disease. However, delayed recovery is most commonly a consequence of the residual effects of drugs administered during anaesthesia. See Chapters 10, 11 and 13–16 for details of specific drugs and their antagonists.

Bleeding from the surgical wound

Early recognition of postoperative bleeding is important so that it can be treated promptly. In cases with a high likelihood of postoperative bleeding, such as animals suffering from coagulopathies, close observation during the postoperative period is essential.

Hyperthermia

Hyperthermia during recovery is a frequent side effect of opioid administration, especially in cats; the mechanism responsible is described in Chapter 10. If there is any suspicion that hyperthermia is due to an opioid, its administration should be stopped; in severe cases, partial or complete reversal can be attempted.

Hyperthermia can also occur in large dogs with thick fur, especially during hot weather. These animals should be actively cooled with ice packs and fans and by placing wet towels around the animal. If needed, the fur can be clipped to increase the exposed surface area, but ideally the owner should be informed before this is done. Cold wet towels should not be left in place over the patient as they will actually insulate the patient and worsen hyperthermia. Intravenous administration of cool fluids (crystalloids) should be considered, as well as placing the patient on a relatively cold surface until normothermia has been achieved.

Haemodynamic instability

Electrolyte disturbances and pH changes can cause severe haemodynamic disturbances including hypotension, often in combination with bradycardia. Evaluation of pH and electrolytes, in particular potassium, should be carried out to enable specific and prompt treatment. Tachycardia can be caused by hypovolaemia, which should be treated with intravenous fluids. Other possible reasons for tachycardia during recovery are pain, shivering

and excitement, and are often accompanied by an increase in ABP. Bradycardia in the postoperative period is most commonly drug induced or caused by hypothermia. The patient's peripheral circulation should be assessed to determine whether the slow heart rate is causing poor tissue perfusion. Patients with neurological pathology may have a combination of hypertension and bradycardia (Cushing's reflex); these animals must be assessed for the possibility of increased intracranial pressure. In patients with chronic renal failure and a history of hypertension, continuous monitoring of ABP is required because pain and anxiety can exacerbate haemodynamic problems during recovery from anaesthesia. Treatment to improve oxygenation, ventilation and perfusion will hasten recovery (see Chapters 17, 18 and 21).

Handover from theatre team to postoperative team

The handover from the theatre team to the personnel who will care for the patient postoperatively is a critical process. If information is lost during the handover, this can lead to delay in diagnosing any problems and providing treatment. The use of checklists can be effective in avoiding this loss of information. A sample checklist, modified from human medicine, is provided in Figure 3.10 (Segall *et al.*, 2012).

Patient information
- Name, species, breed, sex
- Age
- Bodyweight
- Pre-existing diseases and diagnosis
- Medical history
- Procedure performed
- Condition of the animal before anaesthesia

Anaesthesia information
- Type of anaesthesia/anaesthetic protocol
- Anaesthesia complications and anaesthetic course (e.g. use of IPPV)
- Intraoperative medications
- Intravenous fluids administered (type and volume)
- Blood products administered (type and amount)
- Estimated blood loss

Surgical information
- Surgical course
- Surgical site information, including dressings, tubes, drains and packing
- Surgical complications and interventions to manage these

Current status
- Assessment of haemodynamic stability
- Oxygenation status
- Body temperature

Postoperative care plan
- Anticipated recovery and problems
- Clear postoperative management plan
- Monitoring plan and range for physiological variables (pulse rate, temperature, respiratory rate)
- Analgesia plan
- Plan for intravenous fluids, antibiotics and other medications
- Plan for feeding
- Plan for special measurements (e.g. urinary output)
- When to call for advice/help

3.10 Information that should be transferred from the surgical/anaesthesia team to staff who will care for the patient postoperatively. IPPV = intermittent positive pressure ventilation.

References and further reading

Barton-Lamb AL, Martin-Flores M, Scrivani PV *et al.* (2013) Evaluation of maxillary arterial blood flow in anesthetized cats with the mouth closed and open. *The Veterinary Journal* **196**, 325–331

Brodbelt DC (2006) The Confidential Enquiry into Perioperative Small Animal Fatalities. PhD thesis, Royal Veterinary College, University of London

Brodbelt DC, Blissitt KJ, Hammond RA *et al.* (2008) The risk of death: the confidential enquiry into perioperative small animal fatalities. *Veterinary Anaesthesia and Analgesia* **35**, 365–373

Brodbelt DC, Pfeiffer DU, Young LE *et al.* (2007) Risk factors for anaesthetic-related death in cats: results from the confidential enquiry into perioperative small animal fatalities (CEPSAF). *British Journal of Anaesthesia* **99**, 617–623

Davis H, Jensen T, Johnson A *et al.* (2013) 2013 AAHA/AAFP fluid therapy guidelines for dogs and cats. *Journal of the American Animal Hospital Association* **49**, 149–159

Dunphy ED, Mann FA, Dodam JR *et al.* (2002) Comparison of unilateral versus bilateral nasal catheters for oxygen administration in dogs. *Journal of Veterinary Emergency and Critical Care* **12**, 245–251

Dyer F, Diesel G, Cooles S and Tait A (2010) Suspected adverse events, 2010. *Veterinary Record* **168**, 610–613

Hofmeister E, Brainard B, Braun C *et al.* (2011) Effect of a heat and moisture exchanger on heat loss in isoflurane-anesthetized dogs undergoing single-limb orthopedic procedures. *Journal of the American Veterinary Medical Association* **239**, 1561–1565

Kafarnik C, Fritsche J and Reese S (2008) Corneal innervation in mesocephalic and brachycephalic dogs and cats: assessment using *in vivo* confocal microscopy. *Veterinary Ophthalmology* **11**, 363-367

Kurz A, Sessler DI and Lenhardt RA (1996) Perioperative normothermia to reduce the incidence of surgical wound infection and shorten hospitalization. Study of Wound Infection and Temperature Group. *New England Journal of Medicine* **334**, 1209–1215

Machon RG, Raffe MR and Robinson EP (1999) Warming with a forced air warming blanket minimizes anesthetic-induced hypothermia in cats. *Veterinary Surgery* **28**, 301–310

Mosing M, German AJ, Holden SL *et al.* (2013) Oxygenation and ventilation characteristics in obese sedated dogs before and after weight loss: a clinical trial. *The Veterinary Journal* **198**, 367–371

Park Y-W, Son W-G, Jeong M-B *et al.* (2013) Evaluation of risk factors for development of corneal ulcer after nonocular surgery in dogs: 14 cases (2009–2011). *Journal of the American Veterinary Medicine Association* **242**, 1544–1548

Redondo JI, Suesta P, Gil L *et al.* (2012a) Retrospective study of the prevalence of postanaesthetic hypothermia in cats. *Veterinary Record* **170**, 206

Redondo JI, Suesta P, Serra I *et al.* (2012b) Retrospective study of the prevalence of postanaesthetic hypothermia in dogs. *Veterinary Record* **171**, 374

Segall N, Bonifacio AS, Schroeder RA *et al.* (2012) Can we make postoperative patient handovers safer? A systematic review of the literature. *Anesthesia and Analgesia* **115**, 102–115

Soto N, Towle Millard HA, Lee RA *et al.* (2014) *In vitro* comparison of output fluid temperatures for room temperature and prewarmed fluids. *Journal of Small Animal Practice* **55**, 415–419

Steinbacher R, Mosing M, Eberspächer E and Moens Y (2010) Der Einsatz von Infusionswärmepumpen vermindert perioperative Hypothermie bei Katzen. *Tierärztliche Praxis* **38**, 15–22

Stiles J, Weil AB, Packer RA *et al.* (2012) Post-anesthetic cortical blindness in cats: twenty cases. *Veterinary Journal* **193**, 367–373

Watson K (1992) Use of Xylocaine pump spray for intubation in cats. *Veterinary Record* **130**, 455

Zimmerman ME, Hodgson DS, Bello NM (2013) Effects of oxygen insufflation rate, respiratory rate, and tidal volume on fraction of inspired oxygen in cadaveric canine heads attached to a lung model. *American Journal of Veterinary Research* **74**, 1247–1251

Chapter 4

The anaesthetic machine and vaporizers

Hatim I.K. Alibhai

Accurate and continuous delivery of gas and vapour mixtures of desired compositions is made possible by the use of an anaesthetic machine and vaporizer. Several manufacturers produce anaesthetic machines for human or veterinary use and, although the equipment is varied, the basic design remains the same and a working knowledge of the basic components will enable familiarity with newer designs.

A standard machine consists of a rigid steel or aluminium framework on rubber antistatic wheels with brakes. Antistatic measures improve flowmeter performance and reduce the risk of explosions when flammable vapours are used. A modern machine designed for human use often comes with a built-in ventilator, circle system and patient monitoring devices. Some machines also use automated patient record-keeping systems.

Anaesthetic machines are designed to suit a wide variety of environments. Compact (portable) or wall rail-mounted machines (Figure 4.1) may be suitable in areas where space is restricted and they may have single or twin positions for vaporizers on the back bar (Figure 4.2). Ceiling- or trolley-mounted machines (Figure 4.3a) are large and heavy with many components, including an integrated array of monitors. Machines intended for use in magnetic environments are made from non-ferrous metals (Figure 4.3b; see also Chapter 29). Modern machines have very easy-to-clean surfaces, drawers, shelves and rails to accommodate specialist accessories. Modern machines are mains powered, have a rechargeable battery and use compressed air or oxygen to drive their ventilators.

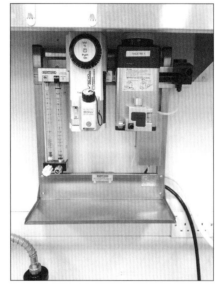

4.2 A wall rail-mounted machine with twin positions for vaporizers on the back bar.

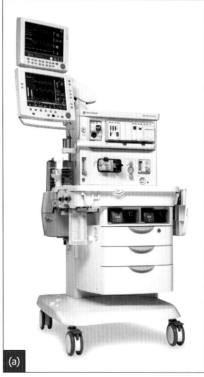

4.3 (a) A modern anaesthetic machine with integrated ventilator and multiparameter monitor. (continues) ▶
(a, Courtesy of GE Medical Systems Ltd)

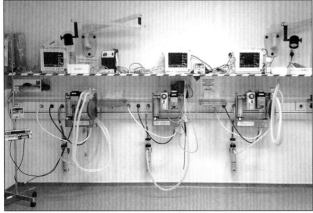

4.1 Three wall rail-mounted anaesthetic machines in a preparation room.

(a)

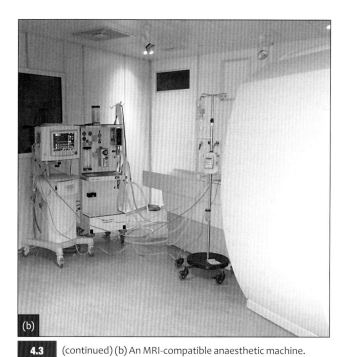

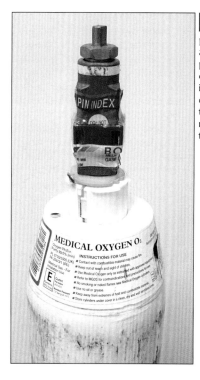

4.4 A size E oxygen cylinder with protective plastic wrapping around the valve block and plastic label showing the contents and other information. The colour-coded plastic discs between the valve block and cylinder neck show when cylinder testing is next due.

4.3 (continued) (b) An MRI-compatible anaesthetic machine.

The basic anaesthetic machine consists of:

- A gas supply
- Pin index system for cylinders
- Pressure gauges
- Pressure-reducing valves
- Secondary pressure regulators
- Flowmeters
- Vaporizers
- Oxygen failure warning device
- Pressure relief valve
- Oxygen flush system
- A common gas outlet
- A multiparameter patient monitor (on modern machines)
- A ventilator (on modern machines).

Gas supplies

The supply of compressed medical gases in any veterinary clinic or hospital takes the form of cylinders or piped gases.

Cylinders

Cylinders in the UK are made of molybdenum steel. Cylinders designed for use in magnetic resonance imaging (MRI) facilities are made from aluminium alloy with special non-ferromagnetic pin index valves. More lightweight cylinders are made from steel or aluminium and have a wrapping of fibreglass in an epoxy resin matrix, and are for use in a home environment. Impact, pressure and tensile tests are carried out by manufacturers every five years; a colour-coded plastic disc around the neck of the cylinder indicates when the next tests are due (Figure 4.4).

Oxygen and medical air are stored in cylinders as compressed gases; oxygen is stored at a pressure of 13,700 kPa. Nitrous oxide and carbon dioxide liquefy at the pressures used to fill the cylinders and therefore most of the gas content is in liquid form. Nitrous oxide is stored in the liquid phase, in equilibrium with its vapour at the top of

the cylinder, at a pressure of 4400 kPa. Cylinders containing liquefied gas are filled to a *filling ratio* (the mass of liquid in the cylinder divided by the mass of water that it could hold); for example, the filling ratio for nitrous oxide is 0.75 in temperate climates and 0.65 in hot climates. This ratio is very important because if the cylinder were overfilled, a small rise in temperature would cause a large rise in pressure and possibly cause the cylinder to rupture. Cylinders with liquefied gas must always be used vertically with the valve uppermost, otherwise liquid will be discharged when the valve is opened.

The pressure in an oxygen cylinder decreases linearly and proportionally as the cylinder empties. With nitrous oxide the pressure gauge will read 'full' until all the liquefied gas has vaporized.

Cylinders are available in sizes A to J: Figure 4.5 shows the capacity of the commonly used ones. Cylinders attached to the anaesthetic machine are size E, while size J is used for cylinder manifolds.

Cylinder identification

Information on cylinder contents is provided on a label (see Figure 4.4), with further information engraved on the side of the valve block. This engraving indicates tare weight, chemical formula of contents, test pressure and dates when tests were carried out.

Cylinders also conform to a colour code in order to prevent accidental misuse of gas or vapour and are painted so

	UK				USA		
	E	F	G	J	E	F	G
Dimensions	34 x 4	36 x 5½	54 x 7	56½ x 9	26 x 4½	51 x 5½	51 x 8½
Oxygen	680	1360	3400	6800	650	2062	5300
Nitrous oxide	1820	3640	9100	18200	1590	5260	13800

4.5 Dimensions (height x outer diameter in inches) and approximate capacity (in litres measured at room temperature and pressure) for various commonly used gas cylinders.
(Data from Ward 1975; Dorsch and Dorsch, 1999)

that their contents can be easily identified. In the UK, oxygen cylinders are painted black with a white shoulder; nitrous oxide, French blue; and carbon dioxide, grey. In North America, the cylinder colours are the same except that oxygen is stored in green or green-and-white cylinders. A new European Standard of cylinder colour coding has been adopted by various EU countries. The Medicines and Healthcare Products Regulatory Agency (MHRA) has approved changes to the colour coding of cylinders in the UK, in line with other EU countries, to reduce the risk of administering the wrong gas to the patient. In future, to distinguish medical from non-medical gas cylinders, all medical gas cylinder bodies will be white. The shoulder colours will not change and these will identify the individual gases (Figure 4.6). Cylinders will also carry the name of the medical gas in large letters on the cylinder body to help identification. For a limited period, oxygen cylinders may have black bodies; these do not have the name 'oxygen' on the body of the cylinder. The programme to convert all compressed medical oxygen cylinders to white bodies will be completed by 2025.

Cylinder storage

Medical gas cylinders should be stored under cover in a specially designed room which must be made of fireproof materials. They must not be subjected to extremes of heat and cold, and should not be stored near flammable materials such as oil or grease, or near any source of heat. Cylinders should be stored away from corrosive chemicals. Storage areas should be kept dry, be well ventilated, provide good access for delivery vehicles and have sound concrete floors. Full and empty cylinders should be stored separately where they cannot fall over and cause injury. Size E and smaller cylinders should be stored horizontally, or vertically in a specially designed trolley (Figure 4.7), whereas size F and larger cylinders (size G and J) should be stored vertically. The layout and racking within the medical gas cylinder store should allow for stock rotation of full cylinders to enable those with the shortest expiry time to be used first. Labels must remain clearly visible at all times and not be removed or covered. Unauthorized labels/tags must not be fitted to cylinders. Large cylinders

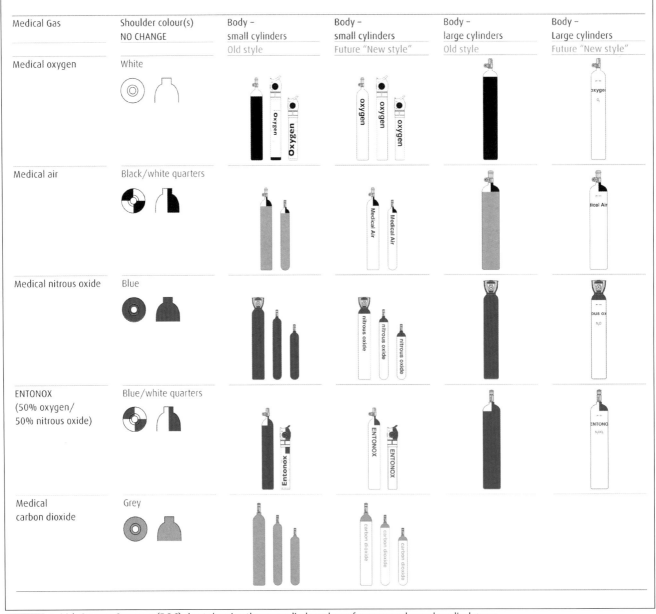

4.6 British Oxygen Company (BOC) chart showing the new cylinder colours for commonly used medical gases. (Courtesy of BOC Healthcare)

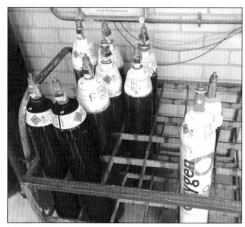

should be transported using a suitable trolley. Do not use oil or grease (or any oil-based products, including hand creams) in the vicinity of medical gas cylinders. If you need to clean the cylinder do not use materials which contain ammonium or chlorine compounds. Do not refill the cylinder or attempt to tamper with the cylinder package.

Smoking and naked flames should be prohibited in the vicinity of a cylinder or in confined spaces where cylinders are stored; clear warning notices to this effect should be posted and clearly visible. Large clear signs (Figure 4.8) should indicate the cylinder storage location and the nature of gases kept there. Cylinders are filled to high pressures and explosions are possible if they are dropped or exposed to high temperatures. The cylinder store must be secure enough to prevent theft or misuse and local emergency services should be advised of the location and contents of the store.

Cylinder valves

Cylinder valves seal and secure the contents within the cylinder. All cylinders come with a plastic wrapping around the valve to prevent dust gathering and blocking the exit port (see Figure 4.4). The cylinder valve is turned on or off with a spindle. The cylinder valves on all gas cylinders, whether they contain flammable or non-flammable gas, are opened by turning the spindle anticlockwise and closed by turning the spindle clockwise.

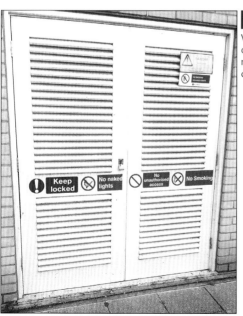

4.8

Warning signs on the door to a medical gas cylinder store.

> **WARNING**
>
> Valves must not be lubricated and must be kept free from carbon-based oils and greases; failure to observe this can result in explosion

Before use, the plastic wrapping of the valve should be removed before connecting the cylinder to the anaesthetic machine. The valve should be opened slowly when the cylinder is attached to the anaesthetic machine to prevent a rapid rise in pressure and associated rise in temperature of the gas in the anaesthetic machine. The cylinder valve should always be opened by two full revolutions. When closing the valve, only sufficient force should be used and the valve should not be over-tightened.

Pin index system

Pin index system valves are fitted to the small cylinders (usually size E) that are commonly connected to anaesthetic machines. This prevents the fitting of a cylinder of the wrong gas to a yoke on the anaesthetic machine. The cylinder valve block bears a specific configuration of holes for each medical gas, which fit on a matching configuration of pins protruding from the yoke on the anaesthetic machine (Figures 4.9, 4.10 and 4.11). This pin index system allows only the correct gas cylinder to be fitted to that yoke. The exit port for the gas will not fit and seal against the Bodok seal (Figure 4.12) on the yoke unless the holes and the pins are aligned. The Bodok seal should be inspected for damage prior to use and spare seals should always be available. It should be kept clean and never be contaminated with oil or grease.

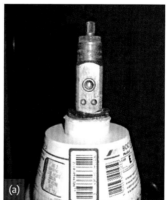 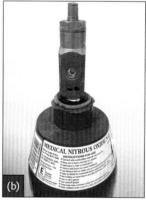

(a) (b)

4.9 Pin indexing on the valve blocks of (a) a size E oxygen cylinder and (b) a size E nitrous oxide cylinder.

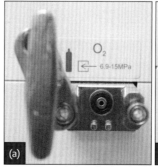 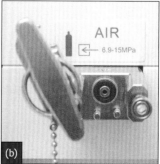

(a) (b)

4.10 Pin-indexed yokes for (a) a size E oxygen cylinder and (b) a size E medical air cylinder.

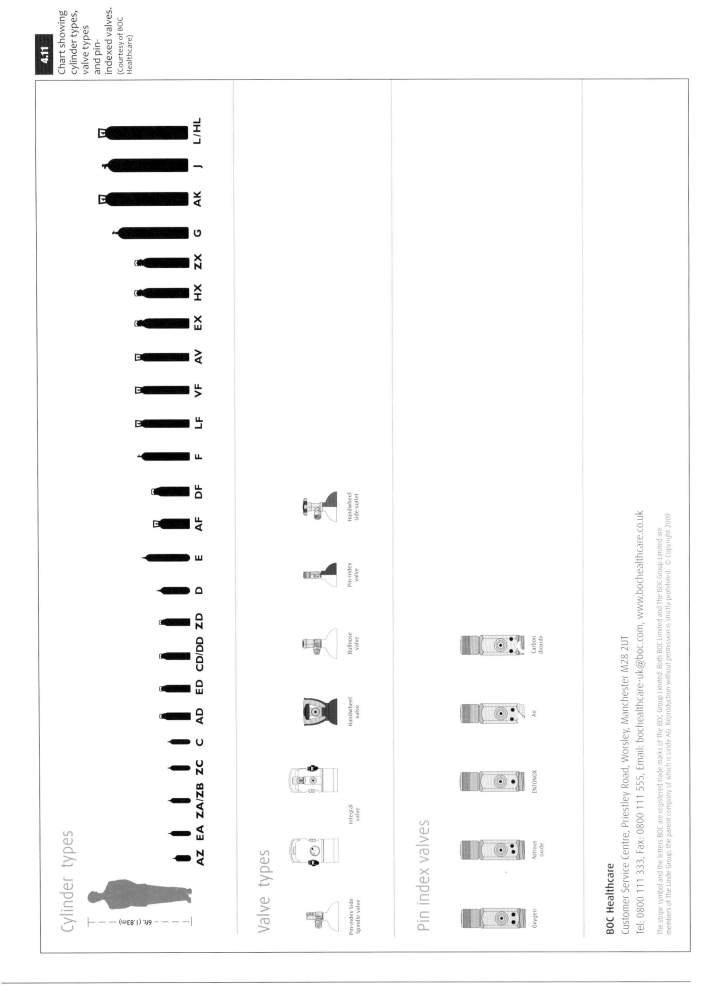

4.11 Chart showing cylinder types, valve types and pin-indexed valves. (Courtesy of BOC Healthcare)

Cylinder types

6ft (1.83m)

AZ EA ZA/ZB ZC C AD ED CD/DD ZD D E AF DF F LF VF AV EX HX ZX G AK J L/HL

Valve types

Pin-index Side Spindle valve   Integral valve   Handwheel valve   Bullnose valve   Pin-index valve   Handwheel side outlet

Pin index valves

Oxygen   Nitrous oxide   ENTONOX   Air   Carbon dioxide

BOC Healthcare

Customer Service Centre, Priestley Road, Worsley, Manchester M28 2UT

Tel: 0800 111 333, Fax: 0800 111 555, Email: bochealthcare-uk@boc.com, www.bochealthcare.co.uk

The stripe symbol and the letters BOC are registered trade marks of The BOC Group Limited. Both BOC Limited and The BOC Group Limited are members of the Linde Group, the parent company of which is Linde AG. Reproduction without permission is strictly prohibited. © Copyright 2009

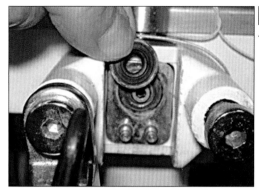

4.12

A Bodok seal.

Cylinder yokes may also be fitted with one-way, spring-loaded check valves. These prevent retrograde gas flow through the inlet nipple of vacant hanger yokes when a pipeline gas source is in use. They also allow changing of empty cylinders by preventing gas transfer from a high-pressure (fresh) cylinder to a low-pressure (used) cylinder. Check valves are difficult to locate within the yokes; their presence is confirmed by removing a cylinder from the yoke under test and allowing an alternative source of the same gas to be turned on. A hiss at the yoke will indicate a malfunctioning or absent check valve. If the function of the check valve is unknown it is safer to close the cylinder that is empty before opening a fresh one.

Pipeline supply

The source of pipeline gas supply can be a cylinder manifold, liquid oxygen storage tank or oxygen concentrators.

Cylinder manifold

Many large veterinary hospitals have cylinder manifolds that supply oxygen, nitrous oxide and medical air. An average cylinder manifold configuration has two banks of gas cylinders (one 'duty' and one 'standby') with a centrally located panel (Figure 4.13), which provides a nominal output of 400 kPa. The changeover from 'duty' to 'standby' bank should ideally be automatic and achieved through a pressure-sensitive device that detects when the cylinders are nearly empty. This changeover also alerts staff to change the cylinders. The arrangement should also contain a manually operated emergency bank with two

cylinders. The total capacity of the bank should be based on one week's supply of gas, with a minimum of two days' supply on each bank and a supply for three days on the spare cylinders held in the manifold room. Nitrous oxide manifolds have heaters fitted to the supply line to prevent it freezing during periods of high demand.

The manifold room should be:

- Constructed from sturdy fireproof material
- Well ventilated
- Ideally located to allow easy delivery and distribution of gases in the hospital
- Well lit
- Temperature regulated
- Used to contain only cylinders for the pipeline supply
- Not used as a general store
- Fitted with warning signs on the outside and inside of the building.

Only suitably trained persons should be allowed to change cylinders and a logbook must be completed when they are changed.

Liquid oxygen storage

When the annual oxygen consumption of a veterinary hospital is considered too great to be supplied via a cylinder manifold, a thermally insulated, double-walled vacuum-insulated evaporator (VIE) is the most economical way to store and supply oxygen (Figure 4.14). This has significant advantages:

- The VIE may be a single main vessel or several reserve vessels all connected to a cylinder manifold containing the secondary backup supply
- It is filled from a remote point, which removes the need for manually handling and connecting large cylinders
- The VIE has an ambient temperature vaporizer to convert cryogenic liquid oxygen to gas, which is delivered to the pipelines through a pressure regulator that maintains the pressure at 400 kPa. A control panel converts the differential pressure between the top and the bottom of the cryotank to an analogue readout and display
- A safety valve, which functions at 1700 kPa, allows gas to escape during periods of low demand. During periods of high demand, a control valve opens, allowing liquid oxygen to evaporate by passing through superheaters.

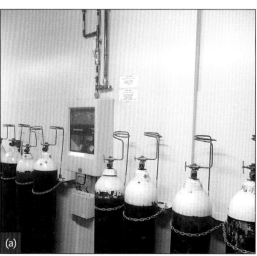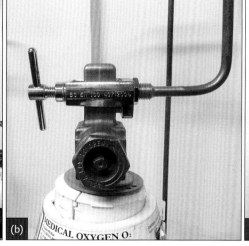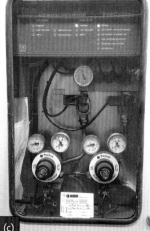

4.13 (a) An oxygen cylinder manifold. (b) Pipeline attached to the valve on a size J oxygen cylinder. (c) Manifold control for the medical gas banks.

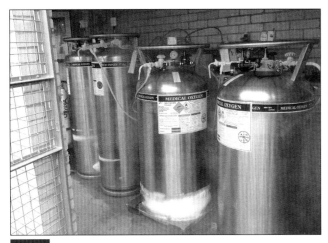

4.14 Vacuum-insulated evaporators for liquid oxygen.

Liquid oxygen is stored at −183°C and at pressures of up to 500–1000 kPa. The storage vessel rests on a weighing balance to measure the mass of liquid oxygen. Modern setups use a telemetry system that provides continuous monitoring for the medical gas supplier and the veterinary hospital. Fresh supplies of liquid oxygen are pumped from a tanker into the vessel, when required. At atmospheric pressure and a temperature of 15°C, liquid oxygen can give 842 times its volume in gas.

Oxygen concentrators

These devices separate oxygen from air by chemical means, and all the currently available models are electrically powered. Oxygen concentrators operate on the principle of adsorption of atmospheric nitrogen and water vapour on to a zeolite (aluminosilicate) sieve at high pressure, and then venting the nitrogen. The adsorption of nitrogen leaves oxygen as the primary remaining gas; small amounts of argon, carbon dioxide, water vapour and other atmospheric constituents are also present. The maximum oxygen concentration achieved is 95% by volume. Most of the modern portable units (Figure 4.15) can supply an oxygen flow of

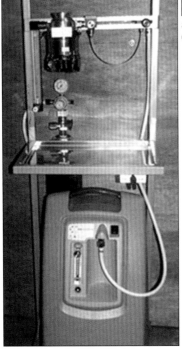

4.15 An oxygen concentrator with an anaesthetic machine. (Courtesy of MSS International Ltd)

0.1–10 l/min. When used with a circle (rebreathing) system, higher gas flows are required to prevent accumulation of argon, which is not removed by the zeolite sieve. These devices are easy to maintain but require filter changes at regular intervals. Low-pressure generators will supply one anaesthetic machine, whereas high-pressure models can be connected to the manifold of an existing pipeline system. To generate oxygen for larger veterinary hospitals, industrial processes are required. These may use much higher pressures and gas flows than single medical units.

Distribution systems

Medical gases are distributed throughout the veterinary hospital at a pressure of 400 kPa, through high-grade copper alloy pipelines (Figure 4.16) designed to achieve a minimum pressure drop from the source to the point of use. Oxygen, nitrous oxide and medical air are the most common gases distributed by pipeline in veterinary hospitals in the UK. All newly installed medical gas pipelines should be inspected and purged according to the laws of the country in which the hospital is located. Before the system is used, a pharmacist is usually employed to check the identity of the gas and its purity and composition. The gases are fed into a labelled and colour-coded pipeline distribution network, which terminates in self-sealing (Schrader) flushed sockets either in the wall (Figure 4.17) or suspended from the ceiling on ceiling-mounted pendants or a hose. Throughout the medical gas network, isolating valves

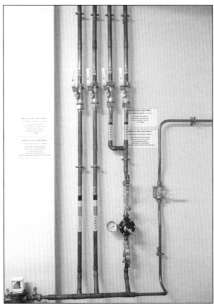

4.16 Gas pipeline leaving the manifold supplying medical gases to the essential areas of a veterinary hospital.

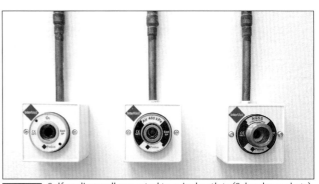

4.17 Self-sealing wall-mounted terminal outlets (Schrader sockets) for oxygen and medical air. Active scavenging is connected to the socket on the right-hand side.

behind breakable glass covers (area valve service units (AVSUs); Figure 4.18) are positioned at various points and can be accessed to isolate the supply to an area in case of fire or emergency. In the UK, a European Standard specifies the dimensioning and construction of the terminal unit and its associated probe. Each socket should have the identity of the gas permanently displayed and accept only a probe of the same identity. A flexible hose connects the terminal outlet to the anaesthetic machine or other medical equipment. Each flexible pipeline has three components:

- The Schrader probe (Figure 4.19a). All the hoses have the same male bayonet fitting. To prevent misconnection to the wrong gas service, the probe for each gas supply has a protruding indexing collar with unique diameter, which fits only the Schrader socket for the same gas
- Flexible hose. Modern hoses are colour-coded for each gas: oxygen is white; nitrous oxide is French blue; medical air is black. Damaged hoses should not be repaired but replaced with new factory-made hoses
- Non-interchangeable screw thread (NIST) for connection to the anaesthetic machine (Figure 4.19b). This ensures that the hose connection is specific to each gas service. The NIST comprises a nut and probe: the probe has a unique profile for each gas, which fits only the union on the machine for that gas. The nut has the same diameter and thread for all services, but can be attached to the

machine only when the probe is engaged. The term NIST is therefore misleading, because the screw thread itself does not determine the unique fit. A one-way valve ensures unidirectional flow. All fittings on the hoses and their connections must be tamper proof.

Alarms

Several different types of alarm are used within the hospital medical gas system; these comprise the main plant alarms and the local alarms. Main/master alarms (Figure 4.20a) provide an indication of plant status and advance warnings that something might be in process of failure. The main plant is connected to a panel that is placed in a strategic area of the hospital where it can be monitored readily. In addition to the analogue indicators on the main plant panel, a visual indicator will appear on each manifold providing more detailed information on the nature of the fault. The alarms indicate whether cylinders require changing or liquid oxygen needs refilling. They also indicate if the reserve is low or if there is a pressure fault within the network.

The local alarm (Figure 4.20b) is more an indication that the problem has already occurred at the point of use. Each local area is monitored by a pressure switch that detects high or low pressure within the pipeline, near an AVSU in the local zone. Alarms are both visual and audible; the audible alarm can be muted for 15 minutes. If the fault has not been rectified during this period, the alarm will repeat until the problem has been resolved. Once the fault is rectified, the alarm will reset itself.

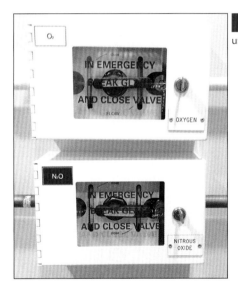

4.18 Area valve service units (AVSUs).

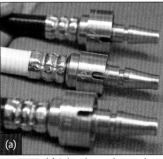
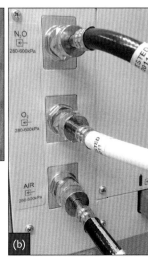

4.19 (a) Schrader probes and hoses for the terminal outlets. From top to bottom: medical air; oxygen; nitrous oxide.
(b) Non-interchangeable screw threads (NISTs) for nitrous oxide, oxygen and medical air, attached to the anaesthetic machine.

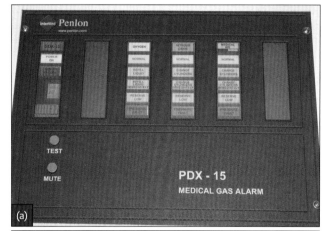

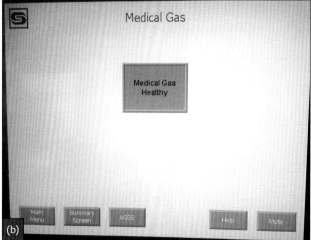

4.20 (a) Master alarm for pipeline medical gas supply to the hospital and (b) local area alarm for medical gases.

The anaesthetic machine

Most anaesthetic machines should have the following features to ensure the safe delivery of anaesthetic gases and vapours:

- Pressure gauges (colour coded for each gas)
- Pressure-reducing valves (pressure regulators)
- Colour-coded flowmeters for oxygen, nitrous oxide and medical air
- Baffling of the oxygen flowmeter so that it is the last gas to be mixed with the other gases (to prevent delivery of a hypoxic mixture to the patient in the event of a cracked flowmeter tube)
- Flow of nitrous oxide is cut off if oxygen pressure is too low (to avoid delivery of a hypoxic gas mixture)
- Pin index system for cylinders and a NIST for pipelines
- An oxygen failure alarm
- At least one reserve oxygen cylinder on machines that use pipeline supply, and two oxygen cylinders on machines that do not use a pipeline supply.

Pressure gauges

These measure the pressure of the gas in the pipeline and cylinders, using Bourdon gauges. The pressure gauges in older machines are mounted above the cylinder yoke (Figure 4.21a) while in modern machines they are mounted on the front panel (Figure 4.21b).

The gauges are labelled, colour coded and calibrated for each gas or vapour. The pressure gauge for oxygen indicates the volume of gas in the cylinder, calculated using Boyle's law ($P \times V = K$, where P represents pressure, V volume and K a constant). For example, a size E cylinder contains 680 litres of gas when filled to 13,700 kPa at 20°C. At the same temperature, a pressure gauge registering 4500 kPa indicates that only 223 litres remain.

The nitrous oxide pressure gauge does not act as the contents gauge; it measures the saturated vapour pressure of gaseous nitrous oxide in equilibrium with its liquid phase. This pressure remains constant until all the liquid has evaporated, after which the pressure falls rapidly. Gas volume in a nitrous oxide cylinder is determined by weighing the cylinder and applying the formula:

Gas present (litres) =
(net – tare) weight (in grams) x 22.4/44

(The tare weight of a nitrous oxide size E cylinder is about 5800–6400 g)

Pressure-reducing valves (pressure regulators)

Pressure-reducing valves (Figure 4.22ab) are used in the anaesthetic machine to:

- Reduce the high pressure delivered from a cylinder, so that sudden surges of pressure cannot be delivered to the patient or damage components of the anaesthetic machine
- Maintain a constant reduced pressure (generally 400 kPa) as the contents of the cylinder are exhausted.

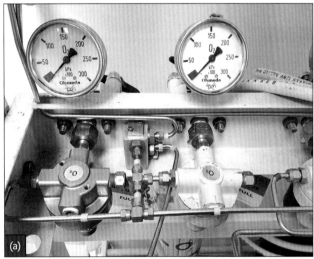

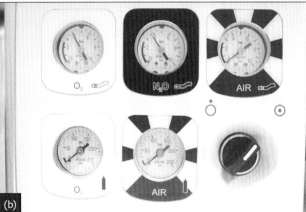

4.21 (a) Pressure gauges for oxygen above the cylinders on an older anaesthetic machine and (b) pressure gauges for oxygen, nitrous oxide and medical air on the front panel of a modern anaesthetic machine.

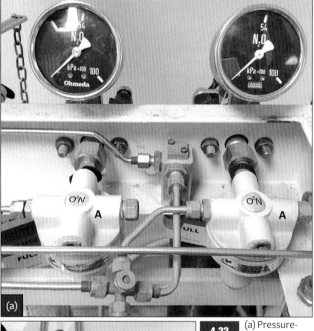

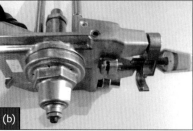

4.22 (a) Pressure-reducing valves (A) for nitrous oxide in an older anaesthetic machine and (b) pressure regulator from a modern Datex Ohmeda Excel 210 machine.
(Courtesy of GE Medical Systems Ltd)

Pressure regulators are positioned between the cylinder and the anaesthetic machine. Machines holding two or more cylinders have one regulator per cylinder. Piped gases are regulated at their source (Figure 4.23). Complex pressure regulators incorporating pressure gauges, regulators, flowmeters and a 'bull-nosed' connector are available for the attachment of pipelines to larger cylinders.

Modern anaesthetic machines have both primary and secondary pressure regulators. Primary regulators are used to reduce high cylinder pressures and thus lower the machine working pressure. Some machines allow cylinder pressure-reducing valves to work at below 400 kPa, thus giving the pipeline preference and allowing pipeline gas to be used instead of cylinder gas. It is preferable to leave the reserve cylinder on, but some cylinders may leak and slowly empty their contents.

Fluctuations in the working pressure of the anaesthetic machine may occur when using oxygen from an auxiliary port (see later) to drive a ventilator, or during peak usage of pipeline gases. For this reason, a secondary pressure regulator is often used to control pipeline pressure surges; when set to a pressure below the anticipated pressure drop, it will smooth out the supply and minimize pressure fluctuations.

All regulators are tested before being installed to withstand pressures of 30 MPa with no disruption and with no variation of their output over a wide flow range. Regulators should be made from good quality metal that is compatible with medical gases (Washenitz *et al.*, 2001). In modern anaesthetic machines, to minimize connections and potential leaks, the NIST connection, cylinder yoke, primary regulator and pressure gauges are housed in a single cast brass block.

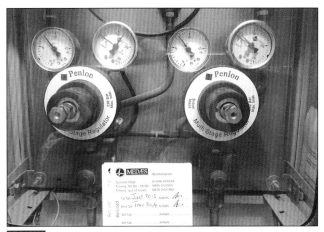

4.23 Piped gases are regulated at their source.

Pressure relief valves (opening at a pressure of 570–700 kPa) are fitted downstream on the anaesthetic machine to allow the escape of gas should the regulators fail; these valves may be spring-loaded so that they open at high pressure and close when the pressure falls. Some may even rupture and need to be replaced by a qualified engineer.

Gas flow measurement and control valves

Control (needle) valves control the gas flow into the flowmeters by manual adjustment. These valves provide the final stage of pressure reduction, and pressures beyond the flowmeters (in the back bar; see below) range from 1–8 kPa. The conventional flowmeter (also called a rotameter) is a tube made of transparent tapered (wider at the top of the flowmeter) glass or plastic, with a lightweight ball or bobbin (e.g. non-rotating H-float, skirted bobbin or non-skirted bobbin) floating on the gas flow (Figure 4.24). The bobbin (or ball) is held in the tube by gas flow passing around it, and the higher the flow, the higher the bobbin rises in the tube. The flows within the tube are both laminar (low flows) and turbulent (higher flows), thus making both the viscosity and density of the gas significant in calibration. The flow is etched on to the tube (in l/min for flows above 1 l/min, and 100 ml/min for lower flows). Gas flow is read from the top of the bobbin; when a ball is used the reading is taken from the centre of the ball. Neoprene washers at either end of the tube make it leakproof. Tubes have different lengths and diameters and are non-interchangeable. Flowmeters are designed to be read in a vertical position. Calibration is done at room temperature and sea level and the margin of error is ±2%. The most common causes of inaccurate flowmeter settings are dirt and static electricity, and contaminated gas supplies may be to blame. This is more likely to be a problem at low flows, when there is a narrow clearance between the bobbin and flowmeter wall. Static electricity builds up over time and can cause the bobbin to stick to the sides of the flowmeter tubing; using an antistatic material coating on the inside and outside of the flowmeter will prevent this. An application of antistatic spray will generally solve the problem of a sticky bobbin.

Flowmeters are calibrated for individual gases; therefore, for example, an oxygen flowmeter would not accurately indicate the flow of nitrous oxide. For this reason the needle valve control knobs are both colour- and touch-coded and bear the name of the gas; the oxygen knob is large, white in colour and has larger ridges than the other knobs (Figure 4.25). In the UK, flowmeters are arranged in a block, with the oxygen flowmeter to the left, nitrous oxide on the right, and the flowmeter for medical air (where fitted) in between these. The flowmeters are arranged vertically and adjacent to each other so that their upper ends discharge into the manifold. In older flowmeter blocks, this resulted in oxygen (instead of nitrous oxide) leaking out if the central flowmeter tube was damaged, resulting in a hypoxic mixture being delivered to the patient. More recent designs of the flowmeter block ensure that oxygen is the last gas to be delivered to the back bar (by baffling the oxygen tube). In the USA and Canada, this problem is solved by placing the oxygen flowmeter to the right of the block and nitrous oxide to the left.

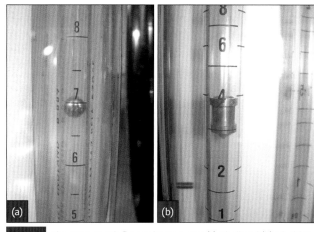

4.24 Flowmeter with flow indicator using (a) a ball and (b) a bobbin.

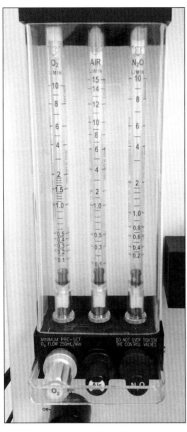

4.25 A flowmeter block. Note the larger size of the oxygen flow control. Oxygen is on the left and nitrous oxide on the right, with medical air in the middle.

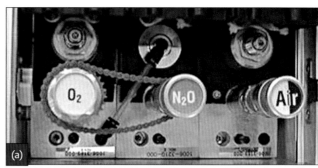

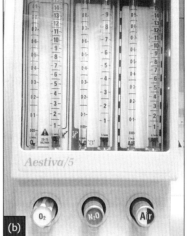

4.26 Hypoxic guard in a GE Healthcare anaesthetic machine. (a) Oxygen and nitrous oxide flowmeter controls are linked by a sprocket and chain. (b) Note the adjacent oxygen and nitrous oxide flowmeters. The photograph also shows 'cascade' flowmeters, which allow accurate measurement of gas flows less than 1 l/min. (Courtesy of GE Medical Systems Ltd)

On some modern machines, it is impossible to deliver nitrous oxide without the addition of a fixed percentage of oxygen; in such machines the interactive nitrous oxide and oxygen controls prevent hypoxic mixtures being delivered to the patient. Machines manufactured by GE Healthcare have a system that delivers a minimum concentration of oxygen (e.g. 25%) and requires the oxygen and nitrous oxide flow control valves to be side by side and linked by a sprocket and chain or cogwheel (Figure 4.26ab). Figure 4.27 shows the Quantiflex MDM, which was one of the earlier machines designed to prevent delivery of hypoxic mixtures.

Low-flow anaesthesia requires flowmeters that can deliver flows accurately below 1 l/min; to achieve this, an arrangement of two flowmeters in series ('cascade' flowmeters) is used (Figure 4.26b). One flowmeter reads to a maximum of 1 l/min, allowing fine adjustment of gas flow. One flow control valve per gas is needed for both the flowmeters.

Some modern anaesthetic units use highly accurate microprocessors to control gas flow. With these machines (e.g. the GE Medical Anaesthesia Delivery Unit), flow is indicated electronically by a numerical display or 'virtual flow tubes' (Figure 4.28). These allow easy identification of gas flows in a darkened theatre and also facilitate export of electronic data to an information system. Thus, electronic flowmeters allow automated recording of fresh gas flows. They are also 5–10 times more accurate than traditional tube flowmeters. In the event of an electrical failure, these machines have a pneumatic backup, which continues the delivery of fresh gas.

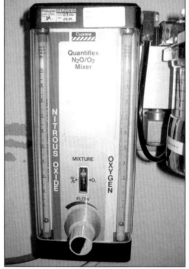

4.27 The Quantiflex MDM. Note that the oxygen flowmeter is on the right and that for nitrous oxide on the left.

Back bar

The back bar supports the flowmeter block, vaporizers and some other components (Figure 4.29). The back bar on older anaesthetic machines has the vaporizer (alone or

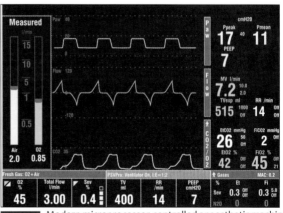

4.28 Modern microprocessor-controlled anaesthetic machines use 'virtual flow tubes'. (Courtesy of GE Medical Systems Ltd)

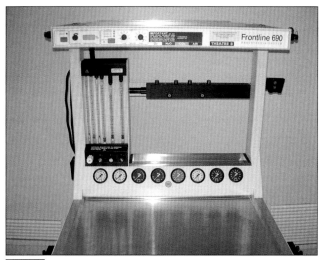

4.29 The back bar, attached to the right of the flowmeter block.

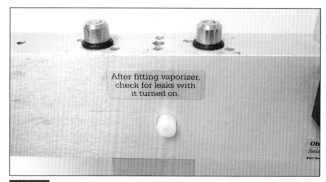

4.30 'Selectatec' station for vaporizer attachment to the back bar.

in series) mounted downstream from the flowmeter block and bolted to the bar with tapered cage mount connector fittings; this makes servicing individual components very difficult. Modern back bars allow greater flexibility in allowing vaporizers to be removed and exchanged with ease for servicing and refilling. The Ohmeda 'Selectatec' fitting is the most popular in the UK (Figure 4.30). The vaporizer assembly has two female ports with a locking mechanism (Figure 4.31), which fit on to two vertically mounted male ports on the Selectatec fitting; between the inlet and the outlet ports is an accessory pin and locking recess. The vaporizers are locked on to the bar by turning a knob. This system prevents the use of older vaporizers on a modern back bar. In order to ensure an airtight seal, O-rings are placed on the male ports on the back bar (Figure 4.31a).

Patients may be at risk of receiving too high a dose of anaesthetic agent if two or more TEC 3 vaporizers can be operated simultaneously on older Selectatec compatible anaesthetic machines without pins designed to prevent the use of TEC 3 vaporizers. Back bars on older

anaesthetic machines should be checked to ensure that pins preventing the fitting of TEC 3 vaporizers have not been removed. If the pins have been removed, they should be replaced with a spring plate assembly incorporating fixed pins. With anaesthetic machines designed to accept more than one TEC 3 vaporizer, it is recommended that only one vaporizer is fitted at a time. Consideration should be given to converting the back bar to a single position, if possible. If there is any possibility that two or more TEC 3 vaporizers could be used together on one back bar, consideration should be given to replacing them with current models featuring safety interlocks. Modern TEC vaporizers (4–7) incorporate an extension rod, which protrudes sideways from the vaporizer when it is turned on: this displaces an equivalent rod in the vaporizer adjacent to it and prevents the adjacent one from being turned on at the same time (Figure 4.32). Dräger anaesthetic machines have a specialized mounting system (Figure 4.33ab) for Dräger vaporizers, with an interlock that prevents two vaporizers from being used simultaneously.

In modern back bars, back pressure from minute volume divider ventilators can damage flowmeters, and a pressure-relief valve (often set at 30–40 kPa) is fitted in the same housing as a non-return valve at the right hand side of the back bar (see later).

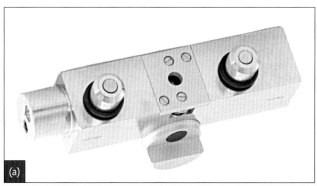

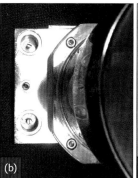

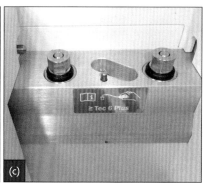

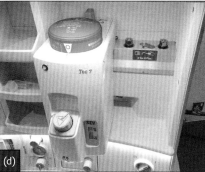

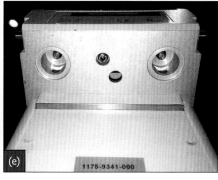

4.31 (a) Selectatec block (compatible with TEC 3, MSS 3 and other Selectatec-compatible vaporizers. Note the O-rings placed on the male ports to ensure an airtight seal when mounted on the back bar). (b) Corresponding TEC 3 vaporizer assembly with two female ports; this assembly is only compatible with older Selectatec fittings that do not have a pin. (c) A modern Selectatec block which will only take modern vaporizers. (Note the pin, which will not allow the use of TEC 3 and MSS 3 vaporizers). (d) A modern Selectatec bar with a TEC 7 vaporizer in place. (e) Corresponding vaporizer assembly showing two female ports, accessory pin and locking recess for a TEC 7 vaporizer.

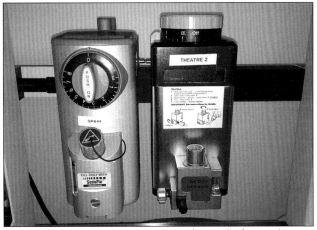

4.32 Safety interlock. An extension rod protrudes from each vaporizer; the rod extends sideways from one vaporizer as it is turned on and immobilizes the equivalent rod on the adjacent vaporizer.

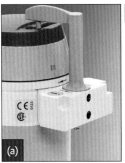

4.33 Dräger mounting system. (a) When the vaporizer dial is moved to the 'Transport' position, the locking lever to the rear of the vaporizer fits into a groove on top of the dial and prevents spillage of liquid anaesthetic agent into the bypass channel during transport. (b) The Dräger Auto Exclusion vaporizer mounting mechanism incorporates a safety interlock preventing two vaporizers from being used simultaneously.
(Courtesy of Dräger Medical UK)

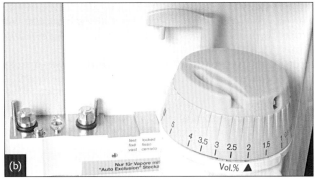

Common gas outlet

All anaesthetic machines have only one common, or fresh, gas outlet (Figure 4.34), which connects the anaesthetic machine to breathing systems, ventilators or oxygen supply devices (e.g. masks). The outlet has a 22 mm male/15 mm female connection. The common gas outlet is either fixed or swivelled; the latter is useful because it reduces the need for the machine to be moved and facilitates breathing system positioning, with reduced risk of hoses kinking. In modern anaesthetic machines with an in-built circle system or a ventilator, there is a switch which allows gas flow to be switched between the in-built circle system and the common gas outlet.

Auxiliary gas sockets

One or more mini-Schrader gas sockets are fitted to modern machines to deliver air or oxygen to gas-driven ventilators (Figure 4.35) and suction units. These sockets have a working pressure of 400 kPa. The sockets should be labelled for their specific gases.

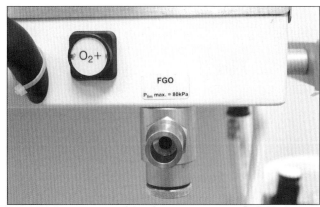

4.34 Common gas outlet and emergency oxygen flush. The latter supplies oxygen directly to the breathing system at a rate of 30–70 l/min. In modern machines, the flush does not have a locking facility (to reduce risk of barotrauma).

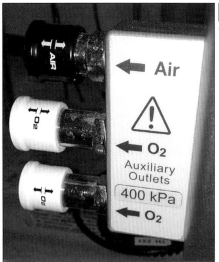

4.35 Auxiliary gas sockets for oxygen and medical air.

Non-return or pressure-relief safety valve

This valve is situated either on the back bar or near the common gas outlet (Figure 4.36). It opens when back pressure exceeds 35 kPa, usually from the use of minute volume divider ventilators. This prevents damage to flow-meters and vaporizers.

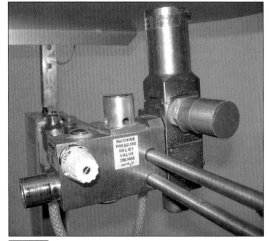

4.36 Pressure-relief valve.

Emergency oxygen flush

The oxygen flush receives oxygen directly from the pipeline or cylinder, thus bypassing the vaporizer (see Figure 4.34). When activated by pressing a button, oxygen is delivered at a high flow of 30–70 l/min at a pressure of 400 kPa. Care should be exercised when using the oxygen flush with patients attached to breathing systems, as it exposes them to risk of barotrauma. In older anaesthetic machines, the flowmeter bypass valve had a locking facility; this is no longer the case in modern anaesthetic machines where the knob is recessed and cannot be accidentally pressed.

Emergency air-intake valve

This is usually situated under the base of the common gas outlet. This valve opens with a loud audible beep when the gas flow from the anaesthetic machine ceases, allowing the patient to breathe room air until flow is restored.

Overpressure valve

This allows release of excessive pressure downstream from the common gas outlet; as the valve opens it also sounds an alarm. This device is useful in testing breathing systems for leaks.

Oxygen failure alarm

Oxygen failure devices are very important on anaesthetic machines because they protect the patient from receiving an inadequate oxygen supply. These devices should not require mains electrical supply or batteries. The current British Standard states that the alarm should be activated when oxygen pressure falls to approximately 200 kPa. Ideally, failing oxygen supply should also prevent nitrous oxide flow and simultaneously sound an alarm, which should be gas driven and depend on the pressure of oxygen alone. Oxygen failure devices may also include visual alarms (Figure 4.37).

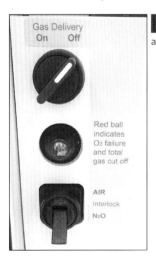

4.37 Visual oxygen failure alarm on a Penlon Prima anaesthetic machine.

Vaporizers

A vaporizer is a device that delivers clinically safe and effective concentrations of anaesthetic vapour. Most inhaled anaesthetics are liquids at room temperature and pressure and therefore need to be vaporized before being delivered to the patient. Molecules of volatile liquid anaesthetic agent escape from the liquid to the vapour phase,

creating a saturated vapour pressure (SVP) on the liquid surface when at equilibrium. The SVP depends only on the physical characteristics of the liquid and its temperature (SVP increases with temperature), but is independent of atmospheric pressure.

The SVP of most volatile anaesthetics is much greater than that needed to produce anaesthesia. For example, the SVP of sevoflurane at 20°C is approximately 160 mmHg, which yields a maximum concentration of 21%; breathing this concentration of sevoflurane would be rapidly fatal. Thus, vaporizers are designed to dilute the saturated vapour of volatile anaesthetics and yield a range of safe and useful concentrations. This dilution can be achieved by:

- Splitting the flow of gas within the vaporizer into two streams. One stream passes through the vaporizer chamber (which contains saturated vapour), while the other stream bypasses the chamber. The ratio between these two flows (the splitting ratio) is dictated by the control dial of the vaporizer; such vaporizers are of the *variable bypass* type. Full saturation in the vaporizing chamber is achieved by the use of wicks, baffles, and by bubbling the gas through the liquid to increase the surface area of contact. Most modern vaporizers use wicks, which may be made of cloth (as in the Fluotec) or metal (as in the Penlon)
- Adding vapour directly to the fresh gas flow. This method is used by *measured flow vaporizers*, e.g. the TEC 6 desflurane vaporizer.

Classification of vaporizers

Gas can be made to flow through a vaporizer in one of two ways:

- Under positive pressure of gas delivered from flowmeters proximal ('upstream') to the vaporizer. This type is called a *plenum vaporizer* (plenum is a term that describes a pressurized chamber). This is the most familiar type, fitted to the back bar of the anaesthetic machine. Resistance to gas flow is relatively high and these are normally referred to as 'out-of-circuit' vaporizers
- Under negative pressure developed distal ('downstream') to the vaporizer. This is known as a *draw-over vaporizer* and the negative pressure is generated by the patient's inspiratory effort. Such vaporizers have a low resistance to gas flow and are normally used 'in-circuit'.

Vaporizer performance

The amount of volatile liquid anaesthetic vaporized depends on:

- The SVP of the anaesthetic agent
- Temperature
- Flow of carrier gas through the vaporizer: the degree of saturation of gas leaving the vaporizing chamber is highly dependent on gas flow (with higher concentrations achieved at lower flows). The problem of flow and temperature dependence is overcome in the design of modern vaporizers
- Carrier gas mixture
- The amount of contact between the liquid and the gases
- Variable vaporizer operational pressures

- The dimensions of the vaporizing chamber
- Movement and tilting of vaporizers: always keep upright. If tilted, liquid anaesthetic may contaminate the bypass channel and expose the next patient to very high vapour concentrations
- Back pressure, e.g. from minute volume divider ventilators.

Plenum vaporizers

Modern plenum vaporizers are often referred to as variable bypass vaporizers which have a much higher internal resistance, requiring a pressurized fresh gas flow above atmospheric pressure. They allow administration of safe, accurate concentrations of volatile anaesthetic agent. Examples include the Ohmeda TEC 3 and TEC 4, GE Healthcare (formerly Ohmeda) TEC 5 and TEC 7, Penlon Sigma Delta, Blease Datum and the Dräger 'Vapor' 2000 series vaporizers. In the UK, MSS International has modified the TEC 3 vaporizers over the past 10 years and made many improvements to the original design to create a more stable vaporizer that gives greater accuracy of output at ±2–5% of dial setting, as well as having a longer period between services. Figure 4.38 summarizes the characteristics of selected plenum vaporizers currently available.

As gas flow increases, it becomes more difficult to achieve full saturation of the gas leaving the vaporizing chamber. Plenum vaporizers maximize the surface area for

Device characteristics	Ohmeda TEC 3	MSS 3	Ohmeda TEC 4	GE Healthcare TEC 5 and TEC 7	Penlon Sigma Delta	Dräger 'Vapor' series 2000	Blease Datum
Agents	Isoflurane Sevoflurane	Isoflurane Sevoflurane	Isoflurane	Isoflurane Sevoflurane	Isoflurane Sevoflurane	Isoflurane Sevoflurane	Isoflurane Sevoflurane
Mounting systems	Cage mount Selectatec[a]	Cage mount Selectatec[a]	Cage mount Selectatec	Selectatec	Cage mount Selectatec	Dräger mount Fixed mount Cage mount Selectatec	Cage mount Selectatec
Interlocking mechanism	None	None	Interlock facility to prevent two vaporizers being used simultaneously	Interlock facility to prevent two vaporizers being used simultaneously	Interlock facility to prevent two vaporizers being used simultaneously	Interlock facility to prevent two vaporizers being used simultaneously	Interlock facility to prevent two vaporizers being used simultaneously
Filling systems	Funnel fill Keyed filler	Funnel fill Keyed filler	Funnel fill Keyed filler	Funnel fill Keyed filler Quik-Fil[b] Easy Fil[c]	Keyed filler Quik-Fil[b]	Dräger Fil Funnel fill Keyed filler Quik-Fil[b] Easy Fil[c]	Funnel fill Keyed filler Quik-Fil[b]
Heat sink	Copper and brass	Copper and brass	Copper and brass	Copper and brass	Aluminium	Copper and brass	Copper and brass
Thermal compensating device	Bimetallic strip	Bimetallic strip	Bimetallic strip	Bimetallic strip	Bimetallic strip	Bimetallic strip	Bimetallic device, central metal alloy rod encased in a brass jacket
Wick-area for vaporization	Cloth wick	Cloth wick	Cloth wick	Helical wick (Teflon)	Sintered polyethylene coiled into a spiral. The wick assembly designed as cartridge for ease of cleaning	Tubular wick made of synthetic material and a wick extension	Elongated Teflon wick with a wick extension
Method used to reduce effects of back pressure	Cotton wick	Cotton wick	Cotton wick	Elongated passage for gas flow within the vaporizer prevents 'pumping effect'	Helical damping coil that prevents vapour from tracking back to the vaporizer	Damping chamber which contains a series of baffles within the vaporizer	Elongated passage for gas flow within the vaporizer prevents 'pumping effect'
Bypass chamber protection when tilted	No protection – will allow liquid agent to enter bypass chamber	No protection – will allow liquid agent to enter bypass chamber	Has a baffle system anti-spill feature to prevent leakage if vaporizer is accidentally tilted over	Has a baffle system anti-spill feature to prevent leakage if vaporizer is accidentally tilted over	When not connected to machine, control dial can be turned on and if vaporizer tilted, liquid agent may enter bypass chamber	Maximum angle of tilt during transport (control dial at 'T'): any position and angle; during operation: 30°	When not connected to machine, control dial can be turned on and if vaporizer tilted, liquid agent may enter bypass chamber
Service interval	1 year	3 years	1 year	TEC 5 – 3 years TEC 7 is factory service free, eliminating the need for scheduled service	10 years	Lifetime calibration – no factory overhaul, no recalibration	10 years

4.38 Some characteristics of selected plenum vaporizers available in the UK. [a] Cannot be used in series on the back bar. [b] Quik-Fil; Abbott. [c] Easy Fil; GE Healthcare.

vaporization by using wicks, baffles, cowls or nebulizers. Teflon or metal wicks create a network of channels, allowing the liquid agent to spread by capillary action over a much larger surface area. Incoming gas is then directed through the vaporization chamber via channels created by metal baffles (Figure 4.39). Modern plenum vaporizers produce an accurate concentration of agent at flows between 0.25 and 15 l/min. The concentration of anaesthetic agent in the vaporization chamber is known (from its SVP), and when this gas is mixed with the anaesthetic-free bypass gas, the concentration of anaesthetic in the gas leaving the vaporizer is also known. The proportion of the total gas flow passing through the vaporizing chamber is controlled by a dial which accurately indicates the concentration of anaesthetic delivered by the vaporizer.

Changes in ambient temperature, as well as heat loss via latent heat of vaporization, can cause changes in the temperature of the anaesthetic agent. A decrease in agent temperature results in a fall in SVP and a consequent decrease in the output of anaesthetic agent. In order to overcome this problem, vaporizers are constructed using dense metals with high thermal conductivity and specific heat capacity (the latter providing a heat sink). The modern TEC series vaporizers are temperature compensated and adjustments to the splitting ratio are made by use of a bimetallic strip or an aneroid bellows: as the temperature falls, more gas flows through the vaporization chamber.

When a vaporizer is purchased, performance data (in graphical form) are provided indicating its actual output (compared to control dial settings) over a range of temperatures and gas flows; it is important to consult these before use (Figure 4.40). For example, at flows less than 1 l/min, the splitting ratio may alter and affect vaporizer output.

Measured flow vaporizers

Measured flow vaporizers have a separate, independent stream of vapour-carrying gas that is added to the fresh gas flow. To deliver an accurate agent concentration, the vaporizer must measure, and adjust for, fresh gas flow.

1	Vapor inlet
2	Vaporizing chamber-bypass
3	Additional bypass
4	Flow control cone
5	Vapor outlet
6	Vaporizing chamber
7a, 7b	Valves
8	Control dial
9	Saturated wick
10	Temperature compensator

4.39 Internal design of the Dräger Vapor 2000 vaporizer.
(Courtesy of Dräger Medical UK)

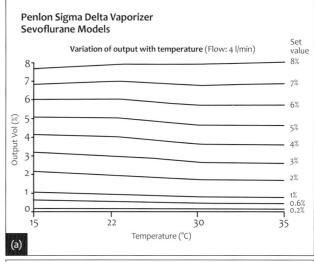

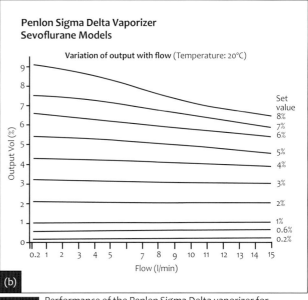

4.40 Performance of the Penlon Sigma Delta vaporizer for sevoflurane over a range of (a) temperatures and (b) fresh gas flows. The Sigma Delta Vaporizer is produced by Penlon Ltd, UK (www.penlon.com).

Datex-Ohmeda TEC 6

The GE Healthcare (Ohmeda) TEC 6 (Figure 4.41), is designed for use with desflurane. Desflurane cannot be used with a conventional vaporizer because its high SVP (88.5 kPa at 20°C) and low boiling point (23.5°C) mean that it would not stay in liquid form in the vaporizing chamber. The TEC 6 overcomes this problem by storing the liquid desflurane in a separate chamber and heating it to 39°C by means of an electrical filament raising the SVP to 200 kPa. Desflurane vapour is then added directly to the fresh gas. To provide an accurate desflurane concentration, the quantity of agent added must be proportional to the fresh gas flow. This is automatically adjusted by a variable resistance at the vaporizing chamber outflow, controlled by a differential pressure transducer (Figure 4.42).

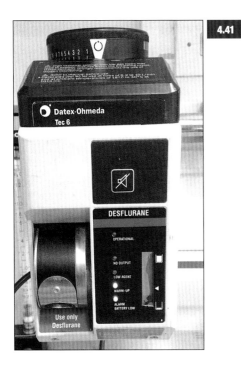

4.41 TEC 6 vaporizer for desflurane.

The delivered concentration of desflurane is adjusted manually via the vaporizer dial, which is linked to a second variable resistance. This dial has an interim stop at 12%; to bypass this, a release bar is depressed, allowing the concentration to be increased to 18%.

Dräger D Vapor

The Dräger D Vapor (Figure 4.43) delivers desflurane and works on a similar principal to the TEC 6. In this vaporizer the agent is heated and the pressure of the desflurane vapour is controlled electronically so as to achieve the desired final output with varying carrier gas flow.

Dräger DIVA

The DIVA (Direct Injection of Vapour Anaesthetic) vaporizer (Figure 4.44) is a measured flow type of device requiring a separate air supply. It is an integral part of the Dräger Zeus anaesthetic machine and forms part of a closed anaesthetic system. It utilizes closed-loop feedback control to determine the amount of volatile agent allowed through a closing valve into a heated vaporization chamber. The flow is directed into the breathing system or to a mixing chamber where it mixes with the fresh gas flow. The control unit monitors the pressure of volatile agent in the vaporizing chamber, the fresh gas flow, and the target expired volatile agent concentration, to determine the amount of volatile agent required to be released to maintain the desired concentration delivered to the patient. By separating delivery of volatile agent from fresh gas flow, quantitative closed-system anaesthesia can be achieved, in which the amount of anaesthetic agent taken up by the patient is monitored and replaced accordingly.

Aladin cassette

The Aladin cassette vaporizer (Figure 4.45) is specifically for use with the GE Healthcare Anaesthesia Delivery Unit (e.g. GE Healthcare Aisys). It consists of two parts: an agent-specific vaporizing chamber (the cassette) and the

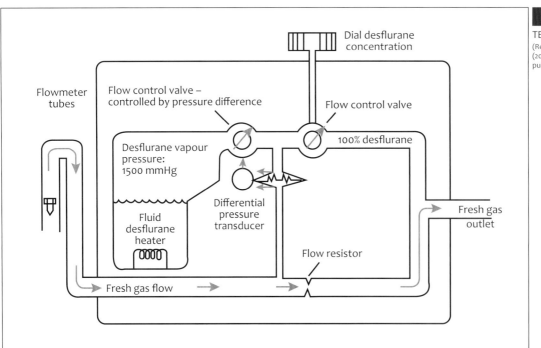

4.42 Schematic diagram of the TEC 6 desflurane vaporizer.
(Reproduced from Eales and Cooper (2007) with permission of the publisher)

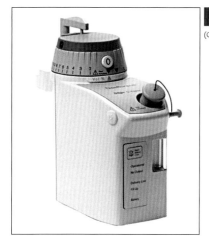

4.43 Dräger D 'Vapor' vaporizer.
(Courtesy of Dräger Medical UK)

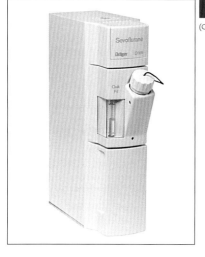

4.44 Dräger DIVA vaporizer.
(Courtesy of Dräger Medical UK)

central processing unit, which is an integral part of the anaesthetic machine. It behaves as both a variable bypass and a measured flow vaporizer. The cassette is a metal box that contains the vaporizing chamber, interspaced with metal plates, which contains a wick. There is a temperature sensor to measure the temperature of the liquid agent, and ball valves at the back of the cassette control the inflow and outflow of the agent. There is a conventional agent-specific filling system.

A valve, controlled by the central processing unit, regulates the gas flow leaving the vaporizing chamber and makes adjustments as required. The fresh gas flow is measured using the principle of a pressure decrease proportional to gas flow over a fixed resistance. Liquid agent temperature is measured in order to calculate vapour pressure; in addition, total pressure within the cassette is measured to allow calculation of vapour concentration (vapour pressure/total pressure). Based on this, the central processing unit adjusts the amount of agent added to the bypass gas, thus providing temperature compensation. Temperature stabilization is provided via the metal plates (which increase heat capacity and conductivity) and a fan beneath the cassette: if agent temperature decreases to 18°C, the fan transfers heat from the workstation's electronics to the cassette. Information on carrier gas composition is fed into the central processing unit, which makes calculations and according adjustments to try to minimize the effect of different carrier gas viscosities. The bypass and vaporizing chamber gas flows reunite in a mixing chamber distinct from the cassette, which overcomes the problems induced by ventilator back pressure (see below).

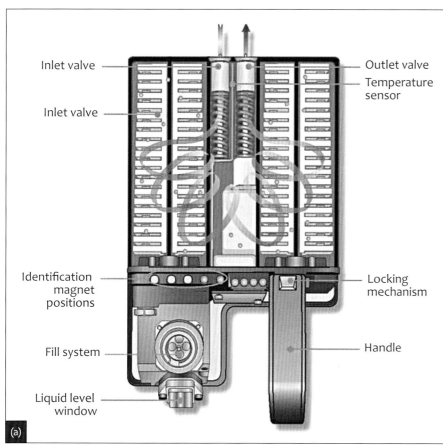

Inlet valve — Outlet valve
Temperature sensor
Inlet valve —
Identification magnet positions —
Fill system —
Liquid level window —
Locking mechanism
Handle

(a)

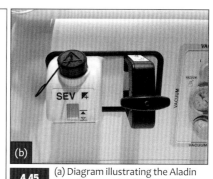

(b)

4.45 (a) Diagram illustrating the Aladin cassette vaporizer's internal design. (b) Aladin cassette vaporizer in place on the anaesthetic machine.
(Courtesy of GE Medical Systems Ltd)

Filling and emptying plenum vaporizers

In older designs, a screw-threaded stopper in the filling port is unscrewed and liquid anaesthetic poured in. This system raises some health and safety concerns, and also allows the possibility of filling the vaporizer with the wrong agent. Therefore, agent-specific filling devices have been developed:

- Key-indexed filling systems: the proximal end of the 'key' will only fit on to the neck of the bottle of a specific agent, while the distal end will only fit into a vaporizer calibrated for that agent (Figure 4.46ab)
- Sevoflurane (Quik-Fil) and desflurane (Saf-T-Fil) are sold in tamper-proof sealed bottles that will only fit into the filler ports on the correct vaporizer (Figure 4.47ab). Dräger uses a similar system (Dräger Fil) for the Vapor range of vaporizers.

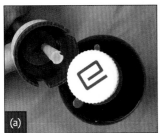
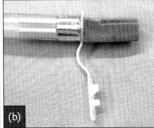

4.46 (a) Proximal end of keyed filler for isoflurane: the grooves on the screw top will only fit on to the collar of an isoflurane bottle. (b) Distal end of the keyed filler for isoflurane: this 'key' will only fit into the filling ports of an isoflurane vaporizer.

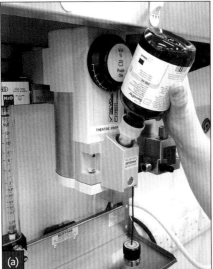
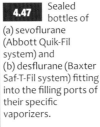

4.47 Sealed bottles of (a) sevoflurane (Abbott Quik-Fil system) and (b) desflurane (Baxter Saf-T-Fil system) fitting into the filling ports of their specific vaporizers.

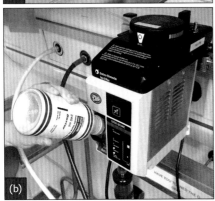

At intervals, vaporizers should be drained when the liquid level is low; any container used to collect the liquid should be suitably marked and the liquid discarded. Longer intervals may be used when the anaesthetic agent does not contain additives or stabilizing agents (e.g. thymol in the case of halothane).

If the wrong agent is put into the vaporizer, proceed as follows:

1. Drain and discard all liquid.
2. Flush the vaporizer with 5 l/min air or oxygen for about 30 minutes with the dial set at 5% (with suitable scavenging attached).
3. Fill with the correct agent and wait about 2 hours to allow for the temperature of the vaporizer to stabilize.

Checking plenum vaporizers before use

Before the gas flow is turned on, vaporizers should be checked to ensure that:

- They contain enough liquid anaesthetic (and are not overfilled)
- The filling port is tightly closed
- The control dial turns smoothly.

Position of vaporizers on the back bar

The Selectatec back bar enables placement and interchange of several vaporizers of different volatile anaesthetic agents on the back bar. If two or more vaporizers are fitted, their relative position is important. In simple terms, the vaporizer for the more volatile agent should be mounted upstream (i.e. closer to the flowmeters). More correctly, vaporizer position depends on the ratio between the SVP and potency (the minimum alveolar concentration – MAC) (see Chapter 15). The vaporizer for the agent with the lowest ratio should be placed upstream and that with the highest ratio downstream (Figure 4.48). The arrangement of sevoflurane–isoflurane (from upstream to downstream) minimizes the potential for vaporizer contamination.

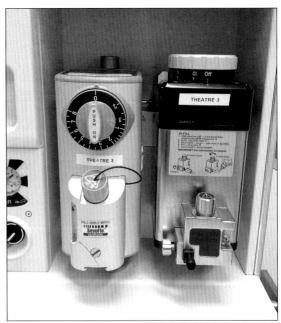

4.48 Correct positioning for sevoflurane and isoflurane vaporizers on the back bar, based on the ratio of saturated vapour pressure (SVP)/minimum alveolar concentration (MAC).

Back pressure

This phenomenon (also known as the 'pumping effect') occurs when pressure from gas-driven ventilators is transmitted in a retrograde fashion to the back bar and vaporizer. This can force gas in the outflow port back into the vaporizing chamber. Saturated gas can be forced back through the vaporizer inlet port and enter the bypass channel, resulting in increased agent delivery. This can be avoided by:

- A one-way valve at the outflow of the vaporizer
- Ensuring that the vaporizing chamber and bypass chamber are of equal volumes so back pressure is transmitted equally to both
- Having a long vaporizer inflow port.

Vaporizer 'in-circuit' anaesthetic machines

The vaporizers used in these machines are referred to as 'draw-over' vaporizers and are placed within the breathing system. They rely on the patient's respiratory effort to draw gas over the vaporizing surface. Examples include the Komesaroff and Stephens' machines; these are basically circle breathing systems (see Chapter 5) with one or more draw-over (low-resistance) vaporizers positioned within the circle. Both isoflurane and sevoflurane can be used in these machines.

The basic design of the Komesaroff machine consists of an oxygen supply, pressure-reducing valve and flowmeter attached to a circle breathing system, which incorporates one or two in-circuit vaporizers (Figure 4.49). The Stephens' machine is similar in design but incorporates a single in-circuit vaporizer and either does not have an integral oxygen supply if wall-mounted or has an oxygen supply when mounted on a mobile stand (Figure 4.50).

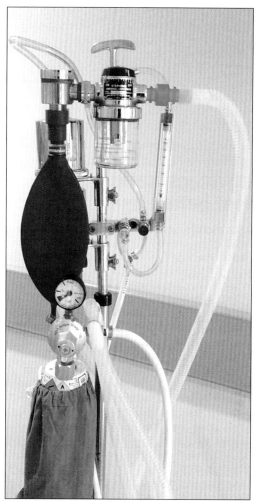

Stephens' anaesthetic machine.

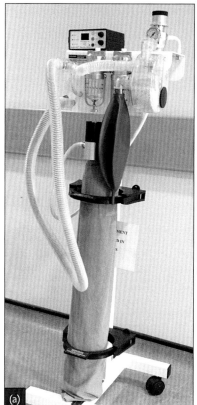

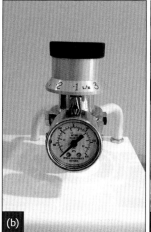

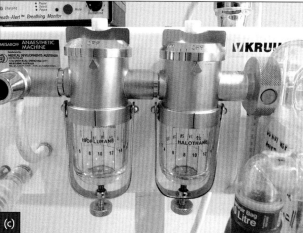

4.49 Komesaroff anaesthetic machine. (a) Complete unit. (b) Flowmeter on the Komesaroff machine, designed for delivering very low flows. (c) Low-resistance draw-over vaporizers for isoflurane and halothane.

These machines are economical to use because of the very low fresh gas flows required, but do need some practice to operate. They are not very accurate and a variable percentage of anaesthetic agent can be administered. Disadvantages include the possibility of anaesthetic overdosage, especially if intermittent positive pressure ventilation is used. In addition, performance of the draw-over vaporizers may be affected by contamination with water vapour condensed from the rebreathed expired gases.

Checking anaesthetic equipment before use

The anaesthetic machine should always be checked before use. The following checklist is adapted from the Association of Anaesthetists of Great Britain and Ireland publication 'Checking Anaesthetic Equipment 2012' (available at www.aagbi.org/sites/default/files/checking_anaesthetic_equipment_2012.pdf; an abbreviated version is available at www.aagbi.org/sites/default/files/checklist_for_anaesthetic_equipment_2012.pdf). The following checks should be made prior to each operating session:

1. Check that the anaesthetic machine is connected to the electricity supply (if appropriate) and switched on. Note that some modern anaesthetic workstations may enter an integral self-test programme when switched on; those functions tested by such a programme need not be retested.
2. Check that all monitoring devices are functioning and have appropriate alarm limits.
3. Check with a 'tug test' that each pipeline is correctly inserted into the appropriate gas supply terminal.
4. Check that the anaesthetic machine is connected to a supply of oxygen and that an adequate supply is available from a reserve oxygen cylinder.
5. Check that adequate supplies of other gases (nitrous oxide, air) are available and connected as appropriate.
6. Check that all pipeline pressure gauges in use on the anaesthetic machine indicate 400–500 kPa.
7. Check the operation of flowmeters (where fitted).
8. Check that each flow valve operates smoothly and that the bobbin moves freely throughout its range.
9. Check that the anti-hypoxia device is working correctly. Note that some veterinary anaesthetic machines may not have such a device.
10. Check the operation of the emergency oxygen bypass control.
11. Check the vaporizer(s):
    - Check that each vaporizer is adequately filled but not overfilled
    - Check that each vaporizer is correctly seated on the back bar and not tilted
    - Check each vaporizer for leaks (with vaporizer on and off) by temporarily occluding the common gas outlet
    - Turn the vaporizer(s) off when checks are completed
    - Repeat the leak test immediately after changing any vaporizer.
12. Check the breathing system to be used (see Chapter 5).
13. Check that the ventilator (if available) is configured appropriately for its intended use (see Chapter 6).
14. Ensure that an alternative means to ventilate the patient's lungs is available (e.g. self-inflating (Ambu) bag and oxygen cylinder).
15. Check that the anaesthetic gas scavenging system is switched on and is functioning correctly.
16. Check that the tubing is attached to the appropriate exhaust port of the breathing system, ventilator or workstation.
17. Check that all ancillary equipment that may be needed is present and working.
18. Check that any suction apparatus is functioning and that all connectors are secure.
19. Record on each patient's anaesthetic chart that the anaesthetic machine, breathing system and monitoring devices have all been checked.

References and further reading

Al-Shaikh B and Stacey S (2013) *Essentials of Anaesthetic Equipment, 4th revised edn.* Elsevier Churchill Livingstone, London

Baum JA (2005) New and alternative delivery concepts and techniques. *Best Practice and Research Clinical Anaesthesiology* **19**, 415–428

Boumphrey S and Marshall N (2011) Understanding vaporizers. *Continuing Education in Anaesthesia, Critical Care and Pain* **11(6)**, 199–203

Clarke KW, Trim CM and Hall LW (2013) Apparatus for the administration of anaesthetics. In: *Veterinary Anaesthesia, 11th revised edn.* Elsevier Saunders, London

Davey AJ and Diba A (2012) *Ward's Anaesthetic Equipment, 6th revised edn.* Elsevier Saunders, London

Dorsch JA and Dorsch SE (1999) *Understanding Anesthesia Equipment, 4th edn.* Lippincott Williams and Wilkins, Philadelphia

Dorsch JA and Dorsch SE (2011) *A Practical Approach to Anaesthesia Equipment, 4th edn.* Lippincott Williams and Wilkins, Philadelphia

Eales M and Cooper R (2007) Principles of anaesthetic vaporizers. *Anaesthesia and Intensive Care Medicine* **8**, 111–115

Ferguson AJ, Filippich LJ, Keates HL (2014) Delivery of sevoflurane to dogs using a Stephens anaesthetic machine. *Veterinary Anaesthesia and Analgesia* **41(1)**, 54–63

Gardner MC and Adams AP (1996) Anaesthetic vaporizers: design and function. *Current Anaesthesia and Critical Care* **7**, 315–321

Laredo FG, Cantalapiedra AG, Agut A, Pereira JL and Murciano J (2001) The Komesaroff anaesthetic machine for delivering sevoflurane to dogs. *Veterinary Anaesthesia and Analgesia* **28**, 161–167

Liu EHC and Dhara SS (1999) Sevoflurane anaesthesia with an Oxford Miniature Vaporiser in vaporiser inside circle mode. *British Journal of Anaesthesia* **82(4)**, 557–560

Love-Jones S and Magee P (2006) Medical gases, their storage and delivery. *Anaesthesia and Intensive Care Medicine* **8**, 2–6

Kelly JM and Kong KL (2011) Accuracy of ten isoflurane vaporisers in current clinical use. *Anaesthesia* **66**, 682–688

Kenny G and Davis PD (2003) *Basic Physics and Measurement in Anaesthesia, 5th edn.* Philadelphia, Butterworth Heinemann.

Middleton B, Stacey S, Thomas R and Phillips J (2012) *Physics in Anaesthesia.* Scion Publishing, Bloxham

Sherwood M (2010) Vapourisation and Vapourisers. *Anaesthesia Tutorial of the Week* **171**. Available at www.aagbi.org/sites/default/files/171-Vapourisation-and-vapourisers.pdf

Sinclair CM, Thadsad MK and Barker I (2006) Modern anaesthetic machines. *Continuing Education in Anaesthesia, Critical Care and Pain* **6(2)**, 75–78

Ward CS (1975) *Anaesthetic Equipment: Physical Principles and Maintenance.* Baillière Tindall, London

Washenitz F, Stoltzfus J, Newton B and Kubinski L (2001) Fire incidents involving regulators used in portable oxygen systems. *Injury Prevention* **7**, i34–i37 (doi:10.1136/ip.7.suppl_l.i34)

Young J and Kapoor V (2013) Principles of anaesthetic vaporizers. *Anaesthesia and Intensive Care Medicine* **14**, 99–102

Chapter 5

Breathing systems and ancillary equipment

Lynne Hughes

Definition and function of breathing systems

Breathing systems are interposed between an anaesthetic machine and a patient, i.e. between the common gas outlet and an endotracheal tube, supraglottic airway device (SGAD) or facemask. They serve to:

- Deliver oxygen and volatile anaesthetic agents from the anaesthetic machine to the patient
- Remove carbon dioxide exhaled by the patient
- Provide a means of ventilating the lungs.

Ancillary functions include delivery of waste anaesthetic gases to a scavenging system and measurement of airway pressures.

Other definitions relating to breathing systems

- *Rebreathing:* inhalation of previously exhaled gases, from which carbon dioxide may have been removed. In some cases this may lead to accumulation of carbon dioxide; however, in the context of anaesthetic breathing systems it is possible for patients to rebreathe either partially or fully without an increase in arterial carbon dioxide tension (hypercapnia). The amount of rebreathing will depend on the fresh gas flow, the apparatus dead space and the design of the breathing system.
- *Apparatus dead space:* the volume of the breathing system occupied by gases that are rebreathed without any change in their composition.
- *Tidal volume:* the volume of gas either inhaled or exhaled in 1 breath. An approximate value in healthy conscious animals at rest is 10–20 ml/kg.
- *Minute volume:* the sum of all gas volumes either inhaled or exhaled in 1 minute. It is calculated by multiplying tidal volume by respiratory rate. An approximate value in healthy conscious animals at rest is 200 ml/kg/min.

Basic components of breathing systems and their function

These features are summarized in Figure 5.1.

Components of breathing systems (and their synonyms)	Functions	Notes
Breathing tubes (limbs)	To convey gases to and from the patient To allow flexibility in positioning of the breathing system To act as a reservoir	May be rubber or plastic Those with a smooth internal bore create less resistance to breathing (less turbulence) Corrugated tubing is capable of expansion
Reservoir bag (breathing bag, rebreathing bag)	To allow accumulation of gas during exhalation To act as a reservoir for inhalation To visualize breathing To provide a method of assisting ventilation To protect the patient from excessive pressure	Should accommodate at least twice the tidal volume of the patient Sizes from 0.5–4 l Ellipsoid shape Open-ended or closed Compliance accommodates any rise in pressure within the system
Carbon dioxide absorbent	To absorb carbon dioxide. This allows complete rebreathing of exhaled gases	See section on breathing systems with carbon dioxide absorption
One-way valves (unidirectional valves)	To ensure that gases flow to the patient in one breathing tube and away from the patient in the other To prevent mixing of fresh gas with carbon dioxide-rich gas	Present in the circle system Valve leaflet/disc may sit horizontally (turret- or dome-type) or vertically
Pressure-relief valve (pop-off valve, scavenging valve, spill valve, expiratory valve, exhaust valve, adjustable pressure-limiting (APL) valve)	To limit the build-up of pressure within the system To release waste gases To allow safe connection to a scavenging system	Most have a lightweight disc on a narrow seating held in place by a spring APL valve limits the maximum pressure in the breathing system
Fresh gas inlet	To connect the breathing system to the common gas outlet on the anaesthetic machine	Attach with 'push and twist' action to avoid accidental disconnection

5.1 Basic components of breathing systems and their function.

Names and classification of breathing systems

The classification of breathing systems is confusing and terminology is complicated. They have been classified in various ways:

- According to their function (open, semi-open, semi-closed, closed)
- Whether they allow rebreathing
- Whether they contain absorbent to remove carbon dioxide
- The systems without carbon dioxide absorption were classified by Mapleson in 1954 (A to F).

For the purposes of this chapter, the most common name for the breathing system will be used and reference will be made to alternative names and classifications. Descriptions of the passage of gas in each system are included in relation to the spontaneously breathing patient only. For further details on classification systems, the mechanical aspects of individual systems and their detailed use during intermittent positive pressure ventilation (IPPV), the reader is directed to a standard textbook on anaesthesia equipment.

In veterinary anaesthesia, the simplest way to describe breathing systems is by grouping them into systems with similarities in their mode of use.

Breathing systems without carbon dioxide absorption

There are some general points to note when using breathing systems *without* carbon dioxide absorption:

- There are no unidirectional valves in any of these systems, with the exception of the pressure-relief valve (also known as the pop-off valve or adjustable pressure-limiting (APL) valve) and, therefore, removal of carbon dioxide from the system is dependent on an adequate fresh gas flow
- The fresh gas flow should not be altered during anaesthesia, unless there is a change in the patient's minute volume
- In order to prevent rebreathing of alveolar gas, all fresh gas flows are based on a multiple of minute volume. Proper function of these systems also requires an end-expiratory pause. If the respiratory pattern alters, and especially if respiratory rate increases during anaesthesia, the fresh gas flow should be recalculated and increased
- When the vaporizer setting is altered, the patient receives the new concentration of anaesthetic agent with the next breath. This makes it possible to alter the depth of anaesthesia rapidly
- Inspired gas is dry and at room temperature, and may contribute to the development of hypothermia, especially in small patients
- High fresh gas flows increase the costs of anaesthesia and also the amount of atmospheric pollution from waste gases
- To increase the efficiency of these systems, a capnograph may be used to monitor inspired carbon dioxide concentrations and the gas flow reduced until rebreathing is detected (see Chapter 7).
- If nitrous oxide is used, the total fresh gas flow may be divided between oxygen and nitrous oxide; the usual oxygen:nitrous oxide ratio is 1:2.

The *T-piece* and the *Bain* systems are functionally similar and require fresh gas flows of 1–2 times the minute volume to flush carbon dioxide from the system. The T-piece is most often used for cats and small dogs, while the Bain is suitable for cats and dogs of all sizes. Both systems may be used for spontaneously breathing patients but are most economical when used for IPPV; this is because IPPV usually provides for rapid inhalation and a long expiratory pause, giving plenty of time for the next tidal volume to be supplied.

The *Magill*, *Lack* and *mini parallel Lack* systems allow partial rebreathing of gas from the patient's anatomical dead space. Thus, a fresh gas flow equal to alveolar ventilation should prevent accumulation of carbon dioxide. However, if these systems are used to provide IPPV, this advantage is lost and gas flows in the order of two to three times the minute volume are required. The Magill and Lack are suitable for medium-sized patients while the mini parallel Lack is recommended for cats and dogs up to 10 kg bodyweight.

T-piece (Mapleson D, E, F)

There are various modifications of the T-piece: either without a bag, Mapleson E (or Ayre's T-piece) or with a bag, Mapleson D (paediatric T-piece) and F (Jackson-Rees modification) (Figure 5.2).

Fresh gas enters the system close to the patient (at a T-junction) and fills the breathing tubing, from where it is inhaled. The exhaled gas passes into the breathing tubing and, during the expiratory pause, is pushed by the continuous flow of fresh gas to the scavenging system, through the tubing itself or via either an open-ended reservoir bag, or an expiratory valve. The tubing thus refills with fresh gas during the expiratory pause, in readiness for the next breath. A high fresh gas flow of 2.5–3 times the minute volume (or approximately 600 ml/kg/min) may be required to prevent rebreathing of alveolar gas (Figure 5.3), although this flow may be reduced (to 1.5–2 times the minute volume) if capnography is used to detect rebreathing. Additional points of interest include:

- There are no one-way valves or carbon dioxide absorbent canisters in this system. Thus, resistance to breathing is low and the system is suitable for small patients. The pressure required to open the APL valve on the paediatric T-Piece (e.g. Intersurgical Infant T-Piece) is small (2–3 cmH$_2$O)
- The requirement for high fresh gas flows makes this system uneconomical in patients greater than 10 kg
- The patient's tidal volume (up to 20 ml/kg), must be accommodated within the breathing tubing and the reservoir bag (if present). If this is not the case, waste gas or air can be entrained during inspiration (Ayre's T-piece and Jackson Rees modification) or the bag could collapse, causing inspiratory resistance (paediatric T-piece)
- In the Jackson Rees modification, waste gas is scavenged through a tail on an open-ended reservoir bag. Extreme care must be taken to ensure that the tail does not become twisted and obstruct the outflow of gas: if this occurs, the high pressures generated within the system can cause a reduction in venous return, pneumomediastinum and/or pneumothorax, possibly resulting in cardiac arrest (see Chapter 31)
- IPPV is possible by partially or intermittently blocking an open-ended reservoir bag, or by partially closing the APL valve on other (Mapleson D) versions

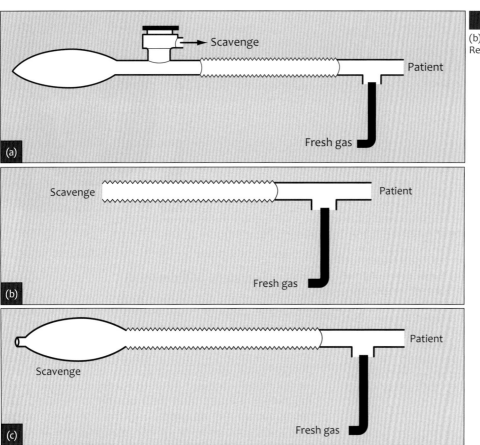

5.2 T-pieces. (a) Paediatric T-piece with APL valve (Mapleson D). (b) Ayre's T-piece (Mapleson E). (c) Jackson Rees modified T-piece (Mapleson F).

Breathing system	Multiple of minute volume	Fresh gas flow (ml/kg/minute)	Size of animal	Suitable for IPPV?
T-piece	2.5–3	500–600	Uneconomical if >10 kg	Yes
Bain	1–2	200–400	Uneconomical if >15–20 kg	Yes
Magill	0.8–1	160–200	Uneconomical if >25–30 kg	Better not to unless gas flow increased
Lack	0.8–1	160–200	Uneconomical if >25–30 kg	Better not to unless gas flow increased
Mini-Lack	1	200	Up to 10 kg	Yes, if gas flow increased to 600 ml/kg/minute
Humphrey ADE, A mode	0.5–0.75	100–150	Up to 10–20 kg	Yes (manual)

5.3 Gas flows and suggested patient size for breathing systems without carbon dioxide absorption. Provided inspired carbon dioxide levels are monitored, gas flows may be reduced further than those stated above. In the Lack system, fresh gas flows of 120 ml/kg/min have not caused rebreathing in dogs greater than 15 kg bodyweight. Note that comments on economy are based on an arbitrary fresh gas flow less than 6 l/min.

- The reservoir bag may look somewhat flat during operation; this is normal as long as breathing does not cause the bag to collapse totally.

Disposable paediatric versions of this system are in common use in veterinary practice. Models with an APL valve (Mapleson D, e.g. Intersurgical Infant T-Piece) are preferable. This ensures that, during routine use, excessive pressures cannot be transmitted to the patient: the APL valve contains an overpressure safety device so that if the valve is accidentally closed, the pressure applied to the patient will not exceed 35 cmH$_2$O. In addition, easy and safe scavenging is possible via a standard scavenging shroud. Disposable systems must be discarded on a regular basis (see below).

The Bain system (Mapleson D)

The Bain is a co-axial (tube within a tube) system, with fresh gas being carried in the inner tube and exhaled gas in the outer tube (Figure 5.4). This system is similar to the T-piece in its mode of action. Before inspiration, fresh gas is delivered from the inner tubing and fills the patient end of the outer tubing, from where it is inhaled and the reservoir bag empties. Exhaled gas passes through the outer tubing to a reservoir bag, a pressure-relief valve and then to the scavenging system. Some mixing of fresh gas and exhaled gas occurs in the outer tubing but, provided fresh gas flow is adequate, no significant rebreathing of carbon dioxide-rich alveolar gas should occur. Fresh gas flows of 1–2 times minute volume are usually adequate for spontaneously breathing animals (200–400 ml/kg/min; see Figure 5.3), although this is highly dependent on an adequate expiratory pause. Gas flow may be lowered further if a capnograph is used to detect rebreathing. As the volume for accommodating fresh gas (the breathing tubing and reservoir bag) is more capacious than in the Ayre's T-piece, the Bain system is suitable for larger patients up to 70 kg if a suitable flowmeter which can deliver the correct gas flow is available. Economics usually limit the use of the Bain for animals <15 kg bodyweight.

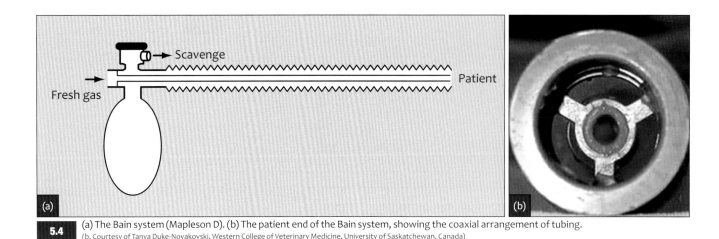

5.4 (a) The Bain system (Mapleson D). (b) The patient end of the Bain system, showing the coaxial arrangement of tubing.
(b, Courtesy of Tanya Duke-Novakovski, Western College of Veterinary Medicine, University of Saskatchewan, Canada)

When used for IPPV, the pressure-relief valve may be closed during lung inflation only and opened immediately following compression of the bag. Alternatively, the valve may remain partially closed at all times. Extreme care should be taken when using the Bain for IPPV, as pressures within the system may build up rapidly when high gas flows are used. High gas flows during IPPV may lead to hypocapnia and are seldom required; fresh gas flow can often be reduced to approximately 70 ml/kg/min during IPPV provided capnography is used.

The Magill system (Mapleson A)

The Magill system consists of a reservoir bag (situated beside the fresh gas inlet), wide-bore breathing tubing and a pressure-relief valve (Figure 5.5). Fresh gas fills the reservoir bag and the breathing tubing before reaching the patient, so that, when the patient inhales, the bag empties. The initial portion of exhaled breath (dead space gas, which does not contain carbon dioxide) passes along the breathing tubing to the partially empty bag, until the pressure increases sufficiently to open the pressure-relief valve. Since the valve is situated close to the patient, alveolar gas containing carbon dioxide is preferentially vented and dead space gas is retained for rebreathing. In the spontaneously breathing patient, the only requirement for fresh gas is to replace alveolar gas: approximately 0.8 times the minute volume (160 ml/kg/min; see Figure 5.3).

The Lack system (Mapleson A)

The Lack system also allows rebreathing of dead space gas and requires a similar fresh gas flow to the Magill (160 ml/kg/min). The system has two lengths of tubing, one for transporting fresh gas to the patient and the other for removing exhaled gas to the scavenging system. The bag is situated between the common gas outlet and the inspiratory tubing. As in the Magill system, when the patient exhales, the first portion of exhaled gas free of carbon dioxide passes into the inspiratory tubing. This, combined with the continuous fresh gas flow, will increase the pressure in the system and push the alveolar portion of the exhaled breath into the expiratory tubing, from where it exits through the pressure-relief valve. There are no unidirectional valves to prevent the patient inhaling gas from both the inspiratory and expiratory tubes, but rebreathing does not occur if the fresh gas flow is adequate. The Lack is available in parallel and co-axial versions (Figure 5.6ab).

The mini parallel Lack (Figure 5.6c) was designed as an alternative to the T-piece for patients <10 kg; the tubing connectors are too narrow for larger patients. The recommended gas flow is 200 ml/kg/min (see Figure 5.3), although this system has been used successfully in cats at lower gas flows (142±47 ml/kg/min) (Walsh and Taylor, 2004).

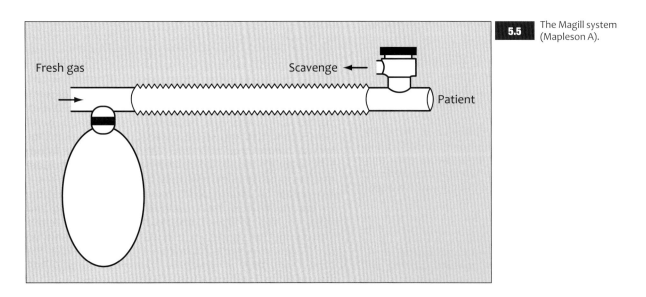

5.5 The Magill system (Mapleson A).

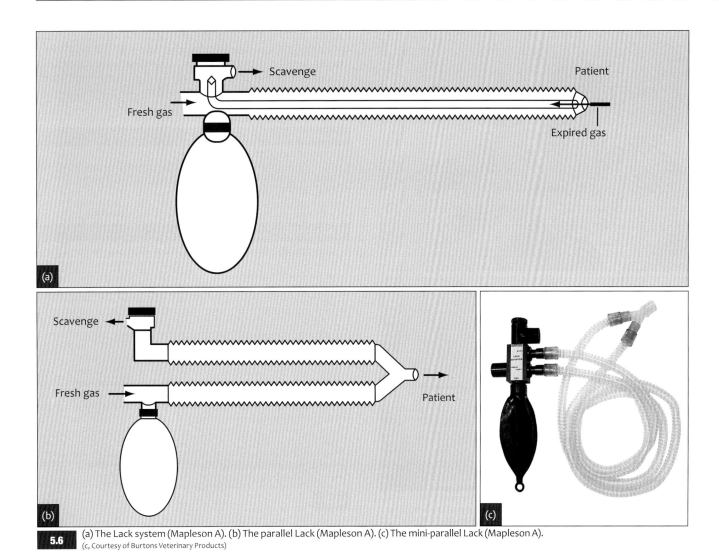

5.6 (a) The Lack system (Mapleson A). (b) The parallel Lack (Mapleson A). (c) The mini-parallel Lack (Mapleson A).
(c, Courtesy of Burtons Veterinary Products)

The Humphrey ADE system

The Humphrey ADE is a versatile breathing system, which may be used in different modes by altering a lever switch (Figure 5.7). The reader is directed to the manufacturer's instructions (Anaequip UK; www.anaequip.com) for detailed descriptions of its use. The notes below are intended to give a summary of the modes of use only.

The main component of the system is the Humphrey block, which attaches to the common gas outlet on an anaesthetic machine. The components are:

- A lever, which can be moved to the upright (A mode) or downward (D or E mode) positions. The lever rotates a metal cylinder within the block with openings that allow the passage of gas into other components
- A pressure-relief valve with a red spindle (to indicate function) and a scavenging shroud. The pressure-relief valve provides a small amount of positive end-expiratory pressure (PEEP) of about 1 cmH$_2$O, which may help to prevent alveolar collapse
- A safety pressure-relief valve, which opens at pressures in excess of 60 cmH$_2$O
- A reservoir bag
- A port for connection to a ventilator
- Two connection ports for lengths of 15 mm smooth-bore breathing tubing. The breathing tubes attach to a Y-connector at the patient end.

When the patient is breathing spontaneously and the lever is in the upright position, the Humphrey ADE may be used in a mode similar to the parallel Lack (Mapleson A). The A mode is more economical than the Lack and gas flows of 100–150 ml/kg/min often prevent rebreathing of alveolar gas. However, a recent study has examined the gas flows required to prevent rebreathing in cats and small dogs, compared to the Bain system (Gale *et al.*, 2015). The mean fresh gas flow that prevented rebreathing was 60 ml/kg/min. This system has also proved suitable for manual ventilation, without altering the gas flow. When the lever is facing downwards and respiration is controlled by a ventilator, the system may be used in a similar way to the paediatric T-piece (Mapleson D or E).

A recent modification is the inclusion of a removable carbon dioxide-absorbent canister, so that the system can be used like a circle system (see below). This further increases efficiency by allowing use of low gas flows, and its use is recommended by the manufacturer in dogs greater than 10–20 kg.

The Humphrey ADE is suitable for use in cats and dogs. The 15 mm smooth-bore tubing has a low internal volume, reduces turbulence, encourages laminar gas flow and does not increase resistance to breathing compared to standard 22 mm corrugated tubing. A smaller reservoir bag (500 ml or 1 l) should be used with cats and small dogs.

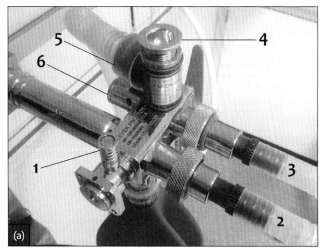

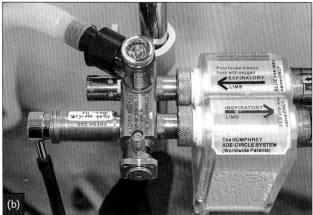

5.7 The Humphrey ADE system. (a) Without canister, with parallel breathing tubing and reservoir bag. The ventilator port is not visible. 1 = lever to select spontaneous or controlled ventilation. The lever is in the 'up' or Mapleson A position for spontaneous ventilation; 2 = inspiratory tubing; 3 = expiratory tubing; 4 = exhaust valve with visible indicator; 5 = scavenging shroud; 6 = safety pressure relief valve. (b) With absorbent canister attached.

(a, Courtesy of Chris Seymour, Royal Veterinary College, London, UK; b, Courtesy of Asher Allison, Animal Health Trust, Newmarket, UK)

Breathing systems with carbon dioxide absorption

In the anaesthetized patient, exhaled gas may be recycled and inhaled, provided the carbon dioxide is removed. The advantages of a breathing system that uses carbon dioxide absorption include:

- Decreased fresh gas requirement (oxygen ± nitrous oxide)
- Decreased use (and expense) of volatile agent
- Decreased environmental pollution
- Decreased loss of heat and moisture from the patient.

The *circle* and *to-and-fro* systems allow rebreathing of exhaled gases from which carbon dioxide has been removed by an absorbent. Fresh gas flow must include oxygen at a rate at least equal to that required for cellular metabolism. Estimates of oxygen requirements in dogs and cats under general anaesthesia vary from 2–7 ml/kg/min. As this figure is dependent on metabolic rate, age, temperature, etc., a safe estimate that also affords ease of calculation is 10 ml/kg/min. These systems are most economical when used for 'low-flow' anaesthesia (see below). Both systems may be used in the spontaneously breathing patient, or may be used to provide IPPV. Unless specifically stated, most systems manufactured for the veterinary market are not suitable for spontaneously breathing patients weighing less than 7–10 kg. The advantages and disadvantages of using these systems are summarized in Figure 5.8.

Advantages
<ul><li>Absorbs carbon dioxide</li><li>Allows rebreathing of exhaled gas, therefore allowing low fresh gas flows to be employed – this results in greater economy</li><li>Warms inspired gas</li><li>Moistens inspired gas</li><li>Low-flow systems result in less environmental pollution</li></ul>

Disadvantages
<ul><li>Channelling or tracking of gases may occur if the canister is not packed correctly or if the granules fragment (particular problem in the to-and-fro system)</li><li>Absorbent presents resistance to breathing</li><li>May generate excessive heat when used for large breed dogs</li><li>Water may collect in the breathing tubes (particular problem in the circle)</li><li>Absorbents may react with some anaesthetic agents to form toxic byproducts (see Figure 5.10)</li><li>Absorbents may generate caustic dust, which may reach the respiratory tract (particular problem in the to-and-fro system)</li><li>Dead space may increase with the duration of the anaesthetic (particular problem in the to-and-fro system)</li><li>May cause 'drag' on the endotracheal tube (particular problem in the to-and-fro system)</li><li>The canister can be bypassed on some machines to allow absorbent to be changed during long anaesthetic periods. The switch must be turned to allow gas to travel through the absorbent afterwards.</li><li>Canister may be difficult to clean</li><li>Canister is prone to leakage</li></ul>

5.8 Advantages and disadvantages of using an absorbent canister.

The circle system

The arrangement of the components of the circle system ensures that gases move in one direction only, in a circular fashion (Figure 5.9ab). Inspired gas is a mixture of fresh gas and previously exhaled gas from which carbon dioxide has been removed. The system contains two unidirectional valves. One allows the patient to inhale only through an inspiratory breathing tube (limb), which connects to the patient at a Y-connector. The other prevents exhaled gas from entering the inspiratory limb; instead it enters the expiratory breathing tube (limb), which is also connected to the Y-connector at the patient end. The other basic components of the system are an absorbent canister, a reservoir bag and a pressure-relief valve. The exact arrangement varies from manufacturer to manufacturer. Some systems include a pressure manometer, which is desirable when carrying out IPPV and when checking the system for leaks (see Chapter 7).

Specific advantages of the circle system include:

- The apparatus dead space is small, provided the unidirectional valves are functioning correctly: mixing of inspiratory and expiratory gases can only occur in the Y-connector
- Removal of carbon dioxide is efficient because the passage of gas in a circular fashion ensures that all exhaled gas must pass through the canister
- The pressure-relief valve is situated remotely from the patient, allowing ease of access
- Caustic dust from the absorbent is unlikely to reach the patient as it will settle in the breathing tube

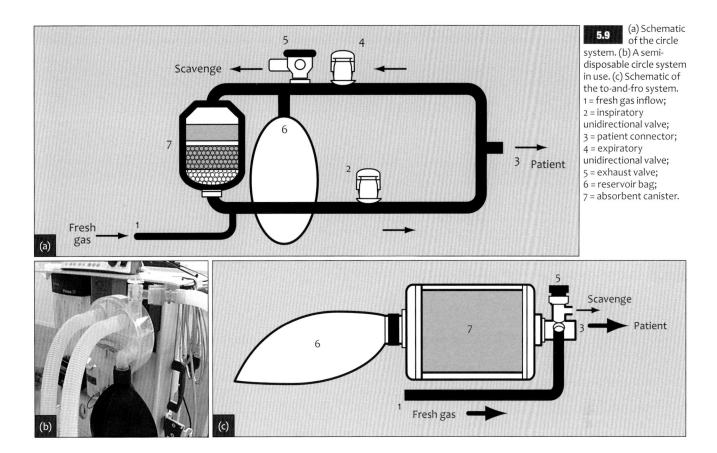

5.9 (a) Schematic of the circle system. (b) A semi-disposable circle system in use. (c) Schematic of the to-and-fro system. 1 = fresh gas inflow; 2 = inspiratory unidirectional valve; 3 = patient connector; 4 = expiratory unidirectional valve; 5 = exhaust valve; 6 = reservoir bag; 7 = absorbent canister.

- The risk of hyperthermia is reduced, as heat generated by the absorption of carbon dioxide may be dissipated by the breathing tubes.

The to-and-fro system

In the to-and-fro system, fresh gas enters the system near the patient. Exhaled gas from the patient passes through a canister containing carbon dioxide absorbent into a reservoir bag, and gas returns to the patient by the same route during inhalation (Figure 5.9c). Excess gas is vented through a pressure-relief valve situated close to the patient connector. This system has several disadvantages when compared with the circle system:

- The canister is usually positioned horizontally and, as the absorbent settles and granules disintegrate, spaces will appear above the absorbent. This allows channelling of gases through spaces with no absorbent, with a resultant reduction in absorption of carbon dioxide
- The canister is situated in close proximity to the patient, increasing the possibility of caustic dust reaching the respiratory tract, especially during IPPV
- The system is bulky and heavy, and exerts considerable drag on the endotracheal tube
- The pressure-relief valve is situated close to the patient, which may be inconvenient during surgery
- As anaesthesia progresses, the absorbent becomes increasingly exhausted from the surface closest to the patient; over time this results in an increase in apparatus dead space
- When used for small patients (<10 kg) a significant portion of alveolar gas may never reach functional absorbent, resulting in rebreathing of carbon dioxide-rich gas.

Substances used to absorb carbon dioxide

The substance most commonly used to absorb carbon dioxide is calcium hydroxide in combination with sodium hydroxide or potassium hydroxide (i.e. soda lime). Various advances in manufacturing have resulted in the addition of other compounds to increase the effectiveness of the absorbent and reduce the production of toxic byproducts, especially with sevoflurane (Figure 5.10).

In soda lime, carbon dioxide is removed from exhaled gases by a chemical reaction. The reaction both requires and generates water – on balance more water is generated than is required. The reaction also generates heat and a pH change. Several steps are involved but they can be summarized as follows:

1. $H_2O + CO_2 \rightarrow H_2CO_3$
2. $2H_2CO_3 + 2NaOH + Ca(OH)_2 \rightarrow CaCO_3 + Na_2CO_3 + 4H_2O + Heat$

Some newer absorbents (e.g. LoFloSorb®, Amsorb®) do not contain sodium or potassium hydroxide and are not, therefore, corrosive. They do not degrade volatile anaesthetic agents, or generate carbon monoxide, Compound A or formaldehyde.

Absorbent materials are granular. The following details are important:

- The size of the granules. A combination of small and large granules is preferable as this minimizes resistance to breathing, increases the surface area for contact and absorption, and decreases caking and channelling
- Granules may fragment, producing dust. If excessive, dust may:
  - Result in increased resistance to breathing

Compound	Properties	Possible problems
Calcium hydroxide	Main component of absorbents	Very soft unless mixed with other substances
Sodium hydroxide	Enhances reactivity and ability to bind water. Usually present in soda lime	If dry, causes degradation of isoflurane, enflurane and desflurane to carbon monoxide, and degradation of sevoflurane to Compound A, formaldehyde and methanol
Potassium hydroxide	As for sodium hydroxide	As for sodium hydroxide. Use now discontinued
Water	14–19% water content of absorbent is required for reaction with carbon dioxide to start	If there is inadequate water, absorbents exhaust quickly, can produce toxic compounds and may absorb anaesthetic agents. Excess water increases resistance and stickiness
Indicators	Acid or base; colour depends on the pH. Used to show when absorbent is exhausted	It is important to be familiar with the expected colour change. Ethyl violet may be deactivated in light
Zeolite	Increases porosity, hardness and water content	May absorb anaesthetic agent if absorbent is very dry
Silica	Overcomes softness of calcium hydroxide	
Calcium chloride and calcium sulphate	Enhance reactivity, are able to bind water and improve hardness	Colour may change if dried out

5.10 Main constituents of carbon dioxide absorbents and their properties.

- Cause caking of granules and channelling of gases through the spaces that are formed
- Reach the patient, where it will cause caustic burns in the respiratory tract
- Settle on valves and other moving parts, causing them to malfunction
- Migrate on to gaskets and rubber seals, causing them to leak.

Modern manufacturing techniques help reduce the quantity of dust produced by absorbents.

Signs of exhaustion of the carbon dioxide absorbent:

- Colour change – the colour varies with the pH indicator used.
- A canister that is cold to the touch when in use.
- Increased inspired carbon dioxide detected by a capnograph.
- Signs of hypercapnia, i.e. increased respiratory rate, heart rate and blood pressure, in association with a bounding pulse and excessive bleeding during surgery.
- Granules that are hard, not crumbly (gloves should be worn when carrying out this test).

Depleted soda lime may appear to regenerate, as the granules dry out when not in use. However, the additional capacity to absorb carbon dioxide is minimal and the indicator usually reverts to the colour indicating that it is exhausted after only a few breaths. Absorbent should be replaced as soon as the indicator colour change is noticed.

Desirable features in the design of an absorbent canister:

- Transparent walls, so that the colour change can be visualized: this is the norm for modern canisters.
- Large cross-sectional area, to decrease resistance and dust migration: this is a feature of most circle absorbers, but not of the to-and-fro.
- Large enough to contain the tidal volume of the patient in the intergranular space: there is variation between manufacturers in the sizes of canisters.
- Situated in the vertical position, to prevent gas channelling through unfilled portions: this is usual in the circle system, but not in the to-and-fro.

Practices that avoid the production of toxic byproducts from absorbents:

- Not allowing the absorbent to dry out, i.e. turning off the anaesthetic machine and/or disconnecting the oxygen supply when not in use, so that gas does not flow through the absorbent for longer than is necessary.
- Turning off the vaporizer when not in use.
- Checking the absorber for excessive heat; heat increases the production of toxic byproducts. Changing the soda lime on time or increasing the gas flow, prevents it from getting too hot.

Precautions for the care and handling of soda lime include:

- Wet soda lime is caustic – avoid touching it (wear gloves), inhaling it (wear a paper or surgical mask) or contact with the eyes.
- Handle the absorbent gently to avoid fragmentation of granules and dust production.
- Reseal the package after opening to prevent the absorbent reacting with air, deactivation of the indicator by light and loss of moisture.
- Store at temperatures above freezing to prevent granules expanding and disintegrating.

F circuit

The universal F circuit (Figure 5.11) is not a complete breathing system in itself: it is a co-axial (tube-within-a-tube) system of breathing tubing in which the inner and outer tubes diverge at one end. The patient is attached at the co-axial end, while the other ends can be connected to the inspiratory and expiratory sides of two one-way valves and a CO_2 absorber canister.

The F circuit is most commonly used as part of a circle system when the diverging ends are attached in the same manner as the traditional lengths of tubing. It is usual for the inner tubing to be the inspiratory limb and the outer tubing the expiratory limb. Characteristics include:

- One length of tubing instead of two attached to the patient. This is more streamlined and less bulky than the two-tube system and may cause less drag on the endotracheal tube

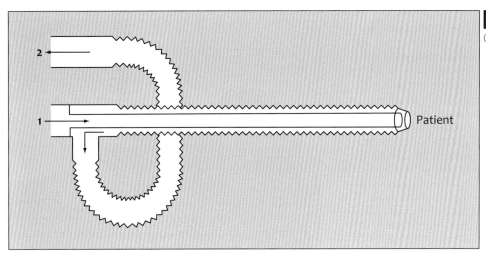

5.11 The F circuit. 1 = fresh gas inflow; 2 = exhaled gas.
(Courtesy of Chris Hughes)

- It is thermally efficient, as heat from the exhaled breath warms the inspired gases
- Water vapour condensing in the outer (expiratory) tube is more likely to cause an obstruction than in the two-tube system.

The F circuit is manufactured in various lengths which are useful for special anaesthetic procedures such as magnetic resonance imaging (MRI).

Low-flow anaesthesia

The circle and to-and-fro systems may be used with low gas flows in veterinary anaesthesia. When considering the minimum fresh gas flow, only the oxygen required for cellular metabolism needs to be supplied, as exhaled gas is rebreathed. Any additional gas must be vented through the pressure-relief valve. These systems are thus economical to run and result in less atmospheric pollution.

Using low-flow anaesthesia in veterinary practice

- Following induction of anaesthesia and endotracheal intubation, a fresh gas flow of 100 ml/kg/min should be provided for 5–10 minutes. The pressure-relief valve should be fully open during this period. The advantages of an initial high flow include purging the system of air (primarily nitrogen) and filling it with fresh gas (oxygen and anaesthetic agent), and also providing sufficient inhaled anaesthetic agent for rapid stabilization of anaesthetic depth.
- Once anaesthetic depth is stabilized, the fresh gas flow may be reduced to approximately 10 ml/kg/min. Alternatively, 0.5–1 l/min is adequate for all dogs weighing less than 50 kg. Moreover, many vaporizers require a fresh gas flow of at least 0.5 l/min to ensure accuracy.

Some general points should be considered when using low-flow anaesthesia:

- The contribution of fresh gas to the overall volume of the breathing system is small; many circle breathing systems used in veterinary practice have a volume in excess of 4 litres. Moreover, exhaled breath usually contains less volatile agent than was inspired by the patient, especially at the beginning of a period of anaesthesia, because of uptake of agent from the lungs. The net result is that the exhaled breath dilutes the effect of the fresh gas and the patient inhales considerably less volatile agent than the vaporizer setting would suggest. The lower the fresh gas flow used and the larger the patient, the greater the discrepancy between the vaporizer setting and the concentration of agent in inspired breath. In addition, this effect is greater with volatile agents that are more readily soluble in blood. The following example illustrates this:
  - The minute volume of a 15 kg dog is approximately 3 l/min (200 ml/kg/min). If the fresh gas flow during the initial high-flow period is 1.5 l/min (100 ml/kg/min), then the diluting effect of the patient's breath is 2:1. However, if the fresh gas flow during the low-flow period is 150 ml/min (10 ml/kg/min), then the fresh gas containing volatile agent is diluted 20:1 by the patient's exhaled breath. This explains why it is difficult to stabilize (or change) the depth of anaesthesia rapidly using volatile agents and a low-flow system. Over time, the patient exhales increasing amounts of volatile agent as uptake decreases, and the difference between the vaporizer setting and inspired concentration of that agent also decreases
- The initial vaporizer setting should be maintained until the required depth of anaesthesia has been achieved. When the gas flow is reduced, a higher vaporizer setting is usually required, for the reasons stated above
- During the course of an uneventful anaesthetic, the vaporizer setting may be increased or decreased by small increments (0.25–0.5%), without varying the gas flow
- If it is necessary to alter the depth of anaesthesia rapidly:
  - The vaporizer setting should be adjusted
  - The gas flow should be increased to 100 ml/kg/min for several minutes with the APL valve open
  - The contents of the reservoir bag may be 'dumped' into the scavenging system, although this is not essential
  - This allows the new vapour setting to wash into the system rapidly. When the required depth of anaesthesia has been achieved, the lower gas flow should again be used
- If nitrous oxide is used in a rebreathing system, care should be taken to provide adequate inspired oxygen. Because oxygen is continuously consumed by the

patient, and nitrous oxide is not, the proportion of oxygen in the system will decrease over time. In the absence of an oxygen analyser, a 1:1 mixture of oxygen:nitrous oxide should be used and oxygen flow should be set at a minimum of 20 ml/kg/min

- If the reservoir bag empties, it should be refilled by increasing the gas flow at the flowmeter. Using the oxygen flush mechanism, which bypasses the vaporizer, will result in dilution of volatile anaesthetic agent; it may also result in rapid, dangerous increases in pressure within the system and within the patient if the APL valve is partially closed
- At the conclusion of anaesthesia, gas flow should again be increased and the contents of the reservoir bag 'dumped' to flush out exhaled anaesthetic agent, which would otherwise recirculate and delay the patient's recovery
- When using a side stream capnograph the gas sampling rate may be as high as 200 ml/min. This should be taken into account when using low flows.

Checking and leak testing of breathing systems

Before use, all breathing systems should be thoroughly checked. This is especially important when a system is used for the first time or following reassembly after cleaning. Checking should comprise the following steps:

1. Inspect the system, checking that:
   - All components are present and assembled correctly
   - There are no obvious holes, obstructions or foreign bodies in tubing
   - The inner tube of co-axial systems is attached at both ends.
2. Attach the breathing system to the common gas outlet with a 'push and twist' action and ensure the connection is secure.
3. Test the system for leaks:
   - Close the pressure-relief valve, or the tail on an open-ended bag
   - Occlude the patient connector with a finger or suitable plug
   - Fill the system with oxygen to a pressure of 30–40 cmH$_2$O
   - In the absence of a pressure gauge, the bag should be filled until it appears to be under pressure and it should be observed for signs of deflation
   - Turn off the oxygen flow and ensure that either the system maintains the set pressure for at least 10 seconds or an oxygen flow <200 ml/min is needed to keep the system filled to this pressure. Open the pressure-relief valve and ensure that the pressure is immediately relieved
   - Remove finger or plug from the patient connector.
4. Check the function of the unidirectional valves on the circle:
   - Occlude the patient end of the breathing system
   - Close the APL valve
   - Partially fill the system with gas
   - Squeeze the rebreathing bag several times and observe that both unidirectional valves open and close freely
   - Open the APL valve (Figure 5.12).

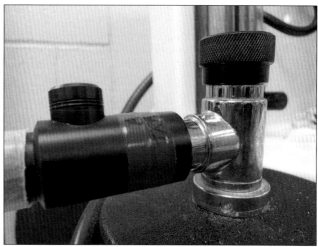

5.12 A spring-loaded valve can be placed on the scavenger side of the APL valve to enable manual intermittent positive pressure ventilation. The button is pressed while squeezing the rebreathing bag and released after the manoeuvre. This device avoids accidentally leaving the APL valve closed.
(Courtesy of Tanya Duke-Novakovski, Western College of Veterinary Medicine, University of Saskatchewan, Canada)

Specific tests are required to check the integrity of the inner tube of co-axial systems (Bain and Lack). Note that these tests must be carried out with care as they can result in disconnection of the inner limb at either end:

- Bain: two tests may be used; an occlusion test and the Pethick test
  - Occlusion test (Foëx Crampton-Smith test): with an oxygen flow of 4 l/min, *briefly* occlude the inner limb (using the tool provided with disposable systems, or with a plunger from a 2 ml syringe) and note that the reservoir bag remains deflated. As this generates considerable back pressure in the anaesthetic machine, the following may also happen:
    - The flowmeter bobbin will drop initially
    - If the machine is fitted with a high-pressure safety valve it will open; if not, the breathing system may be propelled from the common gas outlet
  - Pethick test: occlude the patient end of the breathing system and close the APL valve. Use the oxygen flush to fill the system. Release the occlusion at the patient end and activate the oxygen flush. If the inner tube is intact the reservoir bag should collapse
- Lack: using a suitably sized endotracheal tube, cover the inner tubing at the patient end. Blow down the endotracheal tube; if any movement is observed in the reservoir bag then there is leakage from the inner limb. An alternative method is to occlude both inner and outer tubes at the patient end, with the pressure-relief valve open, then squeeze the reservoir bag: if the inner tube is broken, gas can escape through the pressure-relief valve.

Common hazards caused by breathing systems

There are numerous reports of hazards caused by faulty breathing systems or errors in their use. This section covers the most common faults and errors encountered in veterinary practice, their consequences and main causes:

- Disconnection of the breathing system (with possible resultant hypoxia) caused by:
  - Failure to secure breathing systems using a 'push and twist' action when attaching components. The most common site of disconnection is between the breathing system and the endotracheal tube. This is particularly hazardous during surgery of the head and neck, when the area is covered by drapes
  - Attaching components that are manufactured from different materials. In this case the friction generated will not be as strong as when the two components are made of the same material.
- Increased apparatus dead space (and resultant hypercapnia) caused by:
  - Exhausted absorbent in circle and to-and-fro absorber systems. This may go unnoticed if absorbent at the centre of the canister is fully exhausted while the absorbent around the outside has not changed colour
  - Channelling of gases along the top of an inadequately packed absorbent canister in the to-and-fro system
  - Non-functioning or missing unidirectional valves in a circle system, allowing the mixing of fresh gas with carbon dioxide-containing exhaled gas
  - Inadequate fresh gas flow when using systems without carbon dioxide absorption
  - Use of overlong elbow (or other) connectors between the endotracheal tube and the breathing system, increasing apparatus dead space
  - Disconnection of, or leakage from, the inner tubing in a co-axial Bain system
  - Inadvertent exclusion of carbon dioxide absorbent; this is possible in some older circle systems used for humans.
- Generation of excessive pressure at exhalation (preventing adequate venous return, resulting in barotrauma to the lungs, pneumomediastinum and/or pneumothorax) caused by:
  - Failure to open the pressure-relief valve following leak testing of the breathing system
  - Obstructions of the scavenging outlet, as described above in the open-ended bag of the Jackson-Rees modified T-piece
  - A faulty pressure-relief valve that fails to open. This is most likely if disposable breathing systems are re-used indefinitely or if the valves of re-usable systems are over-tightened
  - Obstruction of the pressure-relief valve with soda lime granules
  - Obstruction or kinking of the breathing tubing or the neck of the bag by other equipment (often a table)
  - The presence of foreign bodies in the breathing system. This has been reported as a manufacturing or packaging fault
  - The presence of large quantities of water in the expiratory limb of a circle breathing system, particularly if the limb hangs off the table in a loop
  - Failure of the expiratory valve on the circle to open.
- Generation of negative pressure at inspiration (and potential pulmonary oedema) caused by:
  - Inadequate fresh gas flow, resulting in an empty reservoir bag when the patient inhales. Some breathing systems incorporate a negative pressure-relief valve, which allows entrainment of air to prevent this
  - Kinking or obstruction of the inspiratory limb of the breathing system, e.g. if wedged between the operating table and anaesthetic machine

  - Excessive 'suction' from an active scavenging system, which empties the reservoir bag
  - Failure of the inspiratory valve on the circle system to open.
- Hyperthermia (potentially resulting in tachycardia, tachyarrhythmias and/or tachypnoea) caused by heat generated during low-flow anaesthesia when using breathing systems with an absorbent. The incidence is increased in giant-breed dogs with a heavy coat, and in high environmental temperatures.

Disposable breathing systems are intended for single use in human anaesthesia. As these systems are not designed for prolonged use, faults will develop over time. It is vital that these systems are checked before every use and that the veterinary practice develops a protocol for discarding them. The most common faults (many of which may have disastrous consequences) include:

- Unidirectional valves that fail to operate – this may be difficult to detect without capnography
- Pressure-relief valves that fail to open
- Cracking, splitting or distortion of the attachment for the common gas outlet
- Holes in the breathing tubing or reservoir bag
- Disconnection of, or leakage from, the inner limb of co-axial systems.

Care and maintenance of breathing systems

For the purposes of this section, breathing systems have been divided into disposable and re-usable. As a general principle, the closer the equipment is to the patient, the greater the need to sterilize or discard it.

Disposable systems (single or limited use)

Disposable systems:

- Should be chosen if it is suspected that a patient has an infectious disease. The system should be discarded after use
- Should be fully checked before every use if re-used; none of the components are designed for repeated use
- If re-used for a limited period, should be discarded on a routine basis (e.g. after a certain number of cases or on a certain date).

Re-usable systems

It is important to adhere to a set routine of thorough cleaning and rinsing, followed by disinfection or sterilization. It is preferable to sterilize re-usable breathing systems fully at regular intervals, using heat or chemical methods appropriate for the material from which they are manufactured. In the intervening periods they should be dismantled, washed in hot soapy water and soaked in a suitable disinfectant solution on a routine (weekly) basis. In addition, moisture collected in the breathing tubing from the circle system should be drained daily. The contents of absorbent canisters should be replaced when a colour change is noticed and not left until the following morning. The absorbent should be changed if desiccation is suspected i.e. if the fresh gas was left on overnight.

All re-usable systems must be checked fully when reassembled.

The medical literature contains several case reports documenting cross-infection of patients by anaesthetic-related equipment. Although there is scant evidence of such incidents in the veterinary field, the potential for trans-mission of infections via this route should not be ignored and procedures should be put in place to minimize the risk.

Endotracheal tubes

Endotracheal tubes may be manufactured from red rubber, PVC or silicone (Figures 5.13 and 5.14), and polyurethane is sometimes used for cuffs. There is generally a pilot balloon, which is used as an indicator that the cuff is inflated. The Murphy eye (Figure 5.13b) is an oval hole opposite the bevel that allows gas to flow through the tube should the bevel become obstructed or be positioned against the wall of the trachea.

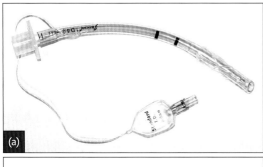

(a)

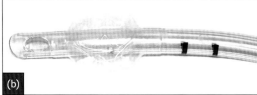

(b)

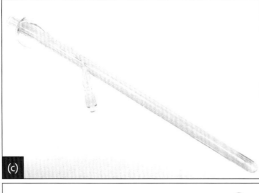

(c)

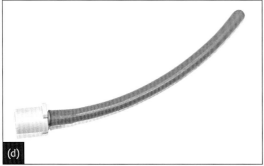

(d)

5.13 Endotracheal tubes. (a) PVC. (b) A PVC tube showing the Murphy eye opposite the bevel. (c) Silicone. (d) Red rubber.
(Courtesy of Asher Allison, Animal Health Trust, Newmarket, UK)

Feature	Red rubber	PVC	Silicone
Durability	May be re-used but will perish over time, especially in sunlight	Disposable	May be re-used
Repair	Cannot be repaired	Cannot be repaired	May be repaired
Available sizes	2–16 mm ID	2–11 mm ID	2–16 mm ID
Withstands autoclave	Yes	No	Yes
Mould to shape when warmed	No	Yes	Yes
Withstands kinking	No, especially when old	Better than red rubber	Better than red rubber
Irritant	Yes	No	No
Expense	Moderate	Inexpensive	Most expensive
Blockages visible	No	Yes	Perhaps
Preformed curve	Yes	Yes	No
Ease of insertion	Easy to insert	Easy to insert	May require stylet to form curve
Self-sealing pilot balloon for cuff inflation	No	Yes	Yes
Types of cuff available	Low-volume, high-pressure	• Low-volume, high-pressure • High-volume, low-pressure	Low-volume, high-pressure

5.14 Comparison of materials used for endotracheal tubes. ID = internal diameter.

Armoured tubes are thick-walled tubes with a spiral wire coil embedded in the wall (Figure 5.15). They are used to prevent kinking during maximal neck flexion, e.g. during some ophthalmic, head and neck surgery, and during cisternal puncture. The part of the tube protruding from the mouth can be bent away from the surgical site without risk of kinking. However, insertion usually requires the use of a stylet, and if the animal bites down on the tube it may become permanently obstructed. In addition, these tubes cannot be shortened because of the wire spiral and because the tube leading to the inflation cuff is integrated into the main tube.

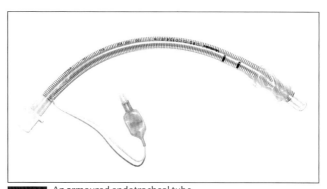

5.15 An armoured endotracheal tube.
(Courtesy of Asher Allison, Animal Health Trust, Newmarket, UK)

There are different cuff types:

- High-pressure, low-volume. These provide superior protection of the airway, although the narrow area of high pressure generated by the profile of the cuff may damage the tracheal mucosa
- Low-pressure, high-volume. Because the region of pressure is spread over a wider area, there is less risk to the tracheal mucosa. However, liquid may pass by the cuff due to the small folds that may develop in the cuff.

When selecting endotracheal tubes:

- Choose the widest diameter that will pass easily through the narrowest part of the airway. However, care must be taken not to damage the larynx or trachea by placing a tube that is too big, and if in doubt a slightly smaller tube should be chosen. Narrow tubes increase resistance to gas flow and therefore increase the work of breathing. It is best to have two or three possible sizes of tube available for every animal. A guide to appropriate sizes is shown in Figure 5.16. Selection of an ETT using the nasal septal width has 21% chance of accuracy while tracheal palpation has 46% accuracy

Sizes (internal diameter) (mm)	Cuffed and/or uncuffed	Approximate lean bodyweight (kg)
2.0, 2.5, 3.0	Cuffed and uncuffed	1–2.5
3.5, 4.0, 4.5	Cuffed and uncuffed	2.5–5
5, 6	Cuffed and uncuffed (size 5)	4–9
7, 8	Cuffed	7–15
9, 10	Cuffed	15–25
11, 12	Cuffed	25–45
14, 16	Cuffed	>40

5.16 Suggested sizes of endotracheal tubes suitable for small animal practice. Note that there is large individual variation in tracheal diameter in dogs and this table is intended as a guideline only. Brachycephalic breeds may have a hypoplastic (narrow) trachea.

- Choose the shortest tube that can be properly secured (see section below). This decreases the work of breathing, decreases the possibility of intubating a main bronchus and decreases apparatus dead space. Tubes (other than armoured tubes; see above) may be cut to the correct length
- Choose a tube with a cuff, as this is preferable in most situations; the cuff will provide superior protection of the airway. Opinions vary on whether cuffs are desirable when intubating cats. The cuffs of modern disposable tubes are manufactured from very thin material that may not restrict the diameter of the airway to the same extent as cuffs on red rubber tubes. A cuff is especially important if:
  - The animal is not fasted, because it is more likely to regurgitate
  - The procedure involves the gastrointestinal tract, upper abdomen or mouth
  - A smaller tube than expected is used.

Technique for intubating cats and dogs

Before inserting an endotracheal tube, the procedure is as follows:

- Inflate the cuff and leave it for 10 minutes to check for leaks (or test under water)

- Ensure the tube is clean and the lumen is patent
- Pre-measure the tube against the patient. It should reach from the incisors to the thoracic inlet when the neck is flexed (Figure 5.17a)
- Ensure there is a 15 mm male connector in place, for attachment to the breathing system
- Lubricate the tube with a water-soluble lubricant (e.g. K-Y Jelly), but do not occlude the bevel or the Murphy eye.

Small animals may be intubated while in lateral, sternal or (more rarely) dorsal recumbency. Occasionally, the patient's pathology dictates which position is best, but most often the choice is the veterinary surgeon's (veterinarian's) personal preference. A trained assistant is of immense benefit when intubating small animals. Cats and dogs are intubated using the following technique (Figure 5.17b):

1. The assistant holds the patient's upper jaw in one hand by means of a bandage tie, taking care not to place fingers in the mouth, and extends the head and neck towards the operator, keeping them straight and in alignment with the spine. Their other hand may be used to help extend the head; it should not be placed under the neck as this will block visualization of the larynx.
2. The operator then grasps the lower jaw, draws out the tongue gently and opens the mouth wide, facilitated by their assistant.

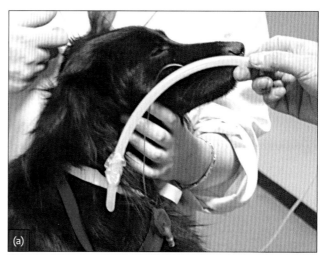

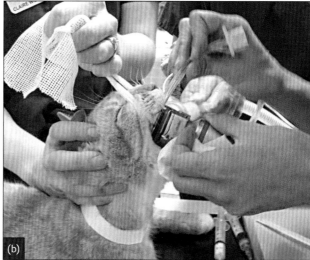

5.17 (a) Premeasuring the length of an endotracheal tube before placement (see text for details). (b) Technique for intubating cats and dogs (see text for details).

3. The laryngoscope (see below) and the tongue should be held in the non-dominant hand and the tip of the laryngoscope placed on the base of the tongue, just rostral to the epiglottis.
4. The laryngoscope should be used to depress the tongue and visualize the larynx (Figure 5.18). It should not be used directly on the epiglottis as it is a delicate structure.
5. As cats are prone to laryngospasm, the larynx should be sprayed with lidocaine at this stage. Wait 30–60 seconds for the spray to desensitize the larynx, and then continue. Oxygen should be administered by facemask or flow-by during this period. Note that the formulation of some dental lidocaine sprays (e.g. Xylocaine®) can cause laryngeal oedema. Moreover, many formulations contain 10 mg lidocaine per spray which is potentially toxic for a small cat. An alternative is to use 1 mg/kg of 2% lidocaine for injection (i.e. approximately 0.2 ml for a 4 kg cat). This can be drawn into an insulin syringe and dropped on to the larynx.

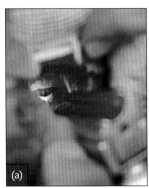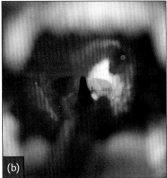

5.18 (a) View of cat larynx. (b) View of dog larynx.
(Courtesy of Asher Allison, Animal Health Trust, Newmarket, UK)

6. The endotracheal tube should be advanced over the epiglottis, keeping to the ventral aspect and depressing the epiglottis. It should then pass through the arytenoid cartilages and vocal folds, into the trachea.
7. In cats, if the larynx is closed when first visualized, wait for inhalation to occur before inserting the tube.
8. Always confirm correct positioning of the tube in the trachea following intubation, using one or two of the following methods:
    *   A capnograph, which will detect exhaled carbon dioxide
    *   A small piece of cotton wool or tissue paper held over the end of the endotracheal tube – this will move when the patient exhales
    *   Visualization of simultaneous movement of the animal's thorax and the reservoir bag on the breathing system
    *   Direct visualization of the tube in the larynx using a laryngoscope
    *   Detection of water vapour on a mirror, the base of the laryngoscope handle or within a clear endotracheal tube
    *   Palpation of the neck to ensure the presence of only one rigid structure.

Following insertion of the endotracheal tube:

1. Secure the tube in place by tying it with a bandage (e.g. white open-weave) to the top or bottom jaw, or behind the ears. The bandage needs to be tied tightly, but must not occlude the lumen of the tube. Ideally, the knot should be around the connector and not the tube.
2. Position the endotracheal tube connector external to the incisors. This ensures that the handler is not bitten when disconnecting or reconnecting the tube.
3. Turn on the oxygen flow.
4. Connect the endotracheal tube to the breathing system, using a 'push and twist' action to prevent accidental disconnection.
5. Inflate the cuff and check for gas leakage. Avoid excessive pressure in the cuff (maximum 25 mmHg or 34 cmH$_2$O) as this will occlude the blood supply to the tracheal mucosa; the use of a manometer is recommended to check the pressure (Briganti et al., 2012). To check for leaks, the following method may be used (note this does not guarantee that appropriate pressure has been applied):
    *   Fill the breathing system with oxygen and briefly close the pressure-relief valve
    *   Inflate the cuff while squeezing the breathing bag and listening for gas leaks from the mouth – this requires an assistant
    *   Stop inflating the cuff immediately when no more leaks are heard
    *   Quickly open the pressure-relief valve on the breathing system
    *   Check the cuff inflation pressure from time to time during the anaesthetic. Most commonly it will deflate. However, nitrous oxide may diffuse into the cuff and cause it to expand.
6. Always disconnect and reconnect the breathing system from the endotracheal tube when turning the patient. This is especially important in cats, which may develop tracheal rupture if the endotracheal tube is twisted within the trachea.

The advantages and complications of using endotracheal tubes, in comparison with facemasks, are shown in Figure 5.19.

Advantages of endotracheal tubes when compared with facemasks
Endotracheal tubes (with an inflated cuff):
• Provide a method of inflating the lungs; facemasks result in inflation of the stomach with gas
• Prevent aspiration of foreign material (saliva, stomach contents, blood, dental debris, etc.) into the lungs
• Result in better maintenance of gas volumes in the breathing system than facemasks. This is particularly important when using a ventilator
• Result in less atmospheric pollution than facemasks
• May be secured with ties; facemasks are difficult to secure

Possible complications of endotracheal intubation
Endotracheal tubes may:
• Be inserted into the oesophagus
• Be inserted into one main bronchus
• Kink or become obstructed
• Become disconnected
• Be bitten by the patient and inhaled
• Damage the trachea or larynx or initiate laryngeal spasm
• Cause tracheal rupture if not disconnected when turning the patient
The cuff may:
• Herniate over the bevel and cause an obstruction
• Deflate during anaesthesia
• Increase in size when nitrous oxide is used
• Cause tracheal necrosis or rupture if over-inflated

5.19 Advantages and possible complications of cuffed endotracheal tubes, compared with facemasks.

Supraglottic airway devices

Laryngeal mask airways (LMAs; Figure 5.20a) and other SGADs were developed in human medicine to overcome the high incidence of haemodynamic changes and laryngeal spasm caused by intubation of the trachea. Their use coincided with the introduction of propofol, a drug that results in reduced laryngeal sensitivity compared to thiopental. Although SGADs have achieved great popularity for relatively short, uncomplicated procedures, the endotracheal tube remains the 'gold standard' for assured protection of the airway. While the use of SGADs has been reported in dogs, cats and rabbits, their benefits in veterinary practice remain unknown. In particular, endotracheal intubation is considerably less difficult in dogs than in humans. The SGAD must not be used in unfasted animals or in patients with a high risk of vomiting or regurgitation.

In 2012, veterinary-specific SGADs were launched for the cat (Cat v-gel®; Figure 5.20bc) and rabbit (Rabbit v-gel®). Initial reports are very encouraging, particularly in rabbit anaesthesia and for short uncomplicated procedures in cats (Crotaz, 2010; Crotaz, 2012; van Oostrom *et al.*, 2013). Advantages of SGADs include:

- Ease and speed of insertion
- No increase in airway resistance
- Lack of irritation and trauma to the larynx and trachea, and simplicity of removal
- Variety of sizes available
- Can be autoclaved and re-used.

Potential disadvantages include:

- Requirement for capnography to ensure correct positioning at all times
- Rotation or displacement of the device if the patient is moved/turned
- Difficulty in ensuring a gas-tight seal if providing IPPV
- Lack of full protection against aspiration in at-risk patients (e.g. dental procedures)
- Lack of access to the mouth for surgery.

Insertion of a SGAD is as follows:

1. Choose an appropriate size (see Wiederstein *et al.*, 2008 for published guidelines on LMAs in dogs and Cat v-gel® manufacturer's information for cats).
2. The device should be lubricated before use and the cuff/balloon deflated.
3. A capnograph should be attached to the device before insertion.
4. The mouth should be checked for debris.
5. Lidocaine may be sprayed on the larynx, although this is not always required.
6. With the head extended and the tongue pulled out, the device is inserted blindly into the mouth, keeping to the centre of the mouth and parallel to the hard palate.
7. The device is advanced towards the larynx until resistance is felt; once clear breath sounds can be heard at the proximal end and exhaled carbon dioxide is detected, the cuff (on an LMA) or balloon (on a Cat v-gel®) should be inflated and the tube secured in place. Further information, including videos demonstrating insertion of the v-gel®, are provided on the manufacturer's website (www.docsinnovent.com).

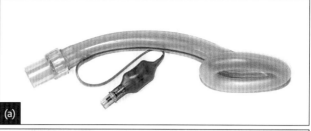

(a)

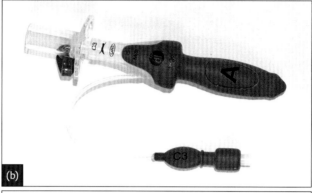

(b)

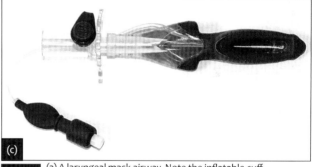

(c)

5.20 (a) A laryngeal mask airway. Note the inflatable cuff surrounding the mask's inner rim. (b) Cat v-gel® supraglottic airway device (dorsal view). Note the inflatable dorsal pressure adjuster (balloon) (A) to increase the sealing pressure if required. (c) Cat v-gel® (ventral view).
(Courtesy of Asher Allison, Animal Health Trust, Newmarket, UK)

Facemasks

Veterinary facemasks are available in a wide range of shapes and sizes to correspond with the diversity in the contours of cats and dogs faces (Figure 5.21). When used for provision of anaesthesia they should cover the nose and mouth, resulting in an airtight seal; care must be taken to avoid trauma to the eyes. The following points are relevant:

- Masks are valuable for preoxygenation and provision of supplemental oxygen to sick patients
- They may be used for induction of anaesthesia using inhaled anaesthetics, although if the seal is inadequate they result in atmospheric pollution
- Masks manufactured from transparent materials are preferable, so that the patient's tongue and mucous membranes, plus any secretions from the patient's nose and mouth, can be visualized
- Masks with a detachable rubber diaphragm provide a good seal around the face but may be poorly tolerated by conscious patients
- Ensure that gases can be vented from the system if the facemask provides a tight seal around the face i.e. use tight-fitting facemasks in conjunction with a breathing system

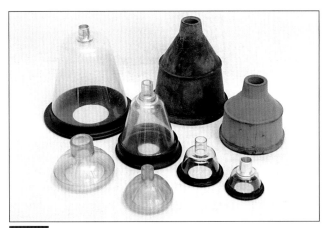

5.21 A selection of facemasks.

- Care should be taken not to exert excessive pressure when applying a mask, as a reduction in venous return from the face will cause oedema of the muzzle. Damage to the eyes may result from the facemask edges pressing against the eyes, or the gas flow may dry the cornea. Ensure adequate lubrication of the eyes
- Dead space should be minimized by using a mask with an appropriate shape, e.g. avoid the use of a conical mask in cats
- Masks are usually well tolerated. However, if previously used, they should be washed well and flushed with oxygen, as they may smell of anaesthetic agent and the patient may resist their application
- Masks do not protect the airway from aspiration of foreign material
- If used for longer than a few minutes, consider using straps to hold the mask in place. Prolonged use of a facemask may result in hyperthermia
- The sampling line from a sidestream carbon dioxide analyser can be used by placing the distal end within the facemask by the nares.

A very low dead space mask (Darvall ZDS; Figure 5.22) has been developed for birds, small mammals and exotics, which delivers inlet gas directly to the patient; this results in more rapid changes in anaesthetic depth. Scavenging of waste anaesthetic gases is also facilitated. This type of mask may be of use for small puppies and kittens which are difficult to intubate.

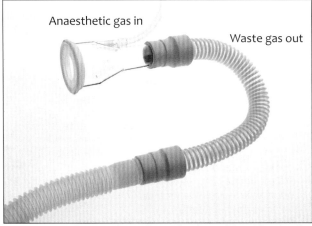

Anaesthetic gas in

Waste gas out

5.22 Darvall ZDS mask. Gas flow within the mask is unidirectional: this results in zero dead space and consequently the animal's nose does not have to fill the mask.
(Courtesy of Colin Dunlop, Advanced Anaesthesia Specialists, Australia)

Laryngoscopes

The main functions of a laryngoscope are to retract the tissues of the pharynx and tongue, providing a clear view of the larynx and thereby facilitating intubation (see section on endotracheal tubes for technique of use). The blade should not be used to depress the epiglottis. A comparison of the different aids available for endotracheal intubation in small animals is shown in Figure 5.23. Laryngoscope blades should always be cleaned and disinfected according to the manufacturers' instructions after each use. Features of laryngoscopes include:

- Detachable blades that are made in several lengths; the most readily available are sizes 00, 0, 1, 2, and 3
- There is a huge array of blade patterns available for anaesthesia in humans. However, only three are commonly used in veterinary patients: the Miller or Wisconsin (straight) and the Macintosh (curved) (Figure 5.24). Personal preference dictates which one is chosen
- The light source may be a tungsten bulb in the blade, or more commonly a fibreoptic bundle from a bulb in the handle. The intensity of fibreoptic light is superior, although the bundle may degrade over time

Laryngoscope (or bright light and tongue depressor)	Endoscope	Bright light and no aids
May be used to depress the tongue	No tongue depression	No tongue depression
Laryngoscope provides better visualization of the larynx and related structures	The light provides excellent visualization of the larynx and related structures	Poor visualization of the larynx
Laryngoscope is useful for demonstrating normal anatomy	Most useful if the larynx is not visible (e.g. pathology of temporomandibular joint)	Should be used only by experienced personnel
Very useful in brachycephalic breeds, Chow Chow and English Bull Terrier		Most reliable in dolichocephalic dogs only
Essential to use as an aid when the patient is suffering from laryngeal pathology (e.g. paralysis, collapse, neoplasia)		No visualization of laryngeal pathology
Handling of the laryngoscope, tongue and endotracheal tube may require a period of training	Most useful if the endoscope will fit through the endotracheal tube, to allow passage of the tube over the endoscope	No additional equipment to handle
Laryngoscope blades designed for use in humans may be awkward for right-handed personnel	Requires expensive equipment	
A variety of sizes and shapes of laryngoscope blades are available, including those designed for veterinary use		

5.23 Comparison of aids for intubation in small animals.

- Blades may be plastic or metal. Metal blades are more expensive but also more robust
- The high ridge on the right-hand side of some blades will impede the view of a right-handed person passing an endotracheal tube into the trachea with their right hand. This problem arises because blades are designed for medical use where humans are intubated supine (in dorsal recumbency) and the ridge is then on the left. A laryngoscope for veterinary use is now available with the ridge on the left-hand side (Advanced Anesthesia Specialists, Australia; Figure 5.24b)
- Boxed sets that contain one handle and up to eight blades are available.

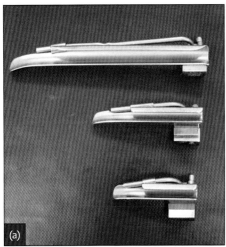

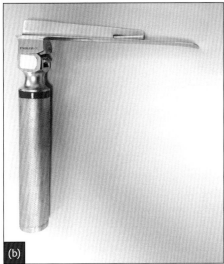

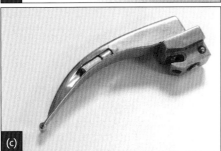

5.24 Types of laryngoscope blade. (a) Miller blades designed for human medical use. (b) A novel laryngoscope blade has been designed for veterinary use with the light source positioned to permit better visualization. (c) Macintosh blade.
(Courtesy of Asher Allison, Animal Health Trust, Newmarket, UK)

Induction chambers

Induction chambers are usually rectangular boxes, constructed of a clear plastic material (Figure 5.25), which allows visualization of the patient in the chamber. Chambers should:

- Have a hinged lid, which can be closed tightly to seal the chamber so it is leak proof
- Have a removable clear partition, allowing the use of a smaller compartment for smaller animals
- Ideally be large enough to allow the patient to lie in lateral recumbency without the neck flexed
- Have at least two ports – one for delivery of volatile anaesthetic agents and oxygen, and the other for scavenging of waste gases.

Induction chambers may also be used as an oxygen cage for very small patients and neonates, although they are most commonly used for gaseous induction of anaesthesia as follows:

1. Fill the chamber with 100% oxygen for 3–5 minutes before turning on the vaporizer.
2. Use a relatively high gas flow to increase the speed of induction of anaesthesia.
3. Watch the patient continuously and remove it from the chamber as soon as it becomes unconscious.
4. There is no need to close the exhaust valve.

The chamber may be used to induce anaesthesia in animals that are difficult to handle, e.g. wild animals or fractious or feral cats, or in tiny animals, where venous access is difficult or intramuscular mass is limited, e.g. small mammals, birds or other exotic pets. While practical in these types of patients, these boxes are not without their disadvantages:

- Pungent anaesthetic gases may cause the patient to struggle and breath-hold. This results in increased concentrations of catecholamines and carbon dioxide in the blood, with the associated risk of cardiac arrhythmias
- They constitute a considerable health and safety hazard, as they result in substantial atmospheric pollution when the lid is opened. A double-box system has been designed for work with laboratory animals, which evacuates all waste anaesthetic gases before the box is opened.

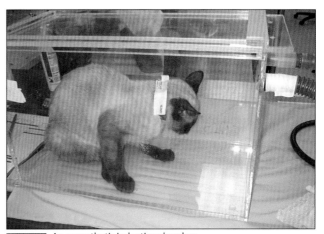

5.25 An anaesthetic induction chamber.
(Courtesy of Tanya Duke-Novakovski, Western College of Veterinary Medicine, University of Saskatchewan, Canada)

Waste anaesthetic gas scavenging systems

Waste anaesthetic gases pose a threat to human health if not removed by an effective scavenging system (see Chapter 15). In addition, legislation in most countries limits exposure to waste gases (see Chapter 1). For these reasons it is essential to install a scavenging system in all veterinary practices.

Waste anaesthetic gases leave most breathing systems via the pressure-relief valve; there is a standard scavenging shroud attached to the valve (30 mm male connector in the UK). This should be connected to 22 mm tubing, which carries the waste gas away from the patient. By convention, the scavenging tubing should be a different colour from that of the breathing system, i.e. blue, green, pink or red (Figure 5.26). Scavenging from the open-ended bag of the Jackson Rees modified T-piece is potentially hazardous (as discussed earlier in this chapter).

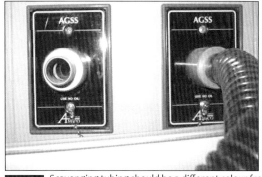

5.26 Scavenging tubing should be a different colour from the breathing tubing.
(Courtesy of Tanya Duke-Novakovski, Western College of Veterinary Medicine, University of Saskatchewan, Canada)

Types of scavenging systems

Active scavenging system

This is the most effective type of scavenging system and it is probable that it will be required by law in many countries in the near future. The components include (Figure 5.27):

- An extractor fan or pump, which generates negative pressure; this is often capable of scavenging gas from several anaesthetic machines at once. It is usually situated above a false ceiling, where the noise nuisance is reduced. It has an outlet to the exterior (i.e. through a wall) and care should be taken in situating this outlet so that it does not in itself pose a health hazard
- A length of non-collapsible tubing connecting the extractor fan to an air break
- An air break receiver (Figure 5.28), which:
  - Is interposed between the extractor fan and the pressure-relief valve
  - Has a visible flow indicator (float), which is activated at flows >80 l/min
  - Prevents transmission of sub-atmospheric (negative) pressure from the extractor fan to the patient by allowing entrainment of air
  - Prevents build up of pressure if the evacuation system fails
  - Has a filter to prevent foreign material blocking the tubing or damaging the fan.
- Coloured, flexible 22 mm tubing leading from the air break to the shroud over the pressure-relief valve on the breathing system.

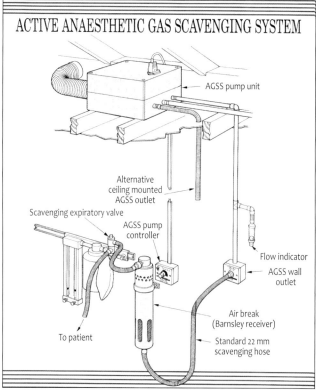

5.27 Components of an active anaesthetic gas scavenging system (AGSS).
(Courtesy of Coltronics Systems)

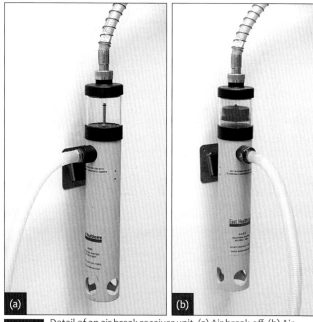

5.28 Detail of an air break receiver unit. (a) Air break off. (b) Air break on.

Active–passive scavenging system

In this system, 22 mm tubing carries waste gas from the expiratory valve on the breathing system to the grille of a ventilation system. The ventilation system must be capable of extracting gas from the room, and must be switched on. Extracted gases must not be recirculated within the building, and care must be taken with the position of the outlet for extracted gases, as in the active system.

Passive scavenging system with absorber

In this system, the scavenging tubing is connected to an activated charcoal container, e.g. Anaesorber (Figure 5.29). The container must be situated below the pressure-relief valve and should not be positioned near a source of heat as vapours may be liberated. The charcoal absorbs volatile agents only (isoflurane, sevoflurane, desflurane) and does *not* absorb nitrous oxide. There is no 'full' indicator, so the container must be weighed daily to ensure it has not exceeded the maximum weight indicated on the canister (usually 1400 g). This requires an accurate weighing scale (±10 g). Correct disposal of the container is essential.

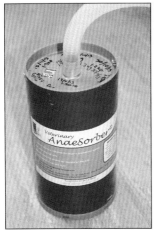

5.29 A veterinary 'Anaesorber' activated charcoal canister with scavenging tubing attached.
(Courtesy of Asher Allison, Animal Health Trust, Newmarket, UK)

Passive scavenging system

In this system the scavenging tubing takes the waste gas to an outlet in a wall or leads out through a window. Such a system has many drawbacks. The total length of the tubing should not be more than 2 m and there should be no constrictions or bends in it, both of which may increase the resistance to expiration. The wall outlet or window opening must be lower than the expiratory valve. The outlet is subject to prevailing wind conditions, and excess negative pressure may be generated or waste gas may be blown back into the building. Care must be taken with the position of the outlet, as in the active system.

Minimizing exposure to waste anaesthetic gases

In addition to installing and using a scavenging system, there are many anaesthetic practices, which, if used *daily*, help to reduce the exposure of personnel to waste anaesthetic gases:

- Leak test all anaesthetic equipment
- Intubate all patients with a cuffed endotracheal tube and inflate the cuff where appropriate
- Avoid the use of facemasks and induction boxes where possible
- Connect the breathing system to the patient and leak test the endotracheal tube before turning on vaporizers
- Use low-flow anaesthesia where appropriate
- Flush the breathing system with oxygen for several minutes before disconnection of the patient
- Cap the breathing system after use (this is more applicable in large animal circle systems)
- Ventilate the recovery area with a minimum of 15–20 air changes per hour, using a system that does not recirculate air

- Fill vaporizers at the end of the day in a well-ventilated area, using a keyed (agent-specific) filler (see Chapter 4)
- Vary the rostering of personnel who fill the vaporizers (Note that pregnant women should not fill vaporizers)
- Carry out regular maintenance of anaesthetic equipment
- Monitor waste anaesthetic gases in the premises every 6 months.

Humidifiers

Humidification of inspired gases is desirable, especially when dry gases are administered at high flows for prolonged periods, and particularly if they bypass the turbinate system in the nares. Without humidification of gases, respiratory secretions become thicker, mucociliary function is reduced and atelectasis may occur. In addition, losses through evaporation are increased, leading to hypothermia.

Two types of humidifiers may be used in veterinary practice:

- *Heat and moisture exchangers and filters* (Figure 5.30) are placed between the endotracheal tube and the breathing system. Their function is to conserve the heat of the exhaled breath and use it to warm the inhaled gases. Porous hygroscopic material absorbs heat from the exhaled gas, allowing water to condense out and be stored in, or adjacent to, the porous material. When the patient inhales, the heat is returned to the inhaled gas and the condensate evaporates. They are most useful when high fresh gas flows are used in systems without carbon dioxide absorption. They are designed for medical use in adult or paediatric patients; they increase dead space and resistance to breathing and should therefore be used with caution in small patients. It is important to follow the manufacturer's directions with regard to patient size. They should be observed frequently for signs of plugging with secretions and must be discarded after use
- *Bubble-through humidifiers* (Figure 5.31) are used in conjunction with supplemental oxygen delivery systems, often in the intensive care setting. A stream of oxygen is passed through a bottle containing sterile water, before reaching the patient. Those in common use do not heat the gas, and most will produce large water droplets, which tend to condense in the delivery system. For maximum efficiency, low gas flows should be used and the gas should be driven below the surface of the water to increase the area available for evaporation.

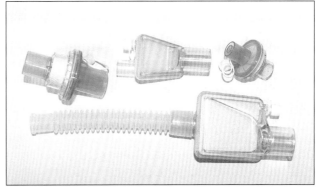

5.30 Heat and moisture exchangers (HMEs) and heat and moisture exchanging filters (HMEFs).
(Courtesy of Asher Allison, Animal Health Trust, Newmarket, UK)

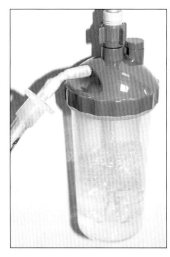

5.31 A bubble-through humidifier, which brings dry oxygen gas to ambient levels of humidity. Dry gas from the flowmeter is directed into the water bottle, where it is broken up into small bubbles, which gain humidity as they rise to the surface of the water.

Valves for applying positive end-expiratory pressure

Positive end-expiratory pressure (PEEP) is sometimes applied to mechanically ventilated patients (see Chapter 6). It helps to prevent alveolar collapse (atelectasis) when lung volume is low (e.g. during thoracotomy) and in patients with pulmonary oedema or loss of surfactant, and so can improve oxygen exchange. Disposable PEEP valves (Figure 5.32a) are available, which are inserted either in the expiratory limb of the breathing system or between the ventilator valve and scavenging tubing (Figure 5.32b). The

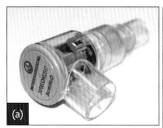
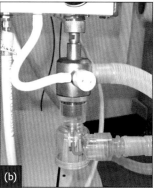

5.32 (a) An Intersurgical® PEEP valve. (b) PEEP valve positioned between a ventilator valve and the scavenging tubing.
(Courtesy of Asher Allison, Animal Health Trust, Newmarket, UK)

Intersurgical® range includes seven colour-coded, fixed-value PEEP valves ranging from 2.5 to 20 cmH$_2$O. The level of PEEP is normally adjusted incrementally, with close monitoring of haemoglobin oxygen saturation, capnography, arterial blood gases and arterial blood pressure.

References and further reading

Al-Shaikh B and Stacey S (2001) *Essentials of Anaesthetic Equipment, 2nd edn.* Churchill Livingstone, New York

Bateman L, Ludders JW, Gleed RD *et al.* (2005) Comparison between facemask and laryngeal mask airway in rabbits during isoflurane anesthesia. *Veterinary Anaesthesia and Analgesia* **32**, 280–288

Briganti A, Portela DA, Barsotti G, Romano M and Breghi G (2012) Evaluation of the endotracheal tube cuff pressure resulting from four different methods of inflation in dogs. *Veterinary Anaesthesia and Analgesia* **39**, 488–494

Crotaz IR (2010) Initial feasibility investigation of the v-gel airway: an anatomically designed supraglottic airway device for use in companion animal veterinary anaesthesia. *Veterinary Anaesthesia and Analgesia* **37**, 579–580

Crotaz IR (2013) An observational clinical study in cats and rabbits of an anatomically designed supraglottic airway device for use in companion animal veterinary anaesthesia. *Veterinary Record* **172**, 606. doi: 10.1136/vr.100668.

Davey AJ and Diba A (2005) *Ward's Anaesthetic Equipment, 5th edn.* Elsevier Saunders, Philadelphia

Dorsch JA and Dorsch SE (2008) *Understanding Anesthesia Equipment, 5th edn.* Lippincott Williams and Wilkins, Philadelphia

Gale E, Ticehurst KE and Zaki S (2015) An evaluation of fresh gas flow rates for spontaneously breathing cats and small dogs on the Humphrey ADE semi-closed breathing system. *Veterinary Anaesthesia and Analgesia* **42**, 292–298

Humphrey D (1983) A new anaesthetic breathing system combining Mapleson A, D and E principles. *Anaesthesia* **38**, 361–372

Lish J, Ko JCH, Payton ME (2008) Two Methods of Endotracheal

Tube Selection in Dogs. *Journal of American Animal Hospital Association* **44**, 236–242

Mitchell SL, McCarthy R, Rudloff E *et al.* (2000) Tracheal rupture associated with intubation in cats: 20 cases (1996–1998). *Journal of the American Veterinary Medical Association* **216**, 1592–1595

Pelligand L, Hammond R and Rycroft A (2007) An investigation of the contamination of small animal breathing systems during routine use. *Veterinary Anaesthesia and Analgesia* **34**, 190–199

van Oostrom H, Krauss MW and Sap R (2013) A comparison between the v-gel supraglottic airway device and the cuffed endotracheal tube for airway management in spontaneously breathing cats during isoflurane anaesthesia. *Veterinary Anaesthesia and Analgesia* **40**, 265–271

Walsh CM and Taylor PM (2004) A clinical evaluation of the 'mini parallel Lack' breathing system in cats and comparison with a modified Ayre's T-piece. *Veterinary Anaesthesia and Analgesia* **31**, 207–212

Wiederstein I and Moen YPS (2008) Guidelines and criteria for the placement of laryngeal mask airways in dogs. *Veterinary Anaesthesia and Analgesia* **35**, 374–382

Wilkes AR (2011) Heat and moisture exchangers and breathing system filters: their use in anaesthesia and intensive care. Part 1 – history, principles and efficiency. *Anaesthesia* **66**, 31–39

Wilkes AR (2011) Heat and moisture exchangers and breathing system filters: their use in anaesthesia and intensive care. Part 2 – practical use, including problems, and their use with paediatric patients. *Anaesthesia* **66**, 40–51

Chapter 6

Automatic ventilators

Richard Hammond and Pamela J. Murison

The role of automatic ventilators

Automatic (mechanical) ventilators enable the provision of intermittent positive pressure ventilation (IPPV) to support ventilation in anaesthetized or heavily sedated patients. An automatic ventilator is an invaluable tool that provides repeated, controlled breaths, so allowing the anaesthetist to attend to other aspects of patient monitoring and support.

In the operating theatre, ventilation is usually performed in anaesthetized patients for limited periods and predominantly in those with normal lung physiology. The ventilators suitable for this situation are therefore relatively basic in design, simple to use and can be sourced easily and relatively inexpensively for general practice use. This chapter describes key aspects of respiratory physiology and ventilator design, and provides practical guidelines for IPPV in cats and dogs.

Indications for IPPV

Intermittent positive pressure ventilation may be used to support any patient with compromised respiratory function. However, there is a marked difference between the role of the ventilator in the intensive care unit (ICU) for support of a patient with pulmonary or central nervous system (CNS) pathology, and its role in the anaesthetized patient.

Among critically ill patients, those requiring IPPV with a specialized ICU ventilator are likely to be those with decreased pulmonary oxygen uptake and subsequent reduced tissue oxygen delivery. In severe or multifactorial disease, these patients may demonstrate concurrent failure of carbon dioxide elimination and consequent hypercapnia (arterial carbon dioxide tension (P_aCO_2) >45 mmHg (6 kPa)) with hypoxaemia (arterial oxygen tension (P_aO_2) ≤60 mmHg (8 kPa)), and require immediate intervention. Patients that are hypoxaemic but have normal or low P_aCO_2 values, as a result of compensatory hyperventilation, may need only oxygen therapy; IPPV is used as a last resort when oxygen supplementation fails to correct the hypoxaemia. An ICU ventilator incorporates computer-based technology that enables provision of many different ventilation modes. Other types of ventilatory support aim to alter specific aspects of the ventilatory process; for example, positive end-expiratory pressure (PEEP) can be applied to correct hypoxaemia, and pressure support ventilation (PSV) can be applied to decrease the work of spontaneous breathing. Further information on ventilation of the critical patient using an ICU ventilator can be found in appropriate texts (e.g. Cairo, 2012).

In contrast, in anaesthetized patients with normal lung physiology and a high inspired oxygen fraction (F_iO_2), respiratory failure is usually due to mild to moderate hypoventilation, which will usually result in hypercapnia without hypoxaemia. Intermittent positive pressure ventilation during anaesthesia is therefore only required to correct hypoventilation (for causes see Figure 6.1) and return P_aCO_2 to within the normal range. Minute volume (respiratory rate × tidal volume) defines the total volume of gas exhaled per minute, which in turn determines the amount of carbon dioxide eliminated from the lungs (assuming inspired gases contain no carbon dioxide and cardiac output remains constant). In these circumstances, automatic ventilation should aim to provide an appropriate minute volume, while minimizing the unwanted effects of IPPV on the animal (see below).

Inability to ventilate
• Open thorax – thoracotomy, thoracoscopy and chest wall trauma
• Neuromuscular blockade
• Phrenic nerve paralysis
• Pneumothorax
• Myasthenia gravis
• Decreased lung or chest wall compliance

Decreased ventilatory drive
• Anaesthetic agents (injectable and volatile)
• Increased intracranial pressure
• Other central nervous system disease – e.g. infarct, encephalopathy
• Hypothermia
• Severe hypoxaemia

6.1 Causes of hypoventilation and indications for intermittent positive pressure ventilation in anaesthetized and high-dependency cases.

When to initiate IPPV

Absolute indications for IPPV during anaesthesia include all causes of alveolar hypoventilation (see Figure 6.1). Relative indications, and the level of hypercapnia at which to initiate IPPV, are controversial. The normal range for P_aCO_2 is considered to be 35–45 mmHg (4.7–6.0 kPa), and some veterinary practitioners would recommend initiation of

IPPV at values above that range in anaesthetized healthy patients. Most anaesthetic agents are non-selective CNS depressants and therefore most anaesthetized patients hypoventilate. Although usually well tolerated in the healthy patient, even mild hypercapnia during anaesthesia can result in acidaemia, hyperkalaemia and reduced myocardial contractility. Hypercapnia and acidaemia contribute to the development of ventricular tachyarrhythmias during anaesthesia with volatile agents. Extreme hypercapnia can also increase vagal tone, inducing a bradycardia which may lead to sinus arrest. This pronounced hypercapnia also produces CNS depression and narcosis, although these are unlikely to occur at P_aCO_2 <95 mmHg (12.7 kPa).

The need for IPPV should therefore be based on a multisystem evaluation, and not simply on the degree of hypercapnia.

Mechanical ventilation definitions and terminology

For an explanation of terminology associated with automatic ventilation, see Figure 6.2.

Term	Definition
Intermittent positive pressure ventilation (IPPV) (= controlled mandatory ventilation, CMV)	Airway pressure is maintained above atmospheric pressure during inspiration and then falls to atmospheric pressure, allowing passive expiration
Positive end-expiratory pressure (PEEP)	Positive (i.e. above atmospheric) pressure is maintained between inspirations delivered by a ventilator. Airway pressure does not return to zero at the end of expiration
Continuous positive airway pressure (CPAP)	Airway pressure is maintained above atmospheric pressure during *spontaneous ventilation*
Intermittent mandatory ventilation (IMV)	This method of ventilation is used for ventilatory support and for weaning patients from ventilators. The patient is allowed to breathe spontaneously, but mechanical breaths are inserted at a preset tidal volume and frequency
Anatomical dead space	The volume of the respiratory tract where no gas exchange occurs, extending from the external nares to the bronchioles
Apparatus dead space	An extension of the anatomical dead space associated with apparatus, e.g. masks or endotracheal tubes extending beyond the nares of the animal
Alveolar dead space	Represented by the volume of the alveoli not taking part in effective gas exchange, i.e. those alveoli that are ventilated but not perfused
Physiological dead space	The sum of alveolar dead space and anatomical dead space
Compliance	A measure of the distensibility of the lungs and of the restriction to expansion imposed by the surrounding structures. Compliance is also defined as the ratio of change in volume for a given change in pressure
Resistance	The pressure difference per unit flow across the airway – not a constant but increases as flow increases

6.2 Definitions of terms associated with mechanical ventilation.

Physiological effects of IPPV

Respiratory effects

During spontaneous ventilation, gases are drawn into the lung during inspiration by a decreasing interpleural pressure. Passive expiration sees a return of the interpleural pressure to baseline, towards atmospheric pressure (Figure 6.3).

In contrast, during IPPV, inspiration occurs by an increase in interpleural pressure, which returns to atmospheric pressure at the end of expiration. The distribution of alveolar ventilation (V_A) and blood perfusion (Q) in the lung depends upon the pressure and volume changes, and is therefore different during spontaneous ventilation compared with IPPV. In a recumbent anaesthetized animal, dependent parts of the lung are less compliant owing to the increased tissue mass surrounding them. Intermittent positive pressure ventilation will preferentially ventilate the more compliant non-dependent lung zones, exacerbating the V_A/Q mismatch already present. In addition, if inflation pressures exceed 30 cmH$_2$O, capillaries in non-dependent lung areas may be compressed, reducing capillary blood flow (and increasing alveolar dead space) and further exacerbating the V_A/Q mismatch.

The main ventilatory determinants of P_aO_2 are F_iO_2, minute volume and mean airway pressure. Mean airway pressure is determined by the duration of inspiration, the inspiratory:expiratory time (I:E) ratio, peak airway pressure and the amount of PEEP, if used. Removal of carbon dioxide is primarily determined by minute volume. High

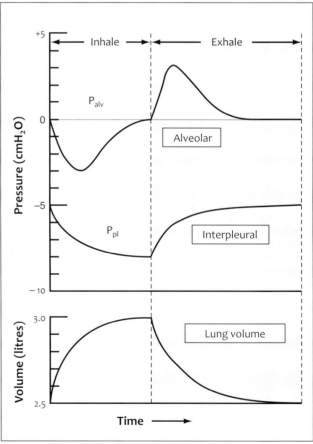

6.3 Thoracic pressures and volumes during spontaneous ventilation. Note that interpleural pressure remains negative during the entire respiratory cycle – a key component of the 'thoracic pump' and the maintenance of cardiac preload.

ventilatory rates with a low tidal volume or low ventilatory rates with a high tidal volume may result in similar minute volumes and consequently similar P_aCO_2.

The ventilator settings should be adjusted so that the ventilatory pattern is as physiological as possible for the individual patient:

- For time- or volume-cycled ventilators, this is achieved by setting the calculated tidal volume first, then observing the chest wall excursion to check that it looks normal for that animal. If possible, the peak airway pressure should be checked to make sure that it does not exceed 20 cmH₂O (12–15 cmH₂O is normally adequate in a healthy animal). The ventilatory rate is then set and adjusted to achieve normocapnia (assessed using either capnometry or blood gas analysis; see Chapter 7). If measurement of carbon dioxide is not available, the rate should be set to just below the normal estimated respiratory rate for that animal; generally IPPV is more effective than spontaneous ventilation and normal ventilatory rates will result in hypocapnia and respiratory alkalosis. Severe hypocapnia (P_aCO_2 <26 mmHg (3.5 kPa)) may result in cerebral vasoconstriction and cerebral hypoxia
- With a pressure-cycled ventilator, the cycling pressure is set and adjusted on the basis of observations of chest wall excursion, as described above. The respiratory rate is then set to achieve normocapnia.

The expiratory phase must be long enough to allow adequate time for exhalation. Too short an expiratory time leads to gas trapping and potential overinflation of the lungs; this is more likely in patients with increased small airway resistance (e.g. feline asthma) or high compliance (e.g. neonates). This is because high minute volume, high lung compliance and high expiratory resistance (from the airway or breathing system) all reduce expiratory time and flow, resulting in auto-PEEP and gas trapping.

Cardiovascular effects

Venous return and adequate preload rely on the maintenance of a pressure gradient between the venous reservoirs and the right atrium of the heart. During IPPV, the elevated intrathoracic pressure is transmitted through the right atrial wall, thus reducing this gradient and consequently reducing venous return. In extreme cases this can mimic cardiac tamponade. Even in less extreme cases, a reduction in ventricular filling (and therefore stroke volume) can alter the amplitude of both pulse oximeter and invasive arterial blood pressure monitoring waveforms, such that a reduced amplitude may be seen during inspiration (Figure 6.4). The reduction in venous return is worsened by long inspiratory times, high mean airway pressures and PEEP. The reduction in right-sided preload reduces right-sided cardiac output, which, in turn, reduces left-sided preload, stroke volume and mean arterial blood pressure. This is more serious in animals with hypovolaemia or with cardiac conditions that are critically dependent on adequate preload (e.g. hypertrophic cardiomyopathy in cats; pericardial effusion). In such cases, evaluation of right-sided preload is invaluable: traditionally, this has been performed by monitoring central venous pressure (see Chapter 7). More recently, however, assessments of a patient's volume status using dynamic indices such as pulse pressure variation (as shown in Figure 6.4) and plethysmographic waveform variation during mechanical ventilation have been used. More information on this developing area is available in recent reviews (Desebbe and Cannesson, 2008; Eyre and Breen, 2010).

Renal and hepatic effects

A reduction in cardiac output results in a baroreceptor-mediated increase in sympathetic tone and release of antidiuretic hormone (arginine vasopressin). Reduced renal perfusion and increased sympathetic drive also stimulate the renin–angiotensin–aldosterone system, resulting in increased renal reabsorption of sodium and water. In addition, reduced preload and atrial stretch also suppress the release of atrial natriuretic peptide, which again increases reabsorption of sodium and water (Pannu and Mehta, 2004).

Reduced mean arterial blood pressure results in a reduced hepatic arterial blood flow. Reduced portal blood flow also results from raised intrathoracic pressure and hepatic venous congestion.

Clinically this means that patients with renal or hepatic dysfunction may be further compromised by IPPV, although this is probably unlikely with the short periods of IPPV used during anaesthesia, especially when haemodynamic function is optimized.

Effects on intracranial pressure and use in traumatic brain injury

Controlled hyperventilation is often used to reduce P_aCO_2 and thereby reduce elevated intracranial pressure (ICP), for example, after a traumatic brain injury (see also Chapter 28). There is an inverse relationship between vascular tone and P_aCO_2, such that hyperventilation results in vasoconstriction of the pial arteries and reduced cerebral blood volume, hence reducing ICP. In humans, however, even short-duration hyperventilation (especially in the first 24 hours after head trauma) may compromise cerebral oxygenation, particularly in areas of the brain that are hypoperfused due to excessive vasoconstriction, leading to reduced oxygen delivery to the tissues (see Chapter 28). Hyperventilation is therefore applied only where there is clear clinical evidence of raised ICP.

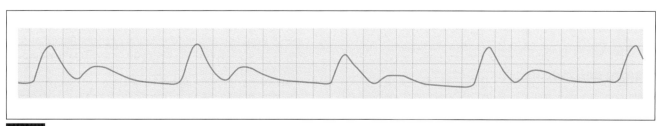

6.4 Invasive arterial blood pressure trace showing the variation in pulse pressure during the respiratory cycle.

Although published data remain equivocal, the following recommendations have been made for the use of IPPV to reduce ICP in veterinary patients with head trauma (Sande and West, 2010):

- If capnometry or arterial blood gas analysis is not available, assessing P_aCO_2 only on the basis of clinical signs (respiratory rate and effort) is not reliable and should not form the basis of clinical decision making regarding whether to intervene with IPPV
- Excessive or prolonged hyperventilation should be avoided (hyperventilation should be applied for a period of minutes only), especially in the first 24 hours of managing the case
- Raised ICP resulting from space-occupying intracranial lesions (as opposed to head trauma) may require more prolonged management with ventilation, including hyperventilation (see Chapter 28).

In cases where raised ICP is a concern, it is important to consider the ventilator settings. A raised intrathoracic pressure during IPPV will reduce jugular venous drainage; the inspiratory phase should therefore be kept short and the maximal inspiratory pressure carefully controlled.

A summary of the potential advantages and disadvantages of IPPV is shown in Figure 6.5.

Advantages
- More accurate control of respiratory variables
- Constant P_aCO_2 contributes to stable plasma pH and potassium concentration
- Regular rhythm depresses ventilation, augments narcosis and improves operating conditions
- Constant tidal volume (in volume-controlled ventilators) allows compliance measurement
- Mechanical ventilator frees anaesthetist for other duties
- Special ventilatory modes may be imposed

Disadvantages
- May reduce venous return and mean arterial blood pressure
- Excessive pulmonary stretch may produce bradycardia
- Unnoticed disconnection/cuff deflation fatal during neuromuscular blockade
- Mechanical failure possible
- Lung trauma more likely if inappropriate variables are set
- Purchase and maintenance costs may be high
- Some mechanical ventilators may be unsuitable for all patient sizes
- Ventilators may become fomites and harbour transmissible respiratory pathogens

6.5 Advantages and potential disadvantages of intermittent positive pressure ventilation in small animal patients. P_aCO_2 = arterial carbon dioxide tension.

Classification of automatic ventilators

There are numerous systems for classifying ventilators. The following descriptions refer to elements that enable a better understanding of the safe and effective use of ventilators and pertain to machines in common use in small animal practice.

Control and cycling

Ventilators are described in terms of how gas is delivered to the patient; they are either *volume controlled* (constant flow delivered), or *pressure controlled* (constant pressure delivered). In addition, volume-controlled ventilators can

be classified as *time cycled*, *volume cycled* or *pressure cycled* according to how the transition (cycling) from the inspiratory phase to the expiratory phase occurs. Understanding the advantages and disadvantages of each cycling method is important for appropriate ventilator selection and set-up for an individual patient. Most ventilators in veterinary use are volume controlled and time cycled: in other words, the flow of gas delivered is constant, the tidal volume is targeted and the pressure delivered is variable and dependent upon lung compliance.

Volume-controlled ventilation with time cycling

The delivered *flow* remains constant during inspiration. Inspiration is terminated once a fixed inspiratory phase time has elapsed. The inspiratory pressure does not normally affect the duration of inspiration. The pressure of the gas being delivered to the patient is variable and increases over the period of inspiration to maintain a constant flow. The rate of increase of airway pressure depends on multiple factors, including the gas flow, airway resistance, compliance of the lungs and the chest wall, and even the density/viscosity of the gases delivered. The operator adjusts the inspiratory flow.

In time-cycled ventilators, the inspiratory phase time is fixed; increasing the inspiratory flow without decreasing the period of inspiration will increase the total delivered tidal volume. In ventilators where the tidal volume is fixed separately and causes cycling (volume cycling; see below), increasing the flow will shorten the inspiratory phase time as the preset tidal volume is reached more quickly. Increasing flows also result in an increased peak airway pressure.

Rarely, machines may allow for the setting of all three variables (inspiratory phase time, flow and tidal volume). In this type of ventilator, if the flow is high enough to deliver the tidal volume before the end of the set inspiratory phase, an inspiratory pause occurs during which there is no inspiratory flow.

Advantages of these ventilators include:

- They are generally simple to operate and set up. The operator sets the appropriate tidal volume for the animal either directly, or indirectly by setting the flow and inspiratory phase time
- The predetermined tidal volume is delivered regardless of changes in resistance and compliance that may occur during anaesthesia (e.g. animal is heavily draped, reducing compliance; mucus in the endotracheal tube reduces its internal diameter and therefore increases resistance). The ventilator compensates for such changes by increasing airway pressure during inspiration to maintain the fixed flow.

Disadvantages of these ventilators include:

- In animals weighing <5 kg, it may be difficult to set an appropriate tidal volume accurately. At the lower end of the control settings, even small changes in the flow may markedly change the delivered tidal volume and result in significant underinflation or overinflation and consequent volutrauma (damage caused to the lung by overinflation)
- If an inappropriately high tidal volume is delivered as a result of having either a long inspiratory phase time or a high flow, the rise in airway pressure may be harmful. Some volume-controlled ventilators have an additional adjustable safety relief valve to avoid high airway

pressures. However, most basic volume-controlled machines do not have a pressure-limiting adjustment, and rely on a high-pressure relief valve with an audible warning sound for prevention of airway trauma. These valves open at a pressure of between 65 and 80 cmH_2O. Even one or two attempted ventilations at these airway pressures may result in volutrauma in patients with highly compliant lungs (e.g. very young animals) because the lungs will be overinflated.

Volume-controlled ventilation with pressure cycling (pressure-limited)

The delivered *flow* remains constant over the period of inspiration. Inspiration is terminated once a targeted airway *pressure* is achieved. The peak inspiratory pressure therefore determines the duration of inspiration. The pressure of the gas being delivered is variable and changes relative to the compliance of the lungs. Inspiratory pressure therefore increases over the period of inspiration to maintain a constant flow. The rate of rise of airway pressure depends on multiple factors including gas flow, airway resistance, compliance of the lungs and chest wall, and even the density/viscosity of the gases delivered. The operator can adjust the inspiratory flow and the peak airway pressure (cycling pressure) but cannot set the tidal volume. High gas flows (especially those where the flow may be turbulent) will shorten the inspiratory phase time because they generate higher pressures and therefore reduce tidal volume.

Advantages of these ventilators include:

- Tidal volume does not have to be calculated. In animals with normal airways, setting the cycling pressure (initially to 10–15 cmH_2O) and adjusting inspiratory flow such that the inspiratory phase time appears to be 'normal' for that patient should provide the correct tidal volume
- The cycling pressure setting will be within the usable range of the ventilator controls and therefore can be set as accurately for a kitten as for a St Bernard. Limitations to animal size will be based on the ability to have a low enough flow. This is not normally a problem
- Volutrauma is less likely because the peak airway pressure is set, and therefore cycling will occur before the lungs are overinflated
- In patients with high airway resistance or low lung compliance due to disease, a higher airway cycling pressure may be needed and can be easily set
- If the effective tidal volume of a patient is reduced during a procedure (e.g. lung lobe removal, lung areas packed off for surgical access or ventilation of one lung), no ventilator adjustment is needed. The ventilator still cycles at the same airway pressure irrespective of changes in tidal volume. This avoids potential overinflation of the remaining functional lung space.

Disadvantages of these ventilators include:

- Tidal volume is unpredictable and may be incorrect where normal cycling pressures are set in animals with abnormal airways
- Changes in resistance or compliance during a procedure (see above) may reduce the delivered volume of gas. In most machines, there is no mechanism to warn of such an occurrence.

Pressure-controlled ventilation with time cycling

These machines are currently rare in veterinary anaesthesia. The delivered *pressure* remains constant over the period of inspiration, which is achieved by delivering a decelerating inspiratory flow as inspiration proceeds. Once the peak inspiratory pressure is reached, flow continues at a gradually reducing rate until the end of the inspiratory phase. Inspiration is terminated at a preset time. This is in contrast to a volume-controlled, pressure-limited machine where flow ceases irrespective of inspiratory phase time once the preset pressure is reached. With a pressure-controlled machine, flow continues once the preset pressure is reached and that pressure is maintained. If tidal volume is reduced it can be restored by increasing the inspiratory phase time rather than peak airway pressure.

Triggering

Triggering describes how the inspiratory phase is initiated.

Time triggering

The expiratory phase time is set by the user, either directly, or indirectly by adjusting either the I:E ratio or the respiratory rate. This method is usually employed during anaesthesia where management of hypoventilation is normally the primary objective and no allowance is made for spontaneous breathing.

Pressure triggering

The inspiratory effort of the patient triggers a positive-pressure breath by creating a decrease in baseline pressure. The ventilatory frequency is set by the animal's inspiratory effort, although in some machines an 'escape rate' may be set in case there is a period of apnoea. Pressure triggering is often used in the ICU in patients with respiratory muscle weakness, inadequate tidal volume and associated atelectasis. It is also used in those situations where the role of the ventilator is not only to correct hypoventilation, for example, during provision of PEEP.

Flow triggering

An advance on pressure triggering is flow triggering, whereby a constant flow is maintained in the breathing circuit. Changes in flow, in response to the animal's spontaneous ventilation attempts, initiate a breath, which reduces the work of breathing compared with pressure triggering.

Practical use of ventilators

Choosing a ventilator for anaesthetic use in small animal practice

The ideal properties of a ventilator suitable for anaesthetic use in small animals are summarized in Figure 6.6. Although no veterinary ventilator fulfils all such requirements, many encompass the key components (as indicated by italicized text in Figure 6.6). The following section describes some commonly available ventilators in use in veterinary practice, their classification, correct set-up and use, and potential hazards. It should be used in conjunction with manufacturers' guidelines where available. The descriptions are not exhaustive, but the principles will be transferable to other machines of similar operation.

General
• Compact, portable, robust and easy to operate
• Economical to purchase, use and maintain

Use
• Maximum inspiratory flow rates of 80 l/min allowing:
• *Variable inspiratory times of 0.5–3.9 seconds*
• *Frequencies of 5–50 breaths/minute*
• *A tidal volume range of 50–1500 ml*
• *A variable I:E ratio (1:1-1:3.5)*
• *The capability to control all the above independently (altering one variable should not affect others)*
• Capable of use with non-rebreathing or rebreathing anaesthetic breathing systems
• Capable of rapid conversion for paediatric use
• Capable of use with air, O₂ mixtures and all anaesthetics
• Capable of humidifying inspired gas
• Should allow 'sigh' breaths and the ability to inflate and hold by the user
• Allow continuous monitoring of airway pressure and of tidal volume

Safety
• Electrically safe, isolated, suppressed and explosion proof
• Have the ability to maintain output even when leaks develop
• Capable of rapid disassembly for easy sterilization
• Capable of using disposable hoses
• Fitted with bacterial filters
• Equipped with a pressure-relief valve
• Fitted with alarms for low pressure and/or circuit disconnection and high pressure and/or pressure overload
• Indicate low expired minute volume and low F_iO_2

6.6 Properties of the ideal ventilator for use in small animals. Key components are in *italics*. F_iO_2 = inspired oxygen fraction; I:E ratio = inspiratory:expiratory time ratio.

Set-up and use of commonly encountered mechanical ventilators in veterinary practice

Pneupac ventiPAC, paraPAC and transPAC

The details in this section also apply to the Penlon Nuffield Series 200.

Classification:

• Volume controlled, time cycled.
• Inspiratory phase is initiated by time (time triggered).

These ventilators are simple, suitable for anaesthesia use, versatile and can be sourced cost-effectively (ex-human medical use). Although some models are designed for ambulatory use and vary in terms of control over inspiratory and expiratory times, these ventilators all work on a similar principle and so are considered together.

The Pneupac ventiPAC is shown in Figure 6.7. The basic unit consists of a control module (Figure 6.7b) and patient valve, which attaches directly to a suitable anaesthetic breathing system (via an adequate length of standard 22 mm diameter corrugated plastic tubing) or to a bellows (bag in bottle) arrangement (Figure 6.7ac). The driving gas may be air or oxygen at 400 kPa, from either an auxiliary gas socket on the anaesthetic machine or a cylinder or pipeline supply. The driving gas should not be able to enter the patient's lungs when the ventilator is attached directly to the breathing system. The control unit comprises a spool valve (Figure 6.7d) and two timers, one to control the inspiratory phase time (A) and the other to control the expiratory phase time (B). The spool valve can be in two positions, one allowing driving gas to pass to the breathing attachment at a rate (controlled by a flow

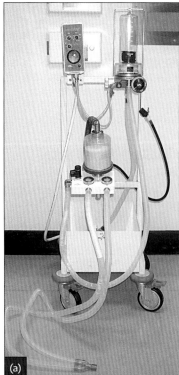
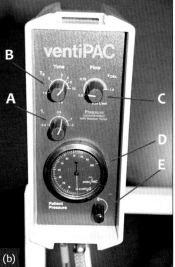
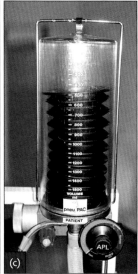
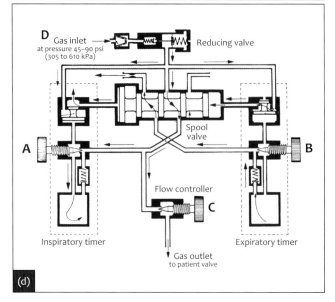

6.7 (a) The Pneupac ventiPAC (*in situ*). (b) Detail of the Pneupac ventiPAC. A = inspiratory phase timer; B = expiratory phase timer; C = flow controller; D = pressure gauge; E = on/off switch. (c) A typical bag-in-bottle arrangement which would be attached to the Pneupac ventiPAC in volume-controlled time-cycled mode. (d) Working principles of the Pneupac ventiPAC. A = inspiratory phase timer; B = expiratory phase timer; C = flow controller; D = gas inlet.

controller; C) for a time that is set by the operator. At the end of inspiration, the spool valve closes and driving gas accumulates in a pneumatic timer until the pressure within it is sufficient to push the spool valve back into the inspiratory position. Pressure applied to the breathing system is indicated by a large gauge on the front of the control unit (D). The patient valve is a simple pneumatic valve at the base of the ventilator, through which the gases pass to the breathing system or bellows. The patient valve directs all gas from the ventilator to the breathing system or bellows during the inspiratory phase, but allows gas returning from the patient to pass to a scavenging port during expiration.

Set-up:

1. Attach driving gas.
2. Estimate the patient's tidal volume based on 10–15 ml/kg. Set the flow and inspiratory phase time settings to achieve this volume. For example, for a 30 kg dog with a tidal volume 350 ml, a flow of 0.3–0.4 l/sec for 1 second will be suitable. Try to make the tidal volume as normal for that animal as possible, judged by adequacy of chest wall excursion.
3. Ensure scavenging is attached to the expiratory port of the patient valve.
4. Connect the hose from the patient valve to the breathing system.
5. Close the adjustable pressure-limiting (APL) valve of the breathing system.
6. Switch on the ventilator (E in Figure 6.7b).
7. Set the expiratory phase time (B) to adjust the number of breaths per minute and hence the minute volume. Ideally it should be adjusted to maintain normal P_aCO_2 based on capnometry or blood gas analysis (see Chapter 7).

Pneupac ventiPAC or Nuffield Series 200 used with a Newton valve

The normal patient valve can simply and quickly be replaced with a Newton valve (Figure 6.8), which converts the ventilator to a 'mechanical thumb' on an Ayre's T-piece or Bain. This makes the ventilator suitable for use in animals weighing less than 10 kg (down to 100 g) because it enables very small tidal volumes to be delivered. The Newton valve connects via a length of 15 mm corrugated tubing to the bag port of a modified Ayre's T-piece, Bain or circle breathing system. At low driving gas flows set on the ventilator, the pressure generated within the valve only partly overcomes the pressure of gas coming from the breathing system; occlusion is partial and tidal volumes are very small. It is analogous to partially occluding the expiratory limb with a thumb. As driving gas flow is increased, occlusion becomes more complete until eventually some driving gas is forced into the tube and the rate of lung inflation is greater than that produced just by the gas flow from the anaesthetic machine.

Set-up:

1. Attach driving gas.
2. Initially, set the inspiratory phase time to be normal for that patient (0.5–1 second).
3. Ensure scavenging system is attached to the expiratory port of the Newton valve.
4. Connect the hose from the patient valve to the breathing system ensuring that the valve on the breathing system is closed.

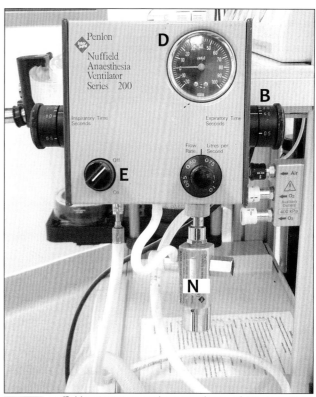

6.8 Nuffield Series 200 anaesthesia ventilator with Newton valve attachment (N), converting this versatile ventilator into a 'mechanical thumb' or pressure generator. B = expiratory phase time dial; D = pressure reading; E = on/off switch.

5. Set the flow to minimum (in case it had been set high during previous use) and switch on the ventilator (E).
6. Starting with the flow on the lowest setting, increase the flow until chest wall excursion appears normal. The pressure reading (D) should be <15 cmH$_2$O.
7. Set the expiratory phase time (B) to adjust the number of breaths per minute (and hence minute volume). Ideally, it should be adjusted to maintain normal P_aCO_2 based on capnometry or blood gas analysis.

Hallowell EMC Model 2000/3000 (and 2002) veterinary ventilator and Surgivet SAV 2500

Classification:

- Volume controlled, time cycled.
- Inspiratory phase is initiated by time (time triggered).

These ventilators have built-in ascending bellows and are designed to attach to the reservoir bag port of a suitable breathing system (Figure 6.9). Both ventilators require a driving gas supply (400 kPa) and a mains power supply. On the Hallowell EMC Model 3000, the controls include inspiratory flow (A) (up to 100 l/min), a variable peak pressure limit (B) (up to 60 cmH$_2$O) and breaths per minute (C). There is also a respiratory 'hold' button (D) for maintaining inflation and overriding cycling. Low breathing-system pressure is indicated by an alarm in the event of disconnection. Three sizes of bellows are available and are interchangeable; this makes the ventilator suitable for tidal volumes from 20 ml to 3 l. The I:E ratio is fixed at 1:2.

A major potential pitfall of this ventilator is that the volume control (A) regulates inspiratory flow directly and is effectively a *minute* volume setting and not a *tidal* volume setting. If the number of breaths per minute is reduced by the operator without a concomitant decrease in the flow

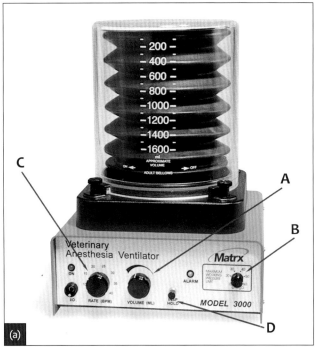

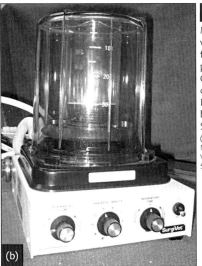

6.9 (a) The Hallowell EMC Model 3000 veterinary ventilator. A = inspiratory flow controller; B = peak pressure controller; C = respiratory rate controller; D = respiratory hold button. (b) The Surgivet SAV 2500 Ventilator. (Courtesy of Tanya Duke-Novakovski, Western College of Veterinary Medicine, University of Saskatchewan, Canada)

4. Connect the corrugated tubing to the breathing system.
5. Close the APL valve on the breathing system and allow the bellows to fill.
6. Switch on power and select breaths per minute.
7. Increase volume setting until each breath is of the correct tidal volume as indicated by excursion of the chest.
8. The rate control is then used to fine tune the tidal volume of each breath.
9. The volume setting is used to control minute volume and is adjusted to maintain normal P_aCO_2 based on capnometry and blood gas analysis.

Vetronic 'Merlin' veterinary ventilator

Classification:

- Volume controlled and either time cycled, pressure cycled or volume cycled.
- Inspiratory phase is initiated either by time (time triggered) or by the patient attempting to breathe when in assist mode (pressure triggered).

This is a highly advanced ventilator specifically designed for veterinary use (Figure 6.10). It is electrically powered and does not require a pressurized gas supply; it uses gases delivered from the anaesthetic machine (or room air) and can deliver tidal volumes in the range of 1–800 ml. The working principle is a precision-controlled piston, which acts like a syringe to generate a driving pressure and can be controlled to within 0.03 ml at low volumes. The manufacturer claims that the Merlin is suitable for animals weighing between 50 g and 70 kg. Inspiratory and expiratory times are between 0.2 and 9 seconds. Maximum airway pressure is 57 cmH$_2$O and negative triggering pressures may be set from 1–10 cmH$_2$O. The maximum flow is relatively low at only 25 l/min. There are audible and visual warnings for high airway pressures, blocked inlets and patient disconnection. A small liquid crystal display (LCD) screen on the ventilator provides information on the patient's tidal volume, minute volume, respiratory rate, I:E ratio, inspiratory and expiratory times and airway pressures, triggering pressure for assist mode, cycling pressure (for pressure-cycled mode) and even a calculated figure for compliance. The Merlin may be used:

- As part of a non-rebreathing system: the ventilator is connected to the common gas outlet of an anaesthetic machine. In this mode, it has a gas flow requirement of at least minute volume. As peak flow into the ventilator exceeds this during piston filling (in the expiratory phase), a reservoir bag must be present between the anaesthetic machine and ventilator
- With a circle system: this is more economical because it allows a lower fresh gas flow from the anaesthetic machine to be used.

In both cases, there must be a one-way valve between the ventilator and the patient on the inspiratory side, to ensure directional gas flow.

It is extremely useful to colour-code the inspiratory and expiratory gas connections and Merlin breathing tubes to facilitate easy and rapid set-up when circle systems are used (Figure 6.10bc).

This ventilator provides a range of operating modes and a wealth of settings not often provided on an anaesthetic ventilator. However, this comes with a greater level of complexity, necessitating more user involvement. The controls are very sensitive and it can be easy to alter the settings inadvertently by knocking against a control knob. The

setting, the tidal volume of each breath will increase. Halving the number of breaths per minute will double the tidal volume, unless the two controls are adjusted in synchrony. The pressure limiter will terminate inspiration, although if this has been set to 60 cmH$_2$O the potential for volutrauma exists.

The Hallowell Model 2002 version is functionally equivalent to the Model 2000, with the exception that there is an additional fine needle valve that may be used to regulate flows from 0 to 20 l/min. This fine control adds to the output of the coarse control and is for 'fine tuning' the tidal volume during ventilation. The ventilator generates a small amount of PEEP (2–3 cmH$_2$O) as the weight of the bellows compresses the gases within. Patients should be able to breathe spontaneously from the bellows when the ventilator is switched off.

Set-up:

1. Attach driving gas.
2. Select and attach appropriate bellows.
3. Set the maximum working pressure limit to 30 cmH$_2$O or less for normal patients.

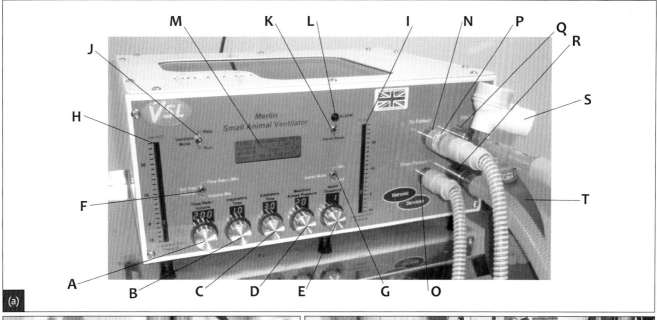

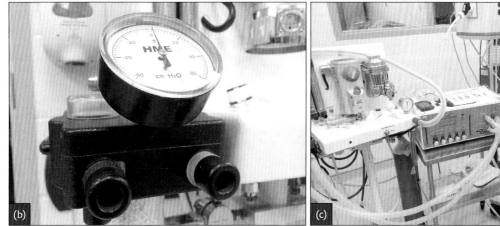

6.10 (a) The Vetronic 'Merlin' veterinary ventilator and controls. A = flow or volume control; B = inspiratory time control (seconds); C = expiratory time control (seconds); D = maximum airway pressure control (cmH$_2$O); E = assist threshold control (cmH$_2$O); F = flow rate/volume selector switch; G = assist mode on/off selector switch; H = LED indicator for expiratory port pressure (cmH$_2$O); I = LED indicator for inspiratory port pressure (cmH$_2$O); J = ventilate mode stop/run selector switch; K = alarm reset switch – non-latching, momentary action only; L = alarm flashing LED indicator; M = main status LCD screen; N = attachment of inspiratory limb of Y-piece; O = attachment of expiratory limb of Y-piece; P = one-way valve; Q = entry for fresh gas (connected to anaesthetic machine); R = exit for gas from ventilator (to scavenging system if used in non-rebreathing mode; to carbon dioxide-absorbent canister if used with a circle system); S = high-pressure relief valve; T = reservoir bag (of appropriate size for patient). (b) Colour coding of inspiratory and expiratory gas connections and Merlin breathing tubes allows easy and rapid set-up when circle systems are used. (c) Set-up for use of the Merlin ventilator with a circle system.

(bc, Courtesy of Tanya Duke-Novakovski, Western College of Veterinary Medicine, University of Saskatchewan, Canada)

highly adjustable nature of the Merlin, coupled with its ability to be used with room air as well as anaesthetic gases, means that it is useful as an ICU ventilator as well as for anaesthetic use, which may be of value in some practices. A PEEP valve for use with the Merlin is also available from the manufacturer (Figure 6.11).

Full details of the operation of this versatile ventilator can be downloaded from the manufacturer's website (www. vetronic.co.uk), and some general tips for its use are shown in Figure 6.12.

Vetronic SAV03 veterinary ventilator
Classification:

- Pressure-cycled 'mechanical thumb'.
- Inspiratory phase is initiated either by time (time triggered) or by the patient attempting to breathe (pressure triggered).

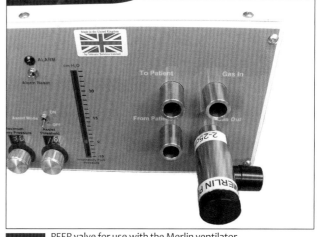

6.11 PEEP valve for use with the Merlin ventilator.
(Courtesy of Keith Simpson, Vetronic UK)

- Ensure set back from the edge of a trolley or table to reduce likelihood of inadvertent interference with setting controls
- Laminate diagrams of set up (or use a photograph) and keep with the ventilator
- Remember to turn the inspiratory time knob completely to the right to access pressure controlled mode
- Remember that when set in 'assist' mode, if no spontaneous efforts to breathe are made, the ventilator will administer intermittent mandatory tidal volumes

6.12 Top tips for using the Merlin ventilator.

Details include:

- Trigger range: 0–40 cmH$_2$O
- Expiratory phase: 1–30 seconds
- Breaths per minute: 2–6.0.

The SAV03 is a mains-powered, pressure-cycled ventilator designed for use in animals up to 10 kg bodyweight (Figure 6.13). The driving gas is taken directly from the anaesthetic machine and delivered via the valve of the ventilator to the endotracheal tube. During inspiration, gas is delivered to the patient until a set airway pressure is reached, at which point the expiratory phase begins. A user-defined delay then elapses before inspiration begins again and the cycle repeats. The peak airway pressure can be adjusted to control tidal volume. This airway pressure is shown on a digital display, together with valve status indicators. The SAV03 is designed for use in very small animals including birds, for which pressure cycling is more suitable.

When not in ventilate mode, the valve remains open and the valve attachment (Figure 6.13b) acts as a T-piece; the patient, attached at P, draws gas from the limb (L). During expiration and the expiratory pause, gas in the limb is replaced by fresh gas (FG) from the anaesthetic machine. In 'IPPV On' mode, the valve is closed in response to attempted ventilation. The negative pressure at which the ventilator is triggered is set by the operator (C in Figure 6.13a). Inspiration is terminated when inspiratory pressure reaches a value set by the operator using the same trigger set control, but before the IPPV mode is switched on. The display (A) indicates the set cycle pressure at this point. The valve then opens and expired gas passes into the limb (L) and thence to the scavenging system. The expiratory phase time is set by the operator (B).

Bird Mark 7 ventilator

Classification:

- Volume controlled, pressure cycled.
- Inspiratory phase is initiated either by time (time triggered) or by the patient attempting to breathe (pressure triggered).

This ventilator (Figure 6.14) is suitable for both small and large animal use depending on the size of the bellows to which it is attached. It is driven by compressed medical air or oxygen at approximately 400 kPa and may be supplied from either the high-pressure oxygen outlet of an anaesthetic machine, or a pipeline supply, or a separate cylinder with regulator. On its own, the ventilator simply produces a flow of gas and it is always used in conjunction with a separate set of bellows. The flow of gas from the Bird pressurizes the space between the bellows and a surrounding canister or 'bottle' (similar to the set-up shown in Figure 6.7c). The bellows, which contain the gases to be delivered to the patient, are compressed by this increase in surrounding pressure. Gas is forced from the bellows via a corrugated tube into the breathing system. Suitable breathing systems include the circle, the Bain (in both of which the attachment to the bellows simply replaces the reservoir bag), a T-piece or the Humphrey ADE in E mode.

The key controls on the Bird include inspiratory flow (up to 70 l/min), peak (and hence cycling) pressure (up to 60 cmH$_2$O), and expiratory phase time (resulting in 4–60 breaths/min). There is also an option to set a triggering pressure (negative 0.5–5.0 cmH$_2$O) at which the ventilator cycles from expiration to inspiration in response to inspiratory effort. This overrides the setting for expiratory phase time. A pressure indicator is also provided.

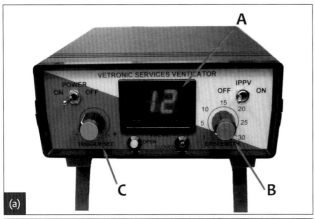

(a)

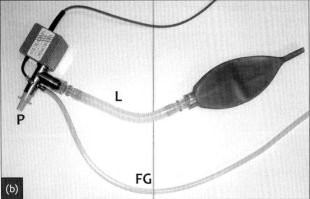

(b)

6.13 (a) The Vetronic SAV03 veterinary ventilator – a pressure-cycled 'mechanical thumb' designed for patients less than 10 kg. A = display; B = expiratory phase time control; C = trigger set control. (b) The Vetronic SAV03 veterinary ventilator valve assembly. FG = fresh gas; L = limb; P = patient attachment.

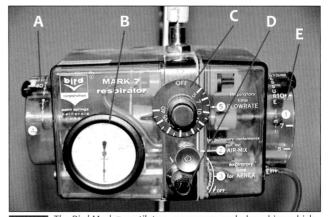

6.14 The Bird Mark 7 ventilator – a pressure-cycled machine which may drive ventilation systems for both small and large animals. A = triggering pressure control; B = pressure indicator; C = flow control; D = expiratory time control; E = inspiratory pressure control.

Set-up:

1. Attach driving gas.
2. Set the inspiratory pressure control (E) to between 15 and 20 cmH$_2$O. This determines the pressure at which the ventilator stops inflating the lungs and is later adjusted in combination with the flow setting to optimize tidal volume.
3. Set the triggering pressure (A) to maximum to prevent patient triggering.
4. Ensure that the expiratory valve assembly on the bellows housing is open and attached to the scavenging system – this allows escape of expired gases in the expiratory phase.
5. Connect the hose from the bellows to the reservoir bag port on the breathing system.
6. Close the APL valve ('pop-off' valve) on the breathing system.
7. Increase or decrease the flow (C) from the ventilator to deliver a tidal volume in a period of time that appears to be normal for that patient.
8. Set the expiratory phase time (D) to adjust the number of breaths per minute and hence minute volume. Ideally, this should be adjusted to maintain a normal P_aCO_2 based on capnometry or blood gas analysis.

Manley MP2/3 and MN2 ventilators

These machines (Figure 6.15) are an old design but are reliable, extremely easy to use and require neither additional driving gas nor a power supply. When purchasing a second-hand machine it is critically important to check the state of the bellows: these devices have both external and internal black rubber bellows that can perish. If there is any sign of such deterioration, the machine should be serviced before first use. The main limitation of these ventilators is that the smallest tidal volume that can be set restricts their use to animals above approximately 13 kg bodyweight.

Classification: These ventilators do not fit into any of the classifications described above. They are best described as minute volume dividers because they take the volume of gas delivered by the anaesthetic machine per minute and deliver it in breaths of a tidal volume set by the operator.

The working principle is explained in Figure 6.15b. The ventilator attaches to the common gas outlet of the anaesthetic machine. This means that all gas from the anaesthetic machine passes into the ventilator. During the expiratory phase, fresh gas accumulates in a set of bellows visible externally on the machine (A). The bellows inflate to a volume set by means of a volume control (B), at which point a mechanism is tripped (C) and the volume in A is delivered to the patient at a fixed pressure set using a sliding weight (D), usually 20 cmH$_2$O. During inspiration, fresh gas from the anaesthetic machine is still flowing and accumulates in a set of internal bellows (E). These bellows inflate to a set volume; when this volume is reached, the expiratory phase is initiated and the gas from E is dumped into bellows A. The degree to which the internal bellows inflate before tripping, controls the inspiratory time and is determined by the setting of the inspiratory phase control. This description may make the device sound complex but in practice the operator normally simply sets the tidal volume on the ventilator and then adjusts the breaths per minute by changing the fresh gas flow on the anaesthetic machine.

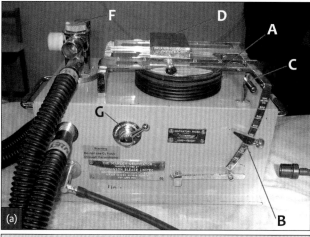

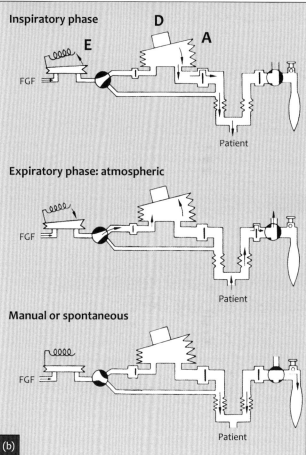

6.15 (a) The Manley MP2, a classic if ageing machine. A = externally visible bellows; B = volume control; C = tidal volume catch for external bellows; D = sliding weight to control pressure of gas delivered; F and G = controls to switch ventilator to automatic mode. (b) Working principles of the Manley MP2. A = externally visible bellows; D = sliding weight; E = internal bellows; FGF = fresh gas flow.

Set-up:

1. Set the estimated tidal volume using the slider (B).
2. Check the weight (D) is approximately at the 20 cmH$_2$O mark.
3. Attach the ventilator to the fresh gas outlet of the anaesthetic machine.
4. Switch the ventilator to automatic at both control knobs F and G.
5. Adjust the fresh gas flow on the anaesthetic machine until the ventilatory rate is suitable to maintain the required P_aCO_2 (as judged by capnometry and blood gas analysis).

Preventing spontaneous breathing during mechanical ventilation

As most anaesthetized patients hypoventilate, spontaneous ventilatory efforts during IPPV ('bucking' or 'fighting' the ventilator) do not tend to occur. If spontaneous breathing attempts are made, they may cause sharp changes (negative and positive) in intrathoracic pressure. This affects the normal thoracic venous pump and may reduce ventilator effectiveness. Strategies to reduce spontaneous ventilatory attempts are listed in Figure 6.16. First of all, however, it is important to ensure that analgesia and anaesthesia are adequate and ventilator set-up is correct.

Strategy	Comment
Increase tidal volume	IPPV activates pulmonary stretch receptors and suppresses spontaneous inspiration. Take care not to exceed a peak airway pressure of 20 cmH$_2$O in healthy patients
Use of neuromuscular blocking agents	See Chapter 16
Use of supplemental CNS depression	Use of low dose of an additional agent will further reduce ventilatory drive (e.g. midazolam 0.2 mg/kg i.v.; ketamine 1–2 mg/kg i.v.; fentanyl 1–5 µg/kg i.v.). Note that these drugs may reduce the requirements for volatile agents

6.16 Strategies to reduce spontaneous ventilatory efforts during intermittent positive pressure ventilation.

Monitoring and supporting the patient during IPPV

All the basic principles of monitoring the anaesthetized patient apply (see Chapter 7). Capnometry is the simplest, most effective non-invasive and reliable way to show ventilatory (and hence ventilator) performance on a breath-by-breath basis. Sidestream spirometry provides valuable information on tidal volume and airway pressure, especially when the patient is covered in drapes, but is rarely available, even in referral hospitals. The other additional focus of monitoring during IPPV should be mean arterial blood pressure, which is the parameter most likely to be compromised by the effects of ventilation, especially where there is reduced cardiovascular reserve (see above).

Ventilators are known fomites in human anaesthetic practice: in-line bacterial filters are widely available and often combined with a heat and moisture exchanger (heat and moisture exchanging filters (HMEFs); see Figure 5.30). They offer low resistance and are cost effective compared with sterilization of the ventilator (where this is possible).

Weaning from automatic ventilation

A reduction of the respiratory rate delivered by the ventilator usually allows a rise in P_aCO_2, which initiates a return to spontaneous ventilation. Alternatively, the patient may be removed from the ventilator and ventilated manually using a suitable breathing system (see Chapter 5) at a reduced rate, until spontaneous ventilation returns. In veterinary practice, weaning from the ventilator most commonly occurs at the end of anaesthesia, when anaesthetic depth and associated CNS depression are declining. Oxygenation should be monitored (with a pulse oximeter) particularly carefully at this time, although with a high F_IO_2 in the healthy patient undergoing some ventilation, this is unlikely to fall. Hypothermia reduces ventilatory drive and attempts to correct this should be initiated at this point, if not already in progress.

References and further reading

Atallah MM, Demian AD, el-Diasty TA et al. (2000) Can we increase hepatic oxygen availability? The role of intentional hypercarbia. Middle East Journal of Anesthesiology 15, 503–514

Cairo JM (2012) Pilbeam's Mechanical Ventilation: Physiological and Clinical Applications, 5th edn. Mosby Elsevier, St Louis

Cannesson M (2011) Non-invasive guidance of fluid therapy. In: Clinical Fluid Therapy in the Perioperative Setting, ed. R Hahn, pp. 103–111. Cambridge University Press, Cambridge

Cullen DJ and Eger EI (1974) Cardiovascular effects of carbon dioxide in man. Anesthesiology 41, 345–349

Davey AJ (2012) Automatic ventilators. In: Ward's Anaesthetic Equipment 6th edn, eds. AJ Davey and A Diba, pp. 231–252. Saunders Elsevier, Philadelphia

Desebbe O and Cannesson M (2008) Using ventilation-induced plethysmographic variations to optimize patient fluid status. Current Opinion in Anaesthesiology 21, 772–778

Dresse C, Joris JL and Hans GA (2012) Mechanical ventilation during anaesthesia: pathophysiology and clinical implications. Trends in Anaesthesia and Critical Care 2, 71–75

Dugdale A (2007) The ins and outs of ventilation 1: Basic principles. In Practice 29, 186–193

Dugdale A (2007) The ins and outs of ventilation 2: Mechanical ventilators. In Practice 29, 272–282

Eichbaum FW and Yasaka WJ (1973) Influence of pulmonary ventilation with oxygen and carbon dioxide-oxygen mixtures upon cardiac arrhythmias. Arquivos Brasileiros de Cardiologia 26, 109–123

Eisele JH, Eger EI and Muallem M (1967) Narcotic properties of carbon dioxide in the dog. Anesthesiology 28, 856–865

Eyre L and Breen A (2010) Optimal volaemic status and predicting fluid responsiveness. Continuing Education in Anaesthesia, Critical Care and Pain 10, 59–62

Kil HK (2000) Hypercapnia is an important adjuvant factor of oculocardiac reflex during strabismus surgery. Anesthesia and Analgesia 91, 1044

Pannu N and Mehta RL (2004) Effect of mechanical ventilation on the kidney. Best Practice and Research: Clinical Anaesthesiology 18, 189–203

Putensen C, Wrigge H and Hering R (2006) The effects of mechanical ventilation on the gut and abdomen. Current Opinion in Critical Care 12, 160–165

Rolf N and Cote CJ (1991) Persistent cardiac arrhythmias in pediatric patients: effects of age, expired carbon dioxide values, depth of anesthesia, and airway management. Anesthesia and Analgesia 73, 720–724

Sande A and West C (2010) Traumatic brain injury: a review of pathophysiology and management. Journal of Veterinary Emergency and Critical Care 20, 177–190

West JB (2008) Pulmonary Pathophysiology: The Essentials, 7th edn. Lippincott, Williams and Wilkins, Philadelphia

Chapter 7

Patient monitoring and monitoring equipment

Stijn Schauvliege

General anaesthesia carries an inherent risk for every patient. Checking the equipment before every anaesthetic (see Chapters 4 and 5) and selecting an appropriate anaesthetic protocol on the basis of a thorough history and preanaesthetic examination of the patient (see Chapter 2) will help to reduce the risk. Nevertheless, cardiovascular and respiratory side effects and other unexpected adverse responses to anaesthesia can always occur. Additionally, individual differences in sensitivity to anaesthetic agents and their side effects exist. Therefore, monitoring of anaesthesia remains fundamentally important, with particular emphasis on anaesthetic depth, cardiovascular and respiratory function and other parameters reflecting general homeostasis. The adequacy of antinociceptive measures should also be regularly assessed.

Central to the monitoring process is the person interpreting the information gathered and making adjustments to patient management where needed. Simple clinical assessments of the patient provide important information, help to distinguish artefactual information from true values displayed by monitors and remain the best method to assess anaesthetic depth in animals (see below). Besides the human senses, equipment is available to evaluate respiratory and cardiovascular function in a more quantitative way, to monitor the patient's response to treatment, and to guide the veterinary surgeon (veterinarian) in the use of the anaesthetic machine and ventilator. Finally, monitors can show the effects of administered drugs or interventions and thus act as a 'teacher' to the veterinary surgeon in his/her role as anaesthetist.

Simultaneous observation of multiple parameters, and integration of all the information obtained from the various observations, is needed to create a complete overview of the patient before any intervention. To facilitate this, it is important that both patient and equipment are easily accessible from one location (Figure 7.1). This allows simultaneous clinical assessment of the patient and the devices used for anaesthesia, such as the breathing system, including reservoir bag and anaesthetic apparatus (flowmeters, vaporizer, ventilator), as well as infusion and monitoring equipment.

An essential component of patient monitoring is the anaesthetic record. This will help the veterinary surgeon to develop a systematic approach to monitoring anaesthesia and to recognize both trends in and correlations between measured parameters. It also acts as a reference for future anaesthesia of the same patient or for retrospective studies. Importantly, the record serves as a medicolegal document which illustrates that the patient has been monitored properly.

Clinical monitoring: use of the human senses

While monitoring equipment offers many advantages, such as objectivity, providing more complete information, allowing continuous measurement and being equipped with automatic alarms, the human senses of the anaesthetist

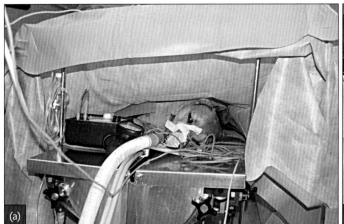
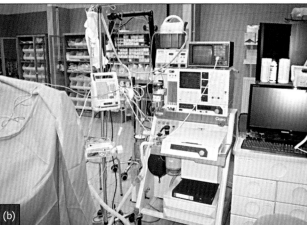

7.1 Ergonomics in theatre. (a) An 'anaesthetic window' allows continuous evaluation of the patient. (b) Strategic positioning of the anaesthetic machine, monitoring equipment, fluids and syringe drivers to facilitate monitoring of the patient and all equipment.

provide invaluable information and are available under all circumstances without the need for specialized equipment. Veterinary surgeons are trained to use their senses when performing a thorough clinical examination, and should apply the same skills to the anaesthetized patient.

Examples of ways veterinary surgeons can use their senses during anaesthetic monitoring are palpation of peripheral pulses (touch), assessment of the depth of anaesthesia (sight), detection of leaks when using volatile anaesthetics (smell) and auscultation of heart and lung sounds by means of an (oesophageal) stethoscope (hearing) (Figures 7.2 and 7.3).

During palpation of peripheral pulses, attention is paid to:

- Pulse rate
- Pulse rhythm
- Vessel 'tone'
- Pulse amplitude and duration
- Synchronicity with the heart rate (based on auscultation or electrocardiography).

The 'tone' of the artery gives an impression of the diastolic arterial blood pressure (ABP) and is mainly influenced by circulating blood volume and the degree of vasoconstriction. The pulse amplitude reflects the difference between systolic and diastolic ABP and correlates

with stroke volume (SV). For example, in the presence of vasodilation and a compensatory increase in SV, palpation of the pulse can sometimes give misleading information: a large pulse amplitude (associated with the SV) is palpable as a clear, 'bounding' pulse, despite a low mean ABP. In such cases arterial tone will also be low, leading to a flaccid artery, but this may be difficult to appreciate in smaller patients.

Finally, the human senses can still be considered the most reliable way to assess anaesthetic depth, by evaluation of the animal's eye position, palpebral reflexes, lacrimation, jaw tone, heart and respiratory rates and autonomic responses to surgical stimulation (Figures 7.4 and 7.5).

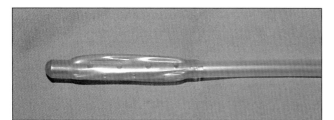

7.2 Tip of an oesophageal stethoscope.

Parameter	Light anaesthesia	Surgical anaesthesia	Deep anaesthesia
Movement	Possible	Possible/absent	Usually absent
Jaw tone	Moderate to strong	Moderate	Absent to moderate
Lacrimation	Moist cornea	Moist cornea	Moist/dry cornea
Eye position	Central	Central	Central
Palpebral reflex	Positive	Positive	Possible
Heart rate	Usually increased	Normal	May be decreased
Respiratory rate	Usually increased	Normal	Usually decreased
Haemodynamic or respiratory alterations in response to surgical stimulation	Present	Usually absent	Absent

7.4 Clinical assessment of anaesthetic depth during maintenance with dissociative anaesthetics.

Parameter	Senses used	Observations to be made
Depth of anaesthesia	Sight Touch Hearing	Palpebral reflexes, pupil size, eye position, lacrimation, movement, heart and respiratory rate Muscle tone (e.g. jaw), pulse rate and strength Heart rate (auscultation or audible signal from ECG, pulse oximeter or Doppler monitor)
Circulation	Sight Touch Hearing	Arterial pressure waveform, capillary refill time, surgical site (bleeding, tissue colour, vessel colour and turgescence) Mucous membrane colour: • pale (anaemia, vasoconstriction) • pink (normal) • red (vasodilation/congestion) • blue (cyanosis) Palpation of peripheral pulses and arterial tone (femoral, metacarpal, metatarsal, dorsal pedal or sublingual artery), skin turgor, skin temperature Cardiac auscultation, signal from pulse oximeter or Doppler monitor
Respiration	Sight Touch Hearing	Movement of chest, abdomen and reservoir bag or ventilator bellows Manual lung inflation (squeeze the reservoir bag with closed pressure-relief valve): enables assessment of pulmonary compliance and inspiratory resistance Auscultation, pitch of pulse oximeter
Temperature	Touch	Skin temperature Temperature of carbon dioxide absorbent (normal increase during absorption of carbon dioxide *versus* no increase when absorbent is exhausted *versus* extreme increase due to presence of dried absorbent)
Leaks from anaesthetic equipment	Sight Touch Hearing Smell	Abnormal shape of capnogram, collapse of reservoir bag, absence of pressure swings on manometer during ventilation in the case of disconnection Pressure in pilot balloon of endotracheal tube Audible leak, e.g. due to underinflated endotracheal tube cuff (can be used as a guide during cuff inflation; see Chapter 5) Odour of volatile anaesthetic

7.3 Parameters that can be monitored during anaesthesia using the senses.

Parameter	Light anaesthesia	Surgical anaesthesia	Deep anaesthesia
Movement	Possible	No	No
Jaw tone	Mild to strong	Relaxed	Relaxed
Lacrimation	Moist cornea	Moist cornea	Dry cornea
Eye position	Central	Rotated	Central
Palpebral reflex	Positive	Negative	Negative
Heart rate	Usually increased	Normal	May be decreased
Respiratory rate	Usually increased	Normal	Usually decreased
Haemodynamic or respiratory alterations in response to surgical stimulation	Present	Usually absent	Absent

7.5 Clinical assessment of anaesthetic depth during maintenance with volatile anaesthetics.

Monitoring equipment

Capnometry and capnography

Capnometry provides real-time information on respiratory rate, end-tidal carbon dioxide and often also inspired carbon dioxide levels. End-tidal carbon dioxide values can be displayed as either concentrations ($FE'CO_2$; %) or partial pressures ($PE'CO_2$; mmHg or kPa).

Capnography is the graphical representation of continuous capnometry throughout the respiratory cycle. The resulting *capnogram* allows easy assessment of the respiratory rhythm because it displays multiple consecutive breaths at the same time. The shape of the capnogram also provides other useful information on, for example, the presence of leaks within the breathing system, increased resistance to breathing or rebreathing of carbon dioxide (see later).

Different measurement techniques are used, but most anaesthetic monitors rely on the principle of absorption of infrared light by the carbon dioxide molecules. This measurement can be performed by a sensor placed directly between the endotracheal tube and the breathing circuit (*mainstream* capnography; Figure 7.6). However, more often the monitor continuously withdraws a sample from

7.6 Mainstream capnography. The analyser transmits a beam of infrared light through the window of the connection piece, which is placed between the endotracheal tube and the Y-piece of the anaesthetic breathing system.

the breathing system at a fixed rate and analyses the sample in a measuring chamber within the monitor itself (*sidestream* capnography; Figure 7.7).

Mainstream capnography has a more rapid response time than sidestream capnography, and is more suitable for patients with fast respiratory rates and very small tidal volumes. However, it requires placement of an endotracheal tube; increases apparatus dead space; is bulky; is prone to malfunctioning as a result of water vapour in the sample; and carries greater risk of either dirt entering, or damage being caused to, the measuring chamber. Newer-generation mainstream capnographs have smaller and much more durable sensors, and low dead-space versions are also available.

With sidestream capnographs, gases are continuously aspirated from the anaesthetic circuit through a sampling line, which is usually attached to a connector positioned between the endotracheal tube and the breathing system. Low dead-space connectors are available for smaller patients (Figure 7.7c). A water trap or paper filter ensures that water vapour is removed from the sample so that dry gases are used for analysis within the monitor (Figure 7.7d). With this technique, there is a delay before changes in carbon dioxide concentration are displayed. This delay depends on the length of the sampling line and the sampling rate of the monitor, but is rarely longer than a few seconds. An advantage of this technique is the ability to position the sampling line at the level of the nares or inside a facemask in non-intubated patients. End-tidal carbon dioxide monitoring via an intranasal catheter has been shown to provide a clinically acceptable alternative to arterial blood gas analysis in healthy sedated dogs (Pang *et al.*, 2007). Most sidestream capnographs allow selection of the sampling rate: typically there is a choice between 50 ml/min and 200 ml/min. A higher sampling rate will reduce the response time of the monitor, but also means that a larger part of the fresh gas flow is 'lost' each minute, unless sampled gas exiting the monitor is returned to the anaesthetic breathing system. However, modern 'microstream' technologies have become available which use a low sampling rate of 50 ml/min without compromising response time (Figure 7.8). If sidestream

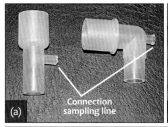
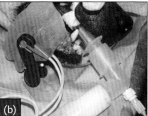

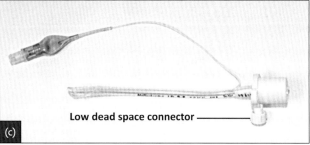

Low dead space connector

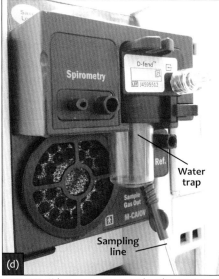

Spirometry

D-fend™

Ref.
Water trap

Sample Gas Out
M-CAIOV

Sampling line

7.7 Sidestream capnography. The monitor continuously withdraws gas through a sampling line, which is attached to the connection piece. (a) Normal connector. (b) Low dead space connector between the endotracheal tube and the Y-piece of the anaesthetic breathing system. (c) Low dead space connector. (d) A water trap filters out water vapour from the sample, to allow infrared analysis of a dry gas sample inside the monitor. Clearly visible is the outlet for the sampled gas.
(c, Courtesy of Asher Allison, Animal Health Trust, Newmarket, UK)

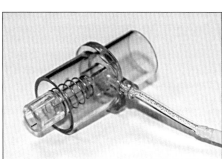
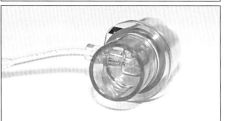

7.8
Microstream capnography connector.
(Courtesy of Asher Allison, Animal Health Trust, Newmarket, UK)

capnography is utilized, exhaust gases from the monitor should be scavenged or returned to the anaesthetic breathing system after analysis has taken place (see Figure 1.1). Further details of scavenging systems can be found in Chapter 5.

The normal capnogram

The typical capnogram is represented in Figure 7.9. There are four distinct phases of the capnogram. Phase I is the *inspiratory baseline*. Normally, the inspired gas mixture does not contain any carbon dioxide, and therefore its carbon dioxide concentration should be zero. During early expiration, gases are exhaled from the patient's airway dead space; these do not contain carbon dioxide, as they have not taken part in any gas exchange. Quite rapidly, however, gases are also exhaled from the alveoli and the expired carbon dioxide level rapidly increases; this is phase II, the *expiratory upstroke*. Phase III is the *expiratory (alveolar) plateau*; during this phase, the carbon dioxide level continues to increase slowly (because of uneven emptying of alveoli) until it reaches a maximum value, the $P_E'CO_2$. During the following inspiration, the carbon dioxide level rapidly decreases again to zero (*inspiratory downstroke*, phase 0).

In obese or pregnant patients, uneven emptying of alveoli may cause an additional rise in the carbon dioxide level at the end of the plateau phase; this extra wave is termed phase IV (Figure 7.10a).

Interpretation of the capnogram

If the capnogram has a normal shape and the tidal volume is high enough to achieve significant alveolar ventilation, the $P_E'CO_2$ can be taken to represent the alveolar tension of carbon dioxide, which usually corresponds well with the arterial carbon dioxide tension (P_aCO_2). In healthy patients, P_aCO_2 is usually 2–5 mmHg higher than $P_E'CO_2$. This relationship may be disturbed when there is a significant degree of alveolar dead-space ventilation; this is relatively rare in healthy small animals. Unlike arterial oxygen tension (P_aO_2), P_aCO_2 and $P_E'CO_2$ are not greatly affected by pulmonary atelectasis. Normal values for P_aCO_2 are between 35 and 45 mmHg (4.7–6.0 kPa).

In normal circumstances, capnometry or capnography thus offers a continuous and non-invasive way to monitor P_aCO_2, which is determined by the balance between alveolar ventilation and carbon dioxide delivery to the lungs. The latter not only depends on carbon dioxide production in the tissues (i.e. metabolism), but also on venous return, which matches cardiac output. This means that three factors determine the value for $P_E'CO_2$:

- Alveolar ventilation
- Metabolism
- Circulation.

When two of these three factors are stable, capnometry provides information on changes in the third factor.

End-tidal carbon dioxide: The most frequent cause of increased $P_E'CO_2$ (>45 mmHg, >6.0 kPa) if there is zero inspired carbon dioxide is hypoventilation, for example due to anaesthesia-induced respiratory depression, which usually responds well to increases in minute volume. Other potential causes are:

- Increased production of carbon dioxide, e.g. malignant hyperthermia, shivering

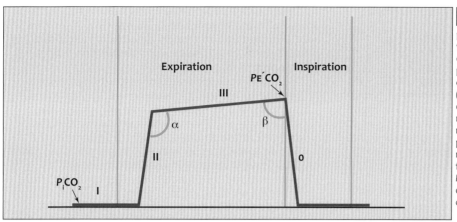

7.9 Normal single-breath capnogram. Note that expiration starts before phase II, because initially dead space gas, which does not contain carbon dioxide, is exhaled. The alpha (α) angle is increased with a partial airway obstruction or when positive end-expiratory pressure is applied. The beta (β) angle increases when there is rebreathing of carbon dioxide or when the monitor response time is long relative to the respiratory cycle time, for example, in small patients with rapid respiratory rates and a relatively low gas sampling rate. See the text for further explanation of the different phases. P_iCO_2 = partial pressure of inspired carbon dioxide; $PE'CO_2$ = partial pressure of end-tidal carbon dioxide.

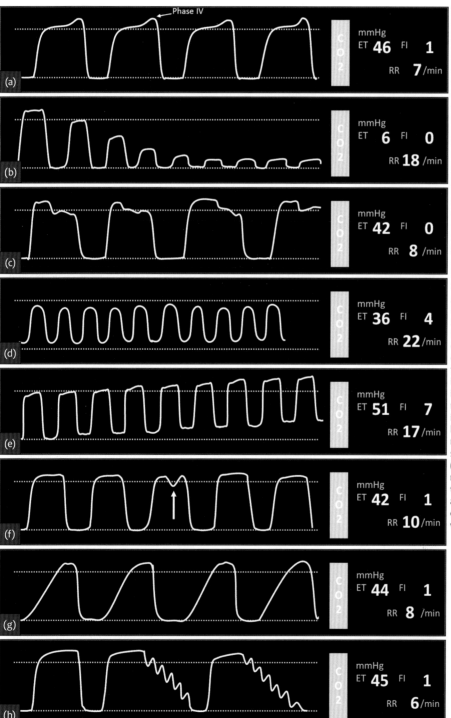

7.10 Capnograms. (a) In some obese or pregnant patients, an additional peak in carbon dioxide concentration (phase IV) can be seen at the end of the plateau phase. A similar capnogram may sometimes be seen when there is a leak in the sampling line or water trap. (b) When ventilation continues during cardiac arrest, the expiratory carbon dioxide concentration quickly decreases over a few breaths, because carbon dioxide produced in the tissues is no longer being transported to the lungs. A similar capnogram can also result from major pulmonary embolism or major reduction in cardiac output. (c) The normal plateau is distorted or absent because of dilution of carbon dioxide by ambient air or fresh gas. This may be caused by a leak (underinflated cuff, leak in the sampling line or water trap) or because the sampling site is too close to the area of fresh gas delivery. In this scenario the $PE'CO_2$ is usually underestimated. (d) When respiratory rate is high and tidal volume and sampling rate (in sidestream capnographs) are low, mixing of gases in the sampling line can cause 'damping' of the capnogram, eventually leading to a sinusoidal shape. (e) A gradual rise in both inspiratory and expiratory carbon dioxide concentrations is typically seen when carbon dioxide absorbent is exhausted or when the fresh gas flow in non-rebreathing systems is insufficient. (f) 'Curare cleft' (arrowed) during intermittent positive pressure ventilation, resulting from spontaneous respiratory effort in a patient recovering from neuromuscular blockade. This may also be seen as a result of manipulation of the thorax or abdomen during surgery. (g) Shallower expiratory upstroke ('shark fin' appearance of capnogram) resulting from expiratory resistance to airflow; this can, for example, be seen in cats with asthma. (h) 'Cardiogenic' oscillations at the end of the plateau may be seen especially when respiratory rate is low.

- Increased cardiac output (this usually causes only a temporary increase)
- Addition of carbon dioxide to the circulation, e.g. capnoperitoneum during laparoscopy.

The most frequent cause of increased $P_E'CO_2$ with increased inspired carbon dioxide is rebreathing of carbon dioxide due either to exhausted carbon dioxide absorbent or a defective exhalation valve in a circle system, or to insufficient fresh gas flow in a non-rebreathing system (see below). Decreased $P_E'CO_2$ can be caused by:

- Hyperventilation
- A significant degree of cardiovascular depression, for example, severe hypovolaemia/hypotension due to blood loss or in profound shock states. When there is a sudden dramatic deterioration in cardiac output (or during cardiac arrest if the animal's lungs are being ventilated mechanically), the $P_E'CO_2$ will very quickly decrease over the course of only a few breaths (Figure 7.10b). This is often the first sign of such events, unless ABP is being monitored continuously by Doppler ultrasonography or by an invasive technique. The $P_E'CO_2$ can also be used to evaluate the efficacy of cardiac compressions in achieving tissue and lung perfusion during cardiopulmonary resuscitation
- Pulmonary embolism causing obstruction of blood flow to a significant part of the lungs
- Reduced metabolism in the tissues, for example, during profound hypothermia.

In specific circumstances, $P_E'CO_2$ values can underestimate P_aCO_2. This is seen:

- During shallow breathing, when predominant ventilation of airway dead space instead of alveoli occurs, resulting in dilution of alveolar gases
- When there is a significant degree of alveolar dead space, for example, in low cardiac output states or pulmonary embolism
- Due to incorrect measurements, for example, in the case of:
  - A leak between the sampling site and the measuring chamber (dilution by ambient air; Figure 7.10c)
  - Dilution by fresh gas when the sampling site is too close to the fresh gas inlet
  - Rapid respiratory rates and low tidal volumes during sidestream capnography with low sampling rates: dispersion of gases in the sampling line results in a 'dampened' or even sinusoidal capnogram with underestimation of $P_E'CO_2$ and overestimation of inspired carbon dioxide (Figure 7.10d).

A complete absence of $P_E'CO_2$ can be caused by:

- Respiratory arrest
- Cardiac arrest
- Technical problems such as a dislodged or malpositioned endotracheal tube (e.g. oesophageal intubation), obstruction of the endotracheal tube or gas sampling line, or disconnection of the endotracheal tube from the sampling connector or mainstream capnography sensor.

Inspiratory carbon dioxide: When the monitor is properly calibrated, an inspired carbon dioxide level above zero indicates rebreathing of previously exhaled carbon dioxide (Figure 7.10e). Causes may be:

- Inadequate fresh gas flow in non-rebreathing systems
- A leak in the inner tube of a Bain system
- Exhausted carbon dioxide absorbent in circle systems
- Inspiratory or expiratory valve dysfunction in circle systems
- Increased apparatus dead space, although this will depend on the site of measurement. Very often the sampling site for sidestream capnography, or the measurement site for mainstream capnography, is between the anaesthetic breathing system and the endotracheal tube. Increases in apparatus dead space between the sampling/measurement site and the patient will not be detected, because the gases from that area will be re-inhaled during the next inspiration, without reaching the sampling/measurement site
- Alternatively, inspired carbon dioxide may falsely appear to be elevated when the respiratory rate is high and the tidal volume small while the sampling rate is low (Figure 7.10d).

Abnormal capnograms: During tachypnoea, the plateau phase of the capnogram becomes shorter and may even disappear. Quite often, breaths become shallower and as a result, the dead space:tidal volume ratio increases. This results in low values for $P_E'CO_2$ despite normal or high P_aCO_2 values because the alveolar gases are diluted by gas from the airway dead space. This can be detected by manually giving the patient a breath of sufficient volume, which results in a higher $P_E'CO_2$ compared to previous breaths, because pure alveolar gas is exhaled at the end of a deeper breath.

The presence of leaks can distort the shape of the capnogram (e.g. irregular or absent plateau phase; Figure 7.10c), especially when they are located close to the sampling site or within the sampling line. Such irregularities in the plateau phase should, however, be distinguished from the results of spontaneous respiratory efforts during mechanical ventilation. A special example of the latter is the 'curare cleft' during neuromuscular blockade (Figure 7.10f). This characteristic dip in the plateau of the capnogram is due to a spontaneous respiratory effort during mechanical ventilation, suggesting recovery from neuromuscular blockade. It can also result from manipulations during surgery that result in movement of the diaphragm or thoracic wall.

When there is partial obstruction to expiratory gas flow, the slope of phase II is less steep than normal and, as a result, the alpha angle (the angle between phases II and III; see Figure 7.9) is increased. A typical example is the 'shark fin' appearance of the capnogram in cats with asthma (Figure 7.10g), but a kinked endotracheal tube or any other cause of reduced expiratory flow can result in similar findings.

'Ripples' on the alveolar plateau and descending limb of the capnogram are usually explained by movement of gas in the airways as a result of cardiogenic oscillations. These are most often observed when respiratory rate is low (Figure 7.10h). Recent evidence suggests that these oscillations of the capnogram arise from pulmonary artery pulsatility rather than from physical transmission of the movement of heartbeats to the lungs (Suarez-Sipmann et al., 2013).

Pulse oximetry

Pulse oximetry is a non-invasive technique that allows real-time determination of the oxygen saturation (S_pO_2) of haemoglobin in arterial blood. The pulse oximeter simultaneously displays the pulse rate. Classic (transmission) pulse oximeters transmit a beam of red and infrared light through a relatively thin layer of tissue, such as the tongue, prepuce or toe web (Figure 7.11), to a receiver in the device. Deoxyhaemoglobin absorbs more red light than oxyhaemoglobin, and the converse is true for infrared light. The pulse oximeter estimates the S_pO_2 on the basis of this difference in absorbance. Although both arterial and venous haemoglobin contribute to the absorption, the pulsatile character of arterial blood flow allows the device to measure arterial saturation selectively. During each pulse the amount of blood flowing underneath the probe (and thus the total absorption of light) increases, which also enables the pulse oximeter to measure the pulse rate.

Reflectance pulse oximeters, in which the light emitter and sensor are placed side by side, are also available (Figure 7.12). When using these devices, the transmitted

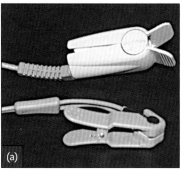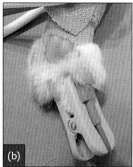

7.11 (a) Transmission pulse oximeters. (b) A relatively thin layer of tissue, such as the toe, is a suitable site for placement of the pulse oximeter.
(b, Courtesy of Marieke de Vries, Davies Veterinary Specialists, Higham Gobion, UK)

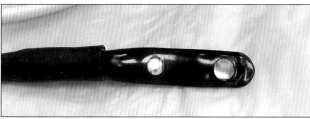

7.12 Reflectance pulse oximeter probe.
(Courtesy of Dr Carolyn McKune, University of Saskatchewan, Canada)

light is reflected from, for instance, subcutaneous tissues and bone and then detected by the receiver. Reflectance pulse oximeters allow measurements to be made from sites of the body where transmission pulse oximetry cannot be applied, for example, on body surfaces such as the forehead in humans, or in the rectum or oesophagus. Under certain conditions, such as hypothermia or peripheral vasoconstriction, measurements from the rectum or oesophagus may also be more reliable than peripheral measurements. These probes are less frequently used than transmission devices in veterinary medicine because the latter are more convenient to use and the intensity of the light detected by the photodiode is lower with reflectance probes, especially in case of pigmentation.

It is important to bear in mind that pulse oximeters measure only S_pO_2 and not P_aO_2. This imposes some limitations, especially in anaesthetized patients breathing an oxygen-enriched gas mixture: in the higher range of the oxyhaemoglobin dissociation curve, at P_aO_2 values above 100 mmHg (13.3 kPa), large changes in P_aO_2 do not cause discernible changes in S_pO_2 (Figure 7.13). As a result, pulmonary disease or atelectasis with right-to-left shunting can significantly reduce P_aO_2 while the S_pO_2 remains high. Only when P_aO_2 falls to values <60 mmHg (8.0 kPa) does S_pO_2 rapidly decrease. Similarly, pulse oximeters provide little or no information on the adequacy of ventilation in hypoventilating patients receiving supplementary oxygen, since normal S_pO_2 values are usually observed. In such circumstances, adequacy of ventilation is better evaluated using capnography and/or blood gas analysis (see below).

Despite these limitations, pulse oximetry remains useful because S_pO_2 is much more important than P_aO_2 in the calculation of the arterial oxygen content. Arterial hypoxaemia is normally defined as a P_aO_2 of ≤60 mmHg (8.0 kPa), which corresponds to an S_pO_2 of ≤90% (Figure 7.13). There is, however, considerable potential for erroneous measurements, which can be caused by:

- Abnormal forms of haemoglobin. The presence of carboxyhaemoglobin leads to falsely high values for S_pO_2, while the presence of methaemoglobin tends to shift the reading towards 80–85%, with the reading becoming closer to these values as the proportion of methaemoglobin increases

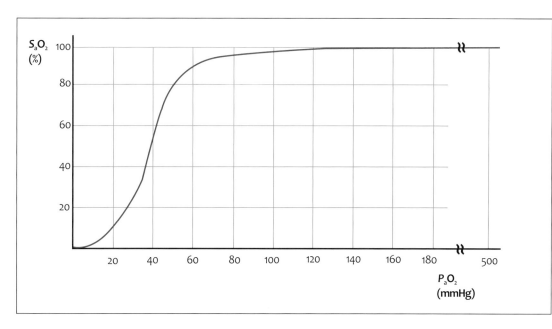

7.13 Oxyhaemoglobin dissociation curve. P_aO_2 = arterial oxygen tension; S_aO_2 = arterial haemoglobin saturation with oxygen.

- Movement artefacts and low perfusion states. Second- and third- generation pulse oximeters have been designed to be less affected by movement and to provide a reading even during low perfusion states. Nevertheless, a poor signal resulting from hypotension, shock, hypothermia or peripheral vasoconstriction (e.g. influence of alpha-2 agonists) will still result in less reliable measurements of S_pO_2 or even failure to register a value. A frequent problem with transmission pulse oximeters is that during use, the signal becomes less clear because of gradual compression of the vessels by the spring of the probe; this results in underestimation of S_pO_2 or a complete loss of signal. Simply moving the probe to a slightly different position usually resolves this problem
- Drying of the tongue. This can result in a weaker or absent signal. On the basis of clinical experience, this can be prevented by using a wet swab between the tongue and the probe (Figure 7.14)
- Pigmentation of the skin or mucous membranes, which may cause underestimation of S_pO_2 or inability of the pulse oximeter to provide a reading
- Use of electrosurgical equipment
- Interference from ambient light, reducing the quality of the signal.

Some pulse oximeters graphically display the signal they receive as a plethysmogram (Figure 7.15). This should closely resemble the arterial pressure waveform; if this is not the case, the reading for S_pO_2 may be unreliable. Similarly, S_pO_2 readings may be unreliable when the displayed pulse rate does not correlate with the true peripheral pulse rate.

Although the technique has some limitations, pulse oximeters give vital information on both oxygenation and circulation in a quick, simple and non-invasive way. They usually also produce an audible sound for each pulse, with a pitch that varies according to the measured value of S_pO_2. This provides information on pulse rate, pulse rhythm and S_pO_2 even at times when the veterinary surgeon is not looking at the display screen of the device.

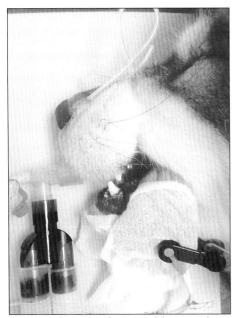

7.14 Placement of a wet swab between the tongue and the pulse oximeter probe may result in better pulse oximeter readings.
(Courtesy of Marieke de Vries, Davies Veterinary Specialists, Higham Gobion, UK)

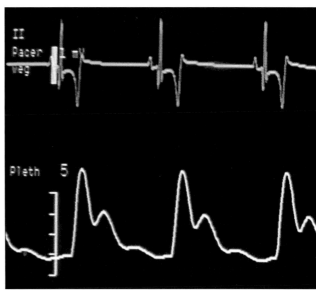

7.15 Plethysmogram (yellow trace). Note the similarity to an arterial pressure trace and the synchrony with the electrocardiogram (green trace).

Blood gas analysis

Blood gas analysis is used to assess:

- Acid–base status
- Adequacy of ventilation
- The ability of the lungs to oxygenate blood.

In traditional bench-top blood gas analysers, the blood sample is aspirated into a circuit, where it is brought into contact with different electrodes. These analysers are expensive, require careful maintenance, and are most often used in larger clinics with a high caseload. However, portable, even hand-held systems, which use disposable cartridges for analysing samples, are also available. Although the cost per analysis is higher with these devices, they are considerably cheaper to purchase and maintain, meaning that they are more economical if a limited number of samples is analysed per day. Depending on the cartridge used, other parameters such as electrolytes, urea, creatinine and/or lactate can be measured simultaneously.

Both arterial and central venous samples can be used for evaluation of acid–base status and ventilation. However, accurate assessment of oxygen uptake in the lungs requires arterial sampling, which can be challenging in very small animals. Possible sites for arterial sampling are the dorsal pedal, femoral, palmar, metatarsal and sublingual arteries in dogs, and the femoral, dorsal pedal and coccygeal arteries in cats. After collection of an arterial blood sample, pressure should be applied to the sampling site for several minutes to avoid haematoma formation. Alternatively, an arterial catheter can be placed for repeated sampling. Venous blood (e.g. for acid–base analysis) is best sampled from the jugular vein. Analysis of lingual venous samples provides clinically acceptable estimations of arterial pH and P_aCO_2 values, but estimation of P_aO_2 is less reliable (Pang et al., 2009).

When collecting either central venous or arterial blood samples, an anaerobic technique and heparinized syringes should always be used, and air bubbles in the sample should be discarded. Arterial blood should be collected slowly, over the course of several breaths, to reduce the influence of variations in P_aO_2 and P_aCO_2 during the respiratory cycle. It is best to analyse samples immediately, because metabolism by leucocytes and erythrocytes will continue within the sample and gases diffuse through the wall of the syringe, both of which will affect the blood gas values. It is often stated that storage of samples in glass syringes and on iced water for a maximum of 1 hour is acceptable, but the magnitude of changes is quite variable and difficult to predict.

Most blood gas analysers measure pH, carbon dioxide tension (PCO_2) and oxygen tension (PO_2). The oxygen saturation of haemoglobin (SO_2) is usually derived from oxyhaemoglobin dissociation curves determined in humans and is not actually measured, except in devices equipped with a co-oximeter. Because of species differences, the calculated value may differ somewhat from the true value, but this difference usually has only limited clinical relevance (Scott et al., 2005). More important, however, is that abnormal forms of haemoglobin are not taken into account. Co-oximetry overcomes this problem by measuring all four types of haemoglobin (oxy-, deoxy-, carboxy- and methaemoglobin). Also, blood gas analysers often calculate values such as base excess, bicarbonate and total carbon dioxide concentration.

Acid–base status

Acid–base status can be assessed by analysing central venous or arterial blood samples. This, coupled with the patient's history, allows detection of respiratory and metabolic acidosis and alkalosis, as well as ongoing compensatory mechanisms (Figure 7.16). When mixed disorders are present, interpretation can be more challenging. Some analysers have the capacity to determine lactate, glucose and electrolyte concentrations (sodium, potassium, chloride and total or ionized calcium), allowing calculation of variables such as anion gap to provide a more complete evaluation of acid–base status.

Disorder	pH	P_aCO_2	Base excess and bicarbonate
Metabolic acidosis	↓	Normal or compensatory ↓	↓
Metabolic alkalosis	↑	Normal or compensatory ↑	↑
Respiratory acidosis	↓	↑	Normal or compensatory ↑
Respiratory alkalosis	↑	↓	Normal or compensatory ↓

7.16 Simplified scheme for interpretation of blood gas results during assessment of acid–base status. The described deviations in pH from normal may be small because of compensatory mechanisms that are activated to maintain homeostasis.

Adequacy of ventilation

Blood gas analysis remains the 'gold standard' for assessing adequacy of ventilation. An increase in P_aCO_2 indicates hypoventilation compared to the amount of carbon dioxide that is being delivered to the lungs; conversely, a decrease in P_aCO_2 indicates hyperventilation. As discussed earlier in this chapter, $P_E'CO_2$, derived by capnography, can be used as a substitute for arterial blood gas analysis, but underestimates P_aCO_2 when there is a significant degree of dead-space ventilation. The normal reference range for PCO_2 in venous blood samples (40–50 mmHg (5.3–6.7 kPa) in dogs; 35–45 mmHg (4.7–6.0 kPa) in cats) is only slightly higher than that for PCO_2 in arterial blood samples (35–45 mmHg (4.7–6.0 kPa) in dogs; 30–40 mmHg (4.0–5.3 kPa) in cats) (Figure 7.17).

Parameter	Unit		Arterial		Venous	
			Mean	95% CI	Mean	95% CI
pH		Dog	7.38	7.38–7.39	7.36	7.36–7.37
		Cat	7.34	7.24–7.44	7.30	7.29–7.31
PCO_2	mmHg	Dog	40	40–41	44	43–45
		Cat	34	27–41	42	33–51
	kPa	Dog	5.3	5.3–5.5	5.9	5.7–6.0
		Cat	4.5	3.6–5.5	5.6	4.4–6.8
PO_2	mmHg	Dog	100	98–101	49	48–51
		Cat	103	88–118	39	27–50
	kPa	Dog	13.3	13.1–13.5	6.5	6.4–6.8
		Cat	13.7	11.7–15.7	5.2	3.6–6.7

7.17 Mean and 95% confidence interval (CI) values for reported arterial and mixed venous (dog; Haskins et al., 2005) or jugular venous (cat; Middleton et al., 1981) values for pH, PCO_2 and PO_2 in healthy awake cats and dogs.

Ability of the lungs to oxygenate blood

Arterial blood gas analysis can also be used to assess the ability of the lungs to oxygenate the blood. It provides more reliable information than pulse oximetry, which is affected by many factors and only provides information on S_pO_2 and not on P_aO_2 (see earlier). When the packed cell volume is simultaneously measured, the values for P_aO_2 and arterial oxygen saturation (S_aO_2) can also be used to calculate the arterial oxygen content (C_aO_2), according to the following equation:

C_aO_2 (ml O_2/dl blood) =
(haemoglobin [g/dl] x S_aO_2 [fraction] x 1.34 [ml/g]) + P_aO_2 (mmHg) x 0.003 ((ml/dl)/mmHg)

This calculation appears somewhat cumbersome, but the equation nicely illustrates the much greater contribution of haemoglobin-bound oxygen than dissolved oxygen (represented by P_aO_2) to the total oxygen content. This means that the main determinants of C_aO_2 are the haemoglobin concentration and S_aO_2. In anaemic patients, C_aO_2 may be dangerously low even if P_aO_2 and S_aO_2 are high, because of the low haemoglobin concentration.

Values for P_aO_2 should always be interpreted alongside the inspired oxygen fraction (F_iO_2). When F_iO_2 is known, the resulting alveolar oxygen tension (P_AO_2) can be calculated using the alveolar gas equation:

P_AO_2 =
F_iO_2 x (atmospheric pressure – 47 mmHg) –
(1.2 x P_aCO_2 [mmHg])

When gas exchange is optimal, P_aO_2 should closely approximate P_AO_2. However, the difference between these values ($P_{[A-a]}O_2$) increases when F_iO_2 becomes higher. The $P_{[A-a]}O_2$ should be <15 mmHg (2 kPa) when F_iO_2 = 21% or <100 mmHg (13.3 kPa) when F_iO_2 = 100%.

A quicker but also useful calculation is the P_aO_2:F_iO_2 ratio. A P_aO_2:F_iO_2 ratio of <300, as well as an increased $P_{[A-a]}O_2$, indicates a significant degree of ventilation–perfusion mismatching and/or right-to-left shunting of pulmonary blood.

Venous oxygenation can also be determined, but mixed venous blood taken from a pulmonary artery catheter is needed for meaningful analysis. By using analysis of venous blood gases in combination with arterial blood gases, a very thorough assessment of oxygen exchange in the lungs and peripheral tissues can be performed, as the results enable calculations to be made of mixed venous oxygen content, oxygen extraction ratio and degree of intrapulmonary shunting. These calculations are mainly performed for research purposes or in critically ill patients. Central venous blood gas values will approximate those of mixed venous blood to a certain degree, but only when the tip of the sampling catheter is either very close to, or within, the right atrium. For clinical purposes, jugular venous samples are usually also regarded as appropriate for analysis.

Arterial blood pressure

Arterial blood pressure (ABP) is one of the most important measures of cardiovascular function available to the veterinary surgeon during anaesthesia. The mean arterial pressure (MAP) is the main factor that overcomes arteriolar resistance, ensuring capillary blood flow. The diastolic arterial pressure (DAP) is mainly determined by the systemic vascular resistance (SVR) and circulating volume. The pulse pressure, which is the difference between systolic arterial pressure (SAP) and DAP, is mainly related to the SV, although factors such as arteriolar tone and elasticity of the arteries are also involved.

Normal ranges in cats and dogs during anaesthesia are 90–120 mmHg for SAP, 55–90 mmHg for DAP and 60–100 mmHg for MAP. In vital organs, the blood flow is autoregulated at MAP values between 60 and 150 mmHg, such that flow through these organs is constant as long as MAP remains within these values. However, if MAP falls below 60 mmHg, perfusion of these organs is likely to become inadequate. It is important to note that ABP is the product of cardiac output and SVR. This means that a normal ABP does not automatically guarantee adequate tissue perfusion: when it results from generalized vasoconstriction combined with a low cardiac output, oxygen delivery to the tissues may be compromised (see Chapter 17). However, hypotension is always pathological.

The ABP can be measured invasively, by means of a catheter directly placed in a peripheral artery, or non-invasively, by means of either the Doppler technique or oscillometry.

Invasive blood pressure measurement

Invasive ABP measurement is reliable and provides continuous information. However, it requires more expensive equipment and placement of an arterial catheter, which can be challenging in smaller patients. An advantage of this technique is that it also allows repeated arterial sampling for blood gas analysis. In dogs, the dorsal pedal artery is most often used, but the palmar, femoral and coccygeal arteries can also be catheterized. In cats, the femoral artery is most commonly used, although the dorsal pedal and coccygeal arteries can also be considered. The catheter is connected to a pressure (usually strain gauge) transducer using non-compliant plastic tubing filled with heparinized saline (1–2 IU/ml). The pressure transducer (Figure 7.18) must be 'zeroed' to atmospheric pressure before use and should be placed at the same height as the right atrium to correct for gravity-induced differences in ABP. Landmarks for estimating the level of the right atrium are the point of the shoulder if the patient is in dorsal recumbency, and the sternum in lateral recumbency. The pressure transducer converts the pressure signal into an electrical signal, which is registered and displayed on a monitor.

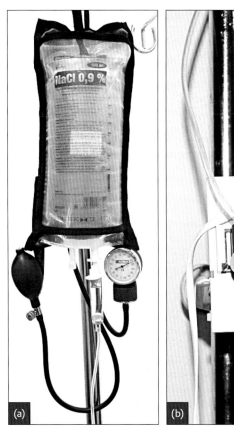

7.18 (a) Continuous flush system used to prevent clot formation and damping of the pressure waveform during invasive arterial blood pressure monitoring. (b) Strain gauge transducer used for blood pressure monitoring.

It is important to avoid the presence of even very small amounts of air in the line connecting the arterial catheter to the transducer, as this will cause significant damping of the waveform (Figure 7.19). Clot formation in the arterial catheter is another potential cause of damping of the pressure trace, but can be avoided by using a pressurized continuous flush system (Figure 7.18a) with heparinized saline. A third potential cause of damping of the waveform is the use of a small catheter (<22 G), for example, in cats. In this case, DAP is usually overestimated and SAP underestimated, while the value for MAP is normally still close to the true value.

The normal ABP waveform is shown in Figure 7.20. During ventricular contraction, blood is ejected into the aorta and peripheral arteries, resulting in the SAP, which forms the peak of the waveform. During ventricular relaxation, the pressure decreases, but once the aortic valve closes, the distended (elastic) aorta contracts, causing a second rise in pressure in the peripheral arteries, which is visible on the arterial pressure trace as the dicrotic notch. The pressure then continues to decline towards the DAP, which is the lowest point of the waveform. Most monitors automatically calculate and display MAP, but if needed it can be calculated manually as:

$$MAP = DAP + \frac{1}{3}(SAP - DAP)$$

The shape of the pressure waveform gives indications of ventricular contractility, cardiac output and SVR. For example, a steep upstroke represents a forceful contraction, while a rapid decrease (narrow wave) and low dicrotic notch are often seen during vasodilation.

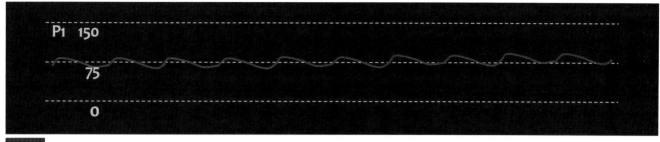

7.19 Damped arterial blood pressure trace.

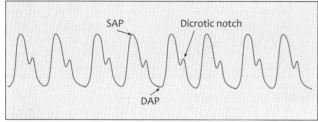

7.20 Arterial blood pressure waveform. DAP = diastolic arterial pressure; SAP = systolic arterial pressure.

Non-invasive blood pressure measurement

Two methods can be used for non-invasive blood pressure measurements in small animals: the Doppler technique and oscillometry. These techniques are easier to perform than invasive measurement; however, they do not allow evaluation of the arterial pressure waveform, are inherently less accurate than the invasive method, and may fail to give a reading in certain circumstances, for example, during hypotension or peripheral vasoconstriction.

Doppler technique: The use of the Doppler technique is shown in Figure 7.21. The technique involves the following steps:

- A cuff, connected to a sphygmomanometer, is placed around an extremity
- A Doppler ultrasound probe is placed on an artery distal to the cuff, such that the pulse waves are clearly audible as a typical 'whoosh' sound. Ultrasound gel should be used to improve the quality of the signal
- The cuff is inflated until the pulses are no longer heard and then gradually deflated

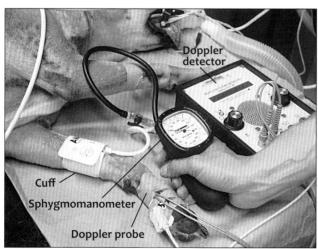

7.21 Doppler monitoring of arterial blood pressure.

- The pressure at which the pulse becomes audible again corresponds to the SAP in dogs. In cats, this technique tends to underestimate SAP and the value measured is usually closer to the MAP (Caulkett *et al.*, 1998)
- The measured pressure must be corrected according to the height of the measurement site (i.e. the cuff) above or below the right atrium: for every 10 cm above the right atrium, the reading will underestimate the true pressure by 7.36 mmHg, while the readings made below the level of the right atrium will be overestimated by 7.36 mmHg for every 10 cm difference.

Doppler measurements can be performed in animals of any size. The equipment required is relatively inexpensive, but the technique requires some operator experience and only provides an estimation of SAP. An advantage, however, is that when the Doppler probe is left in place between measurements, blood flow can be heard continuously. Changes in the pitch of the tone suggest alterations in haemodynamics; irregular rhythms are also audible and can therefore be easily recognized.

Oscillometry: Oscillometric monitors automatically determine ABP by measuring pressure oscillations in a cuff placed around an extremity. These oscillations are detected first at the SAP, have a maximal amplitude at the MAP and suddenly decrease in amplitude around the DAP. Oscillometric monitors can thus determine all three arterial pressures and additionally display the heart rate. However, they may be less reliable or fail to give a reading in smaller patients, especially during hypotension or peripheral vasoconstriction. As with measurements made using the Doppler technique, the values should be corrected according to the height of the measurement site (i.e. the blood pressure cuff) above or below the right atrium.

More recently, so-called 'high-definition oscillometry' has been introduced to the veterinary market. This technology uses a 32-bit processor, allows linear deflation of the cuff and employs a new algorithm specifically designed for animals. These features should improve accuracy and increase the ability of the device to measure blood pressures at high heart rates. Software is available to display or store the data on a personal computer. Conflicting results have, however, been reported for the accuracy and precision of this technique (Chetboul *et al.*, 2010, Wernick *et al.*, 2010, Martel *et al.*, 2013, Rysnik *et al.*, 2013).

For both the Doppler technique and oscillometry, a cuff with a width of 40% of the limb circumference is ideal. A cuff that is too wide will result in underestimation of the pressure, while one that is too narrow will result in overestimation. Care should be taken to ensure that the cuff is placed closely around the extremity but not overtightened, as this can reduce blood flow, leading to underestimation of the pressure. Most cuffs have a mark that should be placed directly over the artery.

Central venous pressure

Central venous pressure (CVP) correlates very closely with right atrial pressure (RAP). It is mainly determined by two factors:

- Venous return, which in turn is determined by:
  - Circulating blood volume
  - Resistance to venous return, which mainly depends on venomotor tone.
- Cardiac output.

Increases in venous return or decreases in cardiac output because of reduced myocardial contractility can both cause an increase in CVP and RAP. Interestingly, however, an increase in CVP tends to reduce venous return and increase cardiac output (by improving right ventricular preload), which may lead to circular reasoning when trying to explain abrupt changes. However, in the absence of acute changes in cardiac output or venomotor tone, RAP gives a measure of the preload of the right ventricle and can be used to guide fluid therapy, as RAP is directly related to circulating blood volume. Conversely, when circulating blood volume and venomotor tone are constant, changes in CVP over a short period of time are usually caused by changes in cardiac function. Measurement of the CVP can thus be useful to differentiate between hypotension caused by hypovolaemia (low CVP) and hypotension caused by cardiac failure (high CVP). More extensive information on CVP is provided in a review by Gelman (2008).

Because the range of normal CVP values is relatively wide (0–6 mmHg or 0–8 cmH$_2$O), single values can be difficult to interpret. Repeated measurements to determine trends will provide more valuable information. Monitoring the response to administration of a fluid bolus can also be of interest: when CVP is low, a transient rise in CVP in response to a fluid bolus, such as 10–20 ml/kg of a crystalloid, suggests hypovolaemia but adequate cardiac function. Subsequent fluid therapy can then be guided on the basis of CVP. In patients with congestive heart failure, a fluid bolus will cause a more pronounced rise in CVP that is sustained for longer (see also Chapter 18).

CVP measurement is mainly performed in critically ill patients who need prolonged fluid therapy and/or are haemodynamically unstable. In most cases, measurements will have already begun before anaesthesia and will be continued afterwards.

To measure CVP, a central venous catheter is usually introduced via the jugular vein and advanced until its tip reaches the thoracic part of the cranial vena cava. Alternatively, a long catheter can be advanced via the femoral or saphenous vein to the thoracic part of the caudal vena cava (peripherally inserted long-stay catheter (Mila®)). If a monitor is available, CVP can then be measured using a pressure transducer in exactly the same way as described above for invasive ABP measurements; this will allow continuous display of the CVP waveform.

If a monitor is not available, CVP can be measured simply by connecting the central venous catheter to a fluid column filled with heparinized saline. When the base of this fluid column is placed at the level of the patient's right atrium, the height of the fluid in the column (in centimetres) represents the CVP (in cmH$_2$O). It may be convenient to replace the fluid column with a pre-filled infusion line, which is connected to the central venous catheter via a three-way stopcock in the infusion set through which fluids are being administered (Figure 7.22). To initiate the measurement with this set-up, the infusion line (representing the fluid column) is held upright and opened to air. The

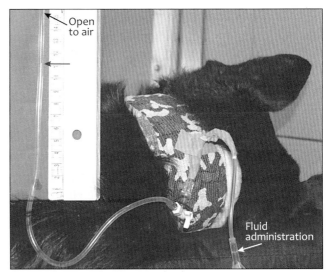

7.22 Central venous pressure (CVP) monitoring. The three-way stopcock is positioned such that fluid administration is discontinued and the open-ended tube (the 'fluid column') is connected to the central venous catheter. The red line represents a pressure of 0 cmH$_2$O, at the level of the right atrium. The red arrow indicates the height of the fluid column and hence the CVP (here, 11.2 cmH$_2$O).

three-way stopcock is then positioned such that fluid administration is discontinued and the 'fluid column' is connected to the central venous catheter. The fluid from the column will initially flow into the patient, until the pressure it exerts because of gravity equalizes with the CVP. At this point, the height of the fluid above the level of the right atrium (in centimetres) is equal to CVP (in cmH$_2$O). Care should be taken to avoid the presence of air bubbles in this system, which may dramatically (but falsely) elevate the reading.

It is important to be aware that because CVP is measured in thoracic veins, changes in intrathoracic pressure in a closed chest, especially during mechanical ventilation, will influence its value. Therefore, measurements should be performed at the end of expiration. Similarly, the use of positive end-expiratory pressure (PEEP) can falsely elevate the readings.

CVP can thus be influenced by many factors, and the values measured can be difficult to interpret. In human medicine, there is a tendency to replace CVP measurement by other indices to guide fluid therapy, such as systolic pressure variation and pulse pressure variation, although these techniques are only applicable during intermittent positive pressure ventilation (see also Chapter 6). The general principle is that ABP and pulse pressure vary between subsequent heartbeats because of changes in intrathoracic pressure (and hence venous return) during the respiratory cycle. The size of these variations depends on the fluid status of the patient and can be used to predict the response to fluid loading. Software is available that continuously calculates these values automatically from ABP measurements (e.g. part of some pulse contour analysis software; see also Chapter 18) or, more recently, even from plethysmographic waveform amplitudes obtained by pulse oximetry.

Electrocardiography

Electrocardiography monitors the electrical activity of the heart. In the normal electrocardiogram (ECG) (Figure 7.23):

- The P wave represents atrial depolarization
- The P–R interval represents the time for conduction through the atria, atrioventricular node and bundle of His

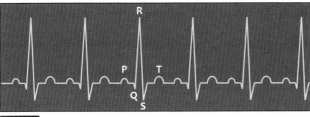

7.23 Normal ECG.

- The QRS complex represents ventricular conduction and depolarization
- The T wave represents ventricular repolarization
- The S–T segment is isoelectric and represents the moment when the ventricles are completely depolarized.

In veterinary anaesthesia, a three-lead system is most often used for electrocardiography. The ECG is recorded between two of the electrodes, with the third electrode serving as the ground electrode. In small animals, the electrodes are usually placed on the paws of the left hindlimb and both forelimbs. Alternatively, the electrodes can be placed in the left inguinal and both axillary regions. If the patient is undergoing surgery that precludes normal placement of the electrodes, a base–apex lead can also be obtained, with one electrode placed dorsal to the heart, the second ventrally (near the apex) and the third peripherally (Figure 7.24). Perfect electrical contact with the skin is needed to obtain reliable results; this can be obtained by using adhesive electrode patches placed on shaved skin or the pads of the feet, transcutaneous needles or crocodile clips. Application of electrode gel is recommended to improve electrical contact. Transoesophageal electrocardiography can also be performed, although this technique is not frequently used in veterinary medicine. With this technique, the leads (Figure 7.25) can be connected to a regular ECG monitor and the signal strength is usually good. The P wave is negative when the leads are more caudal to the atria. Thoracic excursion may cause pronounced wandering of the baseline.

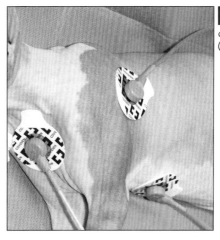

7.24 Alternative placement of a three-lead ECG (base–apex lead).

Although electrocardiography can also be used for other purposes, such as the detection of axis deviation, during anaesthesia it is mainly used to monitor the heart rate and rhythm and to detect changes indicative of electrolyte disturbances and myocardial hypoxia. It is important to remember that a normal ECG does not indicate that ventricular contractions are adequate or even present (e.g. with pulseless electrical activity). On some occasions, the displayed heart rate is incorrect: ECG monitors are normally designed to identify and count the QRS complexes as a measurement of heart rate, but may erroneously also count some or all T waves, especially when these are of relatively large amplitude. The displayed heart rate should therefore be double checked regularly, for example, by comparison with auscultation, pulse palpation, pulse oximetry or arterial pressure trace. Arrhythmias apparent on the ECG should always be distinguished from artefacts, which may be caused by poor electrical contact, movement of the patient or the leads, detachment of electrodes or interference from other electrical devices, especially electrocautery and peripheral nerve stimulators. Further information on common arrhythmias and their treatment can be found in Chapter 21.

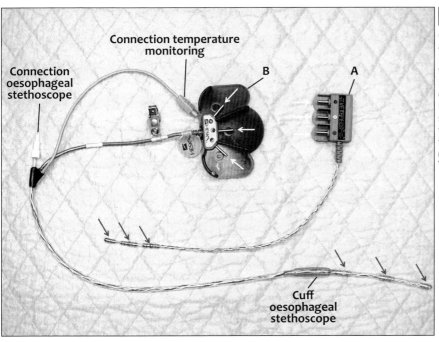

7.25 Probes for transoesophageal electrocardiography in cats or small dogs (A) and medium to large dogs (B). White arrows indicate the cable connectors for normal ECG leads; red arrows indicate the electrodes, which need to be positioned close to the heart. If the probe is inserted too deeply into the oesophagus, the QRS waveform will be inverted. Probe B can also be used as an oesophageal stethoscope and allows measurement of body temperature using an intra-oesophageal thermistor.
(Courtesy of Tanya Duke-Novakovski, Western College of Veterinary Medicine, University of Saskatchewan, Canada)

Connection temperature monitoring

Connection oesophageal stethoscope

B   A

Cuff oesophageal stethoscope

Oxygen analysers

Measurement of the concentration of oxygen within the anaesthetic breathing system helps to avoid delivery of a hypoxic gas mixture to the patient, especially when a mixture of gases, such as oxygen, nitrous oxide and medical air, is used. It is also very useful during low-flow anaesthesia. In healthy anaesthetized patients, a minimal inspired oxygen concentration of 30% should be used. The oxygen concentration can be measured in different ways. For example, in multi-gas monitors, measurement is usually based on the paramagnetic properties of oxygen. However, a simple oxygen sensor (Figure 7.26) utilizing a fuel cell can also be used, for example, in the inspiratory limb of the anaesthetic breathing system. These sensors are relatively expensive and have a limited lifespan which depends on their exposure to oxygen. The lifespan can be increased by avoiding exposure of the sensor to oxygen as much as possible between uses.

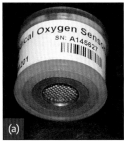
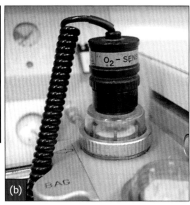

7.26 (a) An oxygen sensor. (b) Oxygen sensor placed in an anaesthetic breathing system.

Depth of anaesthesia

Clinical evaluation of the patient remains the most reliable way to assess anaesthetic depth, and is described in Figures 7.4 and 7.5.

In addition, monitors that measure the inspired and expired concentrations of volatile anaesthetics are available. These devices usually make use of infrared analysis; they can often also measure carbon dioxide concentrations. Measurement of the end-tidal concentration of the inhalant agent (note, *not* the inspired concentration) is a useful aid to the clinical assessment of anaesthetic depth because it reflects the tissue concentration of the agent at its effect site (the brain). However, it should never be used as a replacement for clinical assessments. Simple comparison of the end-tidal concentration of the inhalant agent to the minimum alveolar concentration (MAC) of that specific agent will provide an objective impression of anaesthetic depth. It is generally accepted that 1.2–1.5 x MAC is needed to achieve a surgical depth of anaesthesia if no anaesthetic-sparing drugs have been administered.

In human medicine, recording and analysis of the electroencephalogram (EEG) for assessment of anaesthetic depth is increasingly being used. Examples are the bispectral index (BIS) monitor and evaluation of auditory evoked potentials. EEG monitoring has been described in many animal studies, but to date it has been mainly used for research purposes, and no system is yet available that is sufficiently reliable to be used routinely in clinical veterinary practice.

Spirometry and airway pressures

Spirometry is the measurement of gas flow and volume during breathing. Tidal volume can be measured with simple mechanical systems, such as the Wright's respirometer (Figure 7.27), which are often mounted on the expiratory limb of the anaesthetic breathing system. Some of these devices, for example, the Dräger Volumeter (Figure 7.28), have a built-in timer, which allows determination of minute volume. Electronic spirometers are also available. These simple spirometers are useful for determining whether tidal and minute volumes are within normal limits (7–15 ml/kg and 100–300 ml/kg/min, respectively). However, normal values do not guarantee sufficient alveolar ventilation or normocapnia, since the contribution of dead space volume and the production of carbon dioxide and its delivery to the lungs remain unknown.

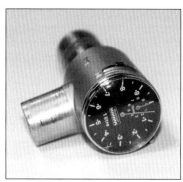

7.27 Wright's respirometer. (Courtesy of Asher Allison, Animal Health Trust, Newmarket, UK)

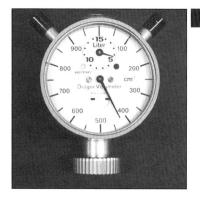

7.28 Dräger Volumeter.

For measurement of gas flow, different techniques can be used, which are often incorporated automatically in modern anaesthetic machines. These are usually based on one of the following mechanisms:

- A pressure drop across a tube with a known resistance to flow. Examples are the Fleisch pneumotachograph and systems using a Pitot tube (Figure 7.29)
- A change in temperature in an electrically heated wire (anemometry)
- The number of revolutions per unit of time of a small turbine (axial turbine flowmetry)
- Ultrasonic changes (ultrasonic flowmeters).

A simple Bourdon gauge (Figure 7.30) can be used to measure the pressure within the breathing system. This is useful in many circumstances:

- During pre-anaesthetic leak tests of the breathing system

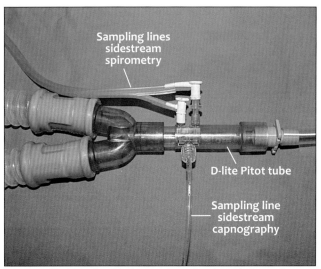

7.29 Pitot tube for sidestream spirometry placed between the Y-piece of the anaesthetic breathing system and the endotracheal tube.

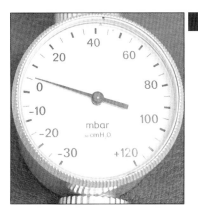

7.30 Bourdon gauge.

- As a guide during manual ventilation and for adjustment of automatic mechanical ventilators
- During mechanical ventilation, the absence of typical pressure swings suggests a major leak or a disconnection between the patient and the anaesthetic machine
- To detect dangerously high airway pressures resulting from incorrect ventilator settings or a closed adjustable pressure-limiting ('pop-off') valve during spontaneous ventilation.

Some devices allow simultaneous measurement of pressure, volume and flow, for example, when sidestream spirometry is performed with D-lite Pitot tubes (GE Healthcare; see Figure 7.29). This allows a very thorough assessment of respiratory function through examination of pressure–volume and flow–volume loops (Figure 7.31).

The pressure–volume loop displays pressure on the X-axis and volume on the Y-axis. The direction of the inspiratory part depends on the type of breathing, that is, spontaneous or mechanical ventilation. The tidal volume can be read on the Y-axis, at the point that corresponds to the highest point of the loop. In normal circumstances, the loop starts at the origin (the zero point where the two axes cross), but when continuous positive airway pressure or PEEP is applied, it starts and ends at a pressure above zero (Figure 7.32a1,b1). The area of the loop is directly proportional to the work of breathing (Figure 7.32c1) and its slope during mechanical ventilation is directly proportional to the compliance of the respiratory system: a very upright

loop indicates that little pressure is needed to deliver a certain tidal volume, and a more horizontal loop indicates that greater pressure was required (Figure 7.32d1).

The flow–volume loop displays volume on the X-axis and flow on the Y-axis (Figure 7.31). The curve is usually plotted with the origin at the right end of the horizontal axis. Inspiration is plotted towards the left (increase in volume) and downwards (flow towards patient), and expiration is plotted to the right (decrease in volume) and upwards (flow towards anaesthetic breathing system). The tidal volume is the difference between the point where the loop crosses the X-axis and its origin. This loop gives a good impression of flow rates during both inspiration and expiration. The early phase of expiration should be characterized by a quick rise to peak flow, followed by a gradual decrease to zero. The shape of this part of the loop is determined by the elastic recoil of the lung and chest wall and by the resistance to expiratory flow, which depends on both patient- and equipment-related factors.

Both pressure–volume and flow–volume loops should start and end at the same point, with a gradual increase in volume during inspiration and a decrease during expiration. A closed loop indicates that the same volume has been exhaled as that inhaled. An open loop, with a lower expired than inspired volume, may be caused by leaks between the site of measurement and the patient's lungs (Figure 7.33a1,a2). Regularly, however, and especially during mechanical ventilation, the expired volume is higher than the inspired volume (Figure 7.33b1,b2). This is not caused by leaks but can be regarded as an erroneous measurement, possibly related to changes in the density (compression during inspiration) and/or temperature of the gases. Irregular loops during mechanical ventilation usually indicate spontaneous respiratory efforts by the patient (Figure 7.33c1,c2). Airway secretions may cause the curves to have a 'rippled' appearance (Figure 7.33d1,d2).

Monitoring neuromuscular blockade

For information on monitoring of neuromuscular blockade, see Chapter 16.

Body temperature

The patient's body temperature often decreases during anaesthesia, as a result of muscle inactivity, reduced metabolic rate, drug-induced peripheral vasodilation and depression of the thermoregulatory centre. Clipping and surgical preparation of the skin, contact of the patient with cold surfaces, exteriorization of intestines during abdominal surgery and air conditioning in the room will all contribute to hypothermia. Hypothermia occurs more rapidly in smaller patients due to their relatively large body surface area:volume ratio. Hypothermia can have pronounced effects on drug metabolism and anaesthetic recovery times, and on immune and cardiovascular function. It is therefore important to take preventive measures, such as insulation of the surgical table, use of warm mattresses (incorporating circulating warm water or conductive fabric) or hot air blankets (see Chapter 3).

On some occasions, however, body temperature may increase during anaesthesia. This may occur when using a circle system with low fresh gas flows in larger-breed dogs, and also in the event of malignant hyperthermia, sepsis, or even as a result of measures taken to prevent hypothermia.

It is therefore important to monitor the patient's body temperature and to take corrective measures when needed. Rectal temperature can be regularly determined using a standard thermometer. Alternatively, monitors are available that measure temperature continuously using a rectal, oesophageal or nasopharyngeal probe that contains a thermistor or thermocouple. A regular thermometer can be carefully inserted into one of the nostrils if no other means of monitoring temperature is available (Figure 7.34).

Nasopharyngeal probes are only reliable when they are in contact with tissue and when there is no gas flow through the nose, and so should be used only in the presence of an endotracheal tube with an inflated cuff. Some warming devices monitor temperature continuously and automatically heat or even cool the patient to obtain the desired preset body temperature. Infrared auricular ther-mometers are also available, but their accuracy (Greer *et al.*, 2007) and precision (Sousa *et al.*, 2011) are reported to be low.

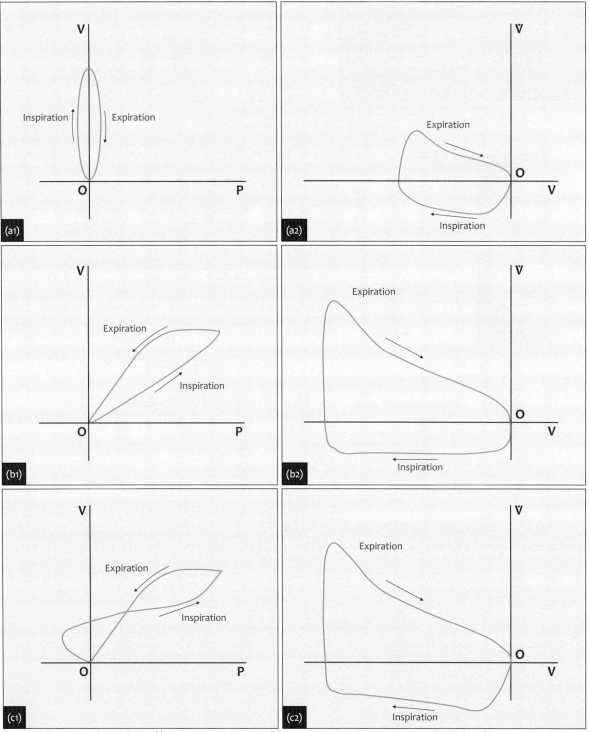

7.31 Spirometry loops during (a) spontaneous breathing, (b) intermittent positive pressure ventilation (IPPV) in a controlled mode and (c) IPPV in an assisted mode. For each type of breathing, (1) pressure (P)–volume (V) and (2) flow($\dot{V}$)–volume (V) loops are shown. During spontaneous breathing, the pressure is negative during inspiration and positive during expiration. During IPPV in a controlled mode, the pressure increases during inspiration and decreases to zero again during expiration. In an assisted mode, the patient generates a negative pressure, triggering the ventilator to deliver a breath, which leads to a positive pressure during the remainder of inspiration. During expiration, the pressure returns to zero.

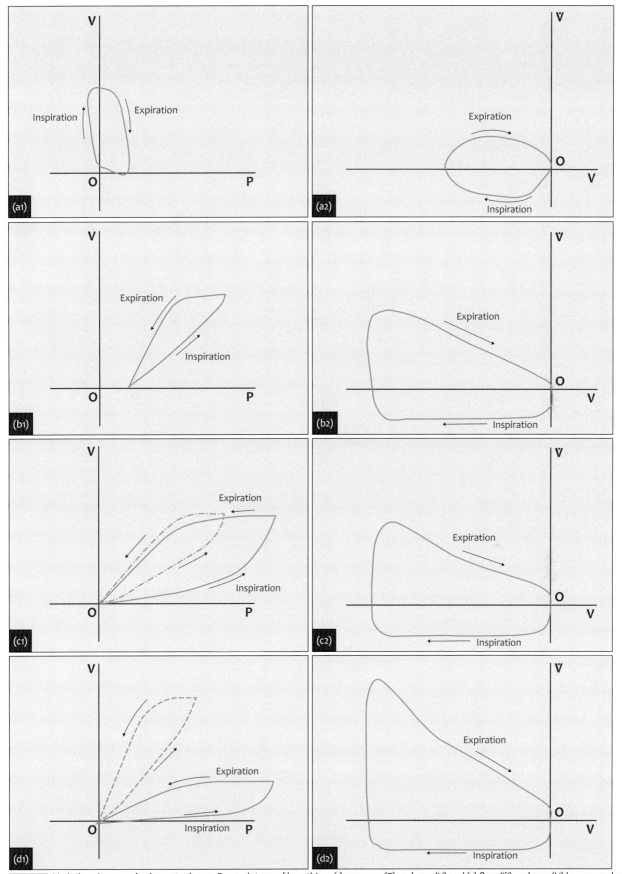

7.32 Variations in normal spirometry loops. For each type of breathing, (1) pressure (P)–volume (V) and (2) flow (V̇)–volume (V) loops are shown. (a) Continuous positive airway pressure with spontaneous breathing, deliberately or because, for example, the adjustable pressure-limiting valve is inadvertently closed. The loop starts and ends at a pressure above zero. Note the more rectangular shape of the pressure–volume loop and the decreased flow during expiration. (b) Intermittent positive pressure ventilation combined with positive end-expiratory pressure. The loop starts and ends at a pressure above zero. Note the somewhat decreased flow during expiration. (c) Increased work of breathing (solid line) compared to the normal curve (dashed line), e.g. in an obese patient. A higher pressure is needed to deliver the same tidal volume. (d) Reduced compliance of the respiratory system (solid line) compared with the normal curve (dashed line) causes the pressure–volume loop to be less steep (closer to the X-axis).

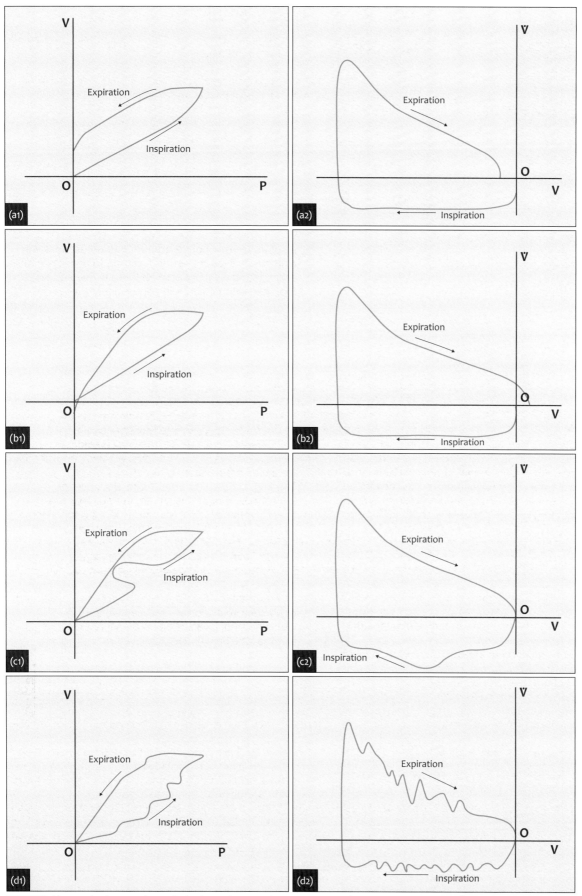

7.33 Abnormal spirometry loops during intermittent positive pressure ventilation. For each type of breathing, (1) pressure (P)–volume (V) and (2) flow (V̇)–volume (V) loops are shown. (a) In the presence of a leak between the sampling site and the patient's lungs the expired volume is lower than the inspired volume. (b) The expired volume is higher than the inspired volume. This artefact is often seen during mechanical ventilation, possibly because of compression of gases by the ventilator during inspiration. (c) Spontaneous respiratory efforts by the patient during intermittent positive pressure ventilation. In this case the inspiratory phase of the loops is distorted. (d) Airway secretions can cause 'ripples' on the spirometry loops.

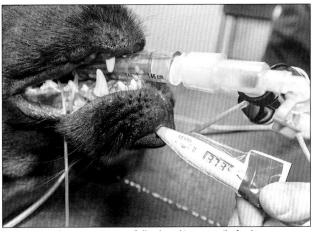

7.34 A thermometer carefully placed in a nostril of a dog.
(Courtesy of Marieke de Vries, Davies Veterinary Specialists, Higham Gobion, UK)

Urine output

Monitoring of urine output is not routinely performed during veterinary anaesthesia, but may be of value in intensive-care patients or in animals with renal or cardiac disease. A pathological decrease in urine output can result from renal disease, cardiovascular failure, hypovolaemia or shock.

Urine output can be monitored by placing an indwelling urinary catheter attached to a sterile collecting system. The collection bag should always be kept below the patient to facilitate urine drainage and avoid retrograde flow. Aseptic technique is essential during placement of the catheter and emptying/replacement of the collection bag, to reduce the risk of urinary tract infections. When inserting the catheter, sterile lubricant should be used to avoid urethral trauma, and care should be taken to avoid bacterial infections. In female patients, after surgical preparation of the perineal region, the catheter is introduced either blindly by palpation of the urethral orifice, or by using a speculum. In males, the penis is extruded from the prepuce to avoid contact of the catheter tip with the prepuce or hairs. In both sexes, the area is best disinfected with, for example, a diluted chlorhexidine solution before the catheter is introduced.

Normal urine production is about 1–2 ml/kg/h in conscious animals. However, it may substantially differ in anaesthetized patients and depends on many factors, such as the health status of the animal, administration of drugs and fluids and the degree of surgical trauma. The volume, colour, odour and turbidity of the urine can provide useful information, as can analysis of urine samples and measurement of specific gravity.

Glucose

Monitoring of blood glucose concentrations is indicated in some patients, for example, in animals with diabetes mellitus or insulinoma (see Chapter 27) and in young animals, which are prone to developing hypoglycaemia in the perioperative period (see Chapter 30). Although simple hand-held devices designed for use in humans can be used, it is preferable to use a veterinary-specific glucometer (AlphaTRAK©). The AlphaTRAK© is more reliable, requires only 0.3–0.6 μl of blood and is calibrated for both feline and canine blood. Further details can be found in Chapter 27.

Guidelines for monitoring

When deciding which monitoring equipment to purchase, there are several factors to consider:

- The practice case load, health status of the patients and types of procedures that are performed. With patients or procedures that have an increased anaesthetic risk, more extensive monitoring will be needed to detect abnormalities rapidly and monitor response to treatment. If magnetic resonance imaging is performed, special (and very expensive) compatible monitoring is needed, because the magnetic field attracts all ferrous materials and disturbs electronic functions (see Chapter 29)
- The anaesthetic technique used. When nitrous oxide or low-flow anaesthesia is used, measurement of the inspired oxygen concentration and the use of pulse oximetry are recommended. During total intravenous anaesthesia (see Chapter 14) there is no need for a monitor that measures the end-tidal agent concentration. Unless an endotracheal tube is placed, capnography is more difficult, although it can be performed using a nasal catheter connected to a sidestream monitor, as mentioned earlier in this chapter
- The organization of the practice. More monitoring equipment will be needed to assist the veterinary surgeon in situations where fewer experienced personnel are available to monitor anaesthesia. It must be stressed, however, that monitors can never replace a dedicated anaesthetist; they may provide incorrect information and should be watched closely (rather than relying on the devices' automated alarms)
- The knowledge of the person responsible for anaesthetic monitoring. A monitoring device is useless if the information it provides is not properly interpreted. Proficiency in clinical monitoring is extremely important even when a comprehensive range of monitoring devices is available, so that both measurement artefacts and equipment failure can be recognized
- Cost-benefit. If no invasive procedures are performed, or no compromised patients (see Chapter 2) anaesthetized, invasive blood pressure monitoring may provide little benefit over noninvasive techniques.

Good practice dictates that a clinical assessment should be performed regularly in all anaesthetized patients, with evaluation of pulse rate, rhythm and quality, respiratory rate and rhythm, capillary refill time, colour of the mucous membranes, palpebral reflexes, eye position, muscle tension and lacrimation. In addition, it is highly desirable to have capnometry/capnography and pulse oximetry available, especially when there is no dedicated person available for monitoring, or during longer procedures. Combined, these two techniques will provide information on the adequacy of ventilation, arterial oxygenation and pulse rate. With longer, more invasive or emergency procedures, ABP measurement and electrocardiography are indispensable. Temperature monitoring is also desirable: at the very least, body temperature should be measured intermittently during longer procedures and at the end of all procedures, so that appropriate measures can be taken for recovery in the event of hypothermia. More advanced monitoring techniques such as blood gas analysis, sidestream spirometry and assessment of urine output are indicated in specific cases.

References and further reading

Cannesson M, Aboy M, Hofer CK and Rehman M (2010) Pulse pressure variation: where are we today? *Journal of Clinical Monitoring and Computing* **25**, 45–56

Caulkett NA, Cantwell SL and Houston DM (1998) A comparison of indirect blood pressure monitoring techniques in the anaesthetized cat. *Veterinary Surgery* **27**, 370–377

Chetboul V, Tissier R, Gouni V *et al.* (2010) Comparison of Doppler ultrasonography and high-definition oscillometry for blood pressure measurements in healthy awake dogs. *American Journal of Veterinary Research* **71**, 766–772

Dalrymple P (2006) Monitoring arterial pressure. *Anaesthesia and Intensive Care Medicine* **7**, 93–94

Dorsch JA and Dorsch SE (2011) *A Practical Approach to Anesthesia Equipment*. Lippincott Williams and Wilkins, Philadelphia

Gelman S (2008) Venous function and central venous pressure: A physiologic story. *Anesthesiology* **108**, 735–748

Greer RJ, Cohn LA, Dodam JR, Wagner-Mann CC and Mann FA (2007) Comparison of three methods of temperature measurement in hypothermic, euthermic and hyperthermic dogs. *Journal of the American Veterinary Medical Association* **230**, 1841–1848

Haskins S, Pascoe PJ, Ilkiw JE *et al.* (2005) Reference cardiopulmonary values in normal dogs. *Comparative Medicine* **55**, 156–161

Hennessey I and Japp A (2007) *Arterial Blood Gases Made Easy, 1st edn.* Churchill Livingstone Elsevier, Edinburgh

Magder S (2006) Central venous pressure: a useful but not so simple measurement. *Critical Care Medicine* **34**, 2224–2227

Martel E, Egner B, Brown SA *et al.* (2013) Comparison of high-definition oscillometry – a non-invasive technique for arterial blood pressure measurement – with a direct invasive method using radio–telemetry in awake healthy cats. *Journal of Feline Medicine and Surgery* **15**, 1104–1113

Middleton DJ, Ilkiw JE and Watson AD (1981) Arterial and venous blood gas tensions in clinically healthy cats. *American Journal of Veterinary Research* **42**, 1609–1611

Pang D, Allaire J, Rondenay Y *et al.* (2009) The use of lingual venous blood to determine the acid-base and blood-gas status of dogs under anaesthesia. *Veterinary Anaesthesia and Analgesia* **36**, 124–132

Pang D, Hethey J, Caulkett NA and Duke-Navakovski T (2007) Partial pressure of end-tidal CO_2 sampled via an intranasal catheter as a substitute for partial pressure of arterial CO_2 in dogs. *Journal of Veterinary Emergency and Critical Care* **17**, 143–148

Rysnik MK, Cripps P and Iff I (2013) A clinical comparison between a non invasive blood pressure monitor using high definition oscillometry (Memodiagnostic MD 15/90 Pro) and invasive arterial blood pressure measurement in anaesthetized dogs. *Veterinary Anaesthesia and Analgesia* **40**, 503–511

Scott NE, Haskins SC, Aldrich J *et al.* (2005) Comparison of measured oxyhaemoglobin saturation and oxygen content with analyzer-calculated values and hand-calculated values obtained in unsedated healthy dogs. *American Journal of Veterinary Research* **66**, 1273–1277

Sousa MG, Carareto R, Pereira-Junior VA and Aquino MC (2011) Comparison between auricular and standard rectal thermometers for the measurement of body temperature in dogs. *Canadian Veterinary Journal* **52**, 403–406

Suarez-Sipmann F, Santos A, Peces-Barba G *et al.* (2013) Pulmonary artery pulsatility is the main cause of cardiogenic oscillations. *Journal of Clinical Monitoring and Computing* **27**, 47–53

Tilley LP, Miller MS and Smith FWK Jr (1993) *Canine and Feline Cardiac Arrhythmias*. Self-Assessment. Williams and Wilkins, Philadelphia

Wernick M, Doherr M, Howard J and Francey T (2010) Evaluation of high definition and conventional oscillometric blood pressure measurement in anaesthetised dogs using ACVIM guidelines. *The Journal of Small Animal Practice* **51**, 318–324

Useful websites

www.capnography.com

Chapter 8

The physiology and pathophysiology of pain

Mary P. Klinck and Eric Troncy

Pain in humans is defined by the International Association for the Study of Pain (IASP) as 'an unpleasant sensory and emotional experience, associated with actual or potential tissue damage, or described in terms of such damage' (IASP, 1979). This definition reflects the multi-dimensional nature of pain and that it is not just a sensory experience. Because the IASP definition relies heavily on the individual describing the pain (i.e. self-reporting), an alternative definition of pain is needed for animals. Molony and Kent (1997) proposed the following definition: 'animal pain is an aversive sensory and emotional experience representing an awareness by the animal of damage or threat to the integrity of its tissues; it changes the animal's physiology and behaviour to reduce or avoid damage, to reduce the likelihood of recurrence, and to promote recovery'.

Pain management in animals has improved over the past 2–3 decades. Previously, there was a tendency both to under-recognize and to under-treat animal pain (Flecknell, 2008). Vertebrate animals share a common anatomy and physiology involved in pain processing; therefore, injuries, diseases and procedures that are painful in humans are likely to be painful in animals. In addition, while physiological adaptive pain can serve a protective function, uncontrolled pain can impede healing and lead to long-term complications.

A variety of pain types are encountered in cats and dogs, including:

- Short-lasting procedural pain (e.g. that due to venepuncture)
- Acute pain associated with injury, illness or surgery
- Chronic pain associated with chronic disease states e.g. osteoarthritis (OA).

Pain is normally proportional to the degree of stimulus, injury or other disease state, but pain and its intensity may also:

- Exceed the stimulus
- Outlast healing or treatment of the inciting cause
- Be present even in the absence of a stimulus.

Such altered pain states tend to be associated with changes in nociceptive processing within the central nervous system (CNS). These changes often play a role in many chronic painful diseases and may explain differences between individuals in the experience of pain intensity produced by similar, detectable pathology (Phillips and Clauw, 2011). In humans, chronic pain may affect the ability to perform certain tasks, and cause sleep disturbance and affective problems such as depression and anxiety (Hadjistavropoulos and Craig, 2002). Comparable sequelae may be present in animals, but are less easily recognized. Understanding the mechanisms of pain helps the practitioner to plan appropriate analgesic protocols and to interpret signs of pain in animals.

Definitions for types of pain

Evolution of definitions

Pain has diverse aetiologies and there is no unifying theory for its various manifestations. Previous definitions of pain were too restrictive, and pain is best described as a combination of various pain types. Most types of pain are in fact of 'mixed origin' and often involve a combination of neuropathic pain with nociceptive and/or inflammatory components; for example, neoplasia can cause mixed pain through a combination of inflammation and the local destruction of tissues and nerves. Many chronic pain states, including those that were previously thought to have purely inflammatory aetiologies (e.g. OA) actually involve mixed pain. It also appears that physiological, protective, nociceptive pain can lead to pathological, deleterious, chronic pain if it is not adequately recognized and treated. Persistent postsurgical pain has characteristics of neuropathic pain (Woolf, 2004; Marchand, 2008), but the contribution of the neuropathic component varies with the type of surgery and probably depends on the degree of surgical nerve injury (Haroutiunian et al., 2013).

Nociceptive (acute) pain

This type of pain is also referred to as physiological, normal, adaptive or protective pain. It occurs when a potentially injurious (noxious) stimulus is applied to the body (Woolf, 2011), and has an intensity and duration proportional to the stimulus (Latremoliere and Woolf, 2009). It usually produces a protective response (e.g. limb withdrawal, behavioural avoidance strategies) and, if no actual injury occurs, stops when the external stimulus is removed. The descriptor 'acute' refers to a pain sensation that is temporary.

An example of nociceptive pain is the pain produced by pinching the skin.

First pain

This is the immediate pain that occurs following the activation of thinly myelinated (rapidly conducting) Aδ nociceptor fibres. It is commonly described by people as sharp, pricking or stabbing in nature (Meintjes, 2012).

Second pain

This is pain associated with the activation of unmyelinated (slowly conducting) C nociceptor fibres, and is therefore perceived after first pain. It is commonly described as slow or burning in nature.

Chronic pain

This term can refer to pain that either outlasts the original tissue injury and the expected healing time or lasts longer than a specified period, generally 3 months. Because of the large differences in life expectancy of different animal species, the first definition may be more applicable for describing chronic pain in animals. Chronic pain is often associated with changes in central pain processing (Phillips and Clauw, 2013).

Inflammatory pain

This type of pain is associated with tissue injury or immune cell activation. Chemical changes in the tissues around the nociceptors either facilitate, or directly cause, nociceptor activation. Pain from a surgical wound and the surrounding tissues is an example of inflammatory pain.

Functional (idiopathic) pain

This is pain that arises in the absence of a detectable tissue or nerve injury; it is therefore difficult to recognize and is rarely diagnosed in animals (Price and Nolan, 2007). It is also called maladaptive or psychogenic pain. Fibromyalgia in humans is associated with functional pain.

Neuropathic pain

This type of pain is initiated or caused by a primary lesion or dysfunction within the nervous system. Secondary changes in both affected and non-affected neurons result in the facilitation or direct activation of nociceptors. Examples of conditions that may be associated with neuropathic pain are diabetic neuropathy and nerve transection (e.g. post-amputation pain).

Processing nociceptive information

The nociceptive pathway consists of peripheral components – nociceptors and their first-order neuron – and complex central components, which consist of second-order and third-order neurons, ascending and descending pain pathways, and internuncial neurons connecting with peripheral nerves to other systems such as viscera and skeletal muscle (Figure 8.1).

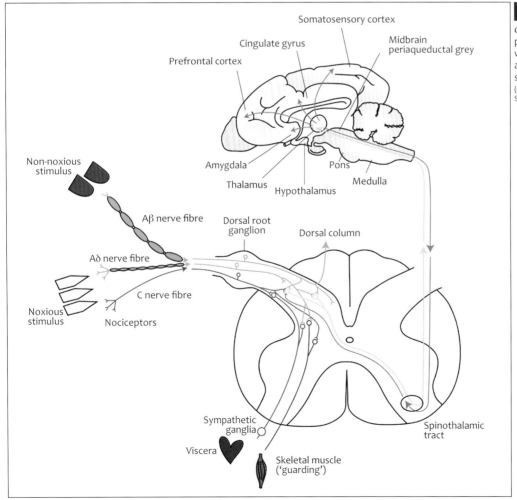

8.1 Diagram illustrating the ascending and descending nociceptive pathways with connections within the spinal cord to the autonomic nervous system and skeletal muscle.
(© Juliane Deubner, University of Saskatchewan, Canada)

The nociceptor and first-order neuron

Nociceptor neurons consist of:

- Specialized, branching, unencapsulated axon terminals in the target tissue (nociceptor)
- An axon (fibre)
- A cell body in the dorsal root ganglion (DRG)
- A central terminal in the dorsal horn of the spinal cord (Figure 8.2a) (Gold and Gebhart, 2010).

They differ from the prototypical neuron, which has a receiving end (dendrite) and a transmitting end (axon) (Figure 8.2b). Instead, nociceptor neurons have a pseudo-unipolar structure, with the cell body connected via a common axonal stalk to both the peripheral and the central terminals; this permits bidirectional transmission of information (Basbaum *et al.*, 2009). The term *dromic* refers to impulse transmission in the normal direction, and *antidromic* is transmission in the opposite direction.

Nociceptor

Nociceptors are present in the skin, muscles, joints and viscera, with the highest numbers being in the skin. They are not found in the brain, except in the meninges (Bear *et al.*, 2007). Their responsiveness varies according to the site and tissue type (Julius and Basbaum, 2001), as well as with the type and strength of the stimulus. For example, cutting and crushing injuries activate nociceptors in the skin, but not necessarily those in the joints, muscle and viscera, while rotation and distension more reliably activate joint and visceral nociceptors. It is important to appreciate that although nociceptors are often called pain-sensing neurons, they merely indicate the presence of potentially harmful stimuli; it is the brain that interprets the signal as painful.

Normal nociceptive processing begins when a potentially injurious stimulus (e.g. mechanical, thermal, electrical or chemical) activates nociceptor cell membrane molecular structures (transducers) (Figure. 8.3). Once triggered, the transducers cause membrane ion channels to open, allowing sodium and calcium ions to move down their respective concentration gradients and resulting in membrane depolarization. If the noxious stimulus is of sufficient amplitude and duration to produce an action potential, an impulse will travel towards the CNS to the dorsal horn of the spinal cord. Flow of potassium ions through membrane channels acts to resist spontaneous depolarization in the resting state; therefore, blockade of potassium channels may also contribute to action potential formation.

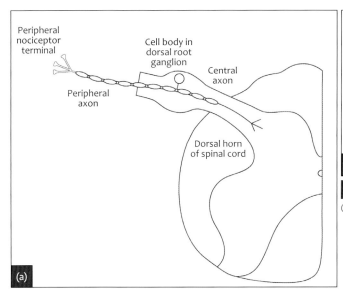

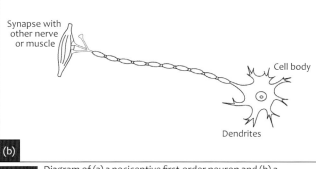

8.2 Diagram of (a) a nociceptive first-order neuron and (b) a prototypical neuron, illustrating structural differences.
(© Juliane Deubner, University of Saskatchewan, Canada)

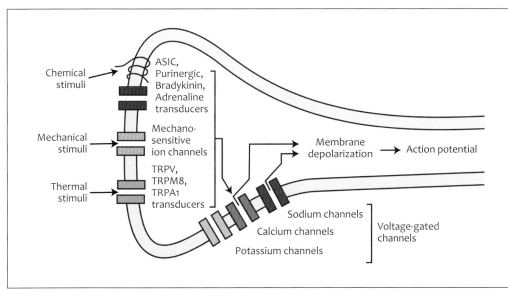

8.3 Diagram of a nociceptor terminal illustrating various transducers sensitive to noxious stimuli and ion channels. Influx of calcium and sodium ions in sufficient concentration will cause an action potential along the nerve axon. Potassium ions are usually inhibitory. ASIC = acid-sensing ion channels; TRP = transient receptor potential.
(© Juliane Deubner, University of Saskatchewan, Canada)

Most nociceptors are polymodal, that is, they respond to multiple types of stimuli. There are also 'silent' nociceptors that become responsive only after they have been sensitized by tissue injury; these have been linked to 'mechanically insensitive afferents' of Type II Aδ (~50%) and C (~30%) fibres (see below) (Dubin and Patapoutian, 2010).

Various channels are associated with stimulus transduction at the nociceptor terminals (see Figure 8.3). These include: mechanosensitive cation channels; purinergic channels (sensitive to adenosine triphosphate (ATP)); acid-sensing ion channels (ASIC); and various transient receptor potential (TRP) ion channels that can detect noxious heat (TRP vanilloid (TRPV) channels, particularly TRPV1) and pressure (TRPV channels), noxious cold (TRP melastatin-8 (TRPM8) and TRPA1 channels), and various chemicals (TRPV1, TRPA1 and TRPM8 channels). Other substances in the tissues (e.g. inflammatory mediators), as well as influences from other channels, can modulate the sensitivity of transduction channels.

Transduction channels can therefore be opened directly (e.g. by protons or capsaicin) or indirectly (via G-protein-coupled receptors and tyrosine kinase receptors). Receptor potentials generated by transduction of noxious stimuli activate voltage-gated ion channels, leading to the generation of an action potential.

First-order neuron

Nociceptive signals are normally transmitted from the periphery to the spinal cord by two types of nociceptive axon fibres: Aδ fibres (thinly myelinated, 1–5 μm diameter) and C fibres (unmyelinated, 0.2–1.5 μm diameter). The Aδ fibres have relatively rapid transmission speeds (~20 m/s) and are responsible for conducting first pain (which should not be confused with 'first'-order neurons). The C fibres have slow transmission speeds (<2 m/s) and are responsible for conducting second pain. The Aδ nociceptors may be classified as:

- Type I: respond to chemical and mechanical stimuli, but have a higher heat threshold compared with Type II unless they are sensitized by tissue injury
- Type II: have a lower heat threshold compared with Type I, but a higher mechanical threshold.

Most C fibres respond to noxious chemical stimuli, such as protons, and to thermal and mechanical stimuli, but some are mechanically insensitive unless they have been sensitized by tissue injury. Peptidergic C fibres release substance P and calcitonin gene-related peptide (CGRP), and have receptors for neural cell derived nerve growth factor (NGF). Non-peptidergic C fibres carry receptors for glial-derived neurotrophic factor. Peptidergic neurons are thought to be involved in inflammatory pain and antidromic 'neurogenic inflammation' (see below) (Chiu et al., 2012). The non-peptidergic neurons may have greater involvement in neuropathic pain (Golden et al., 2010). There is no distinction between Aδ and C fibres in visceral pain, which means that no first and second pain occurs and the pain tends to be poorly localized.

Other sensory neurons (pressure, proprioception) transmit information via large-diameter, myelinated, rapidly conducting Aβ fibres. In the normal state, these Aβ sensory neurons do not transmit pain signals, and their stimulation may even reduce nociceptive transmission: for example, rubbing a painful area can actually reduce pain.

Pharmacological application

Capsaicin (the active component of chilli peppers) can open the TRPV1 channel, but with repeated or prolonged application it causes persistent functional desensitization of the polymodal primary nociceptors associated with TRPV1 activation. Clinically, this mechanism enables the topical application of capsaicin or eugenol (extracted from clove oil), and intrathecal administration of resiniferatoxin (extracted from resin spurge, a cactus-like plant commonly found in Morocco), to be effective.

Capsaicin can therefore be used as a base in which to formulate analgesic molecules. For example, by binding to TRPV1, capsaicin allows the normally ineffective positively charged molecule QX314 (an analogue of lidocaine) to enter neuronal cells and block voltage-gated sodium channels. This mechanism might enable the development of agents that selectively block voltage-gated sodium channels (local anaesthetics, as well as anticonvulsants such as phenytoin or carbamazepine) or N-type calcium channels such as gabapentinoids (gabapentin and pregabalin).

The spinal cord and brain

The spinal cord consists of a central canal filled with cerebrospinal fluid surrounded by the grey matter (divided into the dorsal, lateral and ventral horns) and the more peripheral white matter (Figure 8.4). The dorsal horn is composed of sensory nuclei that receive and process incoming somatosensory information. It is anatomically divided into 10 laminae, based on layer identifications made by the neuroscientist Bror Rexed.

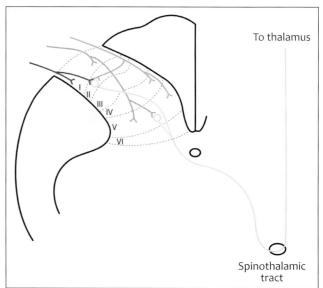

8.4 Diagram of a transverse section of the spinal cord, illustrating the central terminals of the first-order Aβ (green), Aδ (orange) and C (red) neurons within the dorsal horn of the grey matter. The Roman numerals represent the position of the terminals in Rexed's laminae of the spinal cord.

(© Juliane Deubner, University of Saskatchewan, Canada)

Dorsal horn neurons

Nociceptive fibres arriving from the periphery have their cell bodies located either in the DRG of the spinal cord (for neurons innervating most of the body) or in the trigeminal ganglia (for those innervating the head). Their central axonal projections extend into the spinal grey matter to communicate either with second-order neurons located in the dorsal horn, or with the trigeminal subnucleus caudalis in the caudal medulla. Descending pathways have been identified that play a role in pain transmission modulation, mainly through an inhibitory action. Dorsal horn neuron pain signal output therefore depends on the complicated interplay of excitatory inputs and inhibition by spinal interneurons (Kuner, 2010).

Second-order neurons consist of interneurons, neurons of ascending tracts to the brain, intersegmental neurons and projecting neurons, and α-motor neurons involved in reflex withdrawal responses. These connections are partly responsible for muscle guarding of injured sites, withdrawal reflexes and changes within the autonomic nervous system. The Aδ fibres synapse with second-order neurons in Rexed's laminae I and V of the dorsal horn, C fibres synapse in the superficial laminae I and II, and non-nociceptive Aβ fibres synapse in laminae II, IV, and V.

Lamina V contains wide dynamic range (WDR) neurons that respond to both noxious and non-noxious stimulation. The WDR neurons are activated by weak stimuli, but respond with increasing discharge frequency as the intensity of the mechanical stimulus increases. The WDR neurons are important in the descending control of pain, and their sensitization by repetitive nociceptive stimulation plays a key role in the induction of long-term inflammatory and/or neuropathic pain states (Millan, 2002). The WDR neurons also receive visceral input, which explains why visceral pain can be referred to somatic sites, such as the pain in the left arm associated with angina in humans.

Dorsal horn synaptic transmission

Direct excitatory and/or neuromodulatory neurotransmitters are released at synapses in the dorsal horn in quantities proportional to the degree of nociceptor stimulation, to activate receptors on the second-order neuron (Figure 8.5). Glutamate is the main excitatory neurotransmitter (Muir and Woolf, 2001). It acts on the kainate, α-amino-3-hydroxy-5-methyl-4-isoxazolepropionic acid (AMPA) and N-methyl-D-aspartate (NMDA) classes of ionotropic (also known as ligand-gated ion channels) glutamate receptors, and also on metabotropic (G-protein-coupled) glutamate receptors. Other neurotransmitters are also involved, such as substance P, which binds to the neurokinin-1 (NK1) receptor.

Inhibitory substances (Figure 8.6) include gamma-aminobutyric acid (GABA), which decreases neuronal excitability both pre- and postsynaptically through the activation of $GABA_B$ and $GABA_{A,B}$ receptors, respectively. Enkephalin acts in an inhibitory manner on presynaptic voltage-gated calcium channels in the primary afferent nerve terminal. Glycine is primarily inhibitory, but is also required as a co-agonist with glutamate to activate NMDA receptors.

The three main opioid receptors (mu, delta, kappa) and alpha-2 adrenoceptors are co-localized on both pre- and postsynaptic terminals (Riedl *et al.*, 2009). Presynaptic opioid receptor activation is associated with decreased calcium influx and decreased release of neurotransmitter into the synapse (Figure. 8.6). Postsynaptic opioid receptor activation is associated with hyperpolarization (as a result of opening potassium ion channels), which leads to decreased action potential generation and inhibits second-order neuronal activation.

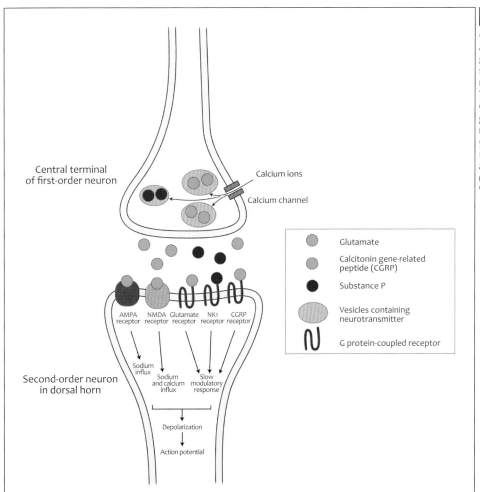

8.5 Diagram of a synapse between first- and second-order nociceptive neurons. Receptors for AMPA and NMDA are ionotropic for glutamate (as is the kainate receptor, not shown on the diagram). The glutamate receptor is metabotropic for glutamate. The metabotropic receptors NK1 and CGRP are for substance P and calcitonin gene-related peptide (CGRP), respectively. AMPA = α-amino-3-hydroxy-5-methyl-4-isoxazolepropionic acid; NK1 = neurokinin-1; NMDA = N-methyl-D-aspartate.
(© Juliane Deubner, University of Saskatchewan, Canada)

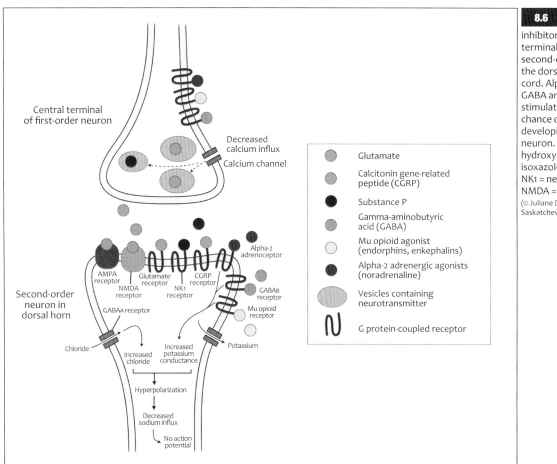

8.6 Diagram showing details of the inhibitory effects between the terminals of first- and second-order neurons within the dorsal horn of the spinal cord. Alpha-2 adrenergic, GABA and mu opioid receptor stimulation decreases the chance of an action potential developing in the second-order neuron. AMPA = α-amino-3-hydroxy-5-methyl-4-isoxazolepropionic acid; NK1 = neurokinin-1; NMDA = N-methyl-D-aspartate.
(© Juliane Deubner, University of Saskatchewan, Canada)

Pharmacological application

Spinal neuronal transmission is the target of many therapeutic interventions, which aim to reduce nociceptive transmission and sensitization processes. Local anaesthetics mainly target the voltage-gated sodium channels. Blocking the sodium channels with anticonvulsants or certain antidepressants inhibits nociceptive conduction and can be useful in the treatment of neuropathic pain. Anticonvulsants can also bind to spinal GABA$_A$ receptors and to cannabinoid receptors to reduce the synaptic release of glutamate.

The anatomical co-localization of opioid and alpha-2 adrenergic receptors at both spinal and supraspinal levels, and the sharing of similar signalling pathways with similar cellular actions, may underlie the mechanism of pharmacological synergism observed with analgesic agents that act at these two receptor types (Chabot-Doré et al., 2014).

Ziconotide, an agent derived from the venom of a Pacific Ocean cone snail, inhibits the N-type calcium channel, which is present throughout the nervous system. When used in humans, to limit adverse effects, ziconotide is administered intrathecally during anaesthesia, but its action within the CNS following recovery from anaesthesia can still generate dizziness, nausea, headache and confusion. Because of this, ziconotide is mainly given to patients with late-stage cancer for analgesia in palliative care.

Glial environment within the dorsal horn

Resident glial cells (astrocytes, oligodendrocytes and microglia) and immigrant T-cells and macrophages infiltrate the dorsal horn following damage to the spinal cord or first-order nociceptive fibres, with subsequent loss of integrity of the blood–CNS barrier. The release of cytokines, excitatory amino acids, neurotrophic factors and prostaglandins (PGs) by microglia can cause hyperexcitability of dorsal horn sensory neurons and central sensitization (Gwak et al., 2012). Dysfunctional glial cells are key contributors in underlying cellular mechanisms contributing to neuropathic pain (gliopathy).

Pharmacological application

Ionic imbalances, neurogenic inflammation and alterations of cell cycle proteins are the predominant neuroanatomical and neurochemical changes that result in glial cell activation and gliopathy. Neuromodulators (anticonvulsants, cannabinoids, gabapentinoids) and anti-inflammatory approaches targeting cytokine release and/or activity can mitigate microglial activation. Anticonvulsants limit the activation of peroxisome proliferator-activated receptors (PPARs) and control microglial activation. Microglial activation can also be decreased by fatty acid-based therapy (n-3 polyunsaturated fatty acids, oleic acid, valproic acid), which reduces the release of pro-inflammatory cytokines involved in PPAR activation, also inducing blockade of voltage-gated sodium channels and a GABAergic effect (Lim et al., 2010; Avila-Martin et al., 2011; Fandel et al., 2013).

Spinocerebral pathways and supraspinal centres

The spinothalamic tract transmits nociceptive information from the dorsal horn of the spinal cord to the brain. Its lateral aspect projects both contralaterally and ipsilaterally to the lateral thalamus and transmits sensory and discriminative information associated with sharp and short-lasting pain. Its medial aspect projects contralaterally to the medial thalamus and is associated with poorly localized, persistent and diffuse pain, the emotional and aversive aspects of pain, and arousal, motivation and motor responses (Lima, 2009). The spinothalamic pathway is the major ascending nociceptive pathway in rodents and primates, but is thought to be less important in carnivores, especially with respect to the spinocervicothalamic tract (Shilo and Pascoe, 2014).

There is some degree of GABA-mediated inhibition of nociceptive transmission in the thalamus. Altered processing of pathways within the thalamus results in the development of a 'thalamo-cortical dysrhythmia', which is recognized as a source of neuropathic pain (Henderson *et al.*, 2013). From the thalamus, nociceptive signals are transmitted to various areas of the brain, including the primary (SI) and secondary (SII) somatosensory cortices, the insular cortex, the anterior (ACG), mid- and posterior cingulate gyrus, the basal ganglia and the frontal motor cortex.

There are also spinal projections that transmit nociceptive information to other parts of the brain, such as the reticular formation, the medulla (including the nucleus of the solitary tract), the pons (including the parabrachial nuclei), the periaqueductal grey (PAG), the hypothalamus, the basal ganglia, the amygdala and the cerebral cortex.

Nociceptive signal transmission therefore occurs via multiple routes, either directly or via multi-synaptic relays. The multitude of brain areas involved in nociceptive processing produces the many aspects of pain, which include sensation and sensory discrimination (SI and SII sensory cortices, insula, lateral thalamus), affective-motivational (emotional) and evaluative-cognitive (learning) effects (amygdala, ACG, mid-cingulate gyrus, insula, basal ganglia), motor responses (motor cortex, basal ganglia), changes in arousal (reticular formation) and autonomic responses (hypothalamus, pons) (Davis and Moayedi, 2013).

Activation in and around SII and the insula are of particular interest, because increased brain metabolism in the SII cortex of cats with OA has been reported (Guillot *et al.*, 2015) (Figure 8.7). These regions are the most strongly activated in response to noxious and innocuous stimuli in neuropathic models compared with controls (Saab, 2012). Greater stimulation was also observed at the level of the thalamus and PAG areas in cats with OA, suggesting the involvement of descending modulatory systems in osteoarthritic cats with chronic pain (Guillot *et al.*, 2015). In addition, electroencephalography has revealed dysfunctional networks in patients that are in pain (Saab, 2012), and the authors of this chapter have found a significantly higher resting electroencephalographic spectral power in cats with OA compared with healthy cats.

Descending pathways and inhibition

Descending fibres influence pain processing and perception in response to a given stimulus, depending on various factors, such as emotional state (e.g. fear, anxiety) and learning. This produces differences in pain experiences for a particular stimulus. The descending modulation of spinal nociceptive processing can be either inhibitory (antinociceptive, endogenous analgesia), for example, for urgent fight-or-flight responses, or facilitatory (pronociceptive). Although various areas of the brain are involved in descending pain modulation, pathways originating in the midbrain are of particular importance; in particular, the PAG and rostroventral medulla (RVM) axis can either inhibit or facilitate dorsal horn pain processing.

The descending modulatory system receives input from the ACG, the anterior insular cortex and the amygdala, allowing influence by affective-motivational and evaluative-cognitive processes. The PAG of the mid-brain has descending inhibitory pathways, which end in enkephalinergic neurons at each spinal segment, producing inhibition of interneurons stimulated by first-order nociceptive fibres. Inhibitory control from the PAG-RVM system preferentially

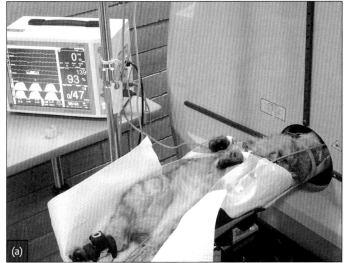
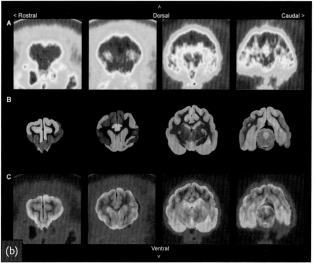

8.7 (a) Increased brain metabolism in the SII cortex as well as the thalamus and PAG of osteoarthritic cats is illustrated in transverse sections of the brain during positron emission tomography/magnetic resonance imaging techniques (Guillot *et al.*, 2015). (b) Four transversal slices of: (A) an osteoarthritic cat brain imaged with [¹⁸F]-fluorodeoxyglucose using a small animal positron emission tomography (PET) scanner; (B) brain regions of interest (ROI) segmented from magnetic resonance (MR) images; (C) PET signal co-registered with MR images. ROI identification from left to right: Slice 1: *salmon*, prefrontal cortex; *aqua*, motor cortex; *purple*, primary somatosensory cortex; *yellow*, anterior cingulate cortex. Slice 2: *purple*, primary somatosensory cortex; *yellow*, anterior cingulate cortex; *dark blue*, insula; *dark red*, secondary somatosensory (SII) cortex. Slice 3: *blue*, thalamus; *dark yellow*, visual cortex. Slice 4: *dark yellow*, visual cortex; *green*, periaqueductal gray (PAG) matter; *orange*, mesencephalon; *light red*, superior temporal cortex.

suppresses nociceptive inputs mediated through C fibres, preserving sensory-discriminative information through sensory A fibres.

Adrenergic and serotonergic pathways descending from the locus coeruleus and nucleus raphe magnus in the brainstem can also activate enkephalinergic neurons in the dorsal horn. There are also (ascending) projections of dopaminergic nociceptive neurons from the substantia nigra in the midbrain to the basal nuclei; dopamine has an analgesic effect in chronic pain. Inhibitory fibres can also be found segmentally in the spinal cord (Woolf and Mannion, 1999), and endogenous opioids (e.g. endorphins, dynorphins and endomorphins) can also be released concurrently with excitatory neurotransmitters (e.g. glutamate) and act on mu, delta and kappa opioid receptors to mediate analgesia. In addition to endogenous opioids, noradrenaline, GABA, serotonin and dopamine, other neurotransmitters involved in antinociceptive pathways include adenosine, somatostatin and cannabinoids.

A commonly used protocol for pain inhibition is based on the diffuse noxious inhibitory control effect, recently renamed conditioned pain modulation. This typically uses two remote painful stimuli, whose interaction generates, in most cases, inhibition of pain (Le Bars et al., 1979). Practical applications in veterinary medicine include the use of nose tongs in cattle, a twitch placed on a horse's upper lip or pinching a skin fold on the neck.

Pharmacological application

The reinforcement of endogenous inhibitory descending modulation using opioid and alpha-2 adrenergic agonists is a popular target for analgesia. Drugs in development include GABA and synthetic cannabinoid agonists. Additional medications found to have central analgesic effects in humans include those with serotonergic and noradrenergic activity, such as tricyclic antidepressants (e.g. amitriptyline), serotonin–noradrenaline reuptake inhibitors (e.g. duloxetine) and, to a lesser extent, selective serotonin re-uptake inhibitors. There is some evidence that these drugs may also act by blocking voltage-gated sodium channels. Tramadol is an example of an analgesic agent that combines opioid, serotonergic and noradrenergic activity.

Altered pain states

Normal pain processing is the result of a carefully maintained equilibrium. When changes occur within nerves or in their environment, that equilibrium is disrupted, producing sensory changes and abnormal pain conditions. Injury to the nervous system can cause both increased and decreased activity, resulting in sensory deficits or loss of sensation, hypersensitivity states, spontaneous pain, and other abnormal sensations.

Signs associated with altered pain states
Allodynia

This is the sensation of pain in response to a normally innocuous stimulus (Figures 8.8 and 8.9). Allodynia may result either from a lowered threshold of nociceptive terminals (as occurs in peripheral sensitization) or from the activation of low-threshold Aβ (sensory) fibres following central sensitization. An example of allodynia is pain in response to light touch, as demonstrated by the

decreased tactile threshold observed in approximately 30% of cats with OA (Guillot et al., 2013).

Hyperalgesia

This refers to an exaggerated pain sensation in response to a normally painful stimulus (Figures 8.8 and 8.9). Hyperalgesia can be classified on the basis of the modality (mechanical, thermal or chemical); in humans, mechanical hyperalgesia is subdivided into either dynamic (evoked by brushing) or static/punctate (evoked by pressure) hyperalgesia. Dynamic hyperalgesia results from central pain responses to Aβ fibre stimulation. An example of hyperalgesia is exaggerated pain in response to a slightly painful procedure such as a skin pinch.

Primary hyperalgesia: Primary hyperalgesia is associated with nociceptor sensitization in the region of an injury, where the nociceptive terminals are exposed to inflammatory mediators. An example of this is the pain felt following surgery in the area of the incision and in the surrounding swelling/bruising.

Secondary hyperalgesia: This refers to hypersensitivity that cannot be explained by sensitization of peripheral nociceptor terminals, because it arises adjacent to, but outside (or even contralateral to), the area where inflammation/injury is present. It provides evidence of central sensitization. An example of secondary hyperalgesia is increased sensitivity to claw trimming in the hindlimb of a dog with hip OA.

Spontaneous pain

As the name implies, spontaneous pain is pain that arises in the absence of a stimulus. This is reported in humans with neuropathic pain, but may be difficult to identify in animals because they are unable to self-report their experience of pain. It may also be difficult to distinguish from paraesthesia or dysaesthesia (see below). A possible manifestation of spontaneous pain in animals is sudden attention to a body part, for example, a tail-docked dog abruptly nibbling at its healed tail stump.

Paraesthesia

This refers to non-painful but abnormal sensations, sometimes described in humans as tickling or tingling. These sensations may result from spontaneous activity in Aβ (sensory) fibres.

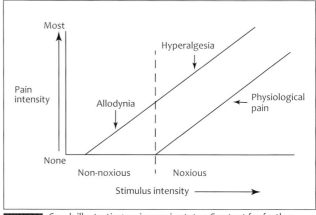

8.8 Graph illustrating various pain states. See text for further details.

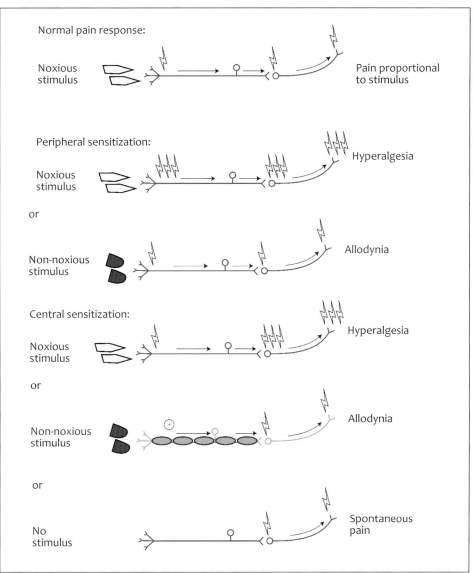

8.9 Diagram illustrating the changes that cause allodynia, hyperalgesia and spontaneous pain.
(© Juliane Deubner, University of Saskatchewan, Canada)

Dysaesthesia

This refers to unpleasant abnormal sensations that may or may not be painful; examples of such sensations reported by humans are burning, shocks, or 'pins and needles'. Dysaesthesia may develop from paraesthesia when central sensitization occurs.

Analgesia

This refers to the absence of pain in response to a normally painful stimulus. By extension, it has been recognized as the treatment of pain, either before (pre-emptive or preventive) or after (curative) it occurs.

Anaesthesia

This refers to an absence of any sensation in response to a stimulus. An example of this is the lack of response to various intensities of hindlimb toe stimulation in a dog with a spinal injury.

Hypoalgesia

This refers to decreased pain sensation in response to a painful stimulus.

Hypoaesthesia

This refers to decreased sensation in response to a stimulus.

Sensitization

Sensitization is defined as a decrease in the threshold and an increase in the magnitude of the response to noxious stimulation. Responsiveness to previously non-noxious stimuli and spontaneous nociceptive signal transmission may both develop.

Peripheral sensitization

Peripheral sensitization is associated with a reduction in the activation threshold and an increase in the responsiveness of peripheral nociceptor terminals (Figure 8.10). The mechanisms by which nociceptors are sensitized include:

- Tissue inflammation secondary to injury, infection, etc., causing changes in the chemical environment of the nociceptor

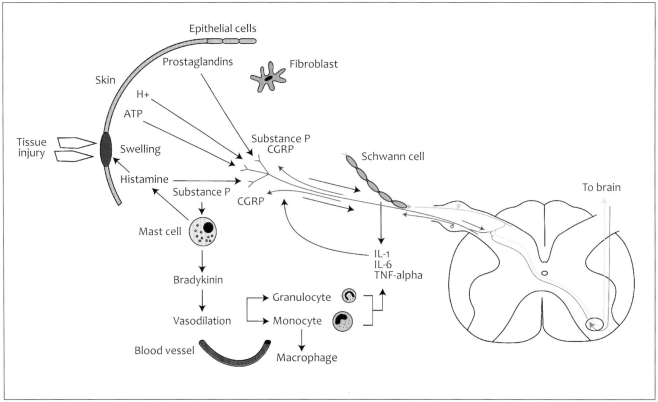

8.10 Diagram showing the action of inflammatory mediators on nociceptors and peripheral sensitization. ATP = adenosine triphosphate; CGRP = calcitonin gene-related peptide; IL = interleukin; TNF = tumour necrosis factor.
(© Juliane Deubner, University of Saskatchewan, Canada)

- Changes in the nociceptive neuron itself, resulting from injury (e.g. altered expression of ion channels)
- Neurogenic inflammation, in which a nociceptive neuron secretes inflammatory substances into its own environment.

Nerve growth factors are implicated in peripheral sensitization states, in that loss of access to these trophic factors after peripheral nerve injury, or their increased production secondary to peripheral inflammation, can increase nociceptor excitability.

Neurogenic inflammation

Peptidergic nociceptive first-order neurons contain substance P and/or CGRP and can release these substances from their peripheral terminals (via antidromic transmission). Both of these substances act directly on vascular endothelial and smooth muscle cells to produce vasodilation and increased capillary permeability. These effects normally contribute to tissue homeostasis, but in injury or sterile inflammation they can produce plasma extravasation and oedema. Both neurotransmitters also sensitize the terminals of injured and adjacent nerves. Nerve growth factor contributes to neurogenic inflammation by promoting increased production of substance P and CGRP in nociceptor neurons.

Nociceptors can release other substances that may also contribute to neurogenic inflammation, including ATP, adrenomedullin, neurokinins, vasoactive intestinal polypeptide (VIP), neuropeptide Y, gastrin-releasing peptide, glutamate, nitric oxide (NO) and cytokines. In addition to vasodilation and plasma extravasation, their release results in the attraction and activation of immune cells; neuropeptides, chemokines and glutamate are chemotactic for neutrophils, eosinophils, macrophages and T cells.

The resulting inflammation sensitizes peripheral nociceptors (see section on inflammatory pain), which then release more immune factors, creating a positive feedback loop. This means that the immune system activation and nociceptor (peripheral) sensitization that occur after injury create the required conditions to prime nociceptive processing, which will lead to central sensitization.

Central sensitization

Central sensitization arises from an increased efficiency of pain signal transmission by nociceptive pathways and can persist following the cessation of nociceptor signalling. It results from intense, prolonged and/or repeated nociceptive input, which may be due to peripheral tissue injury, peripheral nerve injury, or non-injurious noxious stimuli (Figure 8.11). This leads to changes in membrane excitability, synaptic efficacy and/or reductions in inhibition (Latremoliere and Woolf, 2009). Central sensitization therefore represents an uncoupling of the clear stimulus–response relationship with pain, such that, at the extreme, a noxious stimulus may not be necessary for pain to occur. Some individuals appear to be more susceptible to central sensitization than others, and environmental and genetic factors probably contribute to differences between individuals' pain sensitivity and responsiveness to treatment.

Delays in recognition that central sensitization may be responsible for pain in the absence of observable pathology have led to human patients who claimed to be in pain not being taken seriously (Woolf, 2011). This problem is relevant to veterinary surgeons (veterinarians) because animals that respond in an exaggerated manner to relatively benign handling and non-painful procedures may sometimes do so because of this exaggerated processing of pain.

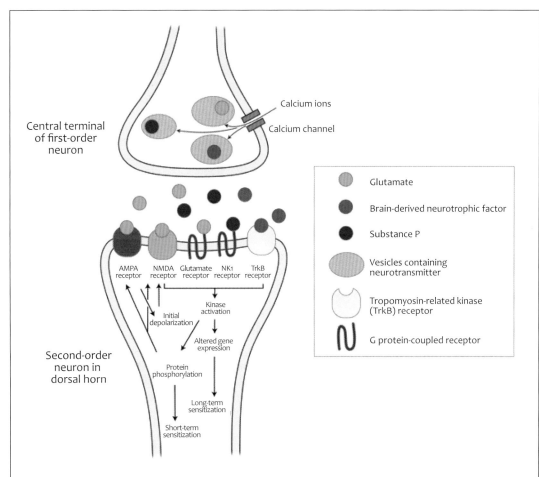

8.11 Central sensitization produces changes within the terminals of the neurons to ensure that nociceptive transmission occurs. See text for further details. AMPA = α-amino-3-hydroxy-5-methyl-4-isoxazolepropionic acid; NK1 = neurokinin-1; NMDA = N-methyl-D-aspartate.

(© Juliane Deubner, University of Saskatchewan, Canada)

Repeated or prolonged nociceptive input from chronic inflammation (e.g. OA) or due to peripheral nerve injury (resulting in increased nociceptor sensitivity or spontaneous activity) will cause central sensitization. After peripheral nerve injury, spinal microglia are activated and accumulate in the dorsal horn around the terminals of the injured neurons; there, they release inflammatory mediators, which further enhance sensitization (Ren and Dubner, 2010). Persistent nociceptive input leads to the activation of protein kinases and phosphorylation of the NMDA receptor, which results in intracellular calcium accumulation. As a consequence, there is increased secretion of excitatory neurotransmitters by nociceptive neurons and increased responsiveness of connecting dorsal horn cells to these neurotransmitters, possibly via increases in dendritic spines, which ensures long-lasting dorsal horn nociceptive transmission (Xu and Yaksh, 2011).

Many parallel signal inputs to dorsal horn neurons can contribute to the initiation of central sensitization, either separately or cooperatively. Dorsal horn neurons normally receive innocuous small-amplitude inputs from low-threshold sensory (Aβ) neurons and from nociceptors outside their receptive fields, in addition to large-amplitude nociceptive inputs. When these low-threshold inputs become capable of activating a dorsal horn neuron, the sensation of pain can be induced by non-nociceptive stimuli, and alterations in receptive fields can develop. In addition, spontaneous activity and temporal summation ('wind-up') of stimuli that would otherwise be subthreshold can occur, so that this repetition of such stimuli generates an increasingly intense response. Once central sensitization has been established, it can then be maintained by a lower-level nociceptive input or by different kinds of non-nociceptive inputs other than those that caused the initial development of central sensitization.

The increased excitability of spinal cord neurons produces heightened clinical pain sensitivity, manifested by a reduced threshold for pain (allodynia), an increased strength and duration of the response to painful stimuli (hyperalgesia), ongoing transmission of pain signals after a stimulus is terminated (after-discharges), and increased peripheral receptor field size, beyond the area of the affected nerve. All of these changes mean that input from neighbouring uninjured tissue can produce pain (secondary hyperalgesia). Patients with central sensitization have lower thermal and mechanical thresholds in a diffuse pattern, which reflects the enlargement of the spinal cord neuron receptive fields. There is a change in nociceptive-specific neurons to become *convergent neurons* – that is, they begin to respond to both innocuous and noxious stimuli. Low-frequency repetition of a fixed-intensity stimulus increases the action potential discharge of dorsal horn neurons followed by after-discharges. This activity-dependent facilitation is called spinal wind-up and, in the presence of spinal plasticity, is associated with temporal and/or spatial summation. Therefore, repeated stimulation results in painful after-sensations that persist after the stimulus is withdrawn, or the rating for the pain (i.e. its intensity) for the last stimulus is greater than the pain rating for the first stimulus, even though the stimuli are exactly the same. There may also be an extension of the receptive field.

Central sensitization also has supraspinal components (Schaible, 2012). For example, microglia in the brainstem are activated after peripheral nerve injury, contributing to supraspinal facilitation of pain signalling. Imaging studies in humans with chronic pain have shown structural changes in various brain regions, although the cause–effect relationship of such changes with pain remains unclear. For example, modifications have been demonstrated in grey matter volume in the prefrontal cortex, insula, ACG and mid-cingulate gyrus, as well as in the thalamus, basal ganglia, SI and SII somatosensory cortices and brainstem; some of these changes resolve following successful pain management. Changes in white matter have also been demonstrated in some pain states, suggesting that in chronic pain there are changes in communication between different areas of the brain.

Possible mechanisms of central sensitization

Some of the mechanisms implicated in central sensitization include altered glutamatergic neurotransmission/ NMDA receptor-mediated hypersensitivity, loss of tonic inhibitory controls, and glial–neuronal interactions. Glutamate, the main excitatory neurotransmitter released by first-order nociceptive neurons, binds to postsynaptic AMPA and kainate ionotropic receptors, causing membrane depolarization. Glutamate also binds to metabotropic glutamate receptors, as well as the normally silent NMDA receptors. The NMDA receptors are activated via a complex cascade of events. Increased AMPA receptor production, phosphorylation (activation) of membrane channels and receptors by tyrosine kinases and activation of intracellular enzymes (e.g. phospholipase A_2) enhance NMDA receptor activity. Full activation of NMDA glutamate receptors also requires the binding of glycine and displacement of a magnesium ion from the calcium channel of this ionotropic receptor; the latter occurs when either substance P, CGRP or AMPA binds to its own receptor on the same membrane. Activation of AMPA/NMDA receptors leads to an increase in intracellular calcium, which results in an increased strength of synaptic connections between nociceptors and dorsal horn neurons.

Substance P and CGRP are involved in transmission between nociceptors and the CNS, and also play a role in central sensitization. Substance P binds to the metabotropic NK1 receptor on second-order neurons, causing long-lasting depolarization. The effect of substance P is potentiated by CGRP receptor stimulation. Synthesis and release of brain-derived neurotrophic factor from nociceptive neurons stimulates tropomyosin-related kinase B receptors, which further activates protein kinases (see Figure 8.11). Wind-up results from activation of NK_1 and CGRP receptors, which permit repeated low-frequency stimuli to produce a cumulative membrane depolarization. Wind-up itself generally lasts only a few seconds.

Bradykinin and serotonin (via 5-HT3 receptors) contribute to central sensitization by increasing synaptic strength, and NO also contributes by activating guanylate cyclase, resulting in increased neuronal excitability and decreased inhibition.

Glycinergic and GABAergic interneurons normally inhibit nociceptive transmission, but this inhibition is lost, possibly through mechanisms including GABAergic neuronal cell death and alterations in potassium–chloride co-transporters, so that GABA receptor activation now depolarizes rather than hyperpolarizes the cell membrane. PGE_2 also acts on spinal excitatory interneurons and projection neurons to cause phosphorylation of glycine receptors, rendering the neurons unresponsive to the inhibitory effects of glycine.

Some forms of activity-dependent plasticity are very brief, others are relatively long-lasting and involve changes in protein phosphorylation and altered gene expression, and some changes are irreversible, with loss of neurons and creation of neuronal sprouting (the formation of new synapses).

With central sensitization, the main therapeutic aim is to block NMDA receptors with the use of drugs such as ketamine, dextromethorphan, amantadine or methadone. Other therapeutic agents include glycine and NK_1 receptor antagonists and inhibitors of neuronal NO synthase or protein kinase. Decreasing presynaptic calcium conductance by administration of gabapentinoids, cannabinoids, opioids or alpha-2 adrenergic agonists reduces neurotransmitter release, thus reducing the transmission of nociceptive information to, and within, the spinal cord neurons and reinforcing endogenous inhibition.

Inflammatory pain

Pain and hypersensitivity resulting from tissue injury are part of a normal protective response. They prevent further damage to an injured area, and promote wound repair by preventing any interference with healing (e.g. by causing the animal to immobilize, and prevent contact with, the affected area). Sensitization of nociceptors is usually reversible; it is normal to have increased nociceptor sensitivity after tissue injury, but this should resolve with healing.

The chemical environment of nociceptor terminals determines their baseline sensitivity and threshold for the generation of action potentials. When tissues are injured, inflammation develops and normally persists until the tissues have healed. Inflammation can alter the chemical environment of the nociceptor, producing a lower threshold for activation, that is, increased sensitivity of both the affected area and adjacent nociceptors exposed to the same chemical changes (see Figure 8.10). Sympathetic postganglionic neurons, Schwann cells, mast cells, basophils, platelets, macrophages, neutrophils, endothelial cells, keratinocytes and fibroblasts also produce mediators that can act on nociceptive neurons following tissue injury.

Inflammatory cytokines including nuclear factor-κB, interleukins (IL-1β, IL-6) and tumour necrosis factor-α (TNF-α) act directly on nociceptors, and promote further inflammation and the production of pro-algesic compounds such as PGs, NGF, bradykinin, and extracellular protons. Substance P and CGRP are both locally released by antidromic activation (the 'local axon reflex'). Other molecules involved in inflammation (serotonin, eicosanoids, thromboxanes, leukotrienes, endocannabinoids, chemokines and extracellular proteases) and mast cell degranulation (histamine, bradykinin) can also sensitize nociceptors. Some inflammatory mediators directly alter neuronal excitability by interacting with membrane ion channels, whereas others (e.g. bradykinin and NGF) act indirectly via metabotropic receptors and secondary messenger cascades. NGF is produced by various cells at inflammatory sites; it alters the expression of membrane channels and receptors such as TRPV1 and voltage-gated sodium channels, and increases the production of substance P and CGRP in DRG neurons.

Neuropathic pain

Neuropathic pain is associated with injury or disease affecting parts of the nervous system, that is, peripheral nerves, DRG or the dorsal root, or the CNS (Mathews, 2008) (Figure 8.12). Some examples of conditions that can produce neuropathic pain in small animals include diabetic neuropathy, amputation or other surgical/traumatic nerve injury and neoplasia. Whereas inflammatory pain may be relieved by eliminating the stimuli that are affecting the inflamed tissue, neuropathic pain may be ongoing. Following nerve injury, a number of changes can occur and may contribute to chronic neuropathic pain: these include changes in the injured nerve itself, in the surrounding nociceptive, sensory and sympathetic nerves, and in glial and Schwann cells.

There may be modifications in the presence, numbers or types of nociceptive neuronal transducers, which include ionotropic and metabotropic receptors. For example, mechanical and/or thermal transducers may appear at or near the cut ends of damaged axons or within the ganglia; certain transducers may be expressed in neurons that do not normally have them; there may be decreases in inhibitory (e.g. opioid) receptors and increases in excitatory (e.g. purinergic) receptors; and there may be changes in the coupling between transducers and signalling pathways. There may also be changes in the expression and/or release of ligands and receptors, and aberrant sources of nociceptor activation may develop.

When a sensory neuron is injured, the number of sodium channels increases both at the site of injury and along the axon and cell body. This results in foci of hypersensitivity and ectopic foci, producing increases in stimulus-evoked pain and in spontaneous pain. There are two main types of sodium channels, tetrodotoxin-sensitive and tetrodotoxin-insensitive, with the insensitive channels normally being found only in nociceptive neurons; however, both types of sodium channels develop in sensory

nerves after they have been injured. Schwann cells can also release TNF-α after nerve injury, which then produces inflammation. Demyelination resulting from injury can also cause hyperexcitability in neurons. In addition, peripheral nerve injury can induce sprouting of Aβ fibres from their usual location in laminae IV and V into laminae I and II of the dorsal horn, which normally receive only C-fibre input. Although C and Aδ fibres may downregulate production of substance P and CGRP following peripheral nerve injury, Aβ fibres begin to produce them, so normally innocuous stimuli can cause release of these neurotransmitters. All of the above changes may result in the interpretation of normally innocuous sensations as painful (allodynia).

Inflammation within a nerve or ganglion can result in alterations to the function and chemistry of a nerve. Inflammation can increase NO because inducible NO synthase is present in neurons and glial cells in the dorsal horn of the spinal cord. NO can sensitize dorsal horn neurons, increase excitatory neurotransmitter output by first-order nociceptive neurons, and increase PG and cytokine production by non-neuronal cells. In addition, PGs released in inflammation (PGE$_2$) can decrease the inhibitory action of glycine, resulting in increased pain sensation.

Neuropathic pain can be associated with an increase in sympathetic nervous system activity. Alpha-1 adrenoceptors develop following injury in both affected and adjacent uninjured nociceptive neurons; alpha-2 adrenoceptors change from being coupled to inhibitory second messenger pathways to being coupled to excitatory pathways, permitting sympathetic nervous system stimulation of nociceptive fibres. Sympathetic axons also sprout in a basket shape around the cell bodies of injured sensory neurons in the DRG.

Peripheral nerve injury can also produce disinhibition of dorsal horn neurons via various mechanisms. Both GABA and opioid receptors are downregulated following injury to afferent nociceptive fibres. In addition, synthesis

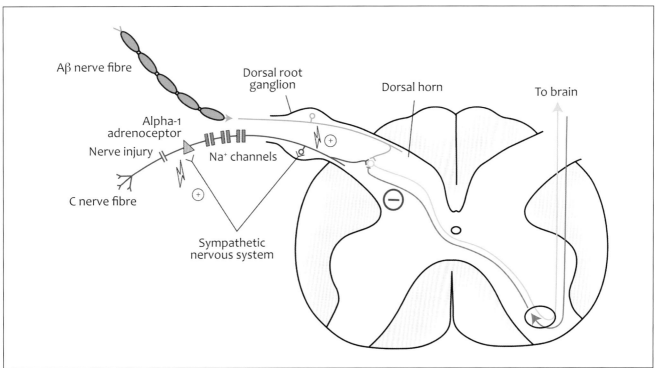

8.12 Neuropathic pain originates from nerve damage and local changes such as increased sympathetic activity and input from Aβ fibres. There is less descending inhibition of nociceptive transmission. Aδ fibres are not shown for clarity.

(© Juliane Deubner, University of Saskatchewan, Canada)

of GABA and glycine may be decreased, production of cholecystokinin (which inhibits opioid receptors) may be increased and inhibitory interneurons may die off, thus altering the normal balance between excitation and inhibition. The result of the decreased inhibitory activity is increased pain sensation.

Neuropathic pain is also associated with decreased thalamic reticular nucleus and SI somatosensory cortex activity, decreased thalamic GABA content and altered functional connectivity between the somatosensory thalamus and various cortical regions associated with pain processing.

Therapeutic targets in the pathophysiology of pain

Analgesic drugs may act at any level in the pain pathway, but an understanding of their mechanisms and sites of action helps to guide selection of an appropriate drug for a given condition. For example, the use of TRPV1 blockade is emerging as a method to stop the transduction and conduction of nociceptive signals.

Local anaesthetics (e.g. lidocaine) provide analgesia by blocking voltage-gated sodium channels, preventing action potential generation in sensory neurons and therefore preventing nociceptive signal transmission from the periphery (see Chapter 11). When administered systemically at low doses, they may also block NMDA receptors in the dorsal horn of the spinal cord, thereby alleviating neuropathic pain (Mathews, 2008). Other compounds target ion channels, such as specific sodium, potassium or calcium channels. In particular, gabapentinoids (gabapentin, pregabalin) that bind to the $\alpha 2\delta 1$ subunit of N-type voltage-dependent calcium channels have been shown to prevent central sensitization (Woolf, 2011; Phillips and Clauw, 2013).

Anti-inflammatory medications include corticosteroids (e.g. prednisolone) and non-steroidal anti-inflammatory drugs (NSAIDs; e.g. carprofen, meloxicam, coxibs). The NSAIDs act by inhibiting cyclo-oxygenases (COX) and block the conversion of arachidonic acid into proinflammatory prostanoids such as PGE_2 (see Chapter 10), which sensitize nociceptor terminals via binding to metabotropic receptors (Julius and Basbaum, 2001). Their use addresses the inflammatory aspect of pain. Removal of inflammatory mediators from affected body parts normalizes the environment surrounding nociceptor terminals, thereby returning their threshold for activation to normal levels. However, COX products are also present in the spinal cord and may interact with the central terminals of nociceptive first-order neurons; for instance, PGE_2 increases the excitability of DRG neurons by altering the activity of tetrodotoxin-resistant sodium channels towards hyperpolarization, and also participates in gliopathy. This suggests that NSAIDs can also have central effects (Schaible, 2012).

Neuropathic pain does not respond to NSAIDs (Woolf and Mannion, 1999) and COX inhibitors are ineffective for central sensitization, unless it was triggered by peripheral inflammation (Woolf, 2011). A related compound, paracetamol (acetaminophen), has analgesic effects that are mediated by inhibitory influences in the dorsal horn, such as reduction of the oxidized form of COX enzymes, interrupting the production of proinflammatory substances, and targeting the cannabinoid pathway (Chiou et al., 2013). This makes paracetamol useful primarily, but not exclusively, for the treatment of inflammatory pain. Therapeutic

blockade of neurogenic inflammation includes the use of anti-cytokines (TNF-α and IL-1β) and NO inhibitors.

Antispasmodic medication (e.g. botulinum toxin) has mechanisms of action including interference with protein transport in neurons and decreased release of glutamate, VIP and neuropeptide Y.

Bisphosphonates reduce bone turnover and osteoclast activity, leading to beneficial effects in the treatment of pain in canine osteosarcoma using zoledronate (Fan et al., 2008) or pamidronate (Fan et al., 2009), or for canine OA using tiludronate (Moreau et al., 2011). The efficacy of tiludronate on pain behaviour and physiological parameters in surgically induced canine OA has been explained by decreased peripheral and central sensitization, as well as by modifications in the release of spinal neuropeptides (Rialland et al., 2014).

Several analgesic drugs have important central effects. Alpha-2 receptor agonists such as dexmedetomidine produce hyperpolarization of spinal projection neurons and inhibition of neurotransmitter release from primary nociceptive afferents, thereby decreasing pain perception (Meintjes, 2012). They show pharmacological synergism with opioid agonists, resulting in potent analgesia (and sedation), which is particularly useful for the treatment of surgical pain (Chabot-Doré et al., 2014).

Mu opioid receptors are most abundant in the PAG of the midbrain and in the substantia gelatinosa of the spinal cord; they act to inhibit neuronal transmission by increasing presynaptic GABA. Both opioid and GABA receptors are found presynaptically on primary sensory neurons and postsynaptically on dorsal horn neurons. There appears to be some functional segregation of opioid receptors at the level of the nociceptor: mu receptors predominate in peptidergic nociceptors, and delta receptors predominate in non-peptidergic receptors. Neuropathic pain may be resistant to opioids (Woolf and Mannion, 1999), and opioids may even induce hyperalgesia in some patients (Phillips and Clauw, 2011).

Antagonists of NMDA such as ketamine and amantadine block the excitatory effects of glutamate and can block central sensitization, as well as alleviate neuropathic pain (Woolf and Mannion, 1999; Woolf, 2011). The use of ketamine infusions is common to counteract or prevent central sensitization (see Chapter 10).

Treatments believed to act by restoring endogenous inhibitory systems include drugs that mimic descending or local inhibitory pathways (alpha-2 adrenergic agonists, opioids, tricyclic antidepressants, serotonin and/or noradrenaline reuptake inhibitors, and GABA agonists such as baclofen) (Woolf and Mannion, 1999).

Pregabalin and gabapentin are also centrally acting analgesics. Their mechanisms of action are unclear, but may involve blocking of N-type voltage-gated calcium channels (Basbaum et al., 2009), presynaptic inhibition of glutamate release (Meintjes, 2012) and inhibition of excitatory synaptogenesis (Kuner, 2010). These drugs seem to be effective both in reducing central sensitization and in some cases of neuropathic pain (Woolf and Mannion, 1999; Woolf, 2011; Phillips and Clauw, 2013).

Non-pharmacological analgesic techniques also exist, including acupuncture, massage, heat and cold therapy, and transcutaneous nerve stimulation. These techniques may provide analgesia in various pain states, including neuropathic pain (Woolf and Mannion, 1999), by activating either segmentary inhibitory control (the gate control theory), and/or descending inhibitory systems (Kuner, 2010). Therapeutic diets including n-3 polyunsaturated fatty acids may have anti-inflammatory and anti-neuropathic properties, and provide another therapeutic option.

Physiological considerations in pain assessment

An understanding of the physiology of pain processing also permits the manifestations of pain to be explained and predicted to some degree. In humans with chronic pain and some neuropathies, quantitative sensory testing (QST) has been recommended (Backonja et al., 2013). QST involves measuring and mapping abnormalities of sensation, including hyperalgesia, allodynia, hypoalgesia or analgesia, and the responses to different types of stimuli (e.g. brush versus punctate mechanical, hot versus cold). These measurements quantify either altered conditioned pain modulation or exacerbated facilitatory pain processing, or both (Tousignant-Laflamme et al., 2008). Although animals cannot make verbal reports of sensation, some degree of QST is possible and can be used to detect peripheral and central sensitization in conditions associated with pain or sensory loss (Lascelles, 2013). For example, central sensitization can be detected using withdrawal reflexes (such as von Frey tests in a laboratory setting) and by identifying allodynia and hyperalgesia in areas that have no demonstrable pathology but surround an injury (Woolf, 2011). Examples of conditions in animals with evidence of central sensitization identifiable using QST are foot rot in sheep (Ley et al., 1995), OA in cats (Guillot et al., 2013), cranial cruciate ligament rupture in dogs (Brydges et al., 2012; Rialland et al., 2014) and ovariohysterectomy in dogs (Lascelles et al., 1997).

While QST shows promise as a pain assessment tool, its standardized clinical use has not yet been established in animals. It is also important to consider that QST focuses on the nociceptive (sensory) aspect of pain, and may not reflect the full pain experience of the individual (including affective-motivational and evaluative-cognitive effects) (Brown, 2012). Moreover, although conditioned pain modulation can be determined in human patients, it is more difficult to evaluate in animals. However, mechanical temporal summation responses are faster in cats with OA compared with responses in healthy cats (Guillot et al., 2014), and central sensitization (assessed by electrical QST) has demonstrated a clear association with clinical signs, such as kinetics or lameness, in OA-affected dogs (Rialland et al., 2014).

Pain has emotional, learning and other behavioural aspects; as a result, spontaneous behaviour and behavioural responses to touch and other interactions can be used to assess pain, either in a relatively unstructured manner or by using validated pain scales (see Chapter 9). If pain scales are used, they must be reliable and valid for the particular species, condition and context before being used for the clinical assessment of pain (Streiner and Norman, 2009). In human patients with pain, neurological tests can detect changes in the structure and function of the brain compared with individuals without pain; however, practical factors may limit the usefulness of such evaluations in animals.

Conclusion

Pain processing is a complex phenomenon that involves sensory, emotional and learning aspects. Injury, disease or surgery affects tissues and/or nerves and results in altered sensation, including pain, which may or may not outlast the healing process. Central sensitization is an important consideration in the treatment of pain. It is likely to be present in many acute and chronic conditions, whether they were initiated by nerve or tissue injury, and it may manifest itself as painful reactions to contact with apparently uninjured body parts. Central sensitization should be considered in any chronic condition where inflammation or nerve pathology exists, and it may explain differences in the intensity of pain between individuals with comparable detectable pathology (e.g. differences in OA pain in the presence of similar joint pathology). Even in animals without obvious injury, abnormalities of sensation may exist. An understanding of the physiological mechanisms involved in different types of pain can help the veterinary surgeon to predict the pain associated with specific conditions and injuries, and to select the most appropriate analgesics. Although evaluation of pain in animals is challenging and lags behind that in humans, partly due to animals' lack of self-reporting, consideration of the sensory, emotional and learning aspects of pain may assist the practitioner in detecting signs of pain during history taking and physical examination. Standardized assessments including validated pain scales, QST, and possibly even neuroimaging hold promise for the future management of pain.

References and further reading

Avila-Martin G, Galan-Arriero I, Gómez-Soriano J et al. (2011) Treatment of rat spinal cord injury with the neurotrophic factor albumin-oleic acid: translational application for paralysis, spasticity and pain. PLoS ONE 6, e26107

Backonja M, Attal N, Baron R et al. (2013) Value of quantitative sensory testing in neurological and pain disorders: NeuPSIG consensus. Pain 154, 1807–1819

Basbaum AI, Bautista DM, Scherrer G and Julius D (2009) Cellular and molecular mechanisms of pain. Cell 139, 267–284

Bear MF, Connors BW and Paradiso MA (2007) The somatic sensory system. In: Neuroscience: Exploring the Brain, 3rd edn, ed. MF Bear, BW Connors and MA Paradiso, pp. 408–422. Lippincott Williams and Wilkins, Baltimore

Brown DC (2012) Quantitative sensory testing: a stimulating look at chronic pain. The Veterinary Journal 193, 315–316

Brydges NM, Argyle DJ, Mosley JR et al. (2012) Clinical assessments of increased sensory sensitivity in dogs with cranial cruciate ligament rupture. The Veterinary Journal 193, 545–550

Chabot-Doré AJ, Schuster DJ, Stone LS et al. (2014) Analgesic synergy between opioid and alpha-2 adrenergic receptors. British Journal of Pharmacology 172, 388–402

Chiou LC, Hu SS and Ho YC (2013) Targeting the cannabinoid system for pain relief? Acta Anaesthesiologica Taiwan 51, 161–170

Chiu IM, von Hehn CA and Woolf CJ (2012) Neurogenic inflammation and the peripheral nervous system in host defense and immunopathology. Nature Neuroscience 15, 1063–1067

Davis KD and Moayedi M (2013) Central mechanisms of pain revealed through functional and structural MRI. Journal of Neuroimmune Pharmacology 8, 518–534

Dubin AE and Patapoutian A (2010) Nociceptors: the sensors of the pain pathway. Journal of Clinical Investigation 120, 3760–3772

Fan TM, Charney SC, de Lorimier LP et al. (2009) Double-blind placebo-controlled trial of adjuvant pamidronate with palliative radiotherapy and intravenous doxorubicin for canine appendicular osteosarcoma bone pain. Journal of Veterinary Internal Medicine 23, 152–160

Fan TM, de Lorimier LP, Garrett LD et al. (2008) The bone biologic effects of zoledronate in healthy dogs and dogs with malignant osteolysis. Journal of Veterinary Internal Medicine 22, 380–387

Fandel D, Wasmuht D, Avila-Martin G et al. (2013) Spinal cord injury induced changes of nuclear receptors PPARα and LXRβ and modulation with oleic acid/albumin treatment. Brain Research 1535, 89–105

Flecknell P (2008) Analgesia from a veterinary perspective. British Journal of Anaesthesia 101, 121–124

Gold MS and Gebhart GF (2010) Nociceptor sensitisation in pain pathogenesis. Nature Medicine 16, 1248–1257

Golden JP, Hoshi M and Nassar MA (2010) RET signalling is required for survival and normal function of nonpeptidergic nociceptors. Journal of Neuroscience 30, 3983–3994

Guillot M, Chartrand G, Chav, R et al. (2015) [18F]-fluorodeoxyglucose positron emission tomography of the cat brain: a feasibility study to investigate osteoarthritis-associated pain. The Veterinary Journal 204, 299–303

Guillot M, Moreau M, Heit M *et al.* (2013) Characterization of osteoarthritis in cats and meloxicam efficacy using objective chronic pain evaluation tools. *The Veterinary Journal* **196**, 360–367

Guillot M, Taylor PM, Rialland P *et al.* (2014) Evoked temporal summation in cats to highlight central sensitization related to osteoarthritis-associated chronic pain: a preliminary study. *PLoS ONE* **9**, e97347

Gwak YS, Kang J, Unabia GC *et al.* (2012) Spatial and temporal activation of spinal glial cells: role of gliopathy in central neuropathic pain following spinal cord injury in rats. *Experimental Neurology* **234**, 362–372

Hadjistavropoulos T and Craig KD. (2002) A theoretical framework for understanding self-report and observational measures of pain: a communications model. *Behaviour Research and Therapy* **40**, 551–570

Haroutiunian S, Nikolajsen L, Finnerup NB and Jensen TS (2013) The neuropathic component in persistent postsurgical pain: a systematic literature review. *Pain* **154**, 95–102

Henderson LA, Peck CC, Petersen ET *et al.* (2013) Chronic pain: lost inhibition. *Journal of Neuroscience* **33**, 7574–7582

International Association for the Study of Pain (1979) The need of a taxonomy. *Pain* **6**, 247–252

Julius D and Basbaum AI (2001) Molecular mechanisms of nociception. *Nature* **413**, 203–210

Kuner R (2010) Central mechanisms of pathological pain. *Nature Medicine* **16**, 1258–1266

Lascelles BDX (2013) Getting a sense of sensations. *The Veterinary Journal* **197**, 115–117

Lascelles BDX, Cripps PJ and Waterman AE (1997) Post-operative central hypersensitivity and pain: the pre-emptive value of pethidine for ovariohysterectomy. *Pain* **73**, 461–471

Latremoliere A and Woolf CJ (2009) Central sensitisation: a generator of pain hypersensitivity by central neural plasticity. *Journal of Pain* **10**, 895–926

Le Bars D, Dickenson AH and Besson JM (1979) Diffuse noxious inhibitory controls (DNIC). II. Lack of effect on non-convergent neurones, supraspinal involvement and theoretical implications. *Pain* **6**, 305–327

Ley SJ, Waterman AE and Livingston A (1995) A field study of the effect of lameness on mechanical nociceptive thresholds in sheep. *Veterinary Record* **137**, 85–87

Lim SN, Huang W, Hall JC *et al.* (2010) The acute administration of eicosapentaenoic acid is neuroprotective after spinal cord compression injury in rats. *Prostaglandins, Leukotrienes, and Essential Fatty Acids* **83**, 193–201

Lima D (2009) Ascending pathways: anatomy and physiology. In: *Science of Pain*, ed. AI Basbaum and C Bushnell, pp. 477–526. Academic Press, Oxford

Marchand S (2008) The physiology of pain mechanisms: from the periphery to the brain. *Rheumatic Disease Clinics of North America* **34**, 285–309

Mathews KA (2008) Neuropathic pain in dogs and cats: if only they could tell us if they hurt. *Veterinary Clinics of North America: Small Animal Practice* **38**, 1365–1414

Meintjes RA (2012) An overview of the physiology of pain for the veterinarian. *The Veterinary Journal* **193**, 344–348

Millan MJ (2002) Descending control of pain. *Progress in Neurobiology* **66**, 355–474

Molony V and Kent JE (1997) Assessment of acute pain in farm animals using behavioural and physiological measurements. *Journal of Animal Science* **75**, 266–272

Moreau M, Rialland P, Pelletier JP *et al.* (2011) Tiludronate treatment improves structural changes and symptoms of osteoarthritis in the canine anterior cruciate ligament model. *Arthritis Research and Therapy* **13**, R98

Muir WW and Woolf CJ (2001) Mechanisms of pain and their therapeutic implications. *Journal of the American Veterinary Medical Association* **219**, 1346–1356

Phillips K and Clauw DJ (2011) Central pain mechanisms in chronic pain states – maybe it is all in their head. *Best Practice and Research: Clinical Rheumatology* **25**, 141–154

Phillips K and Clauw DJ (2013) Central pain mechanisms in rheumatic diseases: future directions. *Arthritis and Rheumatism* **65**, 291–302

Price J and Nolan A (2007) The physiology and pathophysiology of pain. In: *BSAVA Manual of Canine and Feline Anaesthesia and Analgesia, 2nd edn*, ed. C Seymour and T Duke-Novakovski, pp. 79–88. BSAVA Publications, Gloucester

Ren K and Dubner R (2010) Interactions between the immune and nervous systems in pain. *Nature Medicine* **16**, 1267–1276

Rialland P, Otis C, Moreau M *et al.* (2014) Association between sensitisation and pain related behaviours in an experimental canine model of osteoarthritis. *Pain* **155**, 2071–2079

Riedl MS, Schnell SA, Overland AC *et al.* (2009) Coexpression of alpha 2A-adrenergic and delta-opioid receptors in substance P-containing terminals in rat dorsal horn. *Journal of Comparative Neurology* **513**, 385–398

Saab CY (2012) Pain-related changes in the brain: diagnostic and therapeutic potentials. *Trends in Neurosciences* **35**, 629–637

Schaible H-G (2012) Mechanisms of chronic pain in osteoarthritis. *Current Rheumatology Reports* **14**, 549–556

Shilo Y and Pascoe PJ (2014) Anatomy, physiology, and pathophysiology of pain. In: *Pain Management in Veterinary Practice, 1st edn*, ed. CM Egger, L Love and T Doherty, pp. 9–27. John Wiley & Sons, Ames

Streiner DL and Norman GR (2009) Introduction. In: *Health Measurement Scales: A Practical Guide to Their Development and Use, 4th edn*, ed. DL Streiner and GR Norman. Oxford Scholarship, Oxford. doi: 10.1093/acprof:o so/9780199231881.001.0001

Tousignant-Laflamme Y, Page S, Goffaux P *et al.* (2008) An experimental model to measure excitatory and inhibitory pain mechanisms in humans. *Brain Research* **1230**, 73–79

Woolf CJ (2004) Pain: moving from symptom control toward mechanism-specific pharmacologic management. *Annals of Internal Medicine* **140**, 441–451

Woolf CJ (2011) Central sensitisation: implications for the diagnosis and treatment of pain. *Pain* **152**, S2–S15

Woolf CJ and Mannion RJ (1999) Neuropathic pain: aetiology, symptoms, mechanisms, and management. *Lancet* **353**, 1959–1964

WSAVA Global Pain Council (2014) WSAVA Guidelines for Recognition, Assessment and Treatment of Pain. *Journal of Small Animal Practice* **55(6)**, E10–E68

Xu Q and Yaksh TL (2011) A brief comparison of the pathophysiology of inflammatory versus neuropathic pain. *Current Opinion in Anaesthesiology* **24**, 400–407

Chapter 9

Pain assessment methods

Ludovic Pelligand and Sandra Sanchis Mora

Importance of pain assessment and method validation

Pain is often considered to be the fifth vital sign, alongside body temperature, pulse rate, respiratory rate and blood pressure. The recognition and management of pain in animals has gained considerable momentum over the past three decades. Successful recognition and management of pain results in improved patient welfare, lower incidence of chronic refractory pain and greater owner satisfaction (associated with faster recovery and reduced incidence of patient readmission).

However, pain recognition in veterinary patients remains challenging as animals are unable to fully convey what they are experiencing. In humans, the experience of pain includes three recognized components. The first ('sensory-discriminative') component relates to pain intensity, location and duration, and may be objectively quantified in animals. However, the 'affective-motivational' (emotional and aversive aspect of pain) and 'cognitive-evaluative' (evaluation of the consequences of pain for one's quality of life) components can only be, at best, extrapolated from the clinician's or owner's perception.

Veterinary surgeons (veterinarians) evaluating pain may base their judgement on subjective assessment methods (purposely designed pain-scoring scales or tools) or on objective measurements that have been proven to correlate with pain. There are many pain-assessment tools designed for use in humans but only a few have been validated for use in veterinary medicine. The clinical validation of these tools explores their *validity* (the extent to which they actually measure pain), *repeatability* and *sensitivity to change*. Good readability of the material used in applying the tool and the time required to apply the tool are of practical importance in a busy clinic. Pain-assessment tools are validated in a specific animal population (e.g. for acute pain in cats after neutering) and may not be as reliable if applied to other types of pain and patient population.

Objective measures of pain

Objective measures of pain include quantification of physiological and biochemical responses to nociceptive stimuli and measurement of the animal's activity or nociceptive thresholds.

Physiological and neuroendocrine markers

Heart and respiratory rates and arterial blood pressure can be used in the assessment of acute pain. Analysis of trends in these variables is useful in the conscious or anaesthetized patient to recognize the presence of a nociceptive stimulus. However, these changes are not specific enough to differentiate pain from anxiety or fear in conscious patients, or from pre-existing clinical conditions such as hypovolaemia or phaeochromocytoma. Electrophysiological studies (electroencephalography, bispectral index) during anaesthesia and heart rate variability have been explored as potential predictors of nociception and pain in research settings, but their practical applicability in the clinical setting and their specificity for pain remain questionable.

Circulating stress hormones (plasma adrenaline, noradrenaline and cortisol), endogenous endorphins and certain other neuropeptides have been explored as 'biomarkers' of pain. Although none of these are specific enough to identify pain when used alone, they may be useful when integrated into a pain-scoring system. However, the assays for these markers are costly, invasive and of limited use as cage-side tests.

Objective physical measurements of lameness, nociception and activity

For objective evaluation of lameness, a thorough orthopaedic and subjective lameness examination can be augmented by ground reaction force measurement, acquired through the use of a force plate or pressure mats. The use of these instruments is currently restricted to research settings or veterinary referral hospitals because of their cost, the high level of expertise required to acquire and interpret the data, as well as the need to familiarize the animal with these tools in order to standardize the measurement.

Quantitative sensory testing includes assessing the response to mechanical, thermal (heat and cold), vibration and touch stimuli (Lascelles, 2013). Applying gentle fingertip pressure around a painful area is an intuitive and universal, albeit not standardized, method for mechanical threshold testing. An improvised pressure-testing device (or algometer) can be fabricated using a loss-of-resistance syringe (Figure 9.1); if using such a device, it is important to remember that the scale on the syringe does not correspond linearly to the applied force.

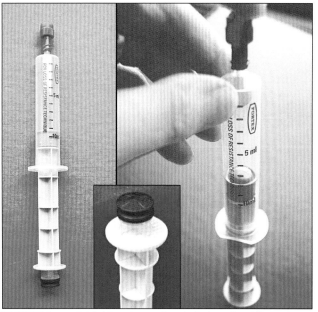

of tactile sensitivity) supported the recognition of allodynia secondary to osteoarthritis in cats (Guillot *et al.*, 2013).

Technological advances and device miniaturization have resulted in two new technologies for the evaluation of nociception. *Infrared thermography* is a non-invasive technique used to confirm findings derived from clinical evaluation. Suspicion of pain identified by any other method could be confirmed with this technology by loss or gain of heat. *Accelerometry* chips embedded on an animal's collar have been shown to record the daily activity of dogs and cats reliably in research settings. This technology is already commercially available (Heyrex® collar) and could be validated for monitoring changes in activity related to musculoskeletal pain in the near future.

Subjective measures of pain

Behavioural assessment

Recognition of pain, whether acute or chronic, is based on the recognition of either expression of new abnormal behaviour or disappearance of normal behaviours. Figure 9.2 summarizes the extensive repertoire of behavioural changes that may be associated with pain. Reflexes such as skin twitch or limb withdrawal following acute nociceptive stimulation are not sufficient to imply the sensation of pain. For this, reflexes must be accompanied by voluntary behaviours evidencing central integration of nociception, such as the animal moving away from the stimulus, turning the head towards the testing site (Figure 9.3) or any form of vocalization. Some animals have learned responses (strategies) to reduce pain or may perform stereotypical activities to cope with it. Reluctance to move or refusal to use the affected limb are examples of behaviours that may manifest as a consequence of acute inflammatory or postoperative pain. Grooming, interaction

9.1 Improvised algometer, made out of a loss-of-resistance syringe and the rubber plunger head of a 5 ml syringe that has a section of exactly 1 cm². Note that the index finger should be kept on the syringe cap to prevent it being propelled off the syringe when pressure builds up during testing.

More sophisticated, handheld thermal or mechanical threshold testing devices have been used in research and could help standardize clinical pain assessment in the future. These precision instruments generate a steady increase in temperature or pressure at the testing site, and are consequently expensive and require user training. Thresholds are highly variable between, but usually consistent within, individual animals. In a recent study, an electronic von Frey aesthesiometer (a modern electronic device for assessment

Characteristics	Behaviours
Body posture and activity	Restlessness and frequent changes in body position, quiet slow breathing, hunched up, guarding or splinting of abdomen, 'praying' position , sitting or lying in an abnormal position, not resting in a normal position (e.g. sternal recumbency or curled up), statue-like appearance, abnormal body part position (e.g. extended head and neck), looking, licking or chewing at the painful area
Locomotor activity	Limping and guarding, reluctance to move or to lie down, stiff, partial or no weight-bearing on injured limb, lameness, slight to obvious limp
Vocalization	Dogs: groaning, whining, whimpering, growling, screaming, howling, barking, crying, none Cats: groaning, growling, purring, meowing, crying, none
Altered facial expression	Dogs: fixed glare, focused, glazed appearance, oblivious Cats: furrowed brow, squinted eyes, depressed
Appetite	Decreased appetite, selective appetite, anorexia
Appearance	Submissive or mentally depressed, protective and aggressive, loss of hair coat, weary, subdued, sad, apprehensive, panicky, nervous, uneasy Dogs: vigilant, timid, fearful Cats: hiding or attempting to escape
Response to manipulation	Aggressive; defensive by protecting the area or by withdrawing to avoid being touched; freezing; looking at the area in question
Urinary and bowel habits	Loss of house training (cats: failure to use the litter tray), change in frequency of defecation/urination
Physiological signs	Tachycardia, tachyarrhythmia, hypertension, hyperthermia, tachypnoea
Possible poor general health or anxiety	Restlessness or agitation, trembling or shaking, tachypnoea or panting, tucked tail or tail flicking (cats), low carriage of tail, depressed or poor response to caregiver, head hanging down, not grooming, appetite decreased/picky/absent, dull, depressed, lying quietly and not moving for hours, stuporous, urinating or defecating and making no attempt to move, recumbent and unaware of surroundings, unwilling or unable to walk, biting or attempting to bite caregivers, weak tail wag (dogs), slow to rise, depressed, ears pulled back, barking or growling (dogs), growling or hissing (cats), sitting in the back of the cage or hiding (cats)

9.2 Pain-associated characteristics and behaviours in cats and dogs.
(Adapted from Mathews, 2000, with permission from *Veterinary Clinics of North America: Small Animal Practice*)

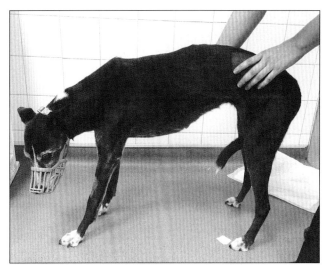

9.4 An 8-year-old, female neutered Lurcher, with a 1-month history of neck pain due to intervertebral disc disease. Note the rigid posture when standing and that the neck is held down. Due to wind-up and anticipation, the patient needed to be muzzled for examination; the unexplained aggressiveness was a behavioural response to pain.

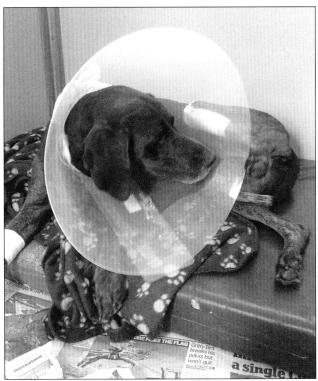

9.3 A 5-year-old, neutered male Pointer, after tibial tuberosity advancement surgery. The dog is looking at the limb and keeping it elevated, which are signs of pain.

with humans (e.g. acceptance of stroking, purring) and mobility (jumping, climbing stairs, exercise) are examples of behaviours that may be affected in chronic pain states.

The ability to hide pain and to appear fit to a predator or competitor despite being injured may have been an evolutionary advantage for some species. This could explain why some animals may not display behavioural changes associated with pain in the same way during a consultation at the veterinary practice as they would at home, in an environment they consider to be safe. Cats may simply hide at the back of their cage and demonstrate no behaviours that would suggest to a casual observer that they are in pain. In dogs, breed differences with regard to expression of pain-related behaviours have been anecdotally reported; for example, small-breed dogs may show exaggerated responses and are considered to be less stoical than some larger breed dogs. Labradors may appear stoical and may not react as obviously to a painful stimulus compared with other breeds. Kittens and puppies tend to communicate pain and discomfort in a more pronounced way than adults.

It is much less straightforward to recognize chronic pain compared with acute pain. Behavioural changes in chronic pain states are less specific, for example, decreased appetite, reduced activity and social interaction, increased time spent asleep and aggression (Figure 9.4). Owners' 'proxy' assessment, made at home, can usefully complement the veterinary surgeon's evaluation, as only the owner will know the animal's normal patterns of behaviours such as sleep and social activity. However, proxy reports may be inaccurate owing to misinterpretation of what constitutes pain or discomfort. In addition, with chronic pain the incidence of behavioural changes may increase so gradually that the owner is not aware of them, and often they are recognized only after a trial of analgesic medication during which the animal's behaviour returns to normal.

Assessment of acute perioperative pain

Pain scales were initially designed for use in humans and have been adapted for veterinary use. Most veterinary pain scales have been designed to assess acute somatic postoperative pain (originating from the skin and deep tissues but not viscera) in dogs and cats (Figure 9.5). They are likely to produce inaccurate results if used for assessment of other types of pain, such as acute visceral pain or chronic pain.

No 'gold standard' exists for assessing pain in animals or for comparing one type of scale or measurement instrument with another. These methods are subjective, prone to error from either underestimating or overestimating the degree of pain and are subject to some variability between different observers using a given scale.

Unidimensional scales
Simple descriptive scale

The simple descriptive scale (SDS) is the most basic form of pain scale. It generally includes four or five categories to choose from, for example, 'no pain', 'mild pain', 'moderate pain' and 'severe pain'. The SDS is intuitive and easy to use; however, it does not provide descriptions of what constitutes each category. The SDS is not sensitive enough to detect small changes in pain behaviour (it has poor resolution) and has not been validated in individual species.

Numerical rating scale

The numerical rating scale (NRS) is an ordinal scale. The observer assigns a numerical score for overall pain intensity. The resolution of the scale is better when it includes more levels for grading the intensity of pain: an NRS ranging from 0 (no pain) to 10 (extreme pain) has better resolution than a scale ranging from 0–4. The NRS has not been validated for linearity: this means that doubling the score does not mean that the pain is twice as severe.

Scale	Description	Cut-off for additional analgesia	Advantages	Disadvantages
SDS	Four or five categories to choose from: no pain; mild pain; moderate pain; severe pain; very severe pain	Not defined	Unidimensional Easy to use	Not species specific and not very sensitive to detect small changes in pain behaviour Does not address the multidimensional aspects of pain Not validated
NRS	Numerical score for pain intensity, usually from 0–10 or 0–100	Not defined	Unidimensional Easy to use	Not species specific and not very sensitive to detect small changes Not validated
VAS	100 mm line with 'no pain' anchored to one end and 'excruciating or unbearable pain' to the other. The distance from the 'no pain' end of the line (measured in mm) is the pain score	Not defined	Unidimensional Easy to use Good for following trends	Not species specific Prone to observer bias
UMPS	Evaluates postoperative pain in dogs on the basis of assessment of behaviour and physiological signs: physiological variables, response to palpation, activity, mental status, posture and vocalization	≥5/27, depending on the individual animal's temperament	Multidimensional Species specific (dogs) Categories are weighted Higher specificity and sensitivity and reduced observer bias	Not validated Does not account for dysphoria and persistent sedation Requires some knowledge of the demeanour of the dog
Colorado Acute Pain Scales	Two different scales for dogs and cats for assessment of acute pain. Three categories are evaluated: behavioural and physiological, response to palpation, body tension Scale for cats available at: www.csuanimalcancercenter.org/assets/files/csu_acute_pain_scale_feline.pdf Scale for dogs available at: www.csuanimalcancercenter.org/assets/files/csu_acute_pain_scale_canine.pdf	≥2/4	Multidimensional Species specific (dogs and cats) Colour scheme and pictures are attractive and easy to use	Not validated, therefore items of the scale are potentially inaccurate
Glasgow CMPS-SF	Assessment involves observation and interaction with the patient (wound palpation and attention to painful area) Available at: http://www.newmetrica.com/cmps	≥6/24 or ≥5/20 for non-ambulatory dogs	Multidimensional Species specific (dogs) Behaviours are listed, weighted and statistically validated in dogs Each descriptor is well defined to avoid misinterpretation Ease of use as it takes only few minutes to complete the short version.	Does not take into account the impact of demeanour/temperament or previous experience of the patient
UNESP-Botucatu MCPS	Ten items are distributed in four dimensions or subscales: vocal expression, physiological variables, protection of the wound area and psychomotor changes Available at: www.animalpain.com.br/assets/upload/escala-en-us.pdf	>7/30	Multidimensional The first validated pain scale to assess postoperative pain in cats. Validated in multiple languages and cultures Descriptors clearly illustrated with online video clips (available at www.animalpain.com.br/en-us/).	Still difficult to assess pain in patients that are either fearful or too friendly Time consuming until assessor is familiar with the scale

9.5 Acute pain assessment scales available for use in small animal practice. CMPS–SF = Composite Measure Pain Scale (short form); MCPS = Multidimensional Composite Pain Score; NRS = numerical rating scale; SDS = simple descriptive scale; UMPS = University of Melbourne Pain Scale; VAS = visual analogue scale.

Visual analogue scale

The visual analogue scale (VAS) consists of a horizontal 100 mm line, anchored at the left end to 'no pain' and at the right end to 'excruciating or unbearable pain' or 'the worst pain possible'. The VAS has been extensively used in humans, where it is generally completed by the patient experiencing the pain. In veterinary practice, the observer examines the animal and places a mark on the line to indicate the amount of pain he/she perceives the animal to be suffering. The distance from the 'no pain' end of the line in millimetres is measured and allocated as the pain score. The VAS is not species specific but is easy to use for monitoring trends (i.e. whether pain is getting worse or improving) and is widely accepted as a sensitive instrument for behavioural pain assessment. However, interobserver variability is higher with the VAS than with

the SDS; therefore assessment should be performed by a single observer who has sufficient experience in assessing pain.

A common modification of the VAS is to add a bar at the midpoint (i.e. 50 mm) to indicate 50% pain intensity, or at other predetermined scores. Defining the 100% score as 'the worst pain possible for this procedure' (rather than simply 'the worst pain possible') increases the scale's sensitivity for pain rated mild to moderate after minor surgical procedures.

The incorporation of a Dynamic and Interactive VAS (DIVAS) assessment was first suggested by Lascelles et al. (1998). In this study, an algometer was used to obtain nociceptive threshold values as an additional tool for assessing pain after ovariohysterectomy in dogs; an alternative standardized stimulus may be applied instead, for example, gentle digital palpation of the wound edges. When performing DIVAS assessment, the observer sequentially:

- Observes the patient from a distance without disturbing it and notes posture and behaviour
- Approaches the animal and interacts with it to see whether previous behaviours are still present or whether new ones emerge
- Palpates the surgical wound or that part of the body from which the pain is suspected to originate, using a standardized instrument or gentle digital palpation
- Writes a few notes under the scale. Attitudes showing that the animal is comfortable should be written under the left half of the scale and behaviours associated with pain should be written under the right half of the scale. The distribution of these notes is used as a visual guide when deciding upon a score
- Takes previous observations as well as potential confounding factors, such as sedation and baseline demeanour, into account in attributing a score.

Multidimensional composite pain scales

Most of the scales described above were designed for acute pain and only evaluate the sensory-discriminative component. They fail to probe the possible affective or cognitive dimensions of pain experience in animals. Pain-scoring tools that include assessment of multidimensional pain experience, described in the following section, represent a significant improvement upon the simpler unidimensional scales. One of the principal objectives of the validation of these scales is to determine a cut-off point beyond which most veterinary surgeons would agree that a patient requires additional rescue analgesia.

University of Melbourne Pain Scale

The University of Melbourne Pain Scale (UMPS) was developed as a multidimensional NRS to evaluate postoperative pain in dogs on the basis of assessments of behaviour and physiological signs (Firth and Haldane, 1999). The scale comprises six categories derived from a review of literature on pain measurement in dogs: physiological variables, response to palpation, activity, mental status, posture and vocalization. The assessor indicates which one (NRS) item from each category best describes the animal being observed; a weighting was assigned to each item according to the developers' subjective perception of how much pain it implied, such that certain behaviours or parameters are considered more important. The UMPS is much more accurate than the VAS, SDS and NRS, and the multiple factors evaluated increase its specificity and sensitivity. Using the UMPS requires knowledge of the demeanour of the dog before anaesthesia and surgery. The disadvantages of this scale are that the behaviours and physiological parameters it covers have not been validated and it does not account for dysphoria and persistent sedation. The scale was designed to assess dogs postoperatively, and therefore the accuracy of the scale for other types of pain or species cannot be evaluated.

Colorado State University Feline and Canine Acute Pain Scales

There are separate Colorado State University pain scales for use in cats and in dogs. For these scales, the observer selects the most appropriate descriptors (by ticking boxes)

for two components: psychological and behavioural signs, and response to palpation. A third component, body tension, is assessed on an SDS. The distribution of ticked boxes suggests an overall pain score from 0–4. This score can be increased or moderated by one-quarter or half a point if the distribution of ticked boxes overlaps two pain scores (Figure 9.6). The patient's analgesia plan should be reviewed if the score is ≥2. A visual prompt of what the animal's demeanour might look like at each level of pain is included to assist the evaluation of the emotional component. Finally, diagrams of left and right profiles of a cat or dog are provided under the scale for mapping of areas that are perceived as tender to palpation, warm or tense. These scales have not been officially validated, but their colour scheme and use of pictures are attractive to the eye and contribute to the popularity of the scales in small animal practice.

Glasgow Composite Measure Pain Scale

The original Glasgow Composite Measure Pain Score (GCMPS) scale was designed on the basis of the McGill Pain Questionnaire (a human pain-scoring instrument) with the aim of capturing the multidimensional experience of pain. The behaviours listed in the scale were chosen by veterinary experts and are weighted for statistical validation in dogs suffering from pain associated with orthopaedic or soft tissue surgeries as well as medical conditions. Each descriptor is clearly defined in an attempt to reduce observer bias.

A short form of the GCMPS (the CMPS-SF; Figure 9.7) was produced as a clinical decision-making tool for dogs with acute pain and is designed to be applied quickly and reliably in a clinical setting. It includes 30 descriptor options within six behavioural categories, including mobility. Within each category, the descriptors are ranked numerically according to their associated pain severity. The person carrying out the assessment chooses the descriptor within each category that best fits the dog's behaviour/condition. When using the CMPS-SF, it is important to carry out the assessment procedure as described on the questionnaire, following the protocol closely. The overall pain score is the sum of the rank scores. The maximum score for the six categories is 24, or 20 if mobility is impossible to assess (in which case this category is omitted). The total CMPS-SF score has been shown to be a useful indicator of analgesic requirements, and the recommended score indicating analgesic intervention is 6/24 or 5/20 (Holton et al., 2001).

UNESP–Botucatu Multidimensional Composite Pain Scale for cats

This is the first pain scale to be validated for postoperative pain in cats (Brondani et al., 2013) and is reproduced in Figure 9.8. It has been validated in multiple languages and cultures. In the English language version, 10 items are distributed in three subscales (described below). Each scale item is ranked numerically and assigned a score from 0–3. The system contains guidelines for evaluation, including a detailed description of the behaviours that should be observed in each scale item. Despite this guidance, initial use of the scale is time consuming for the novice assessor. Due to the multidimensional structure of the instrument, each subscale can be examined separately and when there is difficulty in the assessment of a particular dimension (e.g. blood pressure measurement), that subscale may be omitted.

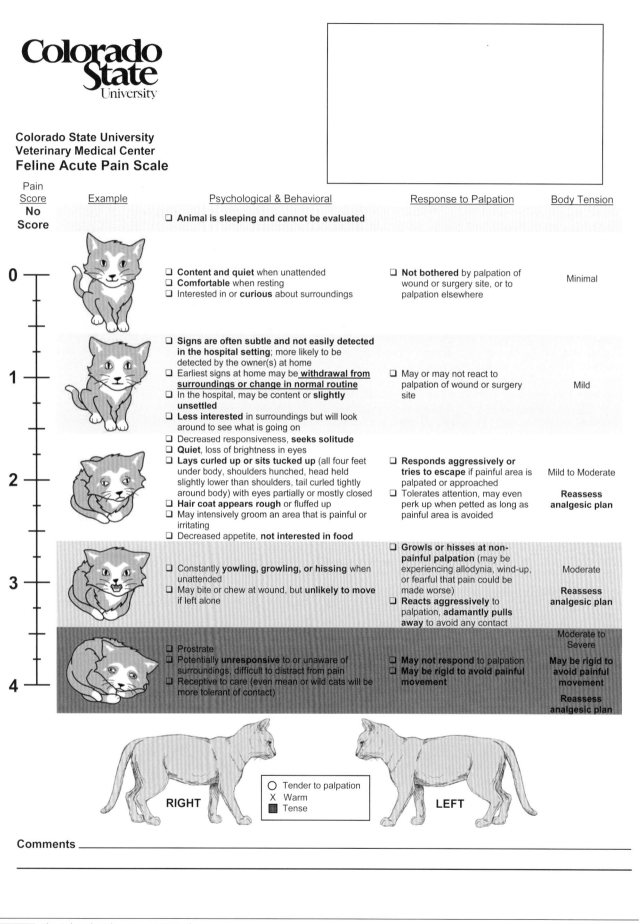

Colorado State University

Colorado State University Veterinary Medical Center
Feline Acute Pain Scale

Pain Score	Example	Psychological & Behavioral	Response to Palpation	Body Tension
No Score		☐ **Animal is sleeping and cannot be evaluated**		
0		☐ **Content and quiet** when unattended ☐ **Comfortable** when resting ☐ Interested in or **curious** about surroundings	☐ **Not bothered** by palpation of wound or surgery site, or to palpation elsewhere	Minimal
1		☐ **Signs are often subtle and not easily detected in the hospital setting**; more likely to be detected by the owner(s) at home ☐ Earliest signs at home may be <u>withdrawal from surroundings or change in normal routine</u> ☐ In the hospital, may be content or **slightly unsettled** ☐ **Less interested** in surroundings but will look around to see what is going on	☐ May or may not react to palpation of wound or surgery site	Mild
2		☐ Decreased responsiveness, **seeks solitude** ☐ **Quiet**, loss of brightness in eyes ☐ **Lays curled up or sits tucked up** (all four feet under body, shoulders hunched, head held slightly lower than shoulders, tail curled tightly around body) with eyes partially or mostly closed ☐ **Hair coat appears rough** or fluffed up ☐ May intensively groom an area that is painful or irritating ☐ Decreased appetite, **not interested in food**	☐ **Responds aggressively or tries to escape** if painful area is palpated or approached ☐ Tolerates attention, may even perk up when petted as long as painful area is avoided	Mild to Moderate **Reassess analgesic plan**
3		☐ Constantly **yowling, growling, or hissing** when unattended ☐ May bite or chew at wound, but **unlikely to move** if left alone	☐ **Growls or hisses at non-painful palpation** (may be experiencing allodynia, wind-up, or fearful that pain could be made worse) ☐ **Reacts aggressively** to palpation, **adamantly pulls away** to avoid any contact	Moderate **Reassess analgesic plan**
4		☐ Prostrate ☐ Potentially **unresponsive** to or unaware of surroundings, difficult to distract from pain ☐ Receptive to care (even mean or wild cats will be more tolerant of contact)	☐ **May not respond** to palpation ☐ **May be rigid to avoid painful movement**	Moderate to Severe **May be rigid to avoid painful movement** **Reassess analgesic plan**

RIGHT   LEFT

○ Tender to palpation
X Warm
■ Tense

Comments _____

_____

9.6 The Colorado Feline Acute Pain Scale.
(Reproduced with permission from Peter W Hellyer, Colorado State University, Veterinary Medical Center, USA)

Short form of the Glasgow Composite Measure Pain Scale

Dog's name _____ Date / / Time _____ Hospital number _____

Procedure or condition_____
_____

In the sections below please circle the appropriate score in each list and sum these to give the total score

A. Look at dog in kennel
Is the dog

(i)
Quiet	0
Crying or whimpering	1
Groaning	2
Screaming	3

(ii)
Ignoring any wound or painful area	0
Looking at wound or painful area	1
Licking wound or painful area	2
Rubbing wound or painful area	3
Chewing wound or painful area	4

In the case of spinal, pelvic or multiple limb fractures, or where assistance is required to aid locomotion, do not carry out section **B** and proceed to **C**. Please tick if this is the case ☐ then proceed to **C**

B. Put lead on dog and lead out of the kennel
(iii)
Normal	0
Lame	1
Slow or reluctant	2
Stiff	3
It refuses to move	4

C. If it has a wound or painful area including abdomen, apply gentle pressure 2 inches round the site
Does it? (iv)
Do nothing	0
Look round	1
Flinch	2
Growl or guard area	3
Snap	4
Cry	5

D. Overall
Is the dog? (v)
Happy and content or happy and bouncy	0
Quiet	1
Indifferent or non-responsive to surroundings	2
Nervous or anxious or fearful	3
Depressed or non-responsive to stimulation	4

Is the dog? (vi)
Comfortable	0
Unsettled	1
Restless	2
Hunched or tense	3
Rigid	4

Total score (i+ii+iii+iv+v+vi) = _____

9.7 The Glasgow Composite Measure Pain Score (short form).
(Reproduced with permission from Jacqueline Reid, University of Glasgow, School of Veterinary Medicine, UK)

Subscale 1: Pain expression (0–12 points)		
Miscellaneous behaviours	Observe and mark the presence of the behaviours listed below A. The cat is lying down and quiet, but moving its tail B. The cat contracts and extends its pelvic limbs and/or contracts its abdominal muscles (flank) C. The cats eyes are partially closed (eyes half closed) D. The cat licks and/or bites the surgical wound	
	• All above behaviours are absent	0
	• Presence of one of the above behaviours	1
	• Presence of two of the above behaviours	2
	• Presence of three or all of the above behaviours	3
Reaction to palpation of the surgical wound	• The cat does not react when the surgical wound is touched or pressed; or no change from pre-surgical response (if basal evaluation was made)	0
	• The cat does not react when the surgical wound is touched, but does react when it is pressed. It may vocalize and/or try to bite	1
	• The cat reacts when the surgical wound is touched and when pressed. It may vocalize and/or try to bite	2
	• The cat reacts when the observer approaches the surgical wound. It may vocalize and/or try to bite. The cat does not allow palpation of the surgical wound	3
Reaction to palpation of the abdomen/flank	• The cat does not react when the abdomen/flank is touched or pressed; or no change from pre-surgical response (if basal evaluation was made). The abdomen/flank is not tense	0
	• The cat does not react when the abdomen/flank is touched, but does react when it is pressed. The abdomen/flank is tense	1
	• The cat reacts when the abdomen/flank is touched and when pressed. The abdomen/flank is tense	2
	• The cat reacts when the observer approaches the abdomen/flank. It may vocalize and/or try to bite. The cat does not allow palpation of the abdomen/flank	3

9.8 The UNESP-Botucatu Multidimensional Composite Pain Scale. Analgesic intervention is recommended when the score is >7 out of a total possible score of 30. (continues)
(Reproduced with permission from Stelio P Luna, School of Veterinary Medicine and Animal Science, UNESP, Brazil)

Subscale 1: Pain expression (0–12 points)		
Vocalization	• The cat is quiet, purring when stimulated, or meows interacting with the observer, but does not growl, groan, or hiss	0
	• The cat purrs spontaneously (without being stimulated or handled by the observer)	1
	• The cat growls, howls, or hisses when handled by the observer (when its body position is changed by the observer)	2
	• The cat growls, howls, hisses spontaneously (without being stimulated or handled by the observer)	3

Subscale 2: Psychomotor change (0–12 points)		
Posture	• The cat is in a natural posture with relaxed muscles (it moves normally)	0
	• The cat is in a natural posture but is tense (it moves little or is reluctant to move)	1
	• The cat is sitting or in sternal recumbency with its back arched and head down; or the cat is in dorsolateral recumbency with its pelvic limbs extended or contracted	2
	• The cat frequently alters its body position in an attempt to find a comfortable posture	3
Comfort	• The cat is comfortable, awake or asleep, and interacts when stimulated (it interacts with the observer and/or is interested in its surroundings)	0
	• The cat is quiet and slightly receptive when stimulated (it interacts little with the observer and/or is not very interested in its surroundings)	1
	• The cat is quiet and 'dissociated from the environment' (even when stimulated it does not interact with the observer and/or has no interest in its surroundings). The cat may be facing the back of the cage	2
	• The cat is uncomfortable, restless (frequently changes its body position), and slightly receptive when stimulated or 'dissociated from the environment'. The cat may be facing the back of the cage	3
Activity	• The cat moves normally (it immediately moves when the cage is opened; outside the cage it moves spontaneously when stimulated or handled)	0
	• The cat moves more than normal (inside the cage it moves continuously from side to side)	1
	• The cat is quieter than normal (it may hesitate to leave the cage and if removed from the cage tends to return; outside the cage it moves a little after stimulation or handling)	2
	• The cat is reluctant to move (it may hesitate to leave the cage and if removed from the cage tends to return; outside the cage it does not move even when stimulated or handled)	3
Attitude	Observe and mark the presence of the mental states listed below **A. Satisfied:** the cat is alert and interested in its surroundings (explores its surroundings), friendly and interactive with the observer (plays and/or responds to stimuli) *The cat may initially interact with the observer through games to distract it from the pain. Carefully observe to distinguish between distraction and satisfaction games **B. Uninterested:** the cat does not interact with the observer (not interested by toys or plays a little; does not respond to calls or strokes from the observer) * In cats which do not like to play, evaluate interaction with the observer by its response to calls and strokes **C. Indifferent:** the cat is not interested in its surroundings (it is not curious; it does not explore its surroundings) * The cat can initially be afraid to explore its surroundings. The observer needs to handle the cat and encourage it to move itself (take it out of the cage and/or change its body position) **D. Anxious:** the cat is frightened (it tries to hide or escape) or nervous (demonstrating impatience and growling, howling, or hissing when stroked and/or handled) **E. Aggressive:** the cat is aggressive (tries to bite or scratch when stroked or handled)	
	• Presence of the mental state A	0
	• Presence of one of the mental states B, C, D, or E	1
	• Presence of two of the mental states B, C, D, or E	2
	• Presence of three or all of the mental states B, C, D, or E	3

Subscale 3: Physiological variables (0–6 points)		
Arterial blood pressure	• 0% to 15% above pre-surgery value	0
	• 16% to 29% above pre-surgery value	1
	• 30% to 45% above pre-surgery value	2
	• > 45% above pre-surgery value	3
Appetite	• The cat is eating normally	0
	• The cat is eating more than normal	1
	• The cat is eating less than normal	2
	• The cat is not interested in food	3

Directions for using the scale

- Initially observe the cat's behaviour without opening the cage. Observe whether it is resting or active; interested or uninterested in its surroundings; quiet or vocal. Check for the presence of specific behaviours (see 'Miscellaneous behaviours' above)
- Open the cage and observe whether the cat quickly moves out or hesitates to leave the cage. Approach the cat and evaluate its reaction: friendly, aggressive, frightened, indifferent, or vocal. Touch the cat and interact with it, check whether it is receptive (if it likes to be stroked and/or is interested in playing). If the cat hesitates to leave the cage, encourage it to move through stimuli (call it by name and stroke it) and handling (change its body position and/or take it out of the cage). Observe when outside the cage, if the cat moves spontaneously, in a reserved manner, or is reluctant to move. Offer it palatable food and observe its response
- Finally, place the cat in lateral or sternal recumbency and measure its arterial blood pressure. Evaluate the cat's reaction when the abdomen/flank is initially touched (slide your fingers over the area) and in the sequence gently pressed (apply direct pressure over the area). Wait for a time, and do the same procedure to assess the cat's reaction to palpation of surgical wound
- To evaluate appetite during the immediate postoperative period, initially offer a small quantity of palatable food immediately after recovery from anaesthetic. At this moment most cats eat normally independent of the presence or absence of pain. Wait a short while, offer food again, and observe the cat's reaction

9.8 (continued) The UNESP-Botucatu Multidimensional Composite Pain Scale. Analgesic intervention is recommended when the score is >7 out of a total possible score of 30.

(Reproduced with permission from Stelio P Luna, School of Veterinary Medicine and Animal Science, UNESP, Brazil)

The first subscale (score 0–12 points) assesses psycho-motor changes and contains four items: posture, comfort, activity and attitude. Attitude is a description of the cat's mental state and is rated as unsatisfied, uninterested in observer, indifferent to surroundings (Figure 9.9), anxious and/or aggressive. The second subscale relates to pain expression (score 0–12 points) and includes the cat's reaction to palpation of the surgical wound, reaction to palpation of the flank, vocalization and expression of miscellaneous validated behaviours. The following behaviours were selected for inclusion in the scale because of their high statistical association with pain: the cat is lying down and quiet, but moving its tail; the cat contracts and extends its pelvic limbs and/or contracts its abdominal muscles (flank); the eyes are partially closed (Figure 9.10); the cat licks and/or bites the surgical wound. The third subscale (score 0–6 points) includes physiological variables such as appetite and changes in systolic blood pressure relative to baseline (blood pressure should be measured before palpation).

Analgesic intervention is recommended when the score is >7 out of a total possible score of 30. Even with this validated system, pain assessment still relies on the assessor's subjective interpretation of the cat's behaviour. The authors of this scale therefore recommend that if a veterinary surgeon considers an animal to be in pain even if the scoring indicates otherwise, the benefit of the doubt should prevail and the animal should receive additional analgesia.

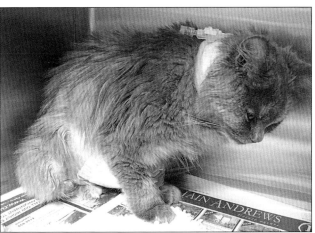

9.9 A 2-year-old, female neutered, Domestic Longhair cat, with postoperative pain following an exploratory laparotomy. The cat presents with a dull look, the head is held below shoulder level and the coat is unkempt; the abdomen was tense on palpation.

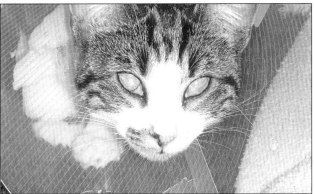

9.10 A 1-year-old, Domestic Shorthair cat recovering from ovariohysterectomy. A glazed look and eyes partially closed (squinted eyes) is one of the miscellaneous behaviours included in the UNESP-Botucatu Multidimensional Composite Pain Scale for assessment of postoperative pain.

As included in these multidimensional scales, response to palpation is a systematic requirement for thorough pain assessment. Additionally, the patient's normal preoperative behaviour and demeanour must be taken into account when response to palpation is assessed.

Assessment of visceral pain

The transmission and perception of visceral pain is different from that of somatic pain. Nociceptive stimulation originating from the gastrointestinal or genitourinary tract is generated by different stimuli, such as inflammation, ischaemia, stretching or dilation. Visceral pain is perceived as dull and is poorly localized with regard to its anatomical origin. It can present as referred pain to muscles, tendons and joints sharing the same dermatome as the stimulated viscera, meaning that the results of clinical examination may be confusing. Manifestations of visceral pain are also different from those associated with somatic pain; they can be as diverse as a change in behaviour (including changes in urinary and bowel habits), nausea and vomiting triggered by autonomic reflexes, or lumbar muscle tension caused by renal colic. Adoption of a 'praying' position (Figure 9.11) is typical with abdominal pain, but does not necessarily mean that the pain is visceral in origin.

Assessment of visceral pain should include a review of the patient's history, diagnostic and laboratory tests and a thorough medical work-up. Again, interaction with the patient and palpation of potentially painful areas could give valuable information. To date, no visceral pain scale has been validated in companion animals.

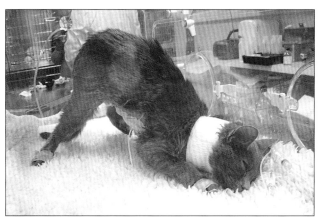

9.11 A 2-year-old, female neutered Domestic Shorthair cat showing a typical 'praying' position. The cat was experiencing abdominal visceral pain due to possible portal hypertension after ligation of a portosystemic shunt.

Assessment of chronic pain

For a more detailed description of the approach to patients suffering chronic pain, see Chapter 12. Chronic pain may have both inflammatory and neuropathic (pain originating from nervous structures themselves) components, or can be associated with neoplasia. Chronic pain is defined as pain that has been present for more than 1 month. As a result, central sensitization and allodynia are likely to be present, and these render the assessment of chronic pain more challenging. A full clinical examination, blood work and imaging studies are essential in these patients. Chronic pain affects the animal's behaviour and quality of life, and these aspects therefore need to be focused upon when evaluating pain related to, for example, osteoarthritis or cancer, or neuropathic pain (Figure 9.12). Objective measures of osteoarthritis-related pain have been used to evaluate loss of function and loss of use of extremities. In osteoarthritic cats, these functional alterations can be measured objectively by force plate analysis, and punctate tactile allodynia can be demonstrated by quantitative sensory testing (Guillot et al., 2013). Proxy assessment by owners and observation of the patient in a familiar and non-stressful environment is used to evaluate behaviours associated with chronic pain and, ultimately, the animal's quality of life. Importantly, questionnaire-based assessments completed by owners often correlate better with objective measures of chronic pain than veterinary surgeons' evaluations.

Several scales, some of them adapted from human medicine, have been devised to evaluate chronic pain in cats and dogs (Figure 9.13), The Glasgow University

Veterinary School Questionnaire (GUV-Quest) has been validated for all types of chronic pain (Reid et al., 2013). Other chronic pain scales focus on canine degenerative joint disease – the Helsinki Chronic Pain Index (Hielm-Björkman et al., 2009) and Canine Brief Pain Inventory (CBPI) – or pain associated with bone cancer (Brown et al., 2009). In cats, the Feline Musculoskeletal Pain Index (FMPI) has been described (Benito et al., 2013). These scales are used to help determine the patient's quality of life and to evaluate whether or not treatment results in improvement in quality of life. There is an urgent need for a reliable tool for assessment of neuropathic related chronic pain in cats and dogs. In one study, a questionnaire originally devised for use in humans was adapted to assess owner-perceived quality of life in dogs with spinal cord injuries (Budke et al., 2008). Owners individually weighted five areas of activities according to how important they believed these were in influencing their dog's quality of life. These areas were mobility, play or mental stimulation, health and companionship, among others.

Problems and pitfalls in pain assessment

It is very important to differentiate pain from fear and anxiety, as well as from other sources of discomfort that may worsen pain perception and the animal's capacity to deal with pain. Sedation is a confounding factor during pain assessment and should be scored concurrently, as many analgesics can also produce sedation (see Chapter 10). For example, when continuous infusions of alpha-2 adrenoceptor agonists are used as part of an analgesic protocol, it can be difficult to determine whether the animal is pain-free and sleeping, or deeply sedated but with insufficient analgesia. Some other clinical scenarios described below may be associated with signs that mimic pain behaviour in the postoperative period; these have to be recognized and differentiated from pain.

Bladder distension can cause discomfort and anxiety, which can result in misinterpretation of clinical signs. Discomfort from other sources should be ruled out and prevented by good nursing practice (e.g. joint pain from malpositioning of a dog with hip dysplasia; placement of Elizabethan collars; cumbersome bandages responsible for 'bandage paralysis' in cats; urge to defecate; in some cases, hunger).

'Emergence delirium', in which recovery from general anaesthesia is accompanied by psychomotor agitation, may be observed after a minor innocuous procedure. This condition is frequently encountered in children and associated with the administration of volatile anaesthetics, especially those agents with low blood solubility (Becker et al. 2013). Emergence delirium should resolve within a few minutes after extubation; the use of gentle care, appeasing voices, dimmed lights and sometimes the administration of an anxiolytic, if there is no contraindication for its use, will help resolve the episode.

Drug-related dysphoria is a possible side effect of opioids in small animal practice. It is very well recognized in human patients, who report depersonalization, hallucinations, unpleasant body sensations, sweating, anxiety and shakiness. A number of reports mention dysphoric states after administration of an opioid to dogs (Hofmeister et al., 2006, Becker et al. 2013) but the incidence of this side effect is unknown. It is also unknown why some

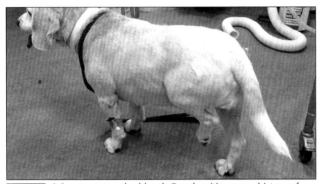

9.12 A 6-year-10-month-old male Beagle with a 5-year history of lameness and allodynia of the left hind cushion. The dog developed neuropathic pain after surgery for removal of fibrotic tissue in that area and remained unresponsive to traditional analgesics. Orthopaedic and neurological examinations were unremarkable with lumbar MRI and EMG within normal limits. Von Frey filament examination showed a low-threshold response (0.6–2 g). The animal responded to the addition of amitriptyline to the treatment.
(Courtesy of Jaime Viscasillas, Royal Veterinary College, Hatfield, UK)

Scale	Relevant information
Glasgow University Veterinary School Questionnaire (GUV-Quest)	Validation: all types of chronic pain Owner's assessment: health-related quality of life of their dog Available at: http://www.newmetrica.com/qol/index.html
Helsinki Chronic Pain Index (HCPI)	Validation: chronic osteoarthritis-associated pain in dogs Owner's assessment: mobility of their dog Available at: www.vetmed.helsinki.fi/english/animalpain/hcpi/HCPI_E2.pdf
Canine Brief Pain Inventory (CBPI)	Validation: dogs with osteoarthritis and appendicular bone cancer Owner's assessment: severity and impact of chronic pain and treatment on their dog Available at: http://www.vet.upenn.edu/research/clinical-trials/vcic/pennchart/cbpi-tool
Feline Musculoskeletal Pain Index (FMPI)	Validation: to differentiate normal cats from cats with degenerative joint disease Owner's assessment: mobility, other behaviours such as eating, interaction and perceived quality of life of their cat Available at: https://cvm.ncsu.edu/research/labs/clinical-sciences/comparative-pain-research/clinical-metrology-instruments/

9.13 Chronic pain scales validated for cats or dogs.

animals become dysphoric with opioids but others do not. The distribution of opioid receptors within the central nervous system could be responsible for the behavioural changes caused by activation of those receptors. Dysphoria can be difficult to differentiate from pain as both have some common behavioural characteristics, such as vocalization, restlessness, lack of awareness of surroundings, hyperaesthesia and uncoordinated agitated activity. As a rule, though, dysphoric patients do not respond to touch and are not calmed by human interaction. Before contemplating the diagnosis of opioid-related dysphoria, it is important to rule out pain first, by physical examination followed by the administration of supplemental analgesia; signs of fear and anxiety should be managed with anxiolytics or sedatives. If the abnormal behaviours persist despite these interventions, opioid dysphoria can be confirmed as a final differential diagnosis by the administration of butorphanol or naloxone while providing other sources of analgesia, such as non-opioid analgesics or local anaesthetic techniques (for the latter, the patient would also have to be sedated or anaesthetized).

Cats receiving buprenorphine may display signs of *euphoria* such as excessive purring, pacing, rubbing, kneading, and rolling on their back. Euphoria occurs at plasma concentrations of buprenorphine lower than those reported to provide analgesia, and these behaviours, which would usually be associated with a comfortable state, have the potential to mask insufficient analgesia if wound palpation is not performed as a means of pain assessment.

Dogs and cats may experience *postoperative nausea* and *vomiting* or *headaches*, as are often reported by humans recovering from procedures under general anaesthesia. Postoperative nausea has not been investigated in companion animals because of animals' inability to self-report and the lack of validated objective measures of nausea, but, if present, nausea could potentially worsen the experience of pain.

Hyperthermia can also have an effect on pain scoring. Cats treated with opioids may become agitated and may also develop hyperthermia; this is most likely after receiving oxymorphone, hydromorphone or fentanyl, but has also been observed with buprenorphine. Hyperthermic cats may appear less lively and look dull – behaviours that are taken as indicators of pain in several scales, as described above.

How frequently should pain be assessed?

The frequency of pain assessment depends upon the severity of the underlying disease and (if applicable) the extent of the surgical procedure. Ideally, an assessment should be performed every 15 minutes during the first hour postoperatively (rewarming and recovery phase), then hourly for the first 4 to 6 hours, or more frequently if the patient is not comfortable. After 6 hours, this frequency can be reduced if the patient is stable and was pain-free during the previous assessment period, although this will also depend on the analgesic drugs used. As a minimum, pain should be reassessed before the next dose of analgesic medication is due.

Conclusion

Several scales or scoring systems for assessing pain exist. None of them are perfect, as they depend upon the scorer's subjective assessment and cannot fully probe the multidimensional nature of pain. A full clinical examination and wound palpation are of paramount importance in the assessment of pain in small animal patients. The benefit of the doubt should always be given in cases where the pain score is low but the overall clinical impression indicates the presence of more severe pain – this highlights one limitation of any pain scale. If there is any doubt, the patient's response to a test dose of analgesic will help provide the answer.

References and further reading

Becker WM, Mama KR, Rao S et al. (2013) Prevalence of dysphoria after fentanyl in dogs undergoing stifle surgery. *Veterinary Surgery* **42**, 302–307

Benito J, Hansen B, DePuy V et al. (2013) Feline Musculoskeletal Pain Index: responsiveness and testing of criterion validity. *Journal of Veterinary Internal Medicine* **27**, 474–482

Brondani JT, Mama KR, Luna SPL et al. (2013) Validation of the English version of the UNESP-Botucatu multidimensional composite pain scale for assessing postoperative pain in cats. *BMC Veterinary Research* **9**, 143

Brown DC, Boston R, Coyne JC et al. (2009) A novel approach to the use of animals in studies of pain: validation of the Canine Brief Pain Inventory in canine bone cancer. *Pain Medicine* **10**, 133–142

Budke CM, Levine JM, Kerwin SC et al. (2008) Evaluation of a questionnaire for obtaining owner-perceived, weighted quality-of-life assessments for dogs with spinal cord injuries. *Journal of the American Veterinary Medical Association* **233**, 925–930

Dobromylskyj P, Flecknell PA, Lascelles BD et al. (2000) Pain assessment. In: *Pain Management in Animals, 1st edn*, ed. PA Flecknell and A Waterman-Pearson, pp. 53–79. W.B. Saunders, London

Firth AM and Haldane SL (1999) Development of a scale to evaluate postoperative pain in dogs. *Journal of the American Veterinary Medical Association* **214**, 651–659

Guillot M, Moreau M, Heitb M et al. (2013) Characterization of osteoarthritis in cats and meloxicam efficacy using objective chronic pain evaluation tools. *Veterinary Journal* **196**, 360–367

Hellyer, P, Rodan I, Brunt J et al. (2007) AAHA/AAFP pain management guidelines for dogs and cats. *Journal of the American Animal Hospital Association* **43**, 235–248

Hielm-Björkman AK, Rita H and Tulamo RM (2009) Psychometric testing of the Helsinki chronic pain index by completion of a questionnaire in Finnish by owners of dogs with chronic signs of pain caused by osteoarthritis. *American Journal of Veterinary Research* **70**, 727–734

Hofmeister EH, Herrington JL and Mazzaferro EM (2006) Opioid dysphoria in three dogs. *Journal of Veterinary Emergency and Critical Care* **16**, 44–49

Holton L, Reid J, Scott EM et al. (2001) Development of a behaviour-based scale to measure acute pain in dogs. *Veterinary Record* **48**, 525–531

Lascelles BD (2013) Getting a sense of sensations. *Veterinary Journal* **197**, 115–117

Lascelles BD, Cripps PJ, Jones A et al. (1998) Efficacy and kinetics of carprofen, administered preoperatively or postoperatively, for the prevention of pain in dogs undergoing ovariohysterectomy. *Veterinary Surgery* **27**, 568–582

Mathews KA (2000) Pain assessment and general approach to management. *Veterinary Clinics of North America: Small Animal Practice* **30**, 729–752

Mich PM and Heyller PW (2008) Objective, categoric methods for assessing pain and analgesia. In: *Handbook of Veterinary Pain Management, 2nd edn*, ed. JS Gaynor and WW Muir, pp. 78–109. Elsevier, St Louis

Moore SA, Hettlich BF and Waln A (2013). The use of an electronic von Frey device for evaluation of sensory threshold in neurologically normal dogs and those with acute spinal cord injury. *Veterinary Journal* **197**, 216–219

Muir WW and Gaynor JS (2008) Pain behaviors. In: *Handbook of Veterinary Pain Management, 2nd edn*, ed. JS Gaynor and WW Muir Elsevier, pp. 62–67. Elsevier, St Louis

Reid J, Wiseman-Orr ML, Scott EM et al. (2013). Development, validation and reliability of a web-based questionnaire to measure health-related quality of life in dogs. *Journal of Small Animal Practice* **54**, 227–233

WSAVA Global Pain Council (2014) WSAVA Guidelines for Recognition, Assessment and Treatment of Pain. *Journal of Small Animal Practice* **55(6)**, E10–E68

Chapter 10

Pain management I: systemic analgesics

Carolyn L. Kerr

Most agents used for analgesia in small animal patients fall into the opioid or non-steroidal anti-inflammatory drug (NSAID) groups. However, *N*-methyl-ᴅ-aspartate (NMDA) antagonists, local anaesthetics and alpha-2 adrenergic agonists are also used to provide analgesia. The different categories of drugs influence pain processing through different mechanisms, and they can therefore be used in combination to maximize analgesia (multimodal analgesia) (see Chapter 8). In the sections below, the general properties of analgesic drugs are reviewed, followed by descriptions of individual drugs within each category. For local anaesthetic agents, see Chapter 11.

Opioid analgesics

The term 'opiate' refers to drugs derived from either opium or thebaine (a derivative of opium); these include morphine, codeine and derived semi-synthetic congeners. Opioid analgesic (or 'opioid') is a general term that refers to any naturally occurring, semi-synthetic or synthetic substance with morphine-like activity. Because opioids can be abused, all countries legally regulate their purchase, storage and use. The level of regulation is dependent on opioid class scheduling and should be understood by veterinary surgeons (veterinarians) for each country, province or state in which they practise (see Chapter 1).

Pharmacology

Morphine is a natural alkaloid derived from the seeds of the opium poppy, *Papaver somniferum*. It is more cost-effective to extract morphine from this source because it is complex and expensive to synthesize. Most other opioids are derived from morphine. There is considerable variability in lipophilicity between different opioids. In general, more lipophilic agents, such as fentanyl, have a shorter duration of action compared with more hydrophilic opioids such as morphine. All opioid analgesics except remifentanil are metabolized in the liver before excretion; the metabolites may possess analgesic properties. Clearance is generally more dependent on hepatic blood flow than on the intrinsic activity of hepatic enzymes.

Most opioids are well absorbed following intramuscular administration. The intravenous route is also suitable for the majority of opioids. However, intravenous administration of some of these drugs can cause mast cell degranulation, histamine release and a significant decrease in systemic arterial blood pressure. Morphine can be administered slowly intravenously with minimal effect on haemodynamics, but pethidine (meperidine) should never be given using the intravenous route of administration. Subcutaneous administration may provide an insufficient duration of analgesia and unreliable efficacy, depending on the opioid and the species being treated. Although most opioids are well absorbed from the gastrointestinal (GI) tract, few are effective when administered by this route because they are extensively metabolized during their first pass through the liver. For some drugs, absorption via the nasal and oral mucous membranes can avert first-pass hepatic metabolism and achieve effective plasma concentrations. Transcutaneous delivery is another suitable approach for long-term administration of some opioids.

The goal of opioid administration is to achieve target tissue concentrations associated with analgesia. Because tissue concentrations are difficult to measure, plasma concentration is measured instead and the elimination half-life is calculated to estimate the duration of action and dosing intervals. However, plasma concentration does not accurately reflect drug concentration at the site of action, and therefore there may be a considerable discrepancy between the plasma concentration and the duration of observable analgesia. It is also possible that an unmeasured active metabolite exists and contributes to analgesia. Recommended dosing intervals are also based on clinical experience and analgesia trials that incorporate measurement of plasma concentration alongside assessment of nociception (pharmacokinetic–pharmacodynamic analysis).

Mechanism of action

The effects of opioid analgesics result from their activity at opioid receptors located within the central nervous system (CNS) and at peripheral sites (ganglia and peripheral nerve endings). Three major classes of opioid receptors mediating analgesia are recognized, designated mu (or MOP), delta (or DOP) and kappa (or KOP). The mu opioid receptor and its subtypes are reviewed elsewhere (Pasternak and Pan, 2013). The pharmacological nomenclature, represented by Greek letters, will be used in this chapter. The other classification stems from the examination of receptor types in molecular biological studies. More recently, a nociceptin/orphanin FQ (NOP) receptor has been characterized as a member of the opioid receptor family; however, it does not bind opioid ligands with high affinity, and its role in analgesia has not been defined.

The mu, delta and kappa receptors differ in their binding properties, functional activity, and distribution. Mu and delta receptors are located both supraspinally and spinally, while kappa receptors are primarily located in the spinal cord. All opioid receptors are coupled to G-proteins and inhibit adenylate cyclase, decreasing the conductance of voltage-gated calcium channels and/or opening inwardly rectifying potassium channels. As a result, neuronal activity is decreased, neurotransmitter release is reduced and/or postsynaptic membranes are hyperpolarized, thereby decreasing the propagation of action potentials and nociceptive information.

Drugs acting on opioid receptors are classified as agonists, partial agonists, mixed agonist–antagonists and antagonists:

- Agonist drugs have high affinity and intrinsic activity for mu receptors. They include morphine, pethidine, hydromorphone, methadone, fentanyl, sufentanil, alfentanil, remifentanil and codeine. Tramadol is a weak mu agonist
- Partial agonists (e.g. buprenorphine) do not have full intrinsic activity at the mu receptor
- Mixed agonist–antagonists (e.g. butorphanol) act as agonists at some receptors and antagonists at others; their affinity and intrinsic activity at the receptor site may vary
- Antagonists (e.g. naloxone) reverse the effects of mu and kappa agonists because of their high affinity and low intrinsic activity.

Analgesic effects

In general, opioids are considered to be more effective for continuous dull pain (C fibre transmission) rather than sharp intermittent pain (Aδ fibre transmission), although it is possible to reduce the intensity of most types of pain rapidly with their use. Within the CNS, opioids specifically act on nerves originating from nociceptors, and have no effect on the nerves for touch, pressure and proprioception. In humans, there is considerable inter-individual variation in opioid requirements for postoperative analgesia. Experimental and clinical studies in animals evaluating the response to thermal and pressure nociceptive stimuli, and using pain scoring systems, also show marked variation in individual responses to analgesia. Therefore, to optimize the effect of opioid treatment, the patient's response should be continuously assessed and treatment adjusted accordingly. Fortunately, opioids can be titrated to effect and have a wide therapeutic index, so doses can be adjusted over a wide range.

The different opioid agents produce characteristic patterns of analgesia, due partly to differences in receptor affinity and receptor distribution (see Chapter 8). In general, mu agonists produce the most profound analgesia and are recommended for moderate to severe pain and for anaesthetic-sparing effects. Mixed agonist–antagonists and partial mu agonists are generally recommended for mild to moderate pain and are suitable for minor surgical procedures. These agents may also have a 'ceiling effect' whereby increasing doses do not increase analgesia beyond a certain level. The relative potency of different opioid agents is generally compared to that of morphine (Figure 10.1). However, potency reflects only the dose required to produce the same magnitude of response, and is not necessarily indicative of overall efficacy in relieving pain.

Tolerance, or the loss of responsiveness to an opioid agonist after continuous short- or long-term exposure, has been described in humans and laboratory animals. Decreased numbers of functional receptors or alterations

Drug	Classification (potency relative to morphine)	Dosage forms	Dose	Duration of effect of one bolus
Morphine	Mu agonist (1)	Injectable: 0.5–50 mg/ml	0.1–1.0 mg/kg slow i.v., i.m. or s.c. Infusion: 0.12–0.34 mg/kg/h	2–6 hours
Pethidine (meperidine)	Mu agonist (0.2–0.3)	Injectable: 10–100 mg/ml	3–5 mg/kg i.m. or s.c.	1–1.5 hours
Methadone	Mu agonist (1)	Injectable: 10 mg/ml	0.1–0.5 mg/kg i.v., i.m. or s.c.	4–8 hours
Hydromorphone	Mu agonist (5)	Injectable: 2–100 mg/ml	0.05–0.2 mg/kg i.v., i.m. or s.c. Infusion: 0.05–0.1 mg/kg/h	4 hours
Fentanyl	Mu agonist (100)	Injectable: 50 and 78.5 μg/ml Transdermal patch: 25, 50, 75 and 100 μg/h Transdermal solution: 50 mg/ml	Injectable: 2–5 μg/kg bolus Infusion rate: • Intraoperative 5–40 μg/kg/h • Postoperative 3–6 μg/kg/h Transdermal: 2–5 μg/kg/h	20–30 minutes
Sufentanil	Mu agonist (500–1000)	Injectable: 50 μg/ml	Infusion: 3–5 μg/kg bolus followed by 2.6–3.4 μg/kg/h i.v.	10–20 minutes
Alfentanil	Mu agonist (10–20)	Injectable: 500 μg/ml	Infusion: 100 μg/kg bolus followed by 30–60 μg/kg/h i.v.	10–20 minutes
Remifentanil	Mu agonist (100–200)	Injectable: 1 mg dried drug/vial (requires dilution)	Infusion: suggest using fentanyl at 3 μg/kg bolus followed by remifentanil at 5–40 μg/kg/h i.v. Diluted to 0.1 mg/ml dilution	Remifentanil has too short a duration of effect for bolus administration
Tramadol	Mu agonist (0.1)	Injectable: 50 mg/ml Tablet: 50 mg	1–4 mg/kg i.v. 3–10 mg/kg orally	6–8 hours
Butorphanol	Mu antagonist–kappa agonist	Injectable: 10 mg/ml	0.2–0.4 mg/kg i.v., i.m. or s.c. Infusion: 0.1–0.2 mg/kg/h	1.5–2 hours
Buprenorphine	Partial mu agonist	Injectable: 0.3 mg/ml	0.01–0.03 mg/kg i.v. or i.m.	4–12 hours
Naloxone	Antagonist	Injectable: 0.4 and 1 mg/ml	0.002–0.04 mg/kg i.v., i.m. or s.c.	30 minutes–1 hour

10.1 Opioid analgesics routinely used in dogs.

in receptor signalling may be responsible for a reduction in the clinical response to an opioid analgesic. The development of tolerance may be agonist dependent (Williams *et al.*, 2013). Evidence to support the development of tolerance to opioid analgesics used in a clinical setting in companion animals has not been documented to date.

Central nervous system effects

Classically, mu receptor agonists produce euphoria and kappa receptor agonists produce dysphoria, but it is now accepted that both euphoria and dysphoria can be observed with all opioids. Euphoria in dogs is described as excessive wakefulness and vocalization. In cats, euphoria is characterized by rolling, grooming, 'kneading' and extreme friendliness. Dysphoria in dogs is typified by agitation, excitement, restlessness, excessive vocalization and disorientation, and can be confused with euphoria. In cats, fearful behaviour, open-mouth breathing, agitation, vocalization, pacing and apparent hallucinations are described. Fortunately, these behaviours can be managed by administering sedatives/tranquillizers and/or opioid antagonists.

In healthy dogs without pain, most mu agonists produce mild to moderate sedation, while the kappa agonists result in either little change or mild sedation. In healthy cats without pain, and in cats with adequate analgesia after surgery, mu agonists can produce mild euphoric behaviour, although a few cats may become dysphoric. In cats or dogs in pain and provided with inadequate opioid analgesia, it is rare for euphoria or dysphoria to occur, and pain behaviours are more likely to be observed.

Mu and kappa agonists potentiate sedation produced by sedatives or tranquillizer drugs when given in combination. High doses of mu agonists such as hydromorphone or fentanyl, in combination with a benzodiazepine, can produce heavy sedation in dogs, and a light plane of anaesthesia in depressed and debilitated dogs.

Respiratory effects

Depression of the central respiratory centre response to hypercapnia and hypoxaemia are well recognized side effects of opioids. At equi-analgesic doses, mu agonists produce a similar degree of respiratory depression. Respiratory depression should be expected when opioids are administered in combination with other CNS depressants, such as volatile anaesthetics, or in patients with respiratory compromise, especially when there is increased work of breathing (e.g. in brachycephalic breeds). It is therefore important to be watchful for severe respiratory depression or apnoea, particularly when the opioid analgesic is administered intravenously, which can result in profound effects. In conscious patients without respiratory compromise, respiratory depression is not clinically significant at recommended doses. Some opioids also suppress the cough reflex, independent of their respiratory depressant effect. Cough suppression is dependent on the individual opioid rather than receptor affinity. For example, both butorphanol and fentanyl are considered to be potent cough suppressants.

A change in respiratory pattern can be observed following opioid administration. In dogs, panting is a frequent observation with full mu agonists, and occurs secondary to a change in the central thermoregulatory set point. In cats, open-mouth breathing may be observed and is probably due to dysphoria.

Cardiovascular effects

At analgesic doses, especially with full mu agonists, decreased heart rate secondary to increased vagal tone is common. However, the resulting bradycardia is responsive to anticholinergics. Rapid intravenous administration of a mu or kappa agonist can result in profound bradycardia. When mu agonists are used alone for analgesia, the decreased heart rate rarely requires treatment. When opioids are administered with volatile anaesthetics, administration of an anticholinergic to correct a low heart rate may significantly improve haemodynamic status. The effect of the opioids on systemic blood pressure is generally minimal when they are administered via recommended routes.

Gastrointestinal effects

The effects of opioids on the frequency of vomiting and defecation are dependent on the specific opioid, route of administration and dose. Vomiting and defecation in dogs without pain are common following administration of the mu agonists morphine and hydromorphone (Wilson *et al.*, 2007; KuKanich *et al.*, 2008). However, when administered to patients in pain, or postoperatively, these side effects are uncommon. In non-painful cats, excessive salivation and emesis may be observed following subcutaneous or intramuscular administration of hydromorphone, but defecation is rarely observed (Steagall *et al.*, 2006; Robertson *et al.*, 2009). The incidence of vomiting is lower in cats and dogs after intravenous injection compared with the intramuscular route. Mu agonists cause direct stimulation of dopamine receptors in the chemoreceptor trigger zone (CRTZ), which is located outside the blood–brain barrier. More lipid-soluble opioids rapidly cross the blood–brain barrier to have an antiemetic action on the vomiting centre. With low doses, slow absorption from depot sites, or more hydrophilic drugs, the opioids do not reach the vomiting centre before they act on the CRTZ. In dogs, vomiting can be reduced if maropitant (an NK1 antagonist) is administered subcutaneously 15–60 minutes before hydromorphone (Kraus, 2013; Kraus, 2014), or acepromazine (an anti-dopaminergic agent) is administered intramuscularly 15 minutes before morphine, hydromorphone or oxymorphone (Valverde *et al.*, 2004).

Decreased gastric emptying time and intestinal propulsive motility have been demonstrated in dogs, and therefore increased GI transit time should be anticipated following opioid administration (see Chapter 24). An increase in pyloric sphincter tone has been reported following administration of some mu agonists, and some authors do not recommend their use before duodenal endoscopy. However, this problem has not been observed in cats (Smith *et al.*, 2004). Similarly, mu agonists increase the tone of the biliary sphincter of Oddi, resulting in a decrease in biliary secretion. Prolonged use of mu agonists in cats or dogs with biliary disease is therefore not generally recommended, although the relative risks and benefits should be considered for each patient.

Ocular effects

The mu agonists produce miosis in dogs, while mydriasis is observed in cats. Miosis is produced through opioid-mediated stimulation of cell bodies in the oculomotor nuclear complex. The miotic effect is a consideration for intraocular surgery, but otherwise appears to have little clinical significance. In cats, mydriasis occurs secondary to an opioid-induced increase in circulating catecholamines. Mydriasis impairs normal vision and increases sensitivity to light; these alterations should be considered when handling and exposing treated cats to light.

Urinary effects

Mu agonists increase urethral sphincter tone and inhibit the voiding reflex. When they are used in anaesthetized patients, the bladder size and tone should be assessed and, if warranted, the bladder expressed before recovery from anaesthesia. Mu agonists increase anti-diuretic hormone (ADH) (vasopressin) release and kappa agonists cause diuresis by decreasing ADH release. These effects should be considered when hydration is assessed by monitoring a patient's urine output, particularly when opioids are being administered long term (Anderson and Day, 2008). Due to the potential for urinary retention, perioperative epidural administration of a long-acting opioid such as morphine is not recommended in patients undergoing cystotomy or bladder repair unless postoperative urinary catheterization is used.

Thermoregulation

In dogs, opioids decrease the thermoregulatory set point in the CNS and cause panting. When opioids have been used perioperatively in dogs, it is common to observe decreased body temperature (Monteiro et al. 2008). In cats, however, postoperative hyperthermia is a potential adverse effect of opioids (Gellasch et al., 2002; Niedfeldt and Robertson, 2006; Posner et al., 2010). Hyperthermia appears to be dose related, with higher doses being associated with a greater probability of hyperthermia. The body temperature at extubation was inversely correlated to the degree of hyperthermia, such that the coldest cats at extubation reached the highest temperatures during recovery (Posner et al., 2007). The mechanism underlying this observation is not yet known. Body temperature should be closely monitored in cats after opioid administration. While opioid antagonist administration can restore body temperature to normal, alternative means of restoring normothermia are recommended in postoperative patients. These include: the removal of any external warming devices; increasing airflow over the patient by using a fan; intravenous administration of a balanced electrolyte solution; and use of low doses of acepromazine (0.01–0.02 mg/kg i.v.).

Opioid receptors appear to be involved in shivering. Intravenous administration of agents with mu agonist activity, such as tramadol, have been used in humans to limit postoperative shivering unrelated to hypothermia, where increased metabolic oxygen demand may increase cardiopulmonary workload (Mohta et al., 2009).

Auditory sensitivity

Certain opioids, such as fentanyl, increase noise sensitivity in cats and dogs, and the environment should be as quiet as possible.

Opioid mu agonists

Morphine

Morphine has a high affinity for mu receptors and mild affinity for kappa and delta receptors. It is relatively hydrophilic compared with more potent mu agonists. Rapid intravenous (15 second) administration is associated with increased plasma histamine concentrations, causing vasodilation and decreased blood pressure in dogs (Guedes et al., 2007a). However, systemic arterial blood pressure has been shown to increase for a brief period in dogs receiving morphine (1 mg/kg i.v. over 1 minute) (Maiante et al., 2009). Clinically, the cardiovascular effect of intravenous morphine is probably dependent on the dose and rate of administration. The less lipophilic nature of morphine makes it suitable to be given via the epidural route (see Chapter 11).

The elimination half-life of intravenous morphine is approximately 60 minutes in dogs (KuKanich et al., 2005a) and 75 minutes in cats (Taylor et al., 2001). Bioavailability is 100% following intramuscular injection (Barnhart et al., 2000). Orally administered sustained- or extended-release formulations have 5–20% bioavailability with considerable individual variability. Reduced bioavailability is attributed to metabolism by the intestinal mucosa and first-pass metabolism in the liver following absorption from the GI tract. Oral formulations are therefore not recommended for use in cats and dogs (Aragon et al., 2008).

In humans, morphine is primarily metabolized to morphine-3-glucuronide (which can produce excitatory effects) and morphine-6-glucuronide (which possesses greater analgesic properties than morphine). Although morphine is rapidly cleared in dogs following intravenous administration, morphine-6-glucuronide does not appear to be a major metabolite (KuKanich et al., 2005a). In cats, the primary mechanism of metabolism is via the formation of sulphate conjugates; the activity of these metabolites is unknown (Taylor et al., 2001).

Using a device to determine thermal and pressure nociceptive thresholds, onset of analgesia following morphine (0.2 mg/kg i.m.) in cats was reported to be 4 hours, with a duration of effect of 2 hours. Using the same model, morphine was found to have lower efficacy relative to hydromorphone or buprenorphine (Taylor et al., 2001). In a more recent study evaluating morphine (0.2 mg/kg s.c.) in cats, only a short-lasting increase in nociceptive thresholds from 45 to 60 minutes was found, while the pressure threshold was increased at 3 to 6 hours after injection (Steagall et al., 2006).

To achieve target serum concentrations for analgesia in dogs, morphine (0.5 mg/kg i.v.) every 2 hours is recommended, although this dosing regimen has not been validated in clinical settings (KuKanich et al., 2005a). A clinical trial using doses of 0.3–0.8 mg/kg i.m. reported good postoperative analgesia following orthopaedic surgery in over 70% of dogs for the 4-hour study period (Taylor and Houlton, 1984). Morphine given at 0.3 mg/kg i.m. for preanaesthetic medication before arthrotomy in dogs resulted in postoperative analgesia for 7 hours (Brodbelt et al., 1997). Following thoracotomy in dogs, doses of morphine of 1.0 mg/kg i.m. or intrapleurally provided similar postoperative pain control to intercostal nerve blocks with bupivacaine (Stobie et al., 1995).

In summary, the duration of effective analgesia is approximately 2–6 hours in cats and dogs at the doses shown in Figures 10.1 and 10.2. This interval is used for repeat dosing, based on patient evaluation. As previously mentioned, high doses of morphine should be combined with a sedative/tranquillizer to prevent dysphoria or euphoria, especially in cats.

A slow intravenous infusion of morphine can be administered either alone, or in combination with other analgesics such as lidocaine and/or ketamine, to produce continuous analgesia (Muir et al., 2003). This technique provides consistent levels of analgesia, minimizes adverse side effects from intermittent boluses, and requires less

Drug	Classification	Dosage forms	Dose	Duration of effect of one bolus
Morphine	Mu agonist	Injectable: 0.5–50 mg/ml	0.1–1.0 mg/kg i.m. or s.c. Infusion: 0.05–0.1 mg/kg/h	2–6 hours
Pethidine (meperidine)	Mu agonist	Injectable: 10–100 mg/ml	3–5 mg/kg i.m. or s.c.	1–1.5 hours
Methadone	Mu agonist	Injectable: 10 mg/ml	0.1–0.3 mg/kg i.v., i.m. or s.c.	4–8 hours
Hydromorphone	Mu agonist	Injectable: 2–100 mg/ml	0.05–0.1 mg/kg i.v., i.m. or s.c.	4 hours
Fentanyl	Mu agonist	Injectable: 50 and 78.5 μg/ml Transdermal: 25 μg/h	Injectable: 5–10 μg/kg bolus Infusion rate: • Intraoperative 2–40 μg/kg/h • Postoperative 2–3 μg/kg/h Transdermal: 4 μg/kg/h	20–30 minutes
Remifentanil	Mu agonist	Injectable: 1 mg dried drug/vial (requires dilution)	Infusion: suggest using fentanyl at 3 μg/kg bolus followed by remifentanil at 5–40 μg/kg/h i.v. Diluted to 0.1 mg/ml dilution	Remifentanil has too short a duration of effect for bolus administration
Tramadol	Mu agonist	Injectable: 50 mg/ml Tablet: 50 mg	1–2 mg/kg s.c. 2–4 mg/kg orally	12 hours
Butorphanol	Mu antagonist–kappa agonist	Injectable: 10 mg/ml	0.2–0.4 mg/kg i.v., i.m. or s.c.	1.5–2 hours
Buprenorphine	Partial mu agonist	Injectable: 0.3 mg/ml	0.01–0.04 mg/kg i.v., i.m. or oral transmucosal (OTM)	4–12 hours
Naloxone	Antagonist	Injectable: 0.4 and 1 mg/ml	0.002–0.04 mg/kg i.v.	30 minutes–1 hour

10.2 Opioid analgesics routinely used in cats.

morphine overall. For example, following laparotomy, dogs were reported to have similar levels of analgesia when receiving morphine either as an infusion (0.12 mg/kg/h i.v.) or at 1.0 mg/kg i.m. every 4 hours. This was despite the infusion group receiving approximately half the total amount of morphine that was used in the intermittent bolus group (Lucas *et al.*, 2001). Plasma concentrations achieved using the infusion technique were also lower than the required concentrations for analgesia reported in other species. Higher infusion rates might be necessary in dogs undergoing more invasive surgery, such as thoracotomy or major orthopaedic interventions (Guedes *et al.*, 2007b). Currently recommended rates of infusion are shown in Figure 10.1. There have been no clinical trials evaluating infusions in cats, but clinically recommended rates are provided in Figure 10.2.

At these recommended doses, morphine produces mild sedation in dogs. Administration with acepromazine or an alpha-2 adrenergic agonist improves the quality of sedation and analgesia in cats and dogs. When administered during inhalational anaesthesia, morphine has an anaesthetic-sparing effect, especially in dogs. The minimum alveolar concentration (MAC) of isoflurane is decreased by 50% using morphine at 2 mg/kg i.v. in dogs, and by 25% using 1 mg/kg i.v. in cats (Steffey *et al.*, 1994; Ilkiw *et al.*, 2002).

Using morphine and atropine for pre-anaesthetic medication in dogs can make duodenal endoscopy more difficult to perform compared with pre-anaesthetic medication with only morphine or pethidine; atropine is therefore not recommended for this procedure (Donaldson *et al.* 1993). Morphine is reported to increase biliary duct pressure and sphincter of Oddi tone more than pethidine, butorphanol or tramadol in humans (Wu *et al.* 2004) and dogs (Shore *et al.* 1971). These effects can be reversed with naloxone or butorphanol (Radnay *et al.*, 1984). The clinical significance of opioid-induced biliary changes is, however, thought to be minimal, particularly in humans (Thompson 2001).

Administration of morphine before anaesthesia in dogs can increase the incidence of gastro-oesophageal reflux, but the clinical significance of this is not clear (Wilson *et al.*, 2005). Administration (intramuscular or subcutaneous) typically induces emesis in non-painful healthy cats and dogs; and the incidence of emesis is lower with the intravenous route. It is rare for emesis to occur when intravenous or intramuscular morphine is administered postoperatively at analgesic doses.

Pethidine (meperidine)

Pethidine is a synthetic mu and kappa agonist with a clinically useful antispasmodic effect. It should only be administered by the intramuscular route because intravenous administration produces a dose-dependent hypotension secondary to histamine release (Thompson and Walton, 1964; Kalthum and Waterman, 1988; Dobromylskyj, 1992). Following intramuscular administration in dogs, it has an elimination half-life of 51 minutes and is not detectable in plasma by 90 minutes (Waterman and Kalthum, 1989a). In cats, the elimination half-life varies widely, but is around 216 minutes (Taylor *et al.*, 2001). Subcutaneous administration is not recommended because pethidine is rapidly metabolized, resulting in low plasma concentrations (Waterman and Kalthum, 1989b). The metabolite norpethidine has weak analgesic properties and can also cause seizures; it is detectable in plasma from 1 hour after intramuscular injection in cats (Taylor *et al.*, 2001). Norpethidine production in dogs is low, but concentrations of the metabolite can reach convulsant levels in cases of accidental pethidine overdose (Golder *et al.*, 2010). Treatment is with conventional anticonvulsants, because naloxone does not reverse the convulsive effects of norpethidine.

Pethidine is not as efficacious as morphine or hydromorphone for treating severe pain. Due to its short duration of action of approximately 45–60 minutes, it is recommended only for procedures associated with mild discomfort (Slingsby and Waterman-Pearson, 2001; Millette et al., 2008). At analgesic doses (3–5 mg/kg), pethidine is associated with mild sedation and a low incidence of vomiting (Wilson et al., 2007). It can therefore be used as a pre-anaesthetic agent to produce light sedation, or where emesis is undesirable, and other full mu agonists can be given to provide 'top-up' analgesia during anaesthesia, if necessary.

Methadone

Methadone is a synthetic, full mu agonist with similar analgesic potency to morphine, but with a longer duration of effect in dogs (Ingvast-Larsson et al., 2010). It is available as a racemic mixture or as the L-enantiomer. The D-enantiomer also has analgesic properties but does not activate opioid receptors, and therefore is not considered an opioid. Methadone is also an NMDA receptor antagonist, and inhibits the reuptake of both serotonin and noradrenaline, which may be advantageous when treating chronic or neuropathic pain. Intravenous, intramuscular and subcutaneous routes of administration are appropriate in cats and dogs. In cats, when methadone was delivered via the buccal mucosal route, plasma concentrations were detectable for 24 hours, suggesting that this route may be clinically useful (Ferreira et al., 2011). In dogs, methadone has very poor enteral bioavailability (KuKanich et al., 2005b).

Methadone is an effective analgesic when used preoperatively for both soft tissue and orthopaedic procedures. In dogs, its analgesic properties are similar to morphine and superior to buprenorphine. In cats, in an experimental study using a nociceptive threshold device, methadone produced analgesia superior to buprenorphine (Steagall et al., 2006). In combination with acepromazine, methadone provided a quality of sedation similar to that observed with morphine in dogs; when used alone, however, methadone produces minimal sedation (Monteiro et al., 2008). Salivation, vocalization and dysphoria have been observed in dogs when methadone is used alone. However, unlike morphine, it rarely induces emesis, and would therefore be useful in cases where vomiting is undesirable (e.g. patients with increased intraocular or intracranial pressure) (Maiante et al., 2009; Ingvast-Larsson et al., 2010).

At equipotent analgesic doses in dogs, methadone is associated with more pronounced haemodynamic changes relative to morphine (Maiante et al., 2009). Following intravenous administration of morphine or methadone in dogs, dose-dependent reductions in heart rate and cardiac index and increases in systemic vascular resistance occur that are similar to those produced by other opioids.

Hydromorphone

Hydromorphone is also a semi-synthetic opioid derived from morphine. It is a full mu agonist and its physiochemical properties are similar to those of morphine, although it has greater lipophilicity. It has five to 10 times the potency of morphine and can be administered intramuscularly, intravenously or subcutaneously. The subcutaneous route gives a longer onset time and shorter duration of action in cats (Robertson et al., 2009). Intravenous administration results in minor increases in plasma histamine concentrations in dogs (Guedes et al., 2007a). The characteristics and efficacy of hydromorphone and oxymorphone are similar, but in some locations hydromorphone is substantially less expensive and has therefore gained popularity.

Following intravenous administration, hydromorphone has a short terminal half-life (<1 hour) and rapid clearance,

and thus needs to be administered often (KuKanich et al., 2008). Similar to morphine, it can be administered as an intravenous infusion to maintain target plasma concentrations for prolonged periods. Investigational products in which hydromorphone is encapsulated into liposomal membranes, allowing slow release over a period of 3 days to 3 weeks, have shown potential for long-term pain control in dogs (Smith et al., 2013).

Similar to other full mu agonists, hydromorphone produces dose-dependent analgesia. When administered intravenously, the onset of analgesia and sedation is more rapid than with morphine. At doses of 0.05–0.1 mg/kg i.m., the duration of analgesic effect is 3–7 hours in cats (Wegner et al. 2004; Wegner and Robertson, 2007). In cats, 0.1 mg/kg i.m. produced an increase in nociceptive threshold within 15 minutes of administration, which lasted 5–7 hours (Lascelles and Robertson, 2004).

Hyperthermia following hydromorphone administration in cats is a potential adverse effect and may occur more commonly than with other opioids (Niedfeldt and Robertson, 2006). Vomiting following intramuscular administration is common (44–100%) in healthy dogs without pain, although it is rare when hydromorphone is administered postoperatively. If maropitant or acepromazine is administered before intramuscular hydromorphone, or if hydromorphone is administered intravenously, the incidence is reduced (Valverde et al. 2004; Kraus 2013, 2014). When hydromorphone is administered in combination with acepromazine, intraocular pressure does not increase in normal dogs; the effect of hydromorphone alone on intraocular pressure in the dog or cat has not been reported (Stephan et al., 2003). In dogs, if an increase in intraocular pressure due to vomiting is undesirable, hydromorphone may be avoided in the pre-anesthetic medication and can be given intravenously once anaesthesia is induced.

Fentanyl

Fentanyl is a synthetic full mu agonist with high potency. It can be administered by the intramuscular, intravenous, subcutaneous or transdermal route. When administered intravenously, the elimination half-life is reported to be 0.75–6 hours in dogs and approximately 2 hours in cats (Kyles et al., 1996; Lee et al., 2000; Sano et al., 2006; KuKanich and Clark, 2012). Clinically, intravenous administration results in a rapid onset (1–2 minutes) and short duration of action (20–30 minutes in dogs). Fentanyl may be administered using a bolus technique to control acute, severe pain (2–5 μg/kg i.v.) or as an infusion. Other routes of administration, such as transmucosal and intranasal, have recently been evaluated in dogs, but further development is required before their clinical use (Little et al., 2008).

In healthy dogs without pain, higher bolus doses (5–10 μg/kg) generally result in recumbency and sedation. Healthy cats without pain given fentanyl 10 μg/kg i.v. are reported to be easy to handle and quiet, with mild signs of euphoria (Robertson et al., 2005a). Plasma concentrations in the range of 1–3 ng/ml are associated with analgesic effects. In cats, the thermal nociceptive threshold was increased for 110 minutes following a 10 μg/kg i.v. bolus of fentanyl. Fentanyl administered as an intravenous bolus produces vagally mediated bradycardia but has minimal direct depressant effects on the myocardium or vasculature. It can also cause respiratory depression in anaesthetized patients.

Transdermal administration of fentanyl can provide prolonged analgesia. Fentanyl patches are available in four different sizes based on the rate of delivery to the systemic circulation across human skin (Figure 10.3). The patch is composed of a drug reservoir, a rate-limiting membrane and an adhesive perimeter for attaching the patch to the skin. The rate of absorption of fentanyl is dependent on the surface area of the patch exposed to skin. Therefore, only partially removing the protective cover will reduce the exposed surface area, lower the rate of fentanyl absorption and result in a lower plasma concentration. The transdermal bioavailability of fentanyl is approximately 64% in dogs and 36% in cats and the dose required for analgesia is approximately 4 μg/kg/h (Kyles *et al.*, 1996; Lee *et al.*, 2000). Several studies have revealed relatively large individual variations in plasma fentanyl concentration. In cats weighing 1.6–4.3 kg, exposure of 50% of a 25 μg/h patch to the skin resulted in plasma concentrations below the theoretical therapeutic value. However, the degree of analgesia in these cats following ovariohysterectomy was comparable to that in cats exposed to the full patch (Davidson *et al.*, 2004). Partial patch exposure in cats weighing <4 kg can be used, but the invasiveness of the procedure and the degree of analgesia required should be considered when selecting the amount of patch exposure, and the degree of analgesia following patch application must be assessed to verify that analgesia is adequate.

Patient bodyweight	Recommended fentanyl patch size
Cats and dogs <10 kg	25 μg/h
Dogs 10–20 kg	50 μg/h
Dogs 20–30 kg	75 μg/h
Dogs >30 kg	100 μg/h

10.3 Recommended fentanyl patch sizes for cats and dogs.

The recommended locations for patch placement include the dorsal or lateral thorax, neck, groin, tarsal area or dorsum (using the area clipped for an epidural injection). An *in vitro* study using canine cadaver skin revealed faster absorption rates from the groin region compared with the thoracic and neck regions, although this has not been tested *in vivo* (Mills *et al.*, 2004).

The area selected should be clipped and the skin cleaned with mild soap (not alcohol), and allowed to dry before patch placement. The protective cover is removed and the patch applied to the skin and held in place for 60 seconds. Transmucosal contact with the patch can result in toxic plasma fentanyl concentrations and therefore, if necessary, a light bandage can be placed over the patch to prevent its disruption or removal. After use, patches should be disposed of by folding the adhesive sides to each other, and returned to the veterinary practice for appropriate biomedical waste disposal.

Following patch application, therapeutic plasma concentrations of fentanyl are reached in approximately 24 hours in dogs and within 12 hours in cats. Plasma fentanyl concentrations are generally maintained within the analgesic range for up to 72 hours following patch application in both species. Removal or replacement of the patch at 72 hours is recommended because plasma concentrations begin to decrease after this time. Once the patch is removed, plasma concentrations decrease to below the analgesic range within 4–6 hours in dogs and 6–20 hours in cats.

Studies have shown that the early postoperative (0–6 hours) analgesic efficacy of transdermal fentanyl in dogs undergoing orthopaedic surgery is equivalent to, or greater than, the analgesia obtained from epidurally administered morphine (Robinson *et al.*, 1999). It provides an analgesic effect after pelvic limb surgery equivalent to systemically administered morphine, but at a greater economic cost (Egger *et al.*, 2007). Following ovariohysterectomy in dogs, epidural morphine can provide better analgesia than transdermal fentanyl but has similar behavioural and analgesic effects to those of systemically administered oxymorphone (Kyles *et al.*, 1998; Pekcan and Koc, 2010). In cats undergoing onychectomy (not permitted in the UK), transdermal fentanyl produced analgesia comparable to butorphanol (Gellasch *et al.*, 2002).

Few adverse effects have been reported with the use of transdermal fentanyl patches (Kyles *et al.*, 1998). Cutaneous irritation at the site of patch placement can be common. Mild sedation, bradycardia and anorexia have been reported in dogs, and hyperthermia, euphoria and dysphoria have been reported in cats. Respiratory depression during patch application has not been shown to be clinically significant in the awake dog. However, plasma fentanyl concentrations which provide analgesia can compound respiratory depression during general anaesthesia. The use of external warming devices such as heating pads and water blankets can dramatically increase fentanyl absorption by increasing skin perfusion and lead to severe respiratory depression.

A transdermal fentanyl solution is now available for use in dogs. Following application of the solution to the interscapular skin, peak plasma concentration is attained within an hour. The formulation provides a depot following its absorption into dermal layers, resulting in maintenance of therapeutic plasma concentration for at least 4 days (Freise *et al.*, 2012a,b). A large, multi-centre clinical trial found this product to provide postoperative analgesia superior to buprenorphine (Linton *et al.*, 2012). Compared with the transdermal patch, the transdermal liquid preparation offers greater ease of application and faster onset of analgesia, and also eliminates the concerns related to patch disposal. Application of the transdermal solution 2–4 hours before surgery is recommended. Veterinary surgeons in countries where the product is available must complete an online training module before accessing the product. Due to the potential for transcutaneous absorption of the product in humans, dogs must be isolated from children for at least 72 hours following transdermal application and dogs >20 kg bodyweight must be hospitalized for a minimum of 48 hours following application.

Sufentanil/alfentanil/remifentanil

Sufentanil, alfentanil and remifentanil are all short-acting, potent derivatives of fentanyl with similar pharmacodynamic effects. In humans, they have fewer side effects with less variability in cardiovascular responses than are observed with fentanyl. Due to their short duration of action, these mu agonists are usually administered as an infusion to provide analgesia during general anaesthesia. They are powerful respiratory depressants and their intraoperative use may require intermittent positive pressure ventilation.

Alfentanil (50 μg/kg i.v.) has been reported to produce brief and transient excitement, mydriasis, a slight increase in systemic blood pressure and approximately 20 minutes of analgesia with sedation in some cats (Pascoe *et al.*, 1993). Alfentanil has been used as an induction agent, as part of balanced anaesthesia protocols and for postoperative analgesia in dogs. The use of anticholinergics is recommended when using high doses of alfentanil (Chambers, 1989).

Sufentanil can be used with or without benzodiazepines for relatively haemodynamically stable induction anaesthesia in debilitated dogs, and as part of a balanced anaesthesia protocol with inhalational or injectable anaesthetics (Hellebrekers and Sap, 1992; Bufalari *et al.*, 2007). A long-acting form of sufentanil that provides sedation and analgesia for approximately 24 hours in dogs may become commercially available in the future (Polis *et al.*, 2004; Slingsby *et al.*, 2006).

Remifentanil is unique in that it undergoes metabolism by non-specific esterases in the blood and does not accumulate with prolonged administration. It has similar potency to fentanyl in humans, but may have only half the potency of fentanyl in dogs (Michelsen *et al.*, 1996). It can be used in dogs and cats with liver or kidney disease to reduce inhalational anaesthetic requirements and to provide perioperative analgesia without prolonging anaesthetic recovery. Remifentanil is only useful postoperatively if the infusion is not disrupted, since its rapid metabolism means that analgesia ceases suddenly once delivery is stopped, even if only for a few minutes.

Codeine

Codeine is a naturally occuring opioid agonist. It exerts its analgesic effects through its parent compound as well as its metabolites, which include morphine. In humans, codeine has an enteral bioavailability of approximately 60% and it is most commonly administered orally. In contrast, in dogs the enteral bioavailability is 4% and the conversion rate to morphine is lower, and therefore the oral route is not recommended (Skingle and Tyers, 1980; KuKanich, 2009). Codeine at a dose of 4 mg/kg s.c. has been shown to be equivalent to morphine 0.2 mg/kg s.c. in dogs. Codeine at 2 mg/kg s.c. produced a similar level of analgesia to tramadol 2 mg/kg s.c. in dogs undergoing mandibulectomy or maxillectomy (Martins *et al.*, 2010). Codeine did not increase thermal nociception threshold in cats when given orally at a dose of approximately 2 mg/kg (Steagall *et al.*, 2015).

Partial agonists
Buprenorphine

Buprenorphine is classified as a high-affinity partial mu agonist and a weak kappa antagonist. Because of this, it needs to occupy a greater fraction of the available pool of functional mu receptors (compared with a full mu agonist) to induce a similar magnitude of response. Its high receptor affinity means that it can displace morphine from mu receptors, and reversal of buprenorphine using naloxone requires higher doses. Buprenorphine can be administered intravenously, intramuscularly and subcutaneously, although the subcutaneous route is less efficacious in cats (Giordano *et al.*, 2010; Steagall *et al.*, 2013). A formulation with a higher concentration of buprenorphine (1.8 mg/ml) is now available in some countries for daily subcutaneous use in cats for up to 3 days, but there are few studies evaluating its efficacy in clinical practice. Buprenorphine has been reported to reach peak concentration 3 minutes after intramuscular injection in cats (Taylor *et al.*, 2001). Its pharmacokinetics are similar in dogs, and some authors advise giving buprenorphine (15 μg/kg i.v.) every 3–4 hours in dogs (Krotscheck *et al.*, 2008).

Buprenorphine has only 3–6% enteral bioavailability in dogs, but it has excellent buccal mucosal bioavailability (100%) in cats, with concentrations peaking by 30 minutes after administration and lasting for 6 hours at a dose of 20 μg/kg (Robertson *et al.*, 2003, 2005b). In dogs, buccal mucosal bioavailability is 30–60%, but new formulations may improve uptake (Abbo *et al.*, 2008; Krotscheck *et al.*, 2010). Studies of a transdermal buprenorphine patch in dogs and cats (Murrell *et al.*, 2007; Pieper *et al.*, 2010) found that it was not effective until 36 hours following patch application, which may limit its use in the perioperative period.

One of the major benefits of buprenorphine is its relatively long duration of action; however, the reported duration of analgesia following parenteral administration varies from 4–12 hours. Its longer onset time of analgesia compared with other opioids such as hydromorphone (ranging from 15–60 minutes, depending on the species, route and stimuli being assessed) is of clinical significance (Wegner *et al.*, 2008; Steagall *et al.*, 2009, 2013). If given for postoperative analgesia, it must be administered pre- or intraoperatively to provide immediate postoperative analgesia.

Doubling the dose of buprenorphine in dogs undergoing ovariohysterectomy has been shown to have no benefit, which may imply a ceiling effect for analgesia, although this requires further investigation (Slingsby *et al.*, 2011). In dogs, buprenorphine (7–20 μg/kg i.m.) has a similar analgesic efficacy to morphine (0.3–0.8 mg/kg i.m.) following orthopaedic surgery, although buprenorphine may not be as reliable as morphine for all dogs having invasive sugery. Interestingly, in cats undergoing surgery, buprenorphine (0.01 mg/kg i.m.) produces increased analgesia for 4–12 hours compared with a duration of only 4–6 hours in cats receiving morphine (0.2 mg/kg i.m.) (Stanway *et al.*, 2002). In a clinical trial evaluating analgesia following ovariohysterectomy in cats, analgesia was equivalent in cats receiving buprenorphine or butorphanol (Polson *et al.*, 2012).

Mixed opioid agonist–antagonists
Butorphanol

Butorphanol has agonist activity at kappa receptors and high-affinity antagonist activity at mu receptors. It is considered to be effective for mild to moderate visceral pain and is used as an analgesic for minor elective surgical procedures. For analgesia, the intravenous, intramuscular or subcutaneous routes of administration are used. An oral formulation is available as an antitussive, but the drug has low enteral bioavailability and high doses are required for analgesia if administered by this route. The duration of analgesia in cats and dogs ranges from 30–120 minutes with intravenous administration (Sawyer *et al.*, 1987; Houghton *et al.*, 1991; Lascelles and Robertson, 2004).

The literature suggests that when used alone in dogs, butorphanol is not an effective analgesic compared with full mu agonists or newer NSAIDs. In dogs following laparotomy, 0.4 mg/kg i.m. provided inadequate postoperative analgesia in half the dogs being studied (Mathews *et al.* 2001). Meloxicam has been shown to provide superior analgesia for 12 hours compared with butorphanol following ovariohysterectomy in dogs (Caulkett *et al.*, 2003). When used as an analgesic for pain associated with orthopaedic procedures in dogs, butorphanol has consistently been demonstrated to result in inadequate analgesia (Mathews *et al.*, 1996).

In experimental studies, butorphanol administered at a dose of 0.1–0.8 mg/kg i.v. increased the thermal threshold in cats in a dose-independent manner for up to 90 minutes. In several clinical trials evaluating its postoperative analgesic efficacy following ovariohysterectomy and/or onychectomy, the results have been less favourable (Al-Gizawiy and Rude, 2004; Carroll et al., 2005; Warne et al., 2013). For example, in cats receiving 0.4 mg/kg butorphanol s.c. before ovariohysterectomy, 60% of the cats required rescue analgesia 20 minutes after recovery from anaesthesia (Warne et al., 2013). Only 44% of cats receiving 0.4 mg/kg butorphanol were assessed as having good or better general impression scores following onychectomy (Carroll et al., 2005). In both of the latter studies, alternative analgesics were found to be superior.

Butorphanol produces mild sedation and is an effective antitussive. Therefore, it is useful as a premedicant for patients undergoing airway examinations and bronchoscopy. It also does not impair the passing of an endoscope through the pyloric sphincter, unlike full mu agonists, and is therefore suitable for patients undergoing duodenal endoscopy. Respiratory depression associated with butorphanol is less profound than with full mu agonists. The degree of respiratory depression is characterized by a 'ceiling effect', as with its analgesic effects, and increasing doses do not increase the degree of respiratory depression and analgesia.

Butorphanol can be used to reverse the effects of full mu agonists (Dyson et al., 1990; MacCrackin et al., 1994). When used in this way, the goal is to reverse the undesirable effects of the full mu agonist and provide kappa receptor-mediated analgesia. It is recommended that 0.1–0.4 mg/kg butorphanol is diluted in a large volume (5–10 ml depending on patient size) of saline and administered intravenously in small increments every 2–5 minutes until adequate reversal has occurred.

Miscellaneous opioid drugs

Tramadol

Tramadol is classified as an atypical, centrally acting opioid. Analgesic effects are produced at mu receptors by the activity of both the parent drug and its metabolites. Tramadol also inhibits serotonin and noradrenaline reuptake, which may contribute to a reduction in nociceptive transmission at the level of the spinal cord. It also has antagonist effects at the muscarinic M_1 receptor. Tramadol is available in oral and parenteral formulations. It is considered a controlled drug in many countries and is under regulatory control as with other opioids.

The enteral bioavailability of tramadol is approximately 65% in dogs and 93% in cats (KuKanich and Papich, 2004; Pypendop and Ilkiw, 2007). It is metabolized in the liver via demethylation and glucuronidation before excretion through the kidney. Cats produce high concentrations of the active metabolite O-desmethyltramadol, which has a high affinity for the mu receptor; in contrast, dogs produce little of this metabolite. Glucuronidation is slower in cats, therefore a lower dose with a longer dosing interval is recommended relative to the dosing regimen for dogs. Bioavailability may be substantially reduced in dogs receiving prolonged treatment, due to either reduced absorption or increased presystemic metabolism of tramadol (Matthiesen et al., 1998).

Pre-emptive administration of tramadol (2.0 mg/kg i.v.) in dogs undergoing elective ovariohysterectomy resulted in similar postoperative analgesia over a 6-hour period to morphine (0.2 mg/kg i.v.) (Mastrocinque and Fantoni, 2003). Tramadol at 4–5 mg/kg orally provided inferior analgesia to that provided by a combination of tramadol and a NSAID following orthopaedic surgery in dogs; the combination is also better for dogs undergoing soft tissue surgery (Davila et al., 2013; Teixeira et al., 2013). Tramadol

should not be administered with a serotonin agonist owing to the potential for serotonin syndrome (see Chapter 2).

Tramadol administered subcutaneously or orally has been shown to increase the thermal nociceptive threshold in a dose-dependent manner in cats (Pypendop et al., 2009). The combination of tramadol (2 mg/kg s.c.) and an NSAID provided effective analgesia for cats undergoing routine ovariohysterectomy (Brondani et al., 2009).

Opioid antagonists

Naloxone

Naloxone is considered to be a full mu and kappa opioid receptor antagonist, with little agonist effect. It can be used to reverse the effects of mu agonists or mixed agonist–antagonists, because it has high affinity for both mu and kappa receptors. However, high doses of naloxone (30 μg/kg) are required to reverse buprenorphine effectively because the latter, a partial mu agonist, has a greater affinity for the mu receptor. When using naloxone to reverse the adverse effects of opioids in an animal that is in pain, it should be administered slowly in small intravenous increments. Ideally, the goal is to reverse the behavioural or respiratory depressant effects of the opioid without reversing its analgesic effect. Naloxone has a rapid onset of action (1–2 minutes), which facilitates such a titration technique. It can also be administered intramuscularly if necessary. The duration of action is reported to be 30–60 minutes, therefore when using naloxone to reverse the effects of long-acting mu agonists, it is important to observe the animal closely for the return of undesirable side effects. For example, when naloxone was used to reverse oxymorphone-induced sedation in dogs, clinical signs of renarcotization appeared 2 hours after naloxone administration (Dyson et al., 1990).

Naltrexone

Naltrexone is a synthetic opioid antagonist that is available in an oral formulation. It is primarily used for the treatment of behavioural disorders in cats and dogs.

Non-steroidal anti-inflammatory drugs

The use of NSAIDs for acute and chronic pain management has become popular with the introduction of newer, less toxic drugs. Although NSAIDs are not reversible and have a much lower therapeutic index than opioids, they have some advantages:

- Long duration of effect
- Anti-inflammatory properties
- No behaviour-modifying effects
- Lack of respiratory and cardiovascular side effects
- Availability in oral formulation
- No regulatory control due to the lack of abuse potential.

NSAIDs are indicated for postoperative pain, inflammatory conditions, osteoarthritis, panosteitis, hypertrophic osteodystrophy, pain from cancer and dental pain. Marked species differences exist in the efficacy and toxicity of NSAIDs, and therefore considerable care must be exercised to ensure appropriate drug and dose selection in cats and dogs.

Pharmacology

Chemically, the NSAIDs are a heterogeneous group of compounds, although they share considerable similarities in their pharmacokinetic and pharmacodynamic properties. Based on their physiochemical properties, they are generally classified into three groups: carboxylic acids; enolic acids and coxibs (cyclo-oxygenase-2 inhibitors). They are all highly protein-bound with a small volume of distribution. NSAIDs have different half-lives between species, so dosing should be based on available drug data for the particular species. The duration of anti-inflammatory effects is considerably longer than the measured plasma half-life. This is because tissue concentrations can remain high for some time after plasma concentration begins to decline. In particular, inflamed tissue has a pH that tends to result in NSAID accumulation at the site of action; this is especially the case for robenacoxib.

Most NSAIDs primarily undergo hepatic metabolism, with the metabolites excreted through the kidney. Entero-hepatic recycling may occur with some NSAIDs, whereby conjugated metabolites excreted in bile are reabsorbed from the GI tract into the circulation. This may result in a prolonged half-life. Cats have a limited ability to metabolize drugs through glucuronidation. This means that the half-life of some NSAIDs may be prolonged in cats, contributing to the risk of toxicity. If the appropriate dose and dosing interval are selected, however, these drugs can be useful for pain management in cats.

Patients with hepatic or renal disease may have greater and more prolonged peak plasma concentrations of the NSAID and its metabolites due to reduced metabolism and/or elimination of the parent drug and metabolites. Therefore, NSAIDs are not recommended in patients with underlying hepatic or renal disease.

Mechanism of action

The majority of desirable and undesirable clinical effects from NSAIDs stem from their inhibitory action on the cyclo-oxygenase (COX) enzyme; COX is responsible for the conversion of arachidonic acid (a byproduct of membrane phospholipids) into prostaglandins (PGE_2, PGF_2, PGD_2), prostacyclin (PGI_2) and thromboxanes (Figure 10.4). These compounds are synthesized throughout the body and have many diverse functions, such as regulation of blood flow in the gastric mucosa, kidney and intestinal tract. Thromboxanes play a key role in platelet aggregation. They are also involved in the initiation and propagation of inflammation, hyperalgesia and allodynia. Prostaglandins are released from injured cells at sites of injury, where they mediate inflammation by causing vasodilation and increased vascular permeability and by promoting neutrophil chemotaxis.

The COX enzyme has two distinct isoforms, COX-1 and COX-2. Conventional NSAIDs, such as aspirin, are non-specific inhibitors of COX and inhibit both COX-1 and COX-2 isoforms. COX-1 was initially thought to be the sole constitutive enzyme, produced in consistent quantities throughout the body and responsible for producing byproducts important for normal homeostatic functions such as regional tissue and organ blood flow, and platelet function. Conversely, COX-2 was thought to be an inducible enzyme, produced in response to stimuli such as cytokines and other mediators released following tissue injury. Therefore, it was hypothesized that drugs that inhibited only the COX-2 isoform would be effective inhibitors of inflammation but would not produce adverse effects. However, COX-2 is also produced constitutively in some

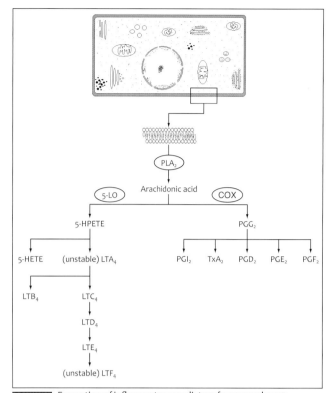

10.4 Formation of inflammatory mediators from membrane phospholipids. COX = cyclo-oxygenase; 5-HETE = 5-hydroxyeicosatetraenoic acid; 5-HPETE = 5-hydroperoxyeicosatetraenoic acid; 5-LO = 5-lipoxygenase; LT = leukotriene; PG = prostaglandin; PGG_2 = endoperoxide; PGI_2 = prostacyclin; PLA_2 = phospholipase A_2; TxA_2 = thromboxane A_2.

tissues such as the CNS, kidney and reproductive tract, and may also play a role in the repair of GI erosions. Therefore, even the newer COX-2-selective NSAIDS are not completely free of adverse effects.

NSAIDs are classified as nonselective, COX-1 selective or COX-2 selective (or preferential) on the basis of relative degree of their inhibition of the COX-1 or COX-2 isoform. The relative inhibition of the two isoforms is determined *in vitro* and is influenced by the techniques used and the species from which the test tissues/cells are derived. Drugs within the coxib category are highly selective COX-2 inhibitors.

Different NSAIDs block the COX enzyme using different mechanisms. Most drugs result in either a competitive, reversible inhibition or a time-dependent inhibition of the active site on the enzyme. Aspirin is an exception, as it forms a covalent bond with the active site of the enzyme, resulting in irreversible inhibition. In addition, some NSAIDs have been shown to inhibit the enzyme lipoxygenase, thereby decreasing formation of leukotrienes in addition to prostaglandins. These NSAIDs are termed 'dual inhibitors', of which an example is tepoxalin.

Analgesic effects

Prostaglandins increase the sensitivity of nociceptors and nociceptive neurons to painful stimuli. High concentrations of prostaglandins in peripheral tissues also result in changes in pathways that transmit nociceptive stimuli within the CNS. NSAIDs block the COX-2 enzyme, limiting the production of prostaglandins and/or leukotrienes in peripheral tissues, and minimizing subsequent alteration of pain-processing pathways. They may also mediate analgesia by inhibiting prostaglandin synthesis within the brain and the dorsal horn of the spinal cord.

Gastrointestinal effects

The COX-1 isoform is responsible for the production of prostaglandins that influence mucosal blood flow, epithelial cell turnover and mucus and bicarbonate secretion in the GI tract. Conventional, non-selective COX inhibitors are liable to produce GI adverse effects including vomiting, diarrhoea, anorexia, abdominal pain and GI ulceration. In severe cases, GI perforation may occur. The risk of adverse GI events is increased with high doses of NSAIDs, prolonged use, multiple NSAID use, underlying GI disease and concurrent glucocorticoid administration. The COX-2-selective drugs are associated with fewer GI side effects, although inappropriate dosing or patient selection can still result in adverse events.

Gastric ulcer prophylaxis may be recommended in some high-risk patients and in patients that have developed clinical signs associated with GI ulcers during NSAID treatment (Figure 10.5). Administration of NSAIDs should be stopped if signs of GI upset are observed and a rest period of at least 1 week should be used when changing from one NSAID to another.

Renal effects

When renal blood flow is reduced, prostaglandins formed locally in the kidney produce afferent arteriolar vasodilation to restore renal blood flow. Prostaglandins are also involved in the control of renin release and tubular function. Both the COX-2 and COX-1 isoforms are constitutively expressed in the kidney, so even the newer COX-2-selective agents may have adverse renal effects. In the well hydrated patient with normal renal function, the probability of NSAID-related renal dysfunction is low. In patients with renal disease or with cardiovascular dysfunction leading to reduced renal blood flow, there is an increased risk of NSAID-induced acute ischaemic renal failure and/or renal papillary necrosis. When administering NSAIDs that are licensed for perioperative use, haemodynamic monitoring and intravenous fluid therapy are still recommended during anaesthesia to detect and prevent periods of low renal blood flow. Some NSAIDs (e.g. meloxicam in humans) have also been reported to prevent prostaglandin-induced inhibition of ADH release, leading to decreased urine output and dilutional hyponatraemia, but renal injury is not present (Liamis et al., 2008).

Effects on coagulation

Inhibition of COX-1 reduces thromboxane production, leading to platelet dysfunction and prolonged bleeding. The non-selective COX inhibitors are therefore not recommended for perioperative use because of the increased risk of intraoperative haemorrhage. Non-selective COX inhibitors should be withdrawn for 10–14 days before elective surgery, to allow adequate time for NSAID elimination and restoration of platelet function. Short-term use of COX-2-selective inhibitors has minimal effect on platelet function in healthy dogs, although long-term use can result in prolonged mucosal bleeding times. However, no association between these agents and clinically significant bleeding disorders has been demonstrated.

Hepatic effects

NSAIDs are metabolized in the liver and hepatotoxicity is a risk following overdose with any of these drugs. Idiosyncratic hepatotoxicity has been reported with numerous different NSAIDs in humans and animals; this toxicity is not dose-dependent and frequently occurs within a few weeks after starting NSAID therapy. Clinical signs of hepatic dysfunction such as vomiting and inappetance are observed, with a marked increase in hepatic enzymes.

Reproductive effects

Prostaglandins are involved in normal labour, closure of the ductus arteriosus in the neonate, ovulation and embryo implantation. The safety of the currently available NSAIDs in respect of the reproductive system is discussed in Chapter 26.

Effects on cartilage

The effects of NSAIDs on cartilage are controversial and appear to depend on the specific NSAID and the method used to evaluate cartilage status. Some NSAIDs decrease proteoglycan synthesis and may contribute to chondrocyte death, while others may have chrondroprotective effects. For the NSAIDs currently licensed for use in dogs for treatment of osteoarthritis, there is no evidence of clinically significant deleterious effects on cartilage, hyaluronate or proteoglycan homeostasis, and some reports suggest they may offer a chondroprotective effect.

Prevention and treatment of ulcers	Drug	Dose	Comments
Prevention of ulcers	Misoprostol (synthetic prostaglandin E1)	Dogs: 2–5 µg/kg orally q12h Cats: 5 µ/kg orally q8h	Reduces incidence of GI ulcers in dogs
	Sulcralfate	Dogs: 0.5–1.0 g orally q8h Cats: 0.25 g orally q8–12h	Can be co-adminstered with misoprostol, but is given 2 hours before or 1 hour after misoprostol
Treatment of ulcers	Sucralfate	Dogs: 1.0–2.0 g orally q8h Cats: 0.5 g orally q8–12h	
	Famotidine	Dogs and cats: 0.5 mg/kg i.v. q12h or 0.5–1.0 mg/kg orally q12–24h	
	Omeprazole	Dogs: 0.5–1.5 mg/kg. i.v. or orally q24h Cats: 0.75–1.0 mg/kg i.v. or orally q24h	
	Ranitidine	Dogs: 2 mg/kg slow i.v., s.c. or orally q8–12h Cats: 2 mg/kg/day continuous i.v. infusion, 2.5 mg/kg slow i.v. q12h or 3.5 mg/kg orally q12h	

10.5 Recommended agents for gastrointestinal ulcer prevention and treatment.

Contraindications for non-steroidal anti-inflammatory drugs

Based on the known side-effects of NSAIDs, these drugs should not be used in patients with the following conditions:

- Impaired renal or hepatic function
- Dehydration or hypovolaemia
- Coagulopathies
- Risk of haemorrhage during surgery
- Animals also receiving other NSAIDs or corticosteroids
- GI ulcers or erosions
- Conditions associated with poor tissue perfusion, such as congestive heart failure
- Pregnant, lactating or breeding animals (see Chapter 26).

When switching from one NSAID to another, a 5–7 day washout interval is recommended in order to prevent adverse drug interactions. If NSAID withdrawal is due to adverse effects, the patient should be fully recovered before starting treatment with an alternative NSAID.

Veterinary approved non-steroidal anti-inflammatory drugs

Several different NSAIDs are currently licensed for use in cats and dogs, while others, although not approved, have been used off-label for many years. Because authorization can change, veterinary surgeons are advised to check the licensing information for their area.

Due to the physiological roles of the different COX isoforms, interest has primarily been given to developing COX-2-specific inhibitors. The selection of a specific NSAID should take into consideration:

- The reported COX-2 selectivity
- The reported efficacy and safety in clinical trials
- A suitable dosing format
- The individual patient's response to the drug.

Suitable doses for use in dogs and cats are shown in Figures 10.6 and 10.7.

Drug	Dosage forms	Dose
Carprofen	Injectable: 50 mg/ml Capsules (not available in UK): 25, 75 and 100 mg Chewable tablets: 20, 50, 100 mg in UK (25, 75, 100 mg in USA and Canada)	4 mg/kg s.c. or i.v. UK: 2–4 mg/kg/day orally in 2 equally divided doses Dose may be reduced to 2 mg/kg/day orally as a single dose after 7 days, subject to clinical response USA and Canada: 4.4 mg/kg orally q24h or 2.2 mg/kg orally q12h
Ketoprofen	Injectable: 100 mg/ml Tablets: 5 and 20 mg	1 mg/kg i.v., i.m., s.c. or orally on day 1, followed by 1 mg/kg i.v., i.m., s.c. q24h for 1–5 days 1 mg/kg orally q24h for 1–5 days In Canada: 2 mg/kg i.v., i.m. or s.c. (single dose) followed by 1 mg/kg orally for up to 4 days
Etodolac	Tablets: 150, 300 and 500 mg	10–15 mg/kg orally q24h
Tolfenamic acid	Injectable: 40 mg/ml Tablets: 6, 20 and 60 mg	4 mg/kg orally or s.c. q24h for 3 days, followed by a minimum of 4 days with no administration, then repeat
Tepoxalin	Tablets: 30, 50, 100, and 200 mg	10–20 mg/kg orally on day 1, followed by 10 mg/kg orally q24h
Meloxicam	Injectable: 5 mg/ml Oral suspension: 1.5 mg/ml	0.2 mg/kg i.v. (not UK) or s.c. on day 1, 0.1 mg/kg i.v. or s.c. on subsequent days 0.2 mg/kg orally on day 1, 0.1 mg/kg orally q24h on subsequent days
Deracoxib	Chewable tablets: 25 and 100 mg	Postoperative: 3–4 mg/kg orally q24h for a maximum of 7 days Chronic treatment: 1–2 mg/kg orally q24h
Firocoxib	Tablets: 57 and 227 mg	5 mg/kg orally q24h
Mavacoxib	Chewable tablets: 20, 30, 75 or 95 mg	2 mg/kg orally on days 1, 14 and 30 followed by once monthly
Robenacoxib	Injectable: 20 mg/ml Tablets: 5, 10, 20, 40 mg	2 mg/kg s.c. 1 mg/kg orally q24h
Cimicoxib	Chewable tablets: 8, 30 or 80 mg	Management of perioperative pain: 2 mg/kg orally 2h before surgery, followed by 2 mg/kg orally q24h for 3–7 days Relief of pain and inflammation associated with osteoarthritis: 2 mg/kg orally q24h for 6 months. For longer-term treatment, regular monitoring should be undertaken by the veterinary surgeon.

10.6 Non-steroidal anti-inflammatory drugs licensed for use in dogs. Clinicians are advised to check current recommendations supplied by the drug distributor for the country of residence.

Drug	Dosage forms	Dose
Carprofen	Injectable: 50 mg/ml	4 mg/kg i.v. or s.c. (single dose only)
Ketoprofen	Injectable: 100 mg/ml Tablets: 5 and 20 mg	2 mg/kg s.c. q24h for a maximum of 3 days 1 mg/kg orally q24h for a maximum of 5 days In Canada: 2 mg/kg s.c. (single dose only) followed by 1 mg/kg orally for up to 4 additional days
Tolfenamic acid	Injectable: 40 mg/ml Tablets: 6, 20 and 60 mg	4 mg/kg orally or s.c. q24h for 3 days, followed by a minimum of 4 days with no administration, then repeat
Meloxicam	Injectable: 2 mg/ml or 5 mg/ml Oral suspension: 0.5 mg/ml	0.2–0.3 mg/kg s.c. followed 24 hours later by 0.05 mg/kg orally q24h for 2 days 0.1 mg/kg orally, followed by 0.05 mg/kg for 1–4 days
Robenacoxib	Injectable: 20 mg/ml Tablets: 6 mg	2 mg/kg s.c. (single dose only) 1 mg/kg orally q24h for up to 6 days

10.7 Non-steroidal anti-inflammatory drugs licensed for use in cats. Clinicians are advised to check current recommendations supplied by the drug distributor for the country of residence.

Carboxylic acids

Carprofen: Carprofen is considered to be a relatively COX-2-selective (preferential) NSAID. It is available in injectable (for the intravenous and subcutaneous routes) and oral formulations. The injectable formulation can be administered perioperatively. In cats and dogs, the oral bioavailability of carprofen is over 90%, and peak plasma concentrations are achieved between 1 and 3 hours after administration. The plasma half-life of injectable carprofen is reported to be 10 hours in dogs. In cats, the plasma half-life is approximately 20 hours, although this may vary considerably (range 9–49 hours). For this reason, repeated administration in cats is not recommended (Parton *et al.*, 2000; Taylor *et al.*, 1996). The prolonged half-life in cats is thought to be due to reduced clearance via hepatic glucuronidation. Time to onset of action following intravenous administration of carprofen is <1 hour and its duration of action in dogs is 12–18 hours (considerably longer than most opioid analgesics) (Dzikiti *et al.*, 2006). In cats, preoperative carprofen administration has been shown to provide postoperative analgesia for the whole 20-hour assessment period (Lascelles *et al.*, 1995; Slingsby and Waterman-Pearson, 2002).

At a dose of 4 mg/kg i.v., carprofen is a very effective postoperative analgesic in dogs undergoing orthopaedic and soft tissue surgery. One study found that its use preoperatively in dogs resulted in superior postoperative analgesia compared with postoperative administration, although both techniques gave good analgesia (Lascelles *et al.*, 1998). The efficacy of carprofen in the immediate postoperative period is unlikely to be as profound as that of potent mu opioid agonists. However, carprofen was shown to be superior to butorphanol in an experimental acute synovitis model (McCann *et al.*, 2004).

Carprofen has been shown to be an effective analgesic for osteoarthritis in numerous studies. It has relatively good GI tolerance when administered to dogs for long periods, and because of its long half-life, once daily administration may provide adequate analgesia. Hepatotoxicity has been reported in dogs following carprofen administration (MacPhail *et al.*, 1998); a large proportion of the dogs were Labrador Retrievers. However, the study did not evaluate the relative breed prevalence of adverse effects, and it is therefore not possible to determine whether a true breed sensitivity exists. Data from the US Food and Drug Administration suggest that the incidence of hepatotoxicity (<0.05%) associated with carprofen is similar to that of other NSAIDs.

Clinically important alterations in renal function have not been demonstrated in dogs given carprofen before anaesthesia (Bergmann *et al.*, 2005). However, maintenance of renal blood flow with fluid therapy, and ensuring adequate systemic arterial blood pressure, is recommended with preoperative administration of any NSAID. Carprofen does not alter serum levels of thromboxane, and has not been shown to have any significant effect on mucosal bleeding time in healthy dogs or in dogs requiring fracture repair (Hickford *et al.*, 2001; Bergmann *et al.*, 2005; Blois *et al.*, 2010). *In vitro* tests have demonstrated alterations in platelet function associated with carprofen, but the clinical significance of these changes has yet to be determined (Mullins *et al.*, 2012).

In cats, carprofen is licensed at a dose of 4 mg/kg s.c., although it has also been shown to be effective at a dose of 2 mg/kg s.c. (Lascelles *et al.*, 1995). It is an effective postoperative analgesic, superior to both pethidine and butorphanol following ovariohysterectomy, and to buprenorphine following orthopaedic surgery (Lascelles *et al.*, 1995;

Al-Gizawiy and Rude, 2004; Mollenhoff *et al.*, 2005). The duration of analgesia is reported to last approximately 20 hours. Carprofen provides a similar degree of analgesia to meloxicam. Due to its variable half-life in cats, long-term use of carprofen is not recommended.

Ketoprofen: Ketoprofen is a non-specific COX inhibitor available in injectable and oral formulations. The injectable formulation can be administered by the intravenous, intramuscular and subcutaneous routes. It has a long duration of effect, despite a relatively short half-life in both cats and dogs and (0.5–1.5 hours), and is therefore administered once every 24 hours. It has been shown to have high oral bioavailability, with rapid absorption from the GI tract.

Ketoprofen has been shown to be an effective postoperative analgesic for dogs undergoing soft tissue and orthopaedic procedures. The quality of analgesia is similar to that provided by carprofen and meloxicam (Grisneaux *et al.*, 1999; Deneuche *et al.*, 2004). Due to its lack of COX selectivity, ketoprofen inhibits platelet aggregation and increases the incidence of GI ulceration compared with placebo. It should only be administered postoperatively to patients with a normal haemostatic profile (Lemke *et al.*, 2002), and should be given for up to 5 days only.

Ketoprofen has also been shown to be an effective postoperative analgesic in cats. It has compared favourably to the opioids buprenorphine and oxymorphone following onychectomy, or onychectomy and neutering (Dobbins *et al.*, 2002). As in dogs, treatment should be limited to a total of 5 days.

Etodolac: Etodolac is a selective COX-2 inhibitor available in an oral formulation. Etodolac is used in dogs for the treatment of inflammation and pain associated with osteoarthritis (Borer *et al.*, 2003). It has an elimination half-life of approximately 14 hours. As with other NSAIDs, GI erosions and bleeding dysfunction have been reported with doses that exceed those recommended.

Tolfenamic acid: Tolfenamic acid is considered a selective COX-2 NSAID, although it also has anti-thromboxane activity. It is available in injectable and oral formulations and is used in cats and dogs for the treatment of postoperative and chronic pain. It is reported to have excellent antipyretic and anti-inflammatory properties, and has a long half-life. Due to its anti-thromboxane activity, it is not recommended for preoperative use or in patients with haemostatic disorders. There have been few clinical studies comparing its analgesic efficacy to other currently available NSAIDs, although it has been shown to provide similar postoperative analgesia to carprofen, ketoprofen or meloxicam following ovariohysterectomy in cats (Slingsby and Waterman-Pearson, 2000).

Enolic acids

Meloxicam: Meloxicam is a COX-2 selective (preferential) inhibitor. It is available in injectable and oral liquid formulations. The injectable formulation is licensed for administration by the intravenous (in some countries) and subcutaneous routes. Injectable meloxicam is used perioperatively. It has a long elimination half-life in dogs (20–30 hours) and cats (11–21 hours), and therefore is administered once a day. Most studies report a 24-hour duration of analgesia in both cats and dogs.

Preoperative or postoperative administration has been shown by several studies to produce effective postoperative analgesia for both soft tissue and orthopaedic surgery in cats and dogs (Mathews *et al.*, 2001; Slingsby and Waterman-Pearson, 2000, 2002; Carroll *et al.*, 2005). The degree of analgesia in the immediate postoperative period is not as effective as that provided by full mu opioid agonists, but is superior to that obtained from buprenorphine or butorphanol (Mathews *et al.*, 2001; Caulkett *et al.*, 2003; Carroll *et al.*, 2005; Gassel *et al.*, 2005). Analgesia from meloxicam is comparable with that provided by perioperative administration of carprofen following ovariohysterectomy in both dogs and cats (Slingsby and Waterman-Pearson, 2000, 2002; Leece *et al.*, 2005). Meloxicam also performed similarly to ketoprofen in dogs following orthopaedic surgery (Deneuche *et al.*, 2004).

No adverse effects on renal function have been demonstrated in dogs when meloxicam is administered preoperatively, even in dogs with periods of mild hypotension; it has also not been shown to impair *in vivo* platelet function or lead to any haemostatic alterations (Fresno *et al.*, 2005; Bostrom *et al.*, 2006).

Meloxicam is also an effective analgesic for chronic osteoarthritis and has been shown to be effective and well tolerated by dogs receiving recommended doses over a long period (Peterson and Keefe, 2004). The most common adverse clinical signs reported in dogs receiving chronic therapy include vomiting, diarrhoea and inappetence. More serious GI complications including perforation have also been reported (Duerr *et al.*, 2004; Luna *et al.*, 2007).

Meloxicam (0.3 mg/kg) was shown to provide good postoperative analgesia in cats for 20 hours after ovariohysterectomy, although all cats still had some incisional tenderness (Gassel *et al.*, 2005). The same dose compared favourably to buprenorphine in cats undergoing ovariohysterectomy, or to butorphanol in cats undergoing onychectomy with or without neutering (Carroll *et al.*, 2005; Gassel *et al.*, 2005).

Meloxicam is also an effective analgesic for cats with osteoarthritis. A prospective study reported analgesic efficacy and minimal side effects with meloxicam administered at a dose of 0.3 mg/kg orally on day 1 followed by 0.1 mg/kg orally q24h for 4 days (Lascelles *et al.*, 2001). The usual protocol for perioperative use consists of an initial dose of 0.2–0.3 mg/kg s.c. or i.v. (some countries only), followed by 0.05 mg/kg q24h orally for 1–5 days. Veterinary surgeons are advised to check the data sheet, as the licensed dose can vary by country (Lascelles *et al.*, 2001; Ingwersen *et al.*, 2012). A retrospective study of 38 cats with degenerative joint disease reported a median maintenance dose of 0.02 mg/kg/day over a prolonged treatment period (median duration of therapy >300 days) (Gowan *et al.*, 2011). Cats should be closely monitored for adverse effects during repeated administration or long-term treatment.

Coxibs

Deracoxib: Deracoxib is a highly selective COX-2 inhibitor used for the treatment of postoperative pain and inflammation associated with orthopaedic surgery or osteoarthritis in dogs (Gordon-Evans *et al.*, 2010). Uniquely among the coxibs, it is reported to inhibit the COX-2 enzyme irreversibly. Deracoxib is currently only available in an oral formulation. This formulation has high bioavailability, and despite its short elimination half-life of approximately 6 hours it is administered every 24 hours.

Deracoxib was shown to be an effective analgesic in an acute synovitis model in dogs, in which it was also superior to carprofen (Millis *et al.*, 2002; Karnik *et al.*, 2006). Deracoxib administered at a dose of 1–2 mg/kg/day for 3 days has been shown to improve postoperative

analgesia following soft tissue surgery (Bienhoff *et al.*, 2012). The efficacy of deracoxib compared with other NSAIDs administered postoperatively remains to be determined.

Despite the COX-2 selectivity of this agent, adverse effects are still possible with its use and dogs should be closely monitored during treatment. The most commonly reported side effects associated with chronic deracoxib administration are vomiting and diarrhoea. GI perforation has also been reported with use at clinical doses (Case *et al.*, 2010; Monteiro-Steagall *et al.*, 2013).

Firocoxib: Firocoxib is available in an oral formulation for the treatment of osteoarthritis and postsurgical pain in dogs. It has good analgesic efficacy, with similar efficacy to other NSAIDs for postsurgical pain in dogs. Its safety profile is also considered to be good. In dogs with osteoarthritis, it has been shown to be superior to carprofen and etodolac (Hanson *et al.*, 2006; Pollmeier *et al.*, 2006).

Mavacoxib: Mavacoxib is a recently developed, highly selective COX-2 inhibitor licensed for use in dogs. Mavacoxib is rapidly absorbed following oral administration. Administration with food increases its enteral bioavailability. Periods between dosing are long (see Figure 10.6) because the elimination half-life is in the range 8–39 days. Robust clinical trials evaluating its efficacy relative to other NSAIDs are not yet available.

Robenacoxib: Robenacoxib is a highly selective COX-2 inhibitor. It is available in an injectable formulation for subcutaneous administration and as a tablet for oral administration. Robenacoxib is used for the treatment of pain associated with chronic osteoarthritis, and orthopaedic and soft tissue surgery in cats and dogs. The drug has a very short residence time in blood, but persists for longer periods at sites of acute inflammation. This profile may theoretically reduce its toxicity, although this remains to be determined in a clinical setting. Bioavailability of the oral formulation is higher in fasted animals and therefore it is recommended not to administer it with a large meal. The analgesic efficacy of robenacoxib following soft tissue and orthopaedic surgery is reported to be similar to that provided by meloxicam or carprofen in dogs, and ketoprofen in cats (Reymond *et al.*, 2012; Edamura *et al.*, 2012; Sano *et al.*, 2012; Gruet *et al.*, 2013). In cats, robenacoxib provided superior postoperative analgesia to buprenorphine following ovariohysterectomy, and was superior to meloxicam following primarily soft tissue surgery (Kamata *et al.*, 2012; Staffieri *et al.*, 2013).

Cimicoxib: Cimicoxib is now available for use in dogs and has an elimination half-life of 3 hours (Kim *et al.*, 2014). Orally adminstered cimicoxib was shown to have similar efficacy to carprofen for orthopaedic and soft tissue surgery (Grandemange *et al.*, 2013).

Non-conventional or adjunctive analgesics

Recommended doses of non-conventional or adjunctive analgesics are shown in Figure 10.8.

Gabapentin

Gabapentin is a structural analogue to the neurotransmitter gamma-aminobutyric acid (GABA). It is primarily

Drug	Dosage forms	Dose
Gabapentin	Capsules: 100, 300 and 400 mg Tablets: 600 and 800 mg	Dog: initial dose of 10 mg/kg orally followed by 10–20 mg/kg orally q8h Cat: initial dose of 10 mg/kg orally followed by 10–20 mg/kg orally q8h
Ketamine	Injectable: 100 mg/ml	Dog: 0.2–1.0 mg/kg i.v. bolus followed by 2–60 µg/kg/minute Cat: 0.2–1.0 mg/kg i.v. bolus followed by 2–60 µg/kg/minute
Lidocaine	Injectable: 20 mg/ml	Dog: 1–4 mg/kg i.v. bolus followed by 1–3 mg/kg/h
Medetomidine	Injectable: 1 mg/ml	Dog: 1–5 µg/kg i.v. or i.m. followed by 1–5 µg/kg/h i.v. Cat: 1–5 µg/kg i.v. or i.m. followed by 1–5 µg/kg/h i.v.
Dexmedetomidine	Injectable: 0.1 mg/ml and 0.5 mg/ml	Dog: 0.5–2.5 µg/kg i.v. or i.m. followed by 0.5–2.5 µg/kg/h i.v. Cat: 0.5–2.5 µg/kg i.v. or i.m. followed by 0.5–2.5 µg/kg/h i.v.
Paracetamol (Acetaminophen)	Injectable: 10 mg/ml Tablets: 500 mg Also available as 400 mg tablet in combination with 9 mg codeine (licensed product in dogs in the UK) Oral suspension: 120 mg/5 ml, 250 mg/5 ml and 500 mg/5 ml	Dog: 10 mg/kg i.v or orally q8–12h Cat: contraindicated ☠

10.8 Non-conventional or adjunctive analgesics used in cats and dogs.

used as an anticonvulsant in humans, although it has been used for both neuropathic pain and postoperative pain following abdominal surgery in humans. The exact mechanism of action is unclear, although it is probably mediated through blockage of N-type voltage-dependent calcium channels on neurons, which results in a decreased release of excitatory neurotransmitters. The terminal half-life of gabapentin is short in cats and dogs.

Although there have been no controlled clinical trials evaluating the analgesic efficacy of gabapentin, it is mainly used to control neuropathic pain in cats and dogs. Gabapentin did not significantly lower pain scores in dogs when used for immediate postoperative analgesia after either hemilaminectomy or forelimb amputation, although dosing may have been inadequate (Wagner et al., 2010; Aghighi et al., 2012). For acute pain or for postoperative use, gabapentin should be used in combination with other analgesics such as opioids or NSAIDs. Its major side effect is sedation. It does not undergo significant hepatic metabolism in cats, but is excreted through the kidney, and therefore should be used only in patients with normal renal function. It is only available in an oral formulation and the recommended dose range is wide (see Figure 10.8).

Ketamine

Ketamine is a non-competitive NMDA receptor antagonist commonly used as an anaesthetic. It is also often used for its analgesic properties. By inhibiting NMDA receptors, ketamine has been shown to reduce the activity of neurons in the spinal cord in response to nociceptive stimuli, and to result in reduced central sensitization (see Chapter 8). Other proposed mechanisms for its analgesic effects include interaction at opioid receptors and/or activation of noradrenergic and serotonergic neurons.

When administered as an intravenous infusion to dogs, ketamine has been shown to reduce the MAC of isoflurane (Pypendop et al., 2007). When given with opioids for 18 hours postoperatively in dogs that had undergone forelimb amputation, pain scores were lower and there was no increase in adverse effects (Wagner et al., 2002). Side effects may include dysphoria, increased blood pressure and possibly ventricular arrhythmias, especially with higher infusion rates.

Lidocaine

When used as an intravenous infusion, lidocaine is thought to inhibit modulatory nociceptive processing. In experimental studies, it has been shown to provide analgesia for neuropathic pain and to possess anaesthetic-sparing effects. Clinically, lidocaine intravenous infusion administered intraoperatively provides some postoperative analgesia (Smith et al., 2004). There are also reports of the use of lidocaine infusions to control pain in dogs refractory to other traditionally used analgesics. In cats, infusions of lidocaine do not increase the nociceptive threshold and may cause hypotension in anaesthetized cats (Pypendop and Ilkiw, 2005; Pypendop et al., 2006). Nausea, occasional vomiting and sedation have been observed in non-painful conscious dogs when prolonged infusions at rates >75 µg/kg/min are given, which may limit the use of this agent (MacDougall et al., 2009). Infusions were otherwise well tolerated in these healthy dogs, but antinociception was not detected. CNS toxicity and seizures are also possible with much higher doses in conscious dogs, and in patients with low hepatic clearance.

Alpha-2 adrenergic agonists

Medetomidine and dexmedetomidine have potent analgesic properties, primarily mediated via alpha-2 adrenoceptors located in the dorsal horn of the spinal cord. These receptors modulate the release of neurotransmitters either responsible for, or facilitating, transmission of nociceptive signals to higher centres. Alpha-2 receptors located in the periphery may also play a role in the mediation of nociception. Alpha-2 adrenergic agonists also have effects on the cardiovascular system (see Chapter 13). In conscious or anaesthetized dogs where sedative and cardiopulmonary effects can be tolerated, low doses of dexmedetomidine can be administered either as a bolus or as an intravenous infusion (Kaartinen et al., 2010; Lervik et al., 2012). Dexmedetomidine infusion was found to be equally as effective as morphine infusion for postoperative pain management in dogs (Valtolina et al., 2009); the authors of this study reported no clinically significant adverse reactions. However, infusion of alpha-2 agonists is associated with significant cardiovascular alterations in dogs, and so the stability of the patient's cardiovascular system should be considered before the use of these agents as an infusion (Grimm *et al*., 2005).

Paracetamol (acetaminophen)

Although it is classified as an NSAID, paracetamol has weak, almost negligible anti-inflammatory properties and it is a weak inhibitor of prostaglandin synthesis. It does, however, have both analgesic and anti-pyretic effects. Recently, other potential mechanisms of action have been proposed:

- Paracetamol may be a prodrug. In the presence of fatty acid amide hydrolase (FAAH), an enzyme found predominantly in the brain and spinal cord, paracetamol, following deacetylation to its primary amine (p-aminophenol) in the liver, is conjugated with arachidonic acid to form N-arachidonoylphenolamine (AM404). The latter compound is an endogenous cannabinoid, which activates cannabinoid-1 (CB1) receptors
- AM404 is also a potent activator of vanilloid subtype 1 (TRPV1) receptors responsible for central and peripheral transmission of pain, and also inhibits COX, nitric oxide and tumour necrosis factor-α
- Activation of descending inhibitory serotonergic pathways also plays a key role in the analgesic action of paracetamol. Its anti-nociceptive effects can be partially inhibited by the co-administration of 5-HT3 receptor antagonists.

Paracetamol may be a useful alternative to other NSAIDs and is available as a preparation for intravenous use. Tablets containing paracetamol in combination with codeine have market authorization in the UK for use in dogs. It is probably underused when there are concerns about the side-effects of 'classical' NSAIDs, and it may be a useful additional agent for neurological pain in dogs (see Chapter 28). As with other NSAIDs, paracetamol is contraindicated in dogs with hepatic dysfunction. Its use in cats is absolutely contraindicated in any circumstance.

References and further reading

Abbo LA, Ko JCH, Maxwell LK et al. (2008) Pharmacokinetics of buprenorphine following intravenous and oral transmucosal administration in dogs. *Veterinary Therapeutics* **9**, 83–93

Aghighi SA, Tipold A, Piechotta M et al. (2012) Assessment of the effects of adjunctive gabapentin on postoperative pain after intervertebral disc surgery in dogs. *Veterinary Anaesthesia and Analgesia* **39**, 636–646

Al-Gizawiy MM and Rude E (2004) Comparison of preoperative carprofen and postoperative butorphanol as postsurgical analgesics in cats undergoing ovariohysterectomy. *Veterinary Anaesthesia and Analgesia* **31**, 164–174

Anderson MK and Day TK (2008) Effects of morphine and fentanyl constant rate infusion on urine output in healthy and traumatized dogs. *Veterinary Anaesthesia and Analgesia* **35**, 528–536

Aragon CL, Read MR, Gaynor JS et al. (2008) Pharamcokinetics of an immediate and extended release oral morphine formulation utilising the spheroidal oral drug absorption system in dogs. *Journal of Veterinary Pharmacology and Therapeutics*, **32**, 129–136

Barnhart MD, Hubbell JAE, Muir WW et al. (2000) Pharamcokinetics, pharmacodynamics, and analgesic effects of morphine after rectal, intramuscular, and intravenous administration in dogs. *American Journal of Veterinary Research* **61**, 24–28

Bergmann HM, Nolte IJ and Kramer S (2005) Effects of preoperative administration of carprofen on renal function and hemostasis in dogs undergoing surgery for fracture repair. *American Journal of Veterinary Research* **66**, 1356–1363

Bienhoff SE, Smith ES, Roycroft LM and Roberts ES (2012) Efficacy and safety of deracoxib for control of postoperative pain and inflammation associated with soft tissue surgery in dogs. *Veterinary Surgery* **41**, 336–344

Blois SL, Allen DG, Wood D et al. (2010) Effects of aspirin, carprofen, deracoxib, and meloxicam on platelet function and systemic prostaglandin concentrations in healthy dogs. *American Journal of Veterinary Research* **71**, 349–358

Booth DA (2001) Control of pain in small animals: opioid agonists and antagonists and other locally and centrally acting analgesics. In: *Small Animal Clinical Pharmacology and Therapeutics*, ed. DA Booth, pp 405–424. W.B. Saunders, Philadelphia

Borer LR, Peel JE, Seewald W et al. (2003) Effect of carprofen, etodolac, meloxicam, or butorphanol in dogs with induced acute synovitis. *American Journal of Veterinary Research* **64**, 1429–1437

Bostrom IM, Nyman G, Hoppe A et al. (2006) Effects of meloxicam on renal function in dogs with hypotension during anaesthesia. *Veterinary Anaesthesia and Analgesia* **33**, 62–69

Brodbelt DC, Taylor PM and Stanway GW (1997) A comparison of preoperative morphine and buprenorphine for postoperative analgesia for arthrotomy in dogs. *Journal of Veterinary Pharmacology and Therapeutics* **20**, 284–289

Brondani JT, Luna SPL, Beier SL et al. (2009) Analgesic efficacy of perioperative use of vedaprofen, tramadol or their combination in cats undergoing ovariohysterectomy. *Journal of Feline Medicine and Surgery* **11**, 420–429

Bufalari A, Di Meo A, Nannarone S et al. (2007) Fentanyl or sufentanil continuous infusion during isoflurane anaesthesia in dogs: clinical experiences. *Veterinary Research Communications* **31**, 277–280

Carroll GL, Howe LB and Peterson KD (2005) Analgesic efficacy of preoperative administration of meloxicam or butorphanol in onychectomized cats. *Journal of the American Veterinary Medical Association* **226**, 913–919

Case JB, Fick JL and Rooney MB (2010) Proximal duodenal perforation in three dogs following deracoxib administration. *Journal of the American Animal Hospital Association* **46**, 255–258

Caulkett N, Read M, Fowler D et al. (2003) A comparison of the analgesic effects of butorphanol with those of meloxicam after elective ovariohysterectomy in dogs. *Canadian Veterinary Journal* **44**, 565–570

Chambers JP (1989) Induction of anaesthesia in dogs with alfentanil and propofol. *Journal of the Association of Veterinary Anaesthetists* **16**, 14–17

Charlton AN, Benito J, Simpson W et al. (2013) Evaluation of the clinical use of tepoxalin and meloxicam in cats. *Journal of Feline Medicine and Surgery* **15**, 678–690

Davidson CD, Pettifer GR and Henry JD (2004) Plasma fentanyl concentrations and analgesic effects during full or partial exposure to transdermal fentanyl patches in cats. *Journal of the American Veterinary Medical Association* **224**, 700–705

Davila D, Keeshen TP, Evans RB et al. (2013) Comparison of the analgesic efficacy of perioperative firocoxib and tramadol administration in dogs undergoing tibial plateau leveling osteotomy. *Journal of the American Veterinary Medical Association* **243**, 225–231

Deneuche AJ, Dufayet C, Goby L et al. (2004) Analgesic comparison of meloxicam or ketoprofen for orthopedic surgery in dogs. *Veterinary Surgery* **33**, 650–660

Dobbins S, Brown NO and Shoefer FS (2002) Comparison of the effects of buprenorphine, oxymorphone hydrochloride, and ketoprofen for postoperative analgesia after onychectomy or onychectomy and sterilization in cats. *Journal of the American Animal Hospital Association* **38**, 507–514

Dobromylskyj P (1992) Severe hypotension and urticaria following the intravenous administration of pethidine in two dogs. *Journal of Veterinary Anaesthesia* **19**, 87–88

Donaldson LL, Leib MS, Boyd C et al. (1993) Effect of preanesthetic medication on ease of endoscopic intubation of the duodenum in anesthetized dogs. *American Journal of Veterinary Research* **54**, 1489–1495

Duerr FM, Carr AP, Bebchuk TN et al. (2004) Challenging diagnosis–icterus associated with a single perforating duodenal ulcer after long-term nonsteroidal antiinflammatory drug administration in a dog. *Canadian Veterinary Journal* **45**, 507–510

Dyson DH, Doherty T, Anderson GI et al. (1990) Reversal of oxymorphone sedation by naloxone, nalmefene, and butorphanol. *Veterinary Surgery* **19**, 398–403

Dzikiti TB, Joubert KE, Venter LF et al. (2006) Comparison of morphine and carprofen administered alone or in combination for analgesia in dogs undergoing ovariohysterectomy. *Journal of the South African Veterinary Medical Association* **77**, 120–126

Edamura K, King JN, Seewald W et al. (2012) Comparison of oral robenacoxib and carprofen for the treatment of osteoarthritis in dogs: a randomized clinical trial. *Journal of Veterinary Medical Science* **74**, 1121–1131

Egger CM, Glerum L, Haag KM et al. (2007) Efficacy and cost-effectiveness of transdermal fentanyl patches for the relief of post-operative pain in dogs after anterior cruciate ligament and pelvic limb repair. *Veterinary Anaesthesia and Analgesia* **34**, 200–208

Ferreira T, Rezende ML, Mama KR et al. (2011) Plasma concentrations and behavioral, antinociceptive, and physiologic effects of methadone after intravenous and oral transmucosal administration in cats. *American Journal of Veterinary Research* **72**, 764–771

Freise KJ, Newbound GC, Tudan C et al. (2012a) Pharmacokinetics and the effect of application site on a novel, long-acting transdermal fentanyl solution in healthy laboratory Beagles. *Journal of Veterinary Pharmacology and Therapeutics* **35**, 27–33

Freise KJ, Savides MC, Riggs KL et al. (2012b) Pharmacokinetics and dose selection of a novel, long-acting transdermal fentanyl solution in healthy laboratory Beagles. *Journal of Veterinary Pharmacology and Therapeutics* **35**, 21–26

Fresno L, Moll L, Peñalba B *et al.* (2005) Effects of preoperative administration of meloxicam on whole blood platelet aggregation, buccal mucosal bleeding time, and haematological indices in dogs undergoing elective oavriohysterectomy. *The Veterinary Journal* **170**, 138–140

Gassel AD, Tobias KM, Egger CM *et al.* (2005) Comparison of oral and subcutaneous administration of buprenorphine and meloxicam for pre-emptive analgesia in cats undergoing ovariohysterectomy. *Journal of the American Veterinary Medical Association* **227**, 1937–1944

Gellasch KL, Kruse-Elliott KT, Osmond CS *et al.* (2002) Comparison of transdermal administration of fentanyl versus intramuscular administration of butorphanol for analgesia after onychectomy in cats. *Journal of the American Veterinary Medical Association* **220**, 1020–1024

Gilmour MA and Lehenbauer TW (2009) Comparison of tepoxalin, carprofen, and meloxicam for reducing intraocular inflammation in dogs. *American Journal of Veterinary Research* **70**, 902–907

Giordano T, Steagall PVM, Ferreira TH *et al.* (2010) Postoperative analgesic effects of intravenous, intramuscular, subcutaneous, or oral transmucosal buprenorphine administered to cats undergoing ovariohysterectomy. *Veterinary Anaesthesia and Analgesia* **37**, 375–366

Golder FJ, Wilson J, Larenza PM *et al.* (2010) Suspected acute meperidine toxicity in a dog. *Veterinary Anaesthesia and Analgesia* **37**, 471–477

Gordon-Evans, WJ, Dunning D, Johnson AL *et al.* (2010). Randomized controlled clinical trial for the use of deracoxib during intense rehabilitation exercises after tibial plateau levelling osteotomy. *Veterinary and Comparative Orthopaedics and Traumatology* **23**, 332–335

Gowan RA, Lingard AE, Johnston L *et al.* (2011) Retrospective case–control study of the effects of long-term dosing with meloxicam on renal function in aged cats with degenerative joint disease. *Journal of Feline Medicine and Surgery* **13**, 752–761

Grandemange E, Fournel S and Woehrlé F (2013) Efficiacy and safety of cimicoxib in the control of perioperative pain in dogs. *Journal of Small Animal Practice* **54**, 304–312

Grimm KA, Tranquilli WJ, Gross DR *et al.* (2005) Cardiopulmonary effects of fentanyl in conscious dogs and dogs sedated with a continuous rate infusion of medetomidine. *American Journal of Veterinary Research* **66**, 1222–1226

Grisneaux E, Pibarot P, Dupuis J and Blais D (1999) Comparison of ketoprofen and carprofen administered prior to orthopedic surgery for control of postoperative pain in dogs. *Journal of the American Veterinary Medical Association* **215**, 1105–1110

Gruet P, Seewald W and King JN (2013) Robenacoxib versus meloxicam for the management of pain and inflammation associated with soft tissue surgery in dogs: a randomized, non-inferiority clinical trial. *BMC Veterinary Research* **9**, 92

Guedes AGP, Papich MG, Rude EP *et al.* (2007a). Comparison of plasma histamine levels after intravenous administration of hydromorphone and morphine in dogs. *Journal of Veterinary Pharmacology and Therapeutics* **30**, 516–522

Guedes AGP, Papich MG, Rude EP *et al.* (2007b) Pharmacokinetics and physiological effects of two intravenous infusion rates of morphine in conscious dogs. *Journal of Veterinary Pharmacology and Therapeutics* **30**, 224–233

Hanson PD, Brooks KC, Case J *et al.* (2006) Efficacy and safety of firocoxib in the management of canine osteoarthritis under field conditions. *Veterinary Therapeutics* **7**, 127–140

Hellebrekers LJ and Sap R (1992) Sufentanil-midazolam anaesthesia in the dog. *Journal of Veterinary Anaesthesia* **19**, 69–71

Hickford FH, Barr SC and Erb HN (2001) Effects of carporfen on hemostatic variables in dogs. *American Journal of Veterinary Research* **62**, 1642–1646

Houghton KJ, Rech RH, Sawyer DC *et al.* (1991) Dose-response of intravenous butorphanol to increase visceral nociceptive threshold in dogs. *Proceedings of the Society for Experimental Biology and Medicine* **197**, 290–296

Ilkiw JE, Pascoe PJ and Tripp LD (2002) Effects of morphine, butorphanol, buprenorphine, and U50488H on the minimum alveolar concentration of isoflurane in cats. *American Journal of Veterinary Research* **63**, 1198–1202

Ingvast-Larsson C, Holgersson A, Bondesson U *et al.* (2010) Clinical pharmacology of methadone in dogs. *Veterinary Anaesthesia and Analgesia* **37**, 48–56

Ingwersen W, Fox R, Cunningham G *et al.* (2012) Efficacy and safety of 3 versus 5 days of meloxicam as an analgesic for feline onychectomy and sterilization. *Canadian Veterinary Journal* **53**, 257–264

Kaartinen JM, Pang DSJ, Moreau M *et al.* (2010) Hemodynamic effects of an intravenous infusion of medetomidine at six different dose regimens in isoflurane-anesthetized dogs. *Veterinary Therapeutics* **11**, E1–E16

Kalthum W and Waterman AE (1988) The pharmacokinetics of intravenous pethidine HCl in dogs: normal and surgical cases. *Journal of the Associaton of Veterinary Anaesthesia* **15**, 39–54

Kamata M, Kind JN, Seewald W *et al.* (2012) Comparison of injectable robenacoxib versus meloxicam for peri-operative use in cats: results of a randomised clinical trial. *The Veterinary Journal* **193**, 114–118

Karnik PS, Johnston S, Ward D *et al.* (2006) The effects of epidural deracoxib on the ground reaction forces in an acute stifle synovitis model. *Veterinary Surgery* **35**, 34–42

Khan SA and McLean MK (2012). Toxicology of frequently encountered nonsteroidal anti-inflammatory drugs in dogs and cats. *Veterinary Clinics of North America: Small Animal Practice* **42**, 289–306

Kim TW, Lebkowska-Wieruszewska B, Owen H *et al.* (2014) Pharmacokinetic profiles of the novel COX-2 selective inhibitor cimicoxib in dogs. *The Veterinary Journal* **200**, 77-81

Kraus BLH (2013) Efficacy of maropitant in preventing vomiting in dogs premedicated with hydromorphone. *Veterinary Anaesthesia and Analgesia* **40**, 28–34

Kraus BLH (2014) Effect of dosing interval on efficacy of maropitant for prevention of hydromorphone-induced vomiting and signs of nausea in dogs. *Journal of American Veterinary Medical Association* **245**, 1015-1020

Krotscheck U, Boothe DM and Little AA (2008) Pharmacokinetics of buprenorphine following intravenous administration in dogs. *American Journal of Veterinary Research* **69**, 722–727

Krotscheck U, Boothe DM, Little AA *et al.* (2010) Pharmacokinetics of buprenorphine in a sodium carboxymethylcellulose gel after buccal transmucosal administration in dogs. *Veterinary Therapeutics* **11**, E1–E8

KuKanich B (2009) Pharmacokinetics of acetaminophen, codeine, and the codeine metabolites morphine and codeine-6-glucuronide in healthy Greyhound dogs. *Journal of Veterinary Pharmacology and Therapeutics* **13**, 15–21

KuKanich B (2013) Outpatient oral analgesics in dogs and cats beyond nonsteroidal antiinflammatory drugs: an evidence-based approach. *Veterinary Clinics of North America: Small Animal Practice* **45**, 1109–1125

KuKanich B, Bidgood T and Knesl O (2012) Clinical pharmacology of nonsteroidal anti-inflammatory drugs in dogs. *Veterinary Anaesthesia and Analgesia* **39**, 69–90

KuKanich B and Clark TP (2012) The history and pharmacology of fentanyl: relevance to a novel, long-acting transdermal fentanyl solution newly approved for use in dogs. *Journal of Veterinary Pharmacology and Therapeutics* **35**, 3–19

KuKanich B, Hogan BK and Krugner-Higby LA (2008) Pharmacokinetics of hydromorphone in healthy dogs. *Veterinary Anaesthesia and Analgesia* **35**, 256–264

KuKanich B, Lascelles BDX, Aman AM *et al.* (2005b) The effects of inhibiting cytochrome P450 3A, p-glycoprotein, and gastric acid secretion on the oral bioavailability of methadone in dogs. *Journal of Veterinary Pharmacology and Therapeutics* **28**, 461–466

KuKanich B, Lascelles BDX and Papich MG (2005a) Pharmacokinetics of morphine and plasma concentrations of morphine-6-glucuronide following morphine administration to dogs. *Journal of Veterinary Pharmacology and Therapeutics* **28**, 371–376

KuKanich B and Papich MG (2004) Pharmacokinetics of tramadol and the metabolite O-desmethyltramadol in dogs. *Journal of Veterinary Pharmacology and Therapeutics* **27**, 239–246

KuKanich B and Papich MG (2009). Opioid analgesic drugs. In: *Veterinary Pharmacology and Therapeutics*, ed. JE Riviere and MG Papich, pp.301–335. Wiley-Blackwell, Iowa

Kyles AE, Hardie EM and Hansen BD (1998) Comparison of transdermal fentanyl and intramuscular oxymorphone on post-operative behaviour after ovariohysterectomy in dogs. *Research in Veterinary Science* **65**, 245–251

Kyles AE, Papich M and Hardie EM (1996) Disposition of transdermally administered fentanyl in dogs. *American Journal of Veterinary Research* **57**, 715–719

Lascelles BDX, Cripps PJ, Jones A *et al.* (1998) Efficacy and kinetics of carprofen, administered preoperatively or postoperatively, for the prevention of pain in dogs undergoing ovariohysterectomy. *Veterinary Surgery* **27**, 568-582

Lascelles BDX, Cripps PJ, Mirchandani S *et al.* (1995) Carprofen as an analgesic for postoperative pain in cats: dose titration and assessment of efficacy in comparison to pethidine hydrochloride. *Journal of Small Animal Practice* **36**, 535–541

Lascelles BDX, Court M, Hardie EM *et al.* (2007). Nonsteroidal anti-inflammatory drugs in cats: a review. *Veterinary Anaesthesia and Analgesia* **34**, 228–250

Lascelles BDX, Henderson AJ and Hackett IJ (2001) Evaluation of the clinical efficacy of meloxicam in cats with painful locomotor disorders. *Journal of Small Animal Practice* **42**, 587–593

Lascelles BDX and Robertson SA (2004) Antinociceptive effects of hydromorphone, butorphanol, or the combination in cats. *Journal of Veterinary Internal Medicine* **18**, 190–195

Lee DD, Papich MG and Hardie EM (2000) Comparison of pharmacokinetics of fentanyl after intravenous and transdermal administration in cats. *American Journal of Veterinary Research* **61**, 672–677

Leece EA, Brearley JC and Harding EF (2005) Comparison of carprofen and meloxicam for 72 hours following ovariohysterectomy in dogs. *Veterinary Anaesthesia and Analgesia* **32**, 184–192

Lemke KA, Runyon CL and Horney BS (2002) Effects of preoperative administration of ketoprofen on whole blood platelet aggregation, buccal mucosal bleeding time, and hematologic indices in dogs undergoing elective ovariohysterectomy. *Journal of the Americian Veterinary Medical Association* **220**, 1818–1822

Lervik A, Haga HA, Ranheim B *et al.* (2012) The influence of a continuous rate infusion of dexmedetomidine on the nociceptive withdrawal reflex and temporal summation during isoflurane anaesthesia in dogs. *Veterinary Anaesthesia and Analgesia* **39**, 414–425

Liamis G, Milionis H and Elisaf M (2008) A review of drug-induced hyponatremia. *American Journal of Kidney Diseases* **52**, 144–153

Linton DD, Wilson MG, Newbound GC *et al.* (2012) The effectiveness of a long-acting transdermal fentanyl solution compared to buprenorphine for the control of postoperative pain in dogs in a randomized, multicentered clinical study. *Journal of Veterinary Pharmacology and Therapeutics* **35**, 53–64

Little AA, Krostscheck U, Boothe DM *et al.* (2008) Pharmacokinetics of buccal mucosal administration of fentanyl in a carboxymethylcellulose gel compared with IV administration in dogs. *Veterinary Therapeutics* **9**, 201–211

Lucas AN, Firth AM, Anderson GA et al. (2001) Comparison of the effects of morphine administered by constant rate intravenous infusion or intermittent intramuscular injection in dogs. Journal of the American Veterinary Medical Association 218, 884–891

Luna SPL, Basilio AC, Steagall PVM et al. (2007) Evaluation of adverse effects of long-term oral administration of carprofen, etodolac, flunixin meglumine, ketoprofen, and meloxicam in dogs. American Journal of Veterinary Research 68, 258–264

MacCrackin MA, Harvey RC, Sackman JE et al. (1994) Butorphanol tartrate for partial reversal of oxymorphone-induced postoperative respiratory depression in the dog. Veterinary Surgery 23, 67–74

MacDougall LM, Hethey JA, Livingston A et al. (2009) Antinociceptive, cardiopulmonary, and sedative effects of five intravenous infusion rates of lidocaine in conscious dogs. Veterinary Anaesthesia and Analgesia 36, 512–522

MacPhail CM, Lappin MR, Meyer DJ et al. (1998) Hepatocellular toxicosis associated with administration of carprofen in 21 dogs. Journal of the American Veterinary Medical Association 212, 1895–1901

Maiante AA, Teixeira Neto FJ, Beier SL et al. (2009) Comparison of the cardio-respiratory effects of methadone and morphine in conscious dogs. Journal of Veterinary Pharmacology and Therapeutics 32, 317–328

Martins TL, Kahvegian MAP, Noel-Morgan J et al. (2010) Comparison of the effects of tramadol, codeine, and ketoprofen alone or in combination on postoperative pain and on concentrations of blood glucose, serum cortisol, and serum interleukin-6 in dogs undergoing maxillectomy or mandibulectomy American Journal of Veterinary Research 71, 1019–1026

Mastrocinque S and Fantoni DT (2003) A comparison of preoperative tramadol and morphine for the control of early postoperative pain in canine ovariohysterectomy. Veterinary Anaesthesia and Analgesia 30, 220–228

Mathews KA (2000) Pain assessment and general approach to management. Veterinary Clinics of North America: Small Animal Practice 30(4), 729–755

Mathews KA, Paley DM, Foster RA et al. (1996) A comparison of ketorolac with flunixin, butorphanol, and oxymorphone in controlling postoperative pain in dogs. Canadian Veterinary Journal 37, 557–567

Mathews KA, Pettifer G, Foster R et al. (2001) Safety and efficacy of preoperative administration of meloxicam, compared with that of ketoprofen and butorphanol in dogs undergoing abdominal surgery. American Journal of Veterinary Research 62, 882–888

Matthiesen T, Wohrmann T, Coogan TP et al. (1998) The experimental toxicology of tramadol: an overview. Toxicology Letters 95, 63–71

McCann ME, Andersen DR, Zhang D et al. (2004) In vitro effects and in vitro efficacy of a novel cyclooxygenase-2 inhibitor in dogs with experimentally induced synovitis. American Journal of Veterinary Research 65, 503–512

Michelsen LG, Salmenperä M, Hug CC Jr et al. (1996) Anesthetic potency of remifentanil in dogs. Anesthesiology 84, 865–872

Millette VM, Steagall PVM, Duke-Novakovski T et al. (2008) Effects of meperidine or saline on thermal, mechanical and electrical nociceptive thresholds in cats. Veterinary Anaesthesia and Analgesia 35, 543–547

Millis DL, Weigel JP, Moyers T et al. (2002) Effect of deracoxib, a new COX-2 inhibitor, on the prevention of lameness induced by chemical synovitis in dogs. Veterinary Therapeutics 3, 453–464

Mills PC, Magnusson BM and Cross SE (2004) Investigation of in vitro transdermal absorption of fentanyl from patches placed on skin samples obtained from various anatomic regions of dogs. American Journal of Veterinary Research 65, 1697–1700

Mohta M, Kumari N, Tyagi A et al. (2009) Tramadol for prevention of postanaesthetic shivering: a randomised double-blind comparison with pethidine. Anaesthesia 64, 141–146

Mollenhoff A, Nolte I and Kramer S (2005) Anti-nociceptive efficacy of carprofen, levomethadone and buprenorphine for pain relief in cats following major orthopedic surgery. Journal of Veterinary Medicine Series A 52, 186–198

Monteiro ER, Figueroa CDN, Choma JC et al. (2008) Effects of methadone, alone or in combination with acepromazine or xylazine, on sedation and physiologic values in dogs. Veterinary Anaesthesia and Analgesia 35, 519–527

Monteiro-Steagall BP, Steagall PVM and Lascelles BDX (2013) Systematic review of nonsteroidal anti-inflammatory drug-induced adverse efffects in dogs. Journal of Veterinary Internal Medicine 27, 1011–1019

Muir WW III, Wiese AJ and March PA (2003) Effects of morphine, lidocaine, ketamine, and morphine-lidocaine-ketamine drug combination on minimum alveolar concentration in dogs anesthetized with isoflurane. American Journal of Veterinary Research 64, 1155–1160

Mullins KB, Thomason JM, Lunsford KV et al. (2012) Effects of carprofen, meloxicam and deracoxib on platelet function in dogs. Veterinary Anaesthesia and Analgesia 39, 206–217

Murrell JC, Robertson SA, Taylor PM et al. (2007) Use of a transdermal matrix patch of buprenorphine in cats: preliminary pharmacokinetic and pharmacodynamic data. Veterinary Record 160, 578–583

Niedfeldt RL and Robertson SA (2006) Postanesthetic hyperthermia in cats: a retrospective comparison between hydromorphone and buprenorphine. Veterinary Anaesthesia and Analgesia 33, 381–389

Parton K, Balmer TV, Boyle J et al. (2000) The pharmacokinetics and effects of intravenously administered carprofen and salicylate on gastrointestinal mucosa and selected biochemical measurements in healthy cats. Journal of Veterinary Pharmacology and Therapeutics 23, 73–79

Pascoe PJ, Ilkiw JE, Black WD et al. (1993) The pharmacokinetics of alfentanil in healthy cats. Journal of Veterinary Anaesthesia 20, 9–13

Pasternak GW and Pan Y-X (2013) Mu opioids and their receptors: evolution of a concept. Pharmacological Reviews 65, 1257–1317

Pekcan Z and Koc B (2010) The post-operative analgesic effects of epidurally administered morphine and transdermal fentanyl patch after ovario-hysterectomy in dogs. Veterinary Anaesthesia and Analgesia 37, 557–565

Peterson KD and Keefe TJ (2004) Effects of meloxicam on severity of lameness and other clinical signs of osteoarthrtis in dogs. Journal of the American Veterinary Medical Association 225, 1056–1060

Pieper K, Schuster T, Levinnois O et al. (2010) Antinociceptive efficacy and plasma concentrations of transdermal buprenorphine in dogs. The Veterinary Journal 187, 335–341

Polis I, Moens Y, Gasthuys F et al. (2004) Anti-nociceptive and sedative effects of surfentanil long acting during and after sevoflurane anaesthesia in dogs. Journal of Veterinary Medicine 51, 242–248

Pollmeier M, Toulemonde C, Fleishman C et al. (2006) Clinical evaluation of firocoxib and carprofen for the treatment of dogs with osteoarthritis. Veterinary Record 159, 547–551

Polson S, Taylor PM and Yates D (2012) Analgesia after feline ovariohysterectomy under midazolam-medetomidine-ketamine anaesthesia with buprenorphine or butorphanol, and carprofen or meloxicam: a prospective, randomised clinical trial. Journal of Feline Medicine and Surgery 14, 553–558

Posner LP, Gleed RD, Erb HN et al. (2007) Post-anesthetic hyperthermia in cats. Veterinary Anaesthesia and Analgesia 34, 40–47

Posner LP, Pavuk AA, Rokshar JL et al. (2010). Effects of opioids and anesthetic drugs on body temperature in cats. Veterinary Anaesthesia and Analgesia 37, 35–43

Pypendop BH and Ilkiw JE (2005) Assessment of the hemodynamic effects of lidocaine administered IV in isoflurane-anesthetized cats. American Journal of Veterinary Research 66, 661–668

Pypendop BH and Ilkiw JE (2007) Pharmacokinetics of tramadol and its metabolite O-desmethy-tramadol in cats. Journal of Veterinary Pharmacology and Theraeutics 31, 52–59

Pypendop BH, Ilkiw JE and Robertson SA (2006) Effects of intravenous administration of lidocaine on the thermal threshold in cats. American Journal of Veterinary Research 67, 16–20

Pypendop BH, Siao KT and Ilkiw JE (2009) Effects of tramadol hydrochloride on the thermal threshold in cats. American Journal of Veterinary Research 70, 1465–1470

Pypendop BH, Solano A, Boscan P et al. (2007) Characteristics of the relationship beteeen plasma ketamine concentration and its effect on the minimum alveolar concentration of isoflurane in dogs. Veterinary Anaesthesia and Analgesia 34, 209–212

Radnay PA, Duncalf D, Novakovic M, et al. (1984). Common bile duct pressure changes after fentanyl, morphine, meperidine, butorphanol, and naloxone. Anesthesia and Analgesia 63, 441–444

Reymond N, Speranza C, Gruet P et al. (2012) Robenacoxib vs. carprofen for the treatment of canine osteoarthritis; a randomized, noninferiority clinical trial. Journal of Veterinary Pharmacology and Therapeutics 35, 175–183

Robertson SA (2005) Assessment and management of acute pain in cats. Journal of Veterinary Emergency and Critical Care 15, 261–272

Robertson SA, Lascelles BDX, Taylor PM et al. (2005b) PK-PD modeling of buprenorphine in cats: intravenous and oral transmucosal administration. Journal of Veterinary Pharmacology and Therapeutics 28, 453–460

Robertson SA, Taylor PA and Sear JW (2003) Systemic uptake of buprenorphine by cats after oral mucosal administration. Veterinary Record 152, 675–678

Robertson SA, Taylor PM, Sear JW et al. (2005a) Relationship between plasma concentrations and analgesia after intravenous fentanyl and disposition after other routes of administration in cats. Journal of Veterinary Pharmacology and Therapeutics 28, 87–93

Robertson SA, Wegner K and Lascelles BDX (2009) Antinociceptive and side-effects of hydromorphone after subcutaneous administration in cats. Journal of Feline Medicine and Surgery 11, 76–81

Robinson TM, Kruse-Elliot KT, Markel MD et al. (1999) A comparison of transdermal fentanyl versus epidural morphine for analgesia in dogs undergoing major orthopedic surgery. Journal of the American Animal Hospital Association 35, 95–100

Sano T, King JN, Seewald W et al. (2012) Comparison of oral robenacoxib and ketoprofen for the treatment of acute pain and inflammation associated with musculoskeletal disorders in cats: a randomised clinical trial. The Veterinary Journal 193, 397–403

Sano T, Nishimura R, Kanazawa H et al. (2006) Pharmacokinetics of fentanyl after single intravenous injection and contant rate infusion in dogs. Veterinary Anaesthesia and Analgesia 33, 266–273

Sawyer DC and Rech RH (1987) Analgesia and behavioral effects of butorphanol, nalbuphine, and pentazocine in the cat. Journal of the American Animal Hospital Association 23, 438–446

Shore JM, Silverman A, Siegel M et al. (1971) Direct observations of the canine sphincter of Oddi. Annals of Surgery 174, 264–273

Skingle M and Tyers MB (1980) Further studies on opiate receptors that mediate antinociception: tooth pulp stimulation in the dog. British Journal of Pharmacology 70, 323–327

Slingsby LS, Murison PJ, Goossens L et al. (2006) A comparison between pre-operative carprofen and long-acting sufentanil formulation for analgesia after ovariohysterectomy in dogs. Veterinary Anaesthesia and Analgesia 33, 313–327

Slingsby LS, Taylor PM and Murrell JC (2011) A study to evaluate buprenorphine at 40 μgkg⁻¹ compared to 20 μgkg⁻¹ as a postoperative analgesic in the dog. *Veterinary Anaesthesia and Analgesia* **38**, 584–593

Slingsby LS and Waterman-Pearson AE (2000) Postoperative analgesia in the cat after ovariohysterectomy by use of carprofen, ketoprofen, meloxicam or tolfenamic acid. *Journal of Small Animal Practice* **41**, 447–450

Slingsby LS and Waterman-Pearson AE (2001) Analgesic effects in dogs of carprofen and pethidine together compared to the effects of either drug alone. *Veterinary Record* **148**, 441–444

Slingsby LS and Waterman-Pearson AE (2002) Comparison between meloxicam and carprofen for postoperative analgesia after feline ovariohysterectomy. *Journal of Small Animal Practice* **43**, 286–289

Smith AA, Posner LP, Goldstein RE *et al.* (2004) Evaluation of the effcts of premedication on gastroduodenscopy in cats. *Journal of the American Veterinary Medical Association* **225**, 540–544

Smith LJ, Bentley E, Shih A *et al.* (2004) Systemic lidocaine infusion as an analgesic for intraocular surgery in dogs: a pilot study. *Veterinary Anaesthesia and Analgesia* **31**, 53–63

Smith LJ, KuKanich B, Kurgner-Higby LA *et al.* (2013) Pharmacokinetics of ammonium sulfate gradient loaded liposome-encapsulated oxymorphone and hydromorphone in healthy dogs. *Veterinary Anaesthesia and Analgesia* **40**, 537–545

Staffieri F, Centonze P, Gigante G *et al.* (2013) Comparison of the analgesic effects of robenacoxib, buprenorphine and their combination in cats after ovariohysterectomy. *The Veterinary Journal* **197**, 363–367

Stanway GW, Taylor PA and Brodbelt DC (2002) A preliminary investigation comparing preoperative morphine and buprenorphine for post-operative analgesia. *Veterinary Anaesthesia and Analgesia* **29**, 29–35

Steagall PVM, Carnicelli P, Taylor PM *et al.* (2006) Effects of subcutaneous methadone, morphine, buprenorphine or saline on thermal and pressure thresholds in cats. *Journal of Veterinary Pharmacology and Therapeutics* **29**, 531–537

Steagall PVM, Mantovani FB, Taylor PM *et al.* (2009) Dose-related antinociceptive effects of intravenous buprenorphine in cats. *The Veterinary Journal* **182**, 203–209

Steagall PVM, Monteiro BP, Lavoie A-M and Troncy E (2015) A preliminary investigation of the thermal antinociceptive effects of codeine in cats. *Journal of Feline Medicine and Surgery* DOI: 10.1177/1098612X14564710 jfms.com

Steagall PVM, Pelligand L, Giordano T *et al.* (2013) Pharmacokinetics and pharmacodynamic modelling of intravenous, intramuscular and muscular and subcutaneous buprenorphine in conscious cats. *Veterinary Anaesthesia and Analgesia* **40**, 83–95

Steffey EP, Baggot JD, Eisele JH *et al.* (1994) Morphine-isoflurane interaction in dogs, swine and Rhesus monkeys. *Journal of Veterinary Pharmacology and Therapeutics* **17**, 202–210

Stephan DD, Vestre WA, Stiles J *et al.* (2003) Changes in intraocular pressure and pupil size following intramuscular administration of hydromorphone hydrochloride and acepromazine in clinically normal dogs. *Veterinary Ophthalmology* **6**, 73–76

Stobie D, Caywood DD, Rozanski EA, *et al.* (1995) Evaluation of pulmonary function and analgesia in dogs after intercostal thoracotomy and use of morphine administered intramuscularly or intrapleurally and bupivacaine administered intrapleurally. *American Journal of Veterinary Research* **56**, 1098–1109

Taylor PM, Delatour P, Landoni FM *et al.* (1996) Pharmacodynamics and enantioselective pharmacokinetics of carprofen in the cat. *Research in Veterinary Science* **60**, 144–151

Taylor PM and Houlton JEF (1984) Post-operative analgesia in the dog: a comparison of morphine, buprenorphine and pentazocine. *Journal of Small Animal Practice* **25**, 437–451

Taylor PM, Robertson SA, Dixon MJ *et al.* (2001) Morphine, pethidine and buprenorphine disposition in the cat. *Journal of Veterinary Pharmacology and Therapeutics* **24**, 391–398

Teixeira RCR, Monteiro ER, Campagnol D *et al.* (2013) Effects of tramadol alone, in combination with meloxicam or dipyrone, on postoperative pain and the analgesic requirement in dogs undergoing unilateral mastectomy with or without ovariohysterectomy. *Veterinary Anaesthesia and Analgesia* **40**, 641–649

Thompson DR (2001) Narcotic analgesic effects on the sphincter of Oddi: A review of the data and therapeutic implications in treating pancreatitis. *American Journal of Gastroenterology* **96**, 1266–1272

Thompson WL and Walton RP (1964) Elevation of plasma histamine levels in the dog following administration of muscle relaxants, opiates, and macromolecular polymers. *Journal of Pharmacology and Experimental Therapeutics* **143**, 131–136

Valtolina C, Robben JH, Uilenreef J *et al.* (2009) Clinical evaluation of the efficacy and safety of a constant rate infusion of dexmedetomidine for postoperative pain management in dogs. *Veterinary Anaesthesia and Analgesia* **36**, 369–383

Valverde A, Cantwell S, Hernández J *et al.* (2004) Effects of acepromazine on the incidence of vomiting associated with opioid administration in dogs. *Veterinary Anaesthesia and Analgesia* **31**, 40–45

Wagner AE, Mich PM, Uhrig SR *et al.* (2010) Clinical evaluation of perioperative administration of gabapentin as an adjunct for postoperative analgesia in dogs undergoing amputation of a forelimb. *Journal of the American Veterinary Medical Association* **236**, 751–756

Wagner AE, Walton JA, Hellyer PW *et al.* (2002) Use of low doses of ketamine administered by constant rate infusion as an adjunct for postoperative analgesia in dogs. *Journal of the American Veterinary Medical Association* **221**, 72–75

Warne LN, Beths T, Holm M *et al.* (2013) Comparison of perioperative analgesic efficacy between methadone and butorphanol in cats. *Journal of the American Veterinary Medical Association* **243**, 844–850

Waterman AE and Kalthum W (1989a) Pharmacokinetics of intramuscularly administered pethidine in dogs and the influence of anaesthesia and surgery. *The Veterinary Record* **124**, 293–296

Waterman AE and Kalthum W (1989b) The absorption and distribution of subcutaneously administered pethidine in the dog. *Journal of the Association of Anaesthetists* **16**, 51–52

Wegner K, Horais K, Tozier NA *et al.* (2008) Development of a canine nociceptive thermal escape model. *Journal of Neuroscience Methods* **168**, 88–97

Wegner K and Robertson SA (2007) Dose-related thermal antinociceptive effects of intravenous hydromorphone in cats. *Veterinary Anaesthesia and Analgesia* **34**, 132–138

Wegner K, Robertson SA, Kollias-Baker C *et al.* (2004) Pharmacokinetic and pharmacodynamic evaluation of intravenous hydromorphone in cats. *Journal of Veterinary Pharmacology and Therapeutics* **27**, 329–336

Williams JT, Ingram SL, Henderson G *et al.* (2013) Regulation of mu-opioid receptors: desensitization, phosphorylation, internalization, and tolerance. *Pharmacological Reviews* **64**, 223–254

Wilson DV, Evans AT and Mauer WA (2007) Pre-anesthetic meperidine: associated vomiting and gastroesophageal reflux during the subsequent anesthetic in dogs. *Veterinary Anaesthesia and Analgesia* **34**, 15–22

Wilson DV, Evans AT and Miller RA (2005) Effects of preanesthetic administration of morphine on gastroesophageal reflux and regurgitation during anesthesia in dogs. *American Journal of Veterinary Research* **66**, 386–390

WSAVA Global Pain Council (2014) WSAVA Guidelines for Recognition, Assessment and Treatment of Pain. *Journal of Small Animal Practice* **55(6)**, E10–E68

Wu SD, Zhang ZH, Jin JZ, *et al.* (2004) Effects of narcotic analgesic drugs on human Oddi's sphincter motility. *World Journal of Gastroenterology* **10**, 2901–2904

Chapter 11

Pain management II: local and regional anaesthetic techniques

Tanya Duke-Novakovski

History

In 1890, the removal of foreign objects from eyes of cattle was made possible using cocaine solution and this event became the first reported use of local anaesthetics in veterinary medicine (Jones, 2002). Adverse stimulatory effects from the systemic absorption of cocaine made this drug unpopular for use, and procaine became the local anaesthetic of choice from 1905 onwards. The use of procaine was, however, limited by its low potency, slow onset, short duration of action, and limited ability to penetrate tissue. Lidocaine was formulated in 1944 and rapidly became a popular choice because of its greater potency, rapid onset and effectiveness for infiltration anaesthesia, local and regional nerve blocks, and for epidural and spinal use. Mepivacaine followed in 1957, and the search for longer acting local anaesthetics brought bupivacaine in 1963. With increasing evidence of cardiotoxicity and fatalities caused by the racemic mixture of bupivacaine, the less toxic isomer levobupivacaine was introduced in the early 1990s. The closely related compound, ropivacaine, was introduced in 1996. More recent developments include packaging local anaesthetics within liposomes and polylactide microspheres to slow their release and increase their duration of action.

Pharmacology and pharmacokinetics

All clinically useful local anaesthetics are either amino-esters or amino-amides. They act by blocking sodium channels and preventing rapid influx of sodium ions into nerve axons (Figure 11.1). This blocks the nerve action potential and propagation of nerve impulse transmission. In myelinated nerve axons, at least three nodes of Ranvier in succession must be blocked for impulse transmission to cease. Local anaesthetic drugs can enter through the cell membrane and/or through open ion channels to reach their binding sites, which are situated at the cytoplasmic end of the channel. Stimulation of the nerve can decrease the time to onset of blockade by allowing more frequent opening of the sodium channels and entry of the drug on to binding sites within the channel. Noxious stimulation will have the same effect of increasing the frequency of channel opening, thus painful areas are more effectively blocked. This is called *use-dependent or frequency-dependent blockade*. The sodium channel is preferentially blocked in the 'open' state, less effectively blocked in the 'inactivated' state and least effectively blocked in the 'closed' state. Nerve axons

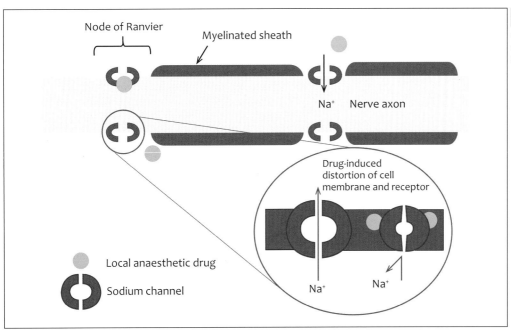

11.1 Diagram of a nerve axon, showing an expanded view of a sodium channel in the open and closed state.

in the periphery of a nerve fibre will come into contact with the local anaesthetic drug first, and so will become blocked before axons in the centre of the fibre. This means that more proximal areas of the body are blocked more effectively than more distal areas. Preganglionic sympathetic nerve fibres (moderately myelinated B fibres) are more sensitive to blockade compared with more heavily myelinated large diameter A fibres. The ability of local anaesthetics to block pain-transmitting non-myelinated C fibres lies somewhere between blockade of A- and B-fibres. Differential blockade is the difference between sensory and motor block, especially noticeable with ropivacaine. The difference is not simply due to the different diameters of nerve bundles or axon types, but may also involve a particular drug affinity for sodium, potassium and even calcium ion channels. The final effects of different local anaesthetic drugs can also vary because there are many types of sodium channels in the body, which can be differentiated on the basis of their unique responses to the substance tetrodotoxin.

The typical structure of a local anaesthetic drug includes a lipophilic group (benzene ring) and a hydrophilic group (tertiary amine). The groups are joined by either an ester (amino-ester) or amide (amino-amide) linkage (Figures 11.2 and 11.3); the type of linkage affects the method of drug metabolism. Based on the chemical structure of the linkage, local anaesthetic drugs are classified as belonging to either the ester or amide groups. The hydrophilic and lipophilic opposite ends of the molecule enable the drug to dissolve within the lipid cell membrane (benzene ring) or enter the cell through the sodium channel to bind with the channel proteins (tertiary amine) (see Figure 11.1). Drugs in the ester group include cocaine, procaine, tetracaine and benzocaine. Amide-linked local

11.3 Chemical structures of three commonly used amide local anaesthetic drugs. Red circles indicate the amide linkage.

11.2 Chemical structures of local anaesthetics from the ester group. Red circles indicate the ester linkage.

anaesthetics include lidocaine, prilocaine, mepivacaine, bupivacaine and ropivacaine.

Plasma cholinesterases break down the amino-ester drugs, except cocaine, which is metabolized in the liver. Amino-amide local anaesthetics are biotransformed by mixed-function oxidase systems in the lung and liver. As a result, amide local anaesthetic drugs are eliminated from the body more slowly and are more likely to accumulate and cause toxicity. Lidocaine is metabolized to several metabolites, including the active metabolite monoethyl-glycinexylidide (MEGX), non-active glycinexylidide and 3-hydroxy-lidocaine. MEGX has anti-arrhythmic properties but can also cause convulsions. In cats, general anaesthesia increases the duration of effect of lidocaine and delays production of MEGX, probably due to lower hepatic perfusion and drug delivery to the liver. This effect is less pronounced in dogs. The metabolite MEGX can be detected within 30 minutes of injecting lidocaine in conscious and anaesthetized cats and conscious dogs.

The pharmacological activity of local anaesthetic molecules depends on a number of physicochemical properties. These include the molecules' lipid solubility, protein binding and their acid dissociation constant, pKa (the pH when equal concentrations of ionized and unionized forms are present). The final pharmacokinetic profile of a drug will depend on all these factors, and drug's interactions with conditions within the injection site (Figure 11.4).

Drug (group)	pKa (at 25°C)	Protein binding (%)	Partition coefficient H-octanol/buffer	Speed of onset	Duration of action
Tetracaine (ester)	8.6	76	221	Slow	Intermediate–long
Procaine (ester)	9.0	6	1.7	Slow	Short
Prilocaine (amide)	7.9	55	25	Rapid	Intermediate
Lidocaine (amide)	7.7	64	43	Rapid	Intermediate
Bupivacaine (amide)	8.1	95	346	Slow	Long
Levobupivacaine (amide)	8.1	96	346	Slow	Long
Ropivacaine (amide)	8.1	94	115	Slow	Long
Mepivacaine (amide)	7.9	77	21	Slow	Intermediate

11.4 Summary of the physicochemical properties of the commonly used local anaesthetics. The higher the pKa, the slower is the onset of action. The higher the partition coefficient, the higher is the potency. The greater the protein binding, the longer is the duration of action.

Lipid solubility

The potency of local anaesthetics is linked to their degree of lipid solubility: more lipid-soluble drugs are more potent because they can penetrate the cell membrane and exert their effect more readily. Greater potency also increases the ability to produce toxic side effects; for example, bupivacaine, which is highly lipophilic, is potent and also more toxic than some other local anaesthetic drugs.

Protein binding

Highly lipophilic drugs also tend to have a higher degree of protein binding, which prolongs their duration of effect. Bupivacaine has a high degree of protein binding.

pKa

Speed of onset of action is thought to be linked to the pKa. All local anaesthetics are weak bases with a pKa in the range 7.7–9.1. This means that at a pH below their pKa, they will accept a proton, become a cation and therefore become less lipophilic. The uncharged, lipophilic base form readily crosses the nerve sheath; the presence of more uncharged molecules speeds the onset of action. Most local anaesthetic molecules have a pKa higher than physiological pH, and therefore more of the drug exists in the cationic (ionized) form. In order to prolong shelf-life the pH of commercial formulations of local anaesthetic is reduced. The addition of bicarbonate to the local anaesthetic speeds the onset of the block by increasing the concentration of unionized molecules. Also, adding bicarbonate to increase the pH will result in less pain on injection (Figure 11.5).

Local anaesthetic drug	Drug volume	Sodium bicarbonate 8.4% volume	Ratio by volume drug:bicarbonate
Lidocaine 2%	1.0 ml	0.1 ml	10:1
Bupivacaine 0.5%	1.0 ml	0.015 ml	67:1
Lidocaine 2% and bupivacaine 0.5% mixture	0.5 ml each = 1.0 ml total	0.1 ml	10:1

11.5 Volumes and ratios of sodium bicarbonate required to alkalize commercial local anaesthetic preparations. Note that overzealous addition of bicarbonate will cause precipitation.
(Data from Davies, 2003)

Disposition of drug

The distribution of the drug around a nerve depends on the volume used, while penetration of the nerve fibre depends on drug concentration. Diluting a local anaesthetic solution will enable injection of an increased volume without increasing the drug dose to a level that may be toxic but the quality of blockade may be adversely affected. Operator skill and the use of technical aids (described later) to enable precise injection of local anaesthetics around the nerve fibres is crucial to achieve a good quality of blockade.

The duration of drug contact with the nerve trunk depends on the vascularity of the tissue: the greater the blood flow through the area of tissue, the faster the drug will be absorbed into the systemic circulation. The order of uptake into the circulation (most rapid first) correlates with vascularity: in humans, intravenous > tracheal > intercostal > epidural > brachial plexus > sciatic > subcutaneous. To prolong the length of action of a local anaesthetic drug, vasoconstrictors are occasionally added to delay absorption into the circulation. Adrenaline is usually used, at a concentration of 1:200,000 (5 µg/ml) or 1:400,000 (2.5 µg/ml). An approximately 1:200,000 adrenaline solution can be made by adding 0.1 ml of a 1 mg/ml (1:1000) commercial preparation of adrenaline to 20 ml of the local anaesthetic drug, or an equivalent ratio. Some local block techniques require the use of local anaesthetics without adrenaline, including those for surgery involving the extremities of the body and for intravenous regional anaesthesia.

Local anaesthetic mixtures

Generally speaking, the combination of two drugs, such as lidocaine and bupivacaine, produces a faster onset of action, but may also shorten the duration of block. The duration of block is shorter than that provided when bupivacaine is used alone, but longer than when lidocaine is used as the sole agent. There may be limited advantages to the combination.

Addition of alpha-2 adrenergic agonists and opioids

Alpha-2 adrenergic agonists are added to local anaesthetics for epidural or spinal use; at these locations, the alpha-2 adrenergic agonist can act upon descending pain pathways. The addition of alpha-2 adrenergic agonists to local anaesthetics for peripheral nerve blocks has also been found to be beneficial (Lamont and Lemke, 2008). Reports have indicated that regional nerve block duration can be doubled through the addition of dexmedetomidine (0.5 μg/ml).

Opioids are also commonly used within the epidural and spinal areas. The addition of opioids to local anaesthetics for peripheral nerve blocks has also been investigated. Buprenorphine, tramadol and pethidine (meperidine) have been found to block sodium channels, and there are reports of these opioids extending the duration of local anaesthetic block in the medical literature. This may be due to sodium channel blocking effects and/or systemic absorption (Bailard *et al.*, 2014).

Adverse effects of local anaesthetics

It is important to recognize the signs of toxicity associated with local anaesthetic drugs to allow prompt treatment. In small patients, it is advisable to use an accurate body-weight for dosage calculations and to decrease the concentration of local anaesthetics in order to increase the volume injected. Ropivacaine is considered to be the least toxic of the longer-acting local anaesthetics, but still requires caution with use and careful calculation of dosage. Mepivacaine also appears to be a good choice with reduced toxic side effects, although these effects have not been fully studied in cats and dogs.

Central nervous system toxicity

In dogs, the bupivacaine plasma concentrations that produce central nervous system (CNS) and cardiovascular system (CVS) toxicity are similar. The mean ± SD dose (and plasma concentrations) that produce convulsant activity in conscious dogs are as follows: lidocaine 20 ± 4.0 mg/kg (47.2 ± 5.4 μg/ml); bupivacaine 4.31 ± 0.36 mg/kg (18.0 ± 2.7 μg/ml); ropivacaine 4.88 ± 0.47 mg/kg (11.4 ± 0.9 μg/ml) (Feldman *et al.*, 1989). In another study, the dose of bupivacaine causing convulsant activity in dogs was reported to be 4.3 mg/kg, and for ropivacaine 4.9 mg/kg (Feldman *et al.*, 1991). Details of safe and toxic doses of local anaesthetic drugs, along with their time to peak onset and duration of effect, are shown in Figure 11.6.

Experimentally, infusions of lidocaine or bupivacaine have been administered to cats until signs of CNS toxicity were observed, and infusions were continued until signs of CVS toxicity were observed (lethal endpoint). Arterial blood pressure decreased earlier in cats receiving lidocaine compared with those receiving bupivacaine. The CVS:CNS toxicity ratio for plasma drug concentration was 4.0 for lidocaine and 4.8 for bupivacaine. The mean ± SD convulsive dose was found to be 11.7 ± 4.6 mg/kg for lidocaine and 3.8 ± 1.0 mg/kg for bupivacaine (Chadwick, 1985).

Signs of CNS toxicity usually manifest before cardiovascular signs, except with bupivacaine. The initial sign is drowsiness, which may be missed in patients that have been sedated. Clinical signs deteriorate to tremors and grand mal seizures as toxicity progresses. Treatment of convulsions is with a gamma-aminobutyric acid A (GABA$_A$) receptor agonist drug: either diazepam (0.2–0.4 mg/kg i.v. or rectally), phenobarbital (2–4 mg/kg i.v., up to 20 mg/kg); pentobarbital (5 mg/kg i.v., up to 20 mg/kg), or propofol (2–4 mg/kg i.v. bolus followed by infusion). The airway should be secured and oxygen and ventilatory support provided.

Cardiovascular toxicity

The adverse effects of local anaesthetics are mediated on the heart and vascular system both directly and through the autonomic nervous system. Local anaesthetics decrease electrical excitability, conduction rate and force of contraction, and cardiac arrhythmias are a common sign of toxicity, especially with bupivacaine. The intense depression of cardiac conducting tissue, and the cardiac arrhythmias produced by bupivacaine, can be difficult to manage if treatment is not started immediately. Lidocaine-induced cardiac depression is not as difficult to treat. Treatment should be directed towards cardiovascular support, with administration of intravenous fluid therapy, oxygen and positive inotropes. Myocardial depression is primarily responsible for hypotension (mean arterial pressure <45 mmHg), and bupivacaine increases myocardial sensitivity to circulating adrenaline (Groban *et al.*, 2001). Cats appear to be especially prone to cardiovascular depression after receiving intravenous lidocaine. In cats, the mean ± SD cardiotoxic dose (complete loss of arterial blood pressure) for lidocaine was reported to be 47.3 ± 8.6 mg/kg, and for bupivacaine 18.4 ± 4.9 mg/kg (Chadwick, 1985). Bupivacaine given at 1.2 mg/kg i.v. is sufficient to cause cardiovascular depression in cats. Bupivacaine-induced cardiac arrhythmias (fibrillation or ventricular tachycardia) can be treated with cardiac massage, bretylium (5–20 mg/kg i.v. over 1–2 minutes), magnesium (0.1–0.3 mg/kg i.v. over 5 minutes), defibrillation (see Chapter 31) or lipid emulsion infusions.

An infusion of 20% lipid emulsion (Liposyn II; Hospira) can be used at a dose of 1.5–3.0 ml/kg administered over 30 minutes to treat toxicity from overdose of local anaesthetics (O'Brien *et al.*, 2010). The mechanism of action is largely unknown, but may be due to reduction of the free drug in plasma by the chylomicrons, simulating a new pharmacological compartment and taking up the local anaesthetic drug; by increasing myocardial calcium concentrations through fatty acids and counteracting the negative inotropic effects of the drug; or by preventing the inhibition of carnitine acyltransferase which transports fatty acids, used for oxidative phosphorylation, into myocardial cells. Care should be taken if intravenous lipids are used as they support bacterial growth, irritate the vasculature and cause some immunosuppression.

Drug	Time to onset of peak effect (minutes)	Duration of effect (hours)	Toxic dose		Maximum safe dose	
Lidocaine	2–5	1–2 with adrenaline <1 without adrenaline	Dog Cat	22 mg/kg i.v. 11 mg/kg i.v.	Dog Cat	10 mg/kg 6 mg/kg
Mepivacaine	2–5	~1.5	Dog	20 mg/kg i.v.	Dog	10 mg/kg
Bupivacaine	5–10	~2	Dog and cat	4 mg/kg i.v.	Dog and cat	2 mg/kg
Ropivacaine	5–10	~2	Dog	5 mg/kg i.v.	Dog	3 mg/kg

11.6 Table indicating time to peak onset and duration of effect, and doses of local anaesthetic drugs in cats and dogs. The duration of action depends on the method of evaluation.

Methaemoglobinaemia

Methaemoglobin is formed when ferrous iron (Fe^{2+}) in haemoglobin is oxidized to the ferric form (Fe^{3+}). This form of haemoglobin is not capable of carrying oxygen or carbon dioxide. Dogs can tolerate methaemoglobin concentrations of less than 20% but at concentrations between 20 and 50% dogs will have signs of fatigue, weakness, dyspnoea and tachycardia. Prilocaine, benzocaine, lidocaine and procaine can cause methaemoglobinaemia. Treatment consists of oxygen therapy and administration of methylene blue (1.5 mg/kg i.v.). Advanced blood gas analysers with co-oximeters (see Chapter 7) can measure the amount of methaemoglobin present in a blood sample.

Tissue toxicity

Local anaesthetic drugs can cause direct tissue irritation and skeletal muscle appears to be the most sensitive to this effect. Injection into a nerve sheath is damaging to the nerve axons and should be avoided. The potent, long-lasting local anaesthetics with high lipid solubility appear to be more likely to cause tissue damage. Recent studies have shown that local anaesthetics may damage chondrocytes. Most of the evidence for damage comes from *in vitro* studies using animal chondrocyte cell lines, but other studies have produced conflicting results. Bupivacaine (0.5%) has been shown to reduce viability in canine cartilage, synovial and osteochondral cell cultures on the second day of contact. There have been few studies examining the long-term effects of a single bolus injection into joints (Baker and Mulhall, 2011). An *in vivo* study found no difference between saline- and bupivacaine-treated joints in dogs. In live dogs, the bupivacaine concentration following injection of 0.5% bupivacaine (1 mg/kg) into joints was found to be too low to cause harm to chondrocytes (Barry *et al.*, 2014). Mepivacaine may become more popular to use in canine joints because it possesses less tissue toxicity (Dutton *et al.*, 2014).

Morphine was considered to be non-toxic to cell cultures, but the preservative methylparaben was shown to reduce the viability of cells by 48%. In an equine monolayer cell culture, viability was reduced to the greatest extent by 0.5% bupivacaine (to approximately 30% viability after 30 minutes' exposure), less so by 2% lidocaine and least by 2% mepivacaine. Ropivacaine was less toxic to bovine chondrocytes than lidocaine and bupivacaine.

Hypersensitivity reactions

Although the number of occurrences of allergic reactions to local anaesthetic drugs is small, ester-linked agents are more likely to produce allergic reactions than are the amide-linked anaesthetics. Amino-esters are derivatives of para-aminobenzoic acid (PABA), a compound that is known to cause hypersensitivity reactions and which is produced during metabolism of the local anaesthetic drug. Methylparaben preservatives in preparations of local anaesthetics have also been implicated in some reactions because they are chemically related to PABA.

Local anaesthetic techniques

The techniques described in this chapter are relatively simple. Additional information can be obtained by consulting the references and further reading section at the end of this chapter.

Skin

Ethyl chloride spray can be used topically to provide short-term anaesthesia of the skin. The spray is used for between 2 and 5 seconds and provides enough analgesia for performing skin biopsies or lancing abscesses. Limitations include the risk of frostbite if applied to large areas, its short duration of effect (<3 minutes) and the flammable nature of ethyl chloride.

A eutectic cream that contains lidocaine and prilocaine and which has good penetration of the dermal layers is also available (EMLA cream). At body temperature, the cream becomes soluble and can be absorbed through skin. The cream is applied to the area to be desensitized and covered with a clean dressing for about 30–40 minutes to prevent the patient licking off the cream. This product is useful in nervous animals before intravenous cannulation, or for intra-arterial catheter placement or arterial blood gas sampling in conscious patients. Methaemoglobinaemia has been reported 1–3 hours after application to a large area or after contact for prolonged periods of time. In humans, a dose of 1–2 g over an area of 10 cm^2 is recommended, with an application time of 1–1.5 hours. In cats treated with 1 g EMLA cream applied to the skin for an hour before jugular vein catheterization, plasma concentrations of lidocaine and prilocaine were undetectable (<0.3 μg/ml) and methaemoglobin levels were comparable to untreated cats. Although the total dose of each drug would be high if given intravenously, the slow absorption from the dermal site and metabolism of the drugs prevents the plasma concentrations rising to toxic levels (Gibbon *et al.*, 2003). EMLA cream should not be applied to mucous membranes.

Transdermal 5% lidocaine patches are licensed for treatment of postherpetic neuralgia in humans. They have been used to decrease pain from surgical incisions by placing them alongside the incision as well as close by other local areas where pain might be elicited. The patches provide analgesia but do not produce numbness or loss of touch sensation. The patches contain an adhesive material with 5% lidocaine content (each patch contains 700 mg lidocaine, or 50 mg lidocaine per gram of adhesive). In dogs, lidocaine patches produce detectable plasma concentrations 12 hours after application, with steady state achieved between 25 and 48 hours and concentrations subsequently declining after 60 hours. Although plasma concentrations of lidocaine are measurable, they do not have clinical effects in dogs (Ko *et al.*, 2007).

Open wounds and infiltration
Splash block

A suitable volume of 2% lidocaine or 0.5% bupivacaine can be used to bathe the wound or incision before closing. The local anaesthetic is left in place for 2 minutes to allow adequate penetration into nerve endings. This method can be used to provide anaesthesia for small wounds to be repaired and postoperative analgesia for surgical incisions (Figure 11.7)

Infiltration anaesthesia

Infiltration anaesthesia can be used in animals where small wounds are to be repaired or skin lesions removed. Local anaesthetic solutions are deposited around the area to be desensitized by multiple intradermal and/or subcutaneous injections. Lidocaine (0.5% to 2%) is often used and the

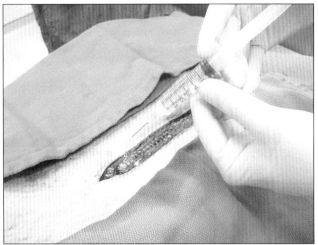

11.7 A 'splash' block being applied on the surgical incision following closure of the linea alba in a dog.

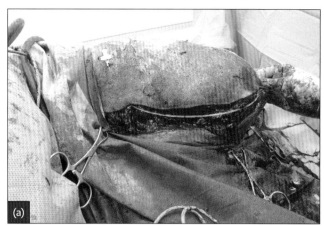

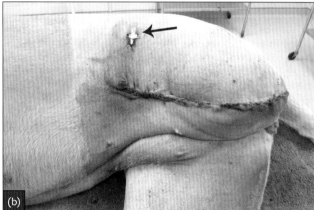

11.8 (a) A diffusion wound catheter placed within the incision used for a hindlimb amputation in a dog. (b) Bupivacaine with bicarbonate was injected through the injection port (arrowed) attached to the catheter for postoperative pain control.

maximum volume available to use should be calculated. After the first needle insertion and deposition of solution, subsequent needle insertions can be made through desensitized tissue, so that the patient feels only the first insertion. It is advisable not to use this block around cancerous lesions or abscesses, because of the risk of spread of cancer cells or bacteria.

The volume of lidocaine to be used depends on the area, but generally 2–5 mg/kg may be used. If adrenaline is used with lidocaine, the total dose can be increased to 5–8 mg/kg. To decrease the concentration and increase the volume, lidocaine can be diluted with sterile saline (but not sterile water). Local anaesthetics with adrenaline should not be injected into tissues supplied by end arteries, such as those of the ears or tail, and should be avoided in dogs with thin skin. It is important to avoid injecting adrenaline-containing solutions subfascially and intra-arterially. Sodium bicarbonate can be added to the lidocaine to reduce pain on injection (see Figure 11.5).

Diffusion catheter (wound soaker catheter)

Long catheters can be implanted during surgery to enable the delivery of local anaesthetics to deeper tissues, depending on the position of the catheter. The catheter should have multiple side-ports to allow infiltration of a larger area of tissue than is possible from a catheter with only one distal opening. A suitable catheter can be made from sterile tubing with side-holes cut, although fenestrated medical-grade silastic catheters are commercially available. Sutures are used to secure the catheter in place on the skin; these are cut before withdrawal of the catheter. Diffusion catheters have been used for several days postoperatively. Strict aseptic technique is required, and a bacterial filter may also be attached to the proximal end of the catheter.

Lidocaine can be used as a continuous infusion, or 0.5% bupivacaine (1–1.5 mg/kg) can be gently infused every 6–12 hours. Bolus bupivacaine is ideal in cats or restless dogs to avoid the need for an infusion set to be attached to the catheter. Infection rates have not been found to be higher in animals treated with use of these catheters. Lidocaine infusion is given at a rate of 2 mg/kg/h and diluted to give a final volume of 5 ml/h in dogs (Abelson *et al.*, 2009; Armitage-Chan, 2013). Situations where diffusion catheters may be used include auricular surgery, sternal split for thoracic surgery, traumatic wounds, injection-site sarcoma removal and amputations (Figure 11.8).

Regional nerve blocks

Most regional nerve blocks are performed in anaesthetized or heavily sedated patients, enabling precise and humane injection. Sterility should be maintained while performing these blocks and the syringe should always be aspirated before injection to check the needle is not within a blood vessel. Although reported elsewhere, this author does not aspirate syringes for epidural techniques in case damage is done to delicate structures within the epidural space. Injections within the neural sheath should be avoided in order to prevent direct nerve toxicity and the possibility of permanent damage to the nerve. The amount of local anaesthetic used will depend on the area of spread required and the size of the patient.

Injections of a local anaesthetic are generally placed using anatomical landmarks, but other technical aids have been introduced to increase precision of injection. An electrical nerve stimulator (or finder) can be used with insulated needles to locate nerves (Figure 11.9). A stimulator used for assessing the quality of skeletal muscle blockade from neuromuscular blocking agents can be used, although accurate use of the scale with currents below 1 mA may be difficult with some older units. Insulated needles tend to be longer than standard hypodermic needles but the insulated area enables the needle to be held safely. The stimulator is set to give repetitive single stimuli at a current of 1 mA. Stimulation of a motor nerve will cause muscle twitching in areas served by the nerve. Direct stimulation of muscle bellies close to the needle point does not indicate that the needle is in close proximity to the nerve. The location of the needle producing greatest muscle twitch distally

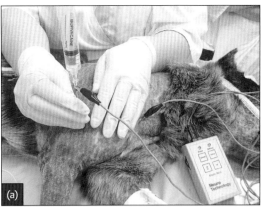
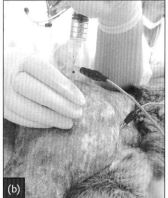
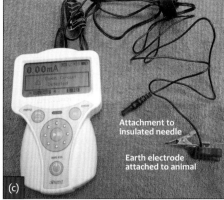

Attachment to
insulated needle

Earth electrode
attached to animal

11.9 (a–b) Use of a nerve stimulator and an insulated needle to perform accurate deposition of local anaesthetic around nerve bundles. These images show a RUMM block being performed with an older unit. New units have electrical current scales which are easier to use and proprietary insulated needles. (c) New model nerve stimulator (Stimpod, Mila International).

indicates the end of the needle is in the proximity of the nerve bundle. Once the nerve has been located, the current should be gradually reduced to 0.4 mA, at which point the contraction of muscle bellies served by the nerve bundle should still be evident. Stimulation at a very low current (<0.4 mA) may indicate penetration of the nerve bundle; if this occurs the needle should be withdrawn slightly before injecting the anaesthetic. Local anaesthetic is then deposited through the needle. If desired, the needle is left *in situ* and after a few minutes, the stimulator can be used again to stimulate the nerve bundle: a diminished or absent response indicates a successful nerve block.

Ultrasonography can also be used to locate nerve trunks because they travel alongside veins and arteries, which can be easily visualized using this technique. An ultrasound probe designed for shallow penetration but enhanced detail will enable the operator to guide the needle to the appropriate position. More details of these techniques can be found in the references listed at the end of the chapter.

Blocks involving the head and neck

Eye and dental blocks: These blocks are described in Chapters 19 and 20, respectively.

Auricular block: This block can be performed to alleviate pain from auricular surgery. It involves blockade of both the great auricular and auriculotemporal nerves (Figure 11.10).

The great auricular nerve (cervical nerve II) can be located by two methods:

- In thinner animals, the hyoid bone from the larynx can be palpated and the head of the hyoid apparatus located where it articulates with the skull
- Alternatively, the nerve can be found through palpation of the site ventral to the wing of the atlas and caudal to the tympanic bulla.

The vertical ear canal can be palpated just rostral to this site, and local anaesthetic is deposited at this point.

The auriculotemporal nerve can be blocked by placing the needle just rostral to the vertical ear canal, on the dorsum of the most caudal part of the zygomatic arch. In effect, the needle is placed rostral to the vertical canal, just opposite the site of the great auricular nerve block.

Difficulty in performing this block may arise when chronic inflammation distorts the ear canal; there is also potential for facial nerve paralysis if the cranial nerve VII is damaged with the injection.

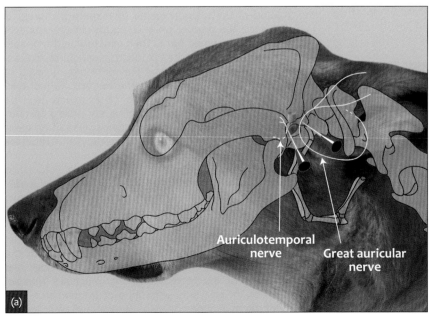

Auriculotemporal
nerve

Great auricular
nerve

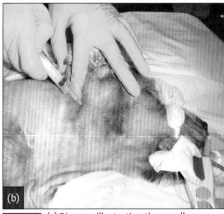

11.10 (a) Diagram illustrating the needle positions to perform the auricular block in a dog. The positions are identical for the cat. (b) Auricular block for a dog undergoing a vertical ear canal ablation.

(a, © Juliane Deubner, University of Saskatchewan, Canada; b, Courtesy of Marieke de Vries, Davies Veterinary Specialists, Higham Gobion, UK)

Infraorbital blocks for rhinoscopy: Bilateral infraorbital nerve blocks within the infraorbital canal (see Chapter 20) can be used before performing rhinoscopy. Even deeply anaesthetized patients can respond to the passage of an endoscope into the nasal cavity, which stimulates sneezing and snorting reflexes. The block should produce a better quality of anaesthesia.

Forelimb blocks

Cervical paravertebral block: This block will provide analgesia to areas below the shoulder, but can also afford some analgesia for forelimb amputation involving removal of the scapula. The dorsal–ventral approach, reported by Lemke and Creighton (2008), is performed by retracting the scapula caudally and palpating the transverse process of cervical vertebra C6. The needle enters the skin from a dorsolateral position to the spine and is advanced until the needle reaches the transverse process. The tip of the needle is then 'walked off' the cranial and caudal borders of the transverse process and local anaesthetic is deposited around the ventral branches of cervical nerves C5 and C6. The needle is then directed caudomedially to the head of the first rib, and two injections are made cranial and caudal to the head of the first rib (C7 and T1).

The author uses an unreported cranial–caudal approach using a spinal or insulated needle, which is inserted parallel to the spinal column to the head of the first rib and then works cranially (Figure 11.11). This technique allows the block to be performed in obese animals in which the landmarks for the dorsal approach may be difficult to palpate. The cranial–caudal approach involves retracting the scapula caudally but also lifting it laterally to enable the needle to pass medially to the shoulder blade. The first block (T1) of four injections is performed by palpating the head of the first rib as it articulates with the vertebra. A quarter of the total dose (maximum 2 mg/kg of 0.5% bupivacaine) is deposited just caudal to the head of the first rib. The needle can be 'walked off' the rib and an attempt made to direct the needle to where the nerve emerges from the vertebral foramen (T1). The second site is just cranial to the head of the first rib and caudal to the lateral prominence of the cervical vertebra (C7); a further quarter of the volume is injected at this site. The needle is then withdrawn slightly to a position just caudal to the lateral prominence of the cervical vertebra C6, and the third quarter of local anaesthetic is administered. For the fourth injection, the same procedure is performed on the next cranial vertebra (C5).

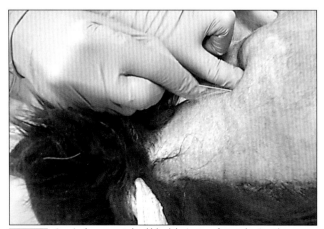

11.11 Cervical paravertebral block being performed using the cranial–caudal approach in a dog about to undergo a humeral fracture repair.

The dorsal–ventral approach is indicated with the green needle and the cranial–caudal approach with the blue needle in Figure 11.12.

Aspiration to check correct needle position should be performed before each injection, because the vertebral arteries are close to the injection sites. The injectate should not be directed into the foramina of the vertebral column and the block should be unilateral, as there is a risk of paralysing the phrenic nerve and causing hypoventilation. Use of an electrical nerve stimulator will increase accuracy of needle placement.

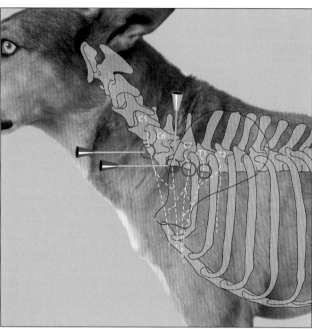

11.12 Approaches to the paravertebral block. The green needle indicates the direction for the dorsal–ventral approach and the blue needles indicate the direction for the cranial–caudal approach. C = cervical; T = thoracic.
(© Juliane Deubner, University of Saskatchewan, Canada)

Brachial plexus block: This block provides analgesia distal to the elbow. A 7.5 cm, 20 or 22G spinal or insulated needle is inserted medial to the shoulder joint and parallel to the vertebral column towards the costochondral junctions. The distal end of the needle should lie caudal to the spine of the scapula (Figure 11.13). Half of the volume of 0.5% bupivacaine (maximum 2 mg/kg) is injected once the needle point is caudal to the spine of the scapula. The remainder is then injected as the needle is withdrawn (aspirating before each injection) to make a 'line' block across the brachial plexus. It may take up to 15 minutes for the block to become evident. To increase the volume of the injectate, the bupivacaine can be diluted by adding a volume of saline equivalent to one-third of the initial volume of bupivacaine. Use of an electrical nerve stimulator increases accuracy and removes the need to dilute the bupivacaine.

Proximal and distal radial/ulnar/median/musculocutaneous block: The radial/ulnar/median/musculocutaneous (RUMM) block involves depositing local anaesthetic around these four nerves. With this block, one injection is made on the lateral side and one on the medial side of the humerus. This block will provide analgesia to areas distal to the elbow. The radial nerve emerges between the medial and lateral heads of the triceps and the brachialis muscle, caudal to the middle and distal third of the humerus. The course of the musculocutaneous, median and ulnar nerves

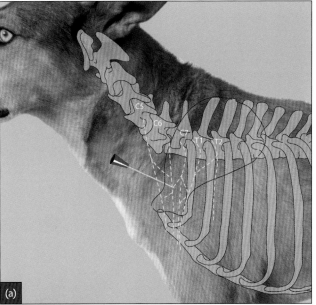

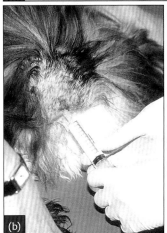

11.13 (a) Diagram illustrating the direction of the needle to perform the brachial plexus block in a dog. The landmarks are the same for the cat. (b) This dog had a fractured radius/ulna and was difficult to handle. Following opioid administration and a brachial plexus block, the dog became friendly and appeared pain-free (Duke *et al.*, 1998). C = cervical; T = thoracic.

(a, © Juliane Deubner, University of Saskatchewan, Canada)

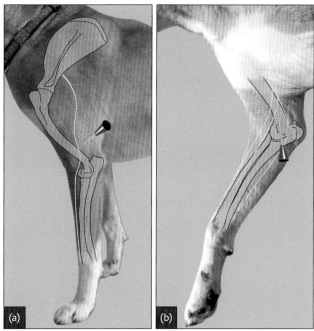

11.14 Diagrams showing the needle positions for performing the RUMM block. (a) The radial nerve is blocked proximal to the elbow on the lateral surface. (b) The musculocutaneous, medial and ulnar nerves are blocked on the medial surface proximal to the elbow. The positions are identical for the cat.

(© Juliane Deubner, University of Saskatchewan, Canada)

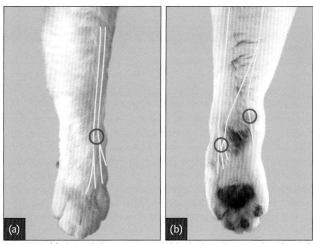

11.15 (a) The radial nerve in a cat is blocked on the cranial surface of the forelimb, and (b) the median and ulnar nerves are blocked on the palmar surface of the forelimb.

(© Juliane Deubner, University of Saskatchewan, Canada)

is adjacent to the brachial artery on the medial side of the limb. Palpation of the brachial pulse will help guide to the correct site for needle insertion. The injection is made around the brachial artery in the mid-humeral area (aspirate before injection to check that the needle has not entered the artery). The block can be performed with the assistance of an electrical nerve stimulator or by using anatomical landmarks and a hypodermic needle. Approximately 0.5–2.0 ml of local anaesthetic is deposited at each site, depending on the size of the animal (Figure 11.14).

For procedures on the distal forelimb, the distal radial/ulnar/median block can be performed in the carpal area. The median and ulnar nerves are blocked by injecting local anaesthetic lateral to the accessory carpal pad (dorsal branch of ulnar nerve), and a larger amount of injectate is deposited transversely in the area between the accessory carpal pad and the dewclaw pad (median and ventral branch of ulnar nerves) to cover the extent of all nerve branches. The radial nerve is blocked at a point dorsomedial to the carpus, just proximal to the carpal joint (Figure 11.15).

Hindlimb blocks

Further information on performing blocks of the lumbar and sacral plexuses, guided by either ultrasonography or an electrical nerve stimulator, are listed in the Further Reading section.

The femoral and sciatic nerves can be blocked to provide analgesia of the pelvic limb from mid-femur distally and are a useful alternative to performing epidural injection (Campoy and Read, 2013). Blocks for the hindlimb have been recently described and reviewed (Gurney and Leece, 2014).

Femoral nerve: The femoral nerve (ventral branches of L4, L5 and L6 spinal nerves) crosses the femoral triangle, and the cutaneous and saphenous nerves branch off the femoral nerve in this region. Within the triangle, the femoral nerve is cranial to the femoral artery and this is the site for injection (Figure 11.16). The nerve is fairly superficial and deep injections are not required.

Sciatic nerve: The sciatic nerve is composed of the ventral branches of L6, L7 and S1 spinal nerves; it emerges between the greater trochanter of the femur and

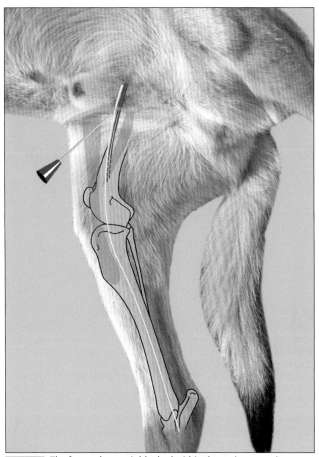

11.16 The femoral nerve is blocked within the groin area as it crosses the femoral triangle.
(© Juliane Deubner, University of Saskatchewan, Canada)

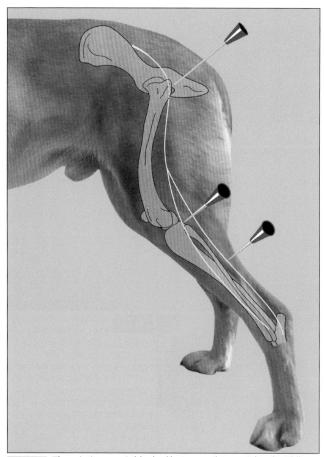

11.17 The sciatic nerve is blocked between the cranial and middle third of a line connecting the greater trochanter and the ischiatic tuberosity. The tibial nerve is blocked deep to the gastrocnemius muscle and the common peroneal nerve is blocked as it passes caudal to the head of the fibula.
(© Juliane Deubner, University of Saskatchewan, Canada)

the ischiatic tuberosity. At this site, the sciatic nerve gives rise to the branches supplying the caudal thigh muscles. The sciatic nerve itself lies between the biceps femoris muscle laterally and the semimembranosus muscle caudomedially. It divides into the tibial nerve medially and the common peroneal nerve laterally; this division can lie anywhere between the level of the hip and just proximal to the stifle. Blocking the sciatic nerve will provide partial analgesia of the stifle and of areas distal to this joint. When a sciatic nerve block is used with a femoral block, the limb will be anaesthetized from mid-femur, including the stifle joint.

The injection point for the sciatic nerve block is between the cranial and middle third of a line connecting the greater trochanter and the ischiatic tuberosity (Figure 11.17). Potential complications include temporary or permanent nerve injury, resulting in knuckling of the hind-paw. If high resistance to injection is felt when performing the injection, the local anaesthetic may be entering the perineural sheath, and can cause nerve toxicity.

Tibial and common peroneal nerves: The tibial and common peroneal nerves can both be blocked to provide local anaesthesia when performing procedures on the distal limb. The tibial nerve can be selectively blocked by passing a needle between the deep and lateral heads of the gastrocnemius muscle between the caudal surface of the tibia and cranial to the muscle bellies. The common peroneal nerve can be blocked as it passes caudal to the fibular head and travels just caudal to the fibula (Figure 11.17).

Lumbosacral epidural (extradural): The epidural and subarachnoid spaces are illustrated in Figure 11.18. Drug options for anaesthesia/analgesia of the hindlimbs include preservative-free 2% lidocaine, 2% mepivacaine, 0.5% bupivacaine or 0.75% ropivacaine, all used at a dose of 1 ml/5 kg (up to a maximum volume of 6 ml). The anaesthetic effect of lidocaine has a duration of approximately 1 hour, while that of bupivacaine or ropivacaine lasts for 2–4 hours. Bupivacaine is most commonly used epidurally; ropivacaine may cause more pronounced hypotension in anaesthetized patients, although they may be able to walk sooner with less ataxia following recovery.

Local anaesthetics can be used either alone or mixed with opioids or alpha-2 adrenergic agonists to provide more effective analgesia. Morphine sulphate (0.1–0.2 mg/kg) without preservative is most commonly added to the local anaesthetic solution, but the final volume should not exceed 1 ml/5 kg (up to a maximum volume of 6 ml). Concentrated formulations of morphine are preferred in order to prevent excessive dilution of the bupivacaine. For example, a 25 kg dog would require a total of 5 ml of 0.5% bupivacaine to extend the block to the thoracolumbar junction. With a 10 mg/ml formulation of morphine, a clinically negligible volume of 0.25 ml of the morphine solution can be added to the 5 ml volume of bupivacaine to give a dose of 0.1 mg/kg morphine. However, if a 1.0 mg/ml morphine solution were to be used, the 2.5 ml of morphine required would excessively dilute the 2.5 ml volume of bupivacaine that could be used, and a 'patchy' block might follow.

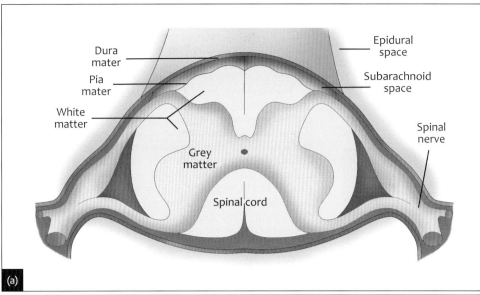

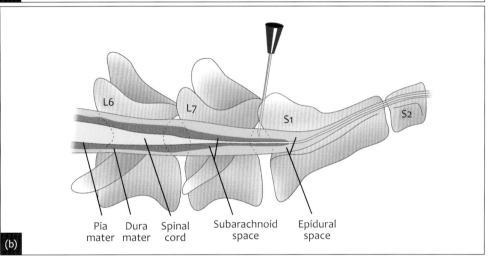

11.18 (a) Cross-section of the spinal cord area depicting the divisions between the epidural and subarachnoid spaces. (b) Sagittal section of the lumbosacral area illustrating needle placement into the epidural space. L = lumbar; S = sacral. (© Juliane Deubner, University of Saskatchewan, Canada)

If epidural opioid analgesia (without local anaesthetic) is required for the trunk and/or forelimbs, concentrations of morphine above 1 mg/ml are diluted with sterile saline (total volume 1 ml/10 kg). Morphine can provide 12–24 hours of analgesia, but onset times vary from 1–2 hours. Other drugs can be substituted and are listed in Figure 11.19.

The side effects of local anaesthetics administered in the epidural space depend on the cranial extent of the block. Hypotension may be observed in anaesthetized patients if the lumbar sympathetic outflow of the autonomic nervous system is blocked. More cranial extension of the block (overdose) causes greater hypotension, respiratory insufficiency, respiratory paralysis and convulsions. Opioids do not cause spinal hypotension but may cause urine retention; therefore, in patients that have received opioids in the epidural space, the bladder should be expressed and urination monitored. Urine retention may be reversible with naloxone or can be treated by catheterization of the bladder. Opioids may rarely cause pruritus or myoclonus; pruritus is reversible with naloxone or the 5-hydroxytryptamine antagonist, ondansetron, but myoclonus may require treatment with $GABA_A$ agonists, for example, propofol infusion.

Epidural injection can be performed with the patient in lateral or sternal recumbency. Positioning the patient in sternal recumbency with the hindlimbs pulled cranially is the easiest position for finding the lumbosacral space. The

Drug	Species	Dose (mg/kg)	Duration of analgesia (hours)	Reference
Pethidine (meperidine)	Cat	5.0	1–2	Tung and Yaksh, 1982
l-Methadone	Cat	1.0	1–2	Tung and Yaksh, 1982
Fentanyl	Cat	0.004	0.3	Duke et al., 1994
Hydromorphone	Cat	0.05	5	Ambros et al., 2009
Morphine	Cat	0.1	10	Pypendop et al., 2008
Buprenorphine	Cat	0.02	24	Steagall et al., 2009
Tramadol	Cat	1.0	6–8	Castro et al., 2009
Morphine	Dog	0.1	12	Pascoe and Dyson, 1993
Oxymorphone	Dog	0.05	7	Vesal et al., 1996
Medetomidine	Cat	0.01	4	Duke et al., 1994
Medetomidine	Dog	0.015	7	Vesal et al., 1996

11.19 Drugs that can be used in the epidural space in cats and dogs. These data are taken from studies in conscious animals. If opioids are mixed with local anaesthetics, ensure that the total volume (1 ml/5 kg) is not exceeded. If local anaesthetics are not used with the opioid, dilute the drug in sterile saline to a total volume of 1 ml/10 kg.

dorsocranial points of the ilium (iliac crests) are palpated with the thumb and middle finger of the non-dominant hand, which allows location of the dorsal spinous process of lumbar vertebra L7 just caudal to an imaginary line drawn between the iliac crests. The index finger is used to locate the lumbosacral junction, which is felt as a depression just caudal to the spinous process of L7. A 2.5 to 7.5 cm, 20 or 22G spinal needle is inserted perpendicular to the line of the dorsum (Figure 11.20).

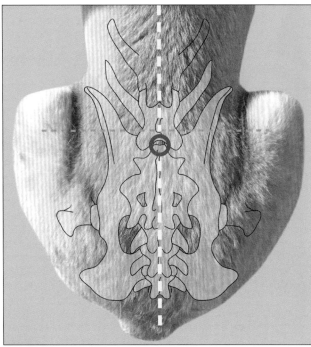

11.20 Diagram illustrating the site for lumbosacral injection, indicated by the red circle. The horizontal blue dashed line illustrates the imaginary line joining the iliac crests, and the yellow dashed line marks the vertebral column.
(© Juliane Deubner, University of Saskatchewan, Canada)

Occasionally, the needle prematurely strikes bone, which indicates that the dorsum of the vertebral column has been struck. The needle can be 'walked off' the dorsal part of the vertebra to the space between L7 and S1. Penetration of the interarcuate ligament and entry into the epidural space may be detected as a popping sensation, although this does not occur in all patients. Further insertion of the needle will meet resistance as the needle reaches the floor of the spinal canal. The stylet is removed at this point. The hub of the needle should be observed for blood or cerebrospinal fluid (CSF). Since the dural sac terminates further caudally in cats and in small or young dogs, CSF may be observed in the hub of the needle. If this occurs, the epidural injection should be either abandoned or retried, or one-quarter to one-third of the originally calculated volume of drug can be administered into the subarachnoid space (spinal or intrathecal injection). Observation of blood means that the ventral venous sinus has been punctured; the needle should be removed, cleaned by flushing with sterile saline, and the injection retried. Care should be taken to ensure that long spinal needles do not penetrate the lumbar disc and enter the pelvic cavity.

To test for correct placement of the needle, an injection of 0.25–0.5 ml of either air or, preferably, sterile saline, can be made, and should meet with no resistance to injection. Air, however, should not be injected into the subarachnoid space. An air bubble can also be introduced into the injectate; compression of the bubble will be observed if any resistance to the injection is encountered (Figure 11.21). 'Loss of resistance' syringes (e.g. Pulsator®) are commercially available and give more precise feedback on the presence or absence of any resistance to injection of the test saline (Figure 11.22).

The 'hanging drop' method can also be used to check correct needle placement. The epidural space can be at sub-atmospheric pressure; because of this difference in pressure, a small amount of saline or injectate placed in the hub of the spinal needle (requires withdrawal of the stylet) will be aspirated into the epidural space once the distal end of the needle enters the epidural space (Figure 11.23). Although this technique may work better in larger dogs, the author has seen it used successfully in a Chihuahua. This technique is not effective in patients positioned in lateral recumbency, because in this position

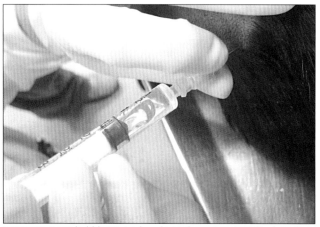

11.21 An air bubble is introduced into the syringe to aid in detecting loss of resistance to injection into the epidural space.

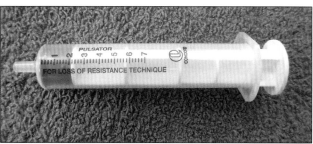

11.22 A loss of resistance syringe for assessing placement of a spinal needle into the epidural space.

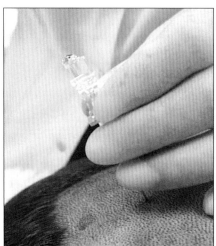

11.23 A hanging drop of sterile saline or injectate can be placed on the hub of the needle; aspiration of the liquid indicates entry of the distal end of the needle into the epidural space.
(Courtesy of Marieke de Vries, Davies Veterinary Specialists, Higham Gobion, UK)

the epidural space is not at sub-atmospheric pressure and placing a drop of fluid in the hub is impractical.

The epidural drugs should be injected into the epidural space over 30–60 seconds, or more slowly if any changes in heart rate are observed or if the patient shows any signs of decreasing depth of anaesthesia.

Epidural catheters with integral wire stiffening or removable stylets can also be placed if long-term administration of analgesics is required (Figure 11.24). The commercial packs that are available contain Tuohy needles, which are suitable for medium- to large-sized dogs. The Tuohy needle should be inserted at an angle of 20 degrees to the vertical in a cranial direction in order to keep the needle lumen free for insertion of a flexible catheter into the epidural space. Take care to avoid pulling the catheter back out with the needle in place or the needle may cut through the catheter. After placement of the catheter, the needle is removed and the catheter taped securely and aseptically in place. A bacterial filter should always be used and strict sterility maintained, and constant supervision of the patient is required.

Contraindications to epidural techniques include distorted anatomy, coagulopathies, septicaemia and skin infections over the puncture site.

Sacrococcygeal epidural block: This block has been used with success in sedated male cats being treated for urinary tract obstruction (O'Hearn and Wright, 2011). Risk of entry into the dural sac is unlikely with this technique. The site of injection is the most cranial moveable joint; this will be either the sacrococcygeal or the first intercoccygeal joint. A 1.6 cm, 25G hypodermic needle is used to enter the epidural space and 0.1–0.2 ml/kg of 2% lidocaine without preservative is injected. There should be no resistance to injection. If the block does not produce enough relaxation to allow passage of a urinary catheter, the block can be repeated once more. This block may also be useful for some cases of dystocia. A peripheral nerve finder will cause the tail to flick with stimulation and is useful to ensure epidural placement.

Blocks applicable to the forelimbs and hindlimbs

Digital nerve block: The digits can be either individually blocked or all blocked, by depositing local anaesthetic alongside the individual digit itself or into the web where the digital nerves bifurcate. The digital nerves run along both lateral and medial surfaces of the digits (Figure 11.25).

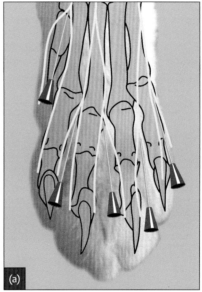

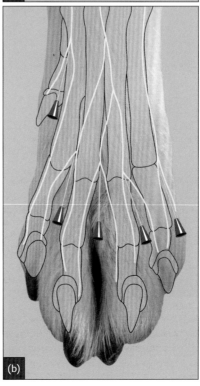

11.25 Diagrams illustrating the needle positions for digital nerve blocks for (a) a cat and (b) a dog. The needle is inserted at the point of bifurcation of the nerves.
(© Juliane Deubner, University of Saskatchewan, Canada)

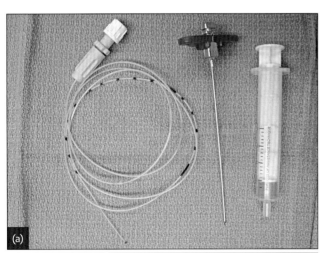

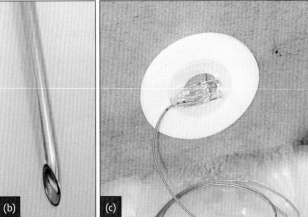

11.24 (a) An epidural catheter and Tuohy needle. (b) The needle has a specially designed end to allow the cranial movement of the catheter. (c) Special patches with clips are available to fix the catheter to the skin.

Intravenous regional analgesia: The application of a tourniquet around a distal limb and intravenous injection of lidocaine distal to the tourniquet provides complete analgesia of the distal limb below the tourniquet for procedures lasting no longer than 60–90 minutes. It is advisable to pre-place an intravenous catheter in a superficial vein (cephalic or saphenous) distal to the tourniquet, as it may be difficult to identify a vein after limb exsanguination (Figure 11.26a). Once the catheter is secured, the tourniquet is loosened. The limb is then exsanguinated either by wrapping it with an Esmarch bandage or by holding it above the level of the heart for a few minutes. Care should be taken not to dislodge the catheter with the Esmarch bandage. The tourniquet is finally tightened enough to obstruct arterial blood flow (a sphygmomanometer cuff can also be used and the pressure in the cuff increased to above systolic blood pressure) or until there is loss of peripheral pulse below the tourniquet. Once the tourniquet is secured, the Esmarch bandage (if used) can be removed. A dose of 2 mg/kg of 2% lidocaine is injected through the catheter with light pressure on the syringe (Figure 11.26b). Analgesia occurs in 5–10 minutes as a result of diffusion of the drug through the tissues. The tourniquet should not be left in place for longer than 90 minutes to avoid complications resulting from deprivation of blood flow.

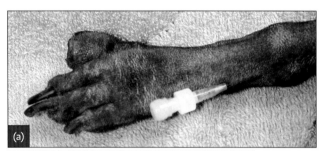

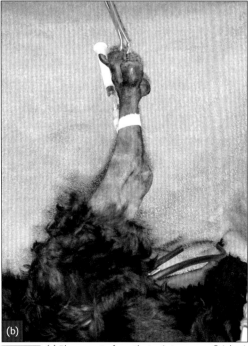

11.26 (a) Placement of a catheter into a superficial vein and application of a tourniquet (not visible in this image) to perform an intravenous regional block in the hindpaw region of an anaesthetized dog for digit removal. (b) The leg is held above heart level for 5 minutes and the tourniquet is tightened until there is loss of a peripheral pulse distal to the tourniquet. Lidocaine is then injected through the pre-placed catheter.

Thoracic area blocks

Intercostal nerve block: This block is often used for relieving pain after a lateral thoracotomy, pleural drainage or rib fractures. Intercostal nerves at two sites, cranial and caudal to the incision or wound, are blocked. The caudal border of the rib close to the intervertebral foramen is located and 0.25–1.0 ml of 0.5% bupivacaine is injected. The volume selected within this range depends on the size of patient. For patients undergoing a sternal split, the author has used a diluted solution of bupivacaine (2 mg/kg total for this block) applied bilaterally to all the intercostal nerves on or ventral to the costochondral junction (Figures 11.27 and 11.28, see Chapter 23).

Interpleural analgesia: Administration of a local anaesthetic agent through a catheter into the pleural cavity can provide analgesia for pain arising from lateral and sternal thoracotomies, rib fractures and chest wall metastases (Figure 11.29). The pleural catheter can be pre-placed during surgery, or a chest drain can be used.

Percutaneous placement requires confirmation of entry into the pleural cavity; this can be achieved through detection of negative pressure. The animal should be sedated and the caudal border of the rib infiltrated with local anaesthetic in order to facilitate catheter insertion. A Tuohy needle is inserted with a drop of sterile saline in the hub of the needle after removal of the stylet. The needle is advanced through the pleura and the saline drop

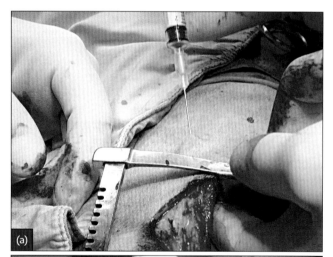

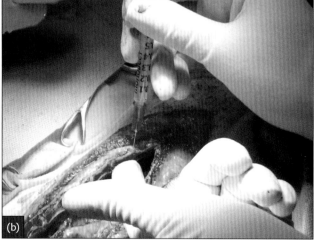

11.27 (a) Placement of an intercostal nerve block in a dog undergoing a lateral thoracotomy. (b) Use of a diluted solution of bupivacaine to allow multiple injections around the intercostal nerves in a cat undergoing a median sternotomy.

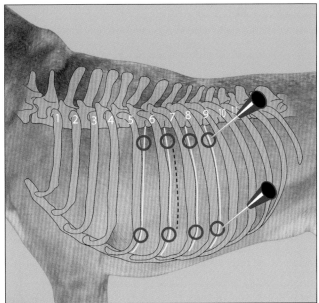

11.28 Diagram illustrating the areas (red circles) where an intercostal block can be performed for a lateral thoracotomy incision (dashed line) or for chest drain placement.
(© Juliane Deubner, University of Saskatchewan, Canada)

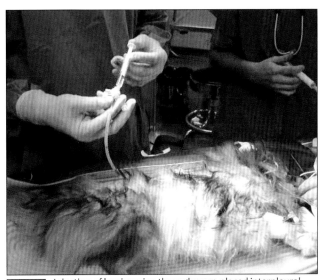

11.29 Injection of bupivacaine through a pre-placed interpleural catheter for administration of an interpleural block in a dog after lateral thoracotomy. The incision is on the left side of the dog.

disappears from the hub as negative pressure within the pleural cavity aspirates the drop into the cavity. A diffusion catheter can be introduced and advanced 3–5 cm beyond the needle tip with minimal resistance, and the needle is then removed. Approximately 1–2 mg/kg of 0.5% bupivacaine is injected through the catheter. There may be some initial discomfort in a conscious patient, but this wanes as the local anaesthetic becomes effective. To overcome the initial discomfort, either some bicarbonate can be added to the bupivacaine, or a small dose of lidocaine may be injected first, followed by the bupivacaine after 20–30 minutes (see Figure 11.5). The patient should be placed with the incision site down for 5 minutes so that the local anaesthetic pools over the incision site. Dogs with a sternal thoracotomy should be placed in sternal recumbency for 5 minutes to allow the drug to exert its maximum effect on the incision. Care should be taken to ensure that the interpleural catheter is not left open to the

atmosphere, otherwise a pneumothorax may be created; constant supervision of the patient is also required. Strict adherence to sterile technique is important to prevent infection. The technique is not recommended for patients with pleural effusions, pleuritis or excessive bleeding into the chest cavity. The potential risk of cardiac toxicity with interpleural administration of lidocaine (1.5 mg/kg) mixed with bupivacaine (1.5 mg/kg) has been shown to be minimal (Bernard *et al.*, 2006). There may be a concern that hypoventilation could occur if the phrenic nerve is accidentally blocked.

Miscellaneous blocks

Intratesticular block

Anaesthetized cats and dogs undergoing orchiectomy appear to benefit from intratesticular lidocaine injections given just before the procedure. A 25 G needle is used and a suitable amount of lidocaine is administered in the centre of each testicle until increased resistance to injection is felt. Approximately 0.1–0.25 ml of 2% lidocaine is used per testicle in cats, with up to 0.5 ml in larger dogs. The author avoids the use of bupivacaine for this block because the testicle is a highly vascular area.

Intra-articular block

For reasons described earlier in this chapter, the administration of local anesthetics intra-articularly may cause some damage to the joint. Administration of local anaesthetic into the joint space is useful, however, for analgesic purposes. The addition of preservative-free morphine to the local anaesthetic, or administration of morphine alone into the joint, has also proven to be effective and can provide analgesia for up to 24 hours. The volumes to be instilled into the joint vary with the capacity of the joint capsule, but over-distension of the capsule should be avoided.

Summary

The provision of local anaesthetic blocks prior to surgery, postoperatively or for critically ill or injured patients is a powerful tool for improving the quality of pain control. When performed correctly, there are observable benefits, such as anaesthetic-sparing properties and improved patient comfort.

References and further reading

Abelson AL, McCobb EC, Shaw S *et al.* (2009) Use of wound soaker catheters for the administration of local anesthetic for post-operative analgesia: 56 cases. *Veterinary Anaesthesia and Analgesia* **36**, 597–602

Ambros B, Steagall PVM, Mantovani F *et al.* (2009) Antinociceptive effects of epidural administration of hydromorphone in conscious cats. *American Journal of Veterinary Research* **70**, 1187–1192

Armitage-Chan E (2013) Use of wound soaker catheters in pain management. *In Practice* **35**, 24–29

Bailard NS, Ortiz J and Flores RA (2014) Additives to local anaesthetics for peripheral nerve blocks: evidence, limitations and recommendations. *American Journal of Health-System Pharmacy* **71(5)**, 373–385

Baker JF and Mulhall KJ (2011) Local anaesthetics and chondrotoxicity: what is the evidence? *Knee Surgery, Sports Traumatology, Arthroscopy* **20**, 2294–2301

Barry SL, Martinez SA, Davies NM *et al.* (2014) Synovial fluid bupivacaine concentrations following single intra-articular injection in normal and osteoarthritic canine stifles. *Journal of Veterinary Pharmacology and Therapeutics* **38(1)**, 97–100

Bernard F, Kudnig ST and Monnet E (2006) Hemodynamic effects of interpleural lidocaine and bupivacaine combination in anaesthetized dogs with and without an open pericardium. *Veterinary Surgery* **35**, 252–258

Campoy L and Read MR (2013) *Small Animal Regional Anesthesia and Analgesia, 1st edn.* Wiley-Blackwell, Ames

Castro DS, Silva, MFA, Shih AC *et al.* (2009) Comparison between the analgesic effects of morphine and tramadol delivered epidurally in cats receiving a standardized noxious stimulation. *Journal of Feline Medicine and Surgery* **11**, 948–953

Chadwick HS (1985) Toxicity and resuscitation in lidocaine- or bupivacaine-infused cats. *Anesthesiology* **63**, 385–390

Davies RJ (2003) Buffering the pain of local anaesthetics: a systemic review. *Emergency Medicine* **15**, 81–88

Duke T (2000) Local and regional anesthetic and analgesic techniques in the dog and cat: Part I, pharmacology of local anesthetics and topical anesthesia. *Canadian Veterinary Journal* **41**, 883–884

Duke T (2000) Local and regional anesthetic and analgesic techniques in the dog and cat: Part II, infiltration and nerve blocks. *Canadian Veterinary Journal* **41**, 949–952

Duke T, Cullen CL and Fowler JD (1998) Anesthesia case of the month. Analgesia for fractures until surgery can take place. *Journal of the American Veterinary Medical Association* **212**, 649–650

Duke T, Komulainen-Cox AM, Remedios AM *et al.* (1994) The analgesic effects of administering fentanyl or medetomidine in the epidural space of cats. *Veterinary Surgery* **23**, 143–148

Dutton TAG, Gurney MA, Bright SR (2014) Intra-articular mepivacaine reduces interventional analgesia requirements during arthroscopic surgery in dogs. *Journal of Small Animal Practice* **55**, 405–408

Feldman HS, Arthur GR and Covino BG (1989) Comparative systemic toxicity of convulsant and supraconvulsant doses of intravenous ropivacaine, bupivacaine, and lidocaine in the conscious dog. *Anesthesia and Analgesia* **69**, 794–801

Feldman, HS, Arthur R, Pitkanen M *et al.* (1991) Treatment of acute systemic toxicity after the rapid intravenous injection of ropivacaine and bupivacaine in the conscious dog. *Anesthesia and Analgesia* **73**, 373–384

Fozzard HA, Lee PJ and Lipkind GM (2005) Mechanism of local anesthetic drug action on voltage-gated sodium channels. *Current Pharmaceutical Design* **11**, 2671–2686

Gibbon KJ, Cyborski JM and Guzinski MV (2003) Evaluation of adverse effects of EMLA (lidocaine/prilocaine) cream for the placement of jugular catheters in healthy cats. *Journal of Veterinary Pharmacology and Therapeutics* **26**, 439–441

Groban L, Deal, DD, Vernon JC *et al.* (2001) Cardiac resuscitation after incremental overdosage with lidocaine, bupivacaine, levobupivacaine, and ropivacaine in anesthetized dogs. *Anesthesia and Analgesia* **92**, 37–43

Gurney MA and Leece EA (2014) Analgesia for pelvic limb surgery. A review of peripheral nerve blocks and the extradural technique. *Veterinary Anaesthesia and Analgesia* **41**, 445–458

Heavner JE (2007) Local anesthetics. *Current Opinions in Anesthesiology* **20**, 336–342

Jones RS (2002) A history of veterinary anaesthesia. *Anales de Veterinaria de Murcia* **18**, 7–15

Ko J, Weil A, Maxwell L *et al.* (2007) Plasma concentrations of lidocaine in dogs following lidocaine patch application. *Journal of the American Animal Hospital Association* **43**, 280–283

Lamont LA and Lemke KA (2008) The effects of medetomidine on radial nerve blockade with mepivacaine in dogs. *Veterinary Anaesthesia and Analgesia* **35**, 62–68

Lemke KA (2000) Local and regional analgesia. *Veterinary Clinics of North America: Small Animal Practice* **32**, 747–763

Lemke KA and Creighton CM (2008) Paravertebral blockade of the brachial plexus in dogs. *Veterinary Clinics of North America: Small Animal Practice* **38**, 1231–1241

McClure HA and Rubin AP (2005) Review of local anaesthetic agents. *Minerva Anestesiologica* **71**, 59–74

Neumann S, Frenz M, Streit F and Oellerich M (2011) Formation of monoethylglycinexylidide (MEGX) in clinically healthy dogs. *Canadian Journal of Veterinary Research* **75**, 317–320

O'Brien TQ, Clark-Price SC, Evans EE *et al.* (2010) Infusion of a lipid emulsion to treat lidocaine intoxication in a cat. *Journal of the American Veterinary Medical Association* **237**, 1455–1458

O'Hearn AK and Wright BD (2011) Coccygeal epidural with local anesthetic for catheterization and pain management in the treatment of feline urethral obstruction. *Journal of Veterinary Emergency and Critical Care* **21**, 50–52

Pascoe PJ and Dyson DH (1993) Analgesia after lateral thoracotomy in dogs: epidural morphine vs. intercostal bupivacaine. *Veterinary Surgery* **22**, 141–147

Pypendop BH, Siao KT, Pascoe PJ *et al.* (2008) Effects of epidurally administered morphine or buprenorphine on the thermal threshold in cats. *American Journal of Veterinary Research* **69**, 983–987

Steagall PVM, Millette V, Mantovani FB *et al.* (2009) Antinociceptive effects of epidural buprenorphine, or medetomidine, or the combination, in conscious cats. *Journal of Veterinary Pharmacology and Therapeutics* **32**, 477–484

Tetzlaff JE (2000) The pharmacology of local anesthetics. *Anesthesiology Clinics of North America* **18**, 217–233

Thomasy SM, Pypendop BH, Ilkiw JE *et al.* (2005) Pharmacokinetics of lidocaine and its active metabolite, monoethylglycinexylidide, after intravenous administration of lidocaine to awake and isoflurane-anesthetized cats. *American Journal of Veterinary Research* **66**, 1162–1166

Tung AS and Yaksh TL (1982) The antinociceptive effects of epidural opiates in the cat: studies on the pharmacology and the effects of lipophilicity in spinal analgesia. *Pain* **12**, 343–356

Vesal N, Cribb PH and Frketic M (1996) Postoperative analgesic and cardiopulmonary effects in dogs of oxymorphone administered epidurally and intramuscularly and medetomidine administered epidurally: A comparative clinical study. *Veterinary Surgery* **25**, 361–369

Chapter 12

Pain management III: chronic pain

Samantha Lindley

Defining chronic pain

There have been many attempts to define pain because the subjective nature of the experience manifests differently between individuals, and it is difficult to describe pain in a way that concisely and accurately encapsulates its purpose, propagation and outcomes. Pain becomes even more nebulous a concept when it is chronic, partly because there is little correlation between the severity of the problem causing the pain and the pain perceived. Indeed, in some cases, there is no lesion present, yet the pain experienced is significant, i.e. the pain has become the disease. This concept can be an intellectual challenge for the clinician, let alone the owner.

> Chronic pain is not simply a continuation of acute pain but is maladaptive, (i.e. of no biological use to the patient), and represents a chronic stressor, with all the damaging physiological changes that accompany chronic stress

After years of struggling with a number of imperfect definitions, the International Association for the Study of Pain (IASP) has concluded that the most appropriate definition of pain in humans is 'whatever the patient says it is'. For the veterinary species we would need to restate this as: 'whatever their behavioural changes, combined with their motivational states, tell us it is'.

Many prey species express their pain in more subtle ways than we may expect, especially when considering the severity of some of the painful conditions they suffer. This trait helps to protect them, but any good stockman, and certainly other animals in the group, can identify the animal that is unwell or in pain because of changes in behaviour. Consider that, if the verbal communication of pain were removed from humans, a wide range of behavioural manifestations of pain would become apparent, including:

- Withdrawal and bad temper
- Becoming more garrulous
- The development of displacement activities
- Engaging in distractions
- Changes of facial expression
- Hypervigilance to sensory stimuli
- Anxiety and depression.

An onlooker would have to be perceptive to understand that any or all of these changes indicate pain in a given individual because humans have long relied on words to give an explanation of such behavioural changes. Animals display a similarly wide range of behavioural manifestations of pain, some of which are not specific to pain and therefore need to be assessed alongside other aspects of the veterinary consultation (Figures 12.1 and 12.2).

Changes in:

- Play – enthusiasm to play and initiation of play, either with the owner or a companion dog
- Exercise tolerance – enthusiasm to go for a walk and to keep walking
- The time spent with the owner – is the dog more 'clingy' or spending more time away from the owner?
- Attitude towards other dogs and/or people – typically dogs in pain may be more wary of, or aggressive towards young, bouncy and/or unfamiliar dogs and children
- Sensitivity to noise – dogs may also be sensitive to other stimuli, but this is harder to ascertain
- The dog's ability to cope when left alone (including separation anxiety)
- The dog's ability to cope with travelling in a car (the animal may be more restless than before or frightened about getting in the car)
- Appetite – although this is not often affected except in severe pain, dogs can have either decreased or, less commonly, increased appetite. However, there may be signs of nausea with spinal pain (increased lip licking, stretching, yawning, eating grass/mud/plants)
- Sleeping position and sleeping generally – dogs may sleep more heavily at night because they are not getting rest in the day, or they may be more restless at night (the latter is more likely to be noticed by the owner)
- General activity
- Enthusiasm towards greeting the owner on their return from an absence
- Acceptance of being groomed/dried and/or petted – either all over the body or in certain areas
- Mood and demeanour

It must be noted that changes in any of these behaviours could be the result of changes in the environment or social situation, such as the loss or illness of a companion dog or owner. These changes cannot be used in isolation to definitively indicate pain and suffering

Specific behaviours strongly suggestive of pain[a]:

- Jumping/startled behaviour
- Restless when trying to sleep
- Excessive licking or chewing of areas of the body
- Panting and/or pacing for no particular reason

Less common signs of pain[a]:

- Compulsive disorders, including polydipsia and polyphagia
- Bizarre fears and anxieties

12.1 Behavioural indicators of pain in dogs. [a]Note that these are changes from the normal behaviour of the animal. An overall confounding factor is present in those patients where the presentation, movement and examination suggests significant long-standing pain and suffering, possibly since the animal was very young. In these cases, pain is 'normal' and so there may be very few noticeable behavioural changes.

Changes in:

- Jumping or accessing elevated areas with ease
- Coat condition – changes in grooming behaviours and allowing grooming by the owner
- Urination/defecation behaviour
- Activity and interaction with the owner
- The time spent with the owner – typically cats in pain will withdraw, but animals that have a strong bond with their owner may seek more attention
- Play and the initiation of play
- Use of a scratching post – presentation of a cat for repeated front claw clipping should cause suspicion that the cat may be reluctant to extend its elbows, assuming all other aspects are constant (i.e. the scratching post has not been changed in either type or position)
- Appetite
- Time spent outside (if relevant)

It must be noted that changes in any of these behaviours could be the result of changes in the environment or social situation, such as the loss or illness of a companion cat or owner. It should be noted that, for cats, changes in the environment are usually much more important than social interactions and may be quite subtle. Behavioural changes cannot be used in isolation to definitively indicate pain and suffering

Specific behaviours strongly suggestive of pain[a]:

- Signs of hyperaesthesia – skin rolling and twitching; attacking certain areas of the body such as the tail/face

Less common signs of pain[a]:

- Compulsive disorders, including polydipsia and polyphagia

12.2 Behavioural indicators of pain in cats. [a]Note that these are changes from the normal behaviour of the animal. An overall confounding factor is present in those patients where the presentation, movement and examination suggests significant long-standing pain and suffering, possibly since the animal was very young. In these cases, pain is 'normal' and so there may be very few noticeable behavioural changes.

Suffering and the components of pain

This chapter deals with the treatment of chronic pain, or rather with the treatment of the *suffering* that chronic pain causes. When treating acute pain, the aim is to provide pain relief while healing and recovery from trauma, injury, disease or surgery takes place. In these circumstances, there is usually an expectation that this recovery *will* take place. For chronic pain, there is no such reliable expectation. There may be no lesion or injury to cure (e.g. a painful limb may have been removed but the (human) patient still perceives it to be painful) or the pathological process may continue relentlessly (e.g. osteoarthritis). In these cases, the aim can be to reduce or remove the pain, but it is more realistic to aim to reduce the suffering associated with the problem.

To make the distinction between pain (the *sensation*) and suffering (the *emotion*) clearer, it can be helpful to consider pain in terms of separate components:

- The *sensory component* is simply the sensation recognized as pain. This sensation is not associated with emotion. A high threshold stimulus excites fast pain fibres (A-δ fibres in skin; type II/III fibres in muscle), causing a reflex movement away from the noxious stimulus and signals the potential for tissue damage to the brain. This reflex protects the body from actual or further damage, and the brain starts to release pain-relieving neurotransmitters. At the point of withdrawal from the noxious stimulus, there is no aversion or suffering

- However, if tissue damage has been caused, the more slowly conducting C-fibres are stimulated and take a multi-synaptic pathway via the limbic system to modulate emotion, giving rise to the feeling of suffering. This motivates the animal to protect the damaged area and avoid such experiences in the future. This is the *emotional component* of pain.

This distinction is helpful, at least in humans, as it allows the components to be examined separately when assessing interventions for the treatment of chronic pain. Human patients may score the sensation of pain similarly before and after a given intervention, but may score their suffering as much improved. In veterinary patients, this distinction guides the clinician towards the correct degree of intervention. For example, a dog with arthritis of the hip may climb stairs more slowly and carefully because it experiences pain as it makes the physical movements of climbing, but there is no hesitation and the dog makes the journey as frequently as it always has done. However, if the prospect of climbing stairs makes the dog hesitate or even refuse, if the dog makes fewer journeys even when the owner is upstairs, if the dog climbs slowly, hugging the wider curve of the stair to minimize turning and if the dog's facial expression conveys anxiety and effort, this is regarded as suffering. Both presentations need to be addressed, but the second is more urgent. There are two further components of pain:

- The *cognitive component*, which is associated with how the patient perceives pain, the associations made with pain, and the conditioned responses
- The *motor component*, which involves the movements and postures associated with pain and the avoidance of pain. This can provide valuable indicators as to the location of the problem (e.g. primary hindlimb dysfunction in a dog which refuses to jump up, climb stairs and pulls itself up with its forelimbs) and how the patient may best be assisted (provision of a ramp or non-slip boots) (Figure 12.3).

These components act together to shape the experience of pain and suffering, and it is often helpful to think of a patient in terms of these components when deciding upon the best interventions. For example, a young Labrador Retriever may present with very painful, end-stage joint disease but no other secondary signs of pain. The patient becomes increasingly lame during very restricted walks, often refuses to walk, will not play and will only get up for food. For this patient, the sensory component is significant and is causing suffering. If the sensory component of pain is removed or limited by

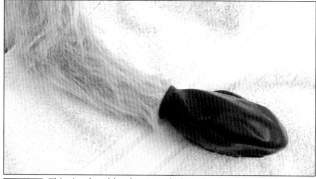

12.3 This simple rubber boot can help patients with difficulty gripping on slippery surfaces.

surgical arthrodesis (or joint replacement), then the suffering is reduced allowing the patient to function. In contrast, another young Labrador Retriever with arthritis may have its activity restricted either on advice or as a result of owner concerns about the condition, and is not allowed to play, interact with other dogs or exercise normally, even though pain is not preventing movement. This patient is also suffering, but the sensory component of pain is not the major cause.

The chronic pain consultation

Veterinary chronic pain clinics, in various forms, have been in existence for approximately 10 years and are growing in popularity. There is no set format for these consultations, but the following approach may be helpful:

- Identify the owner's concerns and expectations
- Identify the problem
- Identify the aim
- Assess the degree of pain
- Classify the components of pain
- Identify the possible sources of pain
- Classify the type of pain for each source
- Decide on treatment
- Plan when to review the patient and give clear outcome measures.

Identify the owner's concerns and expectations

While these concerns and expectations may seem obvious, they are sometimes surprising. Some owners do not realize that their pet is in pain, and are more concerned about weakness or weight gain with reduced exercise tolerance (e.g. owners may be expecting their dog to perform agility when even normal exercise consistently proves a challenge). Identifying concerns early during the consultation will avoid disappointment and misunderstanding later in the process of assessment and treatment.

Identify the problem

The problem may be an obvious disability or lameness, a requirement for post-surgical rehabilitation or a pathological process observed on diagnostic imaging. In addition, the problem may have been identified during a routine examination or on questioning the owner about changes in their pet's habits, particularly in cats. In some cases, the animal may exhibit obvious signs of pain (e.g. crying, restlessness, yelping) but no cause can be found. This is particularly challenging for both the owner and the clinician. It is also difficult for owners to comprehend the absence of a clear lesion when their pet is in pain; some clinicians also find this concept challenging and may start to question the veracity of the information provided by the owner when the patient appears relatively normal in the clinic yet the owner reports marked changes at home or during exercise. In these cases, the pain may be caused by:

- A dynamic lesion – i.e. a problem (such as nerve root impingement) that only occurs when the patient is in a certain position
- Changes in central pain processing – such that very minor trauma is perceived as disproportionately painful

- Central sensitization – part of, but not restricted to, previous causes of pain (see Identify the possible sources of pain, below)
- Myofascial pain – a specific kind of muscle pain that cannot be observed using current imaging techniques (see Identify the possible sources of pain, below).

Identify the aim

It is important that the owner understands the aims of the consultation and how they have been reached. For example, the aim may be to continue trying to positively identify a cause of the pain, or, having tried and failed to identify the cause, the aim may be simply to treat the pain. In the latter, it must be clear whether the aim is to cure the pain or to provide palliative care.

Assess the degree of pain

This is arguably the crux of dealing with chronic pain and is the main focus from which therapeutic decisions are made. If one can assess pain, and more importantly suffering, then it will be relatively straightforward to decide on the appropriate treatment. For instance, a cat in moderate renal failure with osteoarthritis is likely to have non-steroidal anti-inflammatory drugs (NSAIDs) withheld on the grounds they are contraindicated with renal disease, and yet the cat may live for some years with renal problems successfully managed. However, if the same cat is suffering significantly from osteoarthritic pain, such that it does very little but lie in one position all day, then treatment with NSAIDs, in the absence of any workable solution, is likely to be humane. But how to make the decision when the situation is not so extreme or so clear?

Pain scales

There are various pain scales available, but most have been designed for acute pain and cannot be extrapolated for chronic cases. The majority of existing chronic pain scales have been validated for a specific group of patients (e.g. those with orthopaedic conditions), but may be helpful for other groups of patients. A team at Glasgow University has been developing a health-related quality of life scale for dogs, which has been tested for validity, reliability and responsiveness (Reid et al., 2013). This scale is available as an online tool for veterinary practices at www.vetmetrica.com. Behavioural changes in the individual should form part of any pain assessment because changes in response to pain represent suffering. These changes can also be used to assess the relief from suffering following treatment.

A quick rule of thumb, in the absence of any formal scales, is to try to identify at least three outcomes, one of them behavioural, to measure the success of the proposed intervention. For example, if only the degree of lameness is measured, it is possible that this may not change following treatment and the joint may always be painful when fully extended or manipulated. However, if the patient is more enthusiastic about exercise or has started to initiate play, or has stopped being 'grumpy' with other dogs, then this is likely to represent a reduction in suffering.

Triangulation

Triangulation is a system of cross-referencing the information gained from presentation, examination and history in order to increase the probability that the clinician is correct in assuming that the patient is in pain (Figure 12.4). The author uses this system in pain clinics. It is derived from the technique used in navigation to confer greater certainty about one's position and John Webster used the analogy when discussing the difficulty of measuring the intangible areas of science, such as welfare (Webster, 2005). One single variable of behaviour, physiology or husbandry will never be able to accurately predict or measure an animal's welfare, so the greater number of variables that can be assessed, the better.

In terms of measuring chronic pain, triangulation works as follows:

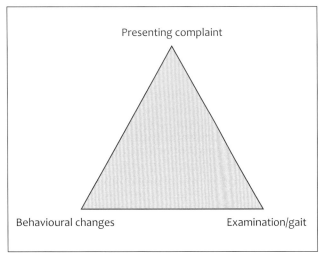

12.4 Triangulation. Assessment of all aspects of the patient's pain will reduce the 'area of uncertainty' (i.e. the area within the triangle) about the degree of patient suffering.

- **Presenting signs/problems** – e.g. the diagnosis of osteoarthritis using radiography does not prove that pain is present or how much suffering is caused by the lesions. However, it is a risk factor for pain and the patient needs to be assessed further
- **Behavioural changes** – these are indicative of suffering when they are caused by pain (e.g. a dog that no longer enthusiastically greets its owner or a cat that no longer goes outside). Behavioural changes can also indicate the degree of suffering (e.g. a dog that has always been highly motivated to exercise may not stop exercising when in pain, but if the dog *will* not exercise because of pain, then it can be concluded that the way the pain affects the dog, i.e. the degree of suffering, is severe). It should also be remembered that behavioural changes may occur for reasons other than pain (see Figures 12.1 and 12.2) and such changes should always be measured against other medical, environmental and social changes
- **Physical examination, including gait and movement** – these are included as one aspect because gait and movement are not relevant to all pain problems. Abnormal gait and lameness may be present without significant suffering and may not change following a successful analgesic intervention. Physical examination is vital, but pain upon examination may reflect the fact that the animal is only in pain when that manipulation or procedure is performed. Conversely, and perhaps more commonly, the examination may reveal little pain when in fact the animal is suffering significantly. In addition to a routine physical examination, central sensitization and myofascial pain should also be assessed (see below).

In terms of the physical examination, there are a number of other points to remember, including:

- The whole animal should be examined, not just the area presumed to be painful
- The examination should begin at the point furthest away from the presumed painful area. This may yield surprising results. For example, a patient with forelimb lameness may be most painful over its back or hindlimbs. In this case, the observed forelimb lameness may be the result of a postural shift from the hindlimbs on to the forequarters
- Arthritic joints with severe signs on radiography may not be painful on palpation or manipulation
- Fully extending or flexing joints to demonstrate pain is not necessarily useful, especially if that joint is not fully flexed or extended during the animal's daily exercise
- Examination of the joints cannot reveal how the joint 'feels' when the animal puts weight on it
- Cats often resent extension of the joint, even if arthritic changes are absent. They also commonly show little swelling, crepitus, joint effusion or other obvious signs of arthritic changes in their joints
- In the dog, manipulation of joints ought to be carried out with the patient in lateral recumbency because if more than one joint or limb is affected, this may make the patient reluctant to have the limb in question moved in such a way that it puts weight on the other limbs, distorting the results of the examination. This is less achievable in cats, although it would still be ideal.

When all aspects of the triangulation process have been assessed, the following can be identified:

- The presenting problem
- The degree of suffering
- Some obvious outcome measures based on behavioural changes, examination findings and gait
- Possible sources of pain (see below).

Classify the components of pain

If possible, the components of pain most significant to the patient should be identified, as this will be a helpful guide to treatment. In many cases it is obvious: for example, with an osteosarcoma it is likely to be the sensory component of pain that leads to suffering. Unless the tumour can be removed, controlling the suffering will be challenging. However, a cat with osteoarthritis of the hips may suffer more from no longer being able to access the places important to it, rather than from the pain itself. In this case, the cognitive and motor components of pain need to be addressed by optimizing the cat's core territory (see below).

Identify the possible sources of pain
Central sensitization

Central sensitization should be identified early in the examination. Arguably, once this has been identified the examination could be considered complete, especially if it is widespread. Central sensitization is often assumed to be synonymous with 'wind-up'. 'Wind-up' is a process involving dynamic changes in dorsal horn neuron excitability, such that the receptive fields of the neurons are modified. It is a physiological process that occurs in response to all pain and usually 'winds-down' over time. However, although the same mechanisms result in central sensitization, this phenomenon is pathological and may be considered as 'wind-up that has not wound down'. It is not an inevitable response to chronic pain and it is not completely understood why it occurs in some individuals and not others, although failure to address acute pain adequately is probably a risk factor.

Central sensitization should be identified by the clinician running their hands lightly over the whole body of the animal. This will identify an adverse response to a previously non-noxious stimulus (i.e. allodynia). The animal may move away, turn to look at the area being touched, or even physically try to stop the examination, and the muscles may fasciculate. The process should be repeated, if the animal tolerates it, to ensure it is a genuine reaction and not just an anxiety response. There may well be clues from the history, such as the patient will no longer tolerate being groomed or even petted, either in certain regions or all over. Hyperalgesia (an exaggerated response to a painful stimulus) is harder to substantiate, but a response to minimal manipulations should not be dismissed as the patient 'being intolerant'.

The examination could arguably be stopped when central sensitization is identified because further assessment will produce distorted responses. The clinician will simply not know whether it is a joint, muscle or the spine that is painful, or even where the focus of the pain may lie. As central sensitization represents a complete separation of the severity of any lesion and the experience of suffering, this must first be 'wound down' before the focal area of pain can be identified.

Focal areas of pain

- Skin – caused by self-trauma or by the disease process itself. Pruritus is a significant source of suffering, even before tissue damage caused by scratching and rubbing.
- Muscle – myositis (usually presented acutely), muscle spasm (usually a feature of acute pain or may arise spasmodically in association with chronic pain) and myofascial pain.
  - Myofascial pain arises from myofascial trigger points (MFTrPs). These are essentially areas of wear and tear or damage in the muscle (usually motor endplate zones). The most popular current hypothesis to explain the development of MFTrPs is that damaged endplates become 'leaky' and, instead of releasing enough acetylcholine to cause normal muscle contraction, release just enough to cause the sarcomeres local to the endplates to contract. These form a distinct 'knot' within the muscle (which becomes a taut band when the muscle is slightly stretched). This contraction compromises the local perfusion of blood, so waste products of muscle metabolism cannot be removed. These toxins accumulate and sensitize the local sensory nerve (hence the painful 'knots' that are commonly found in the postural muscles of the neck, shoulders and hip girdle in humans).
    - Postural strain, blunt trauma, radiculopathies and local pain (e.g. from joints or viscera) can cause trigger points to form. MFTrPs can cause significant pain in their own right (muscular pain often spreads a long way from its source, unlike

tendon or ligament pain), but can also add to the pain of arthritis, intervertebral disc disease and painful visceral disorders (Hong and Simons, 1998).
    - Detection requires a particular palpation technique, and is the reason why most clinicians cannot locate this type of pain. A simple prod moves the denser 'knot' out of the way and it goes undetected. The technique involves rolling a finger or thumb (or all four fingers in the case of large muscles) in contact with the skin over the muscle beneath and across the muscle fibres (because the band runs along the fibres), until a firmer area is discerned. The band is then 'twanged', as though plucking a cello string, and the reaction observed. This reaction can be very significant (even a placid animal may turn to bite).
- Joints – pain arises from inflammation within the joint and joint capsule, from the impingement of bone upon bone within the joint, and from secondary soft tissue changes. Note that the joint pain may have been controlled by NSAIDs, but that the remaining soft tissue pain (especially muscular) is refractory to such therapy. A diagnosis of arthritis may not actually mean that the pain originates from the joint.
- Spine – caused by arthritis, spondylosis or facet joint pain.
- Intervertebral discs – caused by compression of the spinal cord and nervous tissue, or from inflammatory changes in the disc mediated by brain-derived neurotrophic factor (BDNF), glutamate and substance P (Onda et al., 2003). A flare-up of so called 'discogenic' pain may be debilitating without change in cord compression and is also likely to give rise to secondary myofascial pain.
- Viscera – this type of pain is uniquely debilitating and may cause secondary muscular pain in the body wall (usually segmental, i.e. arising in the muscles supplied by the same spinal nerve(s) as the diseased viscera). It is often accompanied by nausea, which is another significant cause of suffering.
- Ear – often intense pain and although initially localized can give rise to secondary muscle pain.
- Teeth – usually accompanied by typical signs such as facial rubbing, dropping food, salivation and backing away from food. Note that rubbing and pawing at the face in the absence of dental disease may be referred pain from muscles in the head and neck.
- Eyes – intense and localized pain.

Classify the type of pain for each source

Classification of the type of pain for each source will guide the clinician to a range of appropriate treatments (Figure 12.5).

- Nociceptive – caused by noxious stimuli threatening tissue damage, arising from structures such as muscles, joints, viscera and skin.
- Neuropathic – this type of pain can be divided into two types:
  - That which arises directly from the nerves or nerve damage/compression/inflammation. Such pain is characterized by sharp, burning, lancinating pain in humans and can be inferred in animals by

Nociceptive pain with no significant suffering or central sensitization

- NSAIDs
- Paracetamol (acetaminophen) (not cats)
- Specific therapy where appropriate (e.g. antibiotics, immunotherapy, gastrointestinal tract support, dietary support)
- Acupuncture
- Physiotherapy/hydrotherapy
- Dietary supplements (e.g. glucosamine/chondroitin, omega-3)
- Pentosan polysulphate

Nociceptive pain with suffering and/or central sensitization

- NSAIDs
- Tramadol[a]
- Paracetamol (acetaminophen) and codeine (not cats)
- Buprenorphine[b]
- Codeine/oxycodone[a]
- Gabapentin[a]
- Amantadine[a]
- Amitriptyline/imipramine[a]
- Acupuncture

Neuropathic pain without central sensitization

- NSAIDs
- Gabapentin[a]
- Amantadine[a]
- Amitriptyline/imipramine[a]
- Buprenorphine[b]
- Codeine/oxycodone[a]

Neuropathic pain with central sensitization

- NSAIDs
- Tramadol[a]
- Buprenorphine[b]
- Codeine/oxycodone[a]
- Gabapentin[a]
- Amantadine[a]
- Paracetamol (acetaminophen) (not cats)
- Acupuncture

12.5 Possible treatments for chronic pain. The therapies listed are not exhaustive nor in order of preference because choices should be made according to individual circumstance, tolerance, contraindications and history. It is assumed that specific treatments should be used in conjunction with analgesia where appropriate. [a] = not licensed for use in animals in the UK; [b] = not authorized for use via the oral transmucosal route. NSAIDs = non-steroidal anti-inflammatory drugs.

jumping/startled behaviour, looking around suddenly at a body area or even the floor where they are lying, running away or sitting down suddenly, attacking a limb or the tail suddenly, and even bizarre behaviours such as not wanting to cross thresholds (real or imaginary)
- That which arises as a result of central sensitization. Such pain is technically neuropathic as it arises from changes in central pain processing, but may be caused by either nociceptive or neuropathic pain.
- Mixed pain – this is commonly encountered and is a combination of nociceptive and neuropathic pain.
- Referred pain – pain is projected from the source to a distant site.
- Sympathetically-mediated pain – it is not known whether this occurs in animals and is still poorly understood in humans. It is characterized by cold, painful areas (usually a limb) and may arise secondary to trauma or apparently spontaneously. There are often changes in hair growth, skin colour and texture, and swelling. As the sympathetic nervous system controls the dilatation/constriction of blood vessels, the term 'sympathetically mediated' is currently in favour, although it is not known whether dysfunction of this system is the cause or the effect.

- Psychogenic pain – this category is both redundant and tautological since all pain is perceived by the brain.

Decide on treatment

Treatment should be decided based on discussion with the owner and concurrent disease(s), taking into account the possible side effects for the patient (and owner). This can be achieved using a simple ABCDE aide memoire (Carmichael, 2006), first devised for orthopaedic patients but useful for all patients with chronic pain.

The 'ABCDE' of treatment

A = Analgesia
B = Bodyweight
C = Control of complications, common sense and comfort
D = Disease modification
E = Exercise

Analgesia

This can be divided into analgesic medications and analgesic interventions. Multimodal analgesia is frequently necessary in chronic pain conditions.

Medications: A list of currently used analgesics is given in Figure 12.6.

Physical techniques: These are challenging to assess in randomized controlled trials because of the difficulties of blinding the patient and owner to a physical technique.

Acupuncture: There are now convincing studies in human medicine for the use of acupuncture in patients with post-operative and post-chemotherapy nausea and vomiting, osteoarthritis of the knee, and migraines and headaches. The National Institute of Health and Care Excellence (NICE) guidelines now include a recommendation for acupuncture for chronic lower back pain and chronic tension headaches and migraines, based on systematic reviews of studies into these conditions. Although there is limited evidence for clinical indications in veterinary species, most of the acute pain studies related to acupuncture in the laboratory have been performed on animals and thus much of the basic science is established (Bowsher, 1998) (Figure 12.7).

While many of the mechanisms involved are known, the resultant analgesia depends upon the responsiveness of the patient to the stimuli and how the needles are used (i.e. the degree of stimulation). Generally, cats and dogs tend to accept the treatment well without sedation. Acupuncture is indicated for arthritic pain, myofascial pain and central sensitization, and appears to be most useful when:

- NSAIDs are contraindicated or no longer sufficiently effective
- There is primary muscle pain
- Secondary muscle pain is causing a significant proportion of the patient's suffering
- There is a need to 'wind-down' central sensitization, except where it is widespread as then needle insertion will be painful
- Nothing else appears effective (occasionally).

Drug action	Dogs: dose/use	Cats: dose/use	Comments
NSAIDs Anti-inflammatory Analgesic	As per datasheets Note: may need to treat for 6 weeks to 'wind-down' chronic pain	Meloxicam is the only NSAID licensed in the UK for chronic use in cats. Dose as per datasheet	Caution in hepatic and renal disease; contraindicated with concurrent corticosteroid therapy
TCAs[a] Enhance noradrenergic transmission via descending inhibitory pathways	Amitriptyline: 1–2 mg/kg orally q12h Imipramine: 0.5 mg/kg orally q8h	Amitriptyline: 0.5–1 mg/kg orally q24h Imipramine: 0.5–1 mg/kg orally q12–24h	Both are bitter and difficult to administer to cats. Antidepressant effects occur at the top end of the dose range and can take 4 weeks; therefore, response to these drugs should not be taken to mean the problem was behavioural – the analgesic effects of these drugs tend to be faster, although this depends on the source of the pain and state of the nervous system. Both drugs require competent renal and hepatic function for clearance. Contraindicated in cardiac dysrhythmia. Note that clomipramine, although a TCA and licensed for separation anxiety in dogs, is not thought to be useful as an analgesic because of its primary serotonergic action
Tramadol[a] Atypical opiate Enhances descending inhibitory pain pathways	2–5 mg/kg orally q12h or 2 mg/kg i.v. once Doses of 2–10 mg/kg orally q6–8h have been quoted, but lower doses (1–2 mg/kg orally q12h) may be effective	2–4 mg/kg orally or 1–2 mg/kg s.c. once Seizures reported in cats at these doses Elimination time is longer in cats, so keep the dose and frequency low	10 mg and 25 mg formulations now available for animal use in the UK. Side effects include vomiting, diarrhoea, sedation, dysphoria and dullness. Seizures have been reported in cats after oral administration at the higher end of the dose range
Gabapentin[a] Membrane stabilizer (binds to calcium channels and inhibits release of excitatory neurotransmitters)	3–10 mg/kg orally q8–12h	3–10 mg/kg orally q8–12h	50 mg tablets now available in the UK. Side effects include sedation, vomiting, diarrhoea, increased drinking, ataxia, stumbling and tripping
Paracetamol (acetaminophen)[a] Analgesic and antipyretic at lower doses Anti-inflammatory at higher doses	10–25 mg/kg orally q12h or 10 mg/kg i.v. q12h Paracetamol with codeine (Pardale V): see datasheet	**Do not use**	
Amantadine[a] NMDA receptor antagonist	2–5 mg/kg orally q24h or 1–2 mg/kg orally q12h	1–4 mg/kg orally q24h	Start low and increase dose. May take 2 weeks to work. Side effects include vomiting and diarrhoea; central nervous system signs of vagueness and apparent disorientation reported to the author
Buprenorphine[b] Opioid: partial mu agonist; kappa antagonist	Oral transmucosal (OTM) dose useful in dogs to cover episodes of pain (0.12–0.2 mg/kg OTM q6–8h)	0.01–0.02 mg/kg OTM q6–8h	Titrate dose to best effect and minimal side effects. Dosages in dogs are often lower and less frequent than quoted – the sedation and dysphoria associated with higher doses are unacceptable and not tolerated by either the owner or patient
Cinchophen plus prednisolone NSAID plus corticosteroid (prednoleucotropin)	25 mg/kg orally q12h	**Do not use**	This combination may give significant pain relief where other analgesics have failed. Arguably the effects must be dramatic to outweigh short- and long-term steroid and NSAID side effects

12.6 Commonly used analgesics for chronic and neuropathic pain. [a] = not licensed for use in animals in the UK; [b] = not licensed for use via the oral transmucosal route. NMDA = N-methyl-D-aspartate; NSAIDs = non-steroidal anti-inflammatory drugs; TCAs = tricyclic antidepressants.

Local effects

- Insertion of an acupuncture needle into the skin and muscles releases vasodilators, nerve growth factor and substance P locally. These are the same neurotransmitters released when the integument is damaged and promote local wound healing where the skin and muscle are compromised

Segmental effects

- Needle insertion stimulates fast pain fibres (i.e. afferent nerves responding to high threshold stimuli). These transmit to the dorsal horn where pain is modulated. This fast pain stimulation triggers the release of metenkephalins from enkephalinergic interneurons in the dorsal horn, and this inhibits slow pain (C-fibre pain) from the pain/injury under treatment. In other words, the acupuncture stimulus competes with the pain stimulus at the dorsal horn

Heterosegmental effects

- The stimulus continues to the brain where it triggers the release of beta-endorphin from the periaqueductal grey matter (PAG), serotonin and noradrenaline (norepinephrine). These act to facilitate descending inhibitory pain pathways, damping down pain at every spinal segment (although the effect is greatest at the segment where the needle is inserted)

Humoral effects

- Release and circulation of endorphins, oxytocin and other neurotransmitters

Effects of multiple treatments

- Subsequent treatments (within 7 days of each other) ramp up the expression of messenger RNA for pre-enkephalin. In other words, the body produces more endorphin over time and this is one reason why acupuncture can continue to work in between treatments and apparently for long periods of time after treatment

12.7

The mechanisms of action of acupuncture.

Physiotherapy: The aim of physiotherapy is to return an animal to function following injury, disease or surgery. There are a number of techniques, including massage, joint mobilization, passive movements and stretches, soft tissue techniques (e.g. soft tissue release, myofascial release and trigger pointing) and therapeutic exercises (Sharp, 2010). While a trained physiotherapist would be the best person to assess and devise a plan for an individual patient, there are some simple techniques that can be used for straightforward problems (Figures 12.8 to 12.12).

Problem	Technique	Comments
Loss of muscle mass and strength in hindlimbs	**Sit to stand:** the patient should start sitting squarely and then be encouraged to stand, usually with the use of a treat or command, so the quadriceps and hamstring muscles are used (Figure 12.9)	If the patient is experiencing pain and struggling to stand, the pain should be controlled first
	Slopes: the patient should be controlled on a lead and walked slowly up a slope so that they use each leg in turn	If the patient is not controlled there will be a tendency to 'bunny hop' up the slope, avoiding using the target muscle groups
	Steps: start with a few wide, shallow steps. With the patient controlled on the lead, walk them slowly up and down the steps, ensuring that each limb is being used to assist ascent and slow descent	If the patient is not controlled there will be a tendency to 'bunny hop' up the stairs, avoiding using the target muscle groups
Restriction of movement in forelimb joints, especially shoulder and elbow Soft tissue injury Requirement for passive joint movement and muscle stretch	**'Shake paws':** the patient should be encouraged to 'give a paw'. The limb is then gently extended and held for 3 seconds before releasing and repeating (Figure 12.10)	Beware of the tendency to pull on the carpus. An alternative technique is to extend the limb by gentle pressure on the caudal aspect of the elbow joint (Figure 12.11). **Do not use this technique if the dog repeatedly jerks the limb**
Restriction of movement in hindlimb joints, especially hip and stifle Soft tissue injury Requirement for passive joint movement and muscle stretch	With the patient in lateral recumbency, gentle caudal pressure on the cranial aspect of the thigh extends the stifle and hip (Figure 12.12)	Some dogs will stretch voluntarily when the flank is stroked. This means that they will stretch the limb naturally and be less inclined to resist the applied pressure. **Do not use this technique if the dog repeatedly jerks the limb**

12.8 Simple physiotherapy techniques. The patient should first be judged to be as pain free as possible. All techniques should be demonstrated by the clinician or nurse and repeated by the owner.

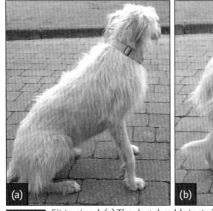 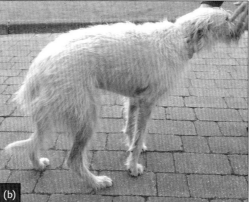 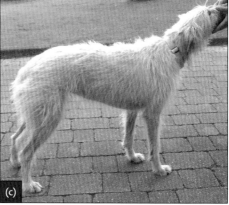

12.9 Sit to stand. (a) The dog should start sitting as squarely as possible. (b) The dog is then encouraged to stand, so that it uses its hindlimb muscles. (c) The dog ends up in a standing position. This exercise can then be repeated.

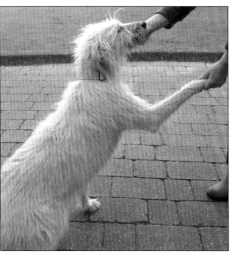

12.10 'Shake paws'. Care should be taken not to pull on the carpus.

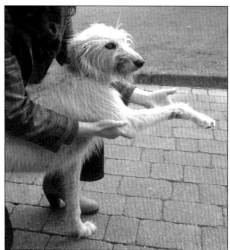

12.11 Elbow extension. This may be a safer technique to stretch the shoulder and major forelimb muscles compared with the 'shake paws' exercise.

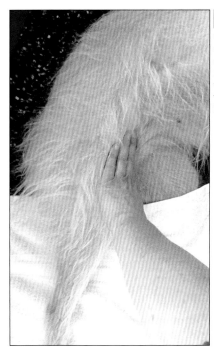

12.12 Hindlimb extension. Gentle pressure on the cranial thigh muscles will extend the hip and stifle. Some dogs will do this voluntarily when the flank or upper thigh area is stroked.

Hydrotherapy: This technique uses the properties of water to help patients regain strength, balance and fitness, and to extend and work joints without concussive pressure. Water provides buoyancy and resistance. Formal hydrotherapy tanks also provide warmth and, when supervised by trained personnel, a controlled environment for graduated exercise and rehabilitation (Figure 12.13). Hydrotherapy is not a panacea and any worsening of the condition after the sessions should be noted. Extending the neck and lordosis of the back to swim may exacerbate an existing problem in patients with spinal problems.

Bodyweight

There is some evidence in humans to suggest that excessive amounts of body fat can contribute to pain and inflammation, and this may also be true in cats and dogs (Ryan *et al.*, 2008). Bodyweight *per se* is not a problem if the animal has well developed muscles and is lean, although this is rarely the case with domestic pets. Owners should be encouraged to monitor weight but also be taught to body score their pet once a month. Underweight and especially cachectic animals will need treatment with appropriate nutrition.

Control of complications, common sense and comfort

Owners are more likely to comply with the treatment plan if they are aware of the potential complications and side effects, know what signs to look out for, and understand the reasons for the frequency of monitoring required (e.g. blood tests). The common sense application of ramps, carts and other strategic aids can be invaluable. Even simple techniques such as applying plastic nail covers to claws susceptible to wear and bleeding can make a difference to both the owner and animal. A working knowledge of such devices, availability of beds, good grooming tools, safe toys and simple forms of mental stimulation are essential for the pain clinic physician (Figure 12.14).

Owners often want to massage their pets. There is plenty of evidence now available regarding the mood benefits of stroking dogs (to humans and dogs alike), but less regarding any specific touch therapies, so the emphasis must be on the animal enjoying the interaction and on it being safe. Animals with allodynia will obviously not enjoy being petted or groomed, so areas that are not painful should be targeted, such as the chest and abdomen. A flat hand technique (i.e. moving the hand and skin together over the underlying tissues) is less likely to cause pain and exacerbate muscle pain than using the fingers to 'knead' and 'press'.

In cats, the single biggest impact on welfare is the quality of its core territory (i.e. the place where it expects to be secure and have access to resources). If the cat is in pain, or if its mobility is restricted, then the ability of the cat to utilize even an ideal core territory is limited. This can have a negative emotional impact on the cat, which in turn exacerbates its suffering. Owners of cats that are in pain or unable to function normally should ensure that their pet has access to the resources listed in Figure 12.15.

Disease modification

A review of nutraceuticals is provided in the *BSAVA Manual of Canine and Feline Rehabilitation, Palliative and Supportive Care*. Essentially, there is still no definitive evidence for the benefits of glucosamine/chondroitin or even omega-3 fatty acids in cats and dogs, although this should not prohibit their use. The current evidence suggests that they are not suitable as sole analgesic agents for arthritis, although there are anecdotal reports of success in some individuals.

Some animals indulge in repetitive types of play such as jumping and twisting, digging or idiosyncratic

Technique	Action	Advantages	Disadvantages
Swimming pool	Swimming: free, controlled by personnel in the pool, or swimming against a forced current	Dogs that enjoy swimming will work hard. Intense exercise. No concussive pressure on joints	Even dogs that enjoy swimming may not like restrictions in small pools. Some animals need hydraulic lifting equipment, which they may resent. Offers better joint flexion than land-based exercise, but not extension. Swimming may increase neck pain. Cats may not tolerate
Underwater treadmill	Patients walk on a treadmill. Height of water and therefore work can be controlled. Action of walking is mimicked. Balance improved	The treadmill offers improved joint flexion and extension compared with land-based exercises. Control over movement is greater. Although still hard work, treadmills are better for elderly or frail patients	Even dogs that enjoy being in water may not accept the restrictions of a small tank. Initial panic when the treadmill starts. Not suitable for cats
'DIY'	Patients swim or walk in local lakes/rivers (or even the bath for small patients)	No expense or travelling for the owner, therefore exercise is likely to be more frequent	Must avoid the patient diving in and scrabbling out of the water. The patient must be dried properly. No advantage of warmth (of water). Little control and graduation of exercise

12.13 Hydrotherapy: techniques and the associated advantages and disadvantages.

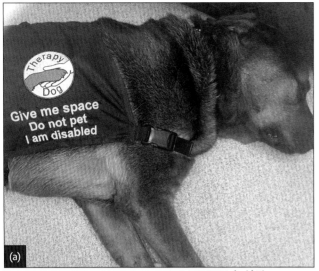
(a)

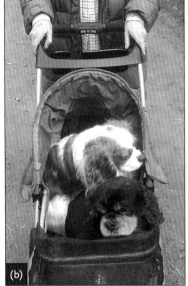
(b)

12.14 (a–b) There are many different devices available to assist animals with mobility problems.
(b, Courtesy of L Lowry)

movements that place an unusual strain on certain areas of the body. Such play may need to be limited or stopped, but replacement activities should be substituted so that the patient does not become under-stimulated and frustrated. Varying and novel food delivery can help mental stimulation, but hide and seek games with toys can also be introduced.

Surgical procedures, such as arthrodesis and joint replacement, will, in some cases such as advanced osteoarthritis, modify disease successfully.

Exercise

Rest is not the panacea for pain. In fact, it is rarely the answer for most painful conditions. Rest induces stiffness, frustration, under-stimulation and loss of muscle strength and bulk. Rest is appropriate for acute conditions (such as a flare-up of osteoarthritis) or conditions where exercise has been demonstrated to worsen the pain, but it is important for owners to recognize that rest is just the beginning of the rehabilitation process and that there is an intention to increase exercise to a level that is acceptable to the owner, satisfying for the patient and conducive to the healing and/or proper palliation of the disease.

Restricted exercise should be varied where possible; all too often, 'short walks' means a 10 minute walk, on concrete, around the block, which is tedious and tiring for all concerned. Variation is stimulating, softer surfaces are often better accepted, and social interaction (where enjoyed) literally takes the mind off pain. The owners should be given clear guidance and realistic aims.

Conclusion

Pain clinics provide an opportunity to help owners struggling to understand their pet's pain, to help the patient to receive the most appropriate and effective analgesia for their condition, and to achieve the best quality of life and enjoyment for both.

Resource	Importance	Achieved by
Height and hiding	Cats will climb and hide in response to fear. Pain causes fear and anxiety. Cats with mobility problems will not be able to access high areas and some hiding places, increasing their anxiety	Create new hiding and high areas or ensure that the cat can reach old favourite areas by providing stepwise access or ramps
Food	Essential	Ensure that the cat does not have to climb or can climb easily to the feeding area, which should be located away from the cat flap, water and busy thoroughfares
Water	Essential, especially for cats on NSAIDs and those with renal compromise and feline lower urinary tract disease (FLUTD). Cats prefer water to be positioned away from the food	Provide multiple water sites at least a room's distance from the food, in wide, shallow non-plastic dishes. Running water may be preferred by some cats and can be provided by water fountains. Ensure that cats with mobility problems never have to walk too far to reach water
Scratching posts	Required for claw health, marking and the release of tension. Cats with elbow arthritis may present frequently for front claw clipping	Provide scratching posts tall enough to allow full stretching, in areas where the cat has shown a preference for scratching. The scratching post should be made of a substrate favoured by the cat and positioned either vertically or horizontally depending on the demonstrated preference of the animal
Play	Pleasure; practice hunting; release of endorphins	Play should be adapted (not abandoned) for cats in pain. Different games should be explored
Access	For cats with access to the outdoors, two entry/exit points are preferred for safety reasons. Ease of moving away from the access point to quickly obtain a vantage point is important for many cats	Ensure that cats with mobility problems can access the entry/exit points with ease and create a stepwise approach to higher areas so they can quickly climb and obtain a vantage point

12.15 Optimizing the core territory for cats in pain or unable to function normally. NSAIDs = non-steroidal anti-inflammatory drugs.

References and further reading

Bowsher D (1998) Mechanisms of acupuncture. In: *Medical Acupuncture: A Western Scientific Approach*, ed. J Filshie and A White, pp. 69–82. Churchill Livingstone, Edinburgh

Carmichael S (2006) Putting theory into practice – best practice management for osteoarthritis. *European Journal of Companion Animal Practice* **16(1)**, 27–31

Chan DL (2010) Immune-modulating dietary components and nutraceuticals. In: *BSAVA Manual of Canine and Feline Rehabilitation, Supportive and Palliative Care*, ed. S Lindley and P Watson, pp. 78–84. BSAVA Publications, Gloucester

Hong CZ and Simons DG (1998) Pathophysiological and electrophysiologic mechanisms of myofascial trigger points. *Archives of Physical Medicine and Rehabilitation* **79**, 863–872

Onda A, Murata Y, Rydevik B *et al.* (2003) Immunoreactivity of brain derived neurotrophic factor in rat dorsal root ganglion and spinal cord dorsal horn following exposure to herniated nucleus pulposus. *Neuroscience Letters* **352**, 49–52

Reid J, Wiseman-Orr ML, Scott EM *et al.* (2013) Development, validation and reliability of a web-based questionnaire to measure health-related quality of life in dogs. *Journal of Small Animal Practice* **54**, 227–233

Ryan VH, German AJ, Wood IS *et al.* (2008) NGF gene expression and secretion by canine adipocytes in primary culture: upregulation by the inflammatory mediators LPS and TNFa. *Hormone and Metabolic Research* **40**, 861–868

Sharp B (2010) Physiotherapy and physical rehabilitation. In: *BSAVA Manual of Canine and Feline Rehabilitation, Supportive and Palliative Care*, ed. S Lindley and P Watson, pp. 90–113. BSAVA Publications, Gloucester

Webster J (2005) *Animal Welfare: Limping towards Eden*. Wiley-Blackwell, Oxford

WSAVA Global Pain Council (2014) WSAVA guidelines for recognition, assessment and treatment of pain. *Journal of Small Animal Practice* **55(6)**, E10–E68

Chapter 13

Pre-anaesthetic medication and sedation

Joanna C. Murrell

The majority of small animal patients are routinely pre-medicated as part of the anaesthetic protocol, yet the importance of pre-anaesthetic medication in the whole process of anaesthesia is often forgotten: the choice of drugs will have a major impact on the characteristics of the ensuing general anaesthetic. The appropriate selection of premedicant drugs can significantly contribute to perioperative analgesia, intraoperative cardiovascular stability and quality of recovery. In order to optimize the advantages of pre-anaesthetic medication, it is important to select drugs and doses on the basis of the needs of the individual patient, rather than to use the same regimen for all animals.

Sedation is often used as an alternative to general anaesthesia for minor procedures. There is a general perception, particularly among pet owners, that sedation is safer and therefore preferable to general anaesthesia. Data generated by the Confidential Enquiry into Perioperative Small Animal Fatalities (CEPSAF), undertaken in the UK between 2002 and 2004, found that risks of death were lower in cats and dogs that were only sedated than in patients undergoing general anaesthesia (Brodbelt et al., 2008). However, the authors acknowledged that the data were confounded by health status and that the conclusion of reduced risks associated with sedation may not be valid. It is important to remember that drugs used for sedation and pre-anaesthetic medication also have cardiovascular and respiratory side effects, and there are fewer options for the monitoring and support of sedated patients compared with animals undergoing general anaesthesia. In this context, general anaesthesia may be safer than profound sedation for many high-risk patients.

The drugs used for pre-anaesthetic medication and sedation are identical and are discussed interchangeably in this chapter. Guides to drug doses are provided in Figure 13.1 (pre-anaesthetic medication) and 13.2 (sedation).

Drug combination		Route of administration	Species	Patient selection
Drug 1	**Drug 2**			
Acepromazine (0.01–0.05 mg/kg)	+ Buprenorphine (20 µg/kg) + Butorphanol (0.2–0.4 mg/kg) + Hydromorphone (0.05–0.15 mg/kg) + Methadone (0.2–0.5 mg/kg) + Morphine (0.2–0.5 mg/kg) + Pethidine (meperidine) (3–5 mg/kg)	i.m. or i.v. i.m. or i.v. i.m. or i.v. i.m. or i.v. i.m. i.m.	Cat and dog	ASA 1–3 patients, depending on assessment of cardiovascular function. Use lower dose of acepromazine in ASA 2–3 patients. Use lower dose range when drugs are given i.v.
Dexmedetomidine (1–10 µg/kg) Use 1–3 µg/kg i.v. Doses up to 10 µg/kg may be used i.m. if profound sedation is required	+ Buprenorphine (20 µg/kg) + Butorphanol (0.2–0.4 mg/kg) + Hydromorphone (0.1 mg/kg) + Methadone (0.1–0.2 mg/kg) + Morphine (0.1–0.2 mg/kg) + Pethidine (3–5 mg/kg)	i.m. or i.v. i.m. or i.v. i.m. or i.v. i.m. or i.v. i.m. i.m.	Cat and dog	ASA 1–2 patients For routine administration of these combinations cardiovascular function should be normal. Exceptions may be made in some circumstances. Use lower end of dose range when drugs are given i.v.
Dexmedetomidine (1–10 µg/kg) Use 1–3 µg/kg i.v. Doses up to 10 µg/kg may be used i.m. if profound sedation is required	+ Diazepam (0.2–0.3 mg/kg) + Midazolam (0.2–0.3 mg/kg)	i.v. i.m. or i.v.	Dog	ASA 1–2 patients For routine administration of these combinations, cardiovascular function should be normal. Exceptions may be made in some circumstances. Useful for non-painful procedures such as diagnostic imaging. Use lower end of dose range when drugs are given i.v.
Midazolam (0.3–0.4 mg/kg)	+ Butorphanol (0.2–0.4 mg/kg) + Hydromorphone (0.05–0.15 mg/kg) + Methadone (0.2–0.5 mg/kg) + Morphine (0.2–0.5 mg/kg) + Pethidine (3–5 mg/kg)	i.m. or i.v. i.m. or i.v. i.m. or i.v. i.m. i.m.	Dog, rarely cat	ASA 3–5 patients Provides good cardiovascular stability. Excitation may occur after i.v. administration; sedation is unreliable if given i.m. Avoid butorphanol if the animal is in pain. Use lower end of dose range when drugs are given i.v.

13.1 Drug combinations used for pre-anaesthetic medication in cats and dogs. ASA = American Society of Anesthesiologists physical status classification; IPPV = intermittent positive pressure ventilation. (continues) ▶

Drug combination		Route of administration	Species	Patient selection
Drug 1	Drug 2			
Midazolam (0.2–0.3 mg/kg)	+ Ketamine (2–5 mg/kg)	i.m. or i.v.	Cat	ASA 2–4 patients. Avoid in patients with hypertrophic cardiomyopathy. Higher dose of ketamine may induce anaesthesia. Use lower end of dose range when drugs are given i.v.
Midazolam (0.3–0.4 mg/kg)	+ Fentanyl (2–5 µg/kg)	i.v.	Cat and dog	ASA 3–5 patients. Provides good cardiovascular stability. Be prepared to induce anaesthesia to allow endotracheal intubation and IPPV if apnoea occurs. Use lower end of dose range when drugs are given i.v.
Zolazepam + tiletamine	Available as a proprietary mixture (Telazol® or Zoletil®). Dose range for pre-anaesthetic medication 3–6 mg/kg	i.m. or i.v.	Cat and dog	As above for midazolam/ketamine mixture. Recovery can be stormy in dogs. Use lower end of dose range when drugs are given i.v.
Alfaxalone (1–3 mg/kg). Use lower dose range in combination with other drugs. Use higher dose s.c.	+ Methadone (0.2–0.5 mg/kg). + Buprenorphine (20 µg/kg). + Butorphanol (0.2–0.4 mg/kg)	i.m. or s.c. i.m. or s.c. i.m. or s.c.	Cat and dog	Volume limits utility in most dogs. Midazolam (0.2–0.3 mg/kg) may be added to this combination to provide increased sedation in anxious or fearful cats and dogs
Morphine (0.2–0.5 mg/kg). Methadone (0.2–0.5 mg/kg). Hydromorphone (0.05–0.1 mg/kg)		i.m. i.m. or i.v. i.m. or i.v.	Cat and dog	ASA 4–5 patients or young animals. Use lower end of dose range when drugs are given i.v.

13.1 (continued) Drug combinations used for pre-anaesthetic medication in cats and dogs. ASA = American Society of Anesthesiologists physical status classification; IPPV = Intermittent positive pressure ventilation.

Drug combination		Route of administration	Species notes	Sedation notes
Drug 1	Drug 2			
Acepromazine (0.03–0.05 mg/kg)	+ Buprenorphine (20 µg/kg). + Butorphanol (0.2–0.4 mg/kg). + Hydromorphone (0.1–0.2 mg/kg). + Methadone (0.2–0.5 mg/kg). + Morphine (0.2–0.5 mg/kg). + Pethidine (meperidine) (4–5 mg/kg)	i.m. or i.v. i.m. or i.v. i.m. or i.v. i.m. or i.v. i.m. i.m.	Cat: use low to mid-dose range of opioids. Dog: higher doses of opioids will provide greater sedation	Will provide light sedation in cats and dogs. Do not expect animals to become recumbent. Use lower end of dose range when drugs are given i.v.
Dexmedetomidine (1–10 µg/kg). Use 1–3 µg/kg i.v. Doses up to 10 µg/kg may be used i.m. if profound sedation is required	+ Buprenorphine (20 µg/kg). + Butorphanol (0.2–0.4 mg/kg). + Hydromorphone (0.1–0.15 mg/kg). + Methadone (0.1–0.2 mg/kg). + Morphine (0.1–0.2 mg/kg). + Pethidine (4–5 mg/kg)	i.m. or i.v. i.m. or i.v. i.m. or i.v. i.m. or i.v. i.m. i.m.	Cat and dog	Higher doses of dexmedetomidine will provide more reliable and profound sedation. Expect animals to become recumbent. Useful for minor invasive painful procedures such as removal of grass seeds from the ear canal. Use lower end of dose range when drugs are given i.v.
Dexmedetomidine (1–10 µg/kg). Use 1–3 µg/kg i.v. Doses up to 10 µg/kg may be used i.m. if profound sedation is required	+ Diazepam (0.3 mg/kg). + Midazolam (0.3 mg/kg)	i.v. i.m. or i.v.	Cat and dog	Higher doses of dexmedetomidine will provide more reliable and profound sedation. Expect animals to become recumbent. Degree of analgesia is less than when dexmedetomidine is combined with an opioid. Use lower end of dose range when drugs are given i.v.
Midazolam (0.4–0.5 mg/kg)	+ Hydromorphone (0.1–0.15 mg/kg). + Methadone (0.2–0.5 mg/kg). + Morphine (0.2–0.5 mg/kg)	i.m. or i.v. i.m. or i.v. i.m.	Dog	Degree of sedation will depend on the health and temperament of the patient. May be able to carry out some invasive procedures if the animal is handled patiently and quietly. Use lower end of dose range when drugs are given i.v.
Midazolam (0.2–0.3 mg/kg)	+ Ketamine (2–5 mg/kg)	i.m. or i.v.	Cat	Expect profound sedation/light general anaesthesia. Use lower end of dose range when drugs are given i.v.

13.2 Drug combinations used for sedation in cats and dogs (see Figure 13.3 for information regarding route of administration). (continues) ▶

Drug combination		Route of administration	Species notes	Sedation notes
Drug 1	**Drug 2**			
Zolazepam + tiletamine	Available as a proprietary mixture (Telazol® or Zoletil®). Dose range for sedation/short-duration general anaesthesia: 9–13 mg/kg	i.m. or i.v.	Cat and dog	As above for midazolam/ketamine mixture. Recovery can be stormy in dogs. Use lower end of dose range when drugs are given i.v.
Alfaxalone (1–3 mg/kg) Use lower end of dose range when administering i.m. or in combination with other drugs. Use higher dose s.c.	+ Buprenorphine (20 µg/kg) + Butorphanol (0.2–0.4 mg/kg) + Methadone (0.2–0.5 mg/kg)	i.m. or s.c. i.m. or s.c. i.m. or s.c.	Cat and dog	Volume limits utility in most dogs. Midazolam (0.2–0.3 mg/kg) may be added to this combination to provide increased sedation in anxious or fearful cats and dogs
Alfaxalone (0.2–0.5 mg/kg i.v.)	+ Butorphanol (0.2–0.3 mg/kg) or midazolam (0.2–0.3 mg/kg)	i.v.	Cat and dog	For (non-painful) diagnostic procedures, start with lower dose, dilute with sterile water for injection or saline to ensure more accurate dosing and have means to intubate within reach
Morphine (0.2–0.5 mg/kg) Methadone (0.2–0.5 mg/kg) Hydromorphone (0.1–0.15 mg/kg)		i.m. i.m. or i.v. i.m. or i.v.	Cat and dog	Mild sedation only. Do not expect animal to become recumbent. Use lower end of dose range when drugs are given i.v.

13.2 (continued) Drug combinations used for sedation in cats and dogs (see Figure 13.3 for information regarding route of administration).

Aims of pre-anaesthetic medication and sedation

- Sedation and anxiolysis: to quieten or immobilize an animal sufficiently to allow a procedure, such as intravenous catheterization, to be carried out. To reduce stress before and during induction of anaesthesia.
- Facilitate animal handling: this increases safety for both patient and personnel during physical restraint.
- Contribute to a balanced anaesthetic technique: to reduce the dose of other anaesthetic agents required for induction and maintenance of anaesthesia.
- Contribute to preventive analgesia: the strategic administration of analgesic drugs can prevent or minimize sensitization of pain pathways as a result of noxious stimulation caused by surgery.
- Counter the side effects of other drugs, e.g. co-administration of anticholinergic agents such as atropine with opioids to prevent bradycardia.
- Contribute to a smooth and quiet recovery.

Pharmacology

The drugs used for pre-anaesthetic medication and sedation in cats and dogs should ideally have the following properties:

- Production of reliable sedation and anxiolysis
- Minimal effects on the cardiovascular and respiratory systems
- Provision of analgesia
- Reversibility.

Unfortunately, no individual drug has all of these characteristics, and therefore combinations of drugs with different properties are employed. Provision of 'balanced' pre-anaesthetic medication and sedation using combinations of drugs with different specific effects allows the dosages of individual drugs to be reduced, minimizing side effects while maximizing the reliability of the sedation achieved. These combinations commonly utilize the synergism that occurs between different groups of sedative drugs, such as between alpha-2 adrenoceptor agonists and opioids, or between phenothiazines and opioids (neuroleptanalgesia).

Route of administration

Drugs are most commonly administered by the intravenous, intramuscular, subcutaneous and oral routes. The oral transmucosal (OTM) route (drug administration into the buccal cavity and absorption across the oral mucous membranes) results in the reliable absorption of some drugs such as buprenorphine in cats, and alpha-2 adrenoceptor agonists in cats and dogs. A transdermal fentanyl solution (Recuvyra™) is licensed for perioperative analgesia in dogs and may therefore be included in pre-anaesthetic medication protocols.

The advantages and disadvantages of each route are shown in Figure 13.3. The route of administration will also influence the time to peak effect; this is shown, along with duration of effect, in Figure 13.4.

Drugs used for pre-anaesthetic medication and sedation

(See Figures 13.1 and 13.2). The classes of drugs commonly used in cats and dogs are:

- Phenothiazines, e.g. acepromazine
- Alpha-2 adrenoceptor agonists, e.g. medetomidine, dexmedetomidine
- Benzodiazepines, e.g. diazepam, midazolam
- Alfaxalone

Route of administration	Advantages	Disadvantages
Intravenous (i.v.)	Reliable drug absorption; allows lower doses of drugs to be administered Immediate onset of action	Animal is not sedated before handling and drug administration – stressful for the animal and animal handlers Some drugs should not be given i.v., e.g. pethidine (meperidine)
Intramuscular (i.m.)	Minimal handling required for administration Drug absorption is more reliable than by subcutaneous route Route of choice for most pre-anaesthetic/sedative drugs	May be painful when drug volume is large Administration may be difficult in very aggressive animals Delay before onset of peak sedation
Subcutaneous (s.c.)	Easy to administer drugs single-handedly Administration of a large volume of drug is not painful	Delay before onset of peak effect is greater than for i.m. route and more variable
Oral transmucosal (OTM)	Non-invasive, so reduces stress to the patient during administration – particularly important in anxious patients Absorption is reliable for some drugs, e.g. dexmedetomidine in cats and dogs and buprenorphine in cats Easy to administer drugs in cats and dogs single-handedly	Difficult to ensure that the total drug dose is absorbed (e.g. spillage from oral cavity if the drug volume is large, or drug may be swallowed) Total drug volume that is practical to administer effectively by this route is limited Efficacy of absorption may be variable between cats and dogs depending on the pH of saliva. Cannot automatically extrapolate doses between the species Limited data describing absorption of drugs used for pre-anaesthetic medication by this route
Oral	Owners are able to administer sedative drugs orally Only oral preparations of acepromazine and diazepam are readily available	Variable onset and duration of action Sedation achieved following oral administration is unpredictable Dose range is unpredictable and dependent on the individual patient
Transdermal fentanyl	Non-invasive and easy to apply	Can only be applied by a veterinary surgeon trained in use of the product (an online training tool is provided by the manufacturer) Suitable for administration only to dogs Precautions must be adopted to prevent spillage or contact with the solution during application (i.e. requires two people – one to restrain the dog and the second to apply the solution) Dogs must be isolated from children for at least 72 hours and dogs >20 kg bodyweight must be hospitalized for a minimum of 48 hours

13.3 Advantages and disadvantages of different routes of administration of pre-anaesthetic sedative drugs.

Drug	Time to peak sedation or effect	Duration of action	Reversible	Analgesia
Acepromazine	35–40 minutes i.m. 10–15 minutes i.v.	4–6 hours	No	No
Dexmedetomidine	15–20 minutes i.m. 2–3 minutes i.v.	Sedation: 2–3 hours Analgesia: 1 hour	Yes – with atipamezole	Yes
Midazolam	10–15 minutes i.m. 5 minutes i.v.	1–1.5 hours	Yes – with flumazenil	No
Diazepam	10–15 minutes i.m. 5 minutes i.v.	2 hours	Yes – with flumazenil	No
Atropine	20–30 minutes i.m. 1–2 minutes i.v.	Vagal inhibition 60–90 minutes	No	No
Glycopyrronium	20–30 minutes i.m. 3–5 minutes i.v.	Vagal inhibition 2–4 hours	No	No
Methadone	20–30 minutes i.m. 2–5 minutes i.v.	2–4 hours	Yes – with naloxone	Yes
Hydromorphone	10–20 minutes i.m. 2–5 minutes i.v.	2–4 hours	Yes – with naloxone	Yes
Morphine	20–30 minutes i.m. 2–5 minutes i.v.	2–4 hours	Yes – with naloxone	Yes
Pethidine (meperidine)	20–30 minutes i.m. Contraindicated i.v.	1–1.5 hours	Yes – with naloxone	Yes
Fentanyl Transdermal fentanyl solution	2–5 minutes i.v. 2–4 hours	10–20 minutes 96 hours	Yes – with naloxone Yes – with naloxone (although will require multiple doses of naloxone or a naloxone infusion)	Yes Yes
Buprenorphine	15–30 minutes i.m. 2–5 minutes i.v. 30–40 minutes OTM (cats)	6 hours	Yes – with naloxone	Yes
Butorphanol	20–30 minutes i.m. 2–5 minutes i.v.	1–1.5 hours	Yes – with naloxone	Yes

13.4 Characteristics of drugs used for sedation and pre-anaesthetic medication. Note that the duration of action of many of these drugs will vary between species and will depend on the dose administered. The times given are approximate guidelines only. OTM = oral transmucosal.

- Opioids, e.g. morphine, methadone, pethidine (meperidine), hydromorphone, oxymorphone, buprenorphine, fentanyl, butorphanol
- Anticholinergics, e.g. atropine, glycopyrronium.

In contrast to previous studies, the CEPSAF study (see above) did not find any association between risk of death and drugs used for pre-anaesthetic medication in cats and dogs.

Phenothiazines

Phenothiazines are dopamine receptor (D_1 and D_2) antagonists, and have calming and mood-altering effects. Acepromazine is the only phenothiazine licensed for pre-anaesthetic medication in small animal practice. It is metabolized in the liver and has a long duration of action (approximately 6 hours in healthy patients). Its use in animals with compromised liver function (e.g. hepatobiliary disease, portosystemic shunts, animals <12 weeks of age) is not recommended.

Sedation

Acepromazine causes sedation and anxiolysis that is initially dose-dependent. Increasing the dose in the range of 0.01–0.1 mg/kg will usually improve sedation, although at doses >0.05 mg/kg a plateau is reached for degree of sedation, cardiovascular side effects are probably more profound and the duration of action is prolonged. In comparison to the sedation produced by alpha-2 adrenoceptor agonists, sedation from acepromazine alone is generally less reliable. However, the quality and reliability of sedation can be improved by combining acepromazine with an opioid (so-called neuroleptanalgesia). Addition of an opioid also provides analgesia, which is advantageous because acepromazine itself has no analgesic properties. Onset of sedation following administration of acepromazine is relatively slow compared with alpha-2 adrenoceptor agonists. In order to maximize sedation, the animal should be left undisturbed for 30–40 minutes after intramuscular administration or 10–15 minutes after intravenous injection. In common with most sedative drugs, animals that appear sedated after receiving acepromazine will often wake up if roused or excited, and therefore quiet handling is necessary.

Other pharmacological effects

Cardiovascular system: Acepromazine is an antagonist at alpha-1 adrenoceptors. Administration can therefore cause peripheral vasodilation and a consequent fall in arterial blood pressure. This is normally tolerated well in healthy animals; however, in animals with shock or cardiovascular disease, acepromazine-induced vasodilation can be clinically significant and can result in cardiovascular collapse. Management of hypotension during anaesthesia after pre-anaesthetic medication with acepromazine can be problematic, and there is some evidence to suggest that crystalloid fluid therapy causes a further decrease in blood pressure by causing further vasodilation (Sinclair and Dyson, 2012). Administration of adrenaline (epinephrine) in this situation is contraindicated due to the risk of adrenaline reversal: in the presence of alpha-1 antagonists such as acepromazine, adrenaline preferentially activates not only beta-2 adrenoceptors in skeletal muscle, resulting in vasodilation and hypotension, but also beta-1 adrenoceptors in the heart, causing tachycardia (Nickerson *et al.*, 1953; Kaul and Grewal, 1970; Hunyady and Johnson, 2006).

Acepromazine also causes a reduction of up to 20% in haematocrit. This is due in part to relaxation of the splenic capsule and sequestration of red blood cells in the spleen, as well as vasodilation of the entire splanchnic vasculature. Acepromazine therefore contributes to the reduction in haematocrit that occurs following induction of anaesthesia, and this should be considered carefully when deciding whether to use acepromazine in anaemic animals.

The effects of acepromazine are long lasting and cannot be antagonized. It is therefore advisable to avoid its use when hypotension or cardiovascular compromise is anticipated as a potential complication of anaesthesia and surgery.

Heart rhythm: Acepromazine is considered to have anti-arrhythmic properties caused primarily by its antagonist effects at alpha-1 adrenoceptors in the heart. The clinical relevance of this effect in small animals is unknown. In the recent CEPSAF study there was a tendency towards a reduced risk of anaesthetic death in animals that had received acepromazine, but this was not statistically significant when other factors contributing to anaesthetic risk, such as health status, age and bodyweight, were taken into consideration.

Respiratory system: Clinical doses of acepromazine have little effect on respiratory function, although higher doses can cause respiratory depression, particularly when given in combination with opioids.

Body temperature: Acepromazine is associated with a fall in body temperature due to a resetting of thermoregulatory mechanisms and increased heat loss caused by peripheral vasodilation. Measures to minimize heat loss and to support body temperature should therefore be initiated immediately after acepromazine administration (see Chapter 3).

Seizure threshold: It has been recommended that acepromazine should be avoided in animals with epilepsy or in those at an increased risk of seizures, such as patients undergoing myelography. However, there are no clinical data in animals to support these recommendations. A small clinical study in dogs that were anaesthetized for myelography found no difference in the incidence of seizures in dogs that received either acepromazine and methadone, or methadone alone as pre-anaesthetic medication (Drynan *et al.*, 2012).

Lower oesophageal sphincter pressure: Acepromazine reduces lower oesophageal sphincter tone in cats and dogs, which may contribute to an increased risk of gastro-oesophageal reflux. However, many factors, such as bodyweight and type of surgical procedure, also contribute to the risk of gastro-oesophageal reflux during anaesthesia, and therefore the clinical relevance of the effect of acepromazine is currently unknown.

Other: Giant breeds of dog are often considered to be 'more sensitive' to the effects of acepromazine. This is probably a reflection of relative overdosing of large dogs when dose is calculated according to bodyweight rather than by using allometric scaling.

Some Boxers are highly sensitive to even small doses of acepromazine, which has been attributed to orthostatic hypotension or vasovagal syncope in this breed; marked sedation associated with a relative bradycardia and hypotension have been reported. Boxers that have a relative bradycardia at pre-anaesthetic examination have a high risk of vasovagal syncope during anaesthesia, and caution should be exercised when anaesthetizing these animals. Although acepromazine is not contraindicated in Boxers, it is not the pre-anaesthetic drug of choice in this breed. A very low dose (≤0.01 mg/kg) is recommended and animals should be monitored carefully after administration.

Acepromazine has an anti-emetic action, and a study in dogs demonstrated that acepromazine given at least 15 minutes before hydromorphone administration decreased the incidence of vomiting (Valverde *et al.*, 2004). This effect is attributed to a depressant effect on the chemoreceptor trigger zone (CRTZ) and vomiting centre.

Acepromazine also has weak anti-histamine effects, so use for pre-anaesthetic medication before intradermal skin testing is not recommended.

Administration of acepromazine during recovery from anaesthesia

Low doses of acepromazine (0.005–0.01 mg/kg i.v.) can be useful to help manage opioid-induced dysphoria in the recovery period in both cats and dogs. In this context, the possible longer duration of action is advantageous compared with using a single dose of dexmedetomidine. Animals should be carefully monitored while sedated, including regular measurement of body temperature, which should be supported if required.

Alpha-2 adrenoceptor agonists

Alpha-2 adrenoceptor agonists are reliable sedative and analgesic drugs. Xylazine was the first to be used in veterinary practice but it has now been largely superseded by medetomidine and dexmedetomidine, which are more selective for the alpha-2 adrenoceptor (the alpha-2:alpha-1 receptor selectivity binding ratios of dexmedetomidine and xylazine are 1620:1 and 160:1, respectively). The agonist effect of xylazine at alpha-1 adrenoceptors in the heart may account for the reduced cardiovascular safety of xylazine compared with medetomidine.

Medetomidine is an equal mixture of two optical enantiomers, dexmedetomidine and levomedetomidine. More recently, dexmedetomidine has received market authorization for sedation and pre-anaesthetic medication of cats and dogs. The proposed advantages of dexmedetomidine over medetomidine include improved analgesia, more predictable sedation and a reduced requirement for metabolism of the drug because only the active enantiomer (dexmedetomidine) is administered. Studies comparing the sedation produced by equipotent doses of medetomidine and dexmedetomidine in cats and dogs have failed to demonstrate a clinical difference between the two drugs; however, due to the efficacy of medetomidine, it would be challenging to detect any additional benefit of using dexmedetomidine. Therefore, despite the clear theoretical pharmacological advantages of dexmedetomidine, the benefit in clinical terms is unknown.

In this chapter, dexmedetomidine is named as the representative example of all licensed alpha-2 adrenoceptor agonists.

Sedation

Sedation after dexmedetomidine administration is profound and dose-related. However, similar to acepromazine, a plateau effect is reached, and beyond this point further increases in dose prolong the duration of effect rather than increasing the intensity of sedation. Synergism between alpha-2 adrenoceptor agonists and opioids or benzodiazepines means that combining dexmedetomidine with either of these drugs produces more profound sedation, allowing the dose of dexmedetomidine to be reduced. This is advantageous because the effects of dexmedetomidine on the cardiovascular and respiratory systems are also dose-dependent. In some circumstances it may be useful to combine dexmedetomidine with acepromazine; this combination (which is not licensed) delivers the advantages of the two drugs at the same time, and can be considered in patients undergoing anaesthetics of long duration (>2–3 hours), or where an extended period of sedation in recovery is desirable (e.g. animals that are very anxious and restless). Alvaides *et al.* (2008) studied the cardiorespiratory and sedative effects of acepromazine (0.05 mg/kg i.v.) given 15 minutes before dexmedetomidine (5 µg/kg i.v.) in dogs. Treatment with acepromazine plus dexmedetomidine did not provide greater intensity of sedation than dexmedetomidine alone, probably reflecting the very profound sedation produced by the latter drug. The cardiorespiratory effects of dexmedetomidine were also unchanged by the addition of acepromazine. The duration of sedation was not investigated in this study.

Characteristics of general anaesthesia following pre-anaesthetic medication with an alpha-2 adrenoceptor agonist

Pre-anaesthetic medication with alpha-2 adrenoceptor agonists has a significant influence on the characteristics of the ensuing anaesthesia. This must be remembered in order to use these drugs safely. The following points should be recognized:

- Significant drug-sparing effect: the dose of induction agent required after pre-anaesthetic medication with dexmedetomidine is dramatically reduced. Failure to recognize this can easily lead to anaesthetic overdose. The concentration of volatile agent required for maintenance of anaesthesia is similarly reduced (by up to 70% for isoflurane)
- Intravenous induction agents must be given slowly and to effect: dexmedetomidine increases the time taken for an intravenously administered induction agent to reach the brain, so it takes longer for the peak central nervous system (CNS) depressant effect of the intravenous agent to become apparent. This can inadvertently lead to anaesthetic overdose if the intravenous agent is given too quickly
- Alpha-2 adrenoceptor agonists have potent analgesic properties: pre-anaesthetic medication with dexmedetomidine can contribute significantly to intraoperative analgesia. This can result in a very stable plane of anaesthesia during the maintenance phase, reducing the fluctuations in depth of anaesthesia associated with changes in the intensity of surgical stimulation.

Other pharmacological effects

Cardiovascular system: Dexmedetomidine typically produces a dose-dependent biphasic effect on blood pressure, comprising an initial increase followed by a return to normal or slightly below normal values. Heart rate is decreased, with normal expected heart rates from 45–60 and 100–115 beats per minute for dogs and cats, respectively. The characteristic changes in cardiovascular function can be divided temporally into two phases. It is important to understand the origin of these changes in order to use alpha-2 adrenoceptor agonists safely and effectively for both sedation and pre-anaesthetic medication.

Phase 1: The immediate response of the cardiovascular system to dexmedetomidine is an increase in blood pressure caused by peripheral vasoconstriction via activation of alpha-2 adrenoceptors located in the peripheral vasculature. The mechanism of vasoconstriction is similar to that caused by activation of the sympathetic nervous system during the 'fight or flight' (stress) response. The increase in blood pressure causes a reduction in heart rate, mediated by the baroreceptor reflex. The duration of vasoconstriction depends on the dose and route of administration, with greater vasoconstriction being produced by higher doses (5–10 µg/kg) given intravenously. Clinically, dogs appear to be more susceptible than cats to the vasoconstrictor effects of dexmedetomidine, with a more profound increase in blood pressure and reduction in heart rate, in response to the same dose.

Phase 2: The peripheral vasoconstriction lasts for approximately 20 minutes after intravenous administration of dexmedetomidine. In Phase 2, blood pressure returns to normal or slightly below normal. Despite the return of blood pressure to approximately normal values, heart rate remains low. This Phase 2 bradycardia is the result of a prolonged reduction in sympathetic nervous system tone, via an effect of dexmedetomidine mediated at presynaptic alpha-2 adrenoceptors located in the CNS.

Heart rhythm: Vagally induced bradyarrhythmias, such as first- and second-degree atrioventricular blocks, are commonly reported in dogs after administration of dexmedetomidine. These can be attributed to the baroreceptor reflex induced by peripheral vasoconstriction and are most likely to occur in the first 20–30 minutes after drug administration (Phase 1). Clinically, first- and second-degree atrioventricular block appear to be less common in cats than dogs. Dexmedetomidine is not, by definition, arrhythmogenic: in standard tests of arrhythmogenicity, an anti-arrhythmic action of the drug has been demonstrated.

Cardiac output: Alpha-2 adrenoceptor agonists cause a reduction in cardiac output. The precise aetiology of this reduction is unknown but it is considered to be multifactorial. The increase in afterload resulting from peripheral vasoconstriction is thought to be a contributing factor. In animals with a healthy, normally functioning cardiovascular system, the reduction in cardiac output is not associated with reduced oxygen delivery to central organs such as the CNS, heart, kidneys and liver. However, in animals with limited cardiovascular reserve, the reduction in cardiac output following dexmedetomidine administration may have detrimental consequences for organ function as oxygen delivery *is* reduced in these patients. Alpha-2 adrenoceptor agonists have a very limited margin of cardiovascular safety and therefore are generally suitable for use for sedation or pre-anaesthetic medication only in animals with a normally functioning cardiovascular system.

Management of extremely low heart rates during anaesthesia following dexmedetomidine: Heart rates during anaesthesia are lower after pre-anaesthetic medication with dexmedetomidine than after other sedative agents

such as acepromazine, but routine administration of anticholinergic agents with dexmedetomidine is not recommended. However, if the heart rate falls below the expected range (45–60 beats per minute for dogs and 100–115 beats per minute for cats) following administration of dexmedetomidine and if clinical monitoring suggests that the bradycardia is having a negative impact on blood pressure, peripheral perfusion and oxygen delivery, or heart rhythm (ventricular escape beats or ventricular premature complexes), action should be taken to increase heart rate. Many other factors can contribute to a low heart rate during anaesthesia, and therefore other causes, such as hypothermia, should also be addressed as appropriate. There are principally three different strategies to manage low heart rates caused by dexmedetomidine during anaesthesia:

- Administration of an anticholinergic
- Administration of a sympathomimetic such as ketamine
- Partial reversal of dexmedetomidine by administration of atipamezole.

There are pros and cons to each of these strategies, and insufficient data from studies are available to give clear clinical recommendations about which is the best option. A suggested guideline is given below, with the advantages and disadvantages of each strategy.

Administration of an anticholinergic: In those cases in which dexmedetomidine is considered to be the primary cause of the low heart rate and there is clear evidence of hypotension, a low dose of an anticholinergic agent (e.g. atropine at 0.0025–0.005 mg/kg slowly i.v.) can be used to shift the heart rate back into the expected normal range. Preferably, atropine should be administered once Phase 1 is over. Administration of an anticholinergic during systemic hypertension carries a high risk of further increasing blood pressure. When the heart has to contract against a high afterload caused by vasoconstriction in Phase 1, the increased myocardial oxygen demand can cause arrhythmias.

Administration of ketamine: Because of its sympathomimetic properties, ketamine is an alternative to administration of an anticholinergic. In Phase 2, when the bradycardia is primarily due to a centrally mediated reduction in sympathetic tone, a low dose of ketamine (0.1–0.2 mg/kg slowly i.v.) can also effectively increase heart rate. Ketamine may also be used as a second-line approach in patients where an anticholinergic has been ineffective. It is important to allow sufficient time for a response to an anticholinergic (3–4 minutes) before ketamine is given.

Administration of atipamezole: Partial reversal of dexmedetomidine by intravenous administration of a low dose of atipamezole, titrated to effect, can be a 'rescue' strategy to increase heart rate either when administration of an anticholinergic or ketamine has been ineffective, or in patients where administration of an anticholinergic is undesirable. A good starting point for administration of atipamezole is to administer half of the pre-anaesthetic dose of dexmedetomidine (i.e. if 5 µg/kg dexmedetomidine was given, administer 2.5 µg/kg atipamezole). It may be necessary to dilute the atipamezole before administration to facilitate accurate dosing. After a period of 2–3 minutes, a second incremental dose of the same magnitude can be given, and this should be repeated as necessary, up to ten times the dose of dexmedetomidine (which would be the licensed reversal dose of atipamezole in dogs) or up to 5 times the dose of dexmedetomidine in cats. The major disadvantage of atipamezole is that the patient may suddenly recover from anaesthesia, due to a decrease in the depth of anaesthesia and the reversal of dexmedetomidine analgesia. The veterinary surgeon (veterinarian) should therefore be prepared to administer an intravenous hypnotic agent (e.g. propofol or alfaxalone) if necessary. Supplementary analgesia may also be required. Ideally, one should wait until the surgery has started before administering atipamezole during Phase 1, as often the stimulus of surgery alone is sufficient to increase heart rate. There are no clinical studies to support the use of atipamezole intraoperatively, and this technique should be used with caution and as a last resort. Atipamezole is not licensed for i.v. use.

Respiratory system: Alpha-2 adrenoceptor agonists produce minimal effects on the respiratory system in healthy animals, and arterial oxygen and carbon dioxide tensions remain within normal limits. Profound sedation after dexmedetomidine can lead to upper airway obstruction in brachycephalic cats and dogs.

Renal system: Urine production is increased due to a reduction in vasopressin and renin secretion. This is not of clinical significance in healthy animals. However, it is good practice to palpate the bladder of the patient before recovery from anaesthesia and express the bladder manually if it is distended, as a full bladder can contribute to a poor recovery from anaesthesia.

Pancreas: Endogenous insulin secretion is reduced with alpha-2 adrenoceptor agonists, leading to a transient hyperglycaemia. This is not of sufficient magnitude to result in an osmotic diuresis in cats and dogs. Use of dexmedetomidine should be considered carefully in animals with pancreatitis, due to the potential for a reduction in splanchnic blood flow, which may result in exacerbation of the pancreatic disease. It should also be used cautiously in patients that are diabetic due to its effects on blood glucose concentration.

Liver: Both hepatic blood flow and the rate of metabolism of drugs by the liver are reduced. This is not of clinical significance in healthy animals, but dexmedetomidine is not the pre-anaesthetic agent of choice in animals with liver disease. Further information on the pragmatic use of dexmedetomidine in animals with liver function abnormalities is provided in Chapter 24.

Body temperature: Although dexmedetomidine has a direct depressant effect on the thermoregulatory centre, peripheral vasoconstriction tends to minimize heat loss. As a consequence it can be easier to maintain normothermia during the perioperative period in animals given dexmedetomidine than in those given acepromazine. Body temperature should be measured as part of routine anaesthetic monitoring and temperature support should be provided if necessary (see Chapter 3).

Intraocular pressure: Dexmedetomidine administered at a dose of 10–15 μg/kg i.v. produces a transient increase in intraocular pressure (IOP) followed by a decrease relative to baseline. These changes in IOP are mediated both indirectly via the effect of dexmedetomidine on blood pressure, and directly via an action at alpha-2 adrenoceptors located pre- and post-junctionally in ocular sympathetic nerve fibres. The increase in IOP caused by alpha-2 adrenoceptor agonists should be taken into consideration when selecting pre-anaesthetic agents in dogs and cats where increased IOP is undesirable (e.g. patients with glaucoma, lens luxation, fragile eyes) (see Chapter 19).

Intracranial pressure: Dexmedetomidine lowers cerebral blood flow via alpha-2 adrenoceptor-mediated vasoconstriction. Hence, it will tend to reduce intracranial pressure (ICP), which may be advantageous in animals with intracranial lesions. However, the potential for dexmedetomidine to induce vomiting, particularly in cats (see below), and to cause respiratory depression at profound levels of sedation (which may elevate arterial carbon dioxide concentrations) should be considered.

Gastrointestinal system: Vomiting is frequently seen in cats and dogs after intramuscular or subcutaneous administration of alpha-2 adrenoceptor agonists due to activation of central alpha-2 adrenoceptors. Vomiting after intravenous administration is less common due to the very rapid onset of sedation following administration by this route. Alpha-2 adrenoceptor agonists are contraindicated in animals with a suspected oesophageal foreign body, where emesis may result in further tissue damage (see Chapter 24). Vomiting will also increase ICP and IOP, and may exacerbate cervical disc disease owing to the posture adopted during vomiting; dexmedetomidine should therefore be used cautiously in patient groups where these are of particular relevance. Dexmedetomidine will also reduce intestinal motility and increase transit time.

Dexmedetomidine and dose selection

In recent years there has been a tendency to use significantly lower doses of dexmedetomidine than those stated in the Summary of Product Characteristics, reflecting the recognition that its cardiovascular effects are dose-dependent, while sedation can be achieved at low doses. Low-dose dexmedetomidine (1–3 μg/kg i.v.) combined with an opioid can produce very reliable sedation in cats and dogs, although concurrent analgesia provided by the alpha-2 adrenoceptor agonist will be of short duration (<20–30 minutes). Similarly, the duration of the dose-sparing effect for maintenance anaesthetic agents will be shorter with lower doses of dexmedetomidine than with higher doses, and therefore careful monitoring of anaesthetic depth is essential. The cardiovascular effects of dexmedetomidine plateau between 5 and 10 μg/kg i.v.: in this dose range the duration of concurrent analgesia will be 30–45 minutes. Sedation from low doses of dexmedetomidine (1–3 μg/kg) given intramuscularly can be unreliable in excitable patients, even when administered in combination with an opioid.

Infusion of dexmedetomidine

Anaesthetic and sedative protocols utilizing dexmedetomidine administered by infusion have also been adopted in recent years. The infusion may be used during anaesthesia after pre-anaesthetic medication with a dexmedetomidine bolus (0.5–2.5 μg/kg i.v.) as part of a balanced anaesthesia protocol, and/or postoperatively to provide sedation and analgesia, particularly in patients that are anxious and restless in the hospital environment. The sedation produced by a dexmedetomidine infusion is described as 'rousable': the patient appears to be well sedated when unstimulated but can still be roused, and dogs can often be walked outside to toilet and maintain mobility. The use of a dexmedetomidine infusion allows administration of a low dose (0.5–2.5 µg/kg/h) that will tend to limit the cardiovascular side effects while still providing prolonged sedation and analgesia. Due to the potency of dexmedetomidine, it is important that a controlled infusion apparatus such as a syringe driver is used. Patients should be carefully monitored to ensure that they remain normothermic and do not develop respiratory obstruction due to excessive sedation. A low-dose (0.5–2.5 µg/kg i.v.) bolus of dexmedetomidine may be useful to manage excitatory phenomena (e.g. emergence from anaesthesia, opioid-mediated dysphoria) in dogs and cats in the immediate postoperative period, although it is important to determine whether poor recovery is due to uncontrolled pain (in which case administration of an opioid is usually indicated) or to the behavioural side effects of anaesthetic drugs.

Reversal of alpha-2 adrenoceptor agonists with atipamezole

Sedation and analgesia produced by alpha-2 adrenoceptor agonists are rapidly reversed by the administration of a specific alpha-2 adrenoceptor antagonist such as atipamezole. Recoveries following intramuscular administration of atipamezole are generally smooth and of good quality. Intravenous administration of atipamezole produces a very rapid, excitable recovery from anaesthesia or sedation; this route is unlicensed and not recommended. It is important to ensure that analgesia is supplemented, if necessary, with different classes of drugs, such as opioids and non-steroidal anti-inflammatory drugs (NSAIDs) before reversal by atipamezole, because atipamezole will also abolish alpha-2 adrenoceptor-mediated analgesia.

The CEPSAF study identified the recovery period to be of relatively high risk because animals are often poorly monitored and observed during recovery. Shortening the length of the recovery period using atipamezole may therefore contribute to improved patient safety. However, when animals are carefully monitored during the recovery period, reversal of dexmedetomidine is not always necessary, particularly if the drug was administered 3–4 hours previously. Monitoring heart rate (i.e. whether the patient is still relatively bradycardic) can be a useful indicator of whether dexmedetomidine administered for pre-anaesthetic medication is still making a significant contribution to sedation in the recovery period.

Yohimbine and tolazoline are commercially available alpha-2 adrenoceptor antagonists in some countries. Compared with atipamezole, these antagonists have a lower alpha-2:alpha-1 receptor selectivity.

MK-467: Concurrent administration of MK-467, a peripherally restricted alpha-2 adrenoceptor antagonist, with dexmedetomidine is under investigation as a new strategy to achieve the centrally mediated, clinically desirable effects of dexmedetomidine (sedation and analgesia) while limiting some of the undesirable cardiovascular side effects. Studies in dogs and other species have shown that co-administration of dexmedetomidine and MK-467 prevents dexmedetomidine-mediated vasoconstriction and therefore prevents reductions in heart rate and cardiac output, but has no effect on the quality of sedation. MK-467 has significant clinical potential to offset the cardiovascular effects of dexmedetomidine and may become available for clinical use in the future.

Patient selection

Dexmedetomidine affords many advantages for pre-anaesthetic medication and sedation in small animals, but in order to use the drug safely and effectively, it should only be used routinely in healthy animals. However, accepted practice relating to selection of patients suitable for dexmedetomidine is changing. There are small populations of animals with specific diseases that may benefit from the physiological effects of dexmedetomidine given in low (1–3 µg/kg i.v.) doses in some circumstances, for example, patients with raised ICP. In human medicine, dexmedetomidine is used preferentially in patients with cardiovascular disease because of the benefits afforded by reductions in heart rate (reduced myocardial oxygen consumption) and sympathetic nervous system tone (reduced risk of catecholamine-induced arrhythmias and myocardial infarction). This principle may translate to small animal patients with some types of myocardial disease such as hypertrophic cardiomyopathy with dynamic ventricular outflow tract obstruction, although there is little clinical evidence to support this practice. Administration of dexmedetomidine to patients with cardiovascular disease should be considered carefully in terms of the effect of the underlying disease on cardiovascular function and the likely impact of the drug on that function. Further discussion of this topic can be found in Chapter 21.

Dexmedetomidine should *not* be used routinely in the following patient groups:

- Cardiovascular disease where an increase in afterload and a reduction in heart rate will be detrimental (e.g. mitral valve regurgitation, dilated cardiomyopathy)
- Systemic disease causing deterioration in cardiovascular function (e.g. toxaemia)
- Severe liver disease
- Geriatric animals: these patients do not have the normal functional organ reserve of healthy adult animals
- Very young animals: the physiological effects of dexmedetomidine in puppies and kittens are poorly documented. Administration of medetomidine in combination with ketamine, midazolam and buprenorphine as part of the Quad protocol (Joyce and Yates, 2011) for early neutering (<6 weeks of age) of kittens is widely used and provides adequate anaesthesia and analgesia for neutering, with a short recovery period (see Figure 13.7). However, routine administration of dexmedetomidine in animals <8–12 weeks of age, particularly without the co-administration of ketamine (which may offset the effects of dexmedetomidine on heart rate), is not currently recommended
- Diabetes mellitus: such patients often have multiple organ disease, which, in combination with the effect of dexmedetomidine on blood glucose concentration, means that dexmedetomidine is not the ideal pre-anaesthetic or sedative drug for these patients.

Routine co-administration of anticholinergic agents (atropine or glycopyrronium) and dexmedetomidine

When alpha-2 adrenoceptor agonists were first introduced into small animal practice, there was a trend for the routine co-administration of anticholinergic agents to offset the bradycardia that ensued. It is now recognized that the routine co-administration of anticholinergic agents with dexmedetomidine is detrimental. The initial reduction in heart rate after dexmedetomidine administration is physiological and a response to an increase in blood pressure. Obtunding this normal physiological response results in tachycardia and greater hypertension. The heart is required to beat faster against a vasoconstricted peripheral vascular bed, increasing myocardial oxygen consumption. There is also less diastolic time for adequate myocardial perfusion, which can lead to ventricular arrhythmias and potential cardiovascular collapse.

Benzodiazepines

Diazepam and midazolam are the benzodiazepines most commonly used in small animal practice. Although they may be used for pre-anaesthetic medication, they are more often used as co-induction agents with ketamine, propofol or alfaxalone. A comparison of the physical properties and pharmacological effects of these two drugs is shown in Figure 13.5. These agents exert their main sedative effects through depression of the limbic system. Their action is thought to be mediated via activation of a specific benzodiazepine receptor, part of the gamma-aminobutyric acid (GABA) receptor complex. GABA is a major inhibitory neurotransmitter in the CNS. These drugs do not have analgesic properties, except to reduce pain associated with skeletal muscle spasm.

Zolazepam is a benzodiazepine derivative available only in combination with tiletamine. This preparation (Telazol® or Zoletil®) is a short-acting anaesthetic agent in cats and dogs. The pharmacological effects of zolazepam and tiletamine are similar to those of ketamine combined with diazepam (see Chapter 14).

Parameter	Midazolam	Diazepam
Preparation	Water soluble, can be injected i.m. and i.v. without causing pain or irritation	Insoluble in water, usually solubilized in propylene glycol, although an emulsion formulation is available Propylene glycol preparation causes pain on injection and thrombophlebitis when given i.v. Unpredictable absorption after i.m. administration
Length of action and metabolism	Metabolized in liver; metabolites are inactive, so midazolam is shorter acting than diazepam with less risk of accumulation	Metabolized in liver; metabolites are active, so there is a risk of accumulation and prolonged action when given repeatedly
Clinical use	Benzodiazepine of choice for use in small animals	Give propylene glycol preparation slowly i.v., preferably with free-running fluids

13.5 Comparison of midazolam and diazepam.

Sedation

Benzodiazepines administered alone produce very mild or no sedation in healthy cats and dogs; they may even cause excitation due to loss of learned inhibitory behaviour and are therefore often given in combination with other sedatives. Many protocols for sedation combine a benzodiazepine with an opioid because both classes of drugs have few negative effects on haemodynamics. Benzodiazepines reduce the concentration of isoflurane required to maintain anaesthesia (minimum alveolar concentration (MAC) sparing effect) in a dose-dependent fashion, although the magnitude of this effect is small compared with that of acepromazine and alpha-2 adrenoceptor agonists. Benzodiazepines also produce centrally-mediated skeletal muscle relaxation.

Other pharmacological effects

Cardiovascular and respiratory systems: Benzodiazepines have minor effects on both of these systems. This is one of their major advantages, and these drugs therefore tend to be used as pre-anaesthetic agents in animals with cardiovascular compromise. Synergism between benzodiazepines and other sedative drugs may enhance the respiratory depression when the drugs are used in combination.

Anticonvulsant effects: Benzodiazepines are commonly used to manage convulsions, particularly as a first-line intervention for animals presenting in status epilepticus. Diazepam may be given rectally to control seizures when intravenous access is not established.

Antagonism of benzodiazepines with flumazenil

The effects of benzodiazepines on the CNS can be effectively reversed by the administration of the benzodiazepine receptor antagonist flumazenil. When given intravenously, it will rapidly reverse all effects of benzodiazepines. Low doses of flumazenil (0.01–0.03 mg/kg) are often adequate to reverse sedation in animals that are slow to recover after receiving high doses of benzodiazepines.

Alfaxalone

Alfaxalone is authorized for induction and maintenance of anaesthesia by the intravenous route in cats and dogs (see Chapter 14). In addition, recent clinical studies have evaluated alfaxalone administered subcutaneously or intramuscularly for sedation or pre-anaesthetic medication in conscious patients where intravenous access could not be achieved (Ramoo et al., 2013; Ribas et al., 2014). Peak sedation was reported to be approximately 30 minutes after subcutaneous administration of 3 mg/kg alfaxalone (combined with butorphanol) to cats, and sedation lasted for approximately 45 minutes. The onset and duration of sedation is shorter following intramuscular administration (10–15 minutes), although this may be a consequence of the lower dose of alfaxalone required when given intramuscularly. As with other sedatives, the reliability of sedation will be greater when alfaxalone is combined with opioids or midazolam, although clinical data on these combinations are sparse. The cardiovascular and respiratory effects of alfaxalone administered subcutaneously or intramuscularly appear to be dose-dependent. The protocol is unsuitable for use in most dogs because of the larger volumes of alfaxalone required to produce reliable sedation (1–2 mg/kg i.m.).

Opioids

Opioids are commonly incorporated into pre-anaesthetic medication protocols to provide analgesia and to improve the reliability and intensity of the sedation provided by the primary sedative drug. The choice of opioid will depend on the degree of analgesia needed, and on both the speed of onset and the duration of action required. Generally, longer-acting opioids such as morphine, methadone, hydromorphone and buprenorphine are used, although intravenous fentanyl combined with midazolam may be used in patients with haemodynamic instability. A transdermal fentanyl solution has recently received market authorization for provision of perioperative analgesia in dogs when moderate to severe pain is expected after surgery. It should be administered 2–4 hours before surgery and has a long duration of action (96 hours). Butorphanol provides poor analgesia compared with that provided by other opioids, but is useful to enhance sedation provided by either acepromazine or dexmedetomidine without inducing panting (e.g. for diagnostic imaging).

Pharmacological effects

A more detailed description of opioid pharmacology can be found in Chapter 10. Analgesic efficacy (i.e. either full or partial mu opioid receptor agonist, or kappa agonist) and the duration of action of different opioids should be taken into account when selecting opioids to administer in pre-anaesthetic medication for painful procedures. The expected duration of action will determine the timing of subsequent opioid doses either intraoperatively or in the postoperative period.

Analgesia: Depending on the opioid chosen, different intensities of analgesia can be obtained. Opioids are a key element of perioperative pain control in small animals. Administration of full mu opioid receptor agonists (e.g. methadone) is recommended when moderate to severe pain is expected following surgery. Buprenorphine is suitable either when mild pain is anticipated, or for more invasive surgeries when a multimodal analgesia technique is used (e.g. locoregional analgesia technique plus NSAID administration).

Sedation: The sedative effect of opioids is usually dose- and drug-dependent. Sedation produced by phenothiazines and alpha-2 adrenoceptor agonists is enhanced when they are combined with opioids. The sedative properties of various opioids may be an important factor in determining choice; for example, methadone generally provides better sedation than buprenorphine and is useful when good sedation is required for healthy, excitable animals. In the author's experience, combinations of transdermal fentanyl solution, administered 2–4 hours before pre-anaesthetic medication, and either acepromazine or dexmedetomidine, administered intramuscularly at an appropriate time point before induction of anaesthesia, produce lighter sedation than that provided by these same sedative drugs when given intramuscularly at the same time as other opioids such as methadone or butorphanol. This is an important consideration, particularly in excitable dogs and other patients where obtaining intravenous access without good sedation is likely to be challenging.

Cardiovascular system: Opioids have few negative effects on haemodynamics. They may cause a reduction in heart rate through stimulation of the vagus nerve, which can be managed by co-administration of an anticholinergic agent if necessary.

Respiratory system: Opioids such as methadone, morphine, pethidine (meperidine) and buprenorphine do not cause clinically significant respiratory depression in animals at the dose rates normally used. However, fentanyl given intravenously with, for instance, midazolam often causes respiratory depression; if using this combination, the veterinary surgeon should therefore be prepared to induce anaesthesia and intubate the trachea promptly so that intermittent positive pressure ventilation can be started if necessary. Transdermal fentanyl solution, administered at the recommended doses, has so far not been associated with respiratory depression in the perioperative period.

Gastrointestinal system: Morphine and hydromorphone given intramuscularly or subcutaneously may directly stimulate the CRTZ and result in vomiting shortly after their administration. Intravenous administration of these opioids is less likely to cause vomiting due to a direct inhibitory action (which precedes stimulation of the CRTZ) on the vomiting centre in the brain. Vomiting is less frequent (or may not occur at all) when morphine or hydromorphone is used postoperatively for management of perioperative pain. Concurrent administration of acepromazine and morphine does not reduce the incidence of vomiting. However, if acepromazine is given intramuscularly 15 minutes before morphine or hydromorphone, the incidence of vomiting is reduced, at least in dogs (Valverde et al., 2004).

Opioids stimulate most sphincters of the gastrointestinal tract, causing an overall action that is constipating when opioids are administered chronically. When animals are anaesthetized for gastrointestinal endoscopy, pyloric constriction after pre-anaesthetic medication with opioids may make passage of an endoscope through the pylorus from the stomach to the duodenum more challenging; further discussion of this topic is provided in Chapter 24. Conversely, morphine (and probably also methadone, hydromorphone and fentanyl) reduces the lower oesophageal sphincter tone in dogs, and has been associated with an increased risk of gastro-oesophageal reflux. However, the factors affecting gastro-oesophageal reflux in dogs and cats are complex, and therefore the influence of opioids alone on the incidence of reflux is unknown.

Other factors determining opioid selection

- Route of administration: pethidine should not be administered intravenously because it causes histamine release. The volume needed for intramuscular injection is relatively large because of the dose required to provide analgesia (3–5 mg/kg) and the concentration of available pethidine solutions (50 mg/ml). Buprenorphine administered subcutaneously provides limited analgesia in cats (this may also be the case in dogs); other opioids may be a better option if subcutaneous administration is unavoidable.
- Duration of action: pethidine and butorphanol have a short duration of action (60–90 minutes) and frequent redosing is therefore needed.
- Contribution to a balanced anaesthesia technique: clinically, opioid receptor agonists reduce the concentration of volatile agent required for maintenance of anaesthesia and may also reduce the required dose of induction agent. This is advantageous even in animals undergoing anaesthesia for non-painful procedures.
- Further requirement for opioids during anaesthesia or in the postoperative period: if full mu opioid receptor agonists are to be administered in the perioperative period, a full mu opioid receptor agonist is recommended for pre-anaesthetic medication.
- Combination with benzodiazepines: when

benzodiazepines are combined with an opioid for pre-anaesthetic medication (e.g. in patients with haemodynamic instability), the sedation provided by a benzodiazepine combined with methadone or hydromorphone is more reliable than that afforded by a benzodiazepine combined with buprenorphine or butorphanol.

Anticholinergic agents

Anticholinergic agents antagonize the muscarinic effects of acetylcholine. Historically, they were used as a routine part of pre-anaesthetic medication to prevent unwanted side effects such as excessive salivation and bradycardia. The two anticholinergic agents commonly used in small animal practice are atropine and glycopyrronium; a comparison of their properties is shown in Figure 13.6.

Aims of pre-anaesthetic medication with an anticholinergic agent are:

- Reduction of salivary and bronchial secretions
- Blockage of the effects of vagal stimulation
- Blockage of the effects of drugs that stimulate the parasympathetic nervous system, such as opioids.

Routine use of an anticholinergic agent as part of pre-anaesthetic medication is unnecessary in current anaesthetic practice. The volatile agents that are in common use do not irritate the airway or cause excessive salivary and bronchial secretions. In addition, pre-emptive administration of an anticholinergic before stimulation of the vagus nerve often causes tachycardia. Although high doses of opioids may cause bradycardia, it is not always necessary to manage this by administration of an anticholinergic. Therefore, anticholinergics are normally given if required during anaesthesia, rather than as part of the pre-anaesthetic medication protocol.

Parameter	Atropine	Glycopyrronium
CNS action	Able to cross the blood–brain barrier	A quaternary ammonium compound and highly polar, therefore limited diffusion across the blood–brain barrier
Routes of administration	i.m., i.v. or s.c. Following i.v. administration, atropine may cause an initial increase in vagal tone associated with a reduction in heart rate. The classic parasympatholytic action occurs secondarily	i.m., i.v. or s.c. Initial increase in vagal tone following i.v. injection is less likely to occur than with atropine
Action on the pupil	Pupil dilation – may impair vision, which can contribute to poor recoveries in cats	No effect on the pupil
Duration of action	Varies between species and is dose-dependent. Vagal inhibition will last for approximately 60–90 minutes	Longer duration of action than atropine Vagal inhibition: lasts 2–4 hours Antisialogogue and gastrointestinal effects effect may persist for up to 7 hours

13.6 Comparison of atropine and glycopyrronium. CNS = central nervous system.

Drug protocols used for pre-anaesthetic medication and sedation

Acepromazine + opioid

- Commonly used in both cats and dogs.
- Degree of sedation is dose-dependent, but usually only light sedation is achieved.
- Sedation is usually inadequate for complex radiography or minimally invasive procedures.
- The cardiovascular effects of acepromazine make it unsuitable for animals that are in shock or patients with severe cardiovascular compromise.
- Use cautiously in animals with reduced liver function as duration of action may be prolonged (>6 hours).

Dexmedetomidine + opioid

- Provides reliable sedation in both cats and dogs; sedation is dose-dependent.
- Suitable for sedation for minor invasive procedures (such as ear examination) and radiography or computed tomography (CT) where the animal needs to be immobile. Be aware that despite being apparently well sedated, animals can be aroused suddenly by noise, movement or noxious stimulation.
- The cardiovascular effects of dexmedetomidine make it unsuitable for use in many patient groups.
- Dexmedetomidine is well absorbed across the oral mucous membranes; this provides a potential alternative route of administration in anxious or aggressive animals.

Dexmedetomidine + benzodiazepine (± opioid)

- More potent sedation than when dexmedetomidine is given alone. The addition of a benzodiazepine and an opioid will increase the reliability of sedation when using low doses of dexmedetomidine (1–3 µg/kg) intramuscularly.
- Useful combination for sedation for procedures such as hip radiography or CT. Be aware that despite being apparently well sedated, animals can be aroused suddenly by noise, movement or noxious stimulation.

Dexmedetomidine + ketamine

- Dexmedetomidine prevents CNS excitation from ketamine.
- Depending on the dose of ketamine administered, this combination will provide heavy sedation/general anaesthesia sufficient for short invasive procedures.
- Addition of an opioid, such as buprenorphine, to this combination will allow the doses of the other drugs to be reduced.
- Recovery from anaesthesia following this combination can be very excitable in dogs.
- The behavioural (excitatory) side effects of ketamine during recovery are present in cats but usually acceptable.
- Following short procedures it is important to wait at least 30–45 minutes before reversing the effects of dexmedetomidine, otherwise the excitatory effects of ketamine are unmasked.

- Medetomidine is used as part of the Quad protocol widely used for early neutering of kittens (Joyce and Yates, 2011; see Figure 13.7).
- Combinations of these agents are well absorbed across the oral mucous membranes; this provides a potential alternative route of administration in anxious or aggressive animals.
- See also Chapter 14 (intravenous anaesthetics).

Bodyweight (kg)	BSA (m²)	Volume of each drug in ml (medetomidine 1 mg/ml; ketamine 100 mg/ml; midazolam 5 mg/ml; buprenorphine 0.3 mg/ml)
0.5	0.07	0.04
1.0	0.1	0.06
1.5	0.14	0.08
2.0	0.17	0.1
2.5	0.19	0.12

13.7 Quad protocol for neutering kittens <6 weeks of age (Joyce and Yates, 2011). The Quad protocol is the administration of medetomidine (600 μg/m²), ketamine (80 μg/m²), midazolam (3 mg/m²) and buprenorphine (180 μg/m²) mixed in the same syringe. Atipamezole is recommended as a reversal agent at 10–50% volume of the previously administered medetomidine, no sooner than 20 minutes after the initial i.m. injection. Note that atipamezole use at 10% volume is unlicensed in cats. BSA = body surface area.

Opioid + benzodiazepine

- Minimal negative effects on the cardiovascular system, so useful for animals with haemodynamic compromise.
- Degree of sedation is dependent on both the dose and the individual patient: animals with severe systemic disease usually become more sedated than healthier patients.
- Intravenous administration produces more reliable sedation than intramuscular administration.
- Midazolam combined with methadone given intravenously generally produces good sedation in dogs. This combination can lead to dysphoria or excitation in a minority of patients, particularly when the midazolam and methadone are mixed in the same syringe. Giving methadone first followed by midazolam 2–3 minutes later is an alternative strategy that makes dysphoria less likely in some animals. Administer agents through a pre-placed intravenous catheter and proceed more quickly to induction of anaesthesia if excitation occurs.
- Midazolam and methadone combinations given intravenously or intramuscularly are not optimal for use in cats; sedation is unreliable and excitation may occur.
- Midazolam combined with fentanyl given intravenously can provide mild sedation in cats and dogs with haemodynamic instability. As with midazolam and methadone combinations, the drugs can be mixed in the same syringe or the fentanyl can be given first followed by midazolam 2–3 minutes later. Administer agents through a pre-placed catheter and be prepared to proceed rapidly to induction of anaesthesia should apnoea occur after administration.
- Very young animals tend to become more sedated than adults.

Benzodiazepine + ketamine

- Benzodiazepine prevents CNS excitation from ketamine.

- Useful for sedating cats when heavy sedation is required.
- With higher doses of ketamine, general anaesthesia can be induced (see Chapter 14).
- The combination provides haemodynamic stability and is useful for cats in which the administration of acepromazine or dexmedetomidine is undesirable. Caution should be exercised in cats with hypertrophic cardiomyopathy; the positive chronotropic effects of ketamine may result in inadequate myocardial perfusion in the presence of a hypertrophic myocardium.
- Difficult to avoid ketamine-induced behavioural changes in recovery. Animals are often disorientated for the first few hours of the recovery period.

Tiletamine + zolazepam (Telazol® or Zoletil®)

- Preparation is an equal mixture (weight to weight) of tiletamine and zolazepam.
- Similar to a combination of ketamine with diazepam or midazolam.
- See above and Chapter 14 for guidelines on clinical use.

Opioid alone

- Can provide good sedation in sick patients or very young animals (<12 weeks age), particularly when given intravenously.
- Methadone or butorphanol generally provide more reliable sedation than buprenorphine or systemic fentanyl in dogs.
- Buprenorphine can provide good sedation in cats with systemic disease, administration by the OTM route is non-invasive and may provide sufficient sedation to obtain intravenous access.
- Sedation from transdermal fentanyl solution alone in dogs is minimal.

Alfaxalone

- Low doses (1–2 mg/kg i.m. or 3 mg/kg s.c.) cause dose-dependent sedation that is sufficient to allow placement of an intravenous catheter.
- Can be combined with an opioid and/or midazolam to increase reliability of sedation (e.g. butorphanol and midazolam or midazolam alone, in patients not in pain, or methadone and midazolam in patients with pain).
- Volume required often restricts intramuscular administration in heavier patients (many dogs).
- Dose-dependent cardiovascular and respiratory system effects of alfaxalone will occur.
- May be useful in cats to provide reliable sedation for achieving intravenous access if acepromazine and dexmedetomidine are contraindicated due to cardiovascular compromise and avoiding ketamine is desirable (e.g. hypertrophic cardiomyopathy).
- Alfaxalone can be given in low doses intravenously to provide sedation for short procedures for cats and dogs.
- Sedation produced by alfaxalone, although dose-dependent, is significant, and the distinction between alfaxalone sedation and alfaxalone anaesthesia is minimal.

- Reducing noise and disturbances in the recovery area is recommended to facilitate a smooth recovery in animals that have been sedated with alfaxalone alone. Muscle twitching is sometimes seen during recovery after sedation with alfaxalone.
- It is good practice to have a laryngoscope and endotracheal tubes at hand in case rapid endotracheal intubation is required after sedation with alfaxalone.

Propofol

- Low doses of propofol administered intravenously can be used to provide sedation in cats and dogs for short procedures.
- Sedation produced by propofol, although dose-dependent, is significant, and the distinction between propofol sedation and propofol anaesthesia is minimal.
- It is good practice to have a laryngoscope and endotracheal tubes at hand in case rapid endotracheal intubation is required after sedation with propofol.

General recommendations to optimize pre-anaesthetic medication in cats and dogs

- Administer drugs at an appropriate time before induction of anaesthesia to synchronize peak sedation and analgesia with induction. Record the time of drug administration in the patient's record and consider redosing if induction of anaesthesia is delayed. This is particularly important for opioids; if the delay exceeds the duration of action of the opioid, redose to ensure adequate analgesia during the procedure.
- Calculate drug doses based on lean bodyweight to avoid overdose in obese patients. Cats and small dogs require larger doses to achieve adequate sedation relative to medium- and large-sized dogs. Dosing on the basis of body surface area prevents both over- and under-dosing in very large and very small patients. Dose conversion charts are available for alpha-2 adrenoceptor agonists. For other drugs, a practical approach is to use the upper end of a recommended dose range for dogs <5 kg bodyweight; conversely, for dogs over 40–45 kg bodyweight, use the lower end of the recommended dose range, or empirically calculate drug dose on a reduced bodyweight (e.g. calculate dose for a bodyweight of 50 kg in a 55 kg dog). In obese animals, estimate lean bodyweight and use the lean bodyweight to calculate drug doses.
- Combine drugs in the same syringe to limit patient handling and pain on injection (when given intramuscularly).
- More reliable sedation and analgesia can be achieved with intramuscular, rather than subcutaneous, injection. Use an appropriate gauge (23–25G) and length (1.6–3.8 cm) of needle depending on the size and body condition score of the animal.
- Consider intravenous administration if a catheter has been pre-placed. Give doses at the low end of the dose range when using the intravenous route. Intravenous administration may be advantageous in high-risk patients where constant observation and monitoring is required (and possible) after drug administration.
- Consider oxygen supplementation after pre-anaesthetic medication in animals with respiratory compromise (e.g. via oxygen tent, facemask).

- Ensure that the animal is kept in a quiet environment following drug administration. Ideally, place cats in dedicated rooms to reduce anxiety and fear and therefore improve the quality of sedation achieved from the drug combination. Darkening the environment can lead to improved sedation.
- Do not disturb the animal until sufficient time has elapsed for drugs to have reached their peak effect, but ensure that animals are observed (remotely) to allow prompt intervention if necessary (e.g. if respiratory obstruction occurs in a heavily sedated brachycephalic cat or dog).
- When the animal is sedated, ensure that it is handled gently and quietly during the procedure or induction of anaesthesia. This helps to prevent sudden arousal from sedation.
- Gently placing cotton wool in the external ear canal of sedated patients and covering the head with a towel/blanket reduces stimulation from environmental stimuli and can ensure that adequate sedation is maintained for a procedure to be carried out, without having to administer further drugs.
- Animals begin to lose heat as soon as they are sedated. Measures to maintain normothermia should therefore be implemented after drug administration (see Chapter 3).

Choosing the right drug combination for each patient

Factors that influence the choice of pre-anaesthetic medication or sedative drugs include:

- American Society of Anesthesiologists (ASA) physical status classification of the patient (see Chapter 2)
- Species and breed of the patient
- Temperament of the patient
- Age of the patient (paediatric, adult or geriatric)
- Reason for anaesthesia and procedure to be carried out
- Degree of pain expected from the procedure, or degree of preoperative pain.

The ASA status can be used as a basis from which protocols for pre-anaesthetic medication and sedation of animals can be introduced into a busy practice, while still taking the needs of individual patients into consideration. The following section describes pre-anaesthetic medication or sedation protocols that are suitable for dogs or cats of different ASA classification status (see also Figures 13.1 and 13.2). It is important to bear in mind that ASA status does not take into account factors such as the patient's age or body condition score and the procedure to be performed. These additional considerations should be mapped on to the guidelines given below and may alter drug selection in some circumstances.

Dogs
ASA 1

- **Combination of either acepromazine or dexmedetomidine with an opioid.** The choice of opioid is primarily determined by the need for intraoperative analgesia. Dexmedetomidine is a potent analgesic, so combining it with buprenorphine, a partial mu opioid receptor agonist, usually provides adequate supplementary intraoperative analgesia, unless very low doses of dexmedetomidine are used (1–3 µg/kg). Methadone or hydromorphone generally produces a greater level of sedation than buprenorphine, particularly when combined with acepromazine, and may therefore be chosen in patients that are very excitable and where moderate sedation is required to achieve intravenous access. The comparative properties of acepromazine and dexmedetomidine are shown in Figure 13.8.

ASA 2

- **Combination of acepromazine and an opioid.**
- **Dexmedetomidine combined with an opioid** is appropriate for some ASA 2 animals, depending on the underlying reason for this ASA classification (see under 'Patient selection' in alpha-2 adrenoceptor agonists section).

ASA 3

- **Acepromazine (low dose) and opioid combination** may be appropriate as long as there is no underlying cardiovascular disease or significant liver dysfunction.
- **Benzodiazepine and opioid combination** is useful for dogs with either cardiovascular disease or systemic abnormalities that affect cardiovascular function. Better sedation can be expected in animals showing more pronounced clinical signs of disease.

ASA 4

- **Benzodiazepine and opioid combination.**
- **Opioid alone** may be appropriate in some dogs, particularly if intravenous access is established. There may be less drug-sparing effect for both induction and maintenance agents compared with that provided by opioid and benzodiazepine combinations.

ASA 5

- **It is unlikely that sedation will be needed.** Low doses of opioids or benzodiazepines before anaesthesia are desirable to reduce anaesthetic doses needed for induction and maintenance of anaesthesia, and an opioid is necessary to provide analgesia before surgery or invasive procedures, but true pre-anaesthetic medication is not usually necessary in very sick patients.

Cats
ASA 1

- **Recommendations are as for dogs.** The profound sedation caused by dexmedetomidine can be advantageous in anxious and frightened cats, where intravenous access can be challenging unless good sedation is achieved. In feral or fear-aggressive cats, the addition of ketamine will ensure heavy sedation or even short-term general anaesthesia. The OTM route can be used for combinations of dexmedetomidine and buprenorphine (with or without ketamine), which can avoid the stress of handling for an intramuscular or subcutaneous injection. Intramuscular or subcutaneous alfaxalone can also be considered, particularly if the animal's health status cannot be determined accurately while fully conscious (e.g. young adult feral cats). Combine with an opioid when low doses of alfaxalone are administered, or if the procedure is expected to cause pain.

ASA 2

- **Recommendations are as for dogs.**

ASA 3

- **Acepromazine and opioid combination.** As with dogs, appropriateness of this combination will depend on evaluation of the cardiovascular system and liver function. The addition of a benzodiazepine to this combination can be helpful to increase sedation in cats that are anxious and frightened.

Characteristics	Acepromazine	Dexmedetomidine
Formulation	Available as 2 and 5 mg/ml solutions; accurate dosing is difficult in small patients unless solution is diluted	Available as a 500 µg/ml and a 100 µg/ml solution to facilitate accurate dosing in cats and dogs <20 kg
Mode of administration	Given as a single dose, repeated at 4–6 hour intervals	Given as a single dose or by constant rate infusion (CRI). In dogs, there is no accumulation over 24 hours when a 1 µg/kg/hour CRI of dexmedetomidine is given
Sedation	Dose-dependent, but less reliable than dexmedetomidine; improved by addition of an opioid	Dose-dependent, reliable sedation; improved by addition of an opioid
Analgesia	No analgesia	Good analgesia, but of short duration (dose-dependent, up to 1 hour)
Cardiovascular system	Vasodilation and possible hypotension, of minimal significance in healthy animals. Reduction in afterload as a result of vasodilation may be beneficial to cardiovascular function in some patients	Dose-dependent decrease in cardiac output that is of minimal significance in healthy animals (when doses up to 10 µg/kg are administered). Significantly reduced margin of safety for the cardiovascular system compared with acepromazine
Respiratory system	Minimal effect	Minimal effect
Drug-sparing effect	Limited (approximately 25%)	Potent drug-sparing effect; improved balanced anaesthesia
Background 'anaesthesia/analgesia'	Limited	Tends to prevent large swings in depth of anaesthesia in response to changing surgical stimulation
Body temperature	Rapid drop in body temperature due to peripheral vasodilation	Fall in body temperature is less rapid due to peripheral vasoconstriction
Reversibility	Not reversible. Length of action approximately 6 hours	Reversible with atipamezole

13.8 Comparison of the pharmacological characteristics of acepromazine and dexmedetomidine.

- **Benzodiazepine and opioid combination.** Unlike in dogs, this combination does not produce reliable sedation in adult cats when given intramuscularly. However, although some cats do not appear to be very well sedated with this combination, they may be remarkably tolerant of intravenous catheter placement.
- **Benzodiazepine and ketamine combination.** This is an alternative to the benzodiazepine/opioid protocol used in dogs. Low doses of ketamine (5 mg/kg) mixed in the same syringe as midazolam (0.3 mg/kg) and administered intramuscularly usually produce profound sedation, allowing easy intravenous access for induction of anaesthesia. Higher doses of ketamine (10 mg/kg i.m.) will produce anaesthesia, allowing intubation and a direct progression to maintenance of anaesthesia with an inhalant agent. Ketamine should be avoided in cats with hypertrophic cardiomyopathy because of its positive chronotropic effects (see Chapters 14 and 21). Pre-anaesthetic medication with ketamine will usually cause behavioural changes during recovery.
- **Alfaxalone** can be administered by the intramuscular or subcutaneous routes. It is advisable to combine alfaxalone with an opioid and/or midazolam to improve sedation when low doses of alfaxalone are administered and to improve the quality of recovery from anaesthesia. Inclusion of an opioid is particularly important if the procedure is expected to cause pain.

ASA 4

- **Benzodiazepine and ketamine combination.**
- **Benzodiazepine and opioid combination.**
- **Opioid alone.** In cats that have a quiet temperament, sedation with an opioid alone (e.g. buprenorphine or methadone) may be adequate to provide mild sedation. This can be useful in cats with hypertrophic cardiomyopathy where ketamine is contraindicated.

ASA 5

- **Recommendations are as for dogs.** Administration of a low dose of a benzodiazepine and an opioid close to the time of induction of anaesthesia will contribute to a balanced anaesthetic technique.

Other specific patient groups

Geriatric animals

Geriatric animals tend to have a higher incidence of concurrent disease than younger animals, which may increase the risk of anaesthesia and affect their ASA physical status classification (see Chapter 30). It is also likely that the normal organ reserve of geriatric animals is decreased compared with that of younger animals. This is particularly relevant for the cardiovascular system: although no abnormalities may be found on pre-anaesthetic examination, cardiovascular function may be decreased under stress, such as during anaesthesia. It is advisable to avoid routine administration of dexmedetomidine to geriatric patients because of this reduced cardiovascular reserve.

Young animals

Cats and dogs older than 12 weeks have normal liver function and can therefore be considered as adults in terms of anaesthetic drug metabolism. In younger patients with immature liver function, the effects of anaesthetic drugs may be prolonged. It is therefore advisable to avoid long-acting agents such as acepromazine in young patients.

There are limited data regarding the use of dexmedetomidine in very young cats and dogs. Medetomidine combined with ketamine, midazolam and buprenorphine has been used successfully for early neutering in kittens (Quad protocol, Joyce and Yates, 2011; see Figure 13.7), although combination with ketamine will counteract the tendency of medetomidine to reduce heart rate. An opioid and benzodiazepine combination can be used very effectively in puppies and kittens, which seem to be more susceptible to the sedative effects of these drugs than adults. An opioid (low dose) administered alone is also suitable, especially in sick animals where sedation will be more profound. (See also Chapter 30.)

Fractious animals

Appropriate drug combinations for sedation and pre-anaesthetic medication of fractious or fearful cats and dogs when intravenous access is not established are shown in Figure 13.9.

Cats: Cats can become fear aggressive in the veterinary practice, particularly if they have had previous negative experiences, such as pain, fear and anxiety associated with being placed in an environment that is noisy or where they have come into eye contact with other cats or dogs. Gentle handling of these cats is a prerequisite to being able to complete a clinical examination or obtain access for administration of sedative drugs. 'Scruffing' a cat to facilitate examination or injection is not recommended in any circumstances. The BSAVA Manual of Feline Practice provides good guidance on how to manage fear aggressive cats in the hospital environment. It is recommended to remove the cat from its basket/home pen and take it to a different quiet room (ideally a room that is used only for cats) for clinical examination and administration of drugs. This prevents the cat forming a negative association between its pen and stressful and painful interventions, and can contribute to the cat feeling less anxious in the ward environment. Following administration of a sedative the cat should be placed back into its basket/pen and left to become sedated, under close observation, with the basket remaining in a quiet undisturbed environment. Covering the cat basket with a towel or blanket can increase the efficacy of the sedative drugs. Care must be taken to ensure that the cat is frequently monitored as it becomes sedated, particularly for signs of vomiting that might lead to respiratory obstruction. Avoid frequently disturbing the cat until it has become sedated, as disturbances can reduce the efficacy of the sedative drugs. Once the cat is adequately sedated it is advisable to place an intravenous catheter immediately, with an extension set attached, so that intravenous access is established before the cat is moved. Should the cat awaken from sedation, further sedative drugs can then be administered intravenously if necessary.

Feral cats can be very challenging to handle and clinical examination before administration of any drugs is often not possible. Judicious use of a crush cage may be indicated to allow administration of drugs to these patients.

Dogs: Many aggressive dogs will allow placement of a muzzle to facilitate examination and handling, although for some animals the muzzle may need to be placed by the owner. However, it is important to be aware of the health and safety implications of asking an owner to place a muzzle on their own dog and to do this only if it is assessed to be safe. Some dogs are easier to handle when removed from their owner; in some circumstances it is therefore

Drug combination		Route of administration	Species	Patient selection
Drug 1	Drug 2			
Dexmedetomidine (10 µg/kg)	+ Butorphanol (0.4–0.5 mg/kg) + Methadone (0.4–0.5 mg/kg) + Hydromorphone (0.1–0.15 mg/kg)	i.m.	Cat and dog	This dose of dexmedetomidine will cause significant cardiovascular depression; best reserved for use in healthy animals (see Chapter 21 for details of use of dexmedetomidine in animals with cardiovascular system disease). Use methadone in animals undergoing painful interventions
Dexmedetomidine (20–40 µg/kg)	+ Buprenorphine (20 µg/kg) Use preservative-free preparation of buprenorphine	OTM	Cat	Use the higher dose of dexmedetomidine in feral cats; the lower dose will usually be sufficient in cats that are only very nervous
Ketamine (5 mg/kg)	+ Midazolam (0.3 mg/kg) and butorphanol (0.3 mg/kg) + Midazolam (0.3 mg/kg) and methadone (0.3 mg/kg) + Midazolam (0.3 mg/kg) and hydromorphone (0.1 mg/kg)	i.m.	Cat	Use methadone in animals undergoing painful interventions. May be a useful alternative to combinations with dexmedetomidine in animals that cannot be examined before drug administration and are of unknown health status. Avoid ketamine in cats with hypertrophic cardiomyopathy
Alfaxalone (2–3 mg/kg)	+ Midazolam (0.2–0.3 mg/kg) and methadone (0.3–0.4 mg/kg) + Midazolam (0.2–0.3 mg/kg) and hydromorphone (0.1 mg/kg) + Midazolam (0.2–0.3 mg/kg) and butorphanol (0.3–0.4 mg/kg)	i.m. or s.c. Use lower dose when administering i.m., use higher dose s.c.	Cat and dog	Volume required limits utility in most dogs. May be a useful combination in cats with hypertrophic cardiomyopathy that are unsuitable for either dexmedetomidine or ketamine administration
Acepromazine (0.1 mg/kg)	+ Midazolam (0.3 mg/kg) and methadone (0.5 mg/kg) + Midazolam (0.3 mg/kg) and hydromorphone (0.1 mg/kg)	i.m. or s.c.	Dog	Produces less reliable sedation than combinations incorporating dexmedetomidine
Sevoflurane		Administer via an induction chamber	Cat	Induction of anaesthesia using sevoflurane can be unpleasant for cats but this technique can be useful if i.m. drug administration proves impossible. Alternatively, it can be used to provide 'top-up' sedation to allow i.v. access in cats that are not adequately sedated after i.m. administration of sedative drugs

13.9 Drug combinations used for sedation and pre-anaesthetic medication of fractious or fearful cats and dogs when intravenous access is not established.

advisable to place a muzzle on the dog in a separate room that is quiet and undisturbed. Ensure that adequate help is available from trained staff to facilitate this process. Often the owner is well placed to report whether the dog is easier to handle when it is with the owner, or when it is on its own. Most dogs are amenable to clinical examination and injection of sedative drugs after placement of a muzzle.

Animals at risk of respiratory obstruction and brachycephalic breeds

Sedation caused by pre-anaesthetic drugs can exacerbate respiratory obstruction caused by anatomical conformation or by laryngeal paralysis, although sometimes this can be offset by the calming effect of sedatives leading to a more normal breathing pattern. These animals must be continuously observed and monitored for respiratory distress after pre-anaesthetic medication or sedation, and provision of supplemental oxygen is advisable. Acute and complete respiratory obstruction is an indication to proceed directly to general anaesthesia. In this situation, opioids and benzodiazepines can be given intravenously after induction of anaesthesia to provide a balanced anaesthetic technique.

Inadequate sedation

In situations where an animal's level of sedation is inadequate for the procedure or to allow intravenous access to be established, the answers to the following questions may be helpful in resolving the problem.

Question 1. Did the animal receive the correct dose of drug?

- Check drug dose: was an adequate dose given for the patient's bodyweight (taking into account allometric scaling)? This knowledge will guide whether a further dose of the same drug is indicated.
- Confirm that the total calculated dose was administered to the patient: it is possible that the total dose was not administered if the patient was difficult to handle during injection. This knowledge will guide whether a further dose of the same drug is indicated.

Question 2. Has there been an adequate waiting period after giving the drug?

- Check that adequate time has elapsed after drug administration: expect to wait up to 25 minutes with drug combinations containing either dexmedetomidine, benzodiazepines or alfaxalone given intramuscularly, or up to 45 minutes following acepromazine combinations given intramuscularly. Ensure the animal remains unstimulated in a quiet environment during this time before removing the patient from the cage/kennel.
- If the patient is obese and/or the drug could have been administered subcutaneously in error, more time will be required until maximum sedation is achieved.
- If too much time has elapsed since the drug was given, so that peak sedation has waned, a repeat dose of drug may be indicated.

Question 3. Is sedation sufficient?

- If yes, placement of an intravenous catheter and carrying out the procedure under general anaesthesia should be considered. Ensure owner consent for general anaesthesia rather than sedation has been obtained.

Options for patient management if intravenous access cannot be established

Consider giving a further dose of the same drug combination:

- Calculate this dose depending on the initial dose administered and the dose range given for the particular drugs in the combination. Be aware that giving multiple small incremental doses is less likely to produce good sedation than giving a single larger top-up dose.
- If the animal is very distressed or anxious, then a further dose of the same drug combination might not produce a deeper level of sedation. Consider postponing the procedure to another day (if possible, based on the animal's health status) and subsequently manage drug administration differently – for example, allow the animal to settle in a quiet environment before giving any drugs, or sedate with the owner present (dogs). Alternatively, choose a different drug combination or dose.

Administer a different drug to deepen sedation:

- Consider alfaxalone or ketamine in cats after prior administration of acepromazine or dexmedetomidine.
- 'Topping up' with a full mu opioid receptor agonist (e.g. methadone) can deepen sedation if butorphanol, pethidine (meperidine) or buprenorphine have been administered previously.
- Cats may be placed in a large induction chamber and anaesthesia induced using a volatile agent, preferably sevoflurane. It is advisable to allow time for the cat to settle in the chamber before starting administration of the volatile agent. Once the cat is anaesthetized, remove it from the chamber, place an endotracheal tube to allow maintenance of anaesthesia with the volatile agent and place an intravenous catheter.

Monitoring and support of the sedated patient

Most of the drugs used for sedation and pre-anaesthetic medication of cats and dogs are associated with varying degrees of cardiovascular and respiratory depression. As well as the direct effects of some drugs on the respiratory system, which may affect any patient, brachycephalic dogs and cats are predisposed to a degree of respiratory tract obstruction after sedation. Sedated animals can also easily become hypothermic due to decreased muscle activity and impairment of the thermoregulatory system. Although it is clear that adequate monitoring and support must be provided for sedated patients, the logistics of this can be difficult. Animals are usually placed in a kennel or cage following administration of sedative drugs, so supplemental oxygen may be difficult to administer. Animals that are being moved between a kennel and diagnostic areas can be difficult to keep warm unless intensive efforts are made such as the use of bubble wrap and bedding to insulate the patient combined with non-electronic heating devices such as wheat bags that have been heated in a microwave. Unless portable monitoring equipment is available, 'kennel-side' monitoring can be difficult. Monitoring and support of sedated patients should begin as early as possible and be continued until the patient is fully awake. The level of support and monitoring provided should be determined by the ASA status classification and breed of the patient and the reason for sedation/pre-anaesthetic medication.

Placement of an intravenous catheter (either before or after administration of sedative drugs) is recommended in all patients undergoing sedation/pre-anaesthetic medication, in order to allow prompt intervention should cardiovascular or respiratory compromise develop. This also provides direct access for intravenous administration of sedative/anaesthetic drugs should it be necessary to prolong sedation or proceed to anaesthesia. It is good practice to monitor and record patient parameters during sedation (in a similar fashion to an anaesthetic record) in order to document changes in cardiovascular and respiratory parameters and body temperature. The drug(s), dose and time of administration should also be recorded.

Monitoring

Monitoring is discussed in greater detail in Chapter 7. Aspects that are most relevant to the premedicated or sedated patient are outlined in the following section.

Depth of sedation/CNS depression

This is useful to assess whether the level of sedation is adequate for the procedure, and should be monitored intermittently throughout the period of sedation and recorded on the patient's record. The following can be assessed:

- Heart and respiratory rate
- Presence of an eyelid/blink reflex
- Response to toe pinch
- Response of the animal to arousal with voice or touch.

Be aware that animals sedated with dexmedetomidine or alfaxalone, particularly when either drug is administered alone, can sometimes show muscle twitching, which does not usually indicate inadequate sedation. In animals that have received dexmedetomidine a further dose of dexmedetomidine to increase the level of sedation rarely abolishes the muscle movements and is inappropriate. In these cases, stimulation of the patient should be reduced as much as possible (e.g. by placing cotton wool in the ears and covering the head with a towel). If the muscle movement is problematic, low-dose propofol or alfaxalone given intravenously can be considered. The administration of a low dose of midazolam (0.2 mg/kg i.v.) can stop muscle twitches in patients that have been sedated with alfaxalone.

Cardiovascular system

The degree of cardiovascular system monitoring will be determined by the cardiovascular status of the patient. Monitoring the pulse rate and pulse quality is mandatory in all animals. Pulse oximetry is useful to monitor oxygen saturation and a probe can easily be placed on the tongue in most lightly sedated animals; other suitable sites include the non-pigmented and hairless vulva or prepuce, the ear pinna or interdigital skin. Pulse oximetry can be unreliable with some monitors following administration of dexmedetomidine because of the peripheral vasoconstriction caused by this agent. Electrocardiographic monitoring is beneficial in higher-risk patients and patients with cardiovascular disease, particularly those with disturbances in heart rhythm.

Respiratory system

Observation of the rate and depth of breathing is mandatory in all sedated animals. In brachycephalic breeds, it is important that the head and neck are kept extended to prevent upper respiratory obstruction from the soft tissues. Placing animals in sternal recumbency also assists in maintenance of a clear airway and maximizes lung function. Monitoring airway gases (inspired and expired carbon dioxide and oxygen concentrations) is possible in animals that are not intubated, depending on the type of capnograph and oxygen monitoring equipment available. With sidestream capnography, the gas sampling tube can be placed in the nasal cavity of the animal; this allows reasonably accurate measurement of expired carbon dioxide concentration. Although severe respiratory depression is unusual after most sedation and pre-anaesthetic medication protocols, always have the means ready to induce anaesthesia and intubate a sedated patient to allow support of ventilation if necessary.

Body temperature

Monitoring body temperature is vital in order to support body temperature adequately in sedated patients. It is practical to use a rectal thermometer.

Blood glucose

It may be appropriate to monitor blood glucose in some patients that may be prone to hypoglycaemia. This is particularly the case for young puppies and kittens that have limited glucose reserves and are therefore at greater risk of hypoglycaemia during sedation and anaesthesia.

Supportive measures

Oxygen

Oxygen can easily be supplemented by using an anaesthetic breathing system and facemask placed on or near the nose of the animal. Pre-oxygenation before induction of anaesthesia will help to prevent hypoxaemia should a period of apnoea occur immediately after induction. Increasing the concentration of oxygen in the inspired gas mixture to >30% in sedated animals breathing room air will prevent hypoxaemia as a result of respiratory depression; ideally, this should be implemented during sedation of all patients. Alternative techniques to increase the inspired oxygen concentration are placing sedated animals in an oxygen cage or administration of oxygen through a nasal catheter. The oxygen cage can be useful for dyspnoeic cats after pre-anaesthetic medication and before induction of anaesthesia, or while an animal is recovering from the effects of sedation. Use of nasal catheters is appropriate for animals that require longer-term sedation and oxygen supplementation, although placement of a nasal catheter is often poorly tolerated by sedated patients.

Support of body temperature

Sedated animals quickly become hypothermic and so preventing a fall in body temperature is important. The following measures can be implemented to help maintain body temperature (see also Chapter 3):

- Ensure adequate ambient temperature
- Provide warm bedding in the kennel/cage of the animal and cover the patient with a blanket
- Ensure that the animal is not lying directly on a cold surface
- Wrap the animal in reflective foil or bubble wrap as insulation
- Place 'hot packs' or latex gloves filled with warm water ('hot hands') around the animal. Be aware that a sedated animal is unable to move away from a heat source that is too hot and capable of causing skin damage
- Use a forced warm air blanket.

Fluid therapy

Indications for fluid therapy during sedation will depend on the reason for sedation and the health status of the animal. It is important to remember that sedated animals are not capable of regulating their own fluid balance and therefore some animals will benefit from supportive fluid therapy. Examples include patients with chronic kidney disease and very young puppies and kittens, which may require support to maintain a normal blood glucose concentration. Higher-risk (ASA 3, 4 and 5) patients for anaesthesia will probably benefit from administration of fluids intraoperatively, and it is therefore good practice to place an intravenous catheter and begin fluid support early, at around the time of pre-anaesthetic medication. This will contribute to optimal stabilization of the patient before induction of anaesthesia.

Summary

Sedation and pre-anaesthetic medication are part of the daily routine in small animal practice. It is important to understand the pharmacology of the different drugs used so that the most appropriate combination for each individual patient can be chosen. Implementation of practice protocols based on ASA physical status classification can be helpful to improve uniformity in a busy clinic, while ensuring that the requirements of individual patients are met. Monitoring and support of sedated patients should be initiated early, and the intensity of this 'peri-anaesthetic' support should be adjusted to the ASA status of the patient and the procedure to be carried out.

References and further reading

Alibhai HI, Clarke KW, Lee YH et al. (1996) Cardiopulmonary effects of combinations of medetomidine hydrochloride and atropine sulphate in dogs. Veterinary Record 138, 11–12

Alvaides RK, Neto FJ, Aguiar AJ et al. (2008) Sedative and cardiorespiratory effects of acepromazine or atropine given before dexmedetomidine in dogs. Veterinary Record 162, 852–856

Brodbelt DC, Blissitt KJ, Hammond RA et al. (2008) The risk of death: the Confidential Enquiry into Perioperative Small Animal Fatalities. Veterinary Anaesthesia and Analgesia 35, 365–373

Clarke KW, Trim CM and Hall LW (2014) Principles of sedation, anticholinergic agents, and principles of premedication. In: Veterinary Anaesthesia, 11th edn, ed. KW Clarke et al., pp. 79–97. W.B. Saunders, London

Drynan EA, Gray P and Raisis AL (2012) Incidence of seizures associated with the use of acepromazine in dogs undergoing myelography. *Journal of Veterinary Emergency and Critical Care* **22**, 262–266

Dugdale A (2010) Small animal sedation and premedication. In: *Veterinary Anaesthesia Principles to Practice, 1st edn*, ed. A Dugdale, pp. 30–45. Wiley-Blackwell, Oxford

Harvey A and Tasker S (2013) *BSAVA Manual of Feline Practice: A Foundation Manual* BSAVA Publications, Gloucester

Honkavaara JM, Restitutti F, Raekallio MR *et al.* (2010) The effects of increasing doses of MK-467, a peripheral alpha₂-adrenergic receptor antagonist, on the cardiopulmonary effects of dexmedetomidine in conscious dogs. *Journal of Veterinary Pharmacology and Therapeutics* **34**, 332–337

Hunt JR, Grint NJ, Taylor PM *et al.* (2013) Sedative and analgesic effects of buprenorphine, combined with either acepromazine or dexmedetomidine, for premedication prior to elective surgery in cats and dogs. *Veterinary Anaesthesia and Analgesia* **40**, 297–307

Hunyady KG and Johnson RA (2006) Anesthesia case of the month. *Journal of the American Veterinary Medical Association* **229**, 1250–1253

Ilkiw JE, Suter CM, Farver TB *et al.* (1996) The behaviour of healthy awake cats following intravenous and intramuscular administration of midazolam. *Journal of Veterinary Pharmacology and Therapeutics* **19**, 205–216

Joyce A and Yates D (2011) Help stop teenage pregnancy! Early-age neutering in cats. *Journal of Feline Medicine and Surgery* **13**, 3–10

Katz J, Clarke H and Seltzer S (2011) Preventive analgesia: quo vadimus? *Anaesthesia and Analgesia* **113**, 1242–1253

Kaul CL and Grewal RS (1970) Is epinephrine reversal a phenomenon purely of α-adrenergic block? *Archives Internationales de Pharmacodynamie et de Therapie* **186**, 363–378

Kuusela E, Raekallio M, Anttila M *et al.* (2000) Clinical effects and pharmacokinetics of medetomidine and its enantiomers in dogs. *Journal of Veterinary Pharmacology and Therapeutics* **23**, 15–20

Lamata C, Loughton V, Jones M *et al.* (2012) The risk of passive regurgitation during general anaesthesia in a population of referred dogs in the UK. *Veterinary Anaesthesia and Analgesia* **39**, 266–274

Murrell JC and Hellebrekers LJ (2005) Medetomidine and dexmedetomidine: a review of cardiovascular and antinociceptive effects in the dog. *Veterinary Anaesthesia and Analgesia* **32**, 117–127

Mutoh T, Nishimura R and Sasaki N (2002) Effects of medetomidine-midazolam, midazolambutorphanol, or acepromazine-butorphanol as premedicants for mask induction of anesthesia with sevoflurane in dogs. *American Journal of Veterinary Research* **63**, 1022–1028

Nickerson M, Henry JW and Nomaguchi GM (1953) Blockade of responses to epinephrine and norepinephrine by dibenamine congeners. *Journal of Pharmacology and Experimental Therapeutics* **107**, 300–309

Pypendop BH and Verstegen JP (1998) Hemodynamic effects of medetomidine in the dog: a dose titration study. *Veterinary Surgery* **27**, 612–622

Pypendop BH and Verstegen JP (1999) Cardiorespiratory effects of a combination of medetomidine, midazolam, and butorphanol in dogs. *American Journal of Veterinary Research* **60**, 1148–1154

Ramoo S, Bradbury LA, Anderson GA *et al.* (2013) Sedation of hyperthyroid cats with subcutaneous administration of a combination of alfaxalone and butorphanol. *Australian Veterinary Journal* **91**, 131–136

Rauser P, Pfeifr J, Proks P *et al.* (2012) Effect of medetomidine-butorphanol and dexmedetomidine-butorphanol combinations on intraocular pressure in healthy dogs. *Veterinary Anaesthesia and Analgesia* **39**, 301–305

Ribas T, Bublot I, Junot S *et al.* (2015) Effects of intramuscular sedation with alfaxalone and butorphanol on echocardiographic measurements in healthy cats. *Journal of Feline Medicine and Surgery* **17**, 530–536

Rishniw M, Tobias AH and Slinker BK (1996) Characterization of chronotropic and dysrhythmogenic effects of atropine in dogs with bradycardia. *American Journal of Veterinary Research* **57**, 337–341

Robinson KJ, Jones RS and Cripps PJ (2001) Effects of medetomidine and buprenorphine administered for sedation in dogs. *Journal of Small Animal Practice* **42**, 444–447

Santos LC, Ludders JW, Erb HN *et al.* (2010) Sedative and cardiorespiratory effects of dexmedetomidine and buprenorphine administered to cats via the oral transmucosal or intramuscular routes. *Veterinary Anaesthesia and Analgesia* **37**, 417–424

Sinclair MD and Dyson DH (2012) The impact of acepromazine on the efficacy of crystalloid, dextran or ephedrine treatment in hypotensive dogs under isoflurane anesthesia. *Veterinary Anaesthesia and Analgesia* **39**, 563–573

Thurmon JC, Tranquilli WJ and Benson GJ (2007) *Lumb & Jones' Veterinary Anaesthesia, 4th edn*. Williams and Wilkins, Baltimore

Valverde A, Cantwell S, Hernandez J *et al.* (2004) Effects of acepromazine on the incidence of vomiting associated with opioid administration in dogs. *Veterinary Anaesthesia and Analgesia* **31**, 102–108

Wilson DV, Evans AT, Carpenter RE *et al.* (2004) The effect of four anaesthetic protocols on splenic size in dogs. *Veterinary Anaesthesia and Analgesia* **31**, 40–45

Chapter 14

Injectable anaesthetics

Sabine B.R. Kästner

Injectable anaesthetics are used either for induction of anaesthesia followed by maintenance with an inhalational anaesthetic agent, or as the sole agent to induce and maintain general anaesthesia. For minor procedures of short duration, a single injection will suffice. Repeated boluses or infusion of an anaesthetic in conjunction with analgesics defines total intravenous anaesthesia (TIVA). Infusion of certain anaesthetics can also be used to control seizures and muscle spasm (e.g. tetanus, status epilepticus) or to provide long-term sedation in intensive care units. For some injectable anaesthetics, there is a dose-dependent transition from sedation to general anaesthesia. Dose rates required for induction and maintenance of anaesthesia depend on the pre-anaesthetic medication given and the individual patient's sensitivity. Slow, incremental dosing of the calculated amount of anaesthetic is therefore recommended to prevent overdosing. For proper administration of potent anaesthetics, it is crucial to choose an appropriately sized syringe; placing small volumes in a large syringe inevitably leads to overdosing. In cats, syringe size rarely needs to exceed 1–2 ml. In the case of very potent, highly concentrated drugs, prior dilution with saline (e.g. 1:10) will improve accuracy of dosing.

Venous access

Secure venous access is necessary for careful and effective administration of anaesthetics. Proper pre-anaesthetic medication and handling usually allows placement of an intravenous catheter without forceful restraint in the majority of cats and dogs.

Catheter site

Accessible veins in the cat and the dog are the cephalic vein on the dorsomedial aspect of the forelimb, and the lateral saphenous vein running across the lateral aspect of the hindlimb above the hock. Catheter fixation can be more difficult on the hindlimbs. In cats, the medial saphenous vein on the medial aspect of the hindlimb is easily localized. In dogs with large, pendulous ears, the auricular veins (Figure 14.1) might be an option for catheterization. For prolonged placement of long venous catheters (central venous catheters) or in very small animals, the external jugular vein can be used.

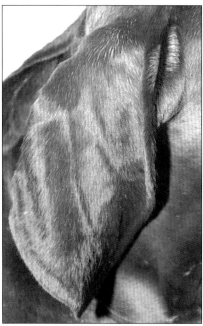

14.1 Marginal auricular veins, such as those observed in this German Shorthaired Pointer, may be suitable for venous catheterization. Avoid the artery which generally courses along the middle portion of the ear pinna.

Catheter types

Various indwelling catheters inserted using an 'over-the-needle' technique are suitable for the peripheral veins; the choice depends on patient size, intended duration of catheter placement and personal preference (Figure 14.2). Because of the flexibility of the neck, short catheters can be easily dislodged from the external jugular vein, and a length of at least 6 cm is required to reduce the risk of this happening. Conventional 'over-the-needle' catheters of this length can be difficult to introduce in the neck area; a Seldinger technique using a guide wire and dilator might be necessary for insertion of a jugular catheter. Commercial catheter kits are available for placement of central venous catheters intended for long-term use.

In well hydrated animals, percutaneous placement of peripheral catheters is possible. In older uncastrated male cats, and dog breeds with very thick skin, initial perforation of the skin with a hypodermic needle is advisable to avoid damage to the catheter tip or kinking of the catheter. In very small animals or in dehydrated, hypovolaemic patients, a cut-down to the vein with prior subcutaneous local anaesthesia might be necessary, or ultrasonography by a skilled operator can be used to locate blood vessels.

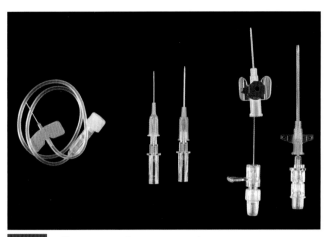

14.2 Different types of intravenous catheters.

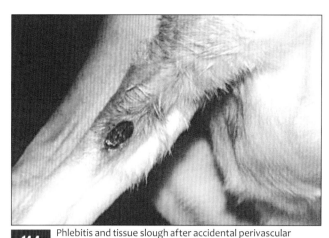

14.4 Phlebitis and tissue slough after accidental perivascular injection of 5% thiopental in a dog.
(Courtesy of Tanya Duke-Novakovski, Western College of Veterinary Medicine, University of Saskatchewan, Canada)

Preparation

Preparation of the catheter area depends on the type of catheter used and intended duration of catheter placement. The hair should be clipped over a sufficiently wide area around the vessel to be catheterized to avoid inadvertent contamination of the catheter during insertion. The clipped area should be prepared with an antiseptic solution (1–2% iodine tincture, iodophors, chlorhexidine or 70% alcohol). When using a cut-down technique or inserting long catheters using guide wires, surgical draping of the area and sterile gloves must be used to avoid contamination. After placement (Figure 14.3a), the catheter is fixed by tape and a covering bandage (Figure 14.3bc) or sutured to the skin. The catheter is flushed with plain saline or heparinized saline (1–2 units heparin/ml) and either capped or attached to a T-connector, or an intravenous fluid infusion immediately instituted to avoid the catheter becoming blocked. To prevent accidental dislodgement of the catheter, the infusion line should also be fixed to the animal's body. For provision of unrestricted access to the vein with concurrent fluid administration, different catheter types with side ports and connecting pieces for multiple infusions are available.

Accidental perivascular injection

Accidental perivascular injection of highly irritant drugs such as thiopental (>2.5% solution) leads to cellulitis, phlebitis or tissue sloughing (Figure 14.4). Immediate infiltration of the

affected area with normal saline will dilute the drug and help to prevent tissue necrosis. Using 2% lidocaine instead of normal saline can neutralize the pH (especially after thiopental), prevent vasospasm, and reduce inflammation and pain. Topical treatment with an ointment dressing containing heparin or an anti-inflammatory drug, in conjunction with systemic therapy using a non-steroidal anti-inflammatory drug, further reduces tissue inflammation.

Anaesthetics

A comparison of the physicochemical and clinical properties of commonly used injectable anaesthetics is given in Figures 14.5 and 14.6.

Barbiturates

Short-acting barbiturates such as thiopental and methohexital have been the 'classic' injectable anaesthetics used in veterinary medicine for several decades. However, with the development of anaesthetic molecules with a better safety index and a better pharmacokinetic profile (i.e. less accumulation), use of barbiturates has dramatically reduced. Barbiturates produce hypnosis with minimal analgesia, and high doses are required to produce surgical anaesthesia when used as the sole anaesthetic agent. Longer-acting barbiturates such as phenobarbital

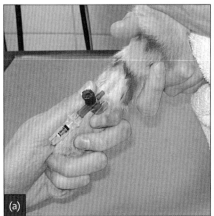
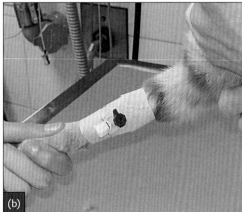
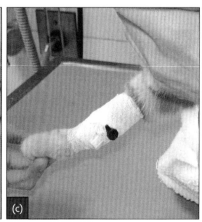

14.3 (a) Insertion of an intravenous catheter into the cephalic vein in a cat. (b) Fixation of the catheter to the limb with tape. (c) An elastic bandage is then applied to cover the tape.

Drug concentration	Physicochemical properties	Induction/recovery	Haemodynamic effects	Respiratory effects	CNS effects	Other
Thiopental 1% (w/v) 2.5% (w/v)	Yellow crystalline powder Solution pH 11–14 Irritating, precipitates with many acidic drugs	Rapid (30 seconds) and smooth induction; not suitable for repeated dosing	HR ↑↑ Tachyarrhythmia MAP ↓ CO ↓↔ SVR ↔	RR ↓ Vt ↓ Apnoea after rapid injection	Cerebral depression Cerebral metabolism ↓ ICP ↓ CBF ↓	IOP ↓ Poor analgesia
Propofol 1% (w/v)	White emulsion pH ~7 Promotes bacterial growth	Smooth induction and recovery, excitatory signs can occur during induction and recovery	HR ↓↑ MAP ↓↓ CO ↓ SVR ↓↓	RR ↓ Vt ↓ Apnoea after rapid injection	Cerebral metabolism ↓ ICP ↓ CBF ↓	IOP ↓ Poor analgesia
Etomidate 0.2% (w/v)	Propylene glycol preparation is hyperosmolar (4640 mOsm/l) White emulsion Promotes bacterial growth	Myoclonus without pre-anaesthetic medication	HR ↔ MAP ↔ ↓ CO ↔ ↓ SVR ↔	RR ↑ Vt ↓ Depression with high doses	Cerebral depression ICP ↓ CBF ↓ CPP ↔	IOP ↓ Adrenal suppression Poor analgesia
Ketamine 1% (w/v) 5% (w/v) 10% (w/v)	Clear, stable solution pH 3.5–5.5	Increased muscle tone, spasms, seizures, excitatory recovery without pre-anaesthetic medication	HR ↑↑ MAP ↑↑ CO ↑ SVR ↔	Apneustic, irregular breathing Apnoea with high doses	Stimulation Cerebral metabolism ↑↑ ICP ↑↑ CBF ↑↑	IOP ↑ Somatic analgesia NMDA receptor antagonist
Ketamine 1–10% (w/v) with either: diazepam 0.5% (w/v) or midazolam 0.5% (w/v)	Mixed immediately before use. Check pharmaceutical compatibility before mixing	Smooth induction Excitatory recovery	HR ↑ MAP ↑ CO ↑ ↔ SVR ↔	Apneustic, irregular breathing More depression than with ketamine alone Apnoea with high doses	Stimulation Cerebral metabolism ↑ ICP ↑ CBF ↑	Somatic analgesia NMDA receptor antagonist
Tiletamine–zolazepam 250 mg/250 mg	Lyophilized powder Solution pH 2–3.5 1:1 mixture	Smooth induction Excitatory recovery, mainly in dogs	HR ↑ ↔ MAP ↑↓ CO ↑ ↔ ↓ SVR ↑ ↔	RR ↓ Vt ↓ Depression with high doses	Stimulation Cerebral metabolism ↑ ICP ↑ CBF ↑	IOP ↑ Somatic analgesia
Alfaxalone 1% (w/v)	Clear stable solution, contains 2-hydroxypropyl-beta cyclodextrin as solubilizer pH ~7	Smooth induction, excitatory signs can occur during recovery	HR ↔ ↑↑ MAP ↓ CO ↓ SVR ↓	RR ↔ ↓ Vt ↓ Apnoea after rapid injection	Cerebral depression	Poor analgesia

14.5 Comparison of some properties of commonly used intravenous anaesthetics. ↑ = mild increase; ↑↑ = moderate increase; ↓ = mild decrease; ↓↓ = moderate decrease; ↔ = no change; CBF = cerebral blood flow; CNS = central nervous system; CO = cardiac output; CPP = cerebral perfusion pressure; HR = heart rate; ICP = intracranial pressure; IOP = intraocular pressure; MAP = mean arterial blood pressure; NMDA = N-methyl D-aspartate; RR = respiratory rate; SVR = systemic vascular resistance; Vt = tidal volume.

Drug	Species	Elimination half-life (minutes)	Total body clearance (Cl_B) (ml/kg/min)	Volume of distribution (Vd_{ss}; Vc) (l/kg)	Reference
Thiopental	Dog Cat	182.4	3.4	0.81 (Vc 0.038)	Ilkiw et al., 1991
Propofol	Dog Cat	90 322 55	58.6 50.1	4.9 6.5 1.3	Nolan et al., 1993 Nolan and Reid, 1993 Adam et al., 1980
Etomidate	Dog Cat	86.4 59.66 173.4	40.1 41.2	Vc 0.108 4.88 (Vc 1.17)	Zhang et al., 1998 McIntosh et al., 2004 Wertz et al., 1990
Ketamine	Dog Cat	61 78.66	39.5 21.33	1.95 2.12	Kaka and Hayton, 1980 Hanna et al., 1988
Alfaxalone	Dog Cat	25–35 52–74	52.9–59.4 14.8–25.1	2.4–2.9 0.325–0.589	Ferré et al., 2006 Heit et al., 2004

14.6 Pharmacokinetic variables of commonly used intravenous anaesthetics (see also Figure 14.12). Vc = volume of the central compartment; Vd_{ss} = volume of distribution at steady state.

and pentobarbital are not used for anaesthesia but may be used for their anticonvulsant and sedative properties. Only the use of thiopental as an anaesthetic agent will be discussed here.

The principal effect of barbiturates is depression of the central nervous system (CNS) by enhancing inhibitory pathways and suppressing excitation at the level of synaptic neurotransmission, mainly by interaction with the gamma-aminobutyric acid (GABA$_A$) receptor. Rapidity of action and dose requirements depend on the amount of the unbound and unionized form of the drug in the bloodstream, because only this form can penetrate cell membranes and enter the CNS. Both a decrease in blood pH and hypoproteinaemia can increase the percentage of free and unionized (active) drug, which means that dose requirements can be dramatically decreased in severely debilitated patients.

Thiopental

Physicochemical properties: Thiopental is a thiobarbiturate. It is a weak organic acid provided as a sodium salt (yellow crystalline powder) in sealed vials. Anhydrous sodium carbonate is added to prevent precipitation of the free acid with atmospheric carbon dioxide. After the powder is reconstituted with sterile water, the solution is very alkaline (pH in the range of 11–14), which makes it extremely irritant at concentrations greater than 2.5%. Reduction of alkalinity of the solution results in precipitation of the free acid. As a result, thiopental does not dissolve well in saline or Ringer's solution and it precipitates with many other acidic drugs. Care must therefore be taken to avoid occlusion of the intravenous line by precipitated thiopental. The prepared solution should be tightly capped so as not to expose it to air, and refrigerated at 5–6°C to prolong shelf-life (approximately 1 week). When the solution becomes turbid, it loses activity and must be discarded.

Clinical properties: Thiopental causes rapid loss of consciousness (approximately 30 seconds) after intravenous injection. The time to onset of action is influenced by the circulation time to the brain, which might be prolonged by sedation (especially with alpha-2 adrenoceptor agonists).

Thiopental is classified as an ultra-short-acting barbiturate and recovery is fast (10–15 minutes) after a single injection. Recovery after a single injection is mainly governed by redistribution of the drug from the bloodstream to other tissues. Initially, well perfused tissues (brain, heart, kidneys) will take up the drug, resulting in a rapid decline in plasma concentration after a single thiopental bolus. A further decrease in plasma thiopental concentration occurs when moderately perfused tissues, such as muscle, take up the drug. At that time, brain concentration begins to fall and recovery occurs. Poorly perfused tissue, such as body fat, will take up thiopental slowly; however, adipose tissue has a high 'storage' capacity for lipid-soluble drugs such as thiopental. Repeated doses of thiopental will lead to an accumulation of the drug, because tissue sites become saturated and liver metabolism is slow. Successive doses lead to a progressive increase in anaesthesia time. Therefore, thiopental is unsuitable for maintenance of anaesthesia as accumulation can lead to serious cardiorespiratory depression and delayed recovery.

Thiopental induces respiratory depression, and induction apnoea commonly occurs after rapid intravenous injection. Thiopental causes dose- and rate-dependent cardiovascular depression (more likely with a high plasma concentration after rapid injection). Peripheral vasodilation and reduction in cardiac output from direct myocardial depression results in hypotension. Tachyarrhythmias (e.g. premature ventricular contractions, transient bigeminy, ventricular tachycardia) are also possible, but usually do not require treatment. In response to hypotension, an increased heart rate helps to maintain cardiac output. Drugs used concurrently (sedatives, opioids) and the animal's body condition will influence the overall effects.

Thiopental should not be used in Greyhounds and other sighthounds. In these breeds, the body disposition (low body fat) and decreased liver metabolism can lead to very high plasma concentrations of thiopental, which can cause severe cardiovascular depression and prolonged recovery. Alternative induction agents (e.g. propofol, alfaxalone, ketamine–benzodiazepine) should be used in sighthounds.

Thiopental reduces the metabolic rate and oxygen requirements of the brain by depressing cellular activity. With the reduction in metabolic demand, a parallel reduction in cerebral blood flow and intracranial pressure (ICP) occurs. A reduction in ICP is desirable for example in patients with head trauma or intracranial tumours (see Chapter 28).

Practical use:
- Use as induction agent or as sole anaesthetic agent for very short procedures only.
- Prepare 1–2.5% solution for small animals (as dilute as possible; consider reasonable injection volume).
- Discard turbid solution.
- Should be administered through an intravenous catheter (perivascular injection leads to tissue necrosis). Flush catheter before and after administration.
- Give to effect (Figures 14.7 and 14.8):
  - Consider pre-anaesthetic medication
  - Consider physical status of the animal
  - Give by slow injection (30–60 seconds)
  - Give half of the calculated dose and await maximum effect, then proceed further with increments until desired effect is achieved (e.g. endotracheal intubation)
  - Decreased blood pH (e.g. azotaemia) and hypoproteinaemia reduce required dose.
- Avoid in severely hypovolaemic patients.
- Avoid in patients with cardiac arrhythmias.
- Poor analgesia (use with analgesic).
- Not the best drug for induction of anaesthesia for Caesarean section (see Chapter 26).
- Not recommended for Greyhounds and other sighthounds.

Non-barbiturates

Propofol

Physicochemical properties: Propofol is a hypnotic alkyl phenol (2,6-diisopropylphenol) with a molecular weight of 178.27 and occurs as an oil at room temperature. It is insoluble in aqueous solutions but highly lipid soluble. To allow intravenous injection, propofol is currently formulated as a white oil-in-water macroemulsion containing Intralipid (1% w/v soya bean oil, 1.2% w/v purified egg phosphatide, 2.25% w/v glycerol). The formulation has a pH of 7 and is a slightly viscous, milky white liquid. Products intended for veterinary use are usually formulated at a concentration of 1% (w/v) but a 2% (w/v) formulation is available as a human medical product.

Drug	Pre-anaesthetic medication	Dose	Comment
Thiopental	– +	20–25 mg/kg i.v. 8–12.5 mg/kg i.v.	Give to effect
Propofol	– +	6–8 mg/kg i.v. 2–4 mg/kg i.v.	Give to effect
Etomidate	– +	1–3 mg/kg i.v. 0.5–2 mg/kg i.v.	High incidence of myoclonus without pre-anaesthetic medication
Ketamine	+ +	2–5 mg/kg i.v. 5–10 mg/kg i.m.	Always with pre-anaesthetic medication Administer i.m. only in very uncooperative dogs
Ketamine and diazepam Ketamine and diazepam Ketamine and midazolam	± ± ±	5 mg/kg i.v. 0.25 mg/kg i.v. 5 mg/kg i.v. 0.5 mg/kg i.v. 5 mg/kg i.v. 0.25 mg/kg i.v.	Mix ketamine (10%) and diazepam (0.5%) at 1:1 (v:v); give 0.05–0.1 ml/kg of this mixture in increments to effect. Lower dose suitable for dogs with gastric dilatation-volvulus Mix ketamine (10%) with midazolam (0.5%) at 1:1 (v/v); give 0.05–0.1 ml/kg of this mixture in increments to effect
Tiletamine–zolazepam	– +	5 mg/kg i.v. 1–2 mg/kg i.v. 4–8 mg/kg i.m.	
Alfaxalone	– +	3 mg/kg i.v. 2 mg/kg i.v.	Give to effect

14.7 Anaesthesia induction doses in the dog. Note that induction doses can vary with type and dose of pre-anaesthetic medication: xylazine and (dex)medetomidine and high-dose opioid pre-anaesthetic medication reduce induction doses by 50–80%. – = without pre-anaesthetic medication; + = with pre-anaesthetic medication.

Drug	Pre-anaesthetic medication	Dose	Comment
Thiopental	– +	10 mg/kg i.v. 2–10 mg/kg i.v.	Give to effect
Propofol	– +	4–8 mg/kg i.v. 4–6 mg/kg i.v.	Give to effect
Etomidate	– +	1–3 mg/kg i.v. 0.5–2 mg/kg i.v.	High incidence of myoclonus without pre-anaesthetic medication
Ketamine	+ +	2–10 mg/kg i.v. 10–20 mg/kg i.m.	Always with pre-anaesthetic medication
Ketamine and diazepam Ketamine and diazepam Ketamine and midazolam	± ± ±	5 mg/kg i.v. 0.25 mg/kg i.v. 5 mg/kg i.v. 0.5 mg/kg i.v. 5 mg/kg i.v. 0.25 mg/kg i.v.	Mix ketamine (10%) and diazepam (0.5%) at 1:1 (v:v); give 0.05–0.1 ml/kg of this mixture in increments to effect Mix ketamine (10%) with midazolam (0.5%) at 1:1 (v/v); give 0.05–0.1 ml/kg of this mixture in increments to effect
Tiletamine–zolazepam	– +	4–5 mg/kg i.v. 1–2 mg/kg i.v. 4–8 mg/kg i.m.	
Alfaxalone	– +	5 mg/kg i.v. 2–3 mg/kg i.v.	Give to effect

14.8 Anaesthesia induction doses in the cat. Note that induction doses can vary with type and dose of pre-anaesthetic medication: xylazine and (dex)medetomidine and high-dose opioid pre-anaesthetic medication reduce induction doses significantly (50–80%). – = Without pre-anaesthetic medication; + = With pre-anaesthetic medication.

The emulsion is an ideal culture medium for bacteria and promotes exponential bacterial growth; because of this, open vials should be used within 24 hours. Aseptic handling of multiple-use vials is essential to avoid contamination. A propofol formulation with a longer broached shelf-life (28 days), PropoFlo Plus™ (PropoFlo 28™ in the USA) or PropoVet™ Multidose, is available. It contains benzyl alcohol (20 mg/ml) as a bacteriostatic preservative. It is licensed for anaesthetic induction and short-term anaesthesia in dogs (and also cats in the UK), but not for prolonged TIVA because the benzyl alcohol may produce toxicity.

Intramuscular injection of propofol does not induce anaesthesia at reasonable dose rates, but inadvertent perivascular injection is non-irritating. Propofol is compatible with 5% dextrose in water if a dilute solution is required, but care has to be taken not to disrupt the emulsion.

Clinical properties: Propofol is primarily a hypnotic agent with a rapid onset (60–90 seconds) and short duration of action after a single dose (approximately 10 minutes). The hypnotic action is mainly mediated by interaction with the $GABA_A$ receptor subunit, potentiating the GABA-induced chloride current.

The half-life of equilibration of propofol between CNS effects and plasma concentration is approximately 2 minutes. Therefore, an injection time of 2 minutes is recommended for administration of induction doses to enable titration to effect and to avoid overdose and apnoea. In dogs, pre-anaesthetic medication with acepromazine reduces the induction dose of propofol; in contrast, such a dose reduction after acepromazine is not observed in cats. However, alpha-2 adrenoceptor agonists with or without opioids reduce propofol requirements significantly in both cats and dogs, and induction doses need to be adjusted in patients that have received these drugs as premedicants.

The pharmacokinetic properties of propofol (see Figure 14.6) contribute to its clinical advantages. After a single bolus injection, blood concentration of propofol decreases rapidly due to redistribution of the drug to highly perfused tissues. After the initial rapid distribution phase, propofol is rapidly metabolized, and further slow distribution to fat occurs. This is followed by prolonged terminal elimination, which reflects slow release from fat, although this has little effect on clinical recovery from anaesthesia. Clearance rates exceed hepatic blood flow, indicating that extra-hepatic metabolism occurs. A high first-pass extraction of propofol in the lung has been demonstrated (Matot et al., 1993). Propofol is metabolized to sulphate and glucuronide conjugates, which are inactive; the conjugates are mainly excreted via the urine. Hepatic and renal disease do not appear to influence propofol pharmacokinetics. In dogs, pre-anaesthetic medication with medetomidine or maintenance of anaesthesia with halothane and nitrous oxide does not alter propofol kinetics to a significant extent (Nolan et al., 1993). In dogs, the propofol doses required to induce anaesthesia seem to decrease with age (Reid and Nolan, 1996).

The rapid metabolism of propofol results in minimal accumulation of the drug after repeated doses. This makes propofol suitable for administration by infusion for maintenance of anaesthesia (i.e. TIVA), with excellent results in dogs. Propofol can still be used in Greyhounds for induction even though recovery can be prolonged after a continuous propofol infusion because of their higher proportion of lean body mass to fat and lower microsomal activity compared with other dog breeds. Cats have a comparatively low capacity for glucuronide conjugation, which is required for metabolism of phenolic compounds. This leads to accumulation of propofol and prolonged recoveries in cats after propofol infusions (TIVA) that last longer than 30 minutes. Infusion times should therefore be limited (Pascoe et al., 2006a). In addition, a propofol infusion lasting more than 30 minutes in cats leads to clinically significant reductions in packed cell volume. Therefore, propofol TIVA in cats should be kept at as low a dose and of as short a duration as possible. In addition, feline haemoglobin is prone to oxidative injury by phenolic compounds. Repeated propofol anaesthesia (more than 3 days consecutively) results in significant Heinz body formation, anorexia, diarrhoea, facial oedema, depression and delayed recovery from anaesthesia (Andress et al., 1995). However, repeated very low doses of propofol for short-term immobilization of cats for radiation therapy were well tolerated (Bley et al., 2007).

The most prominent haemodynamic effect is moderate hypotension due to reductions in cardiac output and systemic vascular resistance, which can become severe in hypovolaemic patients or animals with a low cardiac reserve. Hypotension is most severe 2 minutes after an induction dose of propofol and after rapid injection, and heart rate does not increase in response to hypotension as it does with thiopental. In patients with pre-existing bradycardia (e.g. sick sinus syndrome), refractory bradycardia or asystole can occur. Bradycardia can be severe if a high dose of an opioid is combined with propofol, although severe bradycardia can be prevented by prior administration of an anticholinergic drug. Rapid injection of propofol can result in apnoea, and so equipment for endotracheal intubation should be readily available when administering this drug. Desaturation of haemoglobin, with cyanotic mucous membranes, is often observed after propofol induction.

Respiratory depression with hypercapnia and a decrease in arterial oxygen saturation also occurs after repeated or continuous propofol dosing without apnoea; therefore, oxygen supplementation and availability of equipment for endotracheal intubation is always recommended during prolonged propofol administration, even at very low doses. Surgical anaesthesia with a combination of propofol and a potent opioid very often requires the lungs to be ventilated.

Propofol has both proconvulsant and anticonvulsant properties, mediated by different mechanisms. Propofol has been used successfully for seizure control (Figure 14.9), but paradoxically, excitatory signs such as myoclonus, paddling, opisthotonos and nystagmus can occur during a slow induction period, and to a lesser extent during recovery. Pre-anaesthetic medication reduces the incidence of excitatory signs but cannot completely prevent them. In most cases, excitatory signs cease when administration of inhalational anaesthetics is commenced. Refractory excitations have been treated successfully with ketamine (1 mg/kg i.v.), diazepam (0.2 mg/kg i.v.) or by introducing inhalational anaesthesia with isoflurane or sevoflurane.

Propofol decreases cerebral metabolic requirement for oxygen and cerebral perfusion pressure, and causes a corresponding decrease in ICP (in normal animals and those with intracranial pathology) and intraocular pressure (IOP). The reactivity of cerebral vessels to changes in arterial carbon dioxide tension (P_aCO_2) seems to be maintained during propofol anaesthesia. The lack of cerebrovascular dilation (in contrast to that associated with use of volatile agents) makes propofol TIVA a suitable choice for intracranial surgery in dogs (see Chapter 28).

Propofol has poor analgesic properties and the doses required for induction and maintenance of anaesthesia are significantly reduced by analgesic pre-anaesthetic medications (alpha-2 agonists, opioids).

Propofol readily crosses the placenta and may affect neurological and cardiorespiratory variables in kittens and puppies. It should therefore never be used for maintenance of anaesthesia in cats and dogs undergoing

Drug	Dose	Indication
Diazepam	Repeated boluses (0.2–0.5 mg/kg i.v.) to effect In case of repeated seizures, 0.2–0.5 mg/kg/h CRI to effect. Use diazepam emulsion for CRI; infusion with propylene glycol formulation can induce phlebitis (use long catheter)	Seizure control
Midazolam	Repeated boluses (0.2–0.5 mg/kg i.v.) to effect In case of repeated seizures, 0.3–0.9 mg/kg/h CRI to effect	Seizure control
Propofol	4–6 mg/kg slowly i.v. to effect, then 6–24 mg/kg/h to effect Requires intubation (risk of aspiration) and monitoring of ventilation	In conjunction with phenobarbital for uncontrollable seizures
Fentanyl and diazepam or midazolam	0.5–5 µg/kg/h and 0.2–0.5 mg/kg/h given to effect, alone or in combination with propofol 6–24 mg/kg/h	Long-term sedation for ventilatory support

14.9 Drugs used for long-term sedation and seizure control. CRI = constant rate infusion.

Caesarean section. Clinical experience has shown that propofol is suitable for induction of anaesthesia in the dog before maintenance with inhalational anaesthetics, as long as the animal is haemodynamically stable. An interval of approximately 10 minutes between induction of anaesthesia and delivery of the puppies minimizes respiratory depression by residual propofol effects (see Chapter 26).

Disorders of lipid metabolism could potentially be aggravated by the lipid emulsion formulation of propofol, particularly after long-term infusion. Therefore, propofol should be used with caution in patients with diabetic hyperlipidaemia or pancreatitis. Very low, non-sedative doses can stimulate appetite via disinhibition mechanisms similar to those of benzodiazepines.

Propofol for induction and maintenance of anaesthesia should be titrated to effect, in a similar fashion to a volatile agent, because of the variable influence of pre-anaesthetic medications, concurrent analgesics and surgical stimulation.

Practical use:

- Induction and maintenance agent (see Figures 14.7 and 14.8).
- Can induce pain on injection.
- Keep TIVA in cats as short as possible (<30 minutes).
- Discard open vials after 24 hours (refer to manufacturer's data sheets).
- PropoFlo Plus™ (PropoFlo 28™ in the USA) should not be used for TIVA over several hours (risk of benzyl alcohol toxicity).
- Supplement oxygen when using repeated doses or infusion.
- Surgical anaesthesia with propofol TIVA often requires intermittent positive pressure ventilation (IPPV).
- Give to effect:
  - Consider pre-anaesthetic medication (20–80% reduction in propofol requirement depending on drugs used)
  - Consider physical status of the animal
  - Give by slow or intermittent injection (over 60–120 seconds)
  - Give half of the calculated dose and await maximum effect, then proceed further with increments until desired effect (e.g. deep sedation, endotracheal intubation).
- Poor analgesia (use with analgesic).
- Avoid in hypovolaemic patients.
- Avoid in patients with heart failure.
- Avoid in patients with hyperlipidaemia and pancreatitis.
- Avoid repeated (daily) propofol anaesthesia in cats.
- Can be used for induction of anaesthesia for Caesarean section. Use cautiously in cats for induction only.
- Can be used for induction of anaesthesia in Greyhounds and other sighthounds.

Etomidate

Physicochemical properties: Etomidate is an imidazole derivative with peripheral effects at alpha-2 adrenoceptors (Paris *et al.*, 2003). It exists as a racemate, but only the R(+) isomer has hypnotic activity. Etomidate is water soluble at an acidic pH and becomes lipid soluble at physiological pH. Several formulations of etomidate exist. The 'classic' etomidate 0.2% (v/v) preparation, which appears as a clear solution, contains propylene glycol (35% v/v), has a pH of 6.9 and a high osmolarity (4640 mOsm/l). Perivascular injection of this formulation causes tissue necrosis and phlebitis. It may also induce acute haemolysis after rapid injection or prolonged continuous infusion, mediated by a massive increase in plasma osmolarity.

An Intralipid-containing emulsion (Etomidate-Lipuro®) has a pH of approximately 7 and appears as a slightly viscous, milky white liquid, like propofol. It does not cause irritation when injected perivascularly. The emulsion promotes bacterial growth and therefore open ampoules should be refrigerated and be discarded within 24 hours.

Clinical properties: Etomidate is a hypnotic agent with rapid penetration of the blood–brain barrier. Peak brain concentration is reached within 1 minute of administration. The hypnotic activity of etomidate is related to interaction with the GABA system, by enhancing the effect of GABA after binding to the β3 subunit of the $GABA_A$ receptor. Recovery after a single bolus injection is rapid (10–20 minutes).

After a single bolus injection in cats, etomidate blood concentration initially decreases rapidly, followed by a slower distribution phase and an elimination half-life of approximately 3 hours. Total body clearance rates are high. Etomidate is rapidly hydrolysed to inactive metabolites by hepatic and plasma esterases. Drugs reducing hepatic blood flow (e.g. alpha-2 adrenoceptor agonists) will slow etomidate elimination. The pharmacokinetic profile (see Figure 14.6) would make etomidate suitable for repeated dosing or continuous infusion; however, this is hampered by its potent inhibition of adrenal steroid synthesis (see below).

Etomidate alone produces minimal cardiovascular changes in healthy and hypovolaemic dogs, making it an ideal induction agent in patients with a low cardiac reserve and hypovolaemia. However, etomidate should not be used without pre-anaesthetic medication because of a high incidence of myoclonus and pain on injection (when using the propylene glycol preparation). Therefore, the choice of pre-anaesthetic medication, rather than the etomidate itself, will influence the patient's cardiovascular status. Combinations of etomidate either with diazepam or midazolam, or with fentanyl or other opioids, have been used successfully for induction of anaesthesia in high-risk patients.

Etomidate induces dose-dependent respiratory depression. A slower injection rate results in less profound depression or lower likelihood of induction apnoea, similar to thiopental and propofol.

Etomidate reduces cerebral metabolic oxygen requirements and cerebral blood flow, and decreases elevated ICP. Because of the minimal influence on arterial blood pressure, cerebral perfusion pressure is well maintained. Etomidate also decreases IOP. It has no analgesic properties.

The major drawback or concern with the use of etomidate is its inhibition of adrenal steroid synthesis. The production of cortisol, aldosterone and corticosterone is decreased by inhibition of 11-α and 11-β hydroxylases and the cholesterol side-chain cleavage enzyme. A major adverse effect (Addisonian crisis) can occur after infusion of etomidate: after a single induction bolus, adrenocortical responses and cortisol production are suppressed for 2–6 hours in cats and dogs. The lack of a stress response to anaesthesia and surgery seems to have no detrimental effects in animals after a single intravenous bolus, but care must be taken in animals with pre-existing adrenal insufficiency.

Overall, etomidate is a suitable induction agent for high-risk patients. The high cost, and packaging in single-use glass ampoules, are reasons for its limited use in veterinary practice.

Practical use:

- Induction agent.
- Do not administer repeated boluses or infusions.
- Pain on injection and phlebitis (propylene glycol preparation).
- Refrigerate open ampoules (lipid emulsion).
- Discard open ampoules after 24 hours (lipid emulsion).
- High incidence of myoclonus when used as sole agent.
- Best used with proper pre-anaesthetic medication.
- Give to effect (see Figures 14.7 and 14.8):
  - Consider physical status of the animal
  - Give by slow injection (60 seconds).
- No analgesic properties (use with analgesic).
- Good cardiovascular stability (high-risk patients).
- Avoid in animals with known adrenal insufficiency (unless cortisol supplementation is provided).

Dissociative agents

Ketamine

Physicochemical properties: The phencyclidine derivative ketamine hydrochloride occurs as a white crystalline powder. The commercially available solutions are slightly acidic (pH 3.5–5.5). Ketamine consists of two stereoisomers, S(+) ketamine and R(–) ketamine. The S(+) isomer has about 1.5–3-fold greater hypnotic potency and threefold greater analgesic potency than R(–) ketamine. Compared with the racemic mixture, S(+) ketamine is 1.5–2 times as potent. Racemic ketamine is a mixture of both stereoisomers in equal amounts and is available as 1% (w/v), 5% (w/v) and 10% (w/v) preparations containing the preservative benzethonium chloride. In some countries, S(+) ketamine is available as 0.5% (w/v) and 2.5% (w/v) solutions, marketed as veterinary preparations.

Ketamine solutions are very stable, but should be protected from light and excessive heat. Solutions can be diluted with sterile water or physiological saline for injection. Ketamine can be administered by intramuscular, intravenous, subcutaneous or intraperitoneal injection. It is also effective when given by the transmucosal route (buccal, intranasal, rectal).

Clinical properties: Ketamine penetrates the blood–brain barrier rapidly. After intravenous injection, it has an onset of action of 30–90 seconds in cats and dogs. After intramuscular injection (which is painful due to the low pH of the solution), it is distributed rapidly into body tissues and peak anaesthetic effects occur within 10–15 minutes.

Ketamine induces a dose-dependent alteration in CNS activity that leads to a dissociative state, characterized by profound analgesia and amnesia, with maintained ocular, laryngeal, pharyngeal, pinnal and pedal reflexes, and increased muscle tone. This state of catalepsy is caused (mainly) by inhibition of thalamocortical pathways and stimulation of the limbic system. The neuropharmacology of ketamine is complex and it interacts with multiple binding sites, including *N*-methyl-D-aspartate (NMDA) and non-NMDA glutamate receptors, nicotinic and muscarinic cholinergic, monoaminergic and opioid receptors. In addition, inhibition of voltage-dependent sodium and calcium channels has been described. The antagonism at the NMDA receptor appears to account for the majority of the analgesic, amnesic and psychotomimetic effects.

After an intravenous bolus, racemic ketamine is distributed rapidly, followed by an elimination half-life of approximately 60 minutes in dogs and 80 minutes in cats (see Figure 14.6). Recovery after a single dose occurs mainly by redistribution. Ketamine undergoes high hepatic extraction and is metabolized rapidly by the liver. The main metabolite, norketamine, has about 10–30% of the anaesthetic potency of ketamine. Accumulation of norketamine after repeated doses or infusions of ketamine contributes to prolonged recovery, hallucinatory behaviours and drowsiness. The parent compound and its metabolites undergo glucuronidation and are excreted via the kidney. In cats, unchanged ketamine is also excreted as the active drug via the kidney. Hepatic dysfunction impairs elimination of the drug and prolongs its action considerably.

The main pharmacokinetic difference between racemic ketamine and S(+) ketamine appears to be the higher elimination rate of the S(+) isomer. Complete recovery after S(+) ketamine is faster and less likely to be associated with excitatory effects. However, anaesthesia with either racemic or S(+) ketamine is associated with increased muscle tone, muscle spasm and seizures. Concurrent use of a benzodiazepine or an alpha-2 adrenoceptor agonist is required to reduce these side effects and obtain anaesthesia suitable for surgery. Acepromazine and ketamine can be used together in cats, but this combination is best avoided in dogs because acepromazine does not reliably control ketamine's undesirable effects. Therefore, in a clinical setting, the advantages of S(+) ketamine over racemic ketamine are influenced by the chosen pre-anaesthetic medication.

Ketamine has unique cardiovascular effects. Unlike other intravenous anaesthetics, it stimulates the cardiovascular system, resulting in increased heart rate, arterial blood pressure and cardiac output. These changes in haemodynamic variables are associated with increased myocardial work and oxygen consumption. In a healthy heart, the oxygen supply to the myocardium can increase through coronary vasodilation and increased cardiac output, but a compromised heart (e.g. hypertrophic or ischaemic heart) might not be able to mount such a response. Central stimulation of the sympathetic system is responsible for the cardiovascular stimulation. The concurrent use of sedatives will attenuate the stimulatory effects of ketamine. However, ketamine also has a direct myocardial depressant effect (negative inotropic effect); normally the stimulatory effects predominate, but high intravenous doses can result in transient hypotension. In severely compromised animals, or with concurrent use of other sedatives (e.g. alpha-2 adrenoceptor agonists) or anaesthetics, ketamine may induce cardiovascular depression.

Ketamine has minimal effects on central respiratory drive. After bolus administration of an induction dose, initial respiratory depression occurs, often followed by a so-called 'apneustic' pattern of breathing, characterized by periodic breath-holding on inspiration followed by short periods of hyperventilation. Generally, arterial and tissue oxygenation are well maintained and ketamine produces bronchodilation. Potential respiratory problems can occur in cats and small dogs because ketamine causes increased salivation, leading to upper airway obstruction or endotracheal tube occlusion. Anticholinergics can be administered to reduce salivation. The swallow, sneeze and cough reflexes remain relatively intact after ketamine administration, but 'silent' aspiration can still occur with ketamine anaesthesia.

Due to its excitatory effects on the CNS, ketamine increases cerebral metabolism, cerebral blood flow and ICP. Cerebrovascular responsiveness to carbon dioxide remains intact and therefore reducing P_aCO_2 will attenuate the rise in ICP after ketamine administration. Ketamine has epileptogenic potential and has generally not been recommended for use at high doses in animals with known seizure disorders or in procedures known to have potential to induce seizures (e.g. myelography). However, ketamine has recently also been used as an anticonvulsant in refractory epilepsy in both humans and veterinary patients (Serrano *et al.*, 2006; Gaspard *et al.*, 2013). Ketamine administered alone also increases IOP, and care should be taken when using ketamine for intraocular surgery or open globe injuries. However, these effects are attenuated by concurrent use of benzodiazepines, acepromazine and alpha-2 adrenoceptor agonists. The eyes do not rotate during ketamine anaesthesia, rendering animals prone to corneal drying and ulcers. Recovery from ketamine anaesthesia can be associated with hyperexcitability, because animals become hypersensitive to noise, light and handling.

Ketamine is still licensed for use as the sole anaesthetic agent for cats and non-human primates in some countries. Because of the increased muscle tone, involuntary movements and high incidence of excitation during recovery in cats, it should always be used in combination with a sedative or tranquillizer to offset these side effects (see Figures 14.7 and 14.8). Ketamine is a popular anaesthetic in cats because deep sedation or anaesthesia for short surgical procedures (e.g. castration) can be induced via intramuscular administration – a major advantage in uncooperative, fractious animals (Figure 14.10).

Ketamine readily crosses the placenta. Neurological reflexes in puppies delivered by Caesarean section after anaesthesia induction with ketamine–midazolam are reduced, but induction doses can be used. Unfortunately, diazepam is contra-indicated and the use of benzodiazepines may not be ideal in these patients (see Chapter 26).

The activity of ketamine as a non-competitive antagonist at NMDA glutamate receptors and its ability to produce profound somatic analgesia has expanded the indications for the drug. At sub-anaesthetic doses given in the perioperative period, ketamine may reduce the central 'wind-up' phenomenon (see Chapter 8) and reduce the requirement for postoperative analgesics. In addition, ketamine might be helpful in the treatment of chronic and neuropathic pain, based on its interaction with NMDA receptors. Intravenous infusion of ketamine can be used during inhalational anaesthesia to provide pre-emptive analgesia and reduce the required concentration of the volatile anaesthetic. However, when high infusion rates are used, recovery can be characterized by excitation.

Practical use:

- Induction agent; sole anaesthetic for short surgical procedures (see Figures 14.7, 14.8 and 14.10).

- Effective after intravenous, intramuscular, subcutaneous, intranasal, oral transmucosal or rectal administration.
- Pain can occur after intramuscular injection.
- Increased muscle tone and high incidence of convulsions (dogs) when used alone.
- Combine with benzodiazepine, alpha-2 adrenoceptor agonist or acepromazine.
- Intact eye and laryngeal reflexes.
- Anaesthetic depth difficult to judge.
- Good somatic and superficial analgesia.
- Use eye ointment to prevent corneal drying.
- Cardiovascular stimulation (heart rate and blood pressure increase).
- Do not use in patients with hypertrophic cardiomyopathy.
- Avoid in patients with seizure disorders.
- Avoid in animals with increased ICP (head trauma, tumours).
- Apneustic breathing (apnoea with high doses).
- Recover animal in a quiet, dimmed and heated room.

Tiletamine–zolazepam

Physicochemical properties: Tiletamine is chemically related to ketamine (phencyclidine derivative, cyclohexanone) but has a longer duration of action than ketamine. Zolazepam is a benzodiazepine (diazepinone minor tranquillizer) with muscle relaxant and anticonvulsant effects. Zoletil® (Europe) or Telazol® (USA) is a proprietary combination of zolazepam and tiletamine in a 1:1 ratio (250 mg zolazepam, 250 mg tiletamine). The preparation comes as a lyophilized powder, which can be reconstituted with 5 ml saline, 5% dextrose or sterile water (to give a solution of 50 mg/ml zolazepam, 50 mg/ml tiletamine). The clear solution is acidic (pH 2.0–3.5) and should be discarded if precipitation occurs. The prepared solution can be stored at room temperature for 4 days, or for 14 days when refrigerated. Telazol® is a controlled substance in the USA (under Schedule III).

Clinical properties: Administered alone, tiletamine produces a cataleptic, dissociative state similar to that produced by ketamine. High doses can produce unconsciousness and surgical anaesthesia in cats, but not in dogs, in which tiletamine produces severe convulsions. Zolazepam has anticonvulsant and anxiolytic properties and produces muscle relaxation. As with the benzodiazepine group in general, its sedative effects are unreliable in healthy animals. Zolazepam administered alone

Drugs	Doses	Technique	Indication
Acepromazine Buprenorphine or butorphanol Ketamine	0.02–0.05 mg/kg 0.02 mg/kg 0.2–0.4 mg/kg 20–30 mg/kg	Give acepromazine/opioid combination 15 minutes before ketamine to avoid muscle stiffness	Short surgical procedures (30–40 minutes)
Xylazine Ketamine	1 mg/kg 5–10 mg/kg	Mixed in one syringe	Short surgical procedures (20–30 minutes)
Medetomidine or dexmedetomidine Ketamine	0.04 mg/kg 0.02 mg/kg 5–7 mg/kg	Mixed in one syringe	Short surgical procedures (30–40 minutes)
Medetomidine or dexmedetomidine Butorphanol Ketamine	0.02 mg/kg 0.01 mg/kg 0.1–0.3 mg/kg 5 mg/kg	Mixed in one syringe	Short surgical procedures (30–40 minutes)
Midazolam Ketamine	0.2–0.3 mg/kg 10–20 mg/kg	Mixed in one syringe	Short minor procedures

14.10 Ketamine combinations given by the intramuscular route for short surgical procedures in the cat. Note that combinations with an alpha-2 adrenoceptor agonist can induce vomiting. Administration of oxygen is recommended, whatever combination is used.

causes only minimal CNS depression and has minimal cardiorespiratory effects.

The combination of tiletamine and zolazepam can produce sedation or general anaesthesia in cats and dogs. After intravenous injection, induction of anaesthesia is rapid (60–90 seconds). Onset of action after intramuscular injection varies between 1 and 7 minutes in cats, and between 5 and 12 minutes in dogs. Intramuscular injection can be painful due to the low pH of the solution. Duration of anaesthesia (30–60 minutes) is dependent on the dose used.

In general, complete recovery from tiletamine–zolazepam anaesthesia can be long (4–5 hours) and is smoother in cats than in dogs. In cats, the elimination half-life of zolazepam (4.5 hours) is longer than that of the tiletamine component (2–4 hours) and the recovery phase is influenced by the ongoing effects of tranquilizer. In dogs, the effects of zolazepam wane earlier (half-life 1 hour) than those of tiletamine (half-life 1.2 hours) and the recovery phase is characterized by muscle rigidity, excitation and seizure-like activity. High doses or repeated dosing will prolong and worsen recovery and therefore redosing is not recommended. Animals with renal disease have prolonged anaesthetic duration and recovery periods. Anaesthetic depth is difficult to judge because animals maintain ocular, laryngeal, pharyngeal and pedal reflexes.

Cardiovascular effects of tiletamine–zolazepam in cats and dogs are dose-dependent. In dogs, sinus tachycardia and premature ventricular complexes occur due to sympathetic stimulation, but tiletamine–zolazepam does not change the arrhythmogenic dose of adrenaline. In cats, heart rate responses are variable, but the cardiostimulatory effects of tiletamine–zolazepam should be avoided in cats with hypertrophic cardiomyopathy. At lower doses, the overall haemodynamic state remains stable (blood pressure, cardiac output), whereas at higher doses cardiovascular depression occurs (reduced myocardial contractility, cardiac output and blood pressure).

Respiratory depression with hypoxaemia (when breathing room air) and hypercapnia occurs after intravenous injection and after high intramuscular doses of tiletamine–zolazepam. As with ketamine, hypersalivation is common and can be reduced with atropine or glycopyrronium if necessary.

Like ketamine, tiletamine has excitatory effects on the CNS and increases cerebral metabolism, cerebral blood flow and ICP, and is therefore contraindicated in anaesthetic doses in patients with head trauma or intracranial tumours. Tiletamine increases IOP and is therefore not suitable for intraocular surgery or open globe injuries. In cats, a post-anaesthetic hyperthermic response can occur.

Practical use:

- Induction agent (intravenous).
- Use as sole anaesthetic agent only for diagnostic or minor surgical procedures.
- Effective after intravenous and intramuscular administration.
- Intramuscular induction agent for aggressive dogs and fractious cats (small injection volume).
- Dose recommendations (see Figures 14.7 and 14.8) refer to total drug.
- Pain after intramuscular injection common.
- Intact eye and laryngeal reflexes.
- Anaesthetic depth difficult to judge.
- Do not redose.
- Use eye ointment to prevent drying of the cornea.
- Do not use in patients with hypertrophic cardiomyopathy.

- Avoid in patients with seizure disorders.
- Avoid in animals with increased ICP (head trauma, tumours).
- Apneustic breathing (apnoea with high doses).
- Recover animal in a quiet, dimmed and heated room.
- Pre-anaesthetic medication with acepromazine or an alpha-2 adrenoceptor agonist reduces dose requirements and improves recovery quality.

Steroid anaesthetics
Alfaxalone

Physicochemical properties: The progesterone derivative alfaxalone is a neuroactive steroid. This molecule is insoluble in water and is now formulated with the solubilizing agent 2-hydroxypropyl-beta-cyclodextrin. It is licensed for use in cats and dogs as Alfaxan® and this formulation of alfaxalone will be discussed further. The formulation is a sterile, colourless and clear solution with a neutral pH of approximately 7. Perivascular injection is not painful and does not produce tissue necrosis. This preparation does not cause histamine release, unlike previous formulations. Alfaxan® does not promote bacterial growth, but the manufacturer recommends that any solution remaining in the vial following withdrawal of the required dose should be discarded.

Clinical properties: Neuroactive steroids produce hypnosis and muscle relaxation by enhancing the inhibitory effect of GABA on the GABA$_A$ receptor/chloride channel complex. Anticonvulsive effects are low. Dependent on the dose, either sedation or anaesthesia can be achieved. Intravenous injection leads to rapid relaxation and induction of anaesthesia (30–60 seconds) with dose-dependent duration. Intramuscular injection is effective, with onset of sedation/anaesthesia within 7–10 minutes, but the degree of effect is very variable. Subcutaneous injection has been used to produce sedation in hyperthyroid cats, with maximal effects seen 45 minutes after injection.

Alfaxalone does not show significant plasma protein binding. Glucuronidation processes play a major role in metabolism and excretion of the drug, and hepatic insufficiency will prolong anaesthetic duration. In dogs, alfaxalone is cleared from plasma very rapidly and recovery after an induction dose depends on redistribution (see Figure 14.6). This is reflected by an average duration of anaesthesia (allowing endotracheal intubation) of 6 minutes after a bolus dose of 2 mg/kg and 26 minutes after a bolus dose of 10 mg/kg (Ferré et al., 2006). Alfaxalone produces smooth anaesthesia induction, with excellent muscle relaxation, and dose-dependent changes in cardiovascular and respiratory variables and anaesthetic duration in dogs. At the recommended induction dose (see Figures 14.7 and 14.8), cardiorespiratory parameters return to baseline within 15 minutes. Rapid intravenous injection of alfaxalone can cause induction apnoea. Induction and maintenance of anaesthesia with alfaxalone (2 mg/kg for induction followed by 0.07 mg/kg/min infusion) or propofol (4 mg/kg for induction followed by 0.25 mg/kg/min infusion) for 120 minutes in premedicated (acepromazine and hydromorphone), spontaneously breathing dogs resulted in similar cardiovascular and respiratory changes, with significant hypoventilation (Ambros et al., 2008). Therefore, mechanical ventilation is recommended in TIVA protocols (see later). Recovery after infusion depends more on drug metabolism than redistribution, but cumulative effects in dogs are low.

Pre-anaesthetic medication and dilution of alfaxalone reduces the required induction dose. The recovery phase after alfaxalone induction can be associated with excitatory events, which are attenuated by the use of sedative pre-anaesthetic medication and by recovering the animal in a quiet room. Alfaxalone as an induction agent is suitable for dogs younger than 12 weeks of age (O'Hagan *et al.*, 2012a). Induction of anaesthesia with alfaxalone in dogs for Caesarean section resulted in improved viability (Apgar score) of the puppies during the first 60 minutes after delivery, with no difference in survival rate, compared with propofol induction (Doebeli *et al.*, 2013) (see Chapter 26).

In cats, dose-dependent disposition occurs and elimination is slower than in dogs (Warne *et al.*, 2014). Doses of 5 mg/kg i.v. and 25 mg/kg i.v. resulted in mean anaesthesia times to complete recovery of 44 minutes and 68 minutes, respectively. However, in cats, anaesthetic time increased non-linearly with doses above 5 mg/kg (Heit *et al.*, 2004). Maintenance of anaesthesia with alfaxalone over 60 minutes in cats prolongs the recovery period (Beths *et al.*, 2014). Recovery can be excitable: more paddling during recovery was observed in cats after alfaxalone induction than following propofol induction. The route of administration also affects quality of recovery: more excitation in the recovery phase was observed in cats after intramuscular injection of alfaxalone than after intravenous induction of anaesthesia with alfaxalone. Pre-anaesthetic medication with medetomidine, acepromazine, butorphanol or midazolam reduces the induction dose to 2–3 mg/kg i.v. (see Figure 14.8). Alfaxalone is also suitable as an induction agent for cats younger than 12 weeks of age (O'Hagan *et al.*, 2012b).

The maintenance dose of alfaxalone is approximately 0.1 mg/kg/min (0.01 ml/kg/min) in premedicated dogs and cats, although individual responses may vary. In practical terms, a 10 kg dog would require 10 mg (or 1 ml) for 10 additional minutes of anaesthesia, and a 5 kg cat would require 5 mg (or 0.5 ml) for 10 additional minutes of anaesthesia. Alfaxalone is a poor analgesic, therefore, for painful procedures, appropriate analgesic administration is necessary.

Practical use:

- Induction and maintenance agent in dogs and cats (see Figure 14.13).
- Redosing possible in cats (up to four times) (see Figure 14.14).
- Best used intravenously; also effective after intramuscular injection, but large injection volumes are required in larger animals.

- Give to effect (see Figures 14.7 and 14.8):
  - Dilution reduces induction dose
  - Consider pre-anaesthetic medication (20–50% reduction in induction dose depending on drugs used)
  - Consider physical status of the animal
  - Give by slow injection (over 60 seconds, one-quarter of the dose every 15 seconds).
- Recovery can be excitatory without appropriate pre-anaesthetic medication.
- Poor analgesia (use with analgesic).

Neuroleptanalgesia

The concept of neuroleptanalgesia involves the combination of a neuroleptic agent (butyrophenones, phenothiazines) with a potent opioid analgesic. The combination with benzodiazepines (ataractic agents) is sometimes also referred to as ataractanalgesia. This technique can be used in two ways. At low doses, it is commonly used for sedation and pre-anaesthetic medication via the intramuscular route (see Chapter 13). At high doses, usually given by intravenous injection, the combination can be used to produce sufficient CNS depression to allow endotracheal intubation and moderate surgical stimulation. The excitatory effects of high doses of opioids make this technique unsuitable for healthy cats, although it has been used in severely debilitated cats.

Neuroleptanalgesia is characterized by analgesia, suppression of motor activity, partial suppression of autonomic reflexes and behavioural indifference, but not 'true' unconsciousness as defined by cortical suppression. Neuroleptanalgesia combinations are not suitable for routine induction of anaesthesia in healthy, young animals, because a true anaesthetic state is not reached unless the combination is followed by another anaesthetic agent (volatile or injectable) or unduly high doses are used. However, in high-risk and debilitated patients, sedative–opioid combinations can have a profound effect (Figure 14.11).

The advantages of this technique are a wide safety margin and reversibility (by using an opioid antagonist such as naloxone and the benzodiazepine antagonist flumazenil). The disadvantages are: possible occurrence of panting or marked respiratory depression (requiring IPPV); spontaneous movements; sensitivity to noise and light; and possible postoperative behavioural changes, especially when neuroleptanalgesic combinations are used as the sole anaesthetic agents. Bradycardia related to the high dose of opioid can be treated with an anticholinergic agent (atropine or glycopyrronium).

Drugs	Dose	Maintenance	Comment
Hydromorphone or L-Methadone or Methadone Midazolam/Diazepam	0.05–0.1 mg/kg i.v. 0.5 mg/kg i.v. 1 mg/kg i.v. 0.1–0.2 mg/kg i.v.	Inhalant	Inject in alternate increments until desired effect (intubation) Give opioid first, wait a few minutes, then administer benzodiazepine Do not mix in same syringe (excitement possible)
Fentanyl Midazolam	0.002–0.005 mg/kg i.v. 0.2 mg/kg i.v.	Inhalant	Give opioid first, wait a few minutes, then administer benzodiazepine Do not mix in same syringe
Sufentanil Midazolam	0.003 mg/kg i.v 0.9 mg/kg i.v.	Sufentanil 0.003 mg/kg/h Midazolam 0.9 mg/kg/h	Mix in one syringe, give in increments until intubation possible Used in gastric dilatation–volvulus, endotoxaemic patients Requires IPPV/oxygen Bradycardia possible Reverse midazolam with flumazenil if necessary at end (10–30 µg/kg i.v.)

14.11 Neuroleptanalgesia for induction of anaesthesia in debilitated and old dogs. IPPV = intermittent positive pressure ventilation.

The 'classic' neuroleptanalgesic mixtures contain phenothiazines or butyrophenones such as acepromazine, droperidol or fluanisone, which can lead to significant alpha-1 adrenoceptor blockade (hypotension unresponsive to alpha-1 adrenoceptor agonists such as phenylephrine, adrenaline or noradenaline). Neuroleptanalgesia with benzodiazepines (diazepam, midazolam) has a wide margin of safety, with minimal cardiovascular depression and lack of alpha-1 adrenoceptor blockade. Therefore, combinations of an opioid with a benzodiazepine are well suited for induction of anaesthesia in severely debilitated high-risk patients (see Figure 14.11). The time required to obtain conditions suitable for endotracheal intubation is longer than with other intravenous anaesthetics (>2–3 minutes) so there is an increased risk of aspiration and apnoea can occur, but haemodynamic stability is excellent.

Total intravenous anaesthesia

Total intravenous anaesthesia refers to the induction and maintenance of anaesthesia by intravenous drugs only. An intravenous anaesthetic (usually propofol or alfaxalone) provides hypnosis, muscle relaxation and immobility, whereas analgesia is provided by either an opioid, an alpha-2 adrenoceptor agonist or ketamine. Both the analgesic and the anaesthetic drug can be given by the intravenous route as an infusion. Some anaesthetists prefer to provide the analgesic as part of the pre-anaesthetic medication and supplement it as required. Anaesthesia can be maintained by intermittent boluses of the agents, but a continuous infusion produces a more stable plane of anaesthesia and is more economical in terms of total drug use. Drugs can be given as an intravenous infusion and the rate altered according to requirements (variable rate infusion). A better adjustment of anaesthetic depth and even more drug saving may be achieved with target-controlled infusion (TCI) devices, which deliver a drug to a predicted blood concentration set by the anaesthetist (see later).

Principles of TIVA

Sedation or anaesthesia can be maintained by intermittent drug boluses. This technique is simple and does not require special equipment. The disadvantage of using intermittent drug boluses is the large variation in plasma concentration, and consequently excessive drug effect at the time the bolus is administered and inadequate effect before the next bolus. Continuous infusion results in less variation in plasma concentration, with fewer oscillations in haemodynamic, respiratory and central effects, and thus is safer for the animal.

Pharmacokinetic models can be used to develop dosing regimens for intravenous anaesthetic infusions. Such models are a mathematical description of drug disposition in the body. For detailed accounts of pharmacokinetic principles and models, standard pharmacokinetic textbooks (e.g. Riviere, 2011) should be consulted. The parameters describing the disposition process are usually estimated by administering a known dose of a drug and measuring the resulting plasma concentration at various time points.

Pharmacokinetic variables that are important for intravenous drugs are the *volume of distribution*, *total body clearance* and *elimination half-life* (Figure 14.12). Typically, the drug concentration versus time curve is described as an exponential equation. Depending on the shape of the curve, the equation can have a single exponent (one-compartment model), two exponents (two-compartment model) or three exponents (three-compartment model), which reflect different rates of drug decay at different time points.

Half-lives are derived from the rate of change in drug concentration. Different half-lives are reported, depending on the model. In a one-compartment model, only the elimination half-life occurs; in a two-compartment model, a distribution half-life and an elimination half-life are estimated; in a three-compartment model, there are three half-lives. The disposition of intravenous anaesthetics is usually described by a two- or three-compartment model: a rapid initial decrease in plasma drug concentration (distribution) is followed either by a second, slower distribution phase or directly by the elimination phase. The description of drug disposition by different models for the same drug, and differences in the sensitivity of the analytical technique used to measure drug plasma concentration, contribute to the often large variation in reported elimination half-lives (see Figure 14.6).

After infusion of an intravenous anaesthetic, the offset of effect (recovery) is not merely a function of the elimination half-life; it is also affected by the rate of equilibration between plasma and effect site (brain) and by the duration of infusion. Therefore, the concept of *context-sensitive half-time* has been introduced; this is defined as the time for the plasma concentration to decrease by 50% after

Parameter	Symbol	Description
Distribution half-life Elimination half-life Terminal half-life	$T_{\frac{1}{2}}\alpha$ $T_{\frac{1}{2}}\beta$ r $T_{\frac{1}{2}}\gamma$ or $T_{\frac{1}{2}}$ term	Time required for an amount of drug in plasma to decrease by half. The half-life is dependent on the extent of drug distribution in the body (volume of distribution) and excretion of drug from the body (clearance). About five times the elimination half-life is required to eliminate a drug from the body The number and names of half-lives depends on the pharmacokinetic model used
Total body clearance	Cl_B	Volume of plasma (blood) cleared of a drug per unit time; total body clearance includes all elimination processes (liver, kidney, lung)
Volumes of distribution: Volume of the central compartment Volume of distribution at steady state Volume of distribution at pseudoequilibrium Apparent volume of distribution	Vc Vd_{ss} Vd area Vd (B)	Theoretical or apparent degree of dilution of a drug within the body. A large volume of distribution implies extensive distribution of a drug to tissues. The lower limit is the plasma volume. The highly lipophilic anaesthetics have a very large volume of distribution. Disease states can alter the volume of distribution massively and thereby change dose requirements The volume of the different estimates varies, with Vc < Vd_{ss} < Vd area < Vd (B) Vd_{ss} defines the extent of drug dilution at maximum distribution or when all compartments are in equilibrium; Vc is the volume from which clearance is determined and is used for target-controlled infusion calculations (vascular space)

14.12 Some pharmacokinetic parameters describing drug disposition in the body.

termination of an intravenous infusion designed to maintain a constant plasma concentration. 'Context' refers to the infusion duration. Considerable differences between the elimination half-life after a single intravenous bolus and context-sensitive half-times after different infusion times can be demonstrated for many drugs (e.g. thiopental, ketamine, fentanyl).

Dosing regimens for TIVA consist of a loading dose aimed at achieving an effective concentration of the drug in the plasma, or, better, at the effect site, consistent with anaesthesia. For anaesthesia, the loading dose of a drug is equivalent to an anaesthesia induction dose. With knowledge of the volume of distribution of a drug and the effective plasma concentration, a loading dose can be calculated:

$$\text{Loading dose (LD)} = \text{desired plasma concentration (Cp)} \times \text{volume of distribution (Vd}_{ss})$$

Many different volumes of distribution are reported in pharmacokinetic studies (see Figure 14.12) and there is considerable confusion about which one to use for estimation of a loading dose for a manual infusion regimen. The volume of distribution at steady state (Vd_{ss}) seems to be a very robust estimate because it is independent of any elimination processes and constants, and usually avoids massive over- or under estimation of a loading dose as can occur with other volumes of distribution. For drugs with significant cardiopulmonary effects Vc might even be more appropriate than Vd_{ss}. Plasma

concentration, and thereby anaesthesia, is maintained by a maintenance infusion rate, which compensates for drug 'losses' (via distribution, excretion, metabolism). Therefore, the maintenance dose can be derived from knowledge of the total body clearance of a drug and the desired plasma concentration:

$$\text{Maintenance dose (MD)} = \text{Cp} \times \text{total body clearance (Cl}_B)$$

The ideal drug for TIVA does not accumulate and can be infused at a constant rate over prolonged periods of time. However, distribution processes over time, individual and breed differences in pharmacokinetics and sensitivity to a drug, and surgical stimulation make adjustments of the infusion rate necessary. Therefore, the infusion rate is rarely kept constant throughout the whole anaesthetic, but is adjusted to the animal's needs. A common approach is to keep either the primary analgesic or the injectable anaesthetic at a constant rate and infuse the secondary drug to effect; if necessary both infusion rates can be adjusted (Figures 14.13 and 14.14).

Target-controlled infusion

The idea of TCI systems is to aim for a specific drug plasma concentration, which is known to produce a desired effect. Based on a mathematical (pharmacokinetic–pharmacodynamic) model, the TCI system's microprocessor predicts changes in drug concentration and controls an infusion device. Infusion rates are adjusted automatically by the system to obtain the target drug

Drugs	Induction/loading dose	Maintenance dose	Indication	Infusion
Propofol	4–6 mg/kg	12 mg/kg/h or 2 mg/kg about every 5 minutes as required	Deep sedation	CRI
Propofol	4–6 mg/kg	24–30 mg/kg/h	Non-painful procedures	VRI
Propofol Fentanyl	2–4 mg/kg 0.005 mg/kg	6–12 mg/kg/h 0.03 mg/kg/h	Surgery	VRI CRI
Propofol Fentanyl	2–4 mg/kg 0.005 mg/kg	18 mg/kg/h 0.009–0.018 mg/kg/h	Surgery	CRI VRI
Propofol Alfentanil	2–4 mg/kg 0.005 mg/kg	18 mg/kg/h 0.06–0.3 mg/kg/h	Surgery	CRI VRI
Propofol Remifentanil	2–4 mg/kg No loading	18–30 mg/kg/h 0.018–0.036 mg/kg/h	Surgery	VRI CRI
Propofol Remifentanil	2–4 mg/kg No loading	Plasma target 3–3.5 μg/ml 0.012–0.03 mg/kg/h	Surgery	TCI VRI
Alfaxalone	2–3 mg/kg	7–10 mg/kg/h	Non-painful procedures	VRI
Alfaxalone Buprenorphine	1–3 mg/kg 0.02 mg/kg	4–18 mg/kg/h	Surgery (ovariohysterectomy)	VRI

14.13 Infusion regimens for TIVA in the dog after routine pre-anaesthetic medication. CRI = constant rate infusion; TCI = target-controlled infusion; TIVA = total intravenous anaesthesia; VRI = variable rate infusion.

Drugs	Induction/loading dose	Maintenance dose	Indication	Infusion
Propofol	6–8 mg/kg	12 mg/kg/h or 2 mg/kg every 5 minutes to effect	Deep sedation	CRI
Propofol	6–8 mg/kg	24–30 mg/kg/h	Non-painful procedures	VRI
Propofol and fentanyl or alfentanil or sufentanil	4–6 mg/kg 0.001 mg/kg 0.005 mg/kg 0.001 mg/kg	7.2–18 mg/kg/h 0.006 mg/kg/h 0.03 mg/kg/h 0.006 mg/kg/h	Surgery	VRI CRI CRI CRI
Propofol and remifentanil	6–8 mg/kg No loading	18 mg/kg/h 0.012–0.018 mg/kg/h	Surgery	CRI VRI
Alfaxalone	2–3 mg/kg	4–8 mg/kg/h or 1 mg/kg every 10 minutes to effect	Deep sedation, without endotracheal tube	CRI
Alfaxalone Buprenorphine	3–5 mg/kg 0.02 mg/kg	8–14 mg/kg/h		VRI

14.14 Infusion regimens for TIVA in the cat after routine pre-anaesthetic medication. CRI = constant rate infusion; TIVA = total intravenous anaesthesia; VRI = variable rate infusion.

plasma concentration. With an open, model-based system, the anaesthetist sets the target concentration based on knowledge of drug effects. The plasma target is a calculated number based on a mathematical model and not a measured concentration. Therefore, the performance of TCI systems depends on the pharmacokinetic model (ideally a population-based model) used, and requires careful evaluation. In veterinary anaesthesia, population-based models are lacking and differences between targeted and actual blood concentration can be large. The next step in the development of automated drug-delivery systems is to feed the measured drug effect (e.g. arterial blood pressure measurements, electroencephalography (EEG) traces) back into the system. With such 'closed loop' systems the model is permanently updated based on actual drug effects rather than on drug concentration. With the advent of real-time drug analysers for propofol, feedback based on actual blood concentration might be possible.

Infusion devices

Infusion devices are classified as either controllers or positive displacement pumps. Rate controllers simply control the flow of fluid/drug produced by gravity. Infusion sets with regulating roller clamps come in different sizes, labelled as the number of drops producing 1 ml of fluid. They deliver fluids/drugs with an accuracy of ± 10% depending on the height above ground. To restrict the total volume that can be infused and facilitate standardized dilution, an infusion system with two drip chambers and a burette (Figure 14.15) (SmartSite®; Dosifix®) is useful. Infusion by gravity with an infusion set is a simple way of administering an anaesthetic continuously, but is less accurate than administration with an infusion pump and requires careful calculation and adjustment of the drip rate.

Positive displacement pumps contain an active pumping mechanism. Volumetric infusion pumps (Figure 14.16) work with different delivery mechanisms (bellows, piston, peristaltic, shuttle) and can produce delivery rates of 0.1–1999 ml/h with an accuracy of ± 5%. This type of pump may require special tubing/infusion sets and cannot be used with regular infusion sets.

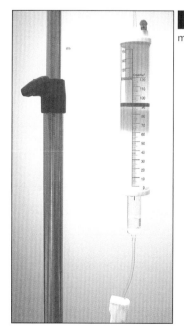

14.15 Infusion system with a burette and a microdrip chamber.

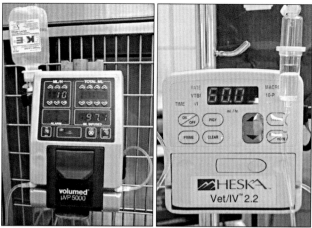

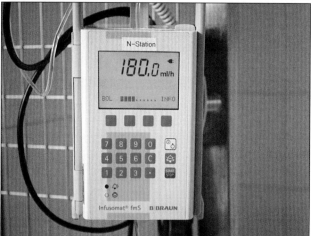

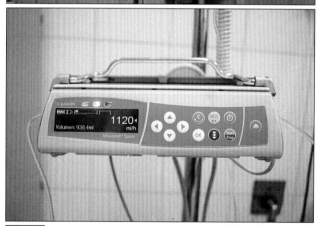

14.16 Volumetric infusion pumps.

Administration of anaesthetics or haemodynamic agents using a drip infusion via roller clamps or a volumetric infusion pump requires dilution of the very potent drugs to obtain dose rates (volume/time) suitable for administration by these systems. This can become prob-lematic, particularly in very small animals. Piston pumps also divide the millilitre dose into portions, which can produce a 'mini-bolus' effect in the patient, especially with diluted drugs that have a very short half-life (e.g. vasopressors).

Syringe pumps (Figure 14.17) that use a stepper motor with a drive screw (syringe drivers) are particularly suitable for the delivery of potent anaesthetics. Rates as low as 0.01 ml/h can be delivered with high accuracy (2–3 %). Many syringe drivers include a calculator feature, which

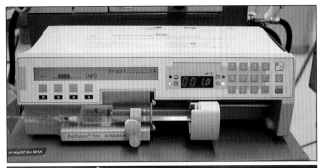

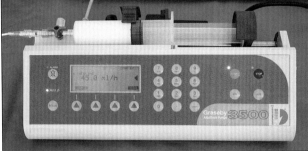

14.17 Syringe drivers.

enables the operator to set the patient bodyweight, the drug concentration and the infusion rate (as dose/weight/time); the device calculates the infusion in volume/unit time. Many pumps allow automatic recognition of syringe size and staged infusions, with programmable loading doses and maintenance infusions. Special tubing is not required with syringe drivers. Syringe drivers can deliver drugs accurately, even to very small patients, and infusion of the anaesthetic can be adjusted independent of fluid administration.

Several modern syringe drivers have inbuilt TCI models for propofol, remifentanil and other drugs in humans. At present, syringe drivers with inbuilt computer software and pharmacokinetic models to run TCIs in dogs and cats are not commercially available. Syringe drivers (Graseby 3400 and 3500; see Figure 14.17) that can be controlled by a custom-built external computer and pharmacokinetic modelling software (Computer Control Infusion Pump (CCIP); University of Hong Kong), have been used to provide a target plasma concentration of various drugs in experimental animal studies and to evaluate TCI protocols for propofol anaesthesia in dogs. Because of the limited availability of infusion hardware and software, as well as the lack of evaluated population-based pharmacokinetic models, the TCI concept is still not ready to be used in veterinary practice.

TIVA protocols

Drugs used for maintenance of anaesthesia must have a pharmacokinetic profile that allows adjustment of anaesthetic depth by changing the infusion rate over prolonged periods of time, without significant accumulation and without significant prolongation of recovery (i.e. short and constant context-sensitive half-time). This means a suitable drug should have rapid onset of effect, short duration of effect and high clearance rates with rapid metabolism to inactive substances and excretion.

Of the currently licensed drugs, propofol is the most suitable and most commonly used for maintenance of anaesthesia by continuous infusion. Alfaxalone can also be used for maintenance of anaesthesia in dogs and for a limited time period in cats. Because both propofol and alfaxalone have poor analgesic properties, it is often combined with fentanyl or one of its derivatives (alfentanil, sufentanil or remifentanil). Medetomidine, dexmedetomidine and ketamine can also be given by infusion (Figure 14.18 and see Chapter 10).

Diagnostic procedures, cast changes and low-invasive surgical procedures might be possible with low dose rates (and a low plasma concentration) of propofol or alfaxalone, at which spontaneous respiration is maintained. However, respiratory depression and hypoxaemia can

Drugs	Induction/loading dose	Maintenance dose	Comment
Morphine	0.15–0.3 mg/kg slow i.v.	0.1–0.2 mg/kg/h	Usually dogs only
Hydromorphone	0.05–0.1 mg/kg i.v.	0.05–0.1 mg/kg/h	Usually dogs only
Fentanyl	0.003–0.005 mg/kg i.v.	0.005–0.04 mg/kg/h	IPPV Bradycardia
Alfentanil	0.003–0.005 mg/kg i.v.	0.03–0.3 mg/kg/h	IPPV Bradycardia
Sufentanil	0.001–0.003 mg/kg i.v.	0.002–0.006 mg/kg/h	IPPV Bradycardia
Remifentanil	None required or use fentanyl (takes 15–30 minutes for remifentanil infusion to reach an effective plasma concentration)	0.012–0.04 mg/kg/h	IPPV Bradycardia
Ketamine	0.3–0.5 mg/kg i.v.	0.12–1.2 mg/kg/h (commonly 0.3 mg/kg/h)	High doses lead to ketamine 'signs' (see text for details)
Medetomidine	0.001–0.002 mg/kg i.m. or i.v.	0.001–0.002 mg/kg/h	Bradycardia
Dexmedetomidine	0.0005–0.001 mg/kg i.m. or i.v.	0.0005–0.001 mg/kg/h	Bradycardia
Lidocaine	Dog: 2 mg/kg i.v. Cat: 0.25 mg/kg slow i.v.	1.5–3 mg/kg/h 0.6–2 mg/kg/h	Haemodynamic depression (hypotension) in cats
Morphine Lidocaine Ketamine (MLK)	Dog: 1–2 ml/kg i.v. Cat: no loading or omit lidocaine	0.2 mg/kg/h morphine 3 mg/kg/h lidocaine 0.6 mg/kg/h ketamine infused at 5 ml/kg/h Postoperative: 1 ml/kg/h	10 mg morphine 150 mg lidocaine 30 mg ketamine in 250 ml saline

14.18 Infusion regimens used in conjunction with inhalational anaesthesia to reduce anaesthetic requirements (partial intravenous anaesthesia). Intermittent positive pressure ventilation (IPPV) becomes necessary.

occur even when spontaneous respiration persists. Therefore, oxygen should be supplemented for all procedures lasting more than 20 minutes and equipment for intubation and IPPV should be readily available. TIVA protocols for prolonged, invasive surgical procedures require concurrent administration of an opioid with high efficacy. With these combinations, spontaneous respiration usually ceases and endotracheal intubation and mechanical ventilation are mandatory.

Various propofol TIVA infusion regimens (see Figure 14.13) have been used with excellent results in dogs for extended procedures (>2 hours), but prolonged recoveries are to be expected in Greyhounds (see earlier). In cats, it seems advisable to restrict the duration of propofol infusions to 30–60 minutes because of cats' increased sensitivity to phenolic compounds and prolonged recoveries after propofol anaesthesia (see Figure 14.14).

Maintenance of anaesthesia with TIVA administered by an infusion pump or a syringe driver does not mean that anaesthesia is automated, without need for intervention. Monitoring of anaesthesia and adjustment of anaesthetic depth by changing infusion rates should be as meticulous as monitoring during inhalational anaesthesia and associated adjustment by changing vaporizer settings.

Balanced anaesthesia

As with propofol TIVA, different analgesic drugs (opioids, medetomidine/dexmedetomidine, ketamine and lidocaine) can be used as continuous infusions in conjunction with volatile agents, resulting in a type of balanced anaesthesia, or partial intravenous anaesthesia (Duke, 2013). The analgesic and anaesthetic-sparing properties of these drugs allow use of reduced concentration of volatile agents and thereby less cardiovascular depression occurs. Dose rates of infusions for balanced anaesthesia techniques using various drugs are given in Figure 14.18. For detailed descriptions of the pharmacology of the single drugs, the reader is referred to Chapters 10 and 13.

References and further reading

Adam HK, Glen JB and Hoyle PA (1980) Pharmacokinetics in laboratory animals of ICI 35 868, a new i.v. anaesthetic agent. *British Journal of Anaesthesia* **52**, 743–746

Ambros B, Duke-Novakovski T and Pasloske KS (2008) Comparison of the anesthetic efficacy and cardiopulmonary effects of continuous rate infusions of alfaxalone-2-hydroxypropyl-beta-cyclodextrin and propofol in dogs. *American Journal of Veterinary Research* **69**, 1391–1398

Andress JL, Day TK and Day D (1995) The effects of consecutive day propofol anesthesia on feline red blood cells. *Veterinary Surgery* **24**, 277–282

Beal MW and Hughes D (2000) Vascular access: theory and techniques in the small animal emergency patient. *Clinical Techniques in Small Animal Practice* **15**, 101–109

Beths T, Reid J, Monteiro AM, Nolan AM and Glen JB (2001) Evaluation and optimisation of target-controlled infusion systems for administering propofol to dogs as part of a total intravenous anaesthetic technique during dental surgery. *Veterinary Record* **148**, 198–203

Beths T, Touzot-Jourde G, Musk G and Pasloske K (2014) Clinical evaluation of alfaxalone to induce and maintain anaesthesia in cats undergoing neutering procedures. *Journal of Feline Medicine and Surgery* **16(8)**, 609–615

Bley CR, Roos M, Price J *et al.* (2007) Clinical assessment of repeated propofol-associated anesthesia in cats. *Journal of the American Veterinary Medical Association* **231**, 1347–1353

Boscan P, Pypendop B, Solano A and Ilkiw JE (2005) Cardiovascular and respiratory effects of ketamine infusions in isoflurane-anesthetized dogs before and during noxious stimulation. *American Journal of Veterinary Research* **66**, 2122–2129

Chamberlin SC, Sullivan LA, Morley PS and Boscan P (2013) Evaluation of ultrasound-guided vascular access in dogs. *Journal of Veterinary Emergency and Critical Care* **23**, 498–503

Clarke KW, Trim CM and Hall LW (2013) *Veterinary Anaesthesia, 11th edn.* Saunders, Edinburgh

Doebeli A, Michel E, Bettschart R, Hartnack S and Reichler IM (2013) Apgar score after induction of anesthesia for canine cesarean section with alfaxalone versus propofol. *Theriogenology* **80**, 850–854

Duke T (2013) Partial intravenous anesthesia in cats and dogs. *Canadian Veterinary Journal* **54**, 276–282

Ferré P, Pasloske K, Whittem T *et al.* (2006) Plasma pharmacokinetics of alfaxalone in dogs after an intravenous bolus of Alfaxan-CD RTU. *Veterinary Anaesthesia and Analgesia* **33**, 229–236

Gaspard N, Foreman B, Judd LM *et al.* (2013) Intravenous ketamine for the treatment of refractory status epilepticus: a retrospective multicenter study. *Epilepsia* **54**, 498–503

Hanna RM, Borchard RE and Schmidt SL (1988) Pharmacokinetics of ketamine HCl and metabolite I in the cat: a comparison of i.v., i.m., and rectal administration. *Journal of Veterinary Pharmacology and Therapeutics* **11**, 84–93

Heit M, Pasloske K, Whittem T, Ranasinghe M and Li Q (2004) Plasma pharmacokinetics of alfaxalone in cats after administration at 5 and 25 mg/kg as an intravenous bolus of Alfaxan-CD RTU. In: *Proceedings of the American College of Veterinary Internal Medicine,* Minneapolis, pp. 849–850

Herbert GL, Bowlt KL, Ford-Fennah V, Covey-Crump GL and Murrell JC (2013) Alfaxalone for total intravenous anaesthesia in dogs undergoing ovariohysterectomy: a comparison of premedication with acepromazine or dexmedetomidine. *Veterinary Anaesthesia and Analgesia* **40**, 124–133

Ilkiw J, Benthuysen J, Ebling W and McNeal D (1991) A comparative study of the pharmacokinetics of thiopental in the rabbit, sheep and dog. *Journal of Veterinary Pharmacology and Therapeutics* **14**, 134–140

Ilkiw J and Pascoe P (2003) Cardiovascular effects of propofol alone and in combination with ketamine for total intravenous anaesthesia in cats. *American Journal of Veterinary Research* **64**, 913–917

Jackson A, Tobias K, Long C, Bartges J and Harvey R (2004) Effects of various anesthetic agents on laryngeal motion during laryngoscopy in normal dogs. *Veterinary Surgery* **33**, 102–106

Kaka J and Hayton W (1980) Pharmacokinetics of ketamine and two metabolites in the dog. *Journal of Pharmacokinetics and Biopharmaceutics* **8**, 193–202

Keates H and Whittem T (2012) Effect of intravenous dose escalation with alfaxalone and propofol on occurrence of apnoea in the dog. *Research in Veterinary Science* **93**, 904–906

Luna S, Cassu R, Castro G *et al.* (2004) Effects of four anaesthetic protocols on the neurological and cardiorespiratory variables of puppies born by caesarean section. *Veterinary Record* **154**, 387–389

Matot I, Neely CF, Katz RY and Neufeld GR (1993) Pulmonary uptake of propofol in cats. Effect of fentanyl and halothane. *Anesthesiology* **78**, 1157–1165

McIntosh MP, Schwarting N and Rajewski RA (2004) *In vitro* and *in vivo* evaluation of a sulfobutyl ether beta-cyclodextrin enabled etomidate formulation. *Journal of Pharmaceutical Sciences* **93**, 2585–2594

Mendes G and Selmi A (2003) Use of a combination of propofol and fentanyl, alfentanil, or sufentanil for total intravenous anesthesia in cats. *Journal of the American Veterinary Medical Association* **223**, 1608–1613

Muir W, Wiese AJ and March PA (2003) Effects of morphine, lidocaine, ketamine, and morphine-lidocaine-ketamine drug combination on minimum alveolar concentration in dogs anesthetized with isoflurane. *American Journal of Veterinary Research* **64**, 1155–1160

Murrell J, Notten RWV and Hellebrekers L (2005) Clinical investigation of remifentanil and propofol for the total intravenous anaesthesia of dogs. *Veterinary Record* **156**, 804–808

Musk GC and Flaherty DA (2007) Target-controlled infusion of propofol combined with variable rate infusion of remifentanil for anaesthesia of a dog with patent ductus arteriosus. *Veterinary Anaesthesia and Analgesia* **34**, 359–364

Musk GC, Pang DSJ, Beths T and Flaherty DA (2005) Target-controlled infusion of propofol in dogs – evaluation of four targets for induction of anaesthesia. *Veterinary Record* **157**, 766–770

Nolan A and Reid J (1993) Pharmacokinetics of propofol administered by infusion in dogs undergoing surgery. *British Journal of Anaesthesia* **70**, 546–551

Nolan AM, Reid J and Grant S (1993) The effects of halothane and nitrous oxide on the pharmacokinetics of propofol in dogs. *Journal of Veterinary Pharmacology and Therapeutics* **16**, 335–342

O'Hagan B, Pasloske K, McKinnon C, Perkins N and Whittem T (2012a) Clinical evaluation of alfaxalone as an anaesthetic induction agent in dogs less than 12 weeks of age. *Australian Veterinary Journal* **90**, 346–350

O'Hagan BJ, Pasloske K, McKinnon C, Perkins NR and Whittem T (2012b) Clinical evaluation of alfaxalone as an anaesthetic induction agent in cats less than 12 weeks of age. *Australian Veterinary Journal* **90**, 395–401

Paris A, Philipp M, Tonner PH *et al.* (2003). Activation of alpha 2B-adrenoceptors mediates the cardiovascular effects of etomidate. *Anesthesiology* **99**, 889–895

Pascoe PJ, Ilkiw JE and Frischmeyer KJ (2006a) The effect of the duration of propofol administration on recovery from anesthesia in cats. *Veterinary Anaesthesia and Analgesia* **33**, 2–7

Pascoe PJ, Raekallio M, Kuusela E, McKusick B and Granholm M (2006b) Changes in the minimum alveolar concentration of isoflurane and some cardiopulmonary measurements during three continuous infusion rates of dexmedetomidine in dogs. *Veterinary Anaesthesia and Analgesia* **33**, 97–103

Pypendop B and Ilkiw J (2005) Pharmacokinetics of ketamine and its metabolite, norketamine, after intravenous administration of a bolus of ketamine to isoflurane-anesthetized dogs. *American Journal of Veterinary Research* **66**, 2034–2038

Ramoo S, Bradbury LA, Anderson GA and Abraham LA (2013) Sedation of hyperthyroid cats with subcutaneous administration of a combination of alfaxalone and butorphanol. *Australian Veterinary Journal* **91**, 131–136

Reid J and Nolan AM (1996) Pharmacokinetics of propofol as an induction agent in geriatric dogs. *Research in Veterinary Science* **61**, 169–171

Riviere JE (2011) *Comparative Pharmacokinetics: Principles, Techniques and Applications, 2nd edn.* John Wiley & Sons

Serrano S, Hughes D and Chandler K (2006) Use of ketamine for the management of refractory status epilepticus in a dog. *Journal of Veterinary Internal Medicine* **20**, 194–197

Strachan FA, Mansel JC and Clutton RE (2008) A comparison of microbial growth in alfaxalone, propofol and thiopental. *Journal of Small Animal Practice* **49**, 186–190

Ueda Y, Odunayo A and Mann FA (2013) Comparison of heparinized saline and 0.9% sodium chloride for maintaining peripheral intravenous catheter patency in dogs. *Journal of Veterinary Emergency and Critical Care* **23**, 517–522

Warne LN, Beths T, Whittem T, Carter JE and Bauquier SH (2015) A review of the pharmacology and clinical application of alfaxalone in cats. *The Veterinary Journal* **203(2)**, 141–148

Wertz E, Benson G, Thurmon J *et al.* (1990) Pharmacokinetics of etomidate in cats. *American Journal of Veterinary Research* **51**, 281–285

Woerlee GM (2008) Gerry's real world guide to pharmacokinetics and other things. Available from www.anesthesiaweb.org/images/real-world-guide/gwoerlee101508a.pdf

Wright M (1982) Pharmacologic effects of ketamine and its use in veterinary medicine. *Journal of the American Veterinary Medical Association* **180**, 1462–1471

Zhang J, Maland L, Hague B *et al.* (1998) Buccal absorption of etomidate from a solid formulation in dogs. *Anesthesia and Analgesia* **86**, 1116–1122

Chapter 15

Inhalant anaesthetic agents

Daniel S.J. Pang

The simplest definition of general anaesthesia, which applies to all anaesthetic agents in current use, is a state of chemically induced, reversible loss of consciousness. Perhaps surprisingly, our understanding of the mechanisms of action of inhalant anaesthetic agents is incomplete. This is in contrast to the majority of injectable anaesthetic agents, for which the gamma-aminobutyric acid A ($GABA_A$) receptor has been identified as a major site of action (see Chapter 14). Current evidence for the mechanisms of action of inhalant anaesthetics has moved away from the once-ubiquitous lipid bilayer theory and instead suggests that interactions with cell membrane proteins play a predominant role, with involvement of a range of receptors and ion channels.

This chapter focuses on the two volatile anaesthetics most commonly used in veterinary practice, isoflurane and sevoflurane. A relatively recent addition to clinical practice, the volatile agent desflurane, is included to highlight relevant differences from isoflurane and sevoflurane. The gaseous general anaesthetic nitrous oxide is described in a separate section. The older inhalational anaesthetic, halothane, is not discussed further in this edition except for comparison with isoflurane and sevoflurane to illustrate pharmacological principles.

The ideal inhalant anaesthetic agent

A list of ideal properties of inhalant anaesthetic agents is useful for assessing current and potential future agents, and to aid in identification of their specific strengths and weaknesses (Figure 15.1). While modern agents have advantages over the older inhalant agents formerly in common use, modern agents continue to cause significant unwanted side effects.

Induction and recovery

Factors determining uptake of inhalant anaesthetic agents and induction time

A range of factors determines the speed with which inhalant anaesthetics are taken up by the body; these affect the speed of both induction and changes in anaesthetic depth during maintenance of anaesthesia. These factors can be broadly divided into those affecting the inspired concentration of agent and those affecting its alveolar concentration.

Factors affecting the inspired concentration of agent

The inspired gas concentration is determined by the vaporizer setting, the fresh gas flow (FGF) and the way in which the breathing system functions. A high FGF promotes a rapid increase in the concentration of anaesthetic agent in the breathing system at the beginning of the anaesthetic period and allows rapid changes in agent concentration in the system during the maintenance phase. This has a greater effect in circle systems, due to rebreathing of gases previously exhaled by the patient. Uptake of

- Chemically stable
  - Unchanged by temperature, ultraviolet light and oxygen
  - Does not react with components of an anaesthetic system, e.g. rubber, metal, plastic
  - Compatible with carbon dioxide absorbent
- Non-flammable
- Favourable physical characteristics
  - Boiling point above room temperature enables simple storage and use in vaporizers
  - Low latent heat of vaporization simplifies vaporizer design
- No environmental hazard
  - To theatre staff in trace concentrations
  - When vented into the atmosphere
- Inexpensive
- High potency
- Allows agent to be given with a high inspired concentration of oxygen
- Low blood solubility
  - Rapid onset of action
  - Rapid offset
  - Depth of anaesthesia altered readily
- Minimal metabolism
  - Recovery is entirely dependent on exhalation
- Minimal toxicity
- No cardiorespiratory side effects
- Analgesic
- Easily administered
  - Non-noxious odour; non-irritant to airways
  - High therapeutic index
  - Simple apparatus required

15.1 Properties of an ideal inhalant anaesthetic agent.

inhaled agent into the body causes the exhaled gases to have a lower agent concentration than that in the FGF and thus dilutes the agent concentration within the system. For this reason, an initially high FGF following connection of a patient to a circle system is recommended (see Chapter 5). By comparison, agent concentrations in non-rebreathing systems such as the Bain or T-piece are minimally affected by FGF provided the flow is appropriate for a given patient. This is because each breath the patient takes should be entirely composed of fresh gas and therefore the inhaled agent concentration reflects the vaporizer setting.

In addition, at the beginning of use, circle systems contain a relatively large volume of room air compared to non-rebreathing systems. This air will slow the rate of increase of agent concentration within the system. Fresh gas must displace the room air present in the system; the rate at which this occurs is a function of both the system volume and the FGF. As the volume of a circle system includes the hoses, the space within the absorbent canister and the reservoir bag, it can take several minutes for agent concentration to increase. In contrast, non-rebreathing systems have a much smaller volume and the inspired concentration of volatile agent almost immediately reflects the vaporizer setting.

Factors affecting alveolar concentration of agent

The alveolar inhalant concentration is important because induction, maintenance and recovery from general anaesthesia depend on an adequate agent effect in the brain and spinal cord; the key sites of action. Alveolar concentration (or, to use the correct terminology, partial pressure) of agent is an approximate reflection of concentration (partial pressure) in the central nervous system (CNS).

As the concentration of inhalant agent in the breathing system increases, the alveolar concentration of agent will also rise. For a given vaporizer setting, the rate of increase of alveolar concentration is determined by the rate of agent uptake into the body and by alveolar ventilation. The rate of agent uptake into the body (the speed at which the agent is removed from the alveoli by the pulmonary circulation) is a function of agent solubility in the blood (and tissues) and alveolar blood flow. The blood solubility of sevoflurane, which has a blood:gas partition coefficient (B:G) of 0.69 at body temperature, is approximately half that of isoflurane (B:G = 1.4). For agents with greater solubility, the rate of increase in alveolar agent concentration is slower because the circulation effectively acts as a sink, rapidly removing the agent as it is added to the alveolar gas from the breathing system by lung ventilation. Therefore, facemask induction of anaesthesia with isoflurane is slower than with sevoflurane (provided other determining factors are equal), as the alveolar concentration of isoflurane will rise more slowly. This principle applies equally to the speed of changes in anaesthetic depth with changes in the vaporizer setting, and to the speed of recovery.

Of the modern inhalant agents, desflurane has the lowest B:G (0.42). This, combined with its potency (relative to nitrous oxide, see below), confers advantages for induction and recovery speed and the ability to alter anaesthetic depth rapidly during surgery (Figure 15.2).

Alveolar blood flow depends on cardiac output, and therefore factors that affect cardiac output will have an effect on agent uptake. In a low cardiac output state (e.g. congestive heart failure) the uptake of agent from the alveoli is lower, which means that alveolar concentration of the agent rises more rapidly. The alveolar concentration of agent, parallels agent concentration in

Agent	Blood:gas partition coefficient[a]	Oil:gas partition coefficient[b]	Saturated vapour pressure at 20°C (mmHg)	Boiling point (°C)
Isoflurane	1.40	98	239	48.5
Sevoflurane	0.69	47	160	58.6
Desflurane	0.42	19	664	23.5
Nitrous oxide	0.47	1.4	3900	−89

15.2 Comparison of physical properties of inhalant anaesthetic agents. [a] The lower the value, the faster are induction and recovery. [b] The higher the value, the more potent the agent and the lower the minimum alveolar concentration (MAC).

the brain, and therefore, changes in depth of anaesthesia occur more rapidly in this state. Conversely, high cardiac output states (e.g. sinus tachycardia) have the opposite effect, and changes in depth of anaesthesia occur more slowly. However, the effect of cardiac output on the uptake of relatively insoluble agents such as isoflurane and sevoflurane is less pronounced compared with the effect on uptake of a more soluble agent such as halothane.

Finally, ventilation determines the speed of anaesthetic induction by controlling the supply of inhalant agent to the alveoli and replacing agent removed by uptake into the body. An increase in ventilation promotes maintenance of alveolar concentration during the period of rapid uptake that occurs at induction, thus ensuring that a large gradient between alveolar and blood concentration is maintained.

Factors determining elimination of inhalant anaesthetic agents and recovery from anaesthesia

Recovery from general anaesthesia occurs when the concentration of inhalant agent in the CNS is sufficiently low to allow consciousness to return. Possible routes of elimination of inhalant agents are through biotransformation (i.e. metabolism) or exhalation. For modern volatile agents such as isoflurane and sevoflurane, recovery is almost entirely mediated through the respiratory system and there is minimal biotransformation. In contrast, for halothane, biotransformation accounts for approximately 25% of elimination. Biotransformation of isoflurane (<1%), sevoflurane (3%) and desflurane (0.02%) occurs in the liver (cytochrome P450 system). In the case of sevoflurane, biotransformation produces measurable amounts of fluoride ions. While fluoride ions could potentially result in nephrotoxicity, the quantities produced do not appear to be clinically relevant. The low level of biotransformation does not preclude the use of sevoflurane or isoflurane in patients with hepatic disease.

The removal of anaesthetic agent by exhalation is driven by the same factors as those determining the rate of induction: the agent concentration in the breathing system and in the blood (and tissues), which in turn is determined by ventilation and agent solubility. Each of these factors contributes to the rate of reduction in anaesthetic agent concentration in the CNS by altering the concentration gradient between the pulmonary circulation and alveoli.

Practical techniques for speeding recovery when using a circle breathing system act by promoting a rapid decrease in agent concentration in both alveoli and breathing system after the vaporizer has been turned off.

These include:

- Increasing the FGF to allow rapid replacement of gas in the breathing system with oxygen
- Increasing minute volume to replace alveolar gas with oxygen
- Emptying the reservoir bag into the scavenging system, which removes the reservoir of inhalational agent that feeds into the circle system to sustain agent concentration.

With non-rebreathing systems, when the vaporizer is turned off, oxygen is delivered directly from the anaesthetic machine; the primary determinant of recovery in these circumstances is ventilation.

The low blood solubility of desflurane means that recovery from general anaesthesia with this agent is rapid. In addition to smaller clinical trials in dogs, large-scale human studies (meta-analyses) have shown faster short-term (time to extubation) and long-term (return to normal function within 24 hours postoperatively) recovery periods compared with sevoflurane and isoflurane. This makes desflurane a popular choice for fast-track outpatient procedures in human medicine.

Anaesthetic periods longer than several hours in duration may result in a slower recovery because the agent is retained in the body. The amount retained depends on both blood and tissue solubility. More soluble agents such as halothane (with a B:G value approximately three times that of sevoflurane) accumulate in body tissues during a long anaesthetic period. At the end of anaesthesia, accumulated agent re-enters the circulation and maintains a small concentration gradient between the cerebral circulation and brain, slowing the reduction of agent concentration in the CNS. However, the relatively lower blood and tissue solubilities of sevoflurane and desflurane, and, to a lesser extent, isoflurane, mean that longer anaesthetic periods with these agents are less likely to be associated with slow recovery.

Potency

The potency of an inhalant anaesthetic agent is expressed as the minimum alveolar concentration (MAC), which is defined as the alveolar concentration of an agent that prevents purposeful movements in 50% of animals when they are exposed to a standardized noxious stimulus at sea level. The concept of MAC allows a standard comparison of the potency of different inhalant anaesthetics. A description of how MAC is measured in a laboratory setting is beyond the scope of this chapter; however, the practical implications are discussed here.

It is apparent from the above definition of MAC that an inhalant agent concentration of 1 MAC will still allow 50% of animals to move in response to a noxious stimulus. To decrease the risk of an animal moving in response to noxious stimulation (e.g. surgical stimulation), a MAC multiple can be used (Figure 15.3). Typically, 1.3 times a given MAC value will prevent movement in approximately 95% of anaesthetized animals. For example, for isoflurane-anaesthetized dogs (MAC 1.3%), an alveolar concentration of 1.7% (1.3 x 1.3%) would prevent movement in approximately 95% of dogs. However, MAC is determined in the absence of other agents. A balanced anaesthetic protocol using sedatives and analgesics will decrease the requirement for inhalant agents (anaesthetic-sparing effect; Figure 15.4). Therefore, when using inhalant anaesthetic agents, close and regular monitoring of anaesthetic depth is an essential part of safe patient management.

Agent	Cat	Dog
MAC isoflurane (%)	1.7	1.3
MAC sevoflurane (%)	3.0	2.3
MAC desflurane (%)	9.8	7.6
MAC nitrous oxide (%)	255	188–222
1.3 x MAC isoflurane (%)	2.2	1.7
1.3 x MAC sevoflurane (%)	3.9	3
1.3 x MAC desflurane (%)	12.7	9.9

15.3 Values of minimum alveolar concentration (MAC) for different inhalant anaesthetic agents, and MAC multiples typically used in the clinical setting, in cats and dogs. Note that the values for MAC are the average values reported in published data and individual variation exists.

Increase in minimum alveolar concentration (MAC)
- Hyperthermia
- Catecholamines/sympathomimetics, e.g. ephedrine
- Hyperthyroidism
- Hypernatraemia

Decrease in minimum alveolar concentration (MAC)
- Hypothermia
- Hypoxaemia
- Hypercapnia (when P_aCO_2 exceeds approximately 95 mmHg)
- Drugs causing CNS depression
- Sedatives[a]
- Injectable anaesthetic agents
- Analgesic agents[ab]
- Pregnancy
- Old age
- Hypotension
- Hypothyroidism

15.4 Factors associated with an increase or decrease in minimum alveolar concentration (MAC), which result in an increase or decrease in concentration of inhalant agent needed to maintain anaesthesia. [a] Potent sedatives and analgesics can result in a profound decrease in MAC, and anaesthetic depth should be closely monitored and adjusted accordingly. Examples include medetomidine, dexmedetomidine, morphine, methadone, fentanyl, epidural bupivacaine. [b] Some analgesic agents also cause CNS depression (sedation), e.g. medetomidine, dexmedetomidine, morphine, methadone. CNS = central nervous system; P_aCO_2 = arterial carbon dioxide tension.

Effects of inhalants on the body

Volatile anaesthetic agents share common adverse effects. They have profound depressant effects on the cardiovascular and respiratory systems. The following section describes the effects of volatile agents when administered alone, to allow direct comparisons between them, although this is seldom the approach used in clinical practice. Additional variables, including systemic disease, the patient's age, surgical stimulation and concurrent use of other drugs, may alter the described effects.

Cerebral effects

Isoflurane and sevoflurane decrease cerebral metabolic rate, which results in a decrease in cerebral oxygen consumption and a subsequent decrease in cerebral blood flow. However, volatile anaesthetics also cause cerebral vasodilation. The overall effect on cerebral blood flow is a balance between the reduced oxygen demand and the cerebral vasodilation, and generally blood flow increases.

Both isoflurane and sevoflurane increase intracranial blood volume (as a result of the increased flow); this is an important consideration when anaesthetizing patients with head trauma or intracranial pathology (see Chapter 28). There is some evidence that sevoflurane may preserve cerebral perfusion better than isoflurane at equipotent values of MAC in healthy dogs. At the same depth of anaesthesia, desflurane is associated with a greater degree of cerebral vasodilation, and therefore it should be used cautiously in patients with increased intracranial pressure.

Cardiovascular effects

Cardiovascular depression is a major side effect of the volatile agents. Isoflurane and sevoflurane cause dose-dependent changes in many of the variables that maintain arterial blood pressure, with resultant hypotension. Both cardiac output and systemic vascular resistance (vascular tone) are reduced as a consequence of decreased myocardial contractility and vasodilation, respectively. As a result, hypotension is one of the most common side effects of volatile agents. In contrast to isoflurane and sevoflurane, desflurane may result in hypotension primarily through reduced myocardial contractility.

The effect of the volatile agents on heart rate is less predictable. Heart rate is influenced by many factors, including vagal tone, concurrent medication, ventilation (hypercapnia and hypoxaemia) and noxious stimulation. In the absence of other agents, heart rate tends to increase, but not to a degree that is sufficient to offset the hypotensive effects of volatile agents resulting from reduced contractility and vasodilation. Desflurane in particular can cause tachycardia when the inspired concentration is rapidly increased, although this response is blunted when potent opioids are also administered.

Monitoring and haemodynamic support are fundamental to ensure adequate organ perfusion and maintenance of normal physiology. In general, mean arterial blood pressure should be maintained at a value between 60 and 150 mmHg for adequate perfusion of vital organs such as the kidneys, heart and brain. The degree of hypotension can be mitigated by reducing the inspired concentration of volatile agent, providing supportive drug and fluid therapy (see Chapters 17 and 18) and limiting the use of intermittent positive pressure ventilation (IPPV), which can reduce venous return. However, the judicious use of IPPV may be necessary to offset respiratory depression and ensuing hypercapnia and respiratory acidosis (see Chapter 6). Lower volatile agent requirements can easily be achieved with the use of systemic opioids and alpha-2 adrenoceptor agonists as part of a balanced anaesthesia protocol, and/or locoregional analgesia (see Chapter 11 and Figure 15.4), or both. Reductions of 30–70% in volatile agent requirements have been reported with the use of powerful opioids such as morphine and fentanyl (see Chapter 10), especially in dogs. Similarly, use of a locoregional anaesthetic technique allows marked decreases in volatile agent requirements because transmission of noxious signals is blocked; in such cases, the required concen–trations to maintain general anaesthesia are close to, or slightly below, the MAC of the agent.

Respiratory effects

In general, administration of volatile agents results in dose-dependent respiratory depression, with consequent hypercapnia. Respiratory depression is caused by a decrease in minute volume (resulting from decreased

respiratory rate and/or tidal volume). Hypoventilation may not be obvious if only the respiratory rate is being monitored, because tidal volume is subjectively evaluated by observation of thoracic excursions or movements of the reservoir bag in the breathing system. The tidal volume tends to decrease initially at lower volatile agent concentrations, before a decrease in respiratory rate occurs. Causes of hypercapnia are multifactorial and include a reduction in respiratory drive (blunted response to carbon dioxide), relaxation of the respiratory muscles, particularly the diaphragm, and a mismatch of ventilated to perfused areas of lung tissue. Hypoxaemia is uncommon because high levels of oxygen are frequently used in the carrier gas for volatile agents. Additional variables can make the effects of volatile agents on ventilation unpredictable; these include obesity, body position, co-existing disease and concurrent medication. Sevoflurane and desflurane tend to have a less depressant effect on minute volume because respiratory rate is better maintained with these agents compared with isoflurane. Given the likelihood of additional factors contributing to respiratory depression, as described above, use of sevoflurane does not, however, guarantee adequate ventilation. In the absence of other agents, respiratory arrest will occur at approximately 2.5 x MAC for isoflurane (end-tidal concentration of 3%) and a little over 3 x MAC for sevoflurane (end-tidal concentration of 7%).

Sevoflurane and isoflurane cause bronchodilation. This can be particularly useful in managing patients at risk of bronchospasm, such as asthmatic cats. When bronchospasm occurs, an increase in the volatile agent concentration can help reverse the problem (see Chapter 22). However, increasing the agent concentration is likely to lead to undesirable cardiopulmonary depression, which can be detrimental.

The odour of sevoflurane is generally better tolerated than that of isoflurane or desflurane. This can be beneficial when attempting induction of anaesthesia by facemask or induction chamber. However, these techniques are associated with several important disadvantages, including workplace pollution and personnel exposure to volatile agent, lack of rapid airway control and potentially increased stress for the patient (and personnel). As soon as the facemask (and anaesthetic) is removed, or the patient removed from the chamber to allow endotracheal intubation, the patient's depth of anaesthesia will invariably lighten, provided they are still breathing. This rapid lightening results in a shorter time available to perform intubation before airway reflexes and jaw tone return, compared to that provided by intravenous anaesthetic agents.

Renal and hepatic effects

Renal and hepatic perfusion is commonly reduced as a result of the hypotension caused by volatile agents. Reduced renal perfusion may manifest as a temporary reduction in urine output postoperatively. In addition, the kidneys may be at increased risk of adverse effects from use of non-steroidal anti-inflammatory drugs (see Chapter 10). Degradation of sevoflurane by carbon dioxide absorbents results in the production of Compound A, which has been associated with renal toxicity in rats; however, there is no evidence that this compound accumulates in a circle system when appropriate fresh gas flows are used (see Chapter 5).

Hepatic dysfunction associated with volatile agents is a combination of direct and indirect effects on the liver.

Direct effects result from hepatocellular dysfunction and a potential reduction in the capacity for drug metabolism. Direct effects are minimal with isoflurane and sevoflurane. Indirect effects result from cardiovascular depression reducing hepatic perfusion and can be corrected with management and support of arterial blood pressure (see Chapters 17 and 24). There is little evidence to support a preference for either isoflurane or sevoflurane in patients with, or at risk of, hepatic dysfunction.

Analgesic effects

Volatile anaesthetic agents are not considered to have analgesic properties. They are 'analgesic' only in the sense that by producing loss of consciousness, they block pain perception, although they do not prevent noxious signals reaching the spinal cord and brain. Following recovery from anaesthesia, a patient is able to perceive the pain resulting from tissue damage that occurred during surgery and adequate analgesia should be part of the anaesthetic protocol (see Chapter 10).

Nitrous oxide

Nitrous oxide differs markedly from other inhaled anaesthetic agents in that it is a gaseous agent that is stored under pressure as a liquid at room temperature (see Chapter 4). It has relatively low potency in comparison to the volatile agents (high MAC value; see Figure 15.3) but is commonly administered for its analgesic properties, thus reducing the requirement for other inhaled agents (anaesthetic-sparing effect). The mechanism of action of nitrous oxide is unclear but its effects appear to be mediated through multiple receptors, including N-methyl-D-aspartate, opioid and alpha-2 adrenoceptors.

Administration

Nitrous oxide has a low B:G partition coefficient (0.47), similar to that of desflurane, which promotes a rapid onset and offset of action. As a result of its low potency, it is usually delivered at a relatively high concentration (approximately 50–70%), which necessitates a decrease in the fraction of inspired oxygen. This mode of use and the physical properties of nitrous oxide favour a rapid increase in anaesthetic depth through two phenomena: the *concentration effect* and the *second gas effect*. The concentration effect is the maintenance of a high concentration of nitrous oxide in the alveoli following uptake. The rapid uptake of nitrous oxide from the alveoli into the pulmonary circulation (nitrous oxide is more soluble than oxygen) leads to a decrease in alveolar volume; as a result, the remaining gases in the alveolus (such as oxygen and a volatile anaesthetic agent) are concentrated in the reduced volume. As ventilation continues, and alveolar volume is refilled, a relatively high concentration of nitrous oxide is maintained while the concentration of volatile anaesthetic agent is augmented (second gas effect). Thus, the second gas effect describes the concentration effect on a second gas, the volatile anaesthetic agent. Together, the concentration effect and second gas effect support high alveolar anaesthetic concentrations, increasing the speed of anaesthetic induction.

These phenomena are also relevant to recovery from anaesthesia, when nitrous oxide is being removed from the body through ventilation. If, at the end of an anaesthetic, the inspired gas is switched from an oxygen–nitrous oxide–volatile agent mixture to air (as happens when an animal is disconnected from the breathing system), there is a risk of diffusion hypoxia. This occurs as a result of a high concentration of nitrous oxide developing in the alveoli at the end of the anaesthetic, which displaces oxygen and dilutes carbon dioxide (which in turn reduces ventilatory drive). It is therefore good practice to deliver a high concentration of oxygen to the patient for 5–10 minutes after nitrous oxide is turned off.

Nitrous oxide is typically administered at a concentration of 50–70%, resulting in an inspired oxygen concentration of 30–50%. Concurrent use of an oxygen analyser and pulse oximeter is recommended when using such gas mixtures.

Clinical use

The anaesthetic-sparing effect of 70% nitrous oxide ranges from 20–40%. This represents a significant reduction in volatile agent requirement, which is beneficial in terms of reducing cardiovascular and respiratory depression.

Nitrous oxide causes mild stimulation of the cardiovascular system, mediated via the sympathetic nervous system. Minute volume is unchanged, with an increased respiratory rate balanced by a decrease in tidal volume. However, hypoxic drive is depressed and therefore close monitoring during the recovery period (when inspired oxygen returns to atmospheric concentration) is essential. Nitrous oxide may predispose to an increase in intracranial pressure in patients with intracranial pathology due to an increase in cerebral metabolic rate and blood flow.

Adverse effects

Nitrous oxide is approximately 20 times more soluble in blood than oxygen and nitrogen. As a result, its use should be avoided where there is the presence of, or potential for, an enclosed gas space, as it will diffuse into that space more rapidly than oxygen and nitrogen can diffuse out (as gases equilibrate). Examples include gastric dilatation–volvulus, air embolism, closed pneumothorax, intestinal obstruction and ophthalmic procedures with a risk of intraocular bubbles.

The use (and abuse) of nitrous oxide has been associated with haemopoietic and neurological abnormalities in both laboratory animals and humans who chronically inhale nitrous oxide. However, the risks of these effects in operating department personnel have largely been removed with the implementation of effective waste gas scavenging systems. It would, however, be prudent to avoid administering nitrous oxide by facemask or chamber to avoid workspace pollution with the gas. Nitrous oxide is not adsorbed by charcoal canisters and scavenging via a scavenging system should be employed.

Cost and use comparison of volatile anaesthetic agents

As the costs of volatile agents change over time and new agents are introduced, it is useful to be able to estimate the cost of using a given agent. Although financial considerations should not be the primary determining factor in drug selection, a cost calculation provides a useful comparison of agents when clinical differences are minimal.

Dion's formula (Dion, 1992) provides an estimate of cost of volatile agent use. It takes into account the molecular weight (M, in grams), cost (C, £/ml) and density (d, g/ml) of the agent. These are combined with the user variables of vaporizer concentration (P, %), fresh gas flow (F, l/min) and duration of anaesthesia (T, minutes) in the following formula:

Cost (£) = $PFTMC/2412d$

The constant 2412 represents the molar volume of a gas at room temperature (21°C). Figure 15.5 provides a comparison of isoflurane, sevoflurane and desflurane at current (2015) costs when delivered in a fresh gas flow of 50 ml/kg/min to a 10 kg dog at vaporizer settings of 1.3 x MAC for 1 hour.

Variable (units)	Isoflurane	Sevoflurane	Desflurane
P (%)	1.7	3	9.9
F (l/min)	0.5	0.5	0.5
T (min)	60	60	60
M (g)	184.5	200.1	168
C (£/ml)	0.10	0.69	0.68
d (g/ml)	1.5	1.5	1.5
Cost (£)	0.26	3.43	9.38

15.5 Cost comparison of isoflurane, sevoflurane and desflurane. C = cost; d = density; F = fresh gas flow; M = molecular weight; P = vaporizer concentration; T = anaesthetic duration.

Workplace exposure

Nitrous oxide can also enter endotracheal tubes cuffs and increase the volume, although the cuffs are relatively compliant. Waste anaesthetic gas is defined as gas that is leaked from the anaesthetic delivery system into the surrounding environment. This includes gas exhaled by patients during recovery. Short-term exposure to high concentrations of volatile agents is associated with headache, irritability, fatigue, nausea, drowsiness, and impaired judgment and coordination.

Engineering controls

These include an appropriate and functional waste anaesthetic gas scavenging system and room ventilation (see Chapter 5), regular maintenance and inspection of anaesthetic equipment and the use of key-indexed vaporizer filling systems (see Chapter 4).

Proper work practice

The lowest suitable fresh gas flow should be used to meet equipment and patient requirements. Induction by facemask or chamber and maintenance of anaesthesia by facemask should be avoided. Anaesthetic machines and breathing systems should be leak-tested daily and the vaporizer and nitrous oxide should be turned off when a patient is not connected to the breathing system. The reservoir bag should be emptied into the scavenging system before disconnection of the patient, and gases sampled for sidestream capnography should also be scavenged.

Small spills of volatile agent evaporate rapidly at room temperature, and often dissipate before they can be cleaned up. In the case of a large spill, such as a broken bottle of agent, the material safety data sheet recommendations should be followed. These typically include: wearing personal protective equipment (PPE: impermeable gloves, laboratory coat, safety glasses), ventilating the spill site if possible, evacuating personnel not wearing PPE from the area, and applying absorbent material suitable for organic chemicals. If absorbent is used, it should be collected and placed in an airtight container, and disposed of according to local regulations.

Monitoring

Volatile agents cannot be detected by smell until a high concentration is present; at the point that they become detectable, unnecessary exposure has already occurred. Monitoring for trace concentrations of agents can be performed periodically to assess personnel exposure. Monitors can sample room air, or personnel can wear badges at shoulder level to indicate respiratory exposure. Badges are sent for analysis and an 8-hour time-weighted average exposure is calculated.

The National Institute for Occupational Safety and Health in the USA goes as far as recommending that hepatic and renal function of personnel should be monitored regularly and medical records monitored for indications of adverse effects that may be associated with exposure to anaesthetic gases.

Training of personnel

All personnel at risk of exposure to anaesthetic gases should receive appropriate training. This includes both information and practical training relating to engineering controls and proper work practice, as well as communicating the health hazards associated with anaesthetic gas exposure.

Environmental considerations

Sevoflurane, isoflurane, desflurane and nitrous oxide are all classed as greenhouse gases. This is due to the significant length of time they remain in the atmosphere and also because their infrared absorption spectra overlap with infrared radiation leaving the earth, thereby reducing its emission into space. The effect on infrared radiation, combined with predicted atmospheric lifetime, is used to calculate a Global Warming Potential (GWP) Index, a widely accepted method of assessing an agent's contribution to climate change. For the volatile agents, the highest to lowest GWP values are desflurane > sevoflurane > isoflurane. Nitrous oxide has a lesser short-term impact but has the potential to contribute for a longer time period as a result of its atmospheric lifetime. Predicted atmospheric lifetimes can be long (isoflurane, 3.2 years; sevoflurane, 1.1 years; desflurane, 14 years; nitrous oxide, 114 years).

While levels of inhalant agents in the atmosphere are low relative to those of carbon dioxide, they can still make a significant contribution to the retention of heat and thus climate change. It has been recommended that potential contributions to climate change be taken into account when selecting anaesthetic agents and introducing new agents to clinical use (Ryan and Nielsen, 2010). A simple and effective way of reducing the use (and therefore emission) of inhalational anaesthetic agents is to use the lowest safe fresh gas flows.

Summary

Inhalant anaesthetic agents are a popular choice for general anaesthesia, but they do have a range of significant adverse effects. The judicious use of balanced anaesthesia techniques and appropriate management can limit the occurrence and impact of adverse effects. Detrimental effects on the health of personnel resulting from chronic exposure to low concentrations of inhalant agents remain unclear, but good working practices and engineering controls can substantially reduce these risks.

Acknowledgements

Thank you to the following people for constructive input: Jessica Paterson, Melanie Prebble.

References and further reading

Burm AGL (2003) Occupational hazards of inhalational anaesthetics. *Best Practice and Research Clinical Anaesthesiology* **17**, 147–161

Dion P (1992) The cost of anaesthetic vapours. *Canadian Journal of Anaesthesia* **39**, 633

Franks NP (2008) General anaesthesia: from molecular targets to neuronal pathways of sleep and arousal. *Nature Reviews Neuroscience* **9**, 370–386

Health and Safety Executive (2014) Workplace exposure limits. www.hse.gov.uk/coshh/basics/exposurelimits.htm

Occupational Safety and Health Administration (2014) Waste anesthetic gases. www.osha.gov/SLTC/wasteanestheticgases/index.html

Ryan SM and Nielsen CJ (2010) Global warming potential of inhaled anesthetics: application to clinical use. *Anesthesia and Analgesia* **111**, 92–98

Sulbaek Andersen MP, Nielsen OJ, Wallington TJ, Karpichev B and Sander SP (2012) Assessing the impact on global climate from general anesthetic gases. *Anesthesia and Analgesia* **114**, 1081–1085

Chapter 16

Neuromuscular blocking agents

Derek Flaherty and Adam Auckburally

Many drugs used for induction or maintenance of anaesthesia provide a degree of skeletal muscle relaxation, but in general this is only mild to moderate at a surgical plane of anaesthesia. More profound muscle relaxation can be achieved in several ways:

- **Increasing the depth of anaesthesia.** Although muscle relaxation will improve with increasing depth of anaesthesia, this is not recommended because of the associated increase in cardiopulmonary depression
- **Local anaesthetic techniques.** By paralysing the motor fibres responsible for maintenance of muscle tone, the use of local anaesthetics can provide profound muscle relaxation (see Chapter 11). However, local anaesthesia may not be applicable or achievable in all cases, and considerable skill is required to perform some regional nerve blocks
- **Centrally acting muscle relaxants.** Benzodiazepines and alpha-2 adrenoceptor agonists both provide moderate to good muscle relaxation. However, because this effect is achieved via a centrally mediated action, they also have numerous other effects, many of which may be undesirable (see Chapter 13)
- **Peripherally acting muscle relaxants.** These are neuromuscular blocking agents (NMBAs) that act at the neuromuscular junction (NMJ) to provide profound skeletal muscle relaxation ('paralysis') throughout the body.

Although other drugs can be considered to be muscle relaxants due to their effects on the central nervous system (CNS) (see above), in general the term 'muscle relaxant' is most often used for NMBAs, and these form the focus of this chapter.

Microanatomy of the neuromuscular junction and physiology of neuromuscular transmission

An understanding of normal neuromuscular transmission is essential for the appropriate use of NMBAs.

Skeletal muscle cells are innervated by myelinated nerve fibres from motor neurons. As each nerve fibre approaches the muscle cell, it loses its myelin sheath. The region of contact between the nerve and the muscle is termed the *motor endplate* (Figure 16.1). Here, the muscle membrane becomes folded, and is separated from the nerve terminal by a distance of approximately 20 nm; this separation is known as the *junctional* (or *synaptic*) *cleft*. Within the nerve terminal there are abundant vesicles containing the neurotransmitter acetylcholine (ACh), and on the crests of the folded muscle membrane lie postjunctional nicotinic ACh receptors.

When an action potential reaches the nerve terminal, ACh storage vesicles in the terminal fuse to the prejunctional membrane and release ACh into the junctional cleft by exocytosis. ACh then diffuses across the cleft to bind to the postjunctional receptors. The receptors comprise a pentameric protein structure, which, when stimulated, undergoes a conformational change to open a transmembrane channel that allows movement of ions across the membrane. Two ACh molecules, binding to two distinct α-subunits of the pentameric structure, are required to open the ion channel. If one subunit is not bound, or is

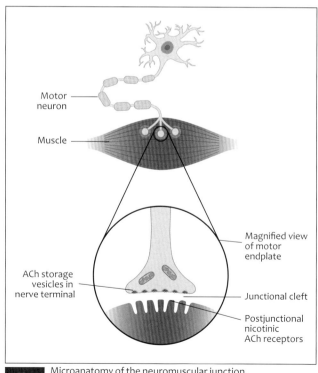

16.1 Microanatomy of the neuromuscular junction.
ACh = acetylcholine.

Motor neuron

Muscle

Magnified view of motor endplate

ACh storage vesicles in nerve terminal

Junctional cleft

Postjunctional nicotinic ACh receptors

BSAVA Manual of Canine and Feline Anaesthesia and Analgesia, third edition. Edited by Tanya Duke-Novakovski, Marieke de Vries and Chris Seymour. ©BSAVA 2016

occupied by another molecule, the channel will not open. The movement of ions through the membrane channel generates an endplate potential, and if enough ion channels are opened, the adjacent muscle membrane depolarizes and an action potential is generated. Within the sarcolemma (muscle membrane), this action potential traverses the T-tubule system and causes release of calcium ions from the sarcoplasmic reticulum, initiating excitation–contraction coupling and subsequent muscle contraction (Figure 16.2).

Acetylcholine remains bound to its receptors for approximately 2 milliseconds, then detaches, and is rapidly hydrolysed into choline and acetate by the enzyme acetylcholinesterase, which is present in the junctional cleft. This terminates the action of ACh on the postjunctional receptors, the transmembrane channel closes and muscle contraction terminates.

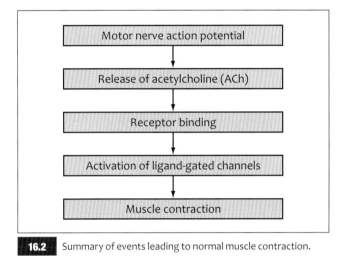

16.2 Summary of events leading to normal muscle contraction.

There are also prejunctional nicotinic ACh receptors, which provide a positive feedback mechanism that augments ACh release during high-frequency nerve stimulation; that is, binding of ACh or an alternative agonist such as suxamethonium (succinylcholine) to these receptors stimulates further ACh release. However, the precise structure and function of the prejunctional receptors is less clearly defined than for those situated postjunctionally.

At physiological frequencies of nerve stimulation, neuromuscular transmission begins to fail only after a minimum of 75% of the postsynaptic ACh receptors have been blocked, and complete failure of transmission occurs with greater than 90% receptor blockade. This so-called neuromuscular 'margin of safety' implies that only 25% of ACh receptors need to be stimulated to induce normal neuromuscular transmission. The major implication of this is that during recovery from use of NMBAs, up to 75% of ACh receptors may still be blocked, with the patient exhibiting no detectable clinical signs, but with a reduced margin of safety.

Mechanism of action of neuromuscular blocking agents

Based on differences in their mechanisms of action, NMBAs can be classified as either *depolarizing (non-competitive)* or *non-depolarizing (competitive)*.

The only depolarizing relaxant used clinically is suxamethonium (succinylcholine), which consists of two molecules of ACh joined together. Because of its structure, administration of suxamethonium causes the generation of an action potential through binding to postsynaptic ACh receptors. However, since suxamethonium is not metabolized by acetylcholinesterase, the drug remains bound to the receptors for a longer period of time than ACh does, until suxamethonium blood concentration has declined sufficiently for the drug to diffuse down its concentration gradient from the NMJ into the plasma, allowing restoration of normal neuromuscular transmission. Plasma degradation of suxamethonium is mediated through the enzyme pseudocholinesterase (plasma cholinesterase; also known as butyrylcholinesterase), which is distinct from acetylcholinesterase. The prolonged binding of suxamethonium to the ACh receptor prevents normal neuromuscular transmission. As a result, the observed clinical effect is one of initial muscle stimulation as a result of the initial action potential, which manifests as widespread transient muscle fasciculations throughout the body, followed by a longer period of muscle flaccidity. This normal pattern of suxamethonium-induced blockade is known as *phase I block* (phase II block is described later).

Non-depolarizing NMBAs have a chemical structure different from that of suxamethonium. Although they also bind to the postsynaptic ACh receptors, they do not induce channel opening and the consequent generation of an action potential. By preventing ACh reaching the receptors, they induce a competitive blockade, resulting in muscle paralysis. Thus, unlike suxamethonium, non-depolarizing relaxants do not produce initial muscle fasciculations before the onset of muscle relaxation. It is not necessary for both α-subunit binding sites within the pentameric receptor structure to be occupied by a non-depolarizing NMBA to result in paralysis; only one site needs to be occupied by the drug and the ion channel will remain closed, even if the other site is occupied by an ACh molecule.

It is important to emphasize that NMBAs are neither anaesthetic nor analgesic. It is therefore possible that, if these agents are used inappropriately, a patient may be paralysed but fully conscious. This must be avoided at all costs by closely monitoring the adequacy of anaesthesia (see later).

Pattern of neuromuscular blockade

As NMBAs paralyse all skeletal muscles within the body, including those responsible for respiration, *it is essential that facilities for controlled ventilation are available whenever these drugs are used.* Not all muscles are equally sensitive to NMBAs. The diaphragm and intercostal musculature in particular are relatively resistant; these are usually the first muscles to recover following administration of an NMBA. However, the muscles around the pharyngeal area are much more sensitive to the effects of NMBAs and take longer to return to normal function. Clinically, patients may appear to be ventilating adequately during recovery from neuromuscular blockade, but may develop upper airway obstruction once the endotracheal tube is removed.

Because the diaphragm and intercostal muscles are less sensitive to NMBAs than other skeletal muscles in the body, attempts have been made to produce muscle relaxation without interference with respiratory function. An example is relaxation of the extraocular muscles to produce a centrally positioned, immobile eye (for ocular surgery) by using low doses of NMBA, while maintaining spontaneous ventilation. This technique appears to avoid the need for either a staff member devoted to manual ventilation of the lungs, or an automatic ventilator (and associated expense). Although some authorities have claimed success with this practice, it involves considerable risk of hypoventilation of the patient, and, in the authors' opinion, should be avoided. As inspired oxygen concentration is often close to 100%, patients are usually able to maintain adequate oxygenation in these circumstances, but may become severely hypercapnic (Sullivan *et al.*, 1998).

Monitoring the neuromuscular junction

When using NMBAs, it is essential to assess the degree of neuromuscular blockade. This is most commonly performed by using a peripheral nerve stimulator (Figure 16.3a). This device delivers a small electrical current (up to 80 mA, depending on the model) through a pair of electrodes attached to the skin overlying a peripheral motor nerve. The ulnar nerve on the medial aspect of the elbow (Figure 16.3b), the peroneal nerve at the lateral head of the fibula (Figure 16.3c) or the dorsal buccal branch of the facial nerve caudoventral to the lateral aspect of the eye (Figure 16.3d) are most often used for stimulation. The response of the muscle groups innervated by these nerves is observed when the nerve stimulator is activated. The negative (black) electrode of the nerve stimulator should be positioned directly over the most superficial part of the nerve, while the positive (red) electrode is placed more proximally along the course of the nerve. The electrodes may be attached directly to the skin, or to subcutaneously placed needles. Although ECG electrode pads are normally used in humans as the interface for attachment of the nerve-stimulating electrodes, they seldom adhere sufficiently well to the skin of dogs and cats to prove reliable. It is important that the electrodes are attached over the nerve rather than the innervated muscle body, otherwise direct electrical stimulation of the muscle may occur, resulting in a muscle response even in the presence of complete neuromuscular blockade. Although techniques such as mechanomyography and electromyography are commonly used to assess the muscle response in research settings, they are too complex to be used clinically, and the veterinary surgeon (veterinarian) usually has to rely on visual and tactile assessment of the evoked muscle response (although clinically useful quantitative methods of assessment are becoming more widely available; see later).

The nerve stimulator should be capable of producing a square-wave pulse, with a constant current of at least 50–60 mA over a 1000 Ω load. The stimulus applied should be supramaximal to recruit all the nerve fibres: in the clinical setting, a supramaximal stimulus is usually achieved by increasing the nerve stimulator to the maximum current output, although lower outputs are probably still supramaximal if the current is being delivered via transcutaneous needles as opposed to ECG electrode pads. However, it is difficult to be sure that the stimulus is genuinely supramaximal merely by direct observation of the muscle response, so it remains customary to set the stimulator to its maximal output even when using needle

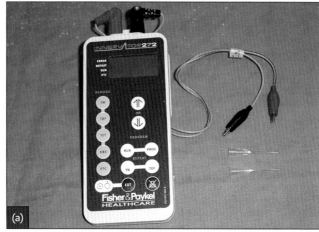

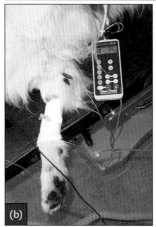
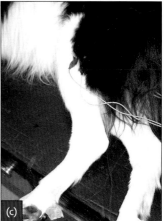

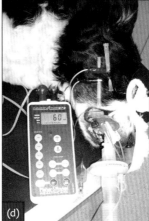

16.3 (a) Peripheral nerve stimulator with needle electrodes. (b) Placement of needle electrodes over the ulnar nerve on the medial aspect of the elbow. (c) Stimulation of the peroneal nerve can be achieved by electrode placement over the lateral head of the fibula. (d) Needle electrodes placed over the dorsal buccal branch of the facial nerve.

electrodes. The disadvantage of using excessive current as the stimulus is that it is proportionally more noxious in minimally anaesthetized animals.

Stimulation patterns

Several different stimulation patterns can be used to assess neuromuscular blockade.

Single twitch

The single twitch is a stimulation pattern that uses a single electrical pulse delivered at a rate between one per second (1 Hz) and one per 10 seconds (0.1 Hz). This pattern is principally used to assess onset of neuromuscular blockade, particularly when NMBAs are used to facilitate endotracheal intubation in humans, and has limited use in veterinary clinical anaesthesia.

Train-of-four

Train-of-four (TOF) is the most common pattern of nerve stimulation, and is used to assess both intraoperative neuromuscular blockade and recovery. Four electrical pulses are applied to the nerve over a 2-second period (i.e. 2 Hz). In the absence of neuromuscular blockade, four distinct muscle twitches will occur (T_1, T_2, T_3 and T_4), each of which is of identical strength (Figure 16.4a). If a non-depolarizing NMBA is then administered, the fourth twitch (T_4) in the TOF will become weaker and eventually disappear, followed by the third twitch (T_3), then the second (T_2) and eventually the first (T_1) if a sufficient dose is given (Figure 16.4bc). This phenomenon of a gradually decreasing muscle response to nerve stimulation during non-depolarizing NMBA-induced relaxation is known as fade (Figure 16.4b). The main cause proposed for the occurrence of fade with non-depolarizing NMBAs is that these drugs also block the prejunctional ACh receptors, thereby reducing the availability of ACh for release during high-frequency nerve stimulation.

Depolarizing NMBAs, in contrast, do not normally 'block' the prejunctional ACh receptors, but initially stimulate them in a similar way to the postjunctional receptors. The increased mobilization of ACh that results from prejunctional receptor stimulation may be partly responsible for the muscle fasciculations seen with depolarizing NMBAs before the onset of muscle relaxation. Given the absence of prejunctional ACh receptor blockade with depolarizing agents, fade is observed only with non-depolarizing agents, or in the presence of abnormal (phase II) suxamethonium blockade (see later). The TOF response to phase I suxamethonium blockade does not exhibit fade; instead, all four twitches are reduced to an equal extent.

With onset of non-depolarizing neuromuscular blockade, T_4 disappears when approximately 75% of ACh receptors are blocked; T_3 when approximately 80% are blocked; T_2 when around 90% are blocked; and loss of T_1 indicates essentially 100% blockade. During recovery, the twitches reappear in reverse order (i.e. T_1 first).

In addition to counting the number of muscle twitches in response to TOF (the 'TOF count') as a means of assessing the degree of neuromuscular blockade, attempts have been made (using mechanomyography in the research setting) to establish a TOF ratio (height of T_4:height of T_1) that indicates recovery of neuromuscular function to a degree that allows the patient adequate muscle strength for control of the airway. In humans, a TOF ratio of at least 0.9 is considered optimal before endotracheal extubation.

A number of studies have demonstrated that visual and tactile assessment of the TOF ratio is able to detect fade only when the TOF ratio is <0.4, implying that a significant degree of neuromuscular blockade may be missed by an observer in the clinical setting. This poor sensitivity of TOF in detecting residual neuromuscular blockade is probably related to the difficulty in comparing the strength of T_4 and T_1, while ignoring the two muscle twitches in between.

Tetanic stimulation

Tetanic stimulation ('tetanus') is defined as a sustained electrical stimulus of 50 Hz (occasionally 100 Hz) for a 5-second period. Because of the high frequency of stimulation, the muscle is unable to respond by producing 50 individual muscle contractions per second, but instead summates to produce one sustained muscle contraction. This pattern of stimulation is painful in the awake and minimally anaesthetized patient. Tetanic stimulation stresses the NMJ sufficiently that neuromuscular blockade can be detected by fade. As with TOF, tetanic fade can only be detected when significant degrees of neuromuscular blockade are present; the absence of obvious fade by visual and tactile assessment is not an indication of adequate neuromuscular transmission. Tetanic stimulation has principally been used to assess recovery from neuromuscular blockade, but due to the potential for severe pain, has largely been superseded by other stimulation patterns.

Double-burst stimulation

Double-burst stimulation (DBS) (Figure 16.5) comprises three short pulses at 50 Hz, followed by either three further 50 Hz pulses ($DBS_{3,3}$) or two 50 Hz pulses ($DBS_{3,2}$). The resultant muscle response is characterized by two individual muscle twitches (D_1 and D_2), which are stronger than those produced by TOF. The ratio of D_2:D_1 in DBS correlates closely with the TOF ratio T_4:T_1. However, it is easier to detect fade with DBS than TOF, because the observer is comparing the strength of two successive twitches, D_2 and D_1, in DBS, but is comparing T_4 with T_1 in TOF, while attempting to ignore T_2 and T_3. Visual and tactile assessment of DBS twitches can detect fade at equivalent TOF ratios <0.6. Thus, although DBS is superior to TOF for detection of residual neuromuscular blockade, it does not completely rule out the presence of residual blockade, since a TOF ratio ≥0.9 is required to ensure adequate neuromuscular recovery. DBS is used to assess recovery from neuromuscular blockade when there is no apparent fade to TOF (Figure 16.6).

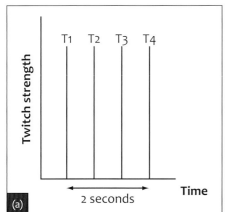
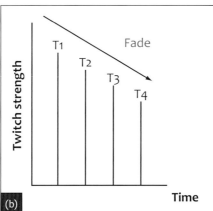
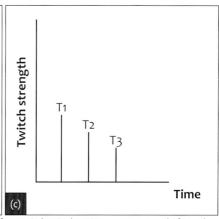

16.4 Train-of-four (TOF) stimulation pattern. (a) Normal animal, no neuromuscular blockade. All four twitches in the TOF are present and of equal strength. (b) Onset of non-depolarizing blockade. Fade is present in the TOF but all twitches are still perceptible. (c) Neuromuscular blockade is now more profound: the fourth twitch in the TOF (T_4) has disappeared and the remaining three twitches are weaker.

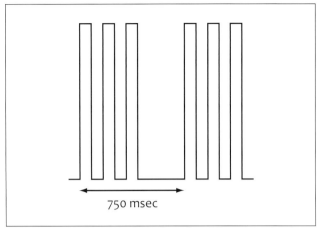

16.5 Double-burst stimulation (DBS$_{3,3}$). Each burst comprises three stimuli at a frequency of 50 Hz with the second burst following 750 milliseconds after the first. In the absence of neuromuscular blockade, this produces two distinct muscle twitches.

Pattern of nerve stimulation	Main use
Single twitch	Assessing onset of blockade
Train-of-four (TOF)	Assessing depth of block Assessing recovery from block
Tetanus	Assessing depth of block Assessing recovery from block
Double-burst stimulation (DBS)	Assessing recovery from block

16.6 Main use of different peripheral nerve stimulation patterns. TOF is the most effective means of assessing depth of neuromuscular blockade. DBS is the most effective means of assessing recovery from neuromuscular blockade (i.e. the most reliable detector of fade).

Use of peripheral nerve stimulation

It is important to emphasize that peripheral nerve stimulation provides an indication *only* of the degree of neuromuscular blockade present – it gives no information on adequacy of anaesthesia. Therefore, a patient may have no response to nerve stimulation, but still be fully conscious.

The nerve stimulator should be placed over an appropriate peripheral nerve (see above), and correct function confirmed by observing muscle twitches during activation of the device, before administration of the NMBA.

Peripheral nerve stimulation serves two useful purposes. Firstly, it has been shown in humans that ideal muscle relaxation for abdominal surgery is achieved when only one or two twitches remain in the TOF (80–90% of receptors blocked). This allows the dose of NMBA to be titrated to achieve suitable surgical conditions. Secondly, at the end of surgery, it enables an assessment of residual neuromuscular blockade. In the absence of a *quantitative* technique of evaluation of blockade (see later), the TOF should have recovered to four equal-strength twitches, and no fade should be detectable on DBS, before the animal is allowed to recover from anaesthesia and the endotracheal tube removed. It is important to recognize that, because individual muscle groups have differing sensitivities to NMBAs (see above), monitoring the response to ulnar nerve stimulation, for instance, will give limited information on the muscles of respiratory function. Consequently, even with apparently adequate recovery of neuromuscular function on nerve stimulation, the patient must be closely observed in the immediate post-anaesthetic period to ensure adequate airway control and ventilation.

Quantitative monitoring of neuromuscular function

Visual and tactile assessment of the motor response to direct nerve stimulation, as described above, provides only a subjective measure of the degree of neuromuscular blockade; that is, it is non-quantifiable. More recently, however, techniques that allow more effective objective assessment of the degree of neuromuscular blockade have been developed. While some of these, such as mechanomyography and electromyography, are largely limited to laboratory-based situations, the technique of acceleromyography has achieved clinical utility.

Acceleromyography uses a small piezoelectric transducer, which is attached to a digit or distal limb of the patient. A current is then passed through the motor nerve supplying that site (in the same way as a 'traditional' peripheral nerve stimulator), producing a muscle response in the innervated area. This muscle movement generates a voltage change in the attached transducer that is proportional to the acceleration developed in the contracting muscle. The force generated by the contracting muscle is calculated automatically by the acceleromyograph on the basis of Newton's second law (force = mass x acceleration), given that the mass of the muscle is constant, and the acceleration has been measured by the machine. Devices based on this concept are now commercially available (e.g. TOF-Watch®) (Figure 16.7). These devices provide a quantitative measure of the TOF ratio and display a numerical value for the ratio, thereby eliminating reliance on visual and tactile assessment of the muscle response. Consequently, they dramatically reduce undiagnosed fade. This allows the clinician to ensure that the TOF ratio is at least 0.9 before the patient's trachea is extubated. In the coming years, it is likely that quantitative measures of neuromuscular blockade will become more common.

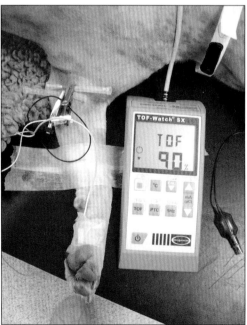

16.7 Acceleromyography using stimulation of the ulnar nerve, with the transducer attached to the palmar aspect of the metacarpus. Note that the leg is fixed in place using tape across the distal antebrachium: this is essential to ensure accuracy of the technique. In this case, the dog was recovering from rocuronium-induced neuromuscular blockade, and the acceleromyograph is displaying a TOF ratio of 90% (0.9), indicating that neuromuscular function has recovered sufficiently to allow endotracheal extubation.

Clinical assessment of recovery from neuromuscular blockade

Although the clinical monitors based on acceleromyography help to identify residual neuromuscular blockade ('curarization') at the end of anaesthesia, they cannot provide an absolute guarantee of adequate neuromuscular function. In addition, these devices are not universally available. Many veterinary anaesthetists still rely on the subjective peripheral nerve stimulation assessment methods described earlier, which at best can only detect TOF ratios <0.6; using such techniques, significant degrees of paralysis may still be present but undetectable.

Since the most serious consequences of residual neuromuscular blockade are hypoventilation and/or loss of airway control, many clinical tests of recovery have focused on assessing tidal volume or minute volume. However, diaphragmatic and intercostal muscle activity may have returned to normal even in the presence of significant degrees of weakness in other muscle groups, since the former are relatively resistant to the effects of NMBAs. As a result, patients may have a normal tidal volume but have limited control of the upper airway musculature, and may be unable to maintain airway patency after tracheal extubation. Thus, the presence of a normal tidal volume during recovery from neuromuscular blockade gives very little information about the degree of residual block in non-respiratory skeletal muscles. Similarly, a normal end-tidal carbon dioxide value on capnography gives no indication of the adequacy of upper airway muscle strength.

Other tests that are occasionally used in humans, such as assessment of vital capacity and maximum negative inspiratory pressure, are more difficult to utilize or interpret in conscious animals. Although maximum negative inspiratory pressure can be measured in anaesthetized animals by occluding the reservoir bag attachment to the breathing system and observing on a manometer the maximum negative pressure generated during inspiration, there is a potential risk of inducing negative-pressure pulmonary oedema with this technique and it is not recommended.

Monitoring adequacy of anaesthesia

Although some studies have suggested that the use of NMBAs may reduce anaesthetic requirements (presumably through reduction in afferent input to the CNS as a result of the loss of normal muscle tone), this is controversial. The animal must always be closely observed for signs of inadequate anaesthesia.

It is more difficult to assess the depth of anaesthesia in animals that have received NMBAs because many of the signs and responses normally monitored during anaesthesia (see Chapter 7) are absent or modified in these patients. For example, while the eye normally rotates ventromedially at surgical planes of anaesthesia in the cat and dog, neuromuscular blockade of the extraocular muscles causes the eye to remain centrally positioned. Similarly, although the presence or absence of the palpebral reflex is often used to quantify the depth of anaesthesia, paralysis of the periocular muscles obliterates this response, and no blinking occurs when the eyelids are stimulated. Paralysis of the respiratory musculature, which makes mechanical ventilation necessary, also abolishes

any alterations in spontaneous ventilatory pattern that might otherwise be observed in response to nociceptive stimulation during a light plane of anaesthesia. Gross movement – the most classical sign of inadequate anaesthesia – is, of course, impossible when NMBAs have been administered.

Assessment of anaesthetic depth in patients that have received NMBAs therefore presents some challenges, but alterations in sympathetic nervous system activity will usually provide a useful guide to the adequacy of anaesthesia and/or analgesia. In general, patients that are too lightly anaesthetized or receiving inadequate analgesia, tend to be tachycardic and hypertensive, although a small number of cases may become bradycardic and hypotensive. In addition, patients may salivate excessively and demonstrate increased tear production and dilation of the pupils. End-tidal carbon dioxide values may also increase and isolated muscle twitching may occur, particularly on the extremities, tongue or oral commissures (Figure 16.8). This muscle twitching can occur even in patients in which there is no response to nerve stimulation. Although various theories have been proposed to explain this apparent anomaly, there is currently no universally accepted explanation. Many modern anaesthetic monitors display information on the end-tidal anaesthetic agent concentration, which provides useful information on approximate anaesthetic depth, and should help to minimize the incidence of inadequate anaesthesia and patient awareness during NMBA use.

Patients that are excessively anaesthetized and have received NMBAs are likely to be hypotensive, and possibly bradycardic. However, too light a plane of anaesthesia must *also* be avoided, and every effort should be made to ensure the adequacy of anaesthesia in patients receiving NMBAs, since it is clearly unacceptable to have a patient aware but immobile.

It is important to reiterate that monitoring of neuromuscular transmission with a peripheral nerve stimulator gives *no* information whatsoever on anaesthetic depth.

- Increase in pulse rate
- Increase in arterial blood pressure
- Salivation
- Lacrimation
- Increase in end-tidal carbon dioxide partial pressure/concentration
- Muscle twitching, especially around the head

16.8 Signs of inadequate anaesthesia during neuromuscular blocking agent (NMBA) use.

Indications for the use of neuromuscular blocking agents

Deep surgical dissection

Neuromuscular blocking agents are extremely useful to relax the abdominal musculature, particularly for dissection deep within the abdomen, for example, nephrectomy and adrenalectomy. However, they will improve surgical conditions even for routine procedures, such as ovariohysterectomy. In addition, NMBAs may reduce the degree of postoperative discomfort by minimizing muscle resistance to abdominal stretching (e.g. by the use of surgical retractors), even though they themselves have no analgesic effects. They are also of value during spinal surgery (e.g. hemilaminectomy) in heavily muscled animals.

Thoracic surgery

Intermittent positive pressure ventilation (IPPV) is mandatory during intrathoracic surgery (see Chapters 6 and 23). Although not required in every case, the use of NMBAs allows a smooth transition from spontaneous to mechanical ventilation.

Dislocations and fractures

Neuromuscular blocking agents facilitate the reduction of dislocated joints. Although controversial, they may also improve surgical conditions during fracture reduction, especially in larger patients; this depends on the degree of muscle fibrosis resulting from the initial trauma.

Ophthalmic surgery

By relaxing the extraocular muscles, NMBAs produce a centrally positioned eye that protrudes slightly. This facilitates delicate ocular surgery. In addition, paralysis of the respiratory musculature means that the patient cannot resist IPPV; 'fighting' or 'bucking' the ventilator would be detrimental because the associated increase in intrathoracic pressure would significantly increase intraocular pressure. Neuromuscular blocking agents have no direct effect on pupillary size in cats or dogs because the iris is composed of smooth muscle, but they cause pupillary dilation in birds, where the ciliary muscle is striated. Further details on anaesthesia for ophthalmic procedures may be found in Chapter 19.

Endotracheal intubation

It is routine practice in cats to apply lidocaine to the larynx before attempting endotracheal intubation: this helps to avoid the development of laryngospasm. However, this technique imposes a time delay between induction of anaesthesia and establishment of a secure airway, because the local anaesthetic requires at least 60 seconds to achieve its peak effect. While this delay is usually well tolerated in healthy cats, those with respiratory impairment (e.g. diaphragmatic rupture) may become severely hypoxaemic during this period.

Relaxation of the larynx may also be achieved by using NMBAs. It is important that an adequate period of preoxygenation (100% oxygen by facemask for 3–5 minutes) is provided before administration of these drugs for the purpose of endotracheal intubation.

Although any NMBA may be used for this purpose, suxamethonium has traditionally been the most common choice because it has the fastest onset time (30–60 seconds). However, given the common side effects of suxamethonium (e.g. painful muscle fasciculations, cardiac arrhythmias), the non-depolarizing relaxant rocuronium may be preferred despite its slightly slower onset time. A number of studies in humans have suggested that when using rocuronium, rapid endotracheal intubation is best accomplished by using higher doses of the drug than those traditionally used for neuromuscular blockade; higher doses shorten the onset time by producing a higher concentration gradient for the drug to diffuse from the blood to the NMJ. In the authors' experience, administration of either suxamethonium or rocuronium to cats, immediately following the anaesthetic induction agent, allows endotracheal intubation in a significantly shorter time than when local anaesthesia is used to desensitize the larynx. In addition, use of an NMBA allows passage of a larger diameter endotracheal tube, since the rima glottidis will open more widely. *This is the only situation where muscle relaxants are administered before securing an airway by endotracheal intubation.*

Individual agents

Neuromuscular blocking agents should only be administered when:

- A patent airway has been established by endotracheal intubation (with the exception of suxamethonium/rocuronium for rapid intubation in cats, as described above)
- A stable plane of anaesthesia has been achieved
- Facilities for IPPV are immediately available
- Facilities for monitoring the degree of neuromuscular blockade are available.

In addition, secure intravenous access should be available throughout the procedure because all NMBAs and associated reversal drugs are administered by this route.

The onset time of NMBAs is inversely proportional to their potency, that is, those that require higher doses (lower potency) have faster onset times. However, this is of minimal clinical significance, as all NMBAs achieve their peak effect over the course of a few (approximately 1–3) minutes.

Many agents have been used to produce neuromuscular blockade over the years, but only those in current clinical use will be considered here.

Depolarizing relaxants
Suxamethonium

Suxamethonium is the only depolarizing agent currently in use. It has the fastest onset time of any muscle relaxant, and is generally relatively short-acting. However, repeated or high doses can lead to a *phase II block* (as opposed to the phase I block usually produced), where the neuromuscular blockade assumes some characteristics of a non-depolarizing block and becomes relatively long-acting. Phase II block can be detected by TOF monitoring because 'fade' develops, a characteristic not normally associated with suxamethonium-induced (phase I) blockade. Phase II block can develop in dogs following even a single dose of the drug, so it is seldom used in this species. The mechanism by which fade occurs during phase II suxamethonium block is not entirely clear, but it may be related to blockade of the prejunctional ACh receptors by the drug, thereby limiting mobilization of ACh to its release sites on the nerve terminal.

Suxamethonium has a number of other side effects that limit its usefulness. In particular, cardiovascular effects can be marked, with either bradycardia or tachycardia arising, as well as arterial hypertension. Cardiac arrhythmias may also occur. Because of the initial muscle fasciculations produced before onset of blockade, suxamethonium is thought to cause muscle damage, and an increase in plasma potassium concentration (by up to 0.5 mmol/l usually) may be observed. This increase may be clinically significant in patients with pre-existing hyperkalaemia, such as cats with urinary obstruction. The muscle fasciculations are associated with significant post-anaesthetic pain in humans, and it is reasonable to presume that this also occurs in animals. Suxamethonium can also increase intraocular pressure through sustained contraction of extra-ocular muscles, and can trigger malignant hyperthermia in susceptible patients, although this is rare.

Since incremental doses of suxamethonium may induce a phase II block, the drug should only be administered as a single dose. No antagonist agent for suxamethonium is available, and the duration of action is principally dictated by plasma cholinesterase levels, which vary widely between patients. As a result of these two factors, suxamethonium has limited use in veterinary anaesthesia, with the main (rare) indication being facilitation of endotracheal intubation in cats.

Dose:

- Dogs: 0.3 mg/kg i.v. provides approximately 25 minutes of relaxation. Not recommended (see above).
- Cats: 3–5 mg i.v. total dose for an adult cat provides approximately 5 minutes of relaxation.

Non-depolarizing relaxants

Non-depolarizing relaxants can be classified on the basis of their chemical structure as either benzylisoquinoline (curariform) derivatives or aminosteroids. The potency of all these agents is inversely related to their onset time; that is, the more potent the agent, the slower its onset. Incremental doses may be given as required, using approximately one-quarter to one-third of the initial dose. Their effects can be reversed with anticholinesterases (see below). Therefore, they offer much greater flexibility in use than suxamethonium. It is important to emphasize that the doses provided below for each drug are guides only, since patients vary widely in their requirements. Use of a peripheral nerve stimulator is the only accurate method of determining the necessary dose and the need for additional increments.

Benzylisoquinolines

Atracurium: Atracurium is degraded in the body both by non-specific esterases and by Hofmann elimination (a spontaneous breakdown process, which is both pH and temperature dependent), and <10% of the drug is excreted unchanged by the liver and kidneys. Consequently, the action of atracurium is independent of renal and hepatic function, and it is generally the NMBA of choice for patients with hepatopathy or nephropathy. Laudanosine, one of the products of Hofmann elimination of atracurium, has been associated with CNS stimulation and precipitation of seizures in the experimental setting. This is unlikely to be relevant clinically unless massive doses of atracurium were to be administered to a patient with concomitant renal and/or hepatic failure, since the plasma concentration of laudanosine observed after clinical doses of atracurium are significantly lower than those which produce these CNS effects. Although atracurium has the potential to release histamine (particularly with high doses given rapidly), this appears to be uncommon in animals. However, the drug is probably best avoided in patients where histamine release may be particularly detrimental, e.g. those with asthma. Due to its temperature dependent spontaneous degradation, atracurium should be stored in a refrigerator.

Dose:

- In cats and dogs, 0.25–0.5 mg/kg i.v. provides approximately 20–40 minutes of relaxation (although it is probably preferable to use doses at the lower end of the range, with increments as necessary). The drug is also suitable for infusion: an initial bolus of 0.25 mg/kg followed by an infusion of 0.4–0.5 mg/kg/h, started immediately after the bolus dose. The infusion should be prepared in 0.9% sodium chloride or 5% dextrose to minimize Hofmann degradation.

Cisatracurium: Cisatracurium is one of 10 stereo-isomers of atracurium. It is eliminated in a similar way by Hofmann degradation, but not by non-specific esterases. Cisatracurium is more potent than atracurium, and has a lower propensity to release histamine. Because of its greater potency, less cisatracurium is required to produce an equivalent degree of neuromuscular blockade, and consequently less laudanosine is produced in comparison with atracurium.

Since histamine release is uncommon in animals following atracurium administration, and since the clinical significance of laudanosine production is probably minimal (see above), the precise advantages of cisatracurium in veterinary anaesthesia are unclear. It may be the relaxant of choice in patients that are at risk from histamine release and additionally have concurrent hepatic disease. The effects of cisatracurium appear to be fairly unpredictable in animals.

Dose:

- Dogs: 0.15 mg/kg i.v. provides approximately 30 minutes of relaxation. Infusion rates of approximately 0.2–0.45 mg/kg/h following the initial bolus dose have also been used successfully.
- Cats: to the authors' knowledge, there are no published reports of the clinical use of cisatracurium in cats.

Mivacurium: Mivacurium is unique among non-depolarizing NMBAs in that it is metabolized by plasma cholinesterase, at a rate of approximately 70–88% that of suxamethonium (in humans). This produces a short duration of neuromuscular blockade. In addition (and unlike suxamethonium), mivacurium can be antagonized readily with anticholinesterases (see below). Although there is very limited information on its clinical use in animals, this agent has provided rapid-onset, medium-duration relaxation in cats. In dogs, however, mivacurium has a long duration of action unless administered at very low doses, although it does appear to be free of significant haemodynamic effects. It would seem, therefore, that mivacurium offers little benefit in animals over the more commonly used NMBAs such as atracurium and vecuronium.

Dose:

- Dogs: 0.01 mg/kg, 0.02 mg/kg and 0.05 mg/kg i.v. provide relaxation for approximately 34, 65 and 151 minutes, respectively.
- Cats: 0.1 mg/kg i.v. provides approximately 25 minutes of relaxation.

Aminosteroids

Vecuronium: Vecuronium has negligible effects on the cardiovascular system, even at high doses. It undergoes hepatic metabolism, with biliary and urinary excretion of both the parent compound and metabolites; the principal metabolite, 3-desacetylvecuronium, has approximately 80% of the potency of vecuronium, and is of longer duration. Prolonged effects of vecuronium may be observed with either hepatic or renal disease. Vecuronium is supplied in a lyophilized form, which is dissolved in sterile water for injection; the resultant solution is stable at room temperature for approximately 24 hours.

Dose:

- In cats and dogs, 0.1 mg/kg i.v. provides approximately 20 minutes of relaxation. Vecuronium can also be administered by intravenous infusion, with an initial bolus dose of 0.1 mg/kg followed immediately by infusion at a rate of 0.1 mg/kg/h.

Pancuronium: Pancuronium is a relatively long-acting NMBA. It can induce tachycardia and hypertension through a vagolytic and mild indirect sympathomimetic action. It is seldom used in current veterinary practice as the preference is now to use shorter-acting NMBAs with fewer cardio-vascular side effects which are administered in increments as required.

Dose:

- In cats and dogs, 0.06 mg/kg i.v. provides approximately 45–60 minutes of relaxation.

Rocuronium: Rocuronium is a short- to intermediate-acting NMBA. It produces minimal cardiovascular side effects, although it occasionally causes mild increases in heart rate and blood pressure. It has the fastest onset among the non-depolarizing agents when used at the higher range of reported doses, being only slightly slower than suxamethonium, but this appears to be its only real advantage over other agents.

Dose:

- Dogs: 0.5–0.6 mg/kg i.v. provides approximately 15–30 minutes of relaxation. An infusion of 0.2 mg/kg/h started immediately after the initial bolus may be used to maintain relaxation.
- Cats: 0.6 mg/kg i.v. provides approximately 15 minutes of relaxation. A higher dose is required if rocuronium is used to achieve endotracheal intubation, and the authors usually use 1.2–1.5 mg/kg i.v. for this purpose.
- There are no reports of the use of this drug by infusion in cats.

Short-acting and long-acting NMBAs

It has been demonstrated in humans that shorter-acting NMBAs are more easily antagonized than longer-acting agents. Therefore, for procedures where relaxation may be required for a relatively long period of time, it is now more common to administer short- or intermediate-duration agents, such as atracurium, rocuronium or vecuronium, and to provide incremental doses as required, rather than to use longer-acting agents such as pancuronium.

Interactions between neuromuscular blocking agents and other drugs

A number of drugs may interact with NMBAs when administered concurrently:

- **Volatile anaesthetic agents.** These potentiate the effects of NMBAs both in terms of dose requirements and duration of action. Although the results of studies vary to some extent, depending on both the species and patient's age, sevoflurane appears more potent or equipotent to isoflurane in this regard, while isoflurane exhibits greater potentiation than halothane. With all the volatile agents, atracurium and vecuronium appear to be potentiated less than pancuronium
- **Injectable anaesthetic agents.** At clinical doses, propofol appears to have minimal effect on the action of NMBAs. Ketamine potentiates all non-depolarizing NMBAs in a dose-dependent manner in a primate model
- **Antibiotics.** Some antibiotics may prolong neuromuscular blockade by mechanisms that vary from agent to agent. Several sites at the NMJ may be affected. The most important antibiotics in this regard are the aminoglycosides, although the effect produced varies depending on the NMBA used, the concentration of the antibiotic achieved *in vivo*, and variability between patients. Close monitoring of the NMJ is certainly recommended if aminoglycosides and NMBAs are used concurrently during anaesthesia. Some studies have shown that administration of calcium salts may be useful to reverse any prolonged blockade that occurs when these agents are used together; however, others have suggested that the use of calcium is inappropriate as its effect will not be sustained (and the patient may therefore redevelop neuromuscular blockade), and also because calcium can antagonize the antibacterial effects of aminoglycosides
- **Anticonvulsants.** The interaction between anticonvulsants and NMBAs is complex and the mechanism by which it occurs is poorly understood. For example, acute administration of phenytoin (in humans) has been shown to augment neuromuscular blockade with rocuronium. Conversely, chronic administration of either phenytoin or carbamazepine appears to produce resistance to all of the aminosteroid NMBAs. Anticonvulsants appear to have minimal effects on the dose requirements and duration of the benzylisoquinolines
- **Histamine (H_2) receptor antagonists.** High-dose oral cimetidine prolongs vecuronium-induced blockade, while intravenous ranitidine has been shown to antagonize atracurium relaxation in rats, but not in humans. The clinical significance of the interaction between muscle relaxants and H_2 antagonists is unclear.

Use of neuromuscular blocking agents in the presence of concurrent disease

The presence of concurrent disease may influence the NMBA chosen, and may also require modification of the dose administered:

- **Renal and hepatic disease.** Atracurium (or cisatracurium) is generally the NMBA of choice for patients with renal or hepatic disease because of its unique method of degradation. Although renal elimination plays only a minor role in terminating the effects of vecuronium, studies in humans have demonstrated an increased duration of action in patients with renal failure
- **Acid–base and electrolyte disturbances.** The effects of acid–base disturbances on NMBAs are extremely

complex and vary between agents, but either potentiation or antagonism of NMBAs may occur. Electrolyte disorders have similarly complex effects, but, generally, hypernatraemia and hypokalaemia will potentiate non-depolarizing agents, while hyponatraemia and hyperkalaemia will antagonize them

- **Burn injuries.** Patients with extensive burns may develop resistance to non-depolarizing NMBAs, while administration of suxamethonium can produce severe hyperkalaemia and ventricular fibrillation. These effects generally occur within approximately 24 hours of the initial injury, and persist until complete healing of the wounds. The mechanism responsible is thought to be proliferation of extrajunctional ACh receptors in association with the burn injury
- **Spinal cord injury.** This may increase sensitivity to non-depolarizing agents, while administration of suxamethonium to these patients can induce hyperkalaemia
- **Myasthenia gravis.** Patients with myasthenia gravis are extremely sensitive to the effects of non-depolarizing NMBAs, and use of a nerve stimulator is mandatory if these agents are used in animals with this condition. An initial dose of approximately one-tenth of the normal dose should be used, and small incremental doses administered as dictated by TOF monitoring
- **Diabetes mellitus.** The duration of action of vecuronium is shorter in dogs with diabetes, as indicated by both tactile and electromyographic monitoring (Clark *et al.*, 2012).

Antagonism of neuromuscular blockade

Recovery from neuromuscular blockade may occur spontaneously, as the plasma concentration of relaxant diminishes (due to metabolism and elimination). This allows the drug to diffuse away from the NMJ, moving down its concentration gradient into the plasma. Alternatively, in the case of non-depolarizing NMBAs, recovery may be hastened by administration of an anticholinesterase. These agents inhibit the effects of the enzyme acetylcholinesterase, which is responsible for the rapid metabolism of ACh following its release. Consequently, anticholinesterases allow accumulation of ACh, which is then able to competitively displace the non-depolarizing NMBA from the postsynaptic ACh receptor, restoring neuromuscular transmission. Anticholinesterases will not reverse classic phase I suxamethonium blockade because the block induced is non-competitive (see earlier); there is some evidence, however, that they may facilitate reversal of a fully-developed phase II suxamethonium block.

Anticholinesterases not only allow ACh to build up at the nicotinic receptors of the NMJ but, in addition, ACh accumulates at postganglionic parasympathetic muscarinic receptors throughout the body. This may produce a number of unwanted side effects, such as bradycardia and cardiac arrhythmias, bronchoconstriction, salivation, defecation and diarrhoea. To prevent these muscarinic effects, anticholinesterases are usually administered in conjunction with antimuscarinic agents, such as atropine or glycopyrronium.

Two anticholinesterases are used clinically for reversal of non-depolarizing NMBA-induced relaxation: neostigmine and edrophonium. Neostigmine has a slow onset but long duration, whereas edrophonium has a more rapid onset but somewhat shorter duration of action. Of the antimuscarinic agents, atropine has a rapid onset and short duration of action, and glycopyrronium has a slow onset and long duration. Therefore, the pharmacokinetic profile of atropine fits more closely with that of edrophonium, while the profile of glycopyrronium fits more closely with that of neostigmine. It is therefore most logical to use either an edrophonium–atropine or neostigmine–glycopyrronium combination for reversal of neuromuscular blockade. A neostigmine–glycopyrronium combination is commercially available (Robinul-Neostigmine). However, even though the pharmacokinetics of neostigmine–glycopyrronium and edrophonium–atropine combinations are the most compatible, it is still not uncommon to see minor muscarinic effects when these combinations are used, particularly mild bradycardia or second-degree atrioventricular block. These effects are, however, usually transient. An edrophonium–atropine combination produces the fewest muscarinic side effects and is the combination of choice in patients where these effects may be detrimental, such as those with significant cardiac disease. Edrophonium is significantly more expensive than neostigmine, so the latter is more commonly used for antagonism of neuromuscular blockade, with edrophonium generally being reserved for specific situations where the more profound muscarinic effects of neostigmine might be problematic.

If a short-acting anticholinesterase (edrophonium) is used with a long-acting NMBA (e.g. pancuronium), there is an increased risk of recurarization in the recovery period; that is, the edrophonium may initially reverse the blockade and restore normal neuromuscular transmission, but because edrophonium is shorter acting than the relaxant, neuromuscular blockade may recur as the edrophonium concentration at the NMJ declines. Thus, if longer-acting NMBAs have been used, neostigmine is the anticholinesterase of choice because of its long duration of action. In addition, neostigmine more reliably antagonizes a more intense blockade than edrophonium. Neostigmine has, however, also been shown to possess neuromuscular-blocking capabilities, particularly if administered in high doses; consequently, the doses described below should not be exceeded.

The greater the TOF count (or TOF ratio if using objective monitoring techniques such as acceleromyography) before reversal, the more likely the success in restoring neuromuscular transmission, and the less likely the occurrence of residual neuromuscular blockade or recurarization during recovery. Consequently, where time allows, it is preferable to wait for restoration of all four twitches in the TOF before administering the antagonist agent. Although it is possible to achieve reversal when only one twitch has reappeared, it is less predictable, requiring higher doses of anticholinesterase, and with a greater potential for residual/re-curarization occurring later.

Inadequate reversal of neuromuscular blockade at the end of anaesthesia risks residual blockade in the recovery period, which may lead to serious consequences for the animal. Numerous studies in humans have demonstrated that patients commonly arrive at the recovery room with significant residual blockade still present, which is responsible for a higher incidence of complications, particularly those involving the respiratory system. The advent of more objective clinical methods for assessment of neuromuscular transmission, such as acceleromyography, may reduce the incidence of residual neuromuscular blockade during the recovery period.

Although reversal is not always required following the use of muscle relaxants, it should certainly be considered when longer-acting NMBAs have been used, or when multiple boluses or infusions of these agents have been delivered. If in doubt as to the patient's state of neuromuscular recovery, it is wise to err on the side of caution and administer an anticholinesterase.

Administration of anticholinesterases

Neostigmine and glycopyrronium are usually mixed in a ratio of 5:1 (2.5 mg neostigmine + 500 µg glycopyrronium/ml in the commercial preparation), with a total dose requirement of 0.01–0.05 mg/kg i.v. neostigmine, depending on the degree of neuromuscular blockade at the time of reversal.

Edrophonium and atropine are usually mixed in a 25:1 ratio (1 mg/kg edrophonium + 40 µg/kg atropine) and given by slow intravenous injection to effect over several minutes.

In preference to mixing the antimuscarinic agent and anticholinesterase in the same syringe, some veterinary surgeons instead administer the antimuscarinic 1–2 minutes before the anticholinesterase to lessen the risk of muscarinic side effects. However, cardiac instability may occur with this approach because the antimuscarinic agent generally induces a transient tachycardia before the heart rate reduces once the anticholinesterase is administered.

It is vital that both ventilatory support and a depth of anaesthesia adequate to prevent awareness are maintained until full reversal of neuromuscular blockade has been achieved. Failure to restore spontaneous ventilation may occur for several reasons (Figure 16.9).

- Ongoing neuromuscular blockade (in absence of a peripheral nerve stimulator):
  - Inadequate antagonism
  - Hepatic/renal disease
  - Acid–base/electrolyte disturbance
- Excessive anaesthetic depth
- Hypocapnia (over-ventilation)
- Hypothermia

16.9 Common causes of failure to restore spontaneous ventilation following the use of neuromuscular blocking agents (NMBAs).

Sugammadex

A specific non-depolarizing NMBA reversal agent, sugammadex, has relatively recently been licensed for use in humans in some countries. This agent is a modified cyclodextrin compound that works in a completely different way to the anticholinesterases. Cyclodextrins have a ring structure with a hydrophilic surface, which makes them water soluble, but with the capability to encapsulate hydrophobic molecules within their central core. Sugammadex was primarily developed as a reversal agent for rocuronium, although it also reverses (slightly less effectively) vecuronium-induced neuromuscular blockade (and, to a much lesser extent, also pancuronium). It is ineffective against benzylisoquinoline NMBAs. Sugammadex is highly efficient at rapidly 'mopping up' aminosteroid NMBA molecules, even during profound (or following prolonged) neuromuscular blockade. Once the rocuronium or vecuronium becomes encapsulated in the central core of the

cyclodextrin molecule, it is no longer able to act at the NMJ. Since sugammadex antagonizes NMBAs without inhibition of acetylcholinesterase, muscarinic effects do not occur, and therefore the concurrent administration of antimuscarinic drugs is unnecessary. Sugammadex is also largely free of any significant side effects of its own.

The ability to rapidly terminate even profound rocuronium-induced blockade (in particular) is a major benefit of sugammadex. In humans, it has been widely used when the anaesthetist has administered rocuronium to facilitate endotracheal intubation but has been subsequently unable to visualize the larynx or pass an endotracheal tube. In this situation, the patient is paralysed and therefore apnoeic, but the anaesthetist may be unable to provide manual ventilation. A number of case reports exist in the human literature of patients being 'rescued' from this 'can't intubate/can't ventilate' scenario by administration of sugammadex, as this agent permits rapid restoration of neuromuscular transmission and spontaneous ventilation. The role of sugammadex as an NMBA reversal agent in other situations is less clearly defined, principally because the drug is extremely expensive; thus, its use can be justified where the patient's life may be at risk, but not for 'routine' situations. Although antagonism of NMBAs using sugammadex has been reported in animals, its high price is likely to dramatically limit its use in veterinary anaesthesia.

References and further reading

Auer U and Mosing M (2006) A clinical study of the effects of rocuronium in isoflurane-anaesthetized cats. *Veterinary Anaesthesia and Analgesia* 33, 224–228

Clark L, Leece EA and Brearley JC (2012) Diabetes mellitus affects the duration of action of vecuronium in dogs. *Veterinary Anaesthesia and Analgesia* 39, 472–479

Clutton RE (1994) Edrophonium for neuromuscular blockade antagonism in the dog. *Veterinary Record* 134, 674–678

Corletto F and Brearley JC (2003) Clinical use of mivacurium in the cat. *Veterinary Anaesthesia and Analgesia* 30, 93–94

Dugdale AHA, Adams WA and Jones RS (2002) The clinical use of the neuromuscular blocking agent rocuronium in dogs. *Veterinary Anaesthesia and Analgesia* 29, 49–53

Fuchs-Buder T (2010) *Neuromuscular Monitoring in Clinical Practice and Research*. Springer-Verlag, Heidelberg

Mosing M, Auer U, West E, Jones RS and Hunter JM (2012) Reversal of profound rocuronium or vecuronium-induced neuromuscular block with sugammadex in isoflurane-anaesthetised dogs. *Veterinary Journal* 192, 467–471

Murphy GS, Szokol JW, Marymont JH et al. (2008) Intraoperative acceleromyographic monitoring reduces the risk of residual neuromuscular blockade and adverse respiratory events in the postanaesthesia care unit. *Anesthesiology* 109, 389–398

Savarese JJ, Miller RD, Lien CA and Caldwell JE (1994) Pharmacology of muscle relaxants and their antagonists. In: *Anesthesia, 4th edn*, ed. RD Miller, pp. 463–468. Churchill Livingstone, New York

Shields M, Giovannelli M, Mirakhur RK et al. (2006) Org 25969 (sugammadex), a selective relaxant binding agent for antagonism of prolonged rocuronium-induced neuromuscular blockade. *British Journal of Anaesthesia* 96, 36–43

Singh YN, Harvey AL and Marshall IG (1978) Antibiotic-induced paralysis of the mouse phrenic nerve-hemidiaphragm preparation, and reversibility by calcium and by neostigmine. *Anesthesiology* 48, 418–424

Smith LJ, Moon PF, Lukasik VM and Erb HN (1999) Duration of action and hemodynamic properties of mivacurium chloride in dogs anesthetized with halothane. *American Journal of Veterinary Research* 60, 1047–1050

Sullivan TC, Hellyer PW, Lee DD and Davidson MG (1998) Respiratory function and extraocular muscle paralysis following administration of pancuronium bromide to dogs. *Veterinary Ophthalmology* 1, 125–128

Chapter 17

Haemodynamic support during the anaesthetic period

Tanya Duke-Novakovski

Arterial blood pressure (ABP) is subject to control by many mechanisms, interacting to provide optimal tissue perfusion under different circumstances. These mechanisms can be classified according to their timeframe of action. Under this system of classification, the mechanism that is most relevant to the period of anaesthesia is control of ABP by the autonomic nervous system (ANS). The response time for the ANS to accommodate tissue perfusion requirements is in the order of seconds to minutes and any changes are easily observed, especially with the aid of monitoring equipment and techniques. This chapter describes the use of drugs which can modify or augment the function of the ANS to enable optimal tissue perfusion.

Review of the autonomic nervous system

Anatomy

The ANS comprises the parasympathetic nervous system (PNS) and sympathetic nervous system (SNS). The PNS is largely responsible for homeostasis, while the SNS directs the stress response for the classic 'fight or flight' reaction. The neural input of the ANS is sometimes called the visceral afferent sensory system; it transmits information on, for example, noxious stimuli, stretch and pressure, to the central nervous system (CNS). These ANS sensory neurons link to the CNS through peripheral nerve fibres, via the vagus nerve and spinal nerves. Visceral input can also be linked to other parts of the nervous system through internuncial neurons in the spinal cord and can trigger responses such as muscle guarding over a painful visceral organ.

The effector (visceral efferent or motor) arm of the ANS consists of a two-neuron pathway, with the synapses between the primary and secondary neurons located in peripherally located ganglia. In the PNS, primary neurons are linked to only a few secondary neurons; this limited branching produces a more localized response. In contrast, within the SNS, linkage of the primary neuron to many secondary neurons enables the response to be more widely distributed through the body. Within the PNS, the primary neuron is long and the ganglia are diffusely located close to the effector organ. Conversely, within the SNS, the primary neuron is short and synapses with the secondary neuron within discrete and easily visualized ganglia located in the sympathetic chains close to the CNS. These motor nerves travel within cranial and spinal nerve bundles.

The PNS effector nerves leave the CNS through the oculomotor (III), facial (VII), glossopharyngeal (IX) and vagus (X) cranial nerves, and through the sacral spinal nerves (S2, S3 and S4). The oculomotor nerve produces pupillary constriction and accommodation of the lens. The facial nerve stimulates the submandibular and sublingual salivary glands, lacrimal glands and mucosal glands of the nose. The glossopharyngeal nerve stimulates the parotid salivary gland. The vagus nerve affects heart rate, gastrointestinal motility and other visceral organ functions, and, with the sacral nerves, serves the body outside the head region.

The primary neurons within the SNS exit the CNS through the ganglia of the sympathetic chain, from where areas of the body beyond the thoracolumbar region are innervated. The vasomotor centre located in the medulla oblongata of the brain controls arterial and venous vasomotor tone; its output is transmitted through the SNS pathways. General anaesthetics can depress the vasomotor centre and cause global vasodilation. Local anaesthetics used for regional blockade can reduce vasomotor tone to the area served by the block, resulting in local vasodilation.

Neurotransmitters

Many of the drugs used in veterinary anaesthesia to support ABP stimulate the receptors of the SNS and are based on a catecholamine structure. Among the catecholamines, dopamine is a common neurotransmitter within the CNS; noradrenaline (norepinephrine) is more commonly found as a neurotransmitter within the SNS; and adrenaline (epinephrine) is secreted by the adrenal glands (Figure 17.1).

Once catecholamines have activated their receptors, their effect is terminated largely by reuptake into the nerve terminal, where they are broken down by monoamine oxidases. The proportion that does not undergo reuptake (approximately 25%) is metabolized in the tissues by catechol-O-methyltransferases, or in the liver. Generally, the primary (preganglionic) neurons of both PNS and SNS ganglia release acetylcholine. The secondary (postganglionic) neurons of the SNS release noradrenaline, while those of the PNS release acetylcholine.

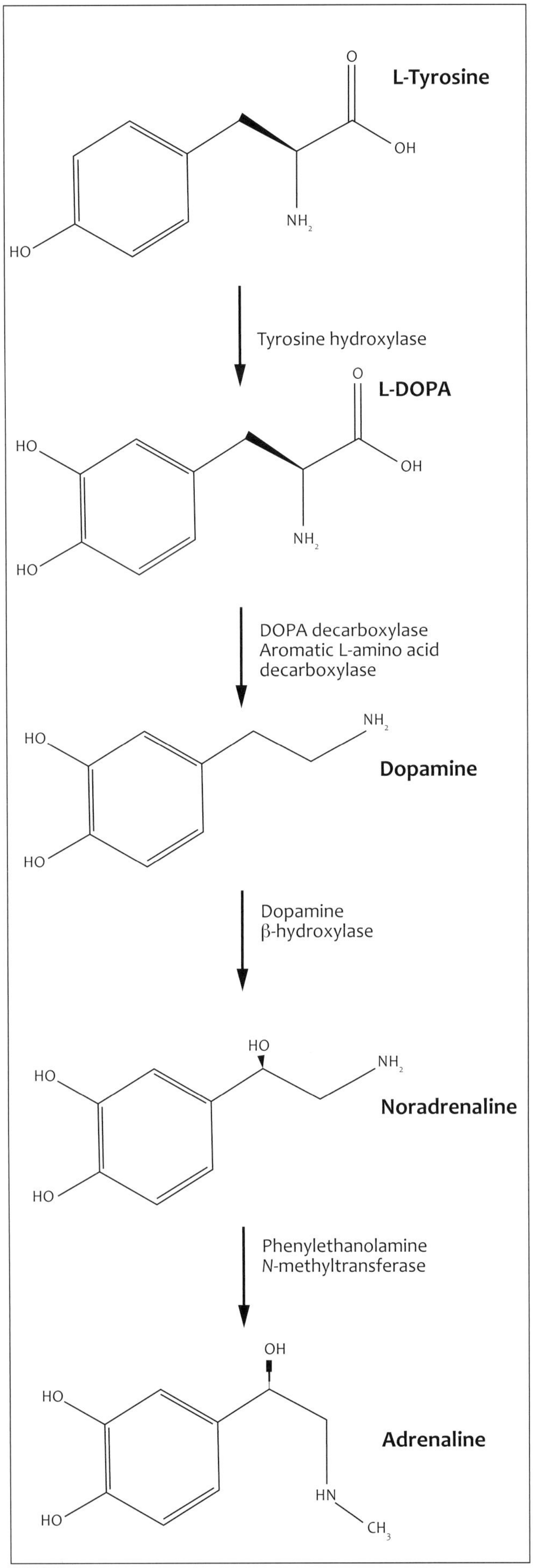

17.1 Metabolic pathway for the synthesis of catecholamines.

L-Tyrosine

Tyrosine hydroxylase

L-DOPA

DOPA decarboxylase
Aromatic L-amino acid
decarboxylase

Dopamine

Dopamine
β-hydroxylase

Noradrenaline

Phenylethanolamine
N-methyltransferase

Adrenaline

Receptors

The neurotransmitters can act on different types of receptor. Many anaesthetic and sedative agents also act upon postganglionic effector organ receptors. Drug effects are covered in Chapters 10, 13, 14 and 15.

Catecholamines activate transmembrane receptors of the G-protein family classified as adrenoceptors. These receptors are further classified into alpha-1 (three subtypes), alpha-2 (three subtypes), and beta-1, beta-2 and beta-3 subtypes. Beta-3 receptors have little role in blood pressure control. Alpha-1 receptors are located within the postsynaptic endplate and are stimulated by noradrenaline. Alpha-2 receptors are located on the effector organ outside the synapses (extrajunctional) and also in a presynaptic position on the postganglionic nerve terminal (Figure 17.2). Alpha-2 receptors are stimulated by noradrenaline and also by adrenaline released from the adrenal glands. Activation of presynaptic alpha-2 receptors limits the release of noradrenaline from the nerve terminal via a negative feedback mechanism. Stimulation of extrajunctional alpha-2 receptors on the effector organ produces the same or a similar effect to stimulation of alpha-1 receptors. However, because of the position of alpha-2 receptors outside the synaptic cleft, they are more easily activated by circulating adrenaline. Adrenaline, which has an elimination half-life of two minutes, produces a longer, more sustained effect than noradrenaline because it is removed predominantly through hepatic metabolism. Circulating noradrenaline arises from the adrenal glands and 'spillover' from the synaptic cleft.

Within vascular tissue, stimulation of alpha-1 and extrajunctional postsynaptic alpha-2 receptors generally produces vasoconstriction. Stimulation of presynaptic alpha-2 receptors decreases vasomotor tone by decreasing the release of noradrenaline from the nerve terminal. Alpha-1 receptors are also present on the great veins and influence the amount of blood pooling in these structures via their effects on vascular tone. Even a small change in the diameter of the great veins can lead to significant changes in cardiac output (CO) by affecting venous return.

Beta-1 receptors are present throughout the heart. Their stimulation results in an increase in contractility (positive inotropy), heart rate (positive chronotropy) and speed of conduction (positive dromotropy). Beta-2 receptors mediate vasodilation of blood vessels within the muscular beds and are activated during times of stress ('fight or flight' response) and physical exertion. During physical exertion, vasodilation within muscle beds offsets the arterial vasoconstriction produced by adrenaline acting within the arterial tree, such that the mean arterial pressure (MAP) does not excessively increase.

In general, alpha receptors are more readily stimulated by noradrenaline compared to adrenaline, and beta receptors are more readily stimulated by adrenaline compared to noradrenaline. This difference reflects the location of the receptors and their activation through mainly neural (noradrenaline) or humoral (adrenaline) means.

The postganglionic PNS neuron releases acetylcholine. Acetylcholine stimulates postsynaptic muscarinic receptors, of which there are three subtypes (M_1, M_2, and M_3). The type of muscarinic receptors present depends on the tissue innervated. Stimulation of the M_2 muscarinic receptors within the atria and sinoatrial and atrioventricular (AV) nodes decreases normal pacing and slows the heart rate (negative chronotropy and dromotropy). The PNS has little effect on vasomotor tone in most tissues.

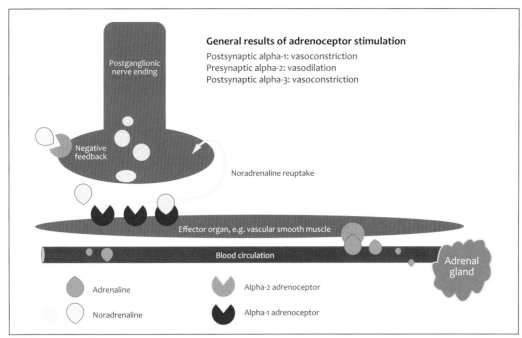

17.2 Diagram of the sympathetic nervous system postganglionic synaptic cleft and surrounding area showing the position of alpha-1 and alpha-2 adrenoceptors.

Blood flow, pressure and perfusion

The vascular system can be thought of as a system of pipes (the blood vessels) with a pump (the heart). The pipes can change in diameter, are not completely 'water-tight' and can be affected by pressure changes outside their walls. The pump can change its rate of pumping, its force of contraction and its distensibility.

The arteries and arterioles are elastic and can store energy during systole and transmit this energy back during diastole to maintain pressure. However, the diastolic pressure does gradually decrease until the subsequent systole increases blood pressure once again. The pressure wave generated (the pulse) rebounds off structures within the arterial tree and generates the typical arterial waveform (Figure 17.3ab). The heart rate maintains the pressure within the system: bradycardia decreases MAP because diastolic arterial pressure (DAP) mathematically contributes more to the calculation of MAP than systolic arterial pressure (SAP).

The MAP is the average blood pressure during one cardiac cycle and can be calculated with the following simple mathematical equation:

$$MAP\ (mmHg) = 1/3\ (SAP - DAP) + DAP$$

More accurately, the MAP is the value at which, on the arterial pulse waveform, the areas above and below that value are equal. The MAP is equivalent to organ perfusion pressure. MAP values below 60 mmHg may compromise organ perfusion.

Cardiac output (CO) is the volume of blood pumped from the left ventricle of the heart in 1 minute. Its value is affected by the heart rate and the volume of blood pumped in one contraction (stroke volume), and it is calculated as follows:

$$CO\ (l/min) = heart\ rate\ (bpm) \times stroke\ volume\ (l)$$

Furthermore, stroke volume depends upon contractility, afterload and venous return. Venous return is affected by

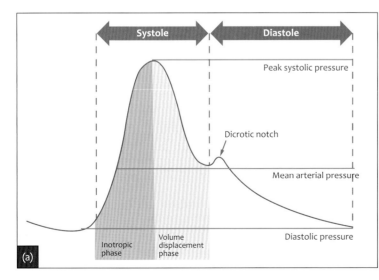

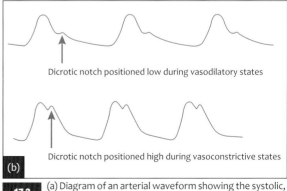

17.3 (a) Diagram of an arterial waveform showing the systolic, mean and diastolic pressures, dicrotic notch, and areas dependent on inotropy and volume displacement. (b) Changes in position of the dicrotic notch during states of vasodilation and vasoconstriction.

factors such as body position, cranial abdominal surgery, the use of intermittent positive pressure ventilation, the volume within the circulation and venomotor tone.

Global oxygen delivery to the tissues (DO_2) is affected by the CO and the quantity of oxygen carried by the blood:

$$DO_2 \text{ (ml/min)} = CO \text{ (l/min)} \times \text{oxygen content (ml/l)}$$

At rest, the vasomotor centre in the CNS maintains tone in vascular tissue at a point midway between full vasoconstriction and full vasodilation. The overall tone of the vasculature is called the systemic vascular resistance (SVR; also known as total peripheral resistance). The SVR can be calculated using the following formula:

$$\text{SVR (dynes.sec.cm}^{-5}) =$$
$$(\text{MAP} - \text{CVP (mmHg)}) \times 80/CO \text{ (l/min)}$$

where CVP is the central venous pressure. Depending on the organ and physiological systems, the diameter of blood vessels may change locally as a result of autoregulation (see later).

Tissue perfusion and MAP are normally optimized for the prevailing conditions within the body. However, if SVR were to increase well above its normal range, as may happen with overzealous administration of alpha-1 adrenergic agonists, blood flow and tissue perfusion would be compromised, especially in areas with a high density of alpha-1 receptors such as the viscera and skin. Using ABP as a guide to tissue perfusion can be misleading in these circumstances: flow requires a pressure difference between points to occur (from higher to lower pressure), but pressure does not require flow. As a result, measurement of pressure for monitoring purposes has the limitation of not providing information on actual blood flow (see Chapter 7). However, since ABP is the primary determinant of organ blood flow, hypotension is always pathological.

Tissue perfusion is better assessed using other indicators such as detection of peripheral pulses, lactate concentration, urine production, acid–base balance and plasma pH. The interrelationships producing optimal tissue perfusion are summarized in Figure 17.4.

Physiology of blood pressure control

Ultra-short-acting control systems

Blood supply at tissue level is usually controlled by the vascular response to accumulated products of metabolism such as potassium and hydrogen ions, adenosine diphosphate and lactate. The endothelium responds to this accumulation of waste metabolites by increasing the catalytic action of endothelial nitric oxide synthase to produce nitric oxide, a potent vascular smooth muscle relaxant. As a result of the vasodilation produced by nitric oxide, more blood flow to the tissue is made possible to remove waste products and to deliver oxygen and nutrients. Nitric oxide has a very short lifespan (nanoseconds) so a continual supply is required.

Individual organs such as the brain and kidney can use a similar and more refined system of organ autoregulation, which ensures a steady blood flow to the whole tissue. Other organ systems which do not have mechanisms of autoregulation, such as the gastrointestinal tract, rapidly become debilitated during periods of hypotension.

Chemoreceptors located on the walls of the aortic arch and carotid body respond to both decreasing partial pressure of oxygen and increasing partial pressure of carbon dioxide to increase SNS tone and increase tissue perfusion. These chemoreceptors also increase ventilatory drive to correct the abnormality in blood gases.

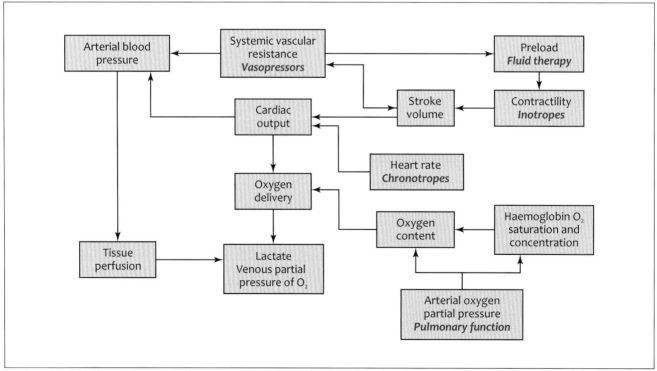

17.4 Simplified diagram showing the interrelationships of cardiopulmonary system homeostasis in order to maintain tissue perfusion and oxygen delivery. The suggested treatment or assessment is indicated in red.

Short-acting control systems
Baroreceptor reflex arc
Baroreceptors located within the aortic arch and bifurcation of the common carotid artery (carotid sinus) detect the amount of stretch produced by the pressure of blood flow. Increasing stretch increases neural traffic (i.e. the number of action potentials) to the vasomotor centre via the glossopharyngeal nerve (carotid sinus baroreceptors) and vagus nerve (aortic arch baroreceptors). Processing within the vasomotor centre is linked to the parasympathetic outflow through the vagus nerve to the atria and sinoatrial and AV nodes of the heart. Increased vagal tone causes a slowing of pacemaker activity when the MAP increases. A decrease in baroreceptor firing reduces vagal tone and allows the heart rate to increase. The cardiac accelerator nerves (lower cervical and upper thoracic spinal nerves) of the SNS also increase heart rate. In this way, CO can be readily modified through neural input/output in a matter of seconds. Baroreceptors are also present in other areas of the body such as the venae cavae, pulmonary veins, atria, ventricles and pericardium.

Use of alfaxalone, propofol or thiopental for induction of anaesthesia depresses the vasomotor centre, causing global vasodilation. The subsequent decrease in ABP is responsible for the increase in heart rate often observed at induction, via the baroreceptor reflex arc. Propofol, however, resets the baroreceptor threshold, so that there is less input to the reflex arc to increase the heart rate compared to the increases observed with alfaxalone and thiopental; this makes propofol a less favourable choice for induction of anaesthesia in patients with circulatory volume deficits.

Long-acting control systems
Long-acting control systems are important for patient management during anaesthesia, but their slow time-course of action makes them less amenable to manipulation while the patient is anaesthetized. Vasopressin is the only drug used to affect these systems during anaesthesia because its onset of action is rapid, and it is often used to provide a higher plasma concentration compared to that found in healthy animals.

Renin–angiotensin–aldosterone system
A reduction in circulating volume causes release of renin from the kidney. Renin cleaves angiotensinogen to inactive angiotensin I. Angiotensin-converting enzyme transforms angiotensin I to active angiotensin II and also increases the breakdown of bradykinin, a compound that causes vasodilation. Angiotensin II is a vasoconstrictor; it also stimulates aldosterone production and antidiuretic hormone (ADH; also called arginine vasopressin) secretion, and increases the sensitivity of catecholamine receptors. Aldosterone is a mineralocorticoid secreted by the adrenal glands that increases reabsorption of sodium and water, and ADH promotes reabsorption of water in the kidney. Antidiuretic hormone is normally secreted in minute amounts; however, if there is a severe decrease of circulating volume, it is secreted in greater amounts to cause vasoconstriction. However, in these circumstances ADH stores usually exhaust after about an hour, and administration of exogenous ADH (vasopressin) is occasionally required in debilitated patients.

Atrial natriuretic peptide
Atrial natriuretic peptide is secreted by atrial cardiac myocytes in response to atrial stretch. This peptide increases loss of sodium ions via the kidney and thus reduces the circulating volume: where sodium goes, water will follow.

Normal ABP in conscious dogs and cats
Normal SAP, MAP and DAP values in dogs and cats are shown in Figure 17.5. In dogs, values are breed specific: retrievers and giant breeds tend to have lower pressures, while sighthounds tend to have a higher pressure range. Normal ABP in cats is not so breed-specific.

Treatment of hypotension during anaesthesia
When faced with a hypotensive patient, assimilating all the available clinical information will help to evaluate the cause of hypotension and direct the veterinary surgeon (veterinarian) towards an appropriate choice of treatment. The cardiovascular effects of drugs used during anaesthesia are shown in Figure 17.6.

Hypotension can be classed as mild (MAP 45–60 mmHg) or severe (MAP <45 mmHg) (Figures 17.7 and 17.8). Mild hypotension usually follows trends and is commonly observed in anaesthetized patients, even healthy animals. Severe hypotension, especially if sudden in onset, requires more aggressive diagnosis and corrective steps. A basic guide to treatment of sudden, profound

Species/breed	Systolic arterial blood pressure (mmHg) (mean ± SD)	Mean arterial blood pressure (mmHg) (mean ± SD)	Diastolic arterial blood pressure (mmHg) (mean ± SD)	Reference
Dog	NA	103 ± 15	NA	Haskins et al., 2005
Dog	135	NA	75	Bodey and Michell, 1996
Greyhound at home with owner	130 ± 12	95 ± 10	80 ± 11	Marino et al., 2011
Greyhound in hospital	154 ± 17	110 ± 14	88 ± 15	Marino et al., 2011
Cat: 1–11 years of age	~125	~88	~67	Bodey and Sansom, 1998
Cat: 11–16 years of age	~160	~93	~67	Bodey and Sansom, 1998
Cat: >16 years of age	~179	~140	~117	Bodey and Sansom, 1998

17.5 Average systemic blood pressures recorded in several studies in conscious dogs and cats. NA = not available; SD = standard deviation.

Drug	Heart rate	Cardiac output	Contractility	Vascular resistance	Blood pressure
Anticholinergic	↑	↑	NC	NC	NC or ↑
Phenothiazine	NC or ↑	NC or ↓	NC or ↓	↓	↓
Benzodiazepine	NC	NC	NC	NC	NC
Alpha-2 adrenoceptor agonist	↓	↓	↓	↑	↑ then ↓
Opioid	↓	↓	NC or ↓	NC or ↓	NC or ↓
Barbiturate	↑	↓	↓	↓	↓
Propofol	NC or ↓	↓	↓	↓	↓
Ketamine	↑	↑	↑	↑	↑
Etomidate	NC or ↑	NC or ↓	NC or ↓	↓	NC
Alfaxalone	↑	↓	↓	↓	↓
Isoflurane	NC	NC or ↓	NC or ↓	NC or ↓	↓

17.6 Summary of the general haemodynamic changes produced by drugs used for sedation and anaesthesia in cats and dogs. NC = no change. See Figure 21.12 for further details of individual drugs.

Mild hypotension (MAP 45–60 mmHg (mild)	Severe hypotension (MAP <45 mmHg) (see also Figure 17.8)
Look for cause Treat bradycardia	Get help, may be life-threatening situation Look for cause Treat bradycardia
Turn down anaesthetic and give analgesics	Turn off anaesthetic, still give oxygen Consider giving ketamine (0.5–1 mg/kg i.v.)
Fluid therapy: 10 ml/kg crystalloids or 2–5 ml/kg colloids over 10–15 minutes	Fluid therapy: 30 ml/kg crystalloids over 10 minutes and/or 5–10 ml colloids over 5–10 minutes
Inotrope: ephedrine/ dobutamine/dopamine	Inotrope: dobutamine/dopamine
Vasopressor: Ephedrine/ dopamine	Vasopressor: Dopamine/noradrenaline/ phenylephrine

17.7 Checklist for managing mild and severe hypotension. Use with the flowchart in Figure 17.9. It can be helpful to classify the degree of hypotension present based on the mean arterial pressure and the rate at which blood pressure decreased. Aggressive or less aggressive treatments are used as depicted in the figure. MAP = mean arterial pressure.

Checklist for sudden/profound hypotension
• Hypoxaemia • Reduction of cardiac contractility • Cardiac arrhythmias • Massive vasodilation (anaphylaxis, inflammatory mediator release) • Massive blood loss • Tension pneumothorax • Closed breathing system exhaust valve • Surgical/physical disruption of venous return • Pulmonary thromboembolism • Electrolyte/pH imbalances

17.8 A list of possible reasons for sudden hypotension. This list is not exhaustive but describes the most common situations. Use with the flowchart in Figure 17.9.

hypotension is provided in Figures 17.9 and 17.10. Note that the flowchart of corrective steps (Figure 17.9) may require other interventions not described, depending on the cause of hypotension.

A combination of haemodynamic states is more common. For example, the use of isoflurane produces vasodilation, while dexmedetomidine may produce brady-cardia and reduce cardiac contractility, but may offset the vasodilation caused by isoflurane. Additionally, chronically

hypertensive patients can become unstable during anaes-thesia and can alternate between periods of profound hypotension and hypertension.

Adequate cortisol concentration is required for proper adrenoceptor function; low concentration may reduce the effectiveness of treatment with catecholamine. Patients on chronic corticosteroid therapy may benefit from supplemental corticosteroid administered during anaesthesia to offset the reduced ability of the adrenal glands to respond to stressful situations such as hypo-tension during anaesthesia.

Problems involving cardiac output
Reduced stroke volume

- Reduced venous return and ventricular filling (treatment: intravenous fluids, alpha-1 adrenoceptor agonists).
- Reduced cardiac contractility (treatment: beta-1 adrenoceptor agonists).

Heart rate

- Bradycardia (treatment: anticholinergics, beta-1 adrenoceptor agonists).
- Heart rates at the low end of normal do not usually affect CO.
- Extreme tachycardia (establish the cause and treat accordingly; see Chapter 31).

Problems involving systemic vascular resistance

- Excessive vasodilation (treatment: intravenous fluids, alpha-1 adrenoceptor agonists, vasopressin).

Anticholinergics

Anticholinergic agents can reverse a vagally-mediated bradycardia by blocking M_2 muscarinic receptors at the postganglionic synaptic junctions in areas of the heart innervated by the vagus nerve. During periods of bradycardia, there is more time for diastolic 'run-off' to occur; therefore DAP and MAP are reduced while SAP

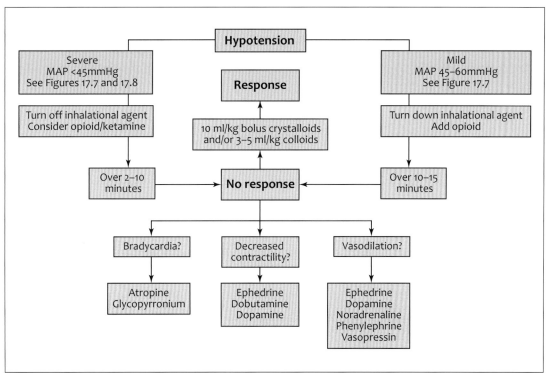

17.9 Flowchart for managing mild and severe hypotension. Use with Figures 17.7 and 17.8.

Drug	Bolus dose (mg/kg)	Infusion dose rate (μg/kg/min)	Route of administration
Atropine	0.02–0.04	NA	i.v. or i.m.
Glycopyrronium	0.005–0.01	NA	i.v. or i.m.
Dopamine	NA	2.0–15.0	i.v.
Noradrenaline	NA	0.1–1.0	i.v.
Adrenaline	0.01–0.10	0.01–0.03	i.v.
Dobutamine	NA	2.0–10.0	i.v.
Phenylephrine	0.002–0.02	1.0–3.0	i.v.
Ephedrine	0.02–0.05	1.0–5.0	i.v.
Vasopressin	0.2–0.6 IU/kg	0.002–0.006 IU/kg/min	i.v.

17.10 Dose rates for drugs used for haemodynamic support. NA = not applicable.

can still be within an acceptable range. For this reason, measuring systolic, mean and diastolic pressure can offer more information on whether bradycardia is causing a problem, compared with measuring systolic pressure alone (Doppler method).

In the first few minutes of action, anticholinergic drugs remove the vagal effect on the sinoatrial node first, followed by removal of vagal tone from the AV node, allowing conduction of impulses to the ventricles. Therefore, when anticholinergics are used to treat a second-degree AV block, more P waves are generated, but not all result in ventricular conduction until the AV node is unblocked. A second-degree AV block may therefore appear to worsen before it gets better, although this is not really the case. Occasionally, and usually with atropine, the heart rate may decrease before increasing to acceptable levels. This response may be due either to other subtypes of muscarinic receptor inhibiting sympathetic tone within the heart, or to a central effect because atropine is capable of crossing the blood–brain barrier.

Occasionally, as a result of removing vagal influence, anticholinergic agents can cause the heart rate to increase rapidly, leading to tachycardia. This usually occurs if the underlying SNS tone is high because of concurrent hypercapnia or another cause. The anticholinergic drug thus 'unmasks' the SNS tone. In such situations the heart rate usually then decreases over a period of approximately 15 minutes.

Atropine

Atropine is a lipophilic molecule (tropane plant alkaloid) and is capable of crossing the blood–brain barrier and placenta. It has a rapid onset of action and its duration of action is approximately 20–40 minutes. Atropine can interfere with ocular lens accommodation and animals treated with this agent should be kept in dim lighting until the pupils are able to constrict; it is contraindicated in patients where ocular drainage is compromised by mydriasis as this can exacerbate glaucoma.

Atropine should be used for life-threatening emergencies because it has a more rapid onset of action than glycopyrronium.

- Bolus dose: 0.02–0.04 mg/kg i.v. or i.m.

Glycopyrronium

Glycopyrronium tends to produce a more controlled increase in heart rate and can have a longer onset time relative to atropine. It is a large, ionized molecule (synthetic quaternary amine) and does not cross the blood–brain barrier or the placenta. Its uptake from intramuscular and especially subcutaneous sites is slow. The lower end of the dose range provided below can be used to treat bradycardia in large dogs, but the higher dose rate is recommended for smaller dogs and cats to achieve a reliable effect (Dyson and James-Davies, 1999). After administration, it can take several minutes for the effect of glycopyrronium to become obvious. Compared with atropine, it is more likely to produce more visible P waves without AV conduction. It is a powerful antisialogogue and dries up salivary and bronchial secretions. These drying effects can last 2–4 hours, whereas the effect on heart rate lasts 1–2 hours.

- Bolus dose: 0.005–0.01 mg/kg i.v. or i.m.

Sympathomimetics

The use of sympathomimetics (inotropes and vasopressors) should complement fluid therapy (see Figure 17.7).

Potent vasopressors can be used both in animals with severe, life-threatening hypotension and in septicaemic patients. Vasopressors are not usually used for mild hypotension, although there is an increasing trend to use these drugs, associated with the increased use of vasodilatory inhalant anaesthetic agents such as isoflurane and sevoflurane. The increased ABP produced by these drugs may not necessarily indicate increased tissue perfusion, which may in fact decrease; for this reason, vasopressors should be used for as short a time as possible.

Inotropes are also commonly used in anaesthetized patients to improve cardiac contractility, and are especially effective in treating hypotension when combined with intravenous fluid therapy.

Most catecholamines are administered to the patient as a continuous intravenous infusion. If necessary, bolus doses can be administered, but this should be done with care otherwise severe hypertension and reflex bradycardia may occur. The half-lives of catecholamines are short (2–3 minutes).

Mixed inotropes and vasopressors

Dopamine: Dopamine is the chemical precursor to noradrenaline and adrenaline (see Figure 17.1). Dopaminergic effects are prominent at low infusion rates; beta-1 adrenergic inotropic and chronotropic effects are produced at mid-range infusion rates; and alpha-1 adrenoceptor stimulation occurs at high infusion rates, producing vasoconstriction. As a result, dopamine can be used as either an inotrope or a vasopressor, depending on the infusion rate. Cardiac arrhythmias may be observed with dopamine, as a result of stimulation of endogenous noradrenaline release within the heart.

Dopamine administered at a mid-range infusion rate increases CO, SVR, MAP and heart rate.

- Low infusion rate (dopaminergic): 2–5 μg/kg/min.
- Mid-range infusion rate (beta-1 adrenergic): 5–10 μg/kg/min.
- High infusion rate (alpha-1 adrenergic): 10–15 μg/kg/min.

Ephedrine: Ephedrine stimulates the release of endogenous noradrenaline, which produces its sympathomimetic action at both alpha and beta adrenoceptors. The final effect is similar to that of giving noradrenaline, although not as profound. This makes ephedrine the ideal drug for correction of mild hypotension, where aggressive treatment is not necessary. As noradrenaline stores are used, the effect of subsequent ephedrine boluses diminishes, although ephedrine also has some direct action on adrenoceptors. Ephedrine decreases renal and splanchnic perfusion, but the reduction in renal perfusion is not as great as that produced by directly acting alpha-1 adrenergic agonists. Ephedrine increases MAP, heart rate and CO. It has a particularly useful vasoconstrictor action on the great veins and increases venous return.

It is possible, although not necessary, to give ephedrine as an infusion. The author has used ephedrine administered at infusion rates lower than those used in the study of Sinclair and Dyson (2012) with some success in patients where hypotension was largely attributed to vasodilation.

- Bolus dose: 0.02–0.05 mg/kg i.v. or i.m.
- Infusion rate: 1–5 μg/kg/min.

Noradrenaline: Noradrenaline stimulates beta-1 adrenoceptors, but not beta-2 adrenoceptors, and increases inotropy and CO. Its effect on alpha-1 adrenoceptors is powerful and dose dependent. Noradrenaline increases SVR, thus limiting any effective increase in CO when given at higher infusion rates. Perfusion of the liver, kidneys, muscles and skin is reduced and therefore the drug should be administered for as short a time as possible. However, its powerful vasoconstrictive effects are useful in patients with vasodilatory shock.

- Infusion rate: 0.1–1.0 μg/kg/min.

Adrenaline: Adrenaline is a powerful inotrope, chronotrope and vasopressor. It is usually reserved for life-threatening situations such as severe hypotension, anaphylactic shock or cardiac arrest. The overall effects are dose dependent, with higher doses stimulating more alpha adrenoceptors in the vascular system. Beta-1 stimulation increases heart rate and CO. Both DAP and MAP may remain constant or decrease due to beta-2-mediated vasodilation within skeletal muscle. Because MAP does not change, the baroreceptor reflex arc is not triggered and bradycardia does not usually occur.

- Bolus dose: 0.01–0.1 mg/kg i.v. or i.m.
- Infusion rate: 0.01–0.03 μg/kg/min.

Inotropes

Dobutamine: Dobutamine is a synthetic catecholamine used to produce dose-dependent increases in CO through beta-1 receptor stimulation. SVR does not usually change or decrease, although coronary artery dilation does occur. There is little risk of cardiac arrhythmias with dobutamine because endogenous noradrenaline is not released. Occasionally, dobutamine causes an increase in heart rate without an appreciable increase in MAP; these patients may be sensitive to the vasodilatory effects of dobutamine and require either lower infusion rates, or more fluid therapy to increase venous return.

- Infusion rate: 2–10 μg/kg/min.

Vasopressors

Phenylephrine: Phenylephrine stimulates alpha-1 adrenoceptors and decreases splanchnic perfusion while increasing SVR. It is useful for treating hypotension mediated through vasodilation and is used in a similar manner to noradrenaline. Vasopressors should not be used aggressively to produce hypertensive states because this may result in shifting of fluid from the circulation via hydrostatic forces, and can cause a condition called vasopressor dependence. The loss of circulating volume to the tissues aggravates the hypotensive state, leading to a continued, but ultimately detrimental, requirement for vasopressor infusion. In this situation, increasing fluid therapy and reducing the alpha-1 agonist infusion is usually required.

Decreased CO can occur through increased afterload (increased MAP and SVR), resulting in a reflex bradycardia.

- Bolus dose: 0.002–0.02 mg/kg i.v.
- Infusion rate: 1–3 μg/kg/min.

Vasopressin: Vasopressin (ADH) is a potent vasoconstrictor whose effect is not mediated via catecholamine receptors. Vasopressin stimulates dedicated vasopressin receptors and thus can have an effect even when treatment with catecholamines fails. The powerful vasoconstrictive effects of vasopressin can decrease the perfusion of the extremities and the viscera; therefore, vasopressin should be used at the lowest effective infusion rate and for as short a period as possible. Vasopressin can be used alongside catecholamines such as dobutamine in extremely debilitated patients.

- Bolus dose: 0.2–0.6 IU/kg.
- Infusion rate: 0.002–0.006 IU/kg/min.

References and further reading

Bodey AR and Michell AR (1996) Epidemiological study of blood pressure in domestic dogs. *Journal of Small Animal Practice* **37**, 116–125

Bodey AR and Sansom DJ (1998) Epidemiological study of blood pressure in domestic cats. *Journal of Small Animal Practice* **39**, 567–573

Duke T and Henke J (2007) Control of blood pressure under anesthesia. Section 2: Pathologic changes in blood pressure. In: *Essential Facts of Blood Pressure in Cats and Dogs, 1st edn*, ed. B Egner, A Carr and S Brown, pp. 109–136. VBS VetVerlag, Buchhandel und Seminar GmbH, Babenhausen, Germany

Dyson DH and James-Davies R (1999) Dose effect and benefits of glycopyrrolate in the treatment of bradycardia in anesthetized dogs. *Canadian Veterinary Journal* **40**, 327–331

Haskins S, Pascoe PJ, Ilkiw JE *et al.* (2005) Reference cardiopulmonary values in normal dogs. *Comparative Medicine* **55**, 156–161

Long KM and Kirby R (2008) An update on cardiovascular adrenergic receptor physiology and potential pharmacological applications in veterinary medicine. *Journal of Veterinary Emergency and Critical Care* **18**, 2–25

Marino CL, Cober RE, Iazbik MC, *et al.* (2011) White-coat effect on systemic blood pressure in retired racing Greyhounds. *Journal of Veterinary Internal Medicine* **25**, 861–865

Sinclair MD and Dyson D (2012) The impact of acepromazine on the efficacy of crystalloid, dextran or ephedrine treatment in hypotensive dogs under isoflurane anesthesia. *Veterinary Anaesthesia and Analgesia* **39**, 563–573

Chapter 18

Fluid therapy and blood transfusion

Adam Auckburally

Fluid therapy is often essential in the perioperative period to optimize and maintain cardiac output, tissue perfusion, electrolyte concentrations and acid–base balance. In recent years, there has been strong interest in the use of 'goal-directed therapy (GDT)' or 'fluid optimization' to avoid tissue oxygen debt and reduce the potential for organ failure. The mechanics of transcapillary water flow have also been re-evaluated to explain some unexpected observations in patients receiving fluids; however, the optimal perioperative fluid rates are still unknown. It is vital that the veterinary surgeon (veterinarian) has adequate understanding of body fluid physiology in order to ensure that each patient receives the correct type and volume of fluid, administered at the correct rate, via an appropriate route.

Fluid distribution and composition within the body

In an adult animal, total body water constitutes approximately 60% of total bodyweight (TBW) (Figure 18.1). This proportion varies with the animal's age, species and body fat content. For example, in neonatal cats and dogs, total body water content is nearer 80% of TBW, and in Greyhounds it is approximately 70% of TBW.

The two main body compartments are the intracellular fluid (ICF) compartment and the extracellular fluid (ECF) compartment. The ICF accounts for two-thirds of total body water content (40% of TBW) and the ECF accounts for the remaining one-third of total body water (20% of TBW). It is difficult to measure ECF volume precisely and reported values may vary. For the purposes of this chapter, the ECF will be taken to represent 20% of TBW. Traditionally, the ECF is subdivided into two compartments: the interstitial fluid (ISF), which includes lymph and the fluid between cells and constitutes three-quarters of the ECF (15% of TBW); and the intravascular compartment, which consists of fluid within blood vessels (plasma) and represents the remaining one-quarter of the ECF (5% of TBW). Transcellular fluid includes cerebrospinal and synovial fluid; it represents approximately 1% of TBW and is usually ignored in fluid therapy calculations.

Solute concentrations also differ between the compartments because solute movement across cell membranes may be restricted or enhanced by various membrane transport systems. Consequently, there are differences in ion composition between the ECF and ICF: in the ICF

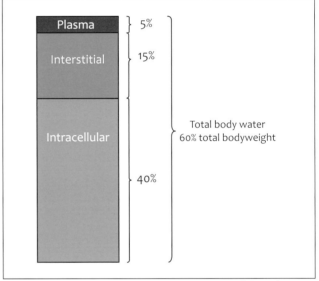

18.1 Body water distribution between the intracellular and extracellular (plasma plus interstitial) fluid compartments. See text for explanation.

the main ions are potassium, magnesium and calcium, whereas within the ECF, sodium and chloride ions predominate. The vascular endothelium is relatively permeable to all solutes and therefore the composition of ISF is similar to that of plasma.

The volume of fluid in each compartment is not fixed, but varies as fluid moves from one compartment to another by osmosis (see below) or is lost in urine, faeces, sweat and from the respiratory tract.

Physical principles and measurements

The physiology of fluid movement between the various body compartments requires an understanding of certain concepts and definitions, which are explained in this section.

Osmosis

Osmosis is the process by which water is drawn across a semipermeable membrane in response to the presence of *osmotically active particles* (Figure 18.2). Osmotically

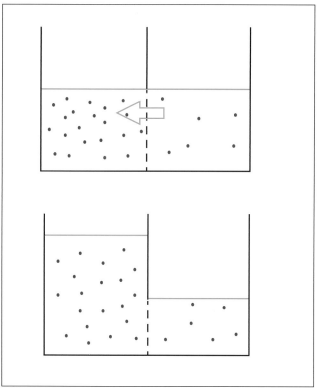

18.2 Osmosis. Direction of arrow indicates the movement of water. The increased number of particles creates an osmotic gradient allowing the movement of water through the semipermeable membrane so that the concentrations of each compartment become equal.

active particles include sodium, potassium and chloride ions and larger molecules such as glucose. Water movement between the body compartments is dictated by differences in the concentration of these solutes. When two compartments are separated by a semipermeable membrane, water will move from the compartment with fewer osmotically active particles to the one with more particles, until the concentration in the two compartments has equalized. *Osmotic pressure* is the theoretical pressure that would have to be applied against the semipermeable membrane to prevent the movement of water by osmosis.

Osmolality and osmolarity

The number of moles of osmotically active particles generated when a compound dissociates in 1 litre of water is expressed in osmoles (Osm) or milliosmoles (mOsm). For example, 1 mole of sodium chloride will dissociate completely in 1 litre of water to generate 1 Osm of both sodium and chloride ions.

Osmolality is the number of osmoles (or milliosmoles) *per kilogram* of solvent. Osmolality is dependent upon the number of particles but not their size, weight or charge. Sodium, potassium, chloride, bicarbonate, urea and glucose together constitute 95% of the total osmolality of plasma. Colligative properties such as freezing point are determined by the osmolality of a solution. Osmometry is the technique used to measure the osmolality of a solution (e.g. plasma, serum, urine or sweat) based on depression of the solution's freezing point. Serum osmolality is approximately 300 mOsm/kg in the dog and 310 mOsm/kg in the cat (DiBartola, 2011).

Osmolality can also be calculated, although all formulae tend to underestimate the true value because they either exclude or estimate unmeasured solutes. One such formula for calculating the osmolality of ECF is as follows:

ECF osmolality (mOsm/kg) =

$2([Na^+] + [K^+]) + ([glucose]/18) + ([BUN]/2.8)$

The values for sodium concentration ($[Na^+]$) and potassium concentration ($[K^+]$) figures in this formula are doubled to account for the major anions that are not included in the calculation (chloride and bicarbonate). Glucose and blood urea nitrogen (BUN) concentrations (denoted in the formula as [glucose] and [BUN], respectively) are divided by constant factors to convert values in mg/dl to mmol/l; this conversion is not necessary if the measured concentrations are already in mmol/l. However, because potassium and BUN are 'ineffective osmoles' (see tonicity, below) and glucose contributes relatively little to the final osmolality, simply doubling the measured sodium concentration ($2 \times [Na^+]$) provides a good approximation of plasma osmolality. The difference between measured and calculated osmolality is known as the *osmolal gap*; the normal range is between 0 and 16 mOsm/kg in the dog. Osmolal gap values for the cat are confusing because the calculated osmolality exceeds the measured value; the reason for this is unclear (DiBartola, 2011). Calculation of the osmolal gap can be useful to detect the presence of unmeasured osmoles, for example, in ethylene glycol toxicity, or in assessment of sodium disorders. In the dog, urine osmolality can be estimated by multiplying the last two digits of the urine specific gravity (USG) by 36 (DiBartola, 2011).

In contrast, *osmolarity* refers to the number of osmoles (or milliosmoles) *per litre* of solution. In practice, however, the terms osmolality and osmolarity are often used interchangeably. They are important to consider when choosing appropriate fluid therapy and for anticipating its effects and potential side effects.

Tonicity

If the membrane dividing two compartments is freely permeable to a particular solute within a solution, the particles of that solute do not exert an osmotic force across the membrane. Tonicity is equivalent to the *effective osmolality* because it ignores particles that do not contribute to fluid shifts. Tonicity can therefore be defined as the osmolality minus the concentration of these ineffective solutes. Tonicity is used to categorize fluids as hypotonic, isotonic or hypertonic, compared with the tonicity of plasma. In the dog, for example, commercially available fluids with effective osmolarity >300 mOsm/l are described as hypertonic, and fluids with effective osmolarity <300 mOsm/l are considered hypotonic.

Oncotic pressure

The vascular endothelium is relatively freely permeable to water and electrolyte molecules but is only selectively permeable to larger molecules such as albumin and globulins. These proteins are osmotically active and therefore exert an osmotic pressure. This is termed the *colloid osmotic pressure* (COP) or *oncotic pressure*, to distinguish it from that exerted by other solutes. Oncotic pressure is important for the maintenance of vascular volume, although it contributes little to the total overall osmolality of plasma. Plasma oncotic pressure can be measured clinically using a colloid osmometer or oncometer; normal values in dogs and cats are approximately 20–25 mmHg (DiBartola, 2011). The ISF also exerts an oncotic pressure because albumin can pass through large pores in blood vessel walls.

Hydrostatic pressure

Hydrostatic pressure is another determinant of fluid movement between the tissues and the intravascular space. Within blood vessels, the hydrostatic pressure is independent of osmotic and oncotic pressures. At the arterial end of a capillary, the hydrostatic pressure is higher than that of the ISF compartment and therefore fluid is 'forced' from the intravascular compartment into the interstitium. At the venous end of a capillary, the intravascular hydrostatic pressure is lower and so will not 'force' as much fluid out of the blood vessel; this allows the oncotic pressure to have more influence over water movement. As a result, the lower vascular pressure at the venous end of the capillary may favour the movement of fluid from the interstitium into the vascular space, although recently this suggestion has been questioned (see Endothelial Glycocalyx Theory, later).

Transcapillary fluid movement

As mentioned above, the ECF can be thought of as being partitioned into the ISF (75%) and intravascular fluid (25%). Intravascular fluid volume is maintained by fluid shifts between these two compartments. The movement of water and solutes occurs at the level of the capillaries. There is a balance between the 'forces' that either favour or oppose movement into the ISF. Pre-capillary hydrostatic pressure and interstitial oncotic pressure together cause movement of water from the intravascular space into the interstitium. Fluid movement from the interstitium back into the intravascular space occurs because of the higher oncotic pressure at the venous end of the capillaries. The balance of 'forces' at the capillary level can be represented diagrammatically and mathematically by the Starling equation (Figure 18.3).

During pathological fluid loss, capillary oncotic pressure increases (concentrating effect) and capillary hydrostatic pressure decreases; together, these changes help to counteract further intravascular volume loss. When hypoproteinaemia is present, fluid shifted into the interstitium may not be resorbed into the capillary because there will be a reduced intravascular oncotic pressure; this may result in tissue oedema formation.

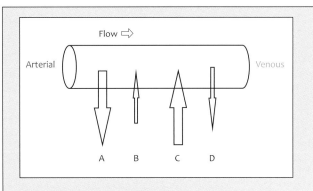

Net filtration = $K_fS[(P_{cap} – P_i) – \sigma(\pi_{cap} – \pi_i)]$

K_f = Filtration coefficient or hydraulic conductance (flow rate of fluid per unit pressure gradient across the endothelium)
S = Surface area of the endothelium
σ = Staverman reflection coefficient (an expression of the permeability of albumin; has a value between 0 and 1, where 0 indicates free passage and 1 indicates total impermeability). This coefficient varies from organ to organ (e.g. 1 in the blood–brain barrier and 0 in hepatic sinusoids). The coefficient also changes in disease processes (e.g. inflammation will push σ towards zero)
P_{cap} = Hydrostatic pressure in the capillary
P_i = Hydrostatic pressure in the interstitium
π_{cap} = Oncotic pressure in the capillary
π_i = Oncotic pressure in the interstitium

18.3 Diagrammatic and mathematical representations of Starling's forces governing transcapillary fluid movement. A = capillary hydrostatic pressure; B = interstitial hydrostatic pressure; C = capillary oncotic pressure; D = interstitial oncotic pressure. The Starling equation can be simplified as: Filtration = (A – B) – (C – D) or hydrostatic pressure difference – oncotic pressure difference.

The Endothelial Glycocalyx Theory

Recent research has led to a re-evaluation of the classical Starling forces of fluid movement. Much of the fluid in the intravascular space is non-circulating. Instead, it is contained within an endothelial glycocalyx layer (EGL), composed of glycoproteins and proteoglycans, which forms an active interface between circulating blood and the vascular endothelium (Figure 18.4). The EGL appears to act as a 'sieve' for plasma proteins and therefore determines the primary oncotic forces that control transcapillary fluid flow through endothelial channels into the sub-glycocalyx layer (SGL). The SGL is virtually protein-free and is referred to as the 'protected region'. Beyond the SGL is the bulk of the interstitium, which contains the

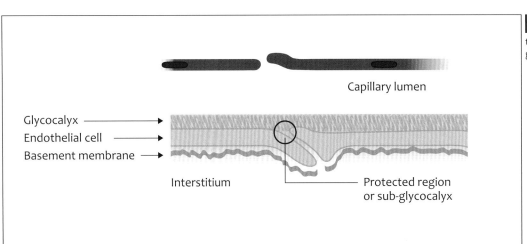

18.4 Schematic representation of the endothelium and the glycocalyx layer in a capillary.

proteins passed from the intravascular space through the large endothelial channels. In areas of high capillary hydrostatic pressure (the arterial end of the capillary bed), the protein concentration in the protected region is very low because proteins do not pass through the EGL at this site. In addition, the physical movement of fluid from the capillary lumen into the interstitium prevents the retrograde diffusion of protein from the interstitium into the protected region. In areas of lower capillary pressure (the venous end of the capillary bed), fluid flow from the capillary lumen through the EGL into the interstitium diminishes towards zero. Proteins are able to diffuse down their concentration gradient from the interstitium into the protected region. This results in increased COP in the protected region, which opposes movement of fluid from the SGL into the capillary, creating a state of minimal fluid movement.

Following on from this model, the Starling hypothesis has been revised, such that forces across the EGL, rather than across the entire endothelial layer, are applied. The revised Starling equation is shown below (Woodcock and Woodcock, 2012):

$$\text{Net filtration} = K_f S[(P_{cap} - P_{sg}) - \sigma(\pi_{cap} - \pi_{sg})]$$

In the modified Starling equation, P_i and π_i (see Figure 18.3) are replaced with P_{sg} and π_{sg}

P_{sg} = Sub-glycocalyx hydrostatic pressure
π_{sg} = Sub-glycocalyx colloid osmotic pressure

The revised hypothesis can be used to explain why *predicted* increases in circulatory volume following infusion of hydroxyethyl starches (HES) are often higher than those clinically observed. Some pathological conditions, such as diabetes mellitus, hyperglycaemia, trauma and sepsis, as well as surgery, are known to cause 'flaking' or 'shedding' of the EGL. This damage allows greater movement of the exogenous colloid (HES) into the interstitium, which promotes tissue oedema and decreases tissue microperfusion; these changes can result in increased morbidity and mortality. Additionally, a large number of controlled and blinded clinical trials in human medicine have demonstrated that administration of colloids to chronically critically ill patients has no benefit, and in fact may even be detrimental compared with administration of crystalloids. Hydrocortisone and sevoflurane have been shown to stabilize and protect the EGL, which may be of clinical relevance (Chappell *et al.*, 2007; Annecke *et al.*, 2012; Woodcock, 2012).

Zero balance

The amount of water (and solute) excreted from the body equals the amount ingested. This concept is used to formulate suggested volumes for daily requirements of sedentary animals in a thermoneutral environment. Changes in activity, environmental temperature and humidity, and pathological states will alter an animal's requirements.

Water is required due to *insensible losses* (through the skin and respiratory tract) and *sensible losses* in urine and faeces. Water production from metabolic processes will contribute to the water load. Sensible losses may be reduced during states of water deprivation, although obligatory urine and faecal losses (to excrete unwanted solutes) will still occur. Approximately one-third of daily water requirements are to replace insensible losses and the remaining two-thirds to replace sensible losses.

Recognition of fluid deficits

Recognizing fluid deficits and being able to quantify not only losses, but also excessive fluid administration, are important when devising an appropriate fluid therapy plan. It is essential to examine the patient thoroughly and use appropriate tests, as discussed in this section, to identify and quantify a fluid deficit or excess.

Patient history

The patient's history can provide information on the type of fluid losses (e.g. vomiting and diarrhoea) and their duration. However, the owner may not recognize that there is a problem until the animal is in a state of collapse. Information should be sought regarding the patient's voluntary water and feed consumption, and the frequency of urination and amount of urine produced.

Physical examination

A thorough physical examination should be performed before any fluid is administered. Particular attention should be paid to the cardiovascular, respiratory and neurological systems. The sympathetic nervous system (SNS) tone will increase as a response to a fluid deficit in a similar way to its response to pain and anxiety. Careful administration of opioids may help to differentiate the cause of the increased SNS tone by alleviating any pain that is present. It is important to distinguish between dehydration and hypovolaemia because loss of circulating volume (hypovolaemia) will require more aggressive treatment. Early recognition of hypovolaemia and prompt administration of fluids will increase the likelihood of the patient recovering from problems associated with fluid loss. However, hypovolaemia and dehydration often co-exist.

Hypovolaemia

Hypovolaemia can be caused by loss of blood and/or loss of water and solutes. It can be categorized as absolute or relative: absolute hypovolaemia refers to loss of volume from the intravascular space (e.g. haemorrhage), whereas relative hypovolaemia refers to either an inappropriate redistribution of fluids across body compartments (burns, severe inflammation), or a pathological vasodilatory state (sepsis, anaphylaxis). Clinical signs of hypovolaemia (Figure 18.5) will be more obvious to both the owner and the veterinary surgeon than the signs of dehydration. Animals with a chronic reduction in body water may appear clinically well but be dehydrated, whereas patients with acute blood loss may present *in extremis* and require immediate fluid resuscitation.

Acute fluid loss reduces cardiac output, leading to various physiological responses (see Chapter 17). Hypotension is detected by baroreceptors in the aorta and

- Increased heart rate
- Weak peripheral pulses and reduced jugular filling
- Pale mucous membranes
- Prolonged capillary refill time
- Increased respiratory rate
- Cool extremities
- Cool core (rectal) temperature
- Depressed mentation
- Reduced urine production

18.5 Clinical signs consistent with the presence of hypovolaemia.

carotid arteries, resulting in inhibition of parasympathetic activity and an increase in sympathetic tone. Heart rate, myocardial contractility and systemic vascular resistance increase. Renin is released from the kidney, resulting in retention of sodium, chloride and water; increased angiotensin II production results in vasoconstriction and maintenance of peripheral vascular resistance; and antidiuretic hormone (vasopressin) is released, which causes vasoconstriction and promotes water reabsorption in the renal collecting ducts.

Patients with severe hypovolaemia will have tachycardia and weak peripheral pulses, cold extremities, pale mucous membranes and a prolonged capillary refill time. If there is poor perfusion of the brain, reduced mentation may be evident.

Dehydration

Loss of water from the interstitium accounts for many of the physical findings in dehydrated patients. However, due to intercompartmental fluid shifts, the water content of the ICF will also be reduced in these patients, and severe dehydration will lead to hypovolaemia. Assessment of dehydration is difficult and subjective, although there are well-reported clinical signs (Figure 18.6). Caution should be exercised when using these signs to estimate the degree of dehydration because factors such as age and body condition can lead to alterations in skin elasticity and ocular fat pad content; these changes may be misinterpreted as evidence of dehydration. In addition, dry mucous membranes can result from open-mouth breathing, while moist mucous membranes can be caused by nausea or recent water intake. Dehydration may not be clinically obvious even with water deficits of up to 16% bodyweight (Hansen and DeFrancesco, 2002). Alterations in plasma sodium concentration may be present, but this will depend on the type of water and/or electrolyte loss responsible for dehydration. Other clinical signs of dehydration may include thirst behaviours, such as the animal standing over an empty water bowl, and general depression.

Laboratory tests

The following laboratory tests are commonly used to assess the state of the circulating volume and the degree of dehydration.

Clinical assessment findings	Estimated percentage dehydration
No clinical signs detectable	<5
Mild loss of skin elasticity, possible drying of oral mucous membranes	5–6
Definite reduction in skin elasticity, dry oral mucous membranes, eyes may start to look sunken, mild increase in capillary refill time	6–8
Skin tenting very obvious, dry oral mucous membranes, sunken eyes, signs of hypovolaemia (rapid heart rate, weak pulses, cool extremities)	8–10
Severe loss of skin elasticity, very dry mucous membranes, obvious sunken eyes, obvious signs of hypovolaemia, altered mentation with possible recumbency, anuria	10–12
Signs of shock, moribund, death imminent	12–15

18.6 Clinical signs that can be used to recognize and estimate the percentage of dehydration.

Packed cell volume and total solids

Measurement of packed cell volume (PCV) and total solids (TS) can be useful to assess volume status but the results must be carefully interpreted:

- The patient's baseline values are usually unknown, and therefore any real change cannot be confirmed unless the measured values are outside the reference range for that species
- Splenic contraction can dramatically increase PCV, while TS can be abnormal in patients with renal or gastrointestinal disease
- Animals with recent haemorrhage will not have dramatic changes in PCV until 3–6 hours after the insult that caused the haemorrhage because of delays in intercompartmental fluid shifts. Changes in TS may be observed sooner; a decrease in TS with a normal PCV may indicate recent haemorrhage
- Elevated PCV and TS generally indicate dehydration, and serial samples to identify trends in these parameters are useful to assess response to treatment.

Urine specific gravity

Specific gravity is measured using a refractometer. Dehydration will lead to increased USG in animals with normal renal function. A reduction in USG following fluid therapy suggests that the deficit in circulating volume is being corrected and, as a result, less water is being reabsorbed by the nephrons. A value of USG >1.045 is highly suggestive of dehydration; if such a value is measured, fluid therapy should be started to correct the value to approximately 1.035 in cats or 1.025 in dogs.

Lactate

Normal blood lactate concentration is <2.0 mmol/l in cats and dogs. Blood samples for lactate measurement should be analysed immediately after collection or placed on ice and analysed within 2 hours because continuing glycolysis in blood cells will falsely elevate the lactate concentration. High blood lactate concentrations have been shown to correlate with poor prognosis for survival in critically ill dogs, especially if the value remains high following aggressive fluid therapy (Stevenson et al., 2007). Accumulation of lactate during dehydration or hypovolaemia is usually a result of poor tissue perfusion, a greater degree of anaerobic metabolism, or poor liver perfusion and consequent poor hepatic metabolism of lactate. While blood lactate concentration is a valuable guide to fluid therapy, it should be used alongside other clinical observations and measurements. Hyperlactataemia produces metabolic acidosis. A pH <7.2 and a base excess (BE) more negative than −7 are considered detrimental and may require treatment. Other causes of hyperlactataemia are discussed in Pang and Boysen (2007), which covers the topic of blood lactate in detail.

Electrolytes

Abnormal plasma electrolyte concentrations can occur with a variety of pathological processes and are covered in detail in the relevant chapters of this book. Fluid therapy can be used to manage many of these abnormalities, but an inappropriate choice of fluid type may worsen electrolyte disturbance. It is, therefore, important to quantify electrolyte disturbances as well as to assess any fluid deficits. The reader is referred to DiBartola (2011) for an in-depth description of electrolyte disorders.

Urea:creatinine ratio

The serum concentrations of urea (BUN) and creatinine can be interpreted as a ratio. A high urea:creatinine ratio (>40–100:1) may be indicative of dehydration (pre-renal azotaemia), but this finding should be interpreted alongside clinical signs and USG. Blood urea concentration is more affected by the animal's hydration status compared to creatinine.

Types of fluid loss

Most pathological states of fluid loss involve loss from the ECF and can be described in one of the following categories.

Hypertonic fluid loss

This is the least common form of fluid derangement, where solute is lost from the ECF. The ECF osmolality decreases relative to that of the ICF, and water moves from the ECF into the ICF to maintain isotonicity. Overall, osmolality decreases in both the ECF and ICF but fluid volume in the ECF (including the circulating volume) decreases and cellular swelling may occur. Excessive sodium loss can occur with kidney disease and some adrenal disorders.

Hypotonic fluid loss

With this form of fluid loss, water is lost from the ECF, which becomes hypertonic relative to the ICF. Water moves from the ICF to the ECF to maintain isotonicity but the osmolality of both compartments increases overall. Increased electrolyte concentrations, especially sodium, within the ICF cause clinical signs such as altered mentation and seizures. Examples are water deprivation and pathological states characterized by high respiratory rates, in which water is lost via the mucosal surfaces (e.g. pneumonia, pyrexia).

Isotonic fluid loss

If isotonic fluid loss occurs, the osmolality of the ECF does not change because water and solute losses are equal. No intercompartmental fluid shifts occur but hypovolaemia is the final outcome. Examples are diarrhoea, 'third space' losses (e.g. trauma) and haemorrhage.

Protein-rich fluid loss

The fluid lost has a similar electrolyte composition to that of the ECF but is rich in protein due to an inflammatory or effusive component (e.g. pleural or peritoneal effusion, protein-losing enteropathy/nephropathy, burns, gastrointestinal sequestration). Oncotic pressure is reduced within the intravascular space, and hypovolaemia follows.

Routes of fluid administration

When planning to administer fluid therapy, the chosen route will depend on the severity of the condition, whether intravenous access is available, clinical skills and the available facilities within the clinic.

Oral

Administration of fluids via the enteral (oral) route is not suitable for patients that require rapid restoration of circulating volume. Water may, however, be administered enterally using feeding tubes and, in conscious patients with a normal gag reflex, by careful syringing. These techniques are described elsewhere (Campbell and Harvey, 2012).

Subcutaneous

This route may be useful in small patients where intravenous access cannot be achieved, and for long-term fluid therapy at home, such as for palliative care. The subcutaneous route is unsuitable for patients with hypovolaemia, where perfusion of the peripheral tissues may be reduced. Fluids given by this route should be relatively isotonic. Fluids with a low sodium concentration or hypotonic solutions should not be administered subcutaneously because water will dissipate throughout all compartments and not correct deficits in circulating volume. Hypertonic fluids will cause water to move to the site of injection and away from other tissues. The sites usually used for subcutaneous injection are the dorsal neck and trunk where loose skin folds are abundant. If large volumes are to be injected, multiple sites can be used. Disadvantages of this route include the possibility of infection at the site(s) of injection and poor or slow response to therapy. A commercially available implantable catheter (Endo-Sof Subcutaneous Catheter; Dechra) is designed for long-term fluid administration and is compatible with animal tissue for up to 12 months. Implantation of such a catheter may be an alternative arrangement to enable owners to administer fluids to their pet at home. Fluids should be warmed to body temperature before injection. When administering the fluid, the animal should be observed carefully for any reaction to the injection and the rate of fluid administration tailored accordingly.

Intravenous

This is generally the route of choice, provided that the intravenous catheter can be closely monitored for complications and dislodgement. Although any available vein can be catheterized, those commonly used are the cephalic, medial and lateral saphenous, jugular and auricular veins. If rapid administration of fluids is desired, a short, large-bore catheter should be used. Long-term catheters are often placed via the Seldinger ('over the wire') technique, which is explained elsewhere (Tefend Campbell and Macintire, 2012). Ultrasound-guided placement of the catheter can also be useful, but requires the veterinary surgeon to be skilled in the technique.

Intraosseous

This route of administration is particularly useful for neonates and other small animals or in any patient with circulatory collapse requiring rapid fluid administration where intravenous access is difficult to obtain. A 16–18G hypodermic needle or spinal needle can be placed into the medullary cavity if the patient has soft cortical bone. Commonly used sites are the greater trochanter of the femur, iliac crest, tibial crest and lateral tuberosity of the humerus. Fluid is taken up rapidly from the dense capillary network within the medullary cavity. For larger animals with dense cortical bone, intraosseous needles are commercially available, such as the EZ-IO Intraosseous Infusion System. This system incorporates the use of a slow power driver to assist with insertion.

Intraperitoneal

Only isotonic fluids should be used with this route. However, these fluids can still precipitate peritonitis, and because of this the intraperitoneal route of administration is not recommended.

Types of fluid

Crystalloids

Crystalloids are aqueous solutions of mineral salts or other water-soluble molecules such as dextrose. Examples include 'normal' or 'physiological' saline (0.9% sodium chloride), Hartmann's solution (compound sodium lactate, CSL), Ringer's solution, lactated Ringer's solution (LRS) and 5% dextrose (D5W). Other electrolyte solutions for intravenous administration, such as potassium chloride, calcium gluconate and sodium bicarbonate are also classified as crystalloids; further information on their use can be found in relevant chapters of this book. Crystalloids can be classified by their tonicity as hypotonic, isotonic or hypertonic. Most fluids for administration by the intravenous or other routes outlined above are isotonic, to prevent osmotically induced damage to erythrocytes and other blood cells. It is wise to store hypotonic and hypertonic fluids separately from isotonic fluids to avoid their accidental infusion. Crystalloids can also be classified by function as either replacement or maintenance fluids. Many different commercial formulations are available (Figure 18.7).

Replacement fluids

Replacement solutions are used to replace lost body water and electrolytes. Examples of this type of fluid include Hartmann's solution and LRS. Some of these solutions are described as 'balanced' which means that their composition is relatively similar to that of fluid in the ECF. Normal saline is classified as a replacement fluid despite its high chloride content but it is not 'balanced' compared with plasma. A replacement fluid will remain in the ECF because of its composition. Its distribution within the ECF will reflect the relative sizes of the sub-compartments; as a result, only 25% of the infused volume will remain in the intravascular space after approximately 30–60 minutes (the remainder will pass into the interstitium).

Replacement fluids are sometimes used for short-term maintenance fluid therapy, but this is not ideal because hypernatraemia and hypokalaemia can develop if the animal has impaired renal function or if the fluids are used for longer periods of time.

Hartmann's solution: This solution is one of the most frequently used crystalloids in clinical practice and has an osmolarity of 279 mOsm/l. Hartmann's solution is probably the best choice for fluid resuscitation (restoration of circulating volume) and for perioperative fluid therapy (see Figure 18.7). The alkalizing effect of Hartmann's solution makes it an ideal choice for patients with concurrent metabolic acidosis (e.g. lactic acidosis), however counter-intuitive this may appear. In these patients, restoration of circulating volume and tissue perfusion is the main goal; rapid administration of Hartmann's solution will restore circulating volume and the liver will clear the increased circulating lactate. In patients with poor hepatic perfusion or severe hepatic dysfunction, the liver's ability to deal with lactate may be impaired; other replacement fluids with an alternative bicarbonate precursor, such as acetate (e.g. Plasma-Lyte®), may be more suitable. Within the body, Hartmann's solution becomes slightly hypotonic once the

Fluid	Fluid class	Osmolarity (mOsm/l)	Sodium (mmol/l)	Potassium (mmol/l)	Chloride (mmol/l)	Calcium (mmol/l)	Magnesium (mmol/l)	Dextrose (g/l)	Buffer (mmol/l)	pH
Canine plasma	–	290–310	145	4	110	2.5	1	–	–	7.407
Feline plasma	–	290–330	155	4	120	2.5	1	–	–	7.386
Dextrose 5% in water	Free water	252	0	0	0	0	0	50	None	4.0
Saline 0.45%	Hypotonic	154	77	0	77	0	0	0	None	5.0
Dextrose 4% in saline 0.18%	Hypotonic	271	30	0	30	0	0	40	None	4.0
Saline 0.9%	Replacement	308	154	0	154	0	0	0	None	5.0
Hartmann's	Replacement	279	131	5	112	2	0	0	Lactate 29	6.5–6.7
Lactated Ringer's	Replacement	272	130	4	109	3	0	0	Lactate 28	6.5
Plasma-Lyte® 148	Replacement	294	140	5	98	0	1.5	0	Acetate 27, Gluconate 23	5.5–6.0
Plasma-Lyte® A	Replacement	294	140	5	98	0	1.5	0	Acetate 27, Gluconate 23	7.4
Normosol®-R	Replacement	294	140	5	98	0	1.5	0	Acetate 27, Gluconate 23	6.6
Plasma-Lyte® M	Maintenance	377	40	16	40	2.5	1.5	50	Acetate 12 Lactate 12	5.5
Normosol®-M	Maintenance	363	40	13	40	0	1.5	50	Acetate 16	5.0
Saline 7.2%	Hypertonic	2464	1232	0	1232	0	0	0	None	5.2
Sodium bicarbonate 8.4%	–	2000	1000	0	0	0	0	0	Bicarbonate 1000	7.0–8.5

18.7 Composition and properties of crystalloid fluids.

lactate has been metabolized. This makes it unsuitable for cases where movement of fluid into the ICF would be detrimental, for example, patients with raised intracranial pressure. Hartmann's solution is unsuitable for infusion alongside blood products because the calcium ions in the fluid counteract the anticoagulant properties of the transfused blood product, which may cause formation of microthrombi. The presence of calcium ions also makes the solution unsuitable for use in hypercalcaemic patients.

Lactated Ringer's solution: LRS contains the same components as Hartmann's solution but at slightly different concentrations. The osmolarity of this solution is very similar to that of Hartmann's (see Figure 18.7). LRS is used for similar conditions and the same caveats apply to its use as to Hartmann's.

Ringer's solution, which does not contain lactate, is used as a laboratory solution.

Normal or physiological saline: Normal or physiological saline (0.9%) has a slightly higher sodium concentration and a much higher chloride concentration compared to plasma (see Figure 18.7). It is described as an acidifying fluid because it dilutes plasma bicarbonate, and the higher chloride concentration may result in a mild hyperchloraemic metabolic acidosis. The decrease in plasma pH is usually well tolerated unless the animal has a pre-existing acidaemia, in which case normal saline is probably not the fluid of choice. Normal saline does not contain potassium ions and infusion can reduce the plasma potassium concentration; electrolyte concentrations should therefore be monitored in hypokalaemic patients. The potassium concentration can decrease soon after starting a saline infusion, and normal saline may be used in patients with hyperkalaemia. However, because normal saline is an acidifying solution, it may actually exacerbate hyperkalaemia by activating the hydrogen/potassium countercurrent transmembrane antiporter system (hydrogen ions in the plasma are exchanged for intracellular potassium ions). In these patients, Hartmann's solution may be a more appropriate choice because its potassium concentration is low enough not to exacerbate the hyperkalaemic state and its alkalizing effect will also be beneficial.

Hyponatraemic patients may be treated with normal saline, but the rate of administration should be limited so that plasma sodium concentration does not increase by more than 0.5 mmol/l/h. Slow correction avoids rapid shifts in sodium concentrations within the various compartments, which have the potential to result in brain dehydration and myelinolysis. Similarly, hypochloraemia may be corrected using normal saline, but the plasma sodium concentration should be monitored while the underlying cause of hypochloraemia is treated. Normal saline is appropriate in hypercalcaemic patients because it has both dilutional and calciuretic effects.

Plasma-Lyte® and Normosol®-R: These fluids are similar in composition and are also comparable to Hartmann's solution, although they both contain slightly higher sodium concentrations, plus magnesium in concentrations similar to that of plasma (see Figure 18.7). They are alkalizing fluids with acetate as the bicarbonate precursor; because of this they are not recommended for treatment of diabetic ketoacidosis unless the patient is already receiving insulin therapy (acetate is a ketone precursor).

Recommended rates for replacement with crystalloids

Hypovolaemia should be treated rapidly to improve patient survival and outcome. It is impossible to quantify the amount of circulatory volume loss on the basis of a physical examination alone, and regular reassessment of the patient and stabilization of vital signs during fluid resuscitation should be used as a guide to determine and optimize the fluid plan. Commonly quoted 'shock doses' of crystalloid fluids originate from the idea that 'one blood volume' should be administered as a bolus; this is stated to be equivalent to 80–90 ml/kg for dogs and 50–60 ml/kg for cats. It is advisable to administer one-quarter of this calculated volume over 10–15 minutes, during which the patient should be continually assessed for improvements in vital signs. If clinical signs of hypovolaemia persist, further (one-quarter) boluses can be given as necessary until vital signs normalize. As mentioned earlier, replacement crystalloids will equilibrate throughout the ECF and only 25% of the amount given will remain in the intravascular space after approximately 1 hour. Co-administration of a colloid (see below) may help to retain fluid in the intravascular space for a longer period.

With active ongoing bleeding (e.g. splenic haemangiosarcoma), fluid resuscitation should be more conservative to prevent dislodgement of clots by the increased blood pressure that will result from administration of fluids. This less aggressive technique is known as 'hypotensive' or 'permissive' resuscitation because the aim is to obtain a mean arterial blood pressure in the range of 40–50 mmHg. This will allow sufficient tissue perfusion but not promote bleeding, and may reduce transfusion requirements. Ideally, blood lost due to haemorrhage should be replaced with transfused whole blood (WB) or packed red blood cells (PRBCs); the latter may be mixed with warm saline immediately before use. Healthy animals can tolerate losses of up to 25% of blood volume, and fluid replacement with crystalloids (with or without colloid) can be used to treat the loss in circulatory volume. The advantages of using crystalloids in this situation include their lower cost, lower risk of adverse reactions and ready availability, which allows prompt administration.

Following fluid resuscitation, any remaining fluid deficits are addressed by delivering fluids at a lower rate. The aim of this phase of treatment is to replace remaining deficits and ongoing losses completely over the following 12–24 hours, at the same time as meeting maintenance requirements. Ongoing contemporaneous losses due, for example, to vomiting, diarrhoea or further haemorrhage must be factored into the calculations for fluid replacement.

A subjective assessment of dehydration can be used to calculate the volume of fluid to be administered. For example, a Labrador weighing 30 kg with estimated 8% dehydration will need 2.4 kg (or 2.4 litres) of fluid. The first quarter of this calculated volume (600 ml) can be given rapidly by the intravenous route while vital signs such as heart and respiratory rates, pulse quality and capillary refill times are monitored. The next quarter to half of the calculated amount (600–1200 ml) is administered over the following 3–4 hours and the remainder, plus extra fluid to compensate for any additional losses, given over the following 4–12 hours, depending on the presence of any complications and the pathology involved. Additional losses may be large, depending on the underlying pathology, and rates of fluid therapy should be adjusted accordingly to maintain stable vital signs. Maintenance requirements can be calculated as described later and are also incorporated into the overall fluid therapy plan.

Maintenance fluids

Maintenance crystalloid fluids are designed to keep the body in zero balance (homeostasis). They provide water and small amounts of electrolytes to replace losses through the sensible (urine and faeces) and insensible (respiratory) routes. These obligatory fluid losses are low in sodium and relatively high in potassium, which is reflected by the composition of the maintenance fluid. As a result, these fluids are hypotonic and dextrose is sometimes added to increase their tonicity and prevent damage to blood cells (resulting from water being drawn into the cells by osmosis). The overall hypotonicity of the fluid once the dextrose has been metabolized makes maintenance fluids unsuitable for replacement purposes. They should not be administered as a bolus, and should not be used until the patient has been stabilized adequately with replacement fluids. Hypertonic maintenance fluids containing dextrose are commercially available (Plasma-Lyte® M and Normosol®-M; see Figure 18.7), but are not licensed for use in animals, and are expensive and have a relatively short shelf-life. However, maintenance solutions can be made in the practice by mixing other fluids together. 'Recipes' for two such fluids are detailed in Figure 18.8.

It is generally more appropriate to encourage the animal to eat and drink as soon as possible, or place a feeding tube through which water can be administered. For those cases where maintenance fluids are necessary, administration rates for maintenance requirements are usually quoted as 2–3 ml/kg/h or 40–60 ml/kg/day. These rates tend to overestimate water requirements in large dogs and underestimate requirements in small dogs and cats, and should be adjusted accordingly. More recent guidelines provide a range of 2–3 ml/kg/h for cats and 2–6 ml/kg/h for dogs (Davis *et al.*, 2013).

Other crystalloids

The commonly used fluids are described here. For other commercially available crystalloid solutions, the reader is directed to other references (DiBartola, 2011).

5% *Dextrose solution:* A solution of 5% dextrose in water provides free water to the body once the dextrose has been metabolized. This fluid is used to replace pure water loss in, for example, a hyperthermic dog with high respiratory water loss. Dextrose solutions do not contain sufficient calories to meet daily energy requirements and should not be used for this purpose. There are alternative nutritional support fluids and techniques available, which are described in the *BSAVA Manual of Canine and Feline Emergency and Critical Care.*

Hypertonic saline: Hypertonic saline (HS) (7.2%) is hyperosmolar (2464 mOsm/l), with an osmolarity approximately eight times that of plasma (see Figure 18.7). Because of its hypertonicity it requires careful infusion. It is not commonly used in small animal practice because colloids are reasonably priced and have more therapeutic advantages.

However, HS can be useful for rapid fluid resuscitation of a severely hypovolaemic animal because its high tonicity enables it to draw water from the intracellular and interstitial compartments to rapidly restore circulating volume. This characteristic is also relevant for treatment of other conditions such as raised intracranial pressure. Only a small volume of HS is required (2–4 ml/kg in cats and 4–7 ml/kg in dogs); this can be given over 10 minutes, which allows rapid resuscitation without the possible risk of peripheral tissue oedema that can occur when large volumes of isotonic crystalloids are given. Experimental data examining the clinical efficacy of HS in small animals are lacking, but results from human studies indicate many potential benefits. These include rapid restoration of arterial blood pressure, improved cardiac contractility, improved tissue microperfusion due to shrinking of erythrocytes (fluid moves out of cells) and reduction of intracranial pressure in patients with intracranial pathology.

HS has some disadvantages resulting from its hyperosmolar nature:

- Its duration of action is only 30 minutes or less
- Hyperchloraemia resulting from infusion of HS can produce hyperchloraemic metabolic acidosis, which may be detrimental to myocardial and cellular enzyme function (although the short duration of action of HS may reduce the clinical significance)
- Plasma potassium and bicarbonate concentrations fall (also not clinically significant unless there is a pre-existing electrolyte derangement)
- Rapid administration can lead to vagally-mediated bradycardia, hypotension and bronchoconstriction
- Vein irritation can occur (HS should be infused into a central vein when possible)
- Intravascular haemolysis is possible and ventricular arrhythmias can occur (the electrocardiogram should be monitored)
- Intracellular dehydration occurs because water has left the ICF; HS administration should be followed by isotonic fluid administration to replace intracellular fluid loss.

High sodium-containing fluids should be used with care in patients with cardiac disease because of the risk of volume overload. Commercial HS should be kept apart from isotonic and hypotonic fluids to prevent accidental administration, because HS can be rapidly fatal if given in large volumes. Hypertonic saline is also available in combination with a colloid (discussed later).

Potassium chloride: This is available in vials containing potassium at a concentration of 2 mmol/ml (= 2 mEq/ml), which must be diluted with other fluids to an appropriate concentration for safe delivery. It is usually added to 0.9% saline or Hartmann's solution to give a final potassium concentration of 20–30 mmol/l. Maximum rates of potassium infusion should never exceed 0.5 mmol/kg/h otherwise clinical signs of hyperkalaemia may follow.

Fluid recipe	Osmolarity (mOsm/l)	Sodium (mmol/l)	Potassium (mmol/l)	Chloride (mmol/l)	Calcium (mmol/l)	Dextrose (g/l)
1 part 0.9% NaCl, 2 parts 5% dextrose. Add 20 mmol KCl per litre of final solution	328	51	20	71	0	33.5
1 part Hartmann's solution, 2 parts 5% dextrose. Add 20 mmol KCl per litre of final solution	317	43	21	56	1	33.5

18.8 Recipes for making maintenance fluids. KCl = potassium chloride; NaCl = sodium chloride. (Data from DiBartola, 2011)

Sodium bicarbonate: This may be used to treat metabolic acidosis caused by loss of bicarbonate. The bicarbonate (HCO_3^-) administered will buffer excess hydrogen ions. However, treatment of metabolic acidosis should aim to deal with the underlying cause rather than simply correct the blood pH, because administration of sodium bicarbonate can be directly harmful. For example, lactic acidosis should be treated with appropriate fluid therapy to restore tissue perfusion, and not with sodium bicarbonate. However, if blood pH is <7.2 or the base excess is more negative than –7 mmol/l, administration of sodium bicarbonate may be necessary to prevent the detrimental effects of acidosis, which comprise: reduced myocardial contractility and arrhythmias; vasoconstriction; right shift of the oxyhaemoglobin dissociation curve; inhibition of cellular glycolysis; central nervous system (CNS) depression; and impaired response to catecholamine administration. Cellular enzyme systems will also be affected by any pH change.

Several preparations of sodium bicarbonate are available, but those commonly used are 4.2% (0.5 mmol/ml Na^+ and 0.5 mmol/ml HCO_3^-) and 8.4% (1 mmol/ml Na^+ and 1 mmol/ml HCO_3^-). Both solutions are very hyperosmolar and ideally should be administered through a central vein. Once sodium bicarbonate has been administered it dissociates:

$$NaHCO_3 \rightleftharpoons Na^+ + HCO_3^-$$

The bicarbonate ions then combine with hydrogen ions to form water and carbon dioxide (CO_2):

$$HCO_3^- + H^+ \rightleftharpoons H_2CO_3 \rightleftharpoons H_2O + CO_2$$

Therefore, when sodium bicarbonate is administered, the animal must have adequate ventilatory ability to 'blow off' excess CO_2, otherwise the lungs must be mechanically ventilated. If ventilation is inadequate and arterial CO_2 is allowed to increase, then a concurrent respiratory and cellular acidosis will develop, which will worsen the acidaemia already present.

To calculate the amount of sodium bicarbonate required, the following equation is generally used:

Sodium bicarbonate required (mmol) =

base deficit x 0.3 x bodyweight (kg)

The factor of 0.3 is used to estimate the ECF volume (0.45 is sometimes used for neonatal animals). One-third to one-half of the calculated amount should be administered slowly (over 15 to 30 minutes), after which the pH should be reassessed. Further aliquots are administered as guided by blood gas analysis, with the aim of raising the blood pH to above 7.2. Alternatively, if blood gas analysis is unavailable, bicarbonate can be administered empirically at 1–2 mmol/kg, but caution must be exercised due to the potential adverse effects.

Side effects of sodium bicarbonate administration include: hypervolaemia and haemodilution due to hypernatraemia; hypercapnia; alkalosis; tetany due to decreased serum ionized calcium concentration; hypokalaemia in response to alkalosis; left shift of the oxyhaemoglobin dissociation curve (less offloading of oxygen at the tissues); and paradoxical CNS acidosis due to diffusion of CO_2 into the cerebrospinal fluid. Bicarbonate solutions should not be administered through the same intravenous catheter as calcium-containing solutions, as the calcium will precipitate out of solution as calcium carbonate.

Colloids

The appropriate use of colloids is a controversial topic in human anaesthesia and critical care. Meta-analyses have shown that colloids are associated with similar or worse outcomes, compared with crystalloids, when they are used for acute volume resuscitation in critically ill human patients (Perel *et al.*, 2009; Zarychanski *et al.*, 2013). They still appear to be useful in veterinary practice, providing the veterinary surgeon is familiar with their pharmacology and avoids their indiscriminate use.

Colloids may be classified as:

- Naturally occurring: plasma and human albumin
- Synthetic: gelatins, dextrans and the HES.

Haemoglobin-based oxygen-carrying (HBOC) solutions are also described as colloids, but will be discussed later in this chapter with blood products. All colloids, except for human albumin, are described as *polydisperse* (made up of particles with different molecular weights (MWs)). The MW can be described in one of two ways: weight averaged MW (Mw_w) and number averaged MW (MW_n). The weight-averaged MW is more influenced by the larger molecules in the system and gives a larger value for the averaged MW than the number averaged MW.

The ratio MWw/MWn gives an index of the degree of polydispersity in the system (Westphal *et al.*, 2009). The degree of polydispersity and number of molecules in the colloid solution determines its COP. The breakdown of the larger molecules into many smaller particles will preserve the COP effect and longevity of the colloid within the circulation. Colloids are primarily used to expand circulating volume and in patients with hypoproteinaemia. They are readily available in different forms, in combination with water and electrolytes (Figure 18.9), and can be administered at the same time as crystalloids to provide sustained blood volume support. Colloids have some potential adverse effects, particularly increased bleeding times. This may be due to simple dilution of proteins involved with coagulation and/or a direct inhibitory effect, but it may limit the maximum safe volume of colloids that can be infused over a 24-hour period.

Infusion of colloids will increase intravascular COP. As a result, water will diffuse from the interstitium into the vasculature and expand the circulating volume; this effect is similar to that of albumin. The volume of expansion may be less than expected due to the effects of the endothelial glycocalyx, as explained earlier. Infusions of colloids may be used concurrently with, or followed by, crystalloids to replenish interstitial and intracellular water deficits. The total volume of colloids that should be given in any 24 hour period is 20 ml/kg for dogs and 10–15 ml/kg for cats, administered in incremental boluses. It is advised to administer one-quarter of the calculated volume initially and evaluate its effect before more colloid is infused.

Metabolism and excretion

Glomerular size selectivity for the excretion of particles of certain size (or MW) is reported to be between 50 and 60 kDa (Ferber *et al.*, 1985; Treib *et al.*, 1999). Particles with lower MWs are freely filtered through the renal glomeruli and removed from the body; as a result their effect will be short lived. Small particles may also 'leak' out of capillaries into the interstitium and may worsen tissue oedema. Larger particles are hydrolysed and then excreted by the kidneys. HES molecules with high substitution (see later)

Fluid	Osmolarity (mOsm l⁻¹)	COP (mmHg)	MW$_n$	MW$_w$	MS	C2:C6 ratio	Sodium (mmol l⁻¹)	Potassium (mmol l⁻¹)	Chloride (mmol l⁻¹)	Calcium (mmol l⁻¹)	Magnesium (mmol l⁻¹)	Dextrose (g l⁻¹)	pH	Manufacturer	Duration (hours)
Canine plasma	290–310	20.8 ± 1.8	NA	NA	NA	NA	145	4	110	2.5	1	–	7.41	NA	NA
Feline plasma	290–330	19.8 ± 2.4	NA	NA	NA	NA	155	4	120	2.5	1	–	7.39	NA	NA
Albumin 5–25%	308–312	20–200	69	69	NA	NA	50–120	<2	50–120	0	0	0	6.4–7.4	various	No data
Gelatin Gelofusine® Gelaspan® Geloplasma® Isoplex® Volplex®	274	34	23.2	30	NA	NA	145–154	0	100–125	1.0	0.9–1.0	0	7.4	B. Braun Fresenius Kabi Beacon	4
Dextran 40 in 5% glucose	255	40	25	40	NA	NA	0	0	0	0		50	4.4	Hospira	3–6
Dextran 40 in 0.9% saline	310	40	25	40	NA	NA	154	0	154	0		0	4.9	Hospira	3–6
Dextran 70 in 7.5% saline (Rescueflow®)	2567	60	39	70	NA	NA	1285	0	1285	0		0	3.5–7.0	Pharmanovia	6–8 hours
Hetastarch 6% in 0.9% NaCl (Hespan®)	310	32		450	0.7	4–5:1	154	0	154	0		0	5.5	Fresenius Kabi	24–36
Hetastarch 6% in LRS (Hextend®)	308	31		670	0.75	4:1	143	1.5	124	2.5		0.99	5.9	Hospira	
Pentastarch 6% (HAES-Steril® 6%) Hemohes® 6%	308–310	32–36	80	200	0.5	5:1	154	0	154	0		0	3.5–7.0	Fresenius Kabi B. Braun	18–24
Pentastarch 10% (HAES-Steril® 10%) Hemohes® 10%	308–310	32	80	200	0.5	5:1	154	0	154	0		0	3.5–7.0	Fresenius Kabi B. Braun	18–24
Tetrastarch (Voluven®)	308	36–37	60	130	0.4	9:1	154	0	154	0		0	4.0–5.5	Fresenius Kabi	18–24
Oxyglobin®	300	42–43	–	200	NA	NA	113	4	113	0		0	7.6–7.9	Dechra	24 +

18.9 Composition and properties of colloids and Oxyglobin®. COP = colloid osmotic pressure; MS = molar substitution; MW$_n$ = number averaged molecular weight; MW$_w$ = weight averaged molecular weight; NA = not applicable.

tend to resist hydrolysis and may be cleared by the reticuloendothelial system; their long-term effect is currently unknown but appears to be clinically insignificant.

Interference with measurement of total solids

Refractometric measurements of TS cannot be interpreted following the administration of colloids. The refractometer values for dextran 70, hetastarch and pentastarch are 45, 45 and 75 g/l, respectively. An oncometer may be required instead to measure oncotic pressure and provide guidance for fluid therapy requirements.

Human albumin

Endogenous albumin provides up to 80% of plasma COP, with the remainder being provided by globulins. Albumin is important not only for the maintenance of intravascular volume but also for the transport of hormones, ions and drug molecules. It also has antioxidant and anti-inflammatory properties. Production of albumin is dependent on plasma COP; a rise in COP results in reduced production. Administration of large volumes of any colloid, which increase COP, may thus reduce the production of endogenous albumin. Albumin is commercially available as a 20% (hyperoncotic) monodisperse solution with a MW of 69 kDa. A large-scale clinical trial in human patients (SAFE study), found no difference in outcome between patients receiving either 0.9% saline or human albumin for fluid resuscitation. There is limited information regarding use of human albumin in veterinary patients, but it is used to treat hypoproteinaemic patients. Dogs may develop a hypersensitivity reaction to human albumin and the risk of anaphylaxis is high, especially in patients receiving repeat infusions; using an in-line transfusion filter may help reduce risk of a reaction (Trow *et al.*, 2008).

Gelatins

Gelatin solutions are manufactured by degrading bovine collagen into polypeptide chains, which are then cross-linked by succinylation (Gelofusine®). These cross-linking reactions either open up the molecule to increase its size or allow the formation of branched chains to increase the weight, both of which improve water retention within the circulation when the product is infused. Both types of gelatin solution are polydisperse and have high numbers of molecules with low MW (30–35 kDa) compared with the MW of starches (70–670 kDa). Gelatin-based colloids are relatively short acting because the molecules are rapidly eliminated by the kidney or metabolized and then excreted. The elimination plasma half-life is reported to be in the region of 8 hours, but clinical effects appear to be shorter (approximately 3 hours) because of the small particle size. Although gelatins are associated with few adverse effects, the incidence of non-allergic anaphylactic reactions appears to be higher than with other types of non-albumin-based colloids; the mechanism of this effect is unclear. Gelatins also prolong bleeding times, but to a lesser extent than colloids with higher MW. In humans there appears to be a direct correlation between the volume of colloid administered and bleeding time. It is therefore important to exercise caution when administering gelatins to a patient with a coagulopathy. Urea-linked gelatin solutions contain significant amounts of calcium and should not be infused in the same administration line as blood products.

Dextran solutions

Dextrans are naturally occurring glucose polymers produced by bacteria. They are polydisperse and many of the particles have a MW below the renal threshold. As a result, the dextrans have a relatively short duration of action. Dextran 40 and Dextran 70 have average MWs of 40 and 70 kDa, respectively. Dextran 70 has a longer duration of action due to the larger average particle size, but Dextran 40, which contains a higher number of small particles, exerts a bigger 'pull' on water. Both solutions will increase intravascular volume by 1–2 times the volume infused, and the effects of Dextran 70 may persist for up to 6 hours. Dextran 40 is available in preparations combined with 5% dextrose or 0.9% saline. Dextran 70 is available in a HS solution marketed as RescueFlow®, which is reported to provide an intravascular volume gain of 2–3 times the infused volume because of the addition of HS. Dextran 70 in other formulations may be difficult to obtain.

The reported advantage of dextrans over other colloids is that they enhance blood flow, especially within the microvasculature. Indications for use include extracorporeal procedures for patients at risk of thrombosis; additionally, low MW dextrans may offer some renal protection (Onen *et al.*, 2003; Eto *et al.*, 2005). Disadvantages include: prolongation of bleeding times due to dilutional coagulopathy and effects on both fibrin and the Factor VIII/von Willebrand factor (vWf) complex (recommended volumes to be infused are therefore lower compared with the starches); and immediate hypersensitivity reactions (although the incidence appears to be no different from that with other colloids).

Hydroxyethyl starches

The acronym 'HES' is used for all types of hydroxyethyl starches. Three important properties of HES are concentration, mean MW and degree of substitution; these determine the longevity, COP and risk of adverse effects. Each type of HES is identified by the use of three numbers, for example, 6% HES 130/0.4. The percentage indicates the concentration of the solution, the second number represents the average MW in kDa, and the third indicates the degree of molar substitution. The duration of action of HES solutions depends upon the particular product used, the species in which it is used and whether it is administered as an infusion or a bolus. However, effects after a bolus injection are likely to last up to 24–48 hours when using the high-MW, high-substitution solutions, but only 4–6 hours when using the smaller MW solutions.

Concentration: The concentration of a HES solution, which is expressed as a percentage, gives an indication of the initial effect on intravascular volume when the colloid is administered. The HES solutions are available as 4%, 6% and 10% concentrations. As an example, 1 litre of a 6% HES solution has the same volume-expansion effect as using 1 litre of whole blood and is termed iso-oncotic ('iso-oncotic' is used to describe colloids, in a similar fashion to 'isotonic' being used to describe crystalloids). A 10% HES solution has a volume-expansion effect exceeding that of the infused volume; the solution is capable of 'pulling' in more water from the interstitial compartment, and is termed hyperoncotic.

Molecular weight: As with other colloids, the MW distribution of the HES solution is important in determining the initial COP exerted and the degradation of the high MW molecules determines the longevity of the solution in circulation. The HES can be classified as high MW (>400 kDa), medium MW (200–400 kDa) and low MW (<200 kDa).

Substitution: The HES colloids are derived from amylopectin, a series of glucose molecules linked together and broken down by amylase. During the manufacture of HES, amylopectin is partially hydrolysed and treated with ethylene oxide, which results in substitution of hydroxyl groups on the glucose rings by hydroxyethyl groups. This substitution takes place at the C2, C3 and C6 positions of the glucose ring, and individual glucose units can each have 0–3 substitutions. Substitution improves the solubility of the molecule and markedly impedes the action of amylase, thereby prolonging the duration of action of the HES. Elimination kinetics are lengthened by higher levels of substitution. Important factors include:

- Molar substitution (MS): This gives a figure for the number of glucose rings per 10 rings that have one or more hydroxyethyl substitutions
- Degree of substitution (DS): This is the probability of finding a hydroxyethyl group on a glucose ring. For example, a DS of 0.6 means there is a 60% chance of finding a substitution; that is, on average, there are six substitutions per 10 glucose rings. The DS has been used to classify HES colloids into hetastarch (0.6–0.7), pentastarch (0.5) and tetrastarch (0.4). The MS and DS are (incorrectly) used interchangeably in the literature
- C2:C6 ratio: Substitution at the C2 atom on a glucose subunit impairs hydrolysis and degradation to a greater extent than substitution at C6. Solutions with ratios >10 may accumulate in the body and increase the risk of coagulopathy.

Adverse effects: The adverse effects of HES colloids are similar to those of the dextrans and gelatins, and are described briefly here.

Allergic and non-allergic anaphylaxis: Amylopectin is derived from vegetable sources (potatoes and maize) and has the potential to induce both allergic and non-allergic anaphylactic reactions in susceptible individuals. Where possible, infusions should be started slowly to observe any potential problems before administering larger volumes.

Coagulopathy: Reductions in Factor VIII and vWf and impaired platelet function occur with HES administration, which can prolong bleeding times. Low MW starches with low substitution ratios appear to have minimal effects on coagulation times.

Tissue deposition: In humans, HES residues have reportedly been found in a variety of tissues up to 54 months following infusion, because some molecules are cleared through the reticuloendothelial system. The clinical significance of this deposition is unknown, although it may explain the pruritus reaction sometimes seen after the administration of colloids in humans.

Renal failure: The HES solutions have been implicated as a cause of acute kidney injury following long-term infusion in septic human patients. Therefore patients at risk of renal injury should be closely monitored if HES is administered. Most of the colloid is excreted by the kidney, and patients with severe renal insufficiency can be susceptible to circulatory volume overload with use of any colloid.

Capillary leak syndrome and colloids

Some colloids, particularly those with a high MW, are thought to be able to plug leaks within capillary walls. This may be important in conditions such as the systemic inflammatory response syndrome, where high MW colloids may reduce the leakage of albumin, which has a smaller MW, into the interstitium and body cavities. Leaked albumin can draw water into these sites to form tissue oedema and protein-rich exudates. Oedema and tissue swelling will compress capillary beds, reducing tissue microperfusion and increasing the diffusion distance for oxygen between capillaries and cells. However, the larger exogenous colloid molecules will eventually be broken down into smaller particles, which can also leak into the interstitium, attract water and promote oedema formation. The normal differences in capillary permeability in different tissue beds influence the distribution of oedema formation in the body. The pulmonary circulation is more permeable to proteins than the systemic circulation in normal circumstances. As a result, the lungs are more susceptible to oedema formation following the administration of a colloid; this may be important in patients with evidence of inflammatory lung disease such as pneumonia. Additionally, the shedding of the EGL that occurs in some disease states may increase the leakage of colloid molecules into the interstitium. Colloids are not necessarily contraindicated in these conditions, and indeed can be valuable in the treatment of hypovolaemia, but they should not be used in an attempt to plug 'leaky' capillaries and prevent tissue oedema. If colloids are used in a patient with capillary leakage, the patient should be monitored for any deterioration in pulmonary function.

Recommended rates and volumes for colloid administration

Rates and volumes of administered colloids will depend on the patient's condition, with hypovolaemic patients requiring more aggressive therapy. Generally, the recommended total volume of a colloid to administer in a 24-hour period is up to 20 ml/kg in dogs and 15 ml/kg in cats. Larger volumes of HES solutions (up to 50 ml/kg) have been administered to experimental animals that had been made hypovolaemic, but adverse effects may be more likely with larger volumes. The rate of administration can vary, but should initially be low, during which the animal should be observed for signs of hypersensitivity reactions. The vital signs should be monitored continuously throughout the infusion. For rapid restoration of blood volume and in the presence of hypovolaemic shock, volumes of 5–20 ml/kg can be administered relatively rapidly to dogs. In cats, lower volumes of only 5 ml/kg are advised for bolus administration because of cats' lower circulating blood volume; a further 5 ml/kg bolus can be administered if necessary up to a total of 15 ml/kg. When treating low COP in normovolaemic patients (hypoproteinaemia), infusion rates are lower to prevent volume overload.

Blood transfusion

While readers are referred elsewhere for detailed information regarding the transfusion of blood products to cats and dogs (Davidow, 2013), this chapter will provide sufficient detail to equip the veterinary anaesthetist with a basic understanding of transfusion medicine for the perioperative management of animals with acute blood loss, anaemia, coagulopathies and hypoproteinaemia. Although blood and blood products are discussed here in the context of fluid therapy, it is important to remember that they contain allogeneic cellular material and proteins, and as such can be highly immunogenic. Additionally, it is possible to transmit infection from the donor to the recipient, which can be life-threatening and even fatal. The availability of blood and its associated products may be limited, although the inception of pet blood banks has improved this situation. Blood and blood products have a short shelf-life, which means that clinics must decide whether or not it is economically viable to store supplies of these products on the premises. Alternatives include having healthy donor animals available, which can be bled if required, or the use of synthetic oxygen-carrying solutions. If blood is stored on the premises, it must be managed appropriately to ensure it remains viable for as long as possible to reduce wastage. The cost of a transfusion can preclude its use even though it may be life-saving. When a patient receives a blood transfusion, this must be clearly indicated in the patient records.

Canine blood types

Blood typing is used to determine which antigens are present on the surface of the red blood cell (RBC). For the dog, a Dog Erythrocyte Antigen (DEA) number is assigned; dogs can be either positive or negative for each antigen. The two subtypes of DEA 1 (DEA 1.1 and 1.2) are the most significant antigens and are most likely to produce an immune response, although there have been reports of transfusion reactions involving DEA 4 and 7. A 'universal donor' would be a dog that is negative for DEA 1.1, 1.2, 4 and 7, although there is no consensus for the definition of a 'universal donor' dog. A newly recognized antigen, *Dal*, is commonly present except in most Dalmatians, and may also be responsible for a significant immunogenic reaction (Blais *et al.*, 2007).

The presence of naturally occurring alloantibodies is uncommon in the dog, and if present, they do not appear to cause significant acute transfusion incompatibility reactions, although they may reduce the lifespan of the donated cells. A DEA 1.1-negative recipient receiving a first transfusion could therefore be given DEA 1.1-positive blood, since it is unlikely that the recipient dog will have naturally occurring alloantibodies reactive to the DEA 1.1 antigen. Following the transfusion, the recipient will produce DEA 1.1 alloantibodies, and if the recipient receives DEA 1.1-positive blood again, an immune-mediated response will then occur. Alloantibodies can be produced in as little as 4 days, although there is wide inter-individual variation in the speed of response. Where possible, DEA 1.1-negative donor blood should be transfused to a DEA 1.1-negative recipient, to prevent formation of alloantibodies.

Feline blood types

Cats are relatively straightforward in terms of blood typing, although finding suitable donors and the practicalities of transfusion in cats are more difficult and there is no 'universal donor' type. The AB blood type system is widely accepted to be of significance, with cats having type A, type B or type AB antigenic components. There appear to be strong geographical and breed-specific differences in the prevalence of the blood types. For example, the most recent study in the UK reported that non-pedigree cats were predominantly type A (68%), with prevalences of 30% for type B and 2% for type AB. Among pedigree cats approximately 82% were type A, 14% type B and 4% type AB (Forcada *et al.*, 2007). In addition, the *Mik* antigen has been reported relatively recently, although its significance is unknown (Weinstein *et al.*, 2007).

In contrast to dogs, cats produce naturally occurring alloantibodies against the antigen they lack without any prior exposure. In clinical terms, this means that all cats must be blood typed before a transfusion. Type AB cats do not produce alloantibodies to either A or B antigens. Transfusion of type A donor blood to a type B recipient can be rapidly fatal due to the presence of strong, naturally occurring haemagglutination antibodies in type B cats. The reaction is less severe in type A cats receiving B donor blood, but the lifespan of the donated cells will be dramatically reduced. It is not recommended to administer canine blood to cats (Bovens and Gruffydd-Jones, 2013).

Blood products

Blood components are often used for therapy. The advantage of using blood components rather than WB is that one 'unit' of blood can be used to treat more than one animal; for example, the RBCs could be given to a dog with acute haemorrhage and the separated plasma used to treat a dog with a coagulopathy. Additionally, component therapy will prevent the administration of blood components that are not required by the recipient. The range of blood products and components that may be available for cats and dogs are described below. Local blood banks can be contacted for their inventory.

Whole blood

Whole blood contains everything collected from the donor (RBCs, white blood cells (WBCs), platelets, proteins and clotting factors), plus anticoagulant. Fresh WB should be infused within 4–6 hours of collection; if not used immediately, it can be stored for up to 28 days at 1–6°C, (note that platelets and WBCs become non-functional following refrigeration). Storage will also rapidly age the RBCs and reduce 2,3-diphosphoglycerate (2,3-DPG) concentrations, which results in a left shift of the oxyhaemoglobin dissociation curve and reduced oxygen delivery to peripheral tissues. As a general rule, 2 ml/kg of WB will increase the recipient's PCV by 1% or haemoglobin concentration ([Hb]) by 3 g/l. A 'unit' of canine WB is typically 450 ml, while a 'unit' of feline blood consists of 45–60 ml, depending on the size of the donor.

Packed red blood cells

These are the RBCs that remain once the plasma has been separated from the collected unit of blood. Packed RBCs are administered to treat anaemia and typically have a PCV of 60–70%. They can be stored for up to 42 days at 1–6°C, depending on the preservative used. PRBCs are useful for treating anaemia in normovolaemic patients, since the lack of plasma proteins reduces the risk of volume overload. As a general rule, 2 ml/kg of PRBCs will increase the recipient's PCV by 2% or [Hb] by 6 g/l. A 'unit' of canine PRBCs is typically 200 ml.

Fresh frozen plasma

Fresh frozen plasma (FFP) is plasma that has been separated from WB and frozen at –30°C within 8 hours following collection. It contains all the clotting factors and is viable for up to 12 months if stored at −30°C. FFP is used to treat coagulopathies but is not recommended for the treatment of hypoalbuminaemia as a large volume (45 ml/kg) of FFP is required to raise the recipient's albumin concentration by only 10 g/l.

Frozen plasma

Frozen plasma (FP) is either:

- Plasma that was frozen more than 8 hours after collection
- The result of thawing and refreezing FFP
- Derived from FFP once this has been frozen for more than 12 months.

It contains clotting factors II, VII, IX and X. It is useful in the treatment of rodenticide toxicity.

Cryoprecipitate

This contains high concentrations of vWf, fibrinogen and clotting factors VIII and XIII. It is used to treat the coagulation disorders that result from a deficiency in these factors.

Cryo-poor plasma or cryosupernatant

This is essentially what remains after removal of the cryoprecipitate. It is used to treat coagulopathies, with the exception of haemophilia A and von Willebrand's disease.

Platelet-rich plasma

Platelet-rich plasma contains separated platelets but it is not commonly used in veterinary practice because it requires careful handling and storage.

Platelet concentrate

Platelets stored in dimethylsulfoxide (DMSO). This product is recommended for the treatment of immune-mediated thrombocytopenia.

Indications for transfusion and transfusion 'triggers'

The patient's clinical condition determines whether a transfusion is necessary. The decision to treat anaemia in the perioperative period will depend on the chronicity of the disease. An animal that is acutely anaemic is more likely to have a reduced chance of survival than an animal in which anaemia has been developing for some time and consequently compensation mechanisms are already established. It is therefore important to assess the patient's history before deciding whether a blood transfusion is really necessary. A patient that has long-standing anaemia and is otherwise clinically well is unlikely to require a blood transfusion before anaesthesia unless haemoglobin concentration is particularly low, whereas an anaemic patient that shows some degree of cardiovascular compromise will almost certainly require blood therapy. The type of blood component required to best treat the patient should also be established and component therapy used wherever possible. For each patient, the risks associated with blood transfusion (infection and transfusion reactions) must be weighed against the potential benefits. Measurement of markers of reduced oxygen delivery, such as blood lactate concentration and jugular venous oxygen saturation, will be helpful to establish whether the degree of anaemia is detrimental. Morbidity and mortality in anaemic patients are increased as a result of reduced oxygen delivery to the tissues; oxygen delivery is dependent on both cardiac output and the oxygen content of blood. The equations used to calculate oxygen delivery and the oxygen content of blood are detailed in Chapter 7.

The veterinary literature contains various recommendations to assist decision making on when to transfuse. For patients with acute haemorrhage, a loss of 20-25% of blood volume is suggested as an indicator that blood transfusion is required (Clarke et al., 2014). Other 'trigger' points that have been recommended for starting blood transfusion include haematocrit values lower than 21–25%, or [Hb] <7 g/dl for an anaesthesized patient (Seeler, 2007).

For reference, current (2008) guidelines from the Association of Anaesthetists of Great Britain and Ireland for transfusion in humans are:

- Transfusion not indicated if [Hb] >10 g/dl
- A strong indication for transfusion if [Hb] <7 g/dl
- Transfusion essential if [Hb] <5 g/dl
- [Hb] of 8–10 g/dl is considered safe even in patients with significant cardiorespiratory disease, but patients showing symptoms should receive a transfusion.

Current (2015) American Society of Anesthesiologists practice guidelines are:

- RBCs should not usually be administered if [Hb] >10 g/dl
- RBCs should usually be administered if [Hb] <6 g/dl
- Determination of whether [Hb] between 6–10 g/dl justifies or requires RBC transfusion should be based on potential or actual ongoing bleeding (rate and magnitude), intravascular volume status, signs of organ ischaemia, and adequacy of cardiopulmonary reserve.

Surgical blood loss during general anaesthesia

Blood loss during surgery can be estimated by:

- Subtracting the quantity of surgical saline used for flushing from the volume of blood and fluids collected in a closed suction jar (or the formula below can be used)

$$\frac{PCV \text{ in jar} \times \text{Volume of fluid in jar (ml)}}{\text{Volume of blood in jar (ml)}} = \text{Patient PCV}$$

- Weighing swabs and subtracting the dry weight of the swabs (1 ml of blood weighs approximately 1.05 g)
- Counting fully soaked swabs (a 10 cm x 10 cm soaked swab will contain 10 ml blood)
- Using the HemoCue® photometer device (Clark et al., 2010).

In anaesthetized patients, blood loss of up to 10% of the circulating volume can be replaced with crystalloids; conscious healthy patients can tolerate losses of this magnitude without requiring fluid replacement. As crystalloids equilibrate throughout the ECF, it has been recommended that the volume of blood lost be replaced with 3–4 times this volume of crystalloids. Recently, however, it has been shown that the volume of crystalloids required may be lower if GDT is used (as described later).

Considerations before blood transfusion

Blood typing

Test kits are available that enable dogs to be rapidly blood typed in the clinic and with a high degree of accuracy. Generally, these tests are for the DEA 1.1 antigen only, but some tests are available for other blood types. Autoagglutination can interfere with the test results and should be ruled out before testing; the test kits contain an autoagglutination saline screen that is intended to eliminate this interference. Another test kit is available that has similar accuracy and filters out autoagglutinated cells (Quick Test; available from Pet Blood Bank UK).

Cats can be blood typed in a similar way using commercially available kits.

Cross-matching

A complete description of blood cross-matching is beyond the scope of this chapter but the veterinary surgeon should be familiar with some of the terminology and concepts used when selecting a blood product. As described above, in recent years new antigens in both cats and dogs have been reported; the practical implication of this new knowledge is that, ideally, cross-matching should be performed whenever a RBC transfusion is necessary. *Agglutination* is the process of RBC 'clumping' initiated by antibodies present in plasma, which link antigenic components on the surface of RBCs. This process can be due either to antibodies present in the recipient animal's plasma that bind to donor RBCs, or *vice versa*. *Autoagglutination* is the process whereby an animal produces autoantibodies to its own RBCs, for example, in immune-mediated haemolytic anaemia.

Cross-matching should be performed where possible to assess compatibility of a transfusion and to reduce the potential risk to the recipient. It can be used in combination with blood typing. It is important to note that cross-matching does not completely remove the risk of a transfusion reaction, as delayed transfusion reactions may occur once the recipient has produced antibodies to the donor RBCs. However, in veterinary practice it is more usual for cross-matching to be performed if the recipient is known to have received a blood transfusion in the past or has an unknown transfusion history. In dogs undergoing a first transfusion, cross-matching is generally unnecessary due to the very low incidence of naturally occurring alloantibodies in this species. Cats should always be cross-matched before transfusion where possible, or blood-typed at the very least, because of the risk of a transfusion reaction associated with naturally occurring alloantibodies (as described above).

Transfusion procedure

1. Ensure secure intravenous access in the recipient. Preferably, there should be a dedicated intravenous line for the blood transfusion. Blood can be administered through an intraosseous catheter if necessary.
2. Check the blood unit label for details of species, type and expiry date. Discoloured blood (brown or purple) is unsuitable for transfusion regardless of the expiry date on the bag.
3. Choose a suitable infusion set with an in-line blood filter to remove debris and clots. The small filters that are present in fluid infusion sets are too small and will clog quickly if used for blood. Small separate filters are available that fit between a syringe and infusion line for

small-volume infusions (e.g. for transfusions in cats). Filters should always be used when transfusing WB, PRBCs or plasma.
4. PRBCs can be mixed with saline (at room temperature or warmed) to reduce viscosity if necessary, depending on the PCV of the transfusion.
5. Blood straight from the refrigerator can be transfused, although this can lead to hypothermia in the recipient if the blood is transfused rapidly. Alternatively, blood can be gently warmed in a water bath up to, but not exceeding, 37°C. Place the bag inside a plastic bag before immersion in the bath to prevent contamination of the ports. Fresh frozen plasma should be gently thawed by leaving the bag at room temperature or placing it in a water bath, again protecting the ports using an outer plastic bag; it should never be thawed in a microwave oven. It is important to handle FFP with care as the bags can crack, rendering the product unusable.
6. Connect the infusion set to the bag in an aseptic fashion to prevent bacterial contamination. Once a closed bag has been punctured it must be used within 24 hours if kept refrigerated.
7. If using a volumetric pump, ensure that the model used is suitable for blood administration as some pumps can fracture cells.
8. Do not administer other fluids through the same line (except 0.9% saline). Calcium-containing fluids can chelate citrate and cause transfused blood to clot, while hypotonic solutions can cause RBC lysis.
9. Calculate the volume of blood to be administered, using the formula given below:

Blood volume required (ml) =

$$k \times \text{Bodyweight (kg)} \times \frac{\text{Required PCV} - \text{Recipient PCV}}{\text{Donor PCV}}$$

(k = circulating blood volume of species; 50–60 ml in cats and 80–90 ml in dogs)
10. Monitor the patient carefully during the first 30 minutes of transfusion. Some clinicians initially use a slow rate of infusion while monitoring for transfusion reactions. Recommended infusion rates are shown in Figure 18.10.
11. Pre-emptive antihistamine administration is generally not recommended.

Transfusion reactions

Reactions to the administration of a blood product can be acute (within 24 hours) or delayed and can range from mild to rapidly fatal. Cardiopulmonary resuscitation may be necessary if a severe transfusion reaction occurs. It is essential that a reaction is detected as soon as possible so that the infusion can be stopped and appropriate treatment given. For this reason, it is important to measure baseline parameters (body temperature, heart and respiratory rates, pulse quality) before starting to transfuse, and to monitor these parameters during transfusion. Reactions can be either immunologically or non-immunologically mediated. Common clinical signs of different types of reaction are listed in Figure 18.11. It should be emphasized that many of these signs will not be evident in the anaesthetized patient. Hypotension should be anticipated and short-acting corticosteroids (e.g. hydrocortisone) and/or antihistamines (e.g. diphenhydramine chlorphenamine) may be beneficial, although there is little compelling evidence to support administration of corticosteroids. Haemolysis occurs due to mismatching of blood types and the destruction of RBCs within the recipient circulation.

Product	Dose	Dose rate
Whole blood	Calculate using the formula: Blood volume required (ml) = k x Bodyweight (kg) x $\frac{\text{Required PCV} - \text{Recipient PCV}}{\text{Donor PCV}}$ (k = circulating blood volume of species; 50–60 ml in cats and 80–90 ml in dogs) As a rough guide, 10–22 ml/kg	Start at a low dose (0.25–0.5 ml/kg/h) then infuse at 1–4 ml/kg/h. The rate can be increased if necessary up to 20 ml/kg/h Complete the infusion within 4 hours
Packed red blood cells	Calculate using the same formula as for whole blood above. As a rough guide, 6–10 ml/kg	Start at a low dose (0.25–0.5 ml/kg/h) then infuse at 1–4 ml/kg/h Complete the infusion within 4 hours
Fresh frozen plasma	6–10 ml/kg. Can be repeated	Start at a low dose (0.25–0.5 ml/kg/h) then increase up to 6 ml/kg/h Complete the infusion within 4 hours
Oxyglobin®	15–30 ml/kg Lower in cats	Maximum 10 ml/kg/h Use much lower rates for normovolaemic animals Rates should be even lower for cats since they are at greater risk of volume overload; rates of 0.5–2 ml/kg/h have been suggested

18.10 Recommended infusion rates of blood products.

Acute haemolysis	Acute hypersensitivity	Bacteraemia
Mentation changes: depression, recumbency, vocalization, seizures	Anxiety and agitation	Tremors
Urination, defecation, vomiting	Vomiting	Vomiting
Apnoea or tachypnoea	Dyspnoea and tachypnoea	Tachypnoea
Tachycardia and arrhythmias	Urticaria, pruritus, erythema, facial swelling	Hypotension, tachycardia
Haemoglobinaemia and haemoglobinuria	Pyrexia	Pyrexia

18.11 Common clinical signs of transfusion reactions.

Other adverse effects of blood transfusion may include: circulatory overload; hypothermia (if cold blood is transfused); hypocalcaemia (citrate toxicity); transmission of pathogens (feline immunodeficiency virus, feline leukaemia virus, *Babesia*); coagulopathy; and air embolism.

Haemoglobin-based oxygen-carrying solutions

Oxyglobin® is currently the only available HBOC solution. It consists of ultrapurified polymerized bovine haemoglobin (130 mg/ml) in modified LRS. The composition and properties of the solution are listed in Figure 18.10. Oxyglobin® is a useful product because it can be stored at room temperature for up to 3 years provided it is kept within its impermeable foil pouch. It is currently available in 60 ml and 125 ml bags. Once the outer pouch has been broached, oxidization of haemoglobin occurs through the plastic bag, causing the formation of methaemoglobin. Toxic levels of methaemoglobin can develop, and because of this an opened bag must be discarded after 24 hours. Oxyglobin® has a p50 (the point of 50% saturation of haemoglobin with oxygen) of 38 mmHg (5.1 kPa). Normal p50 values are 30 mmHg (4 kPa) in dogs and 36 mmHg (4.8 kPa) in cats. This means that the oxyhaemoglobin dissociation curve for Oxyglobin® is shifted to the right and oxygen is more easily offloaded to the tissues. Tissue perfusion may be enhanced due to the lower viscosity of Oxyglobin® compared with blood. Oxyglobin® has been shown to cause vasoconstriction, possibly through a nitric oxide scavenging mechanism. This may be beneficial in patients with pre-existing vasodilation, but it may also cause an increase in afterload and reduce cardiac output. Oxyglobin® has a half-life in the region of 30–40 hours.

Currently, Oxyglobin® is only approved for single-infusion use in dogs, although there is evidence that it can be used successfully in cats and other species. This product is perhaps of most use in cats because blood transfusion requires a suitable donor. Oxyglobin® lacks the cell membranes responsible for the antigenic reaction to transfusion; therefore, pre-infusion testing is unnecessary and the product is potentially suitable for multiple transfusions (although this should be carried out with caution). Antibodies to Oxyglobin® have been demonstrated following multiple transfusions, but these antibodies do not appear to produce significant clinical signs or affect its oxygen-carrying ability. Oxyglobin® can be administered using fluid infusion sets and pumps. It does not need to be filtered but should be infused via a dedicated intravenous catheter.

Adverse effects associated with Oxyglobin® include: discolouration (yellow or brown) of mucous membranes, sclera, urine, faeces and skin; hypervolaemia due to the potent colloid effects of the product (which is hyper-oncotic, with a COP of 37 mmHg), especially in normo-volaemic patients; pulmonary oedema if infusion rates are higher than recommended, especially in cats (see Figure 18.10); mild decrease in PCV after transfusion due to haemodilution; and dilutional coagulopathy.

Following the administration of Oxyglobin®, urine dip-stick measurements (pH, glucose, ketones and proteins) will be inaccurate while there is gross discolouration of urine. The measured (*versus* calculated) haemoglobin concentration remains accurate. Colorimetric analysis of serum biochemistry will be inaccurate following infusion; the manufacturer of the analyser should be contacted for specific details as the degree of interference will depend on the analyser used. Optical methods of measuring pro-thrombin time and activated partial thromboplastin time will also be inaccurate. The TS measured by using a refractometer will increase.

Equipment for fluid therapy and blood transfusion

Volumetric fluid pumps and syringe drivers are now more commonly found in general practice, although the use of free-running fluid infusion sets is also still appropriate and may be advantageous where pumps cannot be used, for example, in magnetic resonance imaging rooms. Before use with the patient, all lines must be purged with fluids to avoid accidental administration of large volumes of air.

Standard infusion sets deliver a relatively accurate volume of fluid. The number of drops/ml is stated on the packaging and varies with the manufacturer. The fluid rate, however, will be affected by hydrostatic pressure (bag height above the catheter). A set providing 10–20 drops/ml is useful for dogs larger than 10 kg bodyweight and sets delivering 60 drops/ml are useful for smaller patients. The formula for calculating the required rate of drops per minute is given below:

$$\frac{\text{Drops/ml provided} \times \text{Fluid rate (ml/kg/h)} \times \text{bodyweight (kg)}}{60}$$
= Drops/min

With these infusion sets, it can be easy to deliver excessive volumes of fluids accidentally to small patients. To avoid this problem use:

- A small bag of fluids in small patients (100 or 250 ml bags)
- A fluid reduction chamber (a burette or buretrol set; Figure 18.12)
- A standard intravenous infusion line with an in-line, dial type flow regulator that allows the rate of fluid administration to be set (Dial-A-Flo) (Figure 18.13).

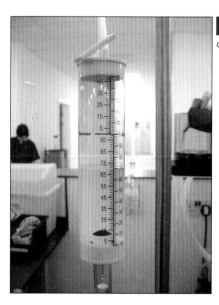

18.12 A burette (sometimes called a buretrol).

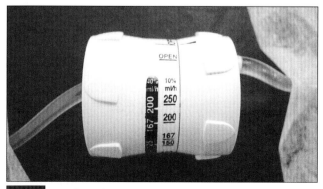

18.13 An in-line infusion rate, dial type flow controller.

Conventional infusion sets may be less likely to allow fluid accumulation in the perivascular tissues if the catheter is dislodged from the vein.

Fluid pumps using peristaltic rollers (linear peristalsis) are also commonly used. The pumps are programmable to set fluid rate (usually ml/h) and the volume to be infused (VTBI), details of which are displayed digitally on screen. The device will also display the total volume infused over time. Some pumps or syringe drivers may have the facility for a 'keep vein open' (KVO) rate which provides a low infusion rate of 1–3 ml/h even when the pump is in standby mode. Pumps allow for the administration of fluid boluses at a set rate over a set time. For example, a 10 ml/kg bolus given to a dog weighing 10 kg can be delivered over 15 minutes by programming a fluid rate of 400 ml/h and a VTBI value of 100 ml. Most pumps are limited to a maximum fluid rate of 999 ml/h. If rapid infusion of fluid to a large patient is necessary, this can be achieved by using a standard infusion set, wide-bore intravenous catheter and a pressure infuser around the fluid bag (Figure 18.14). Using this set-up, a litre of fluid can be quickly administered for rapid volume restoration of, for example, a large-breed dog with gastric dilatation–volvulus.

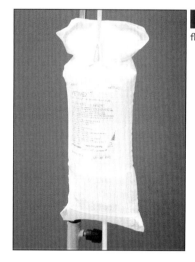

18.14 A pressure infuser placed around a fluid bag.

Disadvantages of fluid pumps include:

- Initial purchase costs
- Requirement for regular servicing and calibration by a trained medical equipment technician
- Staff training costs
- Some pumps require special cassette-type infusion sets (choose pumps using conventional sets)
- Requirement for a power supply
- Rechargeable battery packs need regular replacement
- Pumps may infuse fluids perivascularly if the intravenous catheter is dislodged.

However, many pumps have the advantage of being equipped with 'air-in-line' and 'obstruction' alarms to alert the operator to the presence of unpurged lines and kinked or faulty catheters.

Equipment for the administration of blood and blood products is similar to that used for fluid therapy, although standard blood transfusion sets have an in-line clot filter (Figure 18.15). For cats and small dogs, it is best to administer blood by using a syringe driver because the blood to be transfused is often collected in a 50–60 ml syringe. Separate in-line clot filters are commercially available (e.g. Hemo-Nate®), which fit between the syringe and the infusion line (Figure. 18.16).

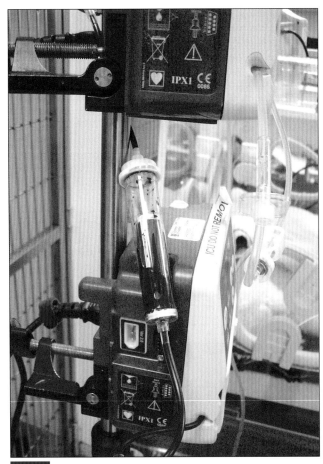

18.15 In-line clot filter for the administration of blood and plasma.

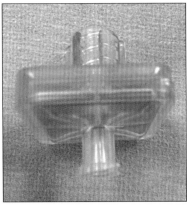

18.16 In-line filter for use with a syringe for administration of small volumes of blood and plasma.

Heating bags of fluids on full power can lead to 'hotspots' within the bag. Fluids should be thoroughly agitated following heating, to ensure that the temperature is consistent throughout the bag, and the temperature checked with an infrared device (e.g. RayTemp® 3). No evidence of changes in fluid composition, including salts, labile substances such as dextrose or leaching of plastics, has been found in fluids that have been warmed using a microwave. In-line fluid warmers are commercially available and are relatively inexpensive (e.g. i-Clam or i-Warm devices; Figure 18.17); these should be positioned as close to the patient as possible.

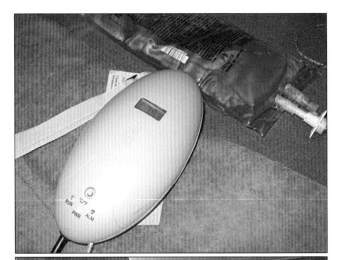

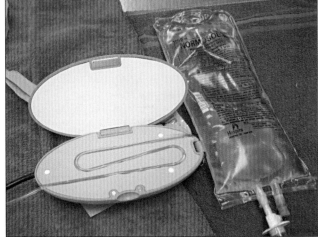

18.17 In-line intravenous fluid warming pod.
(Courtesy of Tanya Duke-Novakovski, Western College of Veterinary Medicine, University of Saskatchewan, Canada)

Miscellaneous considerations

Warming of fluids

Warming the fluid bag in an attempt to prevent hypothermia will be of little use unless the fluid rate is high, since thermal equilibration with room temperature will occur during the time the warm fluid is infused into the patient. Warmed crystalloids are more beneficial when used for surgical lavage. Ideally, crystalloid fluids should be warmed in an incubator, but they can be effectively and safely warmed in a domestic microwave oven if heated at low power settings for longer periods of time.

Labelling and adding drugs to fluid bags

Crystalloids that have been altered in any way (e.g. by adding potassium or other drugs) must be appropriately labelled. Ideally, specific labels that adhere to the bag should be used. It is inadvisable to write directly on to the bag with a permanent ink marker as solvents from the ink may leach through the plastic into the fluid, although tests have shown that PVC seems to be relatively impermeable to a number of inks. A bag of fluids with a drug or electrolyte added should be thoroughly agitated before the fluids are administered, and solutions that have been altered in this way should not be given at high infusion rates to support haemodynamic function.

Fluid therapy for anaesthesia

Infusion of a replacement crystalloid to an animal during general anaesthesia is recommended to:

- Replace fluids that have not been gained because of reduced intake (preoperative fasting)
- Replace ongoing fluid losses (sensible and insensible losses as well as fluids lost due to surgical bleeding)
- Expand intravascular volume to offset vasodilation and diuresis caused by different anaesthetic agents
- Maintain intravenous catheter patency.

The previously recommended maintenance intravenous fluid rate of 10 ml/kg/h has recently been adjusted, based on clinical research in the medical field. The current recommendation is for crystalloids to be given at less than 10 ml/kg/h in euvolaemic patients undergoing lengthy procedures (>1 hour). The 2013 American Animal Hospital Association fluid therapy guidelines advise to start with an administration rate of 5 ml/kg/h in dogs and 3 ml/kg/h in cats and reduce the rate by 25% every hour until the recommended daily maintenance rate is achieved (Davis et al., 2013; see also earlier).

Some medical studies have suggested that administration of high volumes of fluids is beneficial in patients undergoing routine mild to moderate outpatient procedures because of a reduced incidence of postoperative pain (via an unknown mechanism) and reduced nausea and vomiting (due to improved gastrointestinal perfusion). High-risk patients, however, seem to benefit from 're-stricted' fluid therapy regimens and individualized GDT (see later). There is evidence that high volumes of crystalloids may be directly harmful by increasing lung oedema, altering gut function, producing excessive haemodilution, and promoting coagulopathies and damage to the EGL. Current opinion suggests that fluid loading of euvolaemic patients with hypotension will not improve blood pressure, and these patients should instead be treated with sympathomimetics early on to avoid retention of excess water. Treatment of hypotension during anaesthesia usually follows the steps shown in Figure 18.18 (also see Chapter 17). Recently, it has been reported that aggressive perioperative fluid therapy in cats may increase mortality, probably because of the smaller circulating volume and increased risk of volume overload in this species (Brodbelt et al., 2007).

In human patients, it has been shown that restricting water intake for only two hours before general anaesthesia, rather than the traditional 'nil by mouth from midnight', is generally considered safe and may improve outcome by limiting water deprivation and avoiding the need to provide fluid resuscitation. It may be feasible to extrapolate this information to cats and dogs, although there have been no studies to provide supporting evidence.

- Reduce administration of anaesthetic agents if possible
- Administer a fluid bolus: 5–10 ml/kg of the balanced crystalloid fluid being used during the procedure (e.g. Hartmann's solution), given over 15 minutes. Assess the response to the bolus and repeat if required
- If the change following the crystalloid bolus is inadequate, consider administering a colloid bolus (2–5 ml/kg) to provide greater volume expansion for a longer period of time
- If there is no response to fluid therapy, consider supportive drugs such as sympathomimetics

18.18 Steps for treating hypotension during general anaesthesia.

Decisions regarding the type, timing and quantity of fluid administered during anaesthesia will depend on: patient signalment (species and age); patient history (e.g. abnormal fluid losses); electrolyte and acid–base derangements; other biochemical changes such as uraemia or hypoproteinaemia; and any comorbidities such as renal dysfunction or cardiac disease.

Postoperative fluids

The need to continue fluid therapy into the postoperative period will depend on the patient's status, fluid losses during anaesthesia and any problems that arose during anaesthesia, such as persistent hypotension or excessive surgical bleeding. Water should be offered as soon as the patient is able to drink, and the timing will depend upon the speed of recovery.

Monitoring fluid therapy

Once the patient has undergone an initial assessment and fluid therapy has commenced, ongoing patient assessment should be used as a guide to further fluid requirements. Assessment should be performed continuously or at frequent intervals in patients receiving urgent fluid resuscitation such as blood transfusions. In patients having losses replaced over a longer period of time, assessments may be less frequent. For details of fluid therapy monitoring over the longer term, the reader is directed to other resources (DiBartola, 2011). It is important to revise fluid plans on the basis of patient assessment because decisions based on estimations of fluid losses and mathematical formulae are not completely accurate.

Methods of assessment during the perioperative period, which can be used in patients with moderate to severe problems, are described below. However, in order for these assessments to be of value, personnel must understand and be able to use the monitoring equipment; for example, it is useless to measure central venous pressure (CVP) if the results cannot be interpreted correctly.

Fluid therapy endpoints and goal-directed therapy

The term GDT in relation to fluids can be defined and interpreted in various ways, which may cause significant confusion. The 'goals' may vary depending on the monitoring equipment available and the expertise of the veterinary surgeon. Recently, GDT has been used to describe the optimization of stroke volume and cardiac output, and non-invasive monitors using mathematical algorithms that reflect cardiac output and stroke volume have been developed for use in the medical field. Both insufficient and overzealous fluid therapy are known to increase patient morbidity and mortality (Figure 18.19). Early, aggressive fluid resuscitation of critically ill patients may limit tissue hypoxia and progression to organ failure, and improve the overall outcome, but in humans overzealous fluid administration has been associated with more complications, increased length of stay in the intensive care unit and increased mortality.

Traditional methods used to assess fluid status are relatively inaccurate. In human volunteers, it has been shown that healthy, conscious individuals can lose up to 25% of circulating volume without any measurable

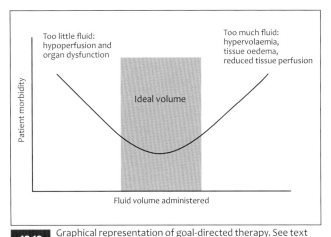

18.19 Graphical representation of goal-directed therapy. See text for explanation.

(Adapted and simplified from Bellamy, 2006)

changes in heart rate or blood pressure, despite significant reductions in stroke volume. However, veterinary surgeons often rely on measurements of heart rate and blood pressure because the sophisticated monitors used for GDT are expensive and impractical for the general practice setting. Despite the drawbacks of the 'traditional' measurements, clinical examination of the patient remains mandatory, and can provide useful information to indicate whether fluid resuscitation is effective (decrease in heart and respiratory rates; improved peripheral pulse quality, mucous membrane colour and capillary refill time). In clinical practice, the goal remains the normalization of vital signs to within the normal range for the size and species of the particular patient. The difference between core body temperature and the temperature of the extremities should decrease as peripheral perfusion improves. For severely compromised animals, changes in mentation should also be observed; animals should become brighter and more responsive to human contact with effective fluid resuscitation.

Urine production is an indirect indicator of renal perfusion, and is normally 1–2 ml/kg/h. As fluids are replaced, urine output should increase over time, and this may be a useful guide to fluid therapy. Urine output can be easily measured if an indwelling urinary catheter is placed, the bladder is expressed or incontinence pads are weighed (assume that 1 ml of urine weighs 1 g). High urine specific gravity may indicate the need for further fluid therapy, while small volumes of dilute urine may indicate impairment of renal perfusion and function. Urine production can also be affected by other factors such as renal disease, trauma and administration of certain drugs, such as opioids.

High blood lactate concentrations may be suggestive of anaerobic metabolism resulting from hypoperfusion. If serial measurements show decreasing lactate concentrations, this indicates appropriate fluid therapy.

Some GDT markers are provided in Figure 18.20.

Parameter	Principle	Advantages	Disadvantages	Goals: dogs	Goals: cats
Arterial blood pressure	Indirect (Doppler or oscillometry) Direct (catheterization of artery)	Quick Inexpensive Can be frequently used	Hypotension, arrhythmias and vasoconstriction may interfere with indirect methods Difficult to place arterial catheter when animal is hypotensive. Catheter-associated risks must be taken into account	SAP 100–120mmHg MAP >60–70 mmHg DAP >40 mmHg	SAP 100–120mmHg MAP >60–70 mmHg DAP >40 mmHg
Central venous pressure	May reflect the state of preload	Trends are useful	Poor correlation between central venous pressure and preload under clinical conditions Can be affected by cardiac function	2–4 cmH₂O increase, which returns to baseline after 15 minutes, following a fluid challenge	2–4 cmH₂O increase, which returns to baseline after 15 minutes, following a fluid challenge
Mixed venous oxygen saturation or oxygen tension	Gold standard measure of oxygen supply and demand	Decreases when delivery of oxygen is compromised or when demand exceeds supply	Ideally requires a pulmonary arterial catheter, but jugular blood sample may be used as an alternative ($S_{cv}O_2$) Interpretation is complex	$S_{cv}O_2$ 70–75% P_vO_2 40 mmHg (5.3kPa) Correlated to mortality in septic dogs ($S_{cv}O_2$: 60–71%)	$S_{cv}O_2$ 70–75% P_vO_2 40 mmHg (5.3kPa)
Arterial or venous lactate concentration	Inadequate oxygen delivery results in anaerobic metabolism and increased production of lactate	Easily measured Inexpensive No training required May be useful as a prognostic indicator in dogs	Blood lactate can be affected by processes other than poor perfusion and results must be interpreted with care, especially in patients with sepsis Blood sampling technique is important and samples should be analysed immediately or kept on ice	Normal lactate <2.0 mmol/l Lactate clearance >10% before and following fluid therapy	Normal lactate <2.0 mmol/l Lactate clearance >10% before and following fluid therapy
Base excess	Marker of metabolic acidosis	Easily measured with blood gas analyser	Must be interpreted with other measurements derived from the blood gas analyser and in conjunction with clinical signs	Cannot be interpreted in isolation. Normal base excess values are 0 ± 4 mmol/l	Cannot be interpreted in isolation. Normal base excess values are 0 ± 4 mmol/l
Urine output	Urine production correlates with renal perfusion	Easy to measure Inexpensive	Can be affected by renal dysfunction and concurrently administered drugs	1–2 ml urine/kg/h USG 1.026	1–2 ml urine/kg/h USG 1.035

18.20 Reference table for goal-directed therapy in dogs and cats. See text for further explanation. DAP = diastolic arterial pressure; MAP = mean arterial pressure; P_vO_2 = venous oxygen tension; SAP = systolic arterial pressure; $S_{cv}O_2$ = central venous oxygen saturation; USG = urine specific gravity.

Monitoring techniques

More sophisticated methods to assess cardiovascular volumes in critically ill or anaesthetized patients receiving fluid therapy are described elsewhere (Marik, 2009; see also Chapter 7).

Arterial blood pressure

Goals for adequate arterial blood pressures during fluid therapy are provided in Figure 18.20 (see also Chapters 7 and 17). In patients that are actively bleeding, hypotensive resuscitation before surgical correction is recommended, as this will prevent large increases in blood pressure, which may dislodge clots and promote further blood loss.

Central venous pressure

Central venous pressure measurement has historically been used to assess preload and volume status. However, clinical trials in humans have shown that CVP is a poor indicator of responsiveness to fluid therapy and does not detect patients who are still hypovolaemic and require more fluid (Marik *et al.*, 2008). A single CVP measurement does not provide reliable information, and trends in CVP are more useful to guide fluid therapy. Measurements of CVP should be made with the patient in the same body position on each occasion and at the end of the expiratory pause to reduce interference by changes in intrathoracic pressure during lung ventilation or spontaneous breathing.

To assess myocardial contractility, CVP is taken to reflect right atrial pressure (RAP), which in turn reflects right ventricular end-diastolic pressure (RVEDP). An increase in CVP can indicate an inability to deal with increased venous return (preload). Figure 18.21 shows an idealized representation of the Frank–Starling curve, which describes this relationship in a normal heart. At low RVEDP (point A on the curve), a small increase in pressure (to point B) as a result of increased preload results in a large change in cardiac output; on the steep part of the curve, the heart has the ability to increase myocardial contraction. The heart is said to have 'recruitable stroke volume' and the patient is likely to respond to a fluid challenge. In contrast, if the heart is unable to deal with a high preload (at point C on the curve) and a fluid challenge is given to increase the RVEDP to point D, there will be little change in cardiac output because the myocardial cells are already at 'maximum stretch'.

Fluids can be given at a high rate and volume until there is less than 10% change in stroke volume in response to a fluid challenge. Unfortunately, stroke volume from the right side of the heart cannot be easily measured, but a continuously elevated CVP (>10 cmH$_2$O) after a fluid challenge (20 ml/kg of a crystalloid) indicates an inability to deal with increased preload, and if this is seen the fluid rate should be slowed or fluids should be stopped. If CVP rises to an acceptable value, this does not necessarily mean that cardiac output is increased. In most circumstances, patients with hypovolaemia will tend to have low CVP values, but these values must be interpreted carefully and in conjunction with other clinical signs and laboratory data. Measurement of CVP requires placement of a central venous catheter; details are given in Chapter 7.

In a hypovolaemic patient with low CVP, a lack of increase in CVP following a fluid challenge usually indicates that more fluid is required and that the response of the heart is on the lowest part of the Frank–Starling curve. A large increase in CVP (>4 cmH$_2$O) following a fluid bolus indicates that either circulating volume (preload) is increased, or that cardiac function is unable to cope with the increased preload and fluid therapy should be reduced or stopped. Optimal circulatory volume resuscitation endpoints using CVP measurements are suggested to be a 2–4 cmH$_2$O increase following a fluid challenge, which returns to previous values after 15 minutes. At this point, it may be considered that blood volume has been restored, but this endpoint should be interpreted in conjunction with other data. CVP should not be allowed to increase to values >15 cmH$_2$O because pulmonary oedema may develop as a result of the higher hydrostatic pressure within the pulmonary circulation.

Lactate and acid–base balance

Normal lactate values and measurement are described earlier and in Figure 18.20. With critically ill patients, initial blood lactate values should be compared with serial measurements made during and after fluid resuscitation. Hyperlactataemia occurs most commonly because of hypoperfusion leading to anaerobic metabolism. Falling blood lactate values suggest successful fluid resuscitation, as lactate is cleared from the circulation and cells become better perfused.

Accurate diagnosis of an acid–base disorder is sometimes complex, especially where mixed disorders are present. In a critically ill patient, having a baseline acid–base measurement will assist the veterinary surgeon in choosing the type of fluid resuscitation to administer, and serial measurements will be useful to guide changes in the fluid therapy plan over time.

Monitoring of mixed venous or jugular blood oxygenation

True mixed venous blood must be taken from a pulmonary artery catheter, but analysis of blood gases and oxygen haemoglobin saturation in a jugular venous sample can be clinically useful. The mixed venous oxygen haemoglobin saturation should be approximately 70% and venous oxygen tension 40 mmHg (5.3 kPa). These values reflect the balance between oxygen supply and consumption. Values lower than normal will reflect increased oxygen extraction by the tissues, which may be due to decreased oxygen delivery resulting from low cardiac output leading

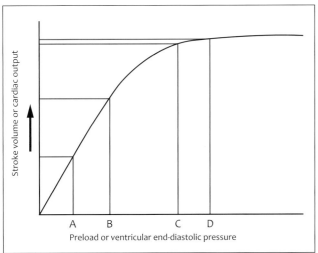

18.21 Idealized Frank–Starling curve demonstrating changes in stroke volume in response to preload. See text for explanation.

to poor tissue perfusion and/or poor pulmonary uptake of oxygen. Tissue hypoperfusion indicates that more aggressive fluid therapy is required.

Cardiac output and pleth variability index

Cardiac output can also be measured to guide fluid therapy; however, details of its measurement are beyond the scope of this chapter. Non-invasive techniques such as Pleth Variability Index (PVI®) are used in the medical field, but the expense of these techniques will probably prevent them from gaining acceptance in veterinary practice. Briefly, the technique of PVI® examines the degree of change in the photoplethysmographic waveform provided by a pulse oximeter during lung ventilation. Greater changes are observed in hypovolaemic states due to decreased venous return. For information on new technological advances in the field of haemodynamic monitoring, readers are directed to information on the PVI®, in the useful websites section at the end of this chapter.

Summary

In the past, the administration of fluids in the perioperative period and in the critical care setting has been largely based on anecdote and/or flawed studies rather than sound evidence. Understanding of body fluid kinetics is rapidly advancing, and recommendations for fluid therapy are changing to keep pace with these developments. Over the next few years, it is likely that equipment to assist in the management of these patients will become available to veterinary surgeons; it is important that clinicians understand the physiological principles behind any new technology that comes into use. Taking a reasoned and logical approach when devising an appropriate fluid therapy plan will improve patient care and is likely to reduce patient morbidity and mortality.

References and further reading

Allen SE and Holm JL (2008) Lactate: physiology and clinical utility. *Journal of Veterinary Emergency and Critical Care* 18, 123–132

American Society of Anesthesiologists (2015) Practice Guidelines for Perioperative Blood Management. *Anesthesiology* 122(2), 241–275

Annecke T, Rehm M, Bruegger D et al. (2012) Ischemia–reperfusion-induced unmeasured anion generation and glycocalyx shedding: sevoflurane versus propofol anesthesia. *Journal of Investigative Surgery* 25, 162–168

Association of Anaesthetists of Great Britain and Ireland (2008) *Blood transfusion and the anaesthetist: red cell transfusion 2* (www.aagbi.org)

Bellamy MC (2006) Editorial: wet, dry or something else? *British Journal of Anaesthesia* 97, 755–757

Blais MC, Berman L, Oakley DA and Giger U (2007) Canine *Dal* blood type: a red cell antigen lacking in some Dalmatians. *Journal of Veterinary Internal Medicine* 21, 281–286

Bovens C and Gruffydd-Jones T (2013) Xenotransfusion with canine blood in the feline species: review of the literature. *Journal of Feline Medicine and Surgery* 15, 62–67

Brodbelt DC, Pfeiffer DU, Young LE and Wood JL (2007) Risk factors for anaesthetic-related death in cats: results from the Confidential Enquiry into Perioperative Small Animal Fatalities (CEPSAF). *British Journal of Anaesthesia* 99, 617–623

Campbell S and Harvey N (2012) Assisted enteral feeding. In: *Advanced Monitoring and Procedures for Small Animal Emergency and Critical Care*, ed. JM Burkitt Creedon and H Davis, pp. 496–512. Wiley Blackwell, Chichester

Chappell D, Jacob M, Hofmann-Kiefer K et al. (2007) Hydrocortisone preserves the vascular barrier by protecting the endothelial glycocalyx. *Anesthesiology* 197, 776–784

Clark L, Corletto F and Garosi LS (2010) Comparison of a method using the HemoCue near patient testing device with a standard method of haemorrhage estimation in dogs undergoing spinal surgery. *Veterinary Anaesthesia and Analgesia* 37, 44–47

Clarke KW, Trim CM and Hall LW (2014) *Veterinary Anaesthesia, 11th edn.* Elsevier Saunders, London

Csete M (2011) Editorial: new molecular players in the great fluid debate. *Anesthesia and Analgesia* 112, 1272–1273

Davidow B (2013) Transfusion medicine in small animals. *Veterinary Clinics of North America: Small Animal Practice* 43, 735–756

Davis H, Jensen T, Johnson A et al. (2013) AAHA/AAFP fluid therapy guidelines for dogs and cats. *Journal of the American Animal Hospital Association* 49, 149–159

DiBartola SP (2011) *Fluid, Electrolyte and Acid-Base Disorders in Small Animal Practice, 4th edn.* Elsevier Saunders, Philadelphia

Doherty M and Buggy DJ (2012) Intraoperative fluids: how much is too much? *British Journal of Anaesthesia* 109, 69–79

Eto N, Kojima I, Uesugi N et al. (2005) Protection of endothelial cells by dextran sulfate in rats with thrombotic microangiopathy. *Journal of the American Society of Nephrology* 16, 2997–3005

Ferber HP, Nitsch E and Förster H (1985) Studies on hydroxyethyl starch. Part II: changes in the molecular weight distribution for hydroxyethyl starch types 450/0.7, 450/0.5, 450/0.3, 300/0.4, 200/0.7, 200/0.5, 200/0.3 and 200/0.1 after infusion in serum and urine of volunteers. *Arzneimittelforschung* 35, 615–622

Forcada Y, Guitian J and Gibson G (2007) Frequencies of feline blood types at a referral hospital in the south east of England. *Journal of Small Animal Practice* 48, 570–573

Hansen B and DeFrancesco T (2002) Relationship between hydration estimate and body weight change after fluid therapy in critically ill dogs and cats. *Journal of Veterinary Emergency and Critical Care* 12, 235–243

King LG and Boag A (2007) *BSAVA Manual of Canine and Feline Emergency and Critical Care, 2nd edn.* BSAVA Publications, Gloucester

Lima A and Bakker J (2005) Non-invasive monitoring of peripheral perfusion. *Intensive Care Medicine* 31, 1316–1326

Magder S (2006) Central venous pressure: a useful but not so simple measurement. *Critical Care Medicine* 34, 2224–2227

Marik PE (2009) Techniques for assessment of intravascular volume in critically ill patients. *Journal of Intensive Care Medicine* 24, 329–337

Marik PE, Baram M and Vahid B (2008) Does central venous pressure predict fluid responsiveness? A systematic review of the literature and the tale of seven mares. *Chest* 134, 172–178

Muir WW and Wellman ML (2003) Hemoglobin solutions and tissue oxygenation. *Journal of Veterinary Internal Medicine* 17, 127–135

Onen A, Cigdem MK, Deveci E et al. (2003) Effects of whole blood, crystalloid, and colloid resuscitation of hemorrhagic shock on renal damage in rats: an ultrastructural study. *Journal of Paediatric Surgery* 38, 1642–1649

Pang DS and Boysen S (2007) Lactate in veterinary critical care: pathophysiology and management. *Journal of the American Animal Hospital Association* 43, 270–279

Perel P, Roberts I and Pearson M (2009) Colloids versus crystalloids for fluid resuscitation in critically ill patients (Cochrane Review). *Cochrane Database of Systematic Reviews*, CD000567

Power I and Kam P (2007) *Principles of Physiology for the Anaesthetist, 2nd edn.* Hodder Arnold, London

Rehm M, Zahler S, Lötsch M et al. (2004) Endothelial glycocalyx as an additional barrier determining extravasation of 6% hydroxyethyl starch or 5% albumin solutions in the coronary vascular bed. *Anesthesiology* 100, 1211–1223

Reinhart K, Perner A, Sprung CL et al. (2012) Consensus statement of the ESICM task force on colloid volume therapy in critically ill patients. *Intensive Care Medicine* 38, 368–383

Rivers E, Nguyen B, Havstad S et al. (2001) Early goal-directed therapy in the treatment of severe sepsis and septic shock. *New England Journal of Medicine* 345, 1368–1377

Seeler DC (2007) Fluid, electrolyte and blood component therapy. In: *Lumb and Jones' Veterinary Anesthesia and Analgesia, 4th edn*, ed. WJ Tranquilli, JC Thurmon and KA Grimm, pp. 183–202. Blackwell Publishing, Ames

Soni N and Bunker N (2010) Transfusion triggers. *Current Anaesthesia and Critical Care* 21, 84–88

Stevenson CK, Kidney BA, Duke T et al. (2007) Serial blood lactate concentrations in systemically ill dogs. *Veterinary Clinical Pathology* 36, 234–239

Tefend Campbell M and Macintire DK (2012) Catheterization of the venous compartment. In: *Advanced Monitoring and Procedures for Small Animal Emergency and Critical Care*, ed. JM Burkitt Creedon and H Davis, pp. 51–68. Wiley-Blackwell, Chichester

Tocci LJ and Ewing PJ (2009) Increasing patient safety in veterinary transfusion medicine: an overview of pretransfusion testing. *Journal of Veterinary Emergency and Critical Care* 19, 66–73

Treib J, Baron JF, Grauer MT and Strauss RG (1999) An international view of hydroxyethyl starches. *Intensive Care Medicine* 25, 258–268

Trow AV, Rozanski EA, Delaforcade AM and Chan DL (2008) Evaluation of use of human albumin in critically ill dogs: 73 cases (2003–2006). *Journal of the American Veterinary Medical Association* 233, 607–612

Weinbaum S, Tarbell JM and Damiano ER (2007) The structure and function of the endothelial glycocalyx layer. *Annual Review of Biomedical Engineering* 9, 121–167

Weinstein NM, Blais MC, Harris K *et al.* (2007) A newly recognized blood group in Domestic Shorthair cats: the *Mik* red cell antigen. *Journal of Veterinary Internal Medicine* **21**, 287–292

West E, Pettitt R, Jones RS, Cripps PJ and Mosing M (2013) Acid-base and electrolyte balance following administration of three crystalloid solutions in dogs undergoing elective orthopaedic surgery. *Veterinary Anaesthesia and Analgesia* **40**, 482–493

Westphal M, James MFM, Kozek-Langenecker S *et al.* (2009) Hydroxyethyl starches: Different products, different effects. *Anesthesiology* **111**, 187–202

Woodcock TE (2012) Editorial: fluid therapy – the basics, reappraised. *Journal of the Intensive Care Society* **13**, 188–190

Woodcock TE and Woodcock TM (2012) Revised Starling equation and the glycocalyx model of transvascular fluid exchange: an improved paradigm for prescribing intravenous fluid therapy. *British Journal of Anaesthesia* **108**, 384–394

Zarychanski R, Abou-Setta AM, Turgeon AF *et al.* (2013) Association of hydroxyethyl starch administration with mortality and acute kidney injury in critically ill patients requiring volume resuscitation: a systematic review and meta-analysis. *Journal of the American Medical Association* **309**, 678–688

Useful websites

American Animal Hospital Association fluid therapy guidelines:
www.aahanet.org/Library/Fluid_Therapy_Guidelines_display.aspx

American Association of Feline Practitioners Practice Guidelines:
www.catvets.com/guidelines/practice-guidelines/fluid-therapy-guidelines

EZ-IO Intraosseous Infusion System:
http://www.arrowzio.com/

Hemo-Nate®:
www.utahmed.com/hemonate.htm

Hospira:
www.hospira.com

Pet Blood Bank UK:
www.petbloodbankuk.org

Pleth Variability Index (PVI®); developments in measuring fluid status in patients.
http://www.masimo.co.uk/pvi/

RayTemp® 3 Infrared Thermometer:
http://thermometer.co.uk/525-raytemp-3-infrared-thermometer.html

RescueFlow®:
www.rescueflow.com

Chapter 19

Ophthalmic surgery

Colette Jolliffe

Patients with ophthalmic disease may require surgery to correct adnexal disease such as entropion, corneal disease, intraocular disease such as cataract, or to remove the globe (enucleation). Patients vary from young, healthy animals with ocular injury or congenital disease to geriatric patients, which may have significant comorbidities.

Factors to consider when planning anaesthesia for an ophthalmic patient

When planning anaesthesia for a patient requiring ophthalmic surgery, the nature of the ocular disease, the surgical procedure, the patient's history and any concurrent disease must all be taken into account. Factors to consider include:

- **Is the animal currently experiencing pain?** Pain should be treated swiftly and appropriately for reasons of animal welfare and practicality. If the animal has a painful eye it may be fearful, aggressive and difficult to handle. Pain may also cause the patient to traumatize the eye further. The anticipated degree of surgical stimulation and the likelihood that the animal will be in pain postoperatively should also be considered
- **Is there a risk that the eye will rupture?** If a lesion is present that weakens the ocular tunic (cornea and sclera), then an increase in intraocular pressure (IOP) could cause the eye to rupture. Such lesions include deep corneal ulceration or a foreign body, descemetocoele and ocular trauma; recent intraocular surgery is another risk factor. Factors that could increase IOP and endanger the eye are discussed in the next section of this chapter. A 'fragile' eye may be extremely painful and the animal must be handled carefully to avoid further ocular damage. Since struggling by the patient and robust physical restraint could both increase IOP, the patient should receive appropriate analgesia and sedation before procedures such as blood sampling and intravenous catheter placement are undertaken. Animals with anterior lens luxation should be handled carefully, as sudden changes in body position or IOP may cause the luxated lens to move posteriorly, complicating the surgery. Other complications of increased IOP in 'fragile' eyes include intraocular haemorrhage or retinal detachment

- **Does the patient have any comorbidities, and is it receiving any medication?** It is important to consider the general health status of the animal and not simply focus on the ocular lesion. Patients with concurrent disease may present considerable challenges for the anaesthetist. In some cases, investigations such as blood tests or radiography may be necessary in order to assess the risks of anaesthesia. A significant proportion of dogs with ocular disease are brachycephalic (Figure 19.1) and these animals may be suffering from brachycephalic obstructive airway syndrome. Geriatric patients may have various comorbidities, including cardiac disease, renal disease, and endocrinopathies. Patients with diabetes mellitus often require treatment of diabetes-related cataracts, and ideally their condition should be stabilized before anaesthesia. Animals that are blind are more likely to be stressed and fearful in a hospital environment compared with patients that have vision, especially if the onset of blindness was acute
- **What is the intended surgical procedure?** Many ophthalmic procedures, for example, adnexal surgery to correct entropion, usually present few anaesthetic challenges. However, some procedures (corneal and intraocular surgery) are facilitated by a central position of the cornea within the palpebral fissure. A centrally positioned eye is normally achieved by the use of

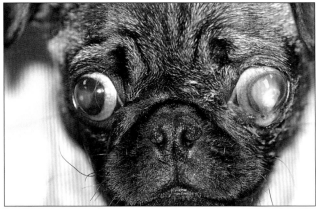

19.1 A young Pug with a deep corneal ulcer. The eye is painful and there is a risk of globe rupture if the intraocular pressure were to increase suddenly. The animal has a significant comorbidity (brachycephalic obstructive airway syndrome) and surgery is likely to require a centrally positioned cornea (achieved by the use of a neuromuscular blocking agent).
(Courtesy of the AHT Comparative Ophthalmology Unit, Newmarket, UK)

neuromuscular blocking agents (NMBAs). Use of these agents necessitates intermittent positive pressure ventilation (IPPV). The position of the animal during surgery may influence the choice of breathing system and endotracheal tube (ETT); for example, an armoured ETT may be useful. Good communication with the surgeon before the procedure and an understanding of the surgeon's requirements are essential when formulating an anaesthesia plan.

Ocular physiology relevant to anaesthesia

Factors influencing intraocular pressure

An increase in IOP can be detrimental in the preoperative period for animals with loss of ocular tunic integrity, and during the intraoperative and postoperative periods for any intraocular surgery. Increased IOP in these circumstances may result in globe rupture, intraocular haemorrhage or retinal detachment. The ability to influence IOP is therefore a very important part of anaesthetic management for ophthalmic surgery. The effect of anaesthesia on IOP in patients with glaucoma is of less concern, but an increase in IOP can adversely affect optic nerve function in such patients. Several factors govern IOP (Figure 19.2).

- Production and drainage of aqueous humour
- Intraocular blood volume (arterial blood pressure, vascular tone, venous drainage)
- Body position
- Extraocular muscle tone
- Rigidity of the ocular tunic (cornea and sclera)
- External pressure
- Drug effects

19.2 Factors governing intraocular pressure.

Aqueous humour production and drainage

Aqueous humour is produced by the ciliary body by processes of active secretion, diffusion and ultrafiltration. It passes from the posterior chamber through the pupil into the anterior chamber. It leaves the anterior chamber at the irido-corneal angle and drains into the scleral venous plexus. The balance between production and drainage of aqueous humour influences IOP because the relatively rigid ocular tunic cannot expand to accommodate an increased volume. Decreased outflow of aqueous humour due to irido-corneal angle abnormalities results in glaucoma. More importantly for the anaesthetist, outflow of aqueous humour is influenced by back pressure from the blood within the scleral venous plexus, which in turn is governed by the jugular venous pressure and central venous pressure (CVP).

Intraocular blood volume

Intraocular blood volume is influenced by intraocular vascular tone (vasoconstriction or vasodilation), arterial blood pressure (ABP), and outflow of blood from the globe. Dilation of ocular blood vessels (especially the choroidal vessels) increases IOP, while vasoconstriction decreases IOP. Intraocular vascular tone is influenced by arterial carbon dioxide and oxygen tensions. Increased arterial carbon dioxide tension (P_aCO_2) causes choroidal vessel vasodilation and an increase in IOP. The P_aCO_2 can be controlled by using IPPV (see Chapter 6) and can be monitored either indirectly by capnography or directly by arterial blood gas analysis (see Chapter 7). Hypoxaemia causes vasodilation of the retinal vessels and a small increase in IOP, which is unlikely to be clinically significant; the effects of hypoxaemia on other organs are far more clinically important than the effect on IOP. Hypoxaemia can be detected using a pulse oximeter, and should be avoided by provision of appropriate oxygen supplementation and ventilation.

Increased ABP can increase IOP; however, the choroidal, retinal and uveal vessels vasoconstrict in response to increased ABP, which tends to reduce intraocular blood volume and IOP. The increased intraocular blood flow resulting from increased ABP is therefore transient, and ABP is of minor importance in the regulation of IOP. An increase in ABP during anaesthesia may be the result of sympathetic stimulation, the cause of which (e.g. inadequate anaesthesia and/or analgesia) should be diagnosed and treated appropriately.

Venous blood drains from the globe through the intra-scleral venous plexus to the jugular veins and the cranial vena cava within the thorax. An increase in jugular venous pressure or CVP will increase intraocular blood volume and therefore IOP.

Jugular venous pressure

Compression of one jugular vein, for example, during jugular venepuncture, causes an insignificant increase in IOP. Compression of both jugular veins, however, as may occur when a dog pulls on its lead while wearing a collar, will cause a significant increase in IOP (Pauli et al., 2006; Klein et al., 2011). Similar effects may result from the use of tight collars, neck bandages, Elizabethan collars, or poor positioning of the patient during general anaesthesia.

Central venous pressure

CVP may be increased if the animal coughs, sneezes, vomits or strains to defecate or urinate. Use of drugs that commonly cause vomiting as a side effect (e.g. morphine) should be avoided when there is risk of globe rupture. Although alpha-2 adrenoceptor agonists may induce vomiting, especially in cats, this potential side effect should be weighed against the risk of trauma to the eye in an uncooperative, aggressive patient. Endotracheal intubation and extubation may induce coughing, which should be avoided in animals with fragile eyes (see later for guidance on reducing the risk of coughing). Inappropriate use of IPPV can increase CVP by increasing intrathoracic pressure during inspiration, resulting in an increase in IOP (McMurphy et al., 2004). Barking and vocalizing also increase CVP.

Body position

Body position may influence scleral and jugular venous pressures. In humans, IOP has been shown to be higher when the patient is supine or positioned with the head lower than the heart. Since the eye-to-heart height difference in quadrupeds is less than that in humans, the gravitational effect of a change in posture is likely to be less significant in cats and dogs (Broadwater et al., 2008). However, a head-down position during anaesthesia should be avoided. A 15-degree head-up position during intraocular surgery has been recommended in humans.

Extraocular muscle tone

The ocular tunic of cats and dogs is sufficiently soft that the extraocular muscles can influence IOP by exerting pressure on the globe. Extraocular muscle tone during intraocular surgery may cause ocular structures to become displaced and distorted, complicating the surgery. Extraocular muscle tone can be decreased by the use of non-depolarizing NMBAs, by maintaining an appropriate plane of anaesthesia, or by a retrobulbar injection of a local anaesthetic (see later). Many veterinary ophthalmologists prefer to use NMBAs for this purpose.

Direct pressure on the globe

Direct pressure on the globe will increase IOP. This may occur inadvertently during ophthalmic examination, especially when the eyelids are stretched laterally (Klein *et al.*, 2011). Care should be taken to avoid putting pressure on the eye during restraint of the patient and while passing an Elizabethan collar over the head. Opening the mouth during tracheal intubation can increase IOP as the coronoid process of the mandible moves into the orbit. Care must be taken when positioning patients for tracheal intubation, as pressure may be exerted on the globe while the maxilla is held; this is especially the case for brachycephalic breeds.

Drug effects on intraocular pressure

Anaesthetic agents may influence IOP via effects on aqueous humour production and outflow, on blood vessels, and on extraocular muscle tone. Traditionally, most anaesthetic drugs were considered to mildly decrease IOP by increasing the outflow of aqueous humour. Researchers have investigated the effects of several sedative drugs, induction agents and drug combinations on IOP, but differences in study design and interpretation of results make it difficult to draw meaningful conclusions. In addition, the use of anaesthetic induction agents without pre-anaesthetic medication in these experimental studies does not reflect normal clinical practice.

Thiopental seems to reduce IOP, whereas propofol, alfaxalone, ketamine and etomidate may all increase IOP. Alpha-2 adrenoceptor agonists cause an initial rise in IOP followed by a fall (Rauser *et al.*, 2012). Most of the increases in IOP associated with these agents are probably not clinically significant, and they seem to be ameliorated by the use of pre-anaesthetic medication or co-induction agents such as opioids, acepromazine, midazolam or diazepam. Ketamine used alone is likely to significantly increase IOP because it causes an increase in extraocular muscle tone. The depolarizing NMBA suxamethonium will also increase extraocular muscle tone initially. Inhalational anaesthetic agents cause small decreases in IOP.

In the author's experience, the most important ways to prevent increased IOP in the perioperative period are to avoid jugular compression and application of direct pressure to the globe, and to prevent the patient vomiting or coughing (Figure 19.3). When there is a risk of globe rupture, careful handling of the patient and (in dogs) the use of a harness rather than a collar or lead are imperative. These measures are more important for IOP than the choice of anaesthetic agents or prevention of increases in ABP and P_aCO_2. Reduction of extraocular muscle tone by the use of NMBAs seems to be helpful for the surgeon during difficult intraocular procedures.

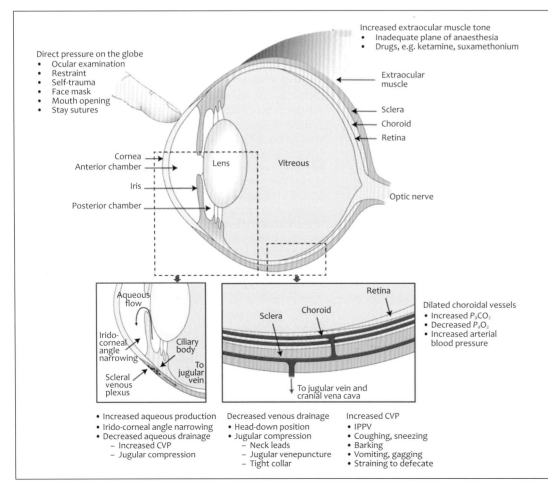

19.3 Management- and anaesthesia-related factors causing increased intraocular pressure. CVP = central venous pressure; IPPV = intermittent positive pressure ventilation; P_aCO_2 = arterial carbon dioxide tension; P_aO_2 = arterial oxygen tension. (© Juliane Deubner, University of Saskatchewan, Canada)

Tear production

The pre-ocular tear film is essential for normal corneal and conjunctival function. It provides lubrication and nutrients to the cornea, as well as a smooth surface to facilitate normal vision. It also aids in the removal of foreign bodies and control of the bacterial flora. Normal function of the pre-ocular tear film depends on adequate tear production and regular blinking to distribute the tears. Many opioid analgesics, sedative drugs and anaesthetic agents, including pethidine (meperidine), fentanyl, butorphanol, morphine, medetomidine, desflurane, isoflurane and sevoflurane, have been shown to reduce tear production. In addition an animal is unable to blink while anaesthetized. A reduction in tear production due to anaesthesia may persist for up to 36 hours (Herring *et al.*, 2000). Tear production is also reduced in critically ill hospitalized dogs (Chandler *et al.*, 2013). Regular corneal lubrication with a tear substitute should be applied from the time of pre-anaesthetic medication and into the recovery period, especially for animals with pre-existing deficits in tear production and those with protruding eyes.

Oculocardiac reflex

The oculocardiac reflex may be triggered by ocular surgery, traction or pressure on the globe, intraocular injection, orbital or maxillofacial injury or surgery, or by any cause of increased intraorbital pressure, including an ocular tumour extending into the orbit (Steinmetz *et al.*, 2012). The reflex can result in bradycardia, bradyarrhythmias and cardiac arrest. The afferent pathway of the reflex is via the long and short ciliary nerves of the ophthalmic nerve, to the trigeminal sensory nucleus; the efferent component is relayed from the vagal nucleus in the brainstem via the vagus nerve to the heart. The reflex is more likely to occur in lightly anaesthetized animals and those with an already high vagal tone. It is less likely to occur in animals that are maintained at an appropriate plane of anaesthesia and provided with good analgesia and muscle relaxation, including neuromuscular blockade (Clutton *et al.*, 1988).

Retrobulbar nerve block has been reported to abolish the oculocardiac reflex (Oel *et al.*, 2014), but a retrobulbar injection itself can increase intraorbital pressure and initiate the reflex. Use of topical local anaesthetic prevented the oculocardiac reflex during corneal surgery in rabbits (Singh *et al.*, 2010).

If the oculocardiac reflex does occur during surgery, the veterinary surgeon (veterinarian) should cease surgical manipulation until the bradycardia is resolved. An anticholinergic agent (atropine 20–40 μg/kg i.v. or glycopyrronium 10 μg/kg i.v.) can be administered if necessary. The incidence of the reflex is too rare to warrant prophylactic use of an anticholinergic agent.

Ocular pain

Sensory innervation of the eye

The optic nerve (cranial nerve II) is a sensory nerve which transmits signals from the light-sensitive retinal cells, through the optic foramen, to the brain. It has no nociceptors and is therefore not involved in ocular pain sensation. The nociceptive innervation to most structures of the eye is provided by the ophthalmic branch of the trigeminal nerve (cranial nerve V). The ophthalmic nerve branches into the nasociliary nerve, the lacrimal nerve and the frontal nerve. The nasociliary branch courses to the orbit and gives rise to the long ciliary nerves, which innervate the globe including the cornea, choroid, ciliary body, iris and bulbar conjunctiva. The lacrimal nerve supplies the lacrimal gland. The frontal nerve innervates the medial part of the upper eyelid. The infratrochlear nerve (a more distal branch of the nasociliary nerve) innervates structures near the medial canthus. The zygomatic branch of the maxillary nerve, which is also derived from the trigeminal nerve, divides into two branches within the orbit: the zygomaticofacial nerve innervates the lower eyelid, lateral canthus and ventrolateral conjunctiva, while the zygomaticotemporal nerve innervates the lateral upper eyelid (Figure 19.4).

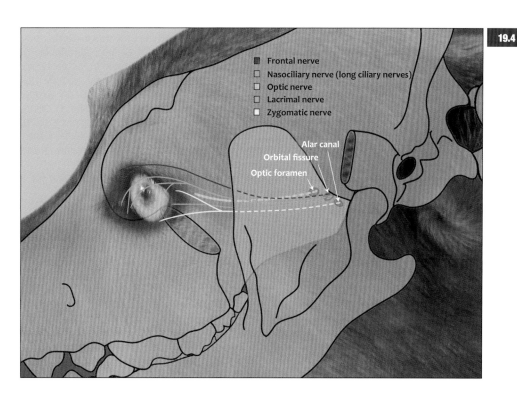

19.4 Sensory innervation of the eye. (© Juliane Deubner, University of Saskatchewan, Canada)

Superficial ocular pain

The need to protect the eye from trauma has resulted in the evolution of a high density of sensory nerve endings in the superficial structures of the eye, and the development of the palpebral and corneal reflexes.

Superficial ocular pain is caused by inflammatory conditions of the cornea and conjunctiva, such as corneal trauma, ulcers and corneal or conjunctival foreign bodies. It is characterized by blepharospasm and lacrimation (Figure 19.5) and can be relieved by the application of a topical local anaesthetic agent (often used to facilitate ocular examination).

Type of ocular pain	Examples of causes	Clinical signs
Superficial	Superficial corneal ulcer, entropion	Blepharospasm, lacrimation, resistance to ocular examination, aggression, depression, anorexia
Deep	Glaucoma, uveitis	Blepharospasm, lacrimation, photophobia, resistance to ocular examination, aggression, depression, anorexia

19.5 Clinical signs of superficial and deep ocular pain.

The cornea and bulbar conjunctiva contain polymodal nociceptors, which respond to various noxious stimuli, including inflammatory mediators released as a result of tissue injury. The corneal epithelium contains abundant nociceptors, while the deeper stroma of the cornea is less densely innervated. This means that superficial corneal lesions are often more painful than deep lesions (Figure 19.6). Brachycephalic cats and dogs have poor corneal sensitivity compared with non-brachycephalic animals, as a result of smaller numbers of corneal sensory nerve endings (Barrett *et al.*, 1991; Kafarnik *et al.*, 2008).

Deep ocular pain

The sclera, iris and ciliary body contain polymodal nociceptors, with the uveal tract (the vascular layer of the eye) being particularly richly innervated. Inflammation of uveal structures causes the pain associated with conditions such as uveitis and acute glaucoma. The deep stroma of the cornea contains pressure receptors, which respond to increased IOP in acute glaucoma (see Figure 19.6). Photophobia is a feature of deep ocular pain (see Figure 19.5) because miosis and lens accommodation may be painful when nociceptors in the iris and ciliary muscle have been sensitized by inflammation. The retina has no nociceptors, but retinal inflammation can be painful due to stimulation of uveal nociceptors by inflammatory mediators. Deep ocular pain is not relieved by the use of topical local anaesthetic agents but can be treated with systemic analgesics such as non-steroidal anti-inflammatory drugs (NSAIDs) and opioids.

Ocular inflammation

Ocular inflammation can occur in response to infection, immune-mediated disease, trauma, stimulation of corneal nociceptors or following surgery. It can have serious consequences, including fibrosis, cataract, glaucoma and retinal detachment. The blood–aqueous barrier consists of endothelial and epithelial layers containing tight junctions that prevent movement of proteins from the blood into the eye. In ocular inflammation, prostaglandins and other

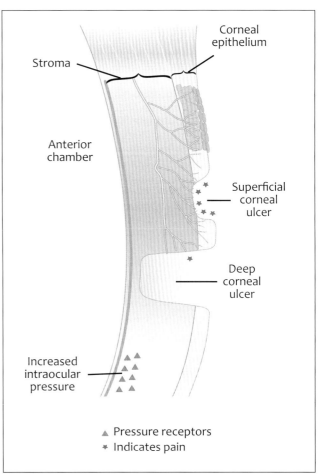

19.6 Diagram of a cross-section of the canine cornea, the sensory nerve supply and how it affects the degree of pain associated with superficial and deep corneal ulcers. The deep stroma of the cornea contains pressure receptors which respond to increased intraocular pressure in acute glaucoma.

inflammatory mediators are involved in the breakdown of the blood–aqueous barrier, which results in an influx of proteins into the anterior chamber (aqueous flare). Inflammatory mediators stimulate polymodal nociceptors in the cornea, conjunctiva, sclera and uvea, while previously silent nociceptors may be triggered by inflammation; stimulation of these various nociceptor types will result in ocular pain. Painful ciliary body contraction and resultant miosis may be triggered by superficial ocular disease via an axonal reflex: stimulation of corneal nociceptors results in ciliary body spasm, miosis, hyperaemia and ocular hypertension, followed by ocular hypotension and aqueous flare. Ciliary body spasm should be treated with topical atropine. Treatment of ocular inflammation is an important part of ocular analgesia and should be considered essential for a successful outcome.

Analgesia for ocular pain

As with any painful condition, alleviation of the underlying cause of the pain is necessary for long-term pain relief. However, treatment of the underlying cause of ocular pain may take time; during this period additional analgesia should be provided for animal welfare and practical reasons. A pre-emptive and multimodal strategy is recommended, as this is more likely to be effective and often allows lower doses of individual drugs to be used.

The different sensitivities of the ocular and extraocular structures to pain should be considered when planning any analgesia strategy. For example, phacoemulsification of a cataract does not appear to be a very painful procedure except during the incision and suturing of the corneal limbus, while an autonomic response to surgical stimulation is often seen during surgery of the cornea, eyelid or uvea (Figure 19.7).

Non-steroidal anti-inflammatory drugs

NSAIDs provide good analgesia and anti-inflammatory effects by inhibiting cyclo-oxygenase enzymes and thus prostaglandin production and the inflammatory cascade (see Chapter 10). They are used in ophthalmology to provide analgesia, to help maintain mydriasis before intraocular surgery and for their anti-inflammatory properties, especially when steroids are contraindicated (e.g. in patients with diabetes mellitus). They can be administered both systemically and topically.

Systemic NSAIDs are long acting, usually requiring once or twice daily dosing. They are therefore useful not only in the perioperative period but also in the days after surgery when the animal has returned home. In dogs, carprofen can reduce breakdown of the blood–aqueous barrier and aqueous flare when administered pre-emptively (Krohne et al., 1998), while tolfenamic acid has been shown to reduce miosis in experimentally induced ocular inflammation (Roze et al., 1996). Other systemic NSAIDs are likely to have similar effects. While NSAIDs can be very useful in the management of ophthalmic disease, it is important to be aware of their adverse effects (see Chapter 10). Because of the associated risk of gastroduodenal ulceration and renal damage, these drugs should not be used in animals with clinical signs of vomiting, diarrhoea or anorexia, or in dehydrated, hypotensive or hypovolaemic patients.

Topical NSAIDs such as ketorolac and flurbiprofen can be used to control miosis and inflammation before and after intraocular surgery, and in the control of ocular inflammatory conditions. These drugs work not only by inhibiting prostaglandin formation but also by a direct effect on corneal nerve endings (Giuliano, 2004). Adverse effects of topical NSAIDs include local irritation, epithelial defects, keratitis and systemic absorption (mainly through the nasal mucosa).

Opioids

Opioids are the mainstay of perioperative analgesia for ophthalmic surgery. They provide good analgesia and sedation and also reduce anaesthetic drug requirements, with few systemic adverse effects. They may be used as part of pre-anaesthetic medication (providing sedation in addition to analgesia), during surgery, and as part of postoperative analgesia. The choice and dose of opioid depends upon the anticipated level of pain caused by the lesion and/or procedure, and the duration of action, licensing and availability of the drug.

Opioids have some adverse effects that may be relevant to ophthalmic patients. Morphine, hydromorphone, oxymorphone and papaveretum are likely to cause vomiting and should not be used in animals at risk of globe rupture; opioids such as methadone, buprenorphine or pethidine are more suitable. Several opioids, including pethidine, fentanyl, butorphanol and morphine, have been shown to cause a significant reduction in tear production (Dodam et al., 1998; Biricik et al., 2004; Mouney et al., 2011), and it is probable that all opioids have this effect. Artificial tears can be used to help prevent sequelae such as corneal ulcers. Opioids tend to cause miosis in dogs and mydriasis in cats. In theory, miosis could prevent

Type of surgery	Examples	Considerations	Pain	Neuromuscular blockade needed?
Adnexal	Hotz-Celsus procedure (entropion correction) Wedge resection	Eyelid swelling postoperatively; use NSAIDs Consider infiltration of local anaesthetic	++	No
Corneal	Keratectomy	Avoid increased IOP perioperatively if corneal lesion is deep	+++	Not essential but facilitates surgery
	Conjunctival graft Corneal graft Corneo-conjunctival transposition	Risk of globe rupture Avoid increased IOP perioperatively	+++	Yes
	Repair of corneal trauma Corneal foreign body removal	Risk of globe rupture Avoid increased IOP perioperatively Assess patient for other injuries	+++	Not essential but facilitates surgery
Intraocular	Phacoemulsification	Animal is usually older Often blind May have diabetes mellitus Avoid increased IOP intra- and postoperatively	+	Yes
	Lendectomy of luxated lens	Often in terriers, may require sedation Risk of lens moving posteriorly: animal must be handled carefully preoperatively Avoid increased IOP intra- and postoperatively	+	Yes
	Uveal tract surgery	Avoid increased IOP intra- and postoperatively	+++	Yes
	Retinopexy	Avoid increased IOP intra- and postoperatively	+	Yes
Removal of the globe	Enucleation Exenteration	Haemorrhage Globe rupture may make surgery more difficult Use retrobulbar anaesthesia or splash block	+++	No

19.7 Common ophthalmic procedures and their anaesthetic considerations. NSAID = non-steroidal anti-inflammatory drug; IOP = intraocular pressure; + = mild; ++ = moderate; +++ = severe.

adequate access during intraocular surgery, however, this does not seem to be a problem in practice, perhaps because topical mydriatic agents are usually applied before intraocular surgery. Mydriasis could increase IOP in animals with glaucoma. Smith *et al.* (2004) reported equal pupil sizes in dogs undergoing general anaesthesia and receiving intravenous infusions of either morphine, lidocaine or saline following topical administration of tropicamide. Topical morphine has been shown to provide analgesia in humans and in experimental studies in dogs and rabbits, but a recent clinical study in cats and dogs with corneal disease was unable to demonstrate such an effect after a single dose (Thomson *et al.*, 2013).

Local anaesthetics

Superficial ocular pain can be alleviated in the short term by the use of topical local anaesthetics formulated for ocular use, such as proxymetacaine (proparacaine); however, these agents are short acting and may interfere with corneal wound healing (Herring, 2013). Topical local anaesthetics can be used to facilitate ocular examination or minor ocular procedures, and during surgery to reduce anaesthetic requirements. Intravenous lidocaine infusion may be useful to provide analgesia for cataract surgery in dogs (Smith *et al.*, 2004).

Miscellaneous treatments

Other drugs may be useful for treating ocular pain, although little has been published on their use in animals. In humans, paracetamol (acetaminophen) is widely used following intraocular surgery, and gabapentin has been used to treat glaucoma-related pain (Kavalieratos and Dimou, 2008). The use of paracetamol in cats is absolutely contraindicated; more information on the use of paracetamol and gabapentin can be found in Chapter 10. Therapeutic contact lenses can also provide analgesia in animals with superficial ocular pain by protecting the superficial corneal nerve endings from the environment.

Local anaesthetic techniques

In canine and feline practice, local anaesthetic techniques are more commonly used as part of a balanced anaesthetic protocol.

Retrobulbar block

The retrobulbar block (RBB) is indicated for enucleation of the globe. It has also been described as part of the anaesthetic technique for phacoemulsification in dogs (Hazra *et al.*, 2008). It provides analgesia by anaesthetizing the ophthalmic branch of cranial nerve V (trigeminal). The eye becomes centrally positioned and proptosed because cranial nerves III (oculomotor), IV (trochlear) and VI (abducens) are also blocked. Mydriasis is produced by effects on the parasympathetic supply to the iris in the oculomotor nerve and ciliary ganglion. The RBB may not provide analgesia for all the structures involved in enucleation, particularly the eyelids, so infiltration of the eyelids with local anaesthetic (see below) may be necessary. Complications of and contraindications for RBB are described in Figure 19.8.

Technique in dogs: Several techniques for RBB in dogs have been described, but the method providing the best distribution of local anaesthetic is the inferior temporal palpebral technique (Accola *et al.*, 2006). A bent 3.8 cm

Complication	Comment
Intravascular injection	Aspirate syringe before injection
Haemorrhage	Retrobulbar haemorrhage may increase IOP
Increased IOP	Caused by pressure on the globe from the needle and from the injectate (or haemorrhage) Not recommended for animals with fragile eyes
Intrathecal injection leading to brainstem anaesthesia	Aspirate syringe before injection
Nerve damage	Do not inject if significant resistance to injection is felt
Oculocardiac reflex	Retrobulbar injection can increase intraorbital pressure and trigger the oculocardiac reflex; however, a successful retrobulbar block should abolish the reflex
Penetration of the globe	With good technique, this should be avoided. More likely where there is significant distortion of normal anatomy
Proptosis and corneal damage	Especially in brachycephalic animals Provide corneal protection and lubrication
Incomplete analgesia	Often analgesia does not include the eyelids. Suturing of the eyelids may induce a response from the patient, necessitating either a deeper plane of anaesthesia or additional analgesia
Seeding of neoplastic cells	Retrobulbar block is not recommended in the presence of intraorbital neoplasia

19.8 Complications and limitations of the retrobulbar nerve block. IOP = intraocular pressure.

22–25G hypodermic needle or a retrobulbar needle (Figure 19.9) can be used to inject a maximum volume of 2 ml of local anaesthetic (not exceeding the maximum safe dose for the patient; see Chapter 11). After clipping and surgical preparation of the skin of the lower eyelid of the anaesthetized patient, the needle is placed at the point where the lateral and middle thirds of the lower eyelid meet (Figure 19.10). The needle is advanced through the skin, along the floor of the orbit and directed dorsomedially, aiming for the orbital cone (Figure 19.11). A 'popping' sensation may be felt as the needle penetrates the orbital fascia. Before injection, the syringe should be aspirated to verify that the tip of the needle is not in a blood vessel or in the meningeal sheath of the optic nerve. If there is any resistance to injection, the tip of the needle may be within a nerve sheath; the needle should be repositioned and the syringe aspirated again before injection. If the RBB is successful, the pupil will become mydriatic and centrally positioned.

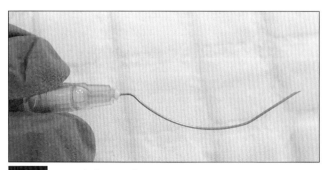

19.9 A retrobulbar needle.

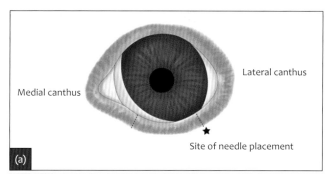

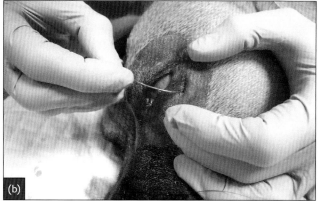

19.10 The inferior temporal palpebral technique for retrobulbar injection. (a) Anatomical landmarks. (b) Needle positioning.
(a, © Juliane Deubner, University of Saskatchewan, Canada)

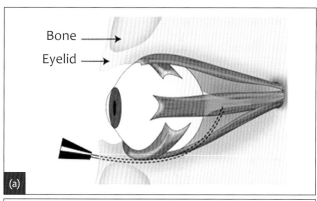

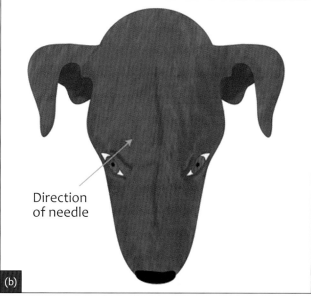

19.11 Diagrams illustrating the inferior temporal palpebral technique for retrobulbar injection. (a) Lateral view. (b) Dorsal view.
(© Juliane Deubner, University of Saskatchewan, Canada)

Technique in cats: Traditionally, the RBB has not been recommended in cats due to anatomical differences from dogs and a lack of published evidence. There is less space around the globe within the orbit and the extraocular muscles are smaller in cats than in dogs, potentially increasing the risk of complications. A recent cadaver study in cats suggested that a ventral approach to the RBB may not be suitable, owing to the smaller skeletal component of the ventral bony orbit compared with dogs (Shilo-Benjamini *et al.*, 2013). More research is required before safe recommendations can be made in cats. A case of brainstem anaesthesia in a cat following inadvertent intrathecal injection has been reported (Oliver and Bradbrook, 2013); this resulted in apnoea, necessitating IPPV, and neurological signs on recovery from anaesthesia, which resolved within 24 hours.

Other techniques

Infiltration of local anaesthetic agents can be useful for eyelid surgery. A splash block can be used for most adnexal procedures; this involves depositing the local anaesthetic solution directly on to the area to be anaesthetized and leaving it in place for a few minutes to enable absorption. This technique can be used following enucleation when an RBB is contraindicated.

A peribulbar block has been recommended for enucleation to anaesthetize the sites of extraocular muscle attachment to the globe. Local anaesthetic (0.1–0.2 ml per site) is injected subconjunctivally, approximately 2 mm from the limbus, at four sites: dorsally, laterally, ventrally and medially (Giuliano and Walsh, 2013). Peribulbar anaesthesia achieved by means of a single injection of lidocaine underneath Tenon's capsule has been evaluated in dogs undergoing phacoemulsification. This technique resulted in adequate extraocular muscle relaxation, mydriasis and analgesia (Ahn *et al.*, 2013).

Intracameral injection of preservative-free lidocaine has also been described as an effective analgesic technique for intraocular surgery in dogs (Park *et al.*, 2010).

Practical considerations and anaesthetic management

Pre-anaesthetic medication

Pre-anaesthetic medication is used to provide sedation and analgesia, to promote a smooth anaesthetic induction and recovery, and to reduce requirements for anaesthetic agents (see Chapter 13). The drugs and doses chosen depend on the health status and temperament, and the presumed requirement for analgesia.

For patients at risk of globe rupture, careful handling and minimizing stress is essential. The potential effects of drugs such as alpha-2 adrenoceptor agonists on IOP are probably less important than the risks of overzealous physical restraint of a stressed animal. Adequate sedation of these patients is recommended to facilitate catheter placement or intravenous anaesthetic injection with only gentle physical restraint. A combination of a low dose of an alpha-2 adrenoceptor agonist and a suitable opioid usually provides good sedation without vomiting (which should be avoided if possible); for example, medetomidine (5–10 μg/kg i.m.) and methadone (0.3–0.5 mg/kg i.m.). The degree of sedation required and the exact dose will depend on the temperament of the animal.

Layout of the operating theatre

Most ophthalmology theatres are arranged so that the head of the animal faces away from the anaesthetist and anaesthetic machine (Figure 19.12). This gives the surgeon more room to work and allows more space for surgical instruments and equipment, but restricts the anaesthetist's access to the head and cranial regions of the patient. This has implications for intravenous access, monitoring of anaesthesia and the choice of breathing system.

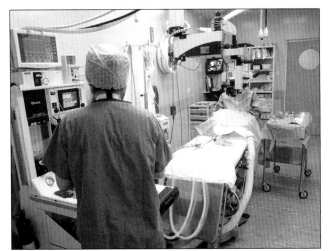

19.12 Typical layout of an ophthalmology operating theatre, showing limited patient access for the anaesthetist.
(Courtesy of Elvira Peeters, Animal Health Trust, Newmarket, UK)

Intravenous access

It is useful to place an intravenous catheter in a pelvic limb vein, such as the lateral or medial saphenous vein in dogs, or the medial saphenous vein in cats (Figure 19.13). This will allow the anaesthetist easy access to the catheter during anaesthesia, facilitating administration of intravenous fluids and drugs.

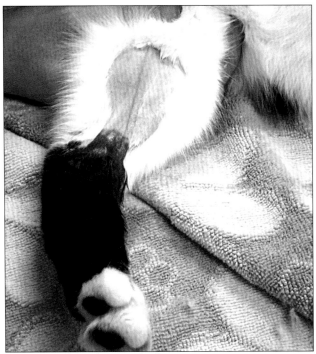

19.13 Medial saphenous vein of a cat.
(Courtesy of Emma Archer, Animal Health Trust, Newmarket, UK)

Anaesthesia induction

Induction of anaesthesia should be smooth, with minimal restraint of the patient, especially for an animal with a 'fragile' eye at risk of rupture. This will be facilitated by the provision of adequate sedation and pre-placement of an intravenous catheter. Induction of anaesthesia with a volatile agent delivered by mask is not recommended as the animal may struggle and the mask may exert pressure on the eyes. The choice of agent(s) depends on the individual patient, the anaesthetist's familiarity with the drug(s), and their availability and cost. Use of ketamine alone significantly increases IOP, which is undesirable in many ophthalmic patients. Although propofol, alfaxalone and etomidate have been shown to increase IOP in experimental studies, this is unlikely to be clinically significant when the drugs are administered after adequate pre-anaesthetic medication.

Endotracheal tube and anaesthetic breathing system

Long tubes for the breathing system may be needed if the patient's head is positioned away from the anaesthetic machine. A right-angled or flexible connector is useful to reduce drag on the ETT and improve access to the head (Figure 19.14), but will increase apparatus dead space. Once the surgical drapes are placed, it is difficult to reach the ETT, and therefore it is essential to ensure that all connections are secure before draping. The ETT must be securely fixed in position; this is usually achieved by tying it to the mandible to prevent the tie hindering surgical access to the eye. The ETT cuff must be adequately inflated, especially if IPPV is being used.

Some ophthalmic procedures are facilitated by positioning the patient in dorsal recumbency with the neck flexed (Figure 19.14). This position can cause either kinking and obstruction of the ETT, or movement of the tip of the ETT into a bronchus. Kinking of the tube can be avoided by careful positioning of the patient and can be detected by monitoring respiratory rate and effort, and by assessment of the capnograph waveform (looking for signs of expiratory resistance). Use of an armoured ETT also helps to prevent kinking (see Chapter 5). Inadvertent bronchial intubation can be avoided by measuring the ETT against the patient before intubation. The distal end of the ETT should be positioned in the cervical trachea, well away from the tracheal bifurcation.

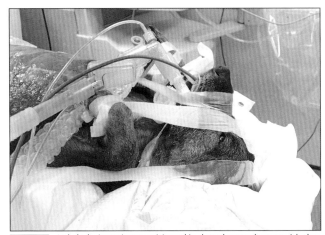

19.14 Ophthalmic patient positioned in dorsal recumbency with the neck flexed. A right-angled connector is being used to improve surgical access to the eye and reduce drag on the endotracheal tube.

Endotracheal intubation

Coughing during endotracheal intubation must be avoided when there is a risk of globe rupture, as coughing will increase CVP and IOP (as described earlier). Coughing may be reduced by administration of opioids, or in dogs by an intravenous bolus of lidocaine (1–2 mg/kg) given 1–5 minutes before intubation. In cats, the use of topical lidocaine on the vocal cords helps to reduce laryngeal responsiveness to intubation. Probably the most reliable way to prevent coughing is to ensure an adequate depth of anaesthesia before attempting intubation.

Globe position

In cats and dogs at a surgical plane of anaesthesia, the globe usually rotates ventromedially, making it difficult to access the cornea. Intraocular surgery and many corneal procedures are greatly facilitated if the cornea is positioned centrally within the palpebral fissure (Figure 19.15). This can be achieved by using stay sutures, retrobulbar injection of a local anaesthetic agent, a deep plane of anaesthesia, or by administering NMBAs that relax the extraocular muscles. A deep plane of anaesthesia is not recommended because of the associated increase in cardiovascular and respiratory depression. The risk of complications associated with RBB must be considered, as the passage of a needle within the orbit and the injection of fluid behind the globe may increase the IOP (see Figure 19.8). Stay sutures can be used but they may distort the anatomy of the eye and complicate the surgical field.

A centrally-positioned cornea is most often achieved by using NMBAs (see Chapter 16 for a detailed discussion of the use of NMBAs). Atracurium, rocuronium and vecuronium are the most commonly used NMBAs in veterinary ophthalmic anaesthesia. Ideally, neuromuscular blockade should be monitored using a peripheral nerve stimulator. The extraocular muscles are more sensitive to the effects of NMBAs, with a faster onset and longer duration of action, compared to the diaphragm and limb muscles (McMurphy *et al.*, 2004). Thus, the cornea may remain centrally positioned with partial neuromuscular blockade, and the effects of the NMBA may be allowed to wear off (as assessed by stimulation of either the ulnar or the peroneal nerve) before the end of the surgical procedure. However, without deep neuromuscular blockade, the extraocular muscles may exert pressure on the globe, distorting the intraocular anatomy and making some surgeries more difficult. Since NMBAs also paralyse the respiratory muscles, IPPV must be provided. Attempts have been made to avoid IPPV by using a low dose of NMBA to produce a central cornea without paralysing the respiratory muscles, but this technique is not recommended because it carries the risk of severe hypoventilation. NMBAs have no hypnotic or analgesic effect, so it is essential to monitor the patient carefully to ensure adequacy of anaesthesia (see Chapter 16).

Non-depolarizing neuromuscular blockade can be antagonized using an anticholinesterase such as edrophonium or neostigmine. Because these drugs can cause significant muscarinic effects (e.g. bradycardia), an anticholinergic agent (atropine or glycopyrronium) is usually co-administered. Concerns that parenteral administration of anticholinergic agents may cause mydriasis and increase IOP seem to be unfounded. However, if it is critical to avoid an increase in IOP, glycopyrronium may be preferable because it does not cause mydriasis or increased IOP at a clinically relevant dose in dogs (Frischmeyer *et al.*, 1993). Sugammadex is a new antagonist designed to reverse the effects of rocuronium; it has no cardiac or ocular effects but it is expensive. The need to antagonize neuromuscular blockade can often be avoided by good communication with the surgeon and careful timing of NMBA administration.

Anaesthesia maintenance and monitoring

An adequate depth of anaesthesia and appropriate analgesia are essential to minimize autonomic responses to surgical stimulation and prevent movement of the patient, which can be disastrous during delicate intraocular surgery. Once the surgical site has been aseptically prepared and drapes placed, it is difficult for the anaesthetist to assess the depth of anaesthesia by using the palpebral reflex, eye position and jaw tone, although the surgeon may assist with this assessment. Neuromuscular blockade paralyses the animal and also prevents assessment of the depth of anaesthesia by means of the palpebral reflex, eye position, jaw tone, respiratory rate or movement of the patient. The anaesthetist must rely on changes in heart rate and ABP to assess the depth of anaesthesia and adequacy of analgesia; if available, expired volatile agent concentration can also be useful. Such assessments can be challenging, and it is one reason why venous access that is easily accessible to the anaesthetist is important. Prompt administration of an intravenous anaesthetic agent may be required if the depth of anaesthesia becomes inadequate.

IPPV can be used with or without neuromuscular blockade, and may be useful during intraocular surgery to prevent increased P_aCO_2, which, if severe, may increase IOP. However, poorly applied IPPV (long inspiratory times and high peak airway pressure) can increase IOP by increasing CVP (McMurphy *et al.*, 2004). Capnography is particularly useful to indirectly monitor P_aCO_2 and adequacy of IPPV, and may also detect disconnection or kinking of the ETT (see Chapter 7).

Monitoring equipment should be placed before draping, preferably on the caudal parts of the animal so

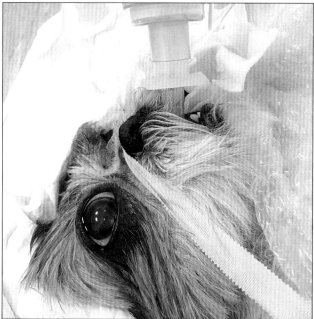

19.15 A central eye. The cornea is positioned centrally within the palpebral fissure following the administration of a neuromuscular blocking agent.
(Courtesy of Fiona Scarlett, Animal Health Trust, Newmarket, UK)

that the anaesthetist has ready access to the devices. For example, a blood pressure cuff can be placed proximal or distal to the hock or on the tail, and the electrodes of a peripheral nerve stimulator can be placed over the peroneal nerve (Figure 19.16). A pulse oximeter probe can be placed on non-pigmented skin on the pelvic limbs, prepuce, vulva or tail if available, since access to the tongue will be difficult. For diabetic patients, it is helpful to clip the skin over a vein on a pelvic limb or the tail to facilitate blood sampling for measurement of glucose concentration during anaesthesia (Figure 19.16).

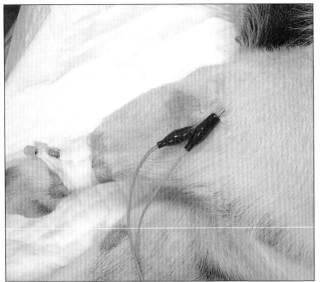

19.16 Electrodes for a peripheral nerve stimulator positioned over the peroneal nerve. An intravenous catheter has been placed in the lateral saphenous vein and the area clipped over the medial saphenous vein for blood sampling, enabling easy access for the anaesthetist.

Extubation and recovery

A smooth and pain-free recovery from anaesthesia is especially important following ophthalmic surgery to help prevent increases in IOP and trauma to the surgery site. Coughing during extubation should be avoided following intraocular surgery or when there is a risk of globe rupture. Before administration of the anaesthetic agent is discontinued, the animal should be moved to a comfortable position, such as lateral recumbency, to help prevent distress during recovery. In patients that have undergone unilateral surgery, the operated eye should be non-dependent. Additional analgesia should be provided as required.

Neuromuscular blockade should be antagonized or can be allowed to wear off provided the level of blockade is closely monitored using a peripheral nerve stimulator or acceleromyography (see Chapter 16). Once muscle function has returned, any non-essential monitoring equipment can be removed. This enables the anaesthetist to concentrate on close observation of the patient and to prepare for extubation.

If IPPV has been used, spontaneous ventilation must resume; this may occur before or after the anaesthetic agent is discontinued. Once spontaneous ventilation is established, the tie securing the ETT to the mandible can be untied (taking care that the ETT is not dislodged accidentally) and the ETT tube cuff deflated. The animal should then be closely observed for signs of recovery

from anaesthesia, and the trachea extubated slightly early, before any coughing occurs, or (in cats) once touching the ear results in twitching of the pinna. This may happen before swallowing occurs. The patient must be carefully observed and ideally positioned with the nose below the poll to help prevent aspiration, at least until the laryngeal reflexes return. Self-trauma to the eye can be prevented by means of good analgesia, an Elizabethan collar, or bandages on the distal limbs. A calm environment and reassurance of the patient may help reduce stress and anxiety during recovery.

For excitable animals that were not well sedated before induction of anaesthesia, or in which the effects of pre-anaesthetic medication may be waning, further sedation may be necessary to ensure a smooth recovery. Options include acepromazine 10 μg/kg i.v. or medetomidine 1 μg/kg i.v. For patients with diabetes, the advantages of providing further sedation and a smooth recovery should be balanced against the need for a rapid return to eating. See also Chapter 27 for anaesthesia of patients with diabetes mellitus.

Care of the contralateral eye

Many drugs used during anaesthesia cause reduced tear production. Combined with inability of the patient to blink, this may result in corneal desiccation and ulceration. It is important to lubricate the contralateral eye and to protect it from physical damage during anaesthesia.

Systemic effects of ophthalmic drugs

Some drugs used in ophthalmic patients may have significant systemic effects. These are discussed below and in Figure 19.17. Topical eye drops can be absorbed across the ocular, nasal or pharyngeal mucosa.

Phenylephrine

Phenylephrine is an alpha-1 adrenoceptor agonist. It is often administered topically before intraocular surgery to induce mydriasis, and intraoperatively to reduce conjunctival haemorrhage. Systemic absorption of phenylephrine can cause systemic vasoconstriction, hypertension and baroreceptor-mediated bradycardia (Herring et al., 2004). In one case report, a cat developed transient arrhythmias and systolic dysfunction following topical application of phenylephrine (Franci et al., 2011). The risk of these effects can be reduced by using a lower concentration of phenylephrine (2.5% rather than 10%) and by minimizing the volume applied. If hypertension and bradycardia occur after phenylephrine administration, an attempt can be made to counteract this by inducing vasodilation (e.g. by administering acepromazine or increasing the concentration of inhalant anaesthetic agent), but usually the effects resolve without treatment.

Topical phenylephrine should be avoided in animals with pre-existing hypertension or cardiac disease related to volume overload. In the author's experience, topical phenylephrine can cause blanching of the tongue and oral mucous membranes (Figure 19.18), which renders pulse oximetry readings inaccurate if measured at the tongue. It is therefore advisable to monitor pulse oximetry at an alternative site following phenylephrine administration.

Drug	Use	Route of administration	Adverse effects	Comments
Atropine (anticholinergic agent)	Mydriasis Paralysis of ciliary muscle	Topical	Tachycardia Salivation Vomiting (cats)	Tachycardia usually of little significance
Butylscopolamine (hyoscine) (anticholinergic agent)	Mydriasis Paralysis of ciliary muscle	Topical	Tachycardia	
Adrenaline (epinephrine) (alpha and beta adrenoceptor agonist)	Mydriasis Haemostasis for intraocular surgery	Intracameral injection	Tachycardia Hypertension Catecholamine-induced arrhythmias	Adverse effects rarely seen
Timolol (non-selective beta adrenoceptor agonist)	Treatment of glaucoma	Topical	Bradycardia Bronchospasm	Contraindications: bradyarrhythmias, heart failure, obstructive pulmonary disease
Carbachol (direct-acting cholinergic agonist)	Treatment of glaucoma Miosis after cataract surgery	Topical Intracameral injection	Bradycardia	
Pilocarpine (direct-acting cholinergic agonist)	Treatment of glaucoma	Topical	Bradycardia	
Acetylcholine (direct-acting cholinergic agonist)	Miosis after cataract surgery	Intracameral injection	Bradycardia	
Apraclonidine (alpha-2 adrenoceptor agonist)	Treatment of glaucoma	Topical	Bradycardia Hypotension Vomiting (cats)	Not used in cats
Brimonidine (alpha-2 adrenoceptor agonist)	Treatment of glaucoma	Topical	Bradycardia Hypotension	

19.17 Systemic effects of some topically or locally applied ophthalmic drugs.

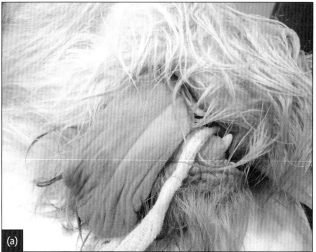
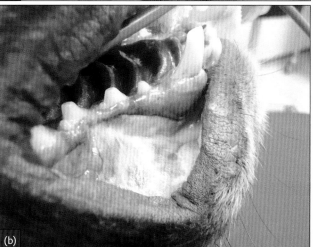

19.18 Blanching of (a) the tongue and (b) oral mucous membranes following ocular administration of phenylephrine drops.
(b, Courtesy of Fiona Scarlett, Animal Health Trust, Newmarket, UK)

Carbonic anhydrase inhibitors

These drugs are used to treat glaucoma by decreasing active secretion of aqueous humour. Inhibition of renal carbonic anhydrase causes decreased bicarbonate reabsorption and retention of chloride by the kidney, resulting in metabolic acidosis, hypokalaemia, hypocalcaemia and hyperchloraemia (Rose and Carter, 1979). Clinical signs of metabolic acidosis include depression, anorexia and hyperventilation (respiratory compensation for the metabolic acidosis). These effects are unlikely to be seen with topically administered drugs (e.g. dorzolamide or brinzolamide), but following oral administration (acetazolamide) the animal's acid–base and electrolyte status should be monitored, and administration of potassium-containing fluid therapy considered. Ideally, metabolic acidosis and electrolyte abnormalities should be corrected before the animal is anaesthetized, but this is difficult if administration of the carbonic anhydrase inhibitor has been continued up to the time of surgery. During anaesthesia, metabolic acidosis (if severe) may predispose to arrhythmias and hypotension. Since anaesthesia causes respiratory depression, the respiratory compensation (hyperventilation) that was present in the conscious patient will not occur, potentially worsening the acidaemia. IPPV may be necessary to normalize the blood pH, and monitoring of acid–base status during anaesthesia is recommended.

Mannitol

Mannitol is an osmotic diuretic used in the emergency management of glaucoma. It increases plasma osmolality and draws water from the eye across the blood–aqueous and blood–vitreous barriers, thus reducing IOP. The initial increase in plasma osmolality can increase blood volume and CVP before ultimately causing dehydration due to the osmotic diuretic effect. Mannitol is therefore contraindicated in animals with cardiac or renal disease and in dehydrated patients.

Ophthalmic effects of drugs used in the anaesthetic protocol

The effects of various anaesthetic, sedative and analgesic drugs on tear production and IOP have been discussed earlier in this chapter. Pupil size may also be influenced by sedative, anaesthetic, analgesic and related drugs. Mydriasis is required for most intraocular procedures but contraindicated for animals with glaucoma. The effects of anaesthesia-related drugs on pupil size do not seem to be clinically significant because different drug combinations and topical mydriatic agents are used before intraocular surgery.

Anticholinergic agents such as atropine and glycopyrronium may be given as part of pre-anaesthetic medication or during anaesthesia to prevent or treat bradycardia. They may also be used in combination with anticholinesterases to prevent bradycardia during antagonism of non-depolarizing NMBAs. When used topically, atropine causes mydriasis and increases IOP by decreasing aqueous outflow. It would be undesirable if parenterally administered atropine or glycopyrronium had the same effect. In one study, intramuscular injection of glycopyrronium at a dose of 10 μg/kg did not alter pupil size or IOP in dogs (Frischmeyer et al., 1993). The same study also found no association between anticholinergic administration and postoperative ocular hypertension in dogs with glaucoma. In humans, parenteral atropine and glycopyrronium have been shown not to affect pupil size or IOP (Cozanitis et al., 1979). Since glycopyrronium does not cross the blood–brain barrier as readily as atropine, it may be preferable to use glycopyrronium when treating bradycardia in patients where mydriasis may be detrimental.

Post-anaesthetic blindness in cats

Blindness in cats following general anaesthesia was poorly understood, and usually attributed to brain ischaemia resulting from anaesthesia-related hypoxaemia or cardiopulmonary depression. Recent research has shown that feline post-anaesthetic blindness is often associated with the use of mouth gags during anaesthesia. In cats, blood supply to the brain, retina and inner ear is provided by the maxillary artery, which passes around the caudal aspect of the mandible and can be compressed during mouth opening. In a retrospective study of 20 cases (Stiles et al., 2012), a mouth gag was used in 16 cases, one had undergone dental surgery without a mouth gag, and three cats had suffered cardiac arrest during anaesthesia. Another study used magnetic resonance imaging to demonstrate compression of the maxillary artery by the angular process of the mandible in some cats when the mouth was held open, resulting in interrupted blood flow (Barton-Lamb et al., 2013). It seems clear that feline post-anaesthetic blindness may sometimes result from brain ischaemia following cardiac arrest, but is more commonly attributable to the use of mouth gags and consequent compression of the maxillary artery. The use of mouth gags to achieve maximal mouth opening is not recommended in cats, and the duration of any procedures requiring wide opening of the mouth should be minimized.

Acknowledgements

The author would like to thank the AHT Comparative Ophthalmology Unit, Elvira Peeters, Emma Archer and Fiona Scarlett, all of the Animal Health Trust, Newmarket, for providing photographs.

References

Accola PJ, Bentley E, Smith LJ et al. (2006) Development of a retrobulbar injection technique for ocular surgery and analgesia in dogs. Journal of the American Veterinary Medical Association 229, 220–225

Ahn J, Jeong M, Lee E et al. (2013) Effects of peribulbar anesthesia (sub-Tenon injection of a local anesthetic) on akinesia of extraocular muscles, mydriasis, and intraoperative and postoperative analgesia in dogs undergoing phacoemulsification. American Journal of Veterinary Research 74, 1126–1132

Barrett PM, Scagliotti RH, Merideth RE, Jackson PA and Alarcon FL. (1991) Absolute corneal sensitivity and corneal trigeminal nerve anatomy in normal dogs. Progress in Veterinary and Comparative Ophthalmology 1, 245–254

Barton-Lamb AL, Martin-Flores M, Scrivani PV et al. (2013) Evaluation of maxillary arterial blood flow in anesthetized cats with the mouth closed and open. Veterinary Journal 196, 325–331

Biricik HS, Ceylan C and Sakar M (2004) Effects of pethidine and fentanyl on tear production in dogs. Veterinary Record 155, 564–565

Broadwater JJ, Schorling JJ, Herring IP, and Elvinger F (2008) Effect of body position on intraocular pressure in dogs without glaucoma. American Journal of Veterinary Research 69, 527–530

Chandler JA, van der Woerdt A, Prittie JE and Chang L (2013) Preliminary evaluation of tear production in dogs hospitalized in an intensive care unit. Journal of Veterinary Emergency and Critical Care 23, 274–279

Clutton RE, Boyd C, Richards DLS and Schwink K (1988) Significance of the oculocardiac reflex during ophthalmic surgery in the dog. Journal of Small Animal Practice 29, 573–579

Cozanitis DA, Dundee JW, Buchanan TA and Archer DB (1979) Atropine versus glycopyrrolate. A study of intraocular pressure and pupil size in man. Anaesthesia 34, 236–238

Dodam JR, Branson KR and Martin DD (1998) Effects of intramuscular sedative and opioid combinations on tear production in dogs. Veterinary Ophthalmology 1, 57–59

Franci P, Leece EA and McConnell JF (2011) Arrhythmias and transient changes in cardiac function after topical administration of one drop of phenylephrine 10% in an adult cat undergoing conjunctival graft. Veterinary Anaesthesia and Analgesia 38, 208–212

Frischmeyer KJ, Miller PE, Bellay Y, Smedes SL and Brunson DB (1993) Parenteral anticholinergics in dogs with normal and elevated intraocular pressure. Veterinary Surgery 22, 230–234

Giuliano EA (2004) Nonsteroidal anti-inflammatory drugs in veterinary ophthalmology. Veterinary Clinics of North America: Small Animal Practice 34, 707–723

Giuliano EA and Walsh KP (2013) The eye. In: Small Animal Regional Anesthesia and Analgesia, 1st edn, ed. L Campoy and MR Read, pp. 103–117. Wiley-Blackwell, Ames, Iowa

Hazra S, De D, Roy B et al. (2008) Use of ketamine, xylazine, and diazepam anesthesia with retrobulbar block for phacoemulsification in dogs. Veterinary Ophthalmology 11, 255–259

Herring IP (2013) Clinical pharmacology and therapeutics. In: Veterinary Ophthalmology, 5th edn, ed. KN Gelatt, BC Gilger and TJ Kern, pp. 423–434. Wiley, Ames, Iowa

Herring IP, Jacobson JD and Pickett JP (2004) Cardiovascular effects of topical ophthalmic 10% phenylephrine in dogs. Veterinary Ophthalmology 7, 41–46

Herring IP, Pickett JP, Champagne ES and Marini M (2000) Evaluation of aqueous tear production in dogs following general anesthesia. Journal of the American Animal Hospital Association 36, 427–430

Kafarnik C, Fritsche J and Reese S (2008) Corneal innervation in mesocephalic and brachycephalic dogs and cats: assessment using in vivo confocal microscopy. Veterinary Ophthalmology 11, 363–367

Kavalieratos CS and Dimou T (2008) Gabapentin therapy for painful, blind glaucomatous eye: case report. Pain Medicine 9, 377–378

Klein HE, Krohne SG, Moore GE, Mohamed AS and Stiles J (2011) Effect of eyelid manipulation and manual jugular compression on intraocular pressure measurement in dogs. Journal of the American Veterinary Medical Association 238, 1292–1295

Krohne SG, Blair MJ, Bingaman D and Gionfriddo JR (1998) Carprofen inhibition of flare in the dog measured by laser flare photometry. Veterinary Ophthalmology 1, 81–84

McMurphy RM, Davidson HJ and Hodgson DS (2004) Effects of atracurium on intraocular pressure, eye position, and blood pressure in eucapnic and hypocapnic isoflurane-anesthetized dogs. American Journal of Veterinary Research 65, 179–182

Mouney MC, Accola PJ, Cremer J *et al.* (2011) Effects of acepromazine maleate or morphine on tear production before, during, and after sevoflurane anesthesia in dogs. *American Journal of Veterinary Research* **72**, 1427–1430

Oel C, Gerhards H and Gehlen H (2014) Effect of retrobulbar nerve block on heart rate variability during enucleation in horses under general anesthesia. *Veterinary Ophthalmology* **17**, 170–174

Oliver JA and Bradbrook CA (2013) Suspected brainstem anesthesia following retrobulbar block in a cat. *Veterinary Ophthalmology* **16**, 225–228

Park SA, Park YW, Son WG *et al.* (2010) Evaluation of the analgesic effect of intracameral lidocaine hydrochloride injection on intraoperative and postoperative pain in healthy dogs undergoing phacoemulsification. *American Journal of Veterinary Research* **71**, 216–222

Pauli AM, Bentley E, Diehl KA and Miller PE (2006) Effects of the application of neck pressure by a collar or harness on intraocular pressure in dogs. *Journal of the American Animal Hospital Association* **42**, 207–211

Rauser P, Pfeifr J, Proks P and Stehlík L (2012) Effect of medetomidine-butorphanol and dexmedetomidine-butorphanol combinations on intraocular pressure in healthy dogs. *Veterinary Anaesthesia and Analgesia* **39**, 301–305

Rose RJ and Carter J (1979) Some physiological and biochemical effects of acetazolamide in the dog. *Journal of Veterinary Pharmacology and Therapeutics* **2**, 215–221

Roze M, Thomas E and Davot JL (1996) Tolfenamic acid in the control of ocular inflammation in the dog: pharmacokinetics and clinical results obtained in an experimental model. *Journal of Small Animal Practice* **37**, 371–375

Shilo-Benjamini Y, Pascoe PJ, Maggs DJ *et al.* (2013) Retrobulbar and peribulbar regional techniques in cats: a preliminary study in cadavers. *Veterinary Anaesthesia and Analgesia* **40**, 623–631

Singh J, Roy S, Mukherjee P *et al.* (2010) Influence of topical anesthetics on oculocardiac reflex and corneal healing in rabbits. *International Journal of Ophthalmology* **3**, 14–18

Smith LJ, Bentley E, Shih A and Miller PE (2004) Systemic lidocaine infusion as an analgesic for intraocular surgery in dogs: a pilot study. *Veterinary Anaesthesia and Analgesia* **31**, 53–63

Steinmetz A, Ellenberger K, März I, Ludewig E and Oechtering G (2012) Oculocardiac reflex in a dog caused by a choroidal melanoma with orbital extension. *Journal of the American Animal Hospital Association* **48**, 66–70

Stiles J, Weil AB, Packer RA and Lantz GC (2012) Post-anesthetic cortical blindness in cats: twenty cases. *Veterinary Journal* **193**, 367–373

Thomson SM, Oliver JA, Gould DJ *et al.* (2013) Preliminary investigations into the analgesic effects of topical ocular 1% morphine solution in dogs and cats. *Veterinary Anaesthesia and Analgesia* **40**, 632–640

Chapter 20

Dental and oral surgery

Lisa Milella and Matthew Gurney

With advanced techniques for dental and oral soft tissue surgery in cats and dogs, the challenge for the anaesthetist is to maintain patient safety while ensuring effective control of pain. This chapter describes the analgesia options for patients undergoing dental or oral surgery, discusses specific concerns relating to different patient groups and potential complications, and outlines factors for veterinary surgeons (veterinarians) to consider in relation to anaesthesia for both standard and more advanced procedures.

Analgesia

The spectrum of patients requiring dental or oral surgery is wide and includes, for example, the traumatized patient with a fractured jaw, the geriatric cat requiring multiple tooth extractions and the patient with oral neoplasia. Despite their varied presentations, these patients have a common requirement for adequate analgesia. Accurate identification of the cause of pain can be challenging in this group of patients because a thorough oral examination may be limited or impossible in the conscious animal. Excellent pain management is essential to help ensure good postoperative nutrition and rehabilitation.

There are no pain scales validated for the assessment of dental and oral pain in small animals (see Chapter 9). Overall patient evaluation (including, where possible, 'proxy' assessments made by the owner of the animal's feeding behaviour and demeanour) therefore plays an important role, both pre- and postoperatively. Pain scales have been adapted for such use (Aguiar et al., 2014).

Opioids and non-steroidal anti-inflammatory drugs (NSAIDs) are the most widely used analgesic agents in patients requiring dental or oral surgery. When combined using multimodal analgesia (MMA) techniques, these drugs are very effective for treating moderate to severe pain (Slingsby and Waterman-Pearson, 2001; Shih et al., 2008). Local anaesthetic agents (see also Chapter 11) prevent transmission of noxious stimuli to the central nervous system (CNS), reducing the requirement for additional intra- and postoperative systemic analgesics. Locoregional anaesthetic techniques can be used as part of an MMA approach and are effective when performed after induction of anaesthesia but before surgery commences. With the use of these techniques, less anaesthetic agent is required to maintain a surgical plane of anaesthesia (balanced anaesthesia), thus decreasing the risk of potential side effects, such as hypotension, produced by volatile agents. In a study evaluating maxillary and inferior alveolar blocks in cats, cats receiving nerve blocks had lower isoflurane requirements during the procedure and lower postoperative pain scores (Aguiar et al., 2014).

Locoregional anaesthetic techniques

The local anaesthetic agents most commonly used in veterinary dentistry belong to the aminoamide group; these include lidocaine, mepivacaine, bupivacaine and ropivacaine. Figure 20.1 shows the recommended doses of these agents. Dental cartridges containing either lidocaine with or without adrenaline (epinephrine), or bupivacaine (Figure 20.2) are available, but injection of a local anaesthetic drug by means of a syringe and needle is equally suitable. For dental patients, bupivacaine (0.2–0.5%) and lidocaine (1–2%) are the most useful concentrations to have available. Consider repeating locoregional nerve blockade postoperatively and before recovery from anaesthesia to improve patient comfort. There is increasing evidence that adding buprenorphine, tramadol or pethidine to the local anaesthetic may prolong duration of analgesia (see Chapter 11).

Bilateral or multiple nerve blocks are often required in these patients. The use of multiple blocks will have a bearing on the volume of agent that can be injected at each

Local anaesthetic agent	Total maximum dose (mg/kg)	Onset of action (minutes)	Duration of action (minutes)
Lidocaine	10 (dogs) 6 (cats)	2–5	60–120
Mepivacaine	10	2–5	90–180
Bupivacaine	2	5–10	180–480
Ropivacaine	3	5–10	180–480

20.1 Local anaesthetic agents used in dental and oral surgery in cats and dogs. The duration of action depends on the method of evaluation.

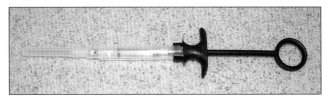

20.2 A dental cartridge containing local anaesthetic.

site, to avoid systemic toxicity. For the selected drug, the maximum safe dose should be calculated and the available volume divided by the number of nerve blocks planned. If there is insufficient volume to provide an effective block at all the sites (e.g. all four quadrants), the drug can be diluted with sterile saline to achieve the required volume. It is important to remember that, when using more than one local anaesthetic agent, toxicity is additive.

If the nerve block is successful, the patient should not react to surgical stimulus. If the patient does react, further analgesia should be provided: fentanyl (1–2 μg/kg i.v.) or ketamine (0.5 mg/kg i.v. or 1–2 mg/kg i.m.) are suitable for this purpose.

Potential complications of locoregional anaesthesia include nerve damage and intravascular injection (Aprea *et al*., 2011). The risk of nerve damage can be minimized by using a fine, short-bevel needle, and avoiding side-to-side movement during needle insertion. If the needle touches

bone, it should be withdrawn and replaced with a fresh needle to avoid the damaged tip snagging on tissue. When blocking a nerve within a bony canal, a smaller volume of anaesthetic agent should be used and injected more slowly, to avoid neuropraxia caused by excessive pressure on the nerve.

Penetration of a blood vessel is a common complication because large blood vessels run alongside the nerves in the neurovascular bundle. Using a fine needle as described above helps to reduce the risk of haematoma formation. The syringe should always be aspirated before injecting the agent to reduce the risk of intravascular injection. The choice of needle length will depend on patient size and the block to be performed.

Figures 20.3 and 20.4 illustrate the various nerve blocks that can be performed in cats and dogs undergoing dental or oral procedures. These blocks are described in turn below.

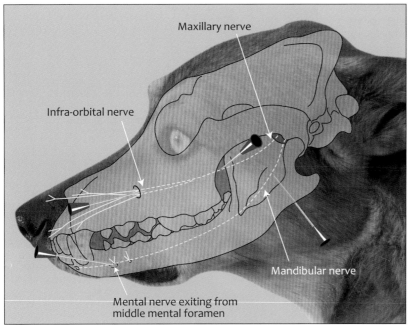

20.3 Diagram illustrating relevant nerves and needle positions for local anaesthetic blocks during dental and oral procedures in the dog.
(© Juliane Deubner, University of Saskatchewan, Canada)

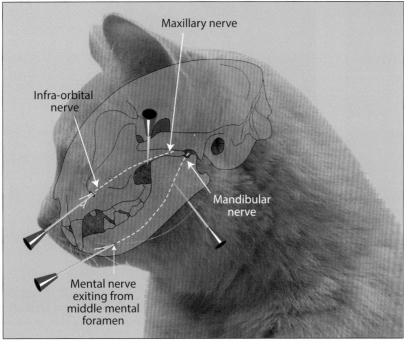

20.4 Diagram illustrating relevant nerves and needle positions for local anaesthetic blocks during dental and oral procedures in the cat.
(© Juliane Deubner, University of Saskatchewan, Canada)

Maxillary nerve block

Area desensitized: This block anaesthetizes the maxillary nerve as it enters the infraorbital canal through the caudal infraorbital foramen. The block produces anaesthesia of all the maxillary teeth, including the last molar, and the oral mucosa, buccal soft tissues and lip on the ipsilateral side.

Indications: Maxillary tooth removal, maxillectomy, mass excision, palate surgery.

Volume used: Maximum volume to inject depends on the individual patient, but approximately 1–2 ml.

Injection site: The block can be performed either intra- or extraorally. The extraoral approach is the preferred method: the needle is inserted below the cranioventral border of the zygomatic arch, between the caudal border of the maxilla and the cranial border of the mandibular ramus (Figures 20.5 and 20.6). Palpating the position of the last molar helps to gauge where to insert the needle. The needle is advanced from this point, parallel to the plane of the hard palate and 1 cm caudal to the lateral canthus. The needle is directed into the pterygopalatine fossa as indicated until bone is contacted. The syringe should then be aspirated before performing the injection.

For the intraoral approach, the needle is inserted behind the last molar, slightly palatal (caudomedial) to the tooth, and advanced at a slight rostral angle towards the caudal infraorbital foramen (Figure 20.7). The nerve may also be approached via the infraorbital canal using an intravenous catheter. When using this approach compared

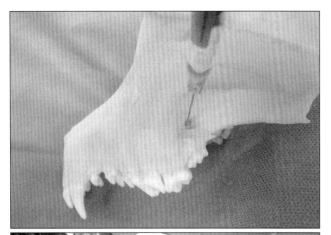

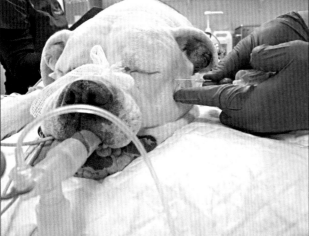

20.5 Extraoral approach for the maxillary nerve block in the dog.

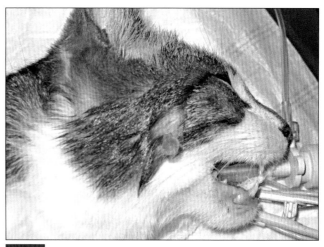

20.6 Extraoral approach for the maxillary nerve block in the cat.

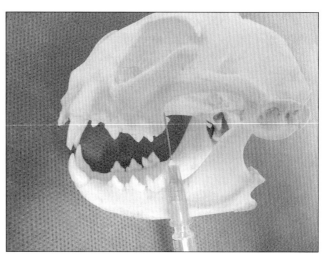

20.7 Intraoral approach for the maxillary nerve block in the cat.

with the extraoral approach in a cadaver study the accuracy of nerve staining was improved and there was no evidence of macroscopic damage (Viscasillas *et al.*, 2013).

Caution: Trauma to the venous plexus in the pterygopalatine fossa can cause haemorrhage. With the intraoral approach in cats catastrophic penetration of the globe is reported (Perry *et al.*, 2015).

Infraorbital nerve block

Area desensitized: At the point of emergence from the infraorbital canal, the maxillary nerve becomes the infraorbital nerve, which provides sensory innervation to the oral mucosa and upper lip rostral to the rostral infraorbital foramen. Deposition of local anaesthetic agent on the nerve as it leaves the infraorbital canal will not anaesthetize the teeth rostral to the foramen. If dental anaesthesia is required, the needle must be inserted into the infraorbital canal, which may cause nerve damage if poor technique is used. A maxillary nerve block may therefore be preferred. If an infraorbital nerve block is to be performed, a 27G needle should be used and care taken not to move the needle excessively.

Indications: Tooth removal, mass excision, surgery of the nostrils.

Volume used: Maximum volume to inject is approximately 0.5–1 ml.

Injection site: The infraorbital nerve exits from the infraorbital foramen, which can be palpated just dorsal to the third premolar, approximately halfway between the zygomatic arch and the root of the canine tooth (Figures 20.8, 20.9). An arterial pulse is often visible intraorally at the foramen. The injection can be made percutaneously but it is more commonly performed intraorally, where it is easier to palpate landmarks. The needle is inserted into the

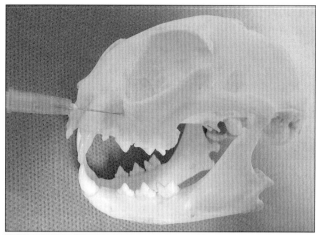

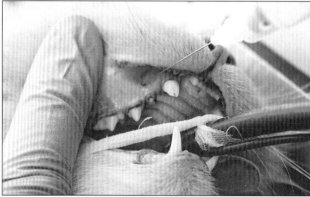

<table><tr><td>**20.9**</td><td>Approach for the infraorbital nerve block in the cat.</td></tr></table>

infraorbital canal through the foramen and advanced caudally, with the needle parallel to the long axis of the maxilla. In cats and brachycephalic dogs, the rostrocaudal dimension of the canal may only be a few millimetres in length, and inserting the needle too far into the canal may result in penetration of the globe. The tip of the needle should be advanced to the point where an imaginary line parallel to the infraorbital canal and a second, perpendicular imaginary line drawn to the lateral canthus transect. The needle should always be pre-measured against the canal before insertion, and the syringe aspirated before injection. There should be no resistance during the injection. A small volume of agent should be used, and injected at low pressure, to avoid neuropraxia. After performing the injection, a finger should be placed and held over the rostral foramen for about 30 seconds to allow the agent to remain *in situ* and to take effect.

Palatine nerve block

Area desensitized: The mucosa of the hard palate. An alternative is a maxillary nerve block.

Indications: Palate surgery. Note that the teeth are not anaesthetized.

Volume used: Maximum volume to inject is approximately 0.1–0.3 ml with a 1 ml syringe.

Injection site: The major palatine nerve runs with the palatine artery to supply the mucosa of the hard palate; it exits the major palatine foramen (this is difficult to palpate because of the thick soft tissue of the palate). Inject halfway between the midline of the palate and the dental arcade at the level of the fourth premolar (Figure 20.10).

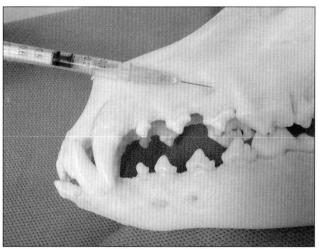

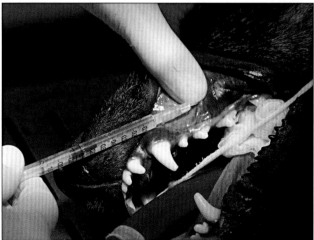

<table><tr><td>**20.8**</td><td>Approach for the infraorbital nerve block in the dog.</td></tr></table>

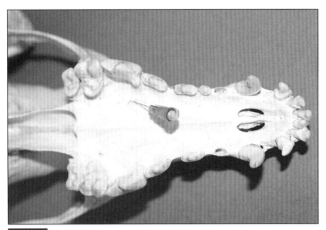

20.10 Approach for the palatine nerve block in the dog.

Caution: Risk of penetrating the artery, and haematoma formation.

Inferior alveolar (mandibular) nerve block

Area desensitized: Hard and soft tissues of the ipsilateral mandible. The mandibular nerve enters the mandible at the level of the mandibular foramen. The nerve divides into three branches: the lingual nerve, the inferior alveolar nerve (the target of this block) and the mylohyoid nerve. If the anaesthetic agent is deposited too far medially and caudally, the lingual and mylohyoid branches may also be affected, which may cause complications arising from loss of sensation to the tongue.

Indications: Mandibular tooth removal, mandibulectomy, mass excision.

Volume used: Maximum volume to inject is approximately 0.5–1.0 ml.

Injection site: The block can be performed either intra- or extraorally. With either approach, the mandibular foramen is palpated on the lingual aspect of the mandible, caudal and ventral to the last molar. It is not always possible to feel the foramen itself but usually the neurovascular bundle can be felt as a soft, string-like structure.

When injecting intraorally, the nerve or foramen is palpated with one hand while the syringe is held in the other hand (Figure 20.11). The needle is advanced in a caudal direction, underneath the mucosa, with the bevel

of the needle positioned towards the bone, to the position of the neurovascular bundle. This is a difficult technique due to limited space, and the extraoral approach is often easier.

For the extraoral approach, the neurovascular bundle is located in the same way as in the intraoral approach. The needle is inserted extraorally, perpendicular and just medial to the body of the mandible, with the bevel facing the mandible (Figure 20.12). In the dog, a useful landmark for this technique is the depression on the caudal border of the ventral mandible (the mandibular notch). The foramen can also be located halfway along an imaginary line drawn between the last molar and the angular process of the mandible. A sufficient volume should be injected to surround the nerve, which is often obvious with direct palpation of the neurovascular bundle during injection.

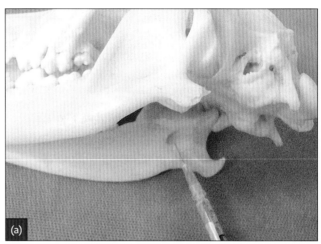

(a)

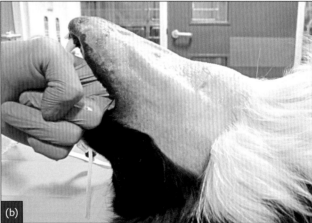

(b)

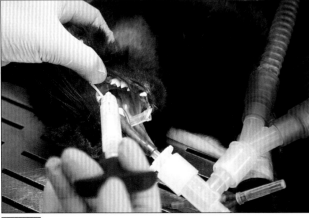

20.11 Intraoral approach for the mandibular nerve block in a cat.

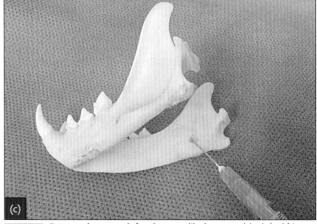

(c)

20.12 Extraoral approach for the mandibular nerve block (a–b) in the dog and (c) in the cat.

Mental nerve block

Area desensitized: When performing this block, superficial injection will anaesthetize the buccal soft tissues and lower lip rostral to the middle mental foramen. If the needle is introduced into the foramen and advanced caudally into the canal, then sensation to the canine and incisor teeth may be blocked; this can be difficult in smaller patients. Care must be taken not to damage the neurovascular bundle when inserting the needle into the canal. The preferred technique is to perform an inferior alveolar (mandibular) block to achieve anaesthesia for the mandibular teeth.

Volume used: Maximum volume to inject is approximately 0.2–0.5 ml with a 1 ml syringe.

Injection site: The middle mental foramen can be palpated through the lip frenulum just rostral to the second premolar, in the upper third area of the mandible (Figure 20.13) Local anaesthetic can be injected at the foramen. The needle can also be introduced carefully into the canal from a rostral to caudal direction and the agent injected slowly. However, in cats and small dogs the canal is often too small to allow insertion of a needle.

Splash block

This term refers to direct application of local anaesthetic agent to the surgical site before closure of the wound. A detailed description of this technique can be found in Chapter 11.

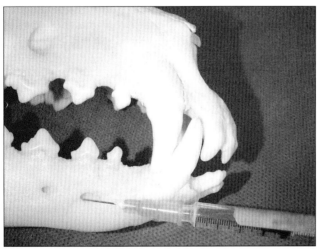

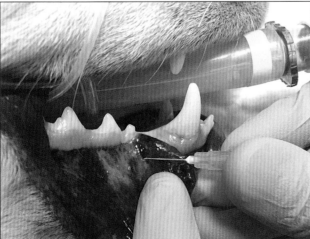

20.13 Approach for the mental nerve block in the dog.

Infiltration anaesthesia

Infiltration anaesthesia can be performed by injection of a local anaesthetic agent into the oral mucosa near the tooth apex. However, this technique is thought to be less effective in cats and dogs compared with humans, as the bone density is much greater in animals.

Intrapulpal injection

If an animal requires dental pulp surgery, the pulp is generally inflamed, which renders this technique ineffective; an appropriate regional block is preferable.

Considerations for different patient groups

Geriatric patients

Owing to the relationship between increasing age and the progression of periodontal and dental diseases, as well as the higher risk of oral neoplasia, geriatric patients often require dental or oral surgery. There is a clear association between age and anaesthetic-related mortality in cats. Geriatric animals may have a low body condition score, and these patients have a higher incidence of concurrent disease. Further information on considerations for geriatric patients can be found in Chapter 30.

Young patients

Young animals may present with cleft palate and dental malocclusions. Palate repair is often delayed until 8–12 weeks of age. Considerations for puppies and kittens include fasting times, maintenance of body temperature and management of blood loss. The reader is referred to Chapters 18 and 30 for further information.

Limited oral opening and airway access

Temporomandibular joint disorders limit oral opening to varying degrees, which makes orotracheal intubation more difficult and sometimes even impossible. Endotracheal tubes (ETTs) can be placed blindly but this technique is not always reliable. Correct placement of the tube always needs to be checked carefully, preferably with the use of capnography. If there is sufficient gape, a small endoscope or, if the opening allows, a laryngoscope can be used to guide an ETT (with or without stylet) into position. Alternatively, the stylet can be placed into the trachea first and the ETT then passed over the stylet (Figure 20.14). A small-diameter endoscope can also be used for this purpose, with the ETT being positioned on the endoscope before it is inserted into the trachea. The ETT is then pushed off the endoscope into position in the trachea. If all other techniques are impossible, a tracheotomy may be required.

Full mouth extractions

With patients requiring a full mouth extraction, careful planning is necessary to ensure provision of excellent analgesia, including the use of locoregional anaesthetic techniques, opioids and NSAIDs (where appropriate). Close attention should be paid to pain assessment. Nutritional support is essential and feeding tube placement is sometimes beneficial.

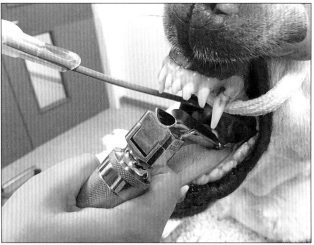

20.14 For difficult endotracheal intubations, a stylet can be used to guide the endotracheal tube into the trachea.

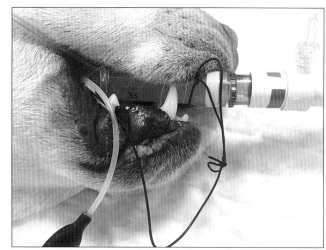

20.15 End of a pharyngeal throat pack secured to the endotracheal tube.

Malnutrition

Chronic dental disease may compromise an animal's nutritional intake, and this is likely to increase the patient's anaesthetic risk. In patients that require extensive dental or oral surgery, it is preferable to place an oesophagostomy feeding tube (necessitating a short anaesthetic period) first, so that nutrition can be optimized and the surgery scheduled for a later date.

Systemic disease

Dental disease may be a manifestation of systemic disease. Examples include patients with diabetes mellitus (see Chapter 27) or renal failure (see Chapter 25).

Secretions

Animals with dental or oral disease may exhibit drooling, dysphagia and oral bleeding. Swabs, cotton buds and a laryngoscope are useful aids for intubation of these patients. Animals with an oronasal fistula may have concurrent rhinitis; these patients are at risk of acquiring aspiration pneumonia or may already have this condition.

Procedural considerations

Airway management

Cuffed ETTs will prevent gross debris entering the airway, but do not prevent all liquid tracking down the trachea. It is important to position the patient in a way that minimizes the risk of fluid aspiration. Care should be taken to avoid fluid running back into the pharynx when the patient is turned, and a pharyngeal pack should always be used. The packing often becomes saturated during surgery, and will need to be changed or squeezed out frequently to avoid seepage of liquid into the airway. If the pharynx is packed too tightly, lingual blood flow may become compromised. The pharyngeal pack can be tied to the ETT so that it is not accidentally left *in situ* at the end of the procedure (Figure 20.15). Alternatively, conforming bandage can be used as packing, leaving a 'tail' of bandage outside the mouth.

Care should be taken when inflating the ETT cuff, especially in cats, as overinflation can cause tracheal

rupture (Hardie *et al.*, 1999). Always disconnect the ETT from the breathing system when turning anaesthetized animals to avoid causing tracheal trauma. Supraglottic airway devices (see Chapter 5) may not provide an adequate seal for dental and oral procedures and additionally may become dislodged, so their use is not recommended for these patients.

Capnography is valuable in ensuring that the airway is patent. The presence of a normal capnogram confirms correct tracheal intubation. This is useful not only immediately after intubation to confirm correct placement, but also during maintenance of anaesthesia to check that the ETT has not become kinked, obstructed, disconnected or removed (see Chapter 7).

Assessment of jaw occlusion is required in the course of certain orthodontic procedures, as well as for jaw fracture repair; however, this assessment is difficult with an ETT in place. Several options are available to provide suitable conditions to assess jaw occlusion:

- Removal of the ETT. This is not ideal because of the risk of debris entering the larynx and trachea, and laryngeal trauma may occur with re-intubation. This is therefore the least desirable option
- Intubation via a pharyngotomy. Use an armoured (wire-reinforced) ETT that will not kink when the tube is bent into position (see Chapter 22)
- Use of a short ETT with an adaptor that fits on to the breathing system end of the tube, thus lengthening the tube. The adaptor is attached to the tube just behind the incisors. It can then be removed (and the more caudal part of the ETT remains intraorally) while jaw occlusion is assessed (Figure 20.16). This is a straightforward technique; however, care must be taken when manipulating the patient's head to avoid accidental disconnection of the adaptor. In addition, when the adaptor is disconnected, it is important to ensure that there is no obstruction of the caudal part of the ETT when the mouth is closed. Adequate scavenging of waste anaesthetic gases is difficult with this technique.

When using cuffed ETTs:

- Check the cuff security before use – deflation of the cuff during the surgery risks aspiration

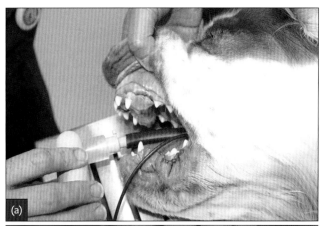

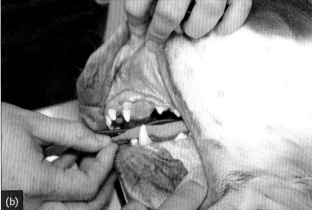

20.16 (a) An adaptor attached to the end of a short endotracheal tube enables assessment of jaw occlusion without the need for extubation. (b) For assessment of jaw occlusion, the adaptor is temporarily removed.

- Using a length of drip tubing to secure the ETT (Figure 20.17) prevents the wicking of blood and fluid that occurs with open-weave bandage (Figure 20.18). Care should be taken to prevent the end of the tubing irritating the eyes
- Always check and clean the oropharynx after removing the pharyngeal pack, using a laryngoscope if necessary, *before* deflating the cuff of the ETT. It is useful to have some form of indicator or reminder to check the oropharynx before extubation.

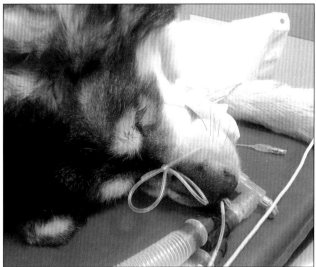

20.17 A length of drip tubing used to secure the endotracheal tube. (Courtesy of Marieke de Vries, Davies Veterinary Specialists, Higham Gobion, UK)

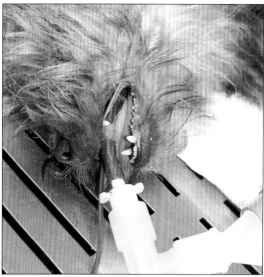

20.18 Open-weave bandage used to secure the endotracheal tube, soaked with blood and fluid.

Preoxygenation for anticipated difficult intubation

Preoxygenation provides a reservoir of oxygen in the lungs should problems arise during endotracheal intubation. The recommended 'gold standard' for preoxygenation is 3–5 minutes of 100% oxygen via a tight-fitting facemask. If the patient does not tolerate the facemask, the diaphragm of the mask can be removed or a 'flow-by' technique can be used.

Duration of procedure

Careful planning is particularly important with long procedures. Analgesia, management of body temperature and patient positioning are priorities.

Diagnostic imaging

During radiography, the patient's position is often changed to enable different projections and care must be taken to ensure that the ETT does not become accidentally disconnected. Movement of the ETT may result in tracheal trauma, and temporary disconnection of the ETT from the breathing system is recommended when changing the patient's body position. If the radiographic examination is prolonged, there is a risk that the patient may lose significant body heat.

Haemorrhage

Blood loss should be anticipated with surgical procedures of the head, especially maxillectomy and mandibulectomy. Iatrogenic damage to the palatine arteries is also a risk with some dental and oral procedures.

Certain breeds or patient groups are predisposed to coagulopathies. These patients should undergo assessment of their coagulation profile before surgery: for example a buccal mucosal bleeding time should be performed in Dobermanns before dental extractions. Methods available for assessing blood loss are discussed in Chapter 18.

Hypothermia

Heat loss will start at the time of pre-anaesthetic medication, when the patient's ability to compensate for heat loss becomes reduced. Body temperature initially falls rapidly and then more slowly in a biphasic manner, reaches a plateau, and eventually rises again in response to the supply of external heat during and after the procedure. Temperature management is an essential part of management of all patients, but special attention should be paid to small, young, geriatric, thin or malnourished animals. Heat loss is potentially greater in dental and oral surgery patients as the mouth is open throughout the procedure, and irrigation water used to cool surgical instruments will also cool the patient. Further details on the prevention and management of hypothermia can be found in Chapter 3.

Use of mouth gags in cats

Spring-held mouth gags can cause cerebral ischaemia and blindness in cats, and their use should be avoided (Stiles *et al.*, 2012; see also Chapter 19). This risk may be compounded by the presence of hypotension and hypoxaemia. The blood supply to the brain in cats is mainly derived from the maxillary artery and it is thought that the extended gag affects flow in this artery. Gags can also cause damage to the teeth, especially if the plane of anaesthesia is inadequate and the animal begins to make chewing movements. Alternative methods, such as using needle caps cut to an appropriate size, should be considered to reduce the force with which the jaw is held open (Figure 20.19).

Pharyngeal stimulation

For procedures involving the pharyngeal area, it is necessary to suppress the gag reflex. This requires an adequate plane of anaesthesia, which is best achieved by using a balanced anaesthetic technique using systemic analgesic drugs and a volatile agent. Neuromuscular blockade may also be appropriate in these circumstances (provided the depth of anaesthesia is confirmed as adequate) as long as intermittent positive pressure ventilation can be provided and the extent of neuromuscular block can be correctly monitored (see Chapter 16). Topical application of a local anaesthetic agent such as lidocaine spray may also be useful in some cases.

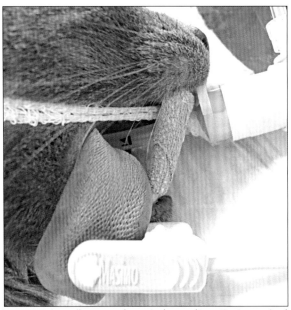

20.19 A needle cap used as a single-use alternative to a spring-held mouth gag to avoid overextension of the jaws.

Soft tissue swelling

Swelling of soft tissues may occur following, for example, tonsillar or lingual surgery. Close monitoring of the patient after extubation of the trachea is important, and equipment and drugs for re-intubation should be available during this high-risk period. Some veterinary surgeons choose to administer corticosteroids to limit inflammation; this precludes the use of NSAIDs for analgesia.

Post-anaesthetic deafness

This has been reported as a complication following dental and ear-cleaning procedures in cats and dogs. Of 62 cases reported, 43 occurred after dental procedures. Geriatric animals were more likely to be affected; no other associations that might indicate risk factors were found. Deafness was permanent (Stevens-Sparks and Strain, 2010).

Patient monitoring

Patient monitoring is covered in detail in Chapter 7. Monitoring equipment is especially useful where access to the patient's head is reduced. A pulse oximeter probe placed on the tongue is likely to be difficult to keep in position if access to the tongue is impeded. Motion during the surgical procedure will affect the accuracy of pulse oximetry; this can be minimized by using modern devices with signal extraction technology, which helps to reduce motion artefact (Shah *et al.*, 2012). If the tongue is inaccessible, some pulse oximeters will work well when applied to non-pigmented skin, toe web, prepuce or vulva.

Pain scoring

Pain should be assessed before the procedure, to help ensure that optimal perioperative analgesia is provided. Pain assessment should be continued postoperatively for as long as deemed necessary. The patient's owners should be encouraged to assess pain in their pet at home (see Chapter 9).

Anaesthesia for routine dentistry

Pre-anaesthetic physical examination

Provided no abnormalities are found on thorough physical examination or in the patient's history, pre-anaesthetic blood testing may be unnecessary. The animal should be examined for dental/oral pain and the ability to open the mouth should be verified. Further details of pre-anaesthetic assessment can be found in Chapter 2.

Pre-anaesthetic medication

Opioid analgesia should form the basis of pre-anaesthetic medication for patients scheduled for dental or oral surgery. Depending on the health status of the patient, opioids can be combined with acepromazine or medetomidine/dexmedetomidine to improve sedation. Drugs that commonly cause salivation, nausea and vomiting may be undesirable for these patients. Nausea and vomiting are common with morphine and hydromorphone, although their occurrence can be reduced by prior administration of acepromazine. Excessive salivation is a rare effect of methadone. Although anticholinergic agents reduce salivation, they are rarely used nowadays as part of pre-anaesthetic medication. See Chapter 13 for further details of pre-anaesthetic medication.

Induction

Choice of anaesthetic induction agent will depend on the clinician's preference and patient status. Both propofol and alfaxalone produce smooth induction of anaesthesia in healthy cats and dogs. Induction using a facemask is not recommended. A laryngoscope with a blade of suitable length should be used to visualize the larynx and facilitate endotracheal intubation, which is mandatory for every dental/oral procedure.

It is important to allow sufficient time for the patient to reach an adequate depth of anaesthesia before starting the oral examination, as stimulation of the gag reflex may induce regurgitation if the animal is too lightly anaesthetized.

Maintenance

Either isoflurane or sevoflurane are suitable options for maintenance of anaesthesia. The most appropriate breathing system for the patient should be selected, with the aim of using the lowest fresh gas flow to minimize heat loss. A heat and moisture exchanger can be used to conserve heat. Analgesic agents should be used as part of a balanced anaesthetic technique, so reducing the concentration of volatile agent needed for maintenance. Intravenous fluids should be administered to ensure adequate circulating blood volume and to support arterial blood pressure. Intravenous access should be maintained throughout the period of anaesthesia.

The recovery period

Ensure that pharyngeal packs are removed and the pharynx is clear before extubation of the trachea. Cats and dogs recovering from anaesthesia should be constantly monitored until they are able to lift the head, and their body temperature is above 35°C. In the early recovery period, attention should be directed towards analgesia, airway protection and patency, fluid therapy and temperature management.

Once the patient has been transferred from the recovery area to the ward, attention should focus on fluid intake (adjust intravenous fluids accordingly) and nutritional support. Pain assessment should be conducted regularly, based on the duration of action of analgesic drugs already being administered.

Anaesthesia for advanced dentistry

In addition to the above considerations for routine dentistry, the following problems should also be considered when planning more advanced dental procedures:

- If the animal is malnourished, attending to nutrition may be necessary before proceeding with dental work. An

American Society of Anesthesiologists (ASA) physical status score of 3 or higher suggests that the patient requires further stabilization before anaesthesia for elective procedures (see Chapter 2)
- A patient in poor body condition because of dental disease may not tolerate intramuscular or subcutaneous injections
- If a long procedure is planned, a repeat dose of opioid should be scheduled according to the duration of action of the drug
- Extensive dental procedures require excellent analgesia. A combination of opioids and locoregional anaesthetic techniques permits maintenance of anaesthesia with a lower concentration of volatile agent (i.e. balanced anaesthesia). Consider using infusions of analgesic drugs to optimize analgesia. In the authors' experience, infusions of either propofol or alfaxalone for maintenance of anaesthesia are suboptimal compared with the use of volatile agents, as intravenous agents tend not to suppress the gag reflex, require concurrent use of opioid or alpha-2 adrenoceptor agonist infusions and prolong recovery from anaesthesia
- Patients may require longer intensive nursing compared with patients undergoing minor dental procedures, and sometimes placement of a feeding tube is required to ensure adequate nutrition after the procedure.

Anaesthesia for oral soft tissue surgery

The principles discussed for routine and advanced dentistry can be applied to anaesthesia for oral soft tissue surgery. In addition:

- If blood loss is anticipated during surgery, baseline laboratory assessment of hydration (packed cell volume, total proteins, urea, creatinine and electrolytes) should be performed in conjunction with clinical assessment of hydration status. Consideration should be given to optimizing the patient's intravascular volume status before surgery (see also Chapter 18)
- If oral neoplasia or a foreign body is suspected, which may make tracheal intubation difficult, mild sedation should be provided as pre-anaesthetic medication. The animal should be observed constantly during this period and intravenous access secured. The choice of opioids should be based on the anticipated level of analgesia required
- Induction of anaesthesia should be swift. A plan should be made in advance in case orotracheal intubation cannot be achieved (see above). Preoxygenation is recommended (see Chapter 22)
- Consideration should be given to a balanced anaesthesia technique employing MMA.

References and further reading

Aguiar J, Chebroux A, Martinez-Taboada F and Leece EA (2014) Analgesic effects of maxillary and inferior alveolar nerve blocks in cats undergoing dental extractions. *Journal of Feline Medicine & Surgery* **17**, 110–116

Aprea F, Vettorato E and Corletto F (2011) Severe cardiovascular depression in a cat following a mandibular nerve block with bupivacaine. *Veterinary Anaesthesia and Analgesia* **38**, 614–618

Brodbelt DC, Pfeiffer DU, Young LE and Wood JL (2007) Risk factors for anaesthetic-related death in cats: results from the confidential enquiry into perioperative small animal fatalities (CEPSAF). *British Journal of Anaesthesia* **99**, 617–623

Brown DC, Bernier N, Shofer F, Steinberg SA and Perkowski SZ (2002) Use of noninvasive dental dolorimetry to evaluate analgesic effects of intravenous and intrathecal administration of morphine in anesthetized dogs. *American Journal of Veterinary Research* **63**, 1349–1353

Gross ME, Pope ER, Jarboe JM *et al.* (2000) Regional anesthesia of the infraorbital and inferior alveolar nerves during noninvasive tooth pulp stimulation in halothane-anesthetized cats. *American Journal of Veterinary Research* **61**, 1245–1247

Hardie EM, Spodnick GJ, Gilson SD, Benson JA and Hawkins EC (1999) Tracheal rupture in cats: 16 cases (1983–1998). *Journal of the American Veterinary Medical Association* **214**, 508–512

Krug W and Losey J (2011) Area of desensitization following mental nerve block in dogs. *Journal of Veterinary Dentistry* **28**, 146–150

Lantz GC (2003) Regional anesthesia for dentistry and oral surgery. *Journal of Veterinary Dentistry* **20**, 181–186

Perry R, Moore D and Scurrell E (2015) Globe penetration in a cat following maxillary nerve block for dental surgery. *Journal of Feline Medicine and Surgery* **17**, 66–72

Shah N, Ragaswamy HB, Govindugari K and Estanol L (2012) Performance of three new-generation pulse oximeters during motion and low perfusion in volunteers. *Journal of Clinical Anaesthesia* **24**, 385–391

Shih AC, Robertson S, Isaza N, Pablo L and Davies W (2008) Comparison between analgesic effects of buprenorphine, carprofen, and buprenorphine with carprofen for canine ovariohysterectomy. *Veterinary Anaesthesia and Analgesia* **35**, 69–79

Slingsby LS and Waterman-Pearson AE (2001) Analgesic effects in dogs of carprofen and pethidine together compared with the effects of either drug alone. *Veterinary Record* **148**, 441–444

Stepaniuk K and Brock N (2008) Hypothermia and thermoregulation during anesthesia for the dental and oral surgery patient. *Journal of Veterinary Dentistry* **25**, 279–283

Stevens-Sparks CK and Strain GM (2010) Post-anaesthesia deafness in dogs and cats following dental and ear cleaning procedures. *Veterinary Anaesthesia and Analgesia* **37**, 347–351

Stiles J, Weil AB, Packer RA and Lantz GC (2012) Post-anesthetic cortical blindness in cats: twenty cases. *Veterinary Journal* **193**, 367–373

Viscasillas J, Seymour CJ, Brodbelt DC (2013) A cadaver study comparing two approaches for performing maxillary nerve block in dogs. *Veterinary Anaesthesia and Analgesia* **40**, 212–219

Woodward TM (2008) Pain management and regional anesthesia for the dental patient. *Topics in Companion Animal Medicine* **23**, 106–114

Chapter 21

Cardiovascular disease

Rebecca Robinson and Kieran Borgeat

The cardiovascular system circulates blood throughout the body, delivering oxygen and nutrients to the tissues and removing waste products, including carbon dioxide. The pulmonary and systemic circulations are arranged in parallel, with approximately 75% of total blood volume in the systemic vasculature. At rest, the majority of the blood is situated within capacitance veins.

Cardiac output (CO; usually expressed in ml/min) is defined as the volume of blood ejected by either the left ventricle (LV) or the right ventricle (RV) per minute. In healthy animals, the cardiovascular system has a large functional reserve and is able to increase CO by up to five times in response to exercise. Direct measurement of CO is technically challenging and rarely used in the clinical setting. However, it is possible to estimate stroke volume (SV; the volume of blood ejected during each cardiac cycle)

by using echocardiography and then calculate CO by multiplying SV (ml) by heart rate (HR; beats/min). For most clinicians, simply considering the factors that influence HR and SV is sufficient to estimate the effect of a particular cardiovascular disease on a patient's CO.

Patients with clinical signs of cardiovascular disease almost invariably have reduced SV, leading to reduced CO despite compensatory physiological mechanisms. Neurohumoral activation, a system that evolved to maintain circulating volume in the face of acute trauma or blood loss, becomes maladaptive in the long term. Chronic activation of the sympathetic nervous system and renin–angiotensin–aldosterone system (RAAS) leads to tachycardia, vasoconstriction, increased extracellular fluid volume, and myocardial remodelling and dysfunction (Figure 21.1).

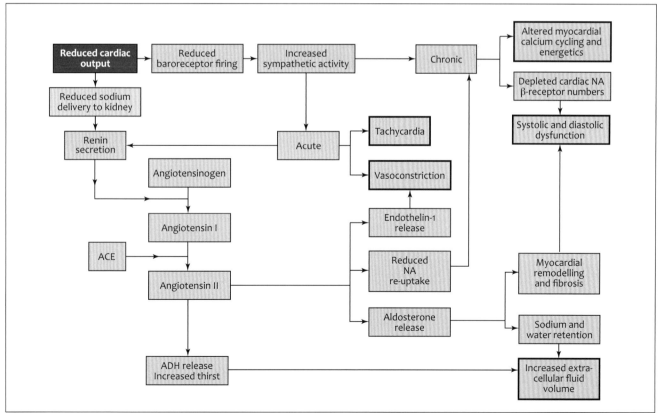

21.1 Flow diagram to illustrate the pathophysiology of congestive heart failure. ACE = angiotensin-converting enzyme; ADH = antidiuretic hormone; NA = noradrenaline (norepinephrine).

Since most anaesthetic agents have effects on autonomic function, vascular tone, HR and myocardial contractility, careful anaesthetic planning is vital before general anaesthesia of patients with cardiovascular disease. A considered approach allows the veterinary surgeon (veterinarian) to select anaesthetic agents that balance the haemodynamic effects of a particular disease, rather than exacerbate them, and to prepare for potential adverse effects. Further details on the autonomic control of the circulation, CO, arterial blood pressure (ABP) and perfusion are provided in Chapter 17.

Systemic considerations in cardiovascular disease

The risks of congestive heart failure (CHF), poor CO and arrhythmias caused by primary cardiovascular disease should be considered before anaesthesia of these patients, as should the chronic effects of cardiovascular disease on other organs. Reduced CO and systemic vasoconstriction lead to a reduced glomerular filtration rate (GFR), which has been associated with increased mortality in human patients with heart failure. Renal insufficiency should be considered in patients with cardiovascular disease, but many animals also have a prerenal azotaemia, which may make the clinical picture less clear. The most useful (albeit insensitive) way to assess GFR clinically is by evaluating routine biochemistry and urine specific gravity. It is impossible, however, to reliably assess urine specific gravity in a patient receiving diuretic treatment, and diuretics may also contribute to a degree of azotaemia. Reduced GFR also affects the pharmacokinetics of renally excreted drugs and leads to prolonged duration of action.

In addition, hepatic congestion due to right-sided CHF may slow the metabolism of drugs by the liver (Figure 21.2).

Circulating noradrenaline (norepinephrine), angiotensin II, aldosterone, antidiuretic hormone (vasopressin) and natriuretic peptides are increased in patients with heart failure. Extracellular fluid volume is also increased and, in extreme cases, hypoalbuminaemia and hyponatraemia may occur due to a dilutional effect. For highly protein-bound drugs, hypoproteinaemia may result in an increased proportion of free, active drug. Neurohumoral activation leads to a proinflammatory state, with increased expression of many inflammatory cytokines, including interleukins (IL-1 and IL-6), and tumour necrosis factor-alpha. In some patients (especially cats), there may be a tendency towards hypercoagulability and a risk of thromboembolism associated with altered haemodynamics during anaesthesia. Patients with advanced heart disease may develop cardiac cachexia, a syndrome that results in a negative energy balance and a loss of lean body mass (Figure 21.3). This is due partly to the proinflammatory state but also to inappetence and malabsorption. The doses of anaesthetic agents administered to patients with significant fluid retention (especially ascites) and/or cachexia should be carefully calculated based on an estimation of lean body mass made by use of body condition and muscle mass scoring systems. Validated World Small Animal Veterinary Association guidelines for condition scoring are available online at www.wsava.org/nutrition-toolkit.

Systemic disease may also have secondary effects on the heart. Cardiac effects of common systemic diseases should be considered when planning to anaesthetize patients with endocrinopathies, gastric dilatation–volvulus (GDV), systemic or pulmonary hypertension (PHT), or conditions that significantly alter blood viscosity (Figure 21.4; see also Chapters 24 and 27).

Parameter	Pathological change due to cardiovascular disease	Overall effect	Practical considerations
Absorption	Poor peripheral perfusion due to reduced cardiac output	Reduced absorption of drugs when administered i.m. or s.c.	Be prepared for a longer onset time and less predictable effects of drugs when administered i.m. or s.c.
	Reduced cardiac output	Alveolar concentrations of volatile anaesthetics increase faster, leading to more rapid alterations in depth of anaesthesia	Greater attention should be paid to vaporizer settings and resultant depth of anaesthesia
Distribution	Reduced cardiac output leading to a reduction in tissue blood flow and slower circulation time	Slower delivery of drugs to the effect site. Potential reduction in volume of distribution	Be prepared for an increased time to effect of i.v. drugs and therefore adjust the time between incremental doses. Drug effects may not be as predictable as in a healthy patient
	Oedema formation	Increase in volume of distribution of water-soluble drugs such as neuromuscular blocking agents	May lead to a decreased patient response to the drug, with unpredictable effects
	Hypoproteinaemia	Reduction in plasma proteins may result in decreased protein binding of drugs and therefore increased fraction of free drug	Drugs that are highly protein bound, such as propofol, thiopental and lidocaine may have a greater therapeutic effect. A reduced dose should be considered and titrated to clinical effect
Metabolism and excretion	Reduced hepatic blood flow with reduced metabolic capacity of the liver	Reduced delivery of drugs to the liver, and therefore reduced metabolism	Drugs may have an extended duration of action. Increased dosing intervals may be required
	Reduced renal blood flow	Reduction in glomerular filtration rate and therefore in renal excretion of drugs	Drugs may have an extended duration of action. Increased dosing intervals may be required

21.2 Possible effects of cardiac disease on the pharmacokinetics of administered drugs.

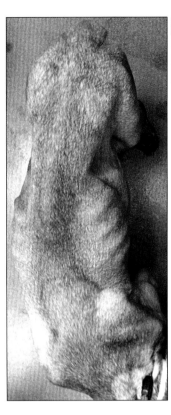

21.3 Profound cardiac cachexia and ascites in a 4-year-old neutered male Dogue de Bordeaux, suffering from atrial fibrillation and right-sided heart failure.

Principles of anaesthesia for the cardiovascular patient

Patients with cardiovascular disease are regularly brought to the clinic for procedures that require anaesthesia. Most commonly, the procedure is not related to the heart disease. In specialist centres, however, veterinary surgeons are more likely to encounter patients that require anaesthesia for specific treatment of congenital cardiovascular disease, for example, balloon dilation of pulmonic stenosis (PS) or occlusion of a patent ductus arteriosus (PDA).

With any general anaesthetic, the aim is to provide unconsciousness, analgesia and muscle relaxation while simultaneously ensuring adequate tissue perfusion. This can be challenging in patients with a compromised cardiovascular system, as the majority of anaesthetic agents cause cardiovascular depression. Although the anaesthetic must be tailored to the individual patient, it is important to remember the essentials underpinning safe anaesthesia and to appreciate some general principles that apply to all patients with cardiovascular disease.

Pre-anaesthetic assessment

Cardiovascular disease is common in cats and dogs. Some acquired and congenital cardiac diseases have particular species and breed predispositions (Figures 21.5

Systemic disease		Possible cardiovascular effects
Thyroid disorders	Hyperthyroidism (especially cats)	Tachycardia, increased myocardial oxygen demand and increased intravascular volume. This may increase preload and the risk of congestive heart failure in patients with previously mild or subclinical cardiac disease
	Hypothyroidism (especially dogs)	Reduced systolic function, sinus bradycardia and atrial fibrillation
Adrenal gland disorders	Hyperadrenocorticism (Cushing's disease)	Systemic hypertension, increased preload and pulmonary thromboembolism
	Hypoadrenocorticism (Addison's disease)	Hypovolaemia reduces preload and may reduce cardiac output. Hyperkalaemia associated with an Addisonian crisis may cause bradycardia and slow conduction (typical ECG changes), with potentially fatal effects
	Phaeochromocytoma	Episodic systemic hypertension, tachycardia, supraventricular and ventricular arrhythmias
Pancreatic disorders	Diabetes mellitus	Associated with a specific cardiomyopathy in humans, but has not been associated with heart disease in cats or dogs
	Pancreatitis	No significant effects reported in animals, but reduced systolic function occurs in humans
Altered blood viscosity	Anaemia (chronic)	Increased circulating volume and myocardial remodelling (four-chamber dilation) through RAAS activation. A haemic murmur relating to reduced blood viscosity may also be present. Anaemic cats are more commonly at risk of heart failure than dogs and should be monitored carefully for a gallop rhythm, tachypnoea or pulmonary crackles. Myocardial changes are reversible once anaemia has resolved
	Erythrocytosis or severe hyperglobulinaemia	Increased afterload and ventricular work, in addition to increased blood volume causing high preload
Hypertension	Systemic	Symmetrical, left ventricular hypertrophy and increased myocardial oxygen demand
	Pulmonary	Right ventricular hypertrophy and dilation, increased myocardial oxygen demand and potentially right heart failure (cor pulmonale)
Other	Sepsis	Reduced systolic function is commonly present in patients with sepsis and should be considered as a contributing factor to hypotension that is not responsive to fluid therapy
	Gastric dilatation–volvulus	Commonly associated with arrhythmias, including ventricular tachycardia, predisposed to by hypotension, autonomic imbalance, electrolyte abnormalities, high sympathetic tone and ischaemia–reperfusion injury. Drug therapy may be necessary, but arrhythmias are usually self-limiting in the perioperative period
	Hypersomatotropism (acromegaly)	Excess growth hormone from pituitary hyperplasia or an adenoma causes left ventricular hypertrophy and left atrial dilation in cats. Probably an underdiagnosed endocrinopathy, and should be considered in patients with poorly controlled diabetes mellitus

21.4 Cardiovascular effects of systemic disease. ECG = electrocardiogram; RAAS = renin–angiotensin–aldosterone system.

and 21.6). Awareness of these predispositions may help to identify cardiovascular disease before the animal undergoes anaesthesia.

A history of coughing is not a strong predictor of CHF and is more likely to indicate airway disease and/or left atrial dilation (Ferasin *et al.*, 2013). However, a history of tachypnoea, dyspnoea, exercise intolerance, syncope or cyanosis (especially if associated with exertion) should prompt consideration of cardiovascular diseases as major differential diagnoses. If an animal's owner reports that the patient has had episodes of collapse, then obtaining a thorough history will assist in determining the presence of neurological and neuromuscular disease apart from causes of true syncope. If specifically hindlimb weakness is reported, an evaluation of the genital mucous membranes during an episode will assist in identifying differential cyanosis, as induced by a right-to-left shunting PDA. The combination of increased respiratory effort during exertion and generalized cyanosis is suggestive of right-to-left shunting cardiac disease. Previous auscultation of an arrhythmia or

Breed	Congenital	Acquired
Afghan Hound		DCM
Airedale Terrier		DCM
Australian Shepherd Dog	PDA	
Beagle	PS	
Bichon Frise	PDA	
Bloodhound	AS	
Border Collie	PDA, VSD	DMVD
Boston Terrier		DMVD
Boxer	AS, PS, tricuspid dysplasia ASD	ARVC, DCM, SSS
Bulldog (English and British)	AS, PS, VSD, Accessory pathway SVT	ARVC (segmental)
Bulldog (French)	AS, PS	
Bullmastiff	AS, PS	DCM, AF, PE (neoplastic)
Cavalier King Charles Spaniel	PDA, PS	DMVD
Cairn Terrier		DMVD SSS
Chihuahua	PDA, PS	DMVD
Chow Chow	PS	
Cocker Spaniel	PDA, PS	DMVD, DCM, SSS
Dalmatian		DCM
Dachshund	PDA	DMVD
Deerhound		DCM
Dobermann		DCM
Dogue de Bordeaux	AS, tricuspid dysplasia	AF, DCM, PE (commonly neoplastic)
English Bull Terrier	Mitral dysplasia, AS	
Fox Terrier	PS, Tetralogy of Fallot	DMVD
German Shepherd Dog	Mitral dysplasia, AS, PDA, inherited ventricular arrhythmia, persistent right aortic arch	DMVD, PE (commonly neoplastic)
Golden Retriever	AS, tricuspid dysplasia, Duchenne's muscular dystrophy	DCM, PE
Great Dane	Tricuspid dysplasia, persistent right aortic arch	DCM, DMVD
Irish Wolfhound		DCM, AF ▶

Breed	Congenital	Acquired
Jack Russell Terrier	PS, PDA	DMVD
Japanese Akita	VSD	
Keeshond	VSD, Tetralogy of Fallot, PDA	
Kerry Blue Terrier	PDA	
Labrador Retriever	PS, PDA, tricuspid dysplasia, Accessory pathway SVT	DCM, PE Isorhythmic AV dissociation
Lakeland Terrier	VSD	
Lhasa Apso		DMVD
Maltese Terrier	PDA	DMVD
Miniature Poodle	PDA	DMVD
Miniature Schnauzer	PS, PDA, VSD, Tetralogy of Fallot	DMVD, SSS
Newfoundland	AS, PDA, PS	DCM
Old English Sheepdog	Tricuspid dysplasia	DCM
Pekingese		DMVD
Pointers	AS, PDA	
Pomeranian	PDA	DMVD
Portuguese Water Dog		DCM (inherited, juvenile)
Pug	AS, His bundle stenosis*	
Rottweiler	AS	
Saint Bernard		DCM, AF
Samoyed	AS, PS	
Scottish Terrier	PS	
Setter (Irish and Gordon)	PDA, Persistent right aortic arch	DMVD, DCM
Standard Poodle	PDA	
Schnauzer	PS	DMVD
Shetland Sheepdog	PDA	
Shih Tzu	PS	DMVD
Springer Spaniel	PDA, VSD	DCM, DMVD, third-degree AV block, atrial standstill
Weimaraner	Tricuspid dysplasia, PPDH	
Welsh Corgi	PDA	
West Highland White Terrier	PS, VSD	SSS, DMVD
Whippet		DMVD
Yorkshire Terrier	PDA, PS	DMVD

21.5 Reported canine breed predispositions to cardiac disease. AF = atrial fibrillation; ARVC = arrhythmogenic right ventricular cardiomyopathy; AS = aortic stenosis; AV = atrioventricular; DCM = dilated cardiomyopathy; DMVD = degenerative mitral valve disease; PDA = patent ductus arteriosus; PE = pericardial effusion; PPDH = peritoneopericardial diaphragmatic hernia; PS = pulmonic stenosis; SSS = sick sinus syndrome/sinus node dysfunction; SVT = supraventricular tachycardia; VSD = ventricular septal defect. *His bundle stenosis has been reported as a post-mortem finding in an experimental colony of related Pugs (James *et al.*, 1975); the clinical implications of this condition are unknown.

Breed	Congenital	Acquired
Abyssinian		DCM
Bengal		HCM
British Blue		HCM
British/American Shorthair		HCM
Burmese	Endocardial fibroelastosis	HCM
Domestic Shorthair/Longhair	VSD	HCM
Maine Coon	DCRV	HCM
Norwegian Forest		HCM
Persian		HCM
Ragdoll		HCM
Siamese and other Oriental		eRCM, HCM
Sphynx		HCM

21.6 Reported feline breed predispositions to cardiac disease. DCM = dilated cardiomyopathy; DCRV = double-chamber right ventricle/infundibular pulmonic stenosis; eRCM = endomyocardial restrictive cardiomyopathy; HCM = hypertrophic cardiomyopathy; VSD = ventricular septal defect.

gallop sound is a strong indicator of cardiac disease, as is a loud (grade IV/VI or above) murmur in dogs.

It is essential to assess the physical examination findings in the context of the individual patient. For example, it may not be appropriate for a calm dog that appears healthy to have a metronomically regular HR of 130 beats/min. This finding may reflect sympathetic activation or an abnormality such as accelerated idioventricular rhythm. Flow murmurs, often described as 'innocent', are common in younger animals. These murmurs occur in early to mid-systole (rather than being holosystolic) and have a point of maximum intensity at the left heart base. They are most often grade I–II/VI and do not have a 'musical' or reverberating quality. They can be dynamic in nature, varying in intensity with HR. Although a newly detected heart murmur in an adult animal is likely to reflect acquired disease, this may not be true in all cases, and the possibility of congenital disease should be borne in mind if a complete history is unavailable. Lower-grade heart murmurs in cats have a relatively low positive predictive value for structural cardiac disease. However, auscultation of a gallop sound or arrhythmia should prompt further investigation, as these findings are much more likely to indicate cardiac disease in any patient. The presence of an arrhythmia in a high-risk breed (such as the Dobermann, Boxer or Great Dane) may confer a greater risk than in other breeds.

If ascites is suspected on abdominal ballottement, the jugular veins should be examined to look for distension, or a positive hepato-jugular reflux, which is suggestive of elevated right atrial pressure and supportive of right heart failure.

Where cardiovascular disease is suspected, a minimum database should include non-invasive systolic blood pressure (using Doppler sphygmomanometry); packed cell volume (PCV) and total protein; urea, creatinine and electrolytes in conjunction with urine specific gravity; and echocardiography. Electrocardiography should be performed if an arrhythmia or inappropriate HR is auscultated or detected on echocardiography, or in a high-risk breed with evidence of structural heart disease. Thoracic radiography should be performed in patients with a history of tachypnoea or dyspnoea, left-to-right shunting cardiac or vascular disease, or where PHT or pulmonary thromboembolism (PTE) is suspected.

Echocardiography

The dimensions of the left atrium (LA) and LV can be assessed echocardiographically from a right-sided approach. This can be performed with the patient in a standing position when right lateral recumbency is either not tolerated or risks decompensation related to stress. The normal LA should have a roughly square appearance in long axis, with an area that would fit approximately twice inside the left ventricular cavity (Figure 21.7a). The normal LV should have a bullet-shaped appearance with a notable apex just off the midline in long axis (Figure 21.7b). The length of the LV lumen should be greater than 1.7 times the diameter at its mid-point. In short axis, an M-mode image may be obtained to assess LV fractional shortening; great care should be taken to position the cursor appropriately within the image (Figure 21.7c). At the heart base, the LA diameter can be assessed; normally this does not exceed 1.5 times the aortic root diameter (Figure 21.7d). It should be noted that echocardiographic measurements rely heavily upon the image plane obtained, position of the cursor and consistency in measurement technique. The inexperienced sonographer may find that subjective assessments are more reliable than absolute measurements. Where measurements are obtained, they should be compared with published reference intervals for the species and breed, where available.

Significant reduction in LV function is usually obvious, but subclinical or 'occult' cardiomyopathy may be more subtle and the clinical picture may be confused where the patient is athletic, sedated or suffering sepsis. LA dilation indicates elevated LA pressure, and the patient should be considered at risk of CHF. A more accurate estimation of cardiac filling pressure can be made using echocardiography; however, this necessitates the use of spectral and tissue Doppler techniques, which are beyond the scope of most practitioners. Where a patient is thought to be at risk of decompensation, and anaesthesia for an elective procedure can be postponed, referral to a veterinary cardiologist should be considered for a more accurate assessment of risk.

Electrocardiography

In dogs, the presence of sinus arrhythmia (Figure 21.8a) on an electrocardiogram (ECG) obtained in the non-sedated patient significantly reduces the likelihood of that patient having CHF. The sympathetic drive associated with heart failure abolishes resting vagal tone, leading to a regular sinus rhythm. Although other influences on HR variability may be present, including breed differences in vagal tone, the detection of sinus arrhythmia before anaesthesia may provide reassurance that current CHF is unlikely in a dog with a newly detected left apical heart murmur.

In contrast, in conscious cats, detection of sinus arrhythmia is more likely to represent a pathological increase in vagal tone. Differential diagnoses for sinus arrhythmia in the non-sedated cat include upper respiratory tract obstruction (including brachycephalic conformation) or inflammation, or gastrointestinal or central nervous system disease.

The presence of a single, isolated ventricular premature complex (VPC) on an ECG may or may not be associated with structural heart disease. Alterations in autonomic tone or a systemic inflammatory response are common causes of monomorphic ventricular arrhythmias (VPCs, bigeminy, trigeminy; Figure 21.8b). These arrhythmias are a frequent finding in the septic or post-coeliotomy patient in the absence of cardiac disease. Increasing complexity of

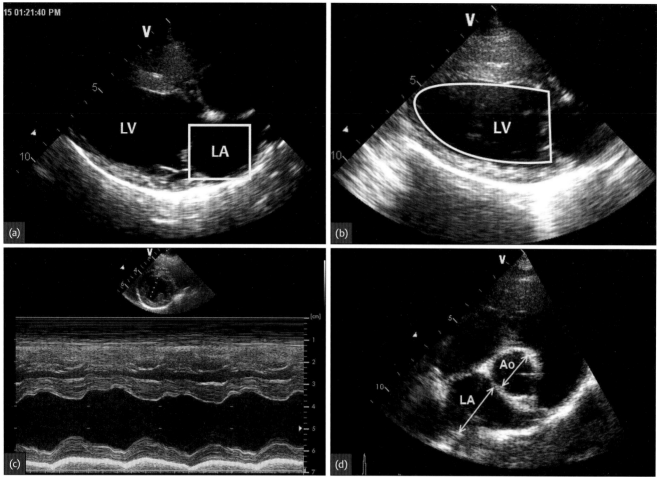

21.7 Normal echocardiographic images of the canine heart. (a) The left atrium (LA) normally has a square appearance in long axis and its area fits approximately twice into the area of the lumen of the left ventricle (LV). (b) The LV has a conical bullet shape with a notable apex off-midline. (c) M-mode assessment of left ventricular dimensions and function. (d) Comparison of the left atrial diameter with aortic root (Ao) diameter, measured in short axis at the heart base.

ventricular arrhythmias (couplets, triplets, paroxysmal ventricular tachycardia (VT); Figure 21.8c) confers an increased likelihood of structural cardiac disease, and a high rate of polymorphic VT may indicate a risk of ventricular fibrillation (VF) and death. However, in breeds that are predisposed to arrhythmic death, such as the Dobermann, Boxer and Great Dane, *any* ventricular ectopy on an ECG should be treated as serious and echocardiography performed. An ambulatory ECG recording (Holter) is recommended in any high-risk breed with an arrhythmia, even in the absence of detectable myocardial remodelling.

Thoracic radiography

If the patient is stable and will tolerate being restrained for conscious radiography, it may be beneficial to look for evidence of cardiomegaly or LA dilation when echocardiography is not available. In a tachypnoeic patient, an interstitial or alveolar pattern in the presence of LA dilation and venous distension is highly suggestive of pulmonary oedema. In cats, pulmonary infiltrates associated with oedema can have a diffuse, nodular appearance, rather than the typical caudodorsal distribution of pulmonary oedema in dogs (Figure 21.9ab). This means that cardiogenic pulmonary oedema may be misinterpreted as metastatic neoplasia in cats. In such cases, repeating radiography after administration of furosemide may show resolution of the lesions, thereby resolving uncertainty regarding their cause.

As basic echocardiography is increasingly accessible in small animal practice, the primary indication for thoracic radiography in a patient without tachypnoea is assessment of the pulmonary vasculature. This can provide valuable clinical information. For example:

- Pulmonary venous distension in a patient with LA dilation suggests elevated LA pressure and a greater risk of left-sided CHF
- A large bulge in the region of the pulmonary artery in a young dog with a loud, left basilar systolic murmur is suggestive of a more severe PS, due to the presence of a post-stenotic dilation
- In patients with a left-to-right shunting cardiovascular anomaly (e.g. PDA), severe overperfusion of the pulmonary vasculature may increase the risk of left-sided CHF (Figure 21.10)
- Abrupt termination of a pulmonary artery, with hyperlucency of the associated lung lobe, is highly suspicious of PTE (Figure 21.11).

Cardiac biomarkers

B-type natriuretic peptide (BNP) is released in response to increased myocardial wall stress. This peptide can be measured in blood, but it is highly labile and degraded by peptidases in plasma. A commercial assay measuring the N-terminals of the peptide (NT-proBNP) is available and is less prone to error than direct measurement of BNP.

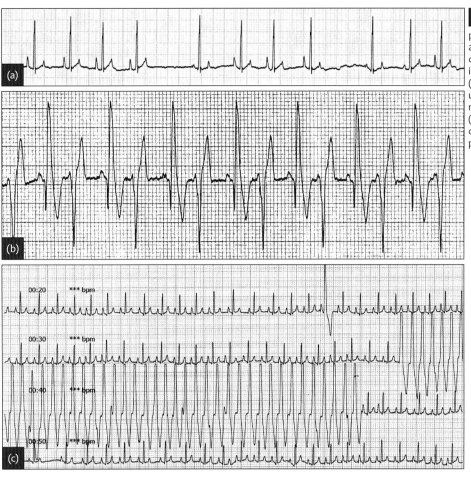

21.8 Common arrhythmias detected electrocardiographically in patients before anaesthesia. (a) Sinus arrhythmia with a wandering pacemaker is common in healthy dogs and is uncommon in dogs with congestive heart failure.
(b) Ventricular bigeminy may suggest underlying myocardial disease but rarely requires specific treatment.
(c) Paroxysmal ventricular tachycardia confers a high index of suspicion regarding primary myocardial disease.

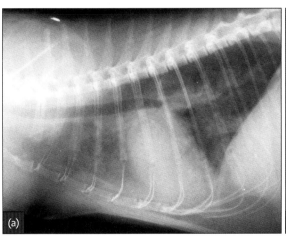
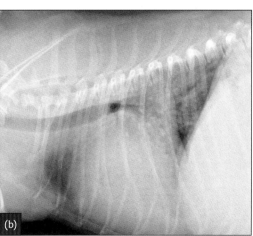

21.9 Lateral thoracic radiographs illustrating the typical distribution of pulmonary oedema in (a) cats and (b) dogs. The diffuse, nodular distribution seen in cats should not be confused with evidence of pulmonary metastasis.

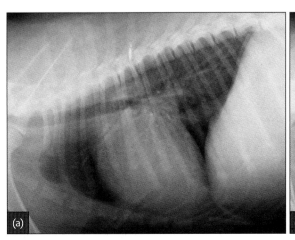
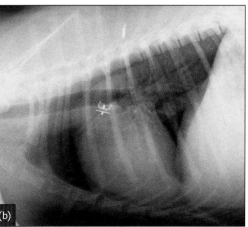

21.10 Lateral thoracic radiographs illustrating the differences in appearance of the pulmonary vasculature, (a) before and (b) after interventional occlusion of a patent ductus arteriosus in a 10-month-old entire female Shetland Sheepdog. After occlusion, the caudodorsal vasculature appears less dense and the cranial lobar vessels are no longer distended. Reduction in left atrial size can also be appreciated.

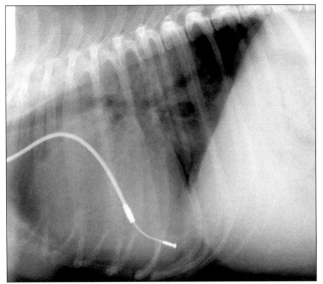

21.11 Right lateral thoracic radiograph from an 11-year-old neutered female Jack Russell Terrier with a pacemaker. Hyperlucency of the apical caudodorsal lung field can be seen, distal to a pulmonary thromboembolus, due to an absence of regional pulmonary blood flow (a Westermark sign). The pacemaker lead can be seen in the right ventricle.

Circulating NT-proBNP concentration is significantly higher in cats and dogs with structural heart disease than in individuals without cardiac disease. The concentration also increases with increasing severity of disease, and distinguishes patients with cardiac (higher concentration) from respiratory (lower concentration) causes of dyspnoea. NT-proBNP is renally excreted, and increased concentrations can occur with hyperthyroidism and PHT. Because of this, mild increases should be interpreted with caution. However, measurement of NT-proBNP is an acceptable method of screening for significant cardiac disease in small animals before elective anaesthesia, if echocardiography is not accessible. A bench-top SNAP test (IDEXX Laboratories) for NT-proBNP has been recently validated in cats for the detection of occult cardiomyopathy (Machen et al., 2014), which will increase the possibility of pre-anaesthetic screening for occult heart disease by measurement of the circulating peptide in cats.

Cardiac troponin I (cTnI) is an intracellular protein of the sarcomere and is specific to myocardial cells. Circulating concentrations of cTnI are normally negligible but increase in response to myocyte stress or necrosis. In humans, the main value of measuring cTnI is in 'patient-side' screening for myocardial infarction. Although increases in circulating troponin in cats and dogs have been shown to help distinguish cardiac from respiratory causes of dyspnoea in an emergency situation and assist the prognostication for cats with cardiomyopathy, the contribution of cTnI measurement to screening for occult heart disease before anaesthesia has not been investigated.

Pre-anaesthetic stabilization

Anaesthesia should be avoided in the newly diagnosed or unstable patient with cardiac problems unless absolutely necessary. In such patients, pre-anaesthetic stabilization should be attempted and elective procedures postponed. Although it is probable that patients with cardiovascular disease will never have normal haemodynamics, the risks of anaesthesia are likely to be lower after stabilization. Ideally, the patient should be stabilized at home, using standard oral therapy for heart failure (furosemide and benazepril in most cats; furosemide, an angiotensin converting enzyme (ACE) inhibitor and pimobendan in most dogs), and should be reassessed before anaesthesia.

It is important to be aware of the side effects of cardiac medication, including hypotension, which may be exacerbated by anaesthetic agents. There is controversy over whether cardiac medications should be administered on the day of anaesthesia. In human medicine, it is generally accepted that patients with good clinical control are more stable throughout anaesthesia. Stopping medication may result in cardiovascular instability and potentially cause rebound effects; therefore, continuing treatment as normal is recommended before anaesthesia. The possible exception is ACE inhibitors, which can cause refractory hypotension; however, ACE inhibitors are likely to have some residual effect even if not administered on the morning of anaesthesia, due to their long elimination half-lives. The authors therefore consider the administration of ACE inhibitors to be acceptable, but the use of other vasodilators, such as acepromazine, should then be avoided to reduce the potential for significant hypotension.

In some cases, extensive stabilization of the patient before anaesthesia is not possible. However, animals with left-sided CHF should receive furosemide (2 mg/kg i.v. up to q1–2 hours for a total of four doses) to achieve control of pulmonary oedema. Pleural effusions should be drained completely if possible. Complete drainage of ascites should be avoided because it can result in electrolyte imbalances and hypoproteinaemia, but, if ascites is severe, partial drainage may reduce pressure on the diaphragm and improve ventilation. Pimobendan can be administered intravenously in dogs (0.15–0.3 mg/kg), and rapidly improves myocardial contractility as well as reducing both afterload and preload. Intravenous pimobendan is recommended before anaesthesia in dogs with left-sided CHF caused by dilated cardiomyopathy (DCM) or degenerative mitral valve disease (DMVD) that have not previously received the drug, or where an oral dose has been missed on the day of anaesthesia.

The frequency and severity of any arrhythmias should be controlled where necessary by stabilization with oral medication at home, and reassessment should be performed before anaesthesia. Holter monitoring may be required for these patients. Where stabilization at home is not possible, acute treatment of arrhythmias may be necessary (see later).

Optimizing haemodynamics

In order to optimize haemodynamics, anaesthesia for the patient with cardiovascular disease should aim to:

- Maintain a 'normal' HR
  - Avoid sudden releases of catecholamines, for example, through stress or excessive noxious or surgical stimulation
  - Avoid situations that may increase vagal tone or induce a vagal reflex
- Avoid depressing myocardial function
- Maintain CO
- Avoid alterations in systemic ABP
- Avoid increasing myocardial workload and therefore oxygen demand
- Maintain oxygen delivery
  - Ensure that an adequate concentration of haemoglobin is present (i.e. ensure that the patient is not anaemic)
  - Ensure adequate provision of oxygen.

Further information may be found in Dugdale (2010a).

Pharmacology

Drugs used to provide analgesia, sedation and anaesthesia often have profound effects on the cardiovascular system, and a working knowledge and understanding of these effects is vitally important. Although these effects are covered in detail in other chapters within this Manual, a useful summary is provided in Figure 21.12.

Type of agent	Drug	CO	Inotropy	HR	MAP	SVR	PVR	CVP	Arrhythmic effects
Sedative agents	Acepromazine	–	o (–*)	o	– –	– –	o	–	Antiarrhythmic properties, possibly due to antagonist action on alpha adrenoceptors
	Medetomidine Dexmedetomidine	– –	o	– – –	Biphasic (+ then –)	Biphasic (+ + then –)	o	+	Bradycardia with high chance of first- or second-degree AV block
	Midazolam	o (+*)	o (–*)	o	o (–*)	o (–*)	o	o	None likely
	Diazepam	o (+*)	o (–*)	o (+*)	o	o	o	o	None likely
Opioids	Butorphanol	o	o	–	–	o	o	o	None likely
	Pethidine	–	–	+	–	o	?	+	None likely
	Morphine	o	o	–	–	o	o	o	Bradycardia with moderate chance of first- or second-degree AV block. Possible tachyarrhythmias due to histamine release after i.v. injection
	Methadone	o (–*)	o	– –	o (+*)	o (+*)	o	o (+*)	Bradycardia with moderate chance of first- or second-degree AV block
	Buprenorphine	–	o	–	o	+	?	?	None likely
	Fentanyl	o	o	– –	–	o	?	o	Bradycardia with moderate chance of first- or second-degree AV block
	Remifentanil	–	–	– –	o	+	?	+	Bradycardia with moderate chance of first- or second-degree AV block
	Alfentanil	–	o	– –	–	–	?	?	Bradycardia with moderate chance of first- or second-degree AV block
	Sufentanil	o	o	– –	–	–	+	o	Bradycardia with moderate chance of first- or second-degree AV block
Induction agents	Thiopental	–	–	+ +	–	o/–	–	–	Possible transient ventricular arrhythmias, e.g. bigeminy
	Propofol	–	–	–	– –	– –	–	o/–	None likely
	Alfaxalone	o	o	+	o (–*)	o	o	o	None likely
	Ketamine	+	–	+	+	+	o	o	Direct myocardial depressant but causes sympathetic stimulation, which may precipitate ectopic rhythms
	Etomidate	o	–	o	o	o	o	o	None likely
Maintenance	Isoflurane	+	–	+ +	– –	– –	o	+	None likely
	Sevoflurane	o/–	o/–	o	– –	–	o	+	None likely
	Desflurane	o/–	o/–	+	– –	– –	o	+	None likely
	Nitrous oxide	o/+	–	o/+	o	o/+	+	+	Causes sympathetic stimulation, which may precipitate ectopic rhythms
Miscellaneous	Lidocaine	o (dogs) – (cats)	o (–*) (dogs) – (cats)	+ (dogs) – (cats)	o (dogs) + (cats)	o (+*) (dogs) + (cats)	o (+*) (dogs) + (cats)	o (dogs) + (cats)	Suppresses ventricular escape beats so caution is advised in cases of AV block. Cats are more susceptible to the cardiovascular toxic effects and its use is not recommended
	Atropine	o/+	o/–	+ + +	o/+	o	?	–	May initially worsen an AV block or bradycardia due to blockade of presynaptic muscarinic receptors, resulting in increased release of acetylcholine ('paradoxical bradycardia')
	Glycopyrronium	o/+	o/–	+ +	o/+	o	?	–	Less likely to cause a worsening of bradycardia than atropine, but this is still possible

21.12 General effects of analgesic, sedative and anaesthetic drugs on the cardiovascular system. These effects may vary depending upon the individual patient and the circumstances. AV = atrioventricular; CO = cardiac output; CVP = central venous pressure; HR = heart rate; MAP = mean arterial blood pressure; PVR = pulmonary vascular resistance; SVR = systemic vascular resistance; o = negligible effects; + = increase on the variable; – = decrease on the variable; * = effect occurs at doses higher than those used clinically; ? = no published information available; o/+ = either no or slight increase; o/– = either no or slight decrease.

Choice of sedation or general anaesthesia

It may often appear attractive to attempt minor procedures with sedation rather than general anaesthesia. However, sedation adequate for appropriate immobilization is often 'heavy' and requires drugs that may have unfavourable cardiovascular effects. Conversely, inadequate sedation can increase patient stress, resulting in higher circulating concentrations of catecholamines, increased myocardial oxygen demand and an increased risk of arrhythmias induced by ischaemia.

General anaesthesia is often safer because it allows endotracheal intubation, which secures the airway and facilitates administration of oxygen. In addition, it is easier to apply monitoring equipment to anaesthetized patients, which enables earlier detection and treatment of problems. Further discussion of these issues can be found in Chapter 13.

Preparation for anaesthesia

Meticulous preparation for anaesthesia is essential; it minimizes the risk of significant complications by enabling the veterinary surgeon to respond rapidly to changes in the patient's status. If it is possible to do so without causing the patient undue stress, an intravenous catheter should be placed before administration of any sedative or anaesthetic drugs. This will allow rapid intravenous access should an emergency situation arise. All the necessary equipment should be organized and checked. Doses of all emergency drugs that may be needed should be calculated and drawn up, ready for use. A custom-made drug calculator (created using Microsoft Excel or similar software) is extremely useful to avoid mistakes in these situations. The induction area should be a quiet, calm environment, but enough personnel should be available to assist in the event that anaesthesia does not proceed as planned.

Pre-anaesthetic medication

Appropriate pre-anaesthetic medication forms part of a balanced anaesthetic protocol. Balanced anaesthesia involves the use of smaller doses of a combination of drugs to achieve the various components of anaesthesia, avoiding the disadvantages of using large doses of any one drug. For patients with cardiac disease, opioids usually form a major part of the anaesthetic protocol. Opioids provide analgesia with some sedation, and help to reduce the adverse cardiovascular effects of anxiety and noxious stimuli.

Pre-anaesthetic medication is best administered in a quiet area, where induction of anaesthesia will also occur, once all the preparations for anaesthesia have been completed. Close monitoring of the patient is then possible and appropriate action can be swiftly taken should the patient's condition deteriorate.

Induction of anaesthesia

Induction is one of the highest-risk phases of the perianaesthetic period. Many induction agents have adverse cardiovascular effects, resulting in myocardial depression and/or vasodilation. Dilation of veins reduces preload and causes a relative hypovolaemia.

Where possible, monitoring equipment should be attached before induction, but only if this does not cause unacceptable patient stress. Preoxygenation is recommended to offset the effects of the hypoventilation invariably caused by induction agents. In healthy dogs, desaturation of haemoglobin during induction can occur within 1–2 minutes; in patients with cardiovascular disease, this is likely to occur more rapidly as a result of compromised oxygen delivery. Preoxygenation, which greatly prolongs the time to desaturation (McNally et al., 2009), should be performed for a minimum of 3 minutes. This is most effectively achieved by using a close-fitting facemask, although some patients may become unacceptably stressed; in such cases, flow-by oxygen may be more appropriate, although this method is less effective.

The choice of drug(s) for induction of anaesthesia is often based on availability and the veterinary surgeon's familiarity with the drug(s). Although a particular induction technique may have certain theoretical benefits, it may not necessarily be safer if it is unfamiliar to the clinician. Drugs that produce fewer cardiovascular side effects include etomidate and potent opioids such as fentanyl. However, if these drugs are not available, or are unfamiliar, the use of 'traditional' induction agents such as propofol or alfaxalone is suitable. These agents may be used as part of a co-induction technique, in which they are combined with a benzodiazepine (e.g. midazolam 0.4 mg/kg i.v.) to reduce dose requirements (Robinson and Borer-Weir, 2013; Hopkins et al., 2014). Further details of drugs used for induction of anaesthesia can be found in Chapter 14.

Endotracheal intubation can cause profound cardiovascular responses, including tachycardia, hypertension and increased myocardial oxygen demand. It is important to attenuate this response by ensuring an adequate depth of anaesthesia before attempting intubation. Application of lidocaine spray to the larynx is useful in both cats and dogs. Excessive anaesthetic depth should also be avoided because of the cardiovascular depressant effects of induction agents.

Maintenance and monitoring of anaesthesia

Balanced, multimodal anaesthetic techniques, using a combination of analgesic, hypnotic and possibly neuromuscular blocking agents, are indicated to minimize the adverse cardiovascular effects caused by any one drug. It is very important to monitor anaesthetic depth closely. In order to maintain optimal haemodynamics, intravenous administration of vasopressors, inotropes, antiarrhythmics and (rarely) vasodilators may be required (Figure 21.13; see also Chapter 17).

As well as standard anaesthetic monitoring techniques, additional monitoring tools can be useful provided their limitations are understood (Figure 21.14; see also Chapter 7). The anaesthetist must be able to interpret the information provided by these tools and act appropriately. However, it is important to remember that such measurements can provide only crude indicators of tissue perfusion: for example, although an adequate mean arterial pressure (MAP) is considered essential, pressure does not directly equate to perfusion. High MAP may result from significant vasoconstriction, which increases systemic vascular resistance (SVR) and reduces tissue perfusion (see Chapter 17).

Generally, spontaneous ventilation is suitable for patients with cardiovascular disease (unless, of course, neuromuscular blocking agents are used). If hypoventilation develops, hypercapnia (and possibly hypoxaemia) can result. Hypercapnia can lead to an increase in circulating concentrations of catecholamines, which increase afterload and myocardial oxygen demand, as well as the

Drug	Mode of action	Dose	Notes and adverse effects
Positive inotropes			
Adrenaline (epinephrine)	Is a mixed beta and alpha adrenoceptor agonist, with slightly greater beta-agonist action This results in an increase in cardiac contractility. There is only mild vasoconstriction as the alpha- agonist action is counteracted to some extent by beta-2 agonist action	0.01–0.10 mg/kg i.v. 0.01–0.03 µg/kg/min i.v.	Generally reserved for CPR due to its non-selectivity of action In some cases, vasoconstriction can lead to an increase in O_2 consumption with an increased sensitivity to hypoxia
Dopamine	Action is primarily through beta-adrenoceptor agonist action, with minimal alpha agonist action at this dose	2.0–15.0 µg/kg/min i.v.	Lower doses activate dopaminergic receptors (D1 and D2) which results in splanchnic vasodilation, natriuresis and diuresis. Arrhythmias and tachycardia are possible. A decrease in P_aO_2 with its use has been observed in humans due to increased cardiac output and pulmonary vasoconstriction
Dobutamine	Increases cardiac contractility with little change in heart rate primarily through beta-1 adrenoceptor agonist action. Has some beta-2 agonist action, preventing an excessive increase in myocardial work, but which may limit its effect on increasing arterial blood pressure	2–10 µg/kg/min i.v. (dogs) 1–5 µg/kg/min i.v. (cats)	Can result in arrhythmias, tachycardia and vasodilation at high doses Can cause seizures in cats
Pimobendan	Inhibits phosphodiesterase III Sensitization of the myocardium to calcium	0.15–0.3 mg/kg i.v. (dogs)	Results in positive inotropic, lusitropic and vasodilatory effects. Calcium sensitization has a positive inotropic effect without increasing myocardial oxygen demand. May result in inhibition of platelet aggregation
Ephedrine	Has a direct beta-adrenoceptor agonist effect. Also has an indirect effect by uptake into presynaptic nerve terminals, resulting in noradrenaline release. It therefore also has some alpha-agonist action	0.02–0.05 mg/kg i.v. 1–5 µg/kg/min i.v.	There is a gradually decreasing effect over time (tachyphylaxis)
Antiarrythmic agents			
Lidocaine	Type 1b antiarrhythmic agent. Blocks Na+ channels, thus decreasing the rate of ventricular depolarization, action potential duration and absolute refractory period. Rapid onset and offset. Particularly affects the Purkinje fibres, so lidocaine is more effective for ventricular arrhythmias	1–2 mg/kg i.v. (maximum of 8 mg/kg within 10 minutes) 25–100 µg/kg/min i.v. (dogs)	Used for sustained ventricular tachycardia or complex ventricular rhythms which are affecting the patient haemodynamically, i.e. causing a reduction in blood pressure. Also indicated in some types of supraventricular tachycardia May increase the defibrillation threshold when used with monophasic defibrillators. Appears to be less of a problem with newer biphasic defibrillators. It is less effective with concurrent hypokalaemia or hypomagnesaemia. Care should be taken with the use of lidocaine in cats as this species is much more sensitive to neuro- and cardio-toxicity of local anaesthetics
Amiodarone	Type 3 antiarrhythmic agent Prolongs the duration of the action potential and refractory period by blocking potassium channels Slows the sinus rate and inhibits AV node conduction	2.5–5 mg/kg slowly i.v. (dogs) 0.03–0.05 mg/kg/min i.v. (dogs)	Can be used for ventricular tachycardia and is sometimes used in an attempt to convert atrial fibrillation Not recommended as an intravenous agent; solvent can result in hypersensitivity reactions including anaphylaxis (solvent free solutions may be imported)
Diltiazem	Type 4 antiarrhythmic agent A calcium channel blocker and so prevents the inward movement of calcium into the myocardium and vascular smooth muscle	0.1–0.25 mg/kg i.v. bolus slowly over 1–2 minutes	Used for cases of supraventricular tachycardia A mild negative inotrope, although vascular smooth muscle is more sensitive to diltiazem then the myocardium, so there is also a decrease in systemic vascular resistance
Esmolol	Type 2 antiarrhythmic agent Ultra-short-acting beta adrenoceptor blocker Cardioselective and primarily blocks beta-1 receptors	0.05–0.5 mg/kg over 5 minutes i.v. 25–200 µg/kg/min i.v.	Used for cases of supraventricular tachycardia due to its negative inotropic and chronotropic effects May precipitate bradycardia and hypotension especially if administered with drugs such as diltiazem or digoxin Caution when using in patients with congestive heart failure, as they may be dependent on beta adrenoceptor stimulation for adequate cardiac function, and their use can lead to fatal pulmonary oedema Renal impairment may be worsened with treatment due to a reduction in glomerular filtration rate

21.13 Medical treatment options for perioperative management of haemodynamics and/or cardiac arrhythmias. AV = atrioventricular; CPR = cardiopulmonary resuscitation; ECG = electrocardiogram; P_aO_2 = arterial oxygen tension; SA = sinoatrial. (continues) ▶

Drug	Mode of action	Dose	Notes and adverse effects
Antiarrythmic agents continued			
Propranolol	Type 2 antiarrhythmic agent Short acting non-selective beta-blocker, blocking both beta-1 and beta-2 receptors	0.02–0.08 mg/kg over 5 minutes i.v. (dogs) 0.02–0.06 mg/kg diluted slowly i.v. (cats)	Used for cases of supraventricular tachycardia due to its negative inotropic and chronotropic effect. There is an overall reduction in myocardial oxygen demand Can also be used to treat hypertension through a reduction in cardiac output, although this should be done after alpha-blockade as propranolol may block the vasodilatory effect of beta-2 receptor stimulation Adverse effects are similar to esmolol, but can also include bronchospasm
Magnesium	Inhibits the release of catecholamines Slows the rate of impulse formation at the SA node and prolongs SA conduction and AV node refractory period	30 mg/kg over 10 minutes i.v. 0.5 mmol/kg/24 hours i.v. (same as 5.2 mg/kg/h i.v.)	Can be used to treat refractory ventricular arrhythmias Can also be used to treat hypertension Magnesium should be given slowly IV and an ECG is recommended during administration (1000 mg is roughly equivalent to 4 mmol)
Atropine	Blocks acetylcholine from acting on the muscarinic acetylcholine receptors Limited effect on the nicotinic acetylcholine receptors Overall effect is to decrease the effects of the parasympathetic system	0.02–0.04 mg/kg i.v., i.m. Can also be administered via the trachea in emergencies	Used for bradycardia, atrioventricular (AV) block and hypotension suspected to be due to high vagal tone. Acts relatively quickly with duration of action of 20–40 minutes. Has the ability to cross the blood–brain barrier Low doses may cause a paradoxical worsening of bradycardia or AV block, but this is usually transient Additional effects include decreased saliva production and respiratory secretions, intestinal motility and decreased respiratory rate with an increased tidal volume
Glycopyrronium	Blocks acetylcholine from acting on the muscarinic acetylcholine receptors Overall effect is to decrease the effects of the parasympathetic system	0.005–0.01 mg/kg i.v., i.m.	Used for bradycardia, AV block and hypotension suspected to be due to high vagal tone. Takes longer to act then atropine, but duration of action is around 2–3 hours Four times more potent then atropine and cannot cross the blood–brain barrier. Additional effects are similar to atropine
Vasoconstrictors			
Dopamine (high dose)	Higher doses result in an increased alpha adrenoceptor agonist action, thus causing vasoconstriction. Agonist actions at beta adrenoceptors still occur.	10–20 µg/kg/min i.v.	The vasoconstriction associated with high dose dopamine may have more negative effects compared with noradrenaline with possible renal, gastrointestinal and cardiac ischaemia
Noradrenaline (norepinephrine)	Major action as an agonist on alpha-1 adrenergic receptors, with a minor agonist action on beta-1 adrenoceptors	0.1–1 µg/kg/min i.v	Vasoconstriction with little increase in heart rate Can cause a reflex bradycardia Increases blood flow to the heart and kidney without tissue ischaemia
Phenylephrine	Alpha-1 adrenoceptor agonist Very little action on other receptors	2–20 µg/kg i.v. 1–3 µg/kg/min i.v	Will cause a reflex bradycardia Increased coronary blood flow but decreased splanchnic blood flow
Metaraminol or Metaradine	Primarily an alpha-1 adrenoceptor agonist with minimal agonist action on beta-1 and beta-2 receptors	0.5–1.0 mg/kg i.m. 0.05–0.2 mg/kg i.v. 0.5–2 µg/kg/min i.v.	Has 1/10th the potency of noradrenaline Not widely used in veterinary medicine Acts directly on alpha-1 adrenoceptors, but also has indirect effects, causing noradrenaline release
Vasopressin	Acts on V_1, V_2 and V_3 receptors, producing more potent vasoconstriction than noradrenaline and phenylephrine	0.2–0.6 IU/kg i.v. 2–6 mU/kg/min i.v No dose established for cats	Low doses cause vasodilation in cerebral, renal, pulmonary and mesenteric vessels Increases water permeability in the renal collecting ducts to help maintain normovolaemia Stimulates aggregation of platelets Stimulates adrenocorticotropic hormone (ACTH) release Not widely used in veterinary medicine, but sometimes used during catecholamine depletion (e.g. sepsis) or in CPR
Vasodilators			
Phentolamine	Acts as an antagonist on alpha-1 adrenoceptors	0.025–0.1 mg/kg i.v 1–2 µg/kg/min i.v.	Can be useful for immediate treatment of increased afterload to reduce cardiac work May result in reflex tachycardia due to a baroreceptor reflex. Excessive hypotension may easily occur. Blood pressure monitoring is required

21.13 (continued) Medical treatment options for perioperative management of haemodynamics and/or cardiac arrhythmias. AV = atrioventricular; CPR = cardiopulmonary resuscitation; ECG = electrocardiogram; P_aO_2 = arterial oxygen tension; SA = sinoatrial. (continues) ▶

Drug	Mode of action	Dose	Notes and adverse effects
Vasodilators continued			
Sodium nitroprusside	Produces more dilation in the venules compared to the arterioles. Sodium nitroprusside is broken down to nitric oxide which results in vascular smooth muscle relaxation and therefore vasodilation	0.5–15 µg/kg/min i.v	Advised not be used for longer than 24 hours due to the build up of thiocyanate: cyanide toxicity is a possibility. Requires protection from UV light as this precipitates its breakdown, liberating cyanide ions. Care is advised in patients with hepatic or renal impairment or those with hyponatraemia, as toxicity is more likely. Blood pressure monitoring is advised during use to help prevent the risk of excessive hypotension
Magnesium	Inhibits release of catecholamines with possible blockade of the sympathetic nervous system	30 mg/kg over 10 minutes i.v. 1000 mg is roughly equivalent to 4 mmol	Can also be used to treat refractory ventricular arrhythmias. Magnesium should be given slowly IV and an ECG is recommended during administration

21.13 (continued) Medical treatment options for perioperative management of haemodynamics and/or cardiac arrhythmias. AV = atrioventricular; CPR = cardiopulmonary resuscitation; ECG = electrocardiogram; P_aO_2 = arterial oxygen tension; SA = sinoatrial.

Equipment	Indication and notes
Anaesthetist	Clinical decision making by the anaesthetist should not be replaced by other monitoring equipment, only supplemented. Anaesthetic depth can be completely assessed only by the anaesthetist; assessment should include inspection of eye position, reflexes and degree of muscle tone. Arterial pulse quality and character should be assessed, in addition to other indicators of perfusion such as mucous membrane colour and capillary refill time. Respiratory rate, depth and character can also be sensitive monitors of status
Thermometer	Normothermia is important in cardiac patients. Hypothermia can precipitate arrhythmias. Hypothermia will decrease ventilation and shift the oxyhaemoglobin curve to the left, thus reducing delivery of oxygen to tissues. Shivering in recovery increases oxygen demand. Enzymatic and cellular action will be decreased, resulting in reduced metabolism of drugs, and impaired coagulation and immune function
Pulse oximeter	Saturation of arterial haemoglobin with oxygen (S_pO_2) should be maintained, especially in patients with right-to-left shunts. The plethysmograph trace can give an indication of pulse quality and tissue perfusion. Variation of amplitude of the plethysmograph trace during intermittent positive pressure ventilation may indicate volume responsiveness (see Chapter 18)
Arterial blood pressure monitor	Monitoring can be either non-invasive (Doppler or oscillometry) or invasive. Monitoring allows haemodynamic responses to anaesthetic agents and surgical stimulation to be monitored
Capnograph	Measures adequacy of ventilation (whether spontaneous or controlled) and provides early warning of reduced cardiac output
Electrocardiography	Allows monitoring of the electrical activity of the heart, thus allowing detection of arrhythmias caused by cardiac or extra-cardiac causes
Central venous pressure (CVP) monitor	Gives information on preload – important for cardiac diseases that are preload dependent or to estimate risk of heart failure due to excessive intravascular volume. CVP changes in response to a fluid bolus provide a crude guide to fluid therapy, which helps to ensure patients do not become overloaded with fluid during anaesthesia
Spirometry	Allows positive pressure ventilation to be optimized, minimizing the risk of excessive inspiratory pressures and tidal volumes, with consequent effects on venous return and cardiac output

21.14 Monitoring equipment useful for the patient with cardiovascular disease.

potential for arrhythmias. Hypoventilation in combination with hypoxaemia may also cause hypoxic pulmonary vasoconstriction, exacerbating reduced oxygen delivery to the tissues. This is especially detrimental in patients with shunting cardiovascular conditions (e.g. Tetralogy of Fallot or a balanced PDA), where the direction of flow through the shunt can become right-to-left, or in patients with pre-existing PHT.

If intermittent positive pressure ventilation (IPPV) is required, it should be performed cautiously, with peak inspiratory pressures not exceeding 15 cmH₂O. Excessive inspiratory pressures and positive end-expiratory pressure can reduce venous return (see Chapter 6). The resultant decrease in CO and hypotension may further compromise tissue perfusion and oxygen delivery.

Fluid balance and intravenous fluid therapy

Fluid therapy is provided during anaesthesia to maintain intravascular volume, CO and oxygen delivery (Kudnig and Mama, 2002). Generally, patients with cardiac disease have an increase in total body water with hypervolaemia,

which leads to increased myocardial work. However, patients being treated for heart failure with vasodilators and diuretics may be relatively hypovolaemic.

In some cases, there may be conflicting requirements, for example, renal azotaemia and CHF, where overzealous use of fluids may precipitate pulmonary oedema. In patients with heart failure, increased preload does not result in increased CO because the myocardial response to increased stretch is abnormal and filling pressure is often chronically high. Conversely, CO can be severely compromised by significant reductions in preload in these patients, or in patients on long-term diuretics.

Cats are at particular risk of decompensation caused by increases in preload as a result of excessive intravenous fluid administration. The rate of fluid administration should be sufficient to replace urinary losses, evaporation from the respiratory tract and open wounds, haemorrhage or third space losses.

In cases of uncomplicated anaesthesia and surgery, fluids administered at 2 ml/kg/h are often adequate. Patients that are actively losing fluid, for example, because of haemorrhage, should have the deficit replaced with crystalloids, colloids or blood products as indicated (see Chapter 18). It is often difficult to monitor the effects of fluid therapy adequately during anaesthesia, but respiratory rate, HR, central venous pressure and ABP may provide indications of hypo- or hypervolaemia. In addition, auscultation (using an oesophageal stethoscope) of pulmonary crackles or a gallop sound may suggest high cardiac filling pressure and a risk of current or imminent CHF resulting from intravenous fluid overload.

The use of fluids with high sodium content is not recommended, as this may exacerbate retention of fluid, increasing preload and risking decompensation. A balanced electrolyte solution, such as lactated Ringer's, is usually suitable. Patients with cardiac disease generally tolerate most synthetic colloids as they can be administered in small volumes. However, due to the greater influence of synthetic colloids on colloid osmotic pressure, the margin for error is smaller compared to crystalloids, and clinicians unfamiliar with colloids may prefer not to use them. Administration of blood products is acceptable but carries a significant risk of volume overload, especially in patients with chronic compensated anaemia. Transfusion of packed red blood cells rather than whole blood may reduce this risk. Cats receiving blood products should be monitored carefully for development of a gallop sound, tachypnoea or pulmonary crackles.

Recovery from anaesthesia

Recovery from anaesthesia is a critical period for any patient, but especially so for those with cardiovascular disease. The patient should be monitored closely until normal homeostasis has re-established, including body temperature, ventilation and haemodynamic variables. Careful attention should be paid to the provision of appropriate analgesia, as pain can result in undesirable sympathetic stimulation, reduced urine output, reduced mobility and inadequate ventilation.

Acquired cardiovascular disease

In dogs, the most common cardiac disease encountered in practice is DMVD (also known as endocardiosis), which accounts for 75% of cases of canine heart disease. In cats, hypertrophic cardiomyopathy (HCM) is common; it has been shown to affect 1 in 7 cats in an unbiased shelter population (Wagner et al., 2010). Both diseases are chronic and may be relatively benign in nature (especially in older animals), but a proportion of cases do result in heart failure. Dilated cardiomyopathy accounts for approximately 10% of canine heart disease, with distinct breed predispositions and differences in disease progression between breeds (see Figure 21.5).

Degenerative mitral valve disease

Chronic pathological changes in the mitral valve cause DMVD, leading to valve prolapse and insufficiency (Figure 21.15). Over time, mitral insufficiency leads to reduced CO and activation of maladaptive compensatory mechanisms. Left-sided heart failure is the end result. Systolic dysfunction is likely to be present in advanced cases of DMVD but is difficult to measure objectively due to severe mitral regurgitation. In the most advanced cases, PHT and

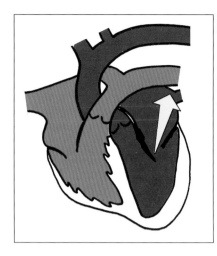

21.15 Schematic diagram illustrating major haemodynamic abnormalities in degenerative mitral valve disease: increased left atrial volume and pressure due to mitral insufficiency.

right-sided heart failure can develop in response to chronically increased pulmonary vascular pressures.

The disease has a long preclinical course, during which a murmur or LA dilation may be present without the development of heart failure. However, dogs with LA dilation are at risk of decompensating in response to intravenous fluid therapy, even in the absence of a prior history of CHF.

Anaesthetic management

Management of patients with DMVD depends upon the severity of mitral regurgitation and LV function. Patients can be considered to have a fixed, low CO unless severely affected, when they will also have poor myocardial contractility.

Bradycardia should be avoided, as a prolonged diastolic interval results in an increased LV end-diastolic volume; as the size of the mitral annulus varies with ventricular size, greater LV volume leads to increased mitral regurgitation. Excessive volume expansion with intravenous fluids can also increase mitral regurgitation in a similar way. Mild increases in HR are desirable to reduce regurgitation, and also improve coronary perfusion by maintaining diastolic aortic pressure. For a detailed explanation of factors affecting myocardial perfusion, see Levick (2010).

The severity of regurgitation in DMVD depends upon the relative difference in two pressure gradients: the first between the LV and LA, and the second between the LV and aorta. A reduction in the pressure gradient between the LV and aorta favours forward flow; therefore, slight reductions in SVR are indicated. Conditions causing vasoconstriction, such as responses to noxious stimuli, should be avoided. Acepromazine can be useful at low doses (10–20 μg/kg either i.v or i.m), although care should be taken to avoid hypotension, particularly if an ACE inhibitor is being administered. The sedative, analgesic and vagolytic actions of pethidine (meperidine) make it an appropriate choice, but other opioids may be more suitable if prolonged analgesia is required. Anticholinergic agents may be needed if bradycardia becomes haemodynamically significant. Alpha-2 adrenoceptor agonists are contraindicated as they cause bradycardia and increase SVR.

Key points:
- Avoid bradycardia, increased SVR and excessive volume expansion
- Aim to decrease SVR slightly to reduce afterload
- Aim for a slight increase in HR above pre-anaesthetic values.

Hypertrophic cardiomyopathy

Left ventricular hypertrophy in the absence of any other cardiac or systemic cause is defined as HCM. Secondary LV hypertrophy should not be confused with HCM, which is a primary disease process. Ventricular hypertrophy and fibrosis leads to LV diastolic dysfunction. This reduces CO, as does outflow tract obstruction caused by myocardial hypertrophy or abnormal mitral valve motion. Maladaptive compensatory mechanisms are activated in response to reduced CO. In more severe disease, LV pressure increases, the LA dilates and LA pressure increases (Figure 21.16), resulting in left-sided CHF. Hypertrophy of the LV is not matched by increased coronary perfusion; myocardial hypoxia contributes to advancing disease and arrhythmogenesis. In cats with reduced function of the LA, pleural effusion may be present instead of, or in addition to, pulmonary oedema (Johns et al., 2012). Cats with HCM and LA dilation are at risk of arterial thromboembolism. This may be the initial presenting sign of the disease in some cats.

Cats with HCM are at risk of decompensation if preload is increased, for example, by intravenous fluid therapy or sympathetic drive. Restrictive and unclassified cardiomyopathies in cats can be considered similar to HCM for the purposes of clinical anaesthesia, but are not usually characterized by outflow tract obstruction.

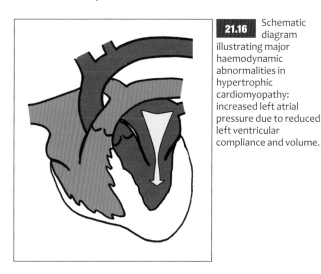

21.16 Schematic diagram illustrating major haemodynamic abnormalities in hypertrophic cardiomyopathy: increased left atrial pressure due to reduced left ventricular compliance and volume.

Anaesthetic management

Minimizing sympathetic activation is crucial to avoid increased HR and myocardial work, as well as increased preload caused by venoconstriction. It is therefore important to ensure that the patient and its environment are as stress-free as possible. A greater degree of sedation than usual may be considered appropriate for these patients.

Tachycardia should be avoided as it increases myocardial work and decreases the available time in diastole for ventricular filling. Maximizing diastolic filling requires maintenance of a normal or slightly reduced pre-anaesthetic HR. Hypovolaemia reduces already compromised ventricular filling and should thus also be avoided. Attempts should be made to minimize outflow tract obstruction, to prevent further reduction in SV. Conditions that worsen obstruction include enhanced contractility, decreased ventricular volume and reduced afterload.

Ketamine is relatively contraindicated in patients with HCM as its sympathomimetic action causes increased myocardial contractility and HR. Acepromazine (5–10 µg/kg)

has been used in HCM patients, but the resultant afterload reduction, as well as the relatively high doses necessary to provide sufficient sedation, are of concern.

Opioids are relatively safe, although pethidine is not recommended in these patients as its vagolytic action can induce tachycardia. Additionally, pethidine cannot be given intravenously because it causes histamine release and vasodilation. Low doses of alpha-2 adrenoceptor agonists (for example, medetomidine or dexmedetomidine 5–7 µg/kg i.v. or i.m.) may have beneficial haemodynamic effects in cats with preclinical HCM; this is particularly the case when administered by slow intravenous injection. Alpha-2 agonists provide good sedation, thus minimizing patient stress, and produce bradycardia, which will increase ventricular filling time. Although overall CO is reduced, myocardial oxygen demand also decreases, which may benefit ischaemic or fibrotic myocardial tissue. Alpha-2 agonists also increase SVR and reduce the severity of dynamic LV outflow tract obstruction (Lamont et al., 2002). The availability of an antagonist is also an advantage if complications occur. However, profound bradycardia can increase preload and risk CHF. Because of this, use of alpha-2 agonists in cats with preclinical HCM and LA dilation remains controversial.

If drug therapy is required to maintain normotension, pure alpha-1 adrenoceptor agonists such as phenylephrine are ideal, as they specifically increase SVR and do not increase myocardial contractility.

> **Key points:**
> - Minimize sympathetic activation and thus increased myocardial oxygen demand and preload
> - Avoid hypovolaemia and ensure adequate intravascular volume
> - Avoid decreased afterload by maintaining SVR.

Dilated cardiomyopathy

Dilation of the LV and reduced systolic function in the absence of another identifiable cardiac or systemic cause is defined as DCM. Secondary causes of LV dilation and reduced systolic function should not be confused with DCM, which is a primary idiopathic myocardial disease. Reduced systolic function reduces CO (Figure 21.17), leading to the activation of neurohumoral compensation. Altered LV geometry leads to mitral annular stretch, causing mitral regurgitation, which further reduces CO.

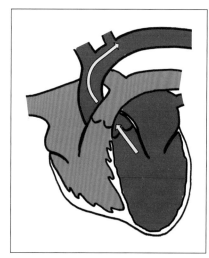

21.17 Schematic diagram illustrating major haemodynamic abnormalities in dilated cardiomyopathy: poor systolic function, reduced cardiac output and eccentric left ventricular hypertrophy.

Despite this, the majority of dogs with DCM do not have an audible heart murmur (Martin *et al.*, 2009). Eventually, LA pressure increases and left-sided heart failure results. Patients can have bilateral CHF if both ventricles are affected by the disease. A long preclinical course, often referred to as 'occult' DCM, is common. Prospective clinical data suggest that Dobermanns with occult DCM benefit from treatment with pimobendan (Summerfield *et al.*, 2012), and this should be considered before anaesthesia.

Differences between breeds in the natural history of DCM are well known. Dobermanns, Boxers and Great Danes have a more aggressive disease, characterized by frequent ventricular arrhythmias, and a high proportion of dogs suddenly die. Newfoundlands and Irish Wolfhounds have a slower disease progression, with a higher prevalence of atrial fibrillation (AF) and a lower incidence of sudden death. The severity of arrhythmias in DCM can be evaluated using ambulatory (Holter) ECG recording and is recommended as part of routine anaesthetic planning for dogs with DCM.

DCM is rarely diagnosed in cats, since the taurine content of commercial feline diets has been increased in the past three decades. However, occasional cases of idiopathic DCM are diagnosed in cats and should be approached in a similar way to dogs with the disease.

Anaesthetic management

Dogs with DCM have the potential for sudden anaesthetic death. Appropriate pre-anaesthetic stabilization of these patients is therefore required. Poor CO should be optimized by intravenous administration of positive inotropes such as dobutamine. Although a formulation of pimobendan is now available for intravenous use, it is currently licensed only as a single dose before initiation of oral medication. DCM causes a reduced SV, which can be only minimally increased. As a result, maintenance of CO is dependent upon HR and bradycardia should be avoided.

Arrhythmias such as AF and ventricular ectopy are common in patients with DCM. As these patients already have reduced CO, arrhythmias may require prompt treatment. Dogs with DCM are at risk of developing AF in response to high vagal tone induced by anaesthesia. Administration of lidocaine in the immediate period after such an event can convert the patient back to sinus rhythm (Moïse *et al.*, 2005; Pariaut *et al.*, 2008).

Preload needs to be maintained in dogs with occult DCM to maintain filling of the dilated LV. Monitoring of central venous pressure can be useful to guide fluid therapy, if appropriate. Intermittent positive pressure ventilation (IPPV) should be used cautiously, with minimal inspiratory and positive end-expiratory pressures to avoid causing further reductions in venous return, which may compromise LV filling.

Opioid-based protocols are useful for pre-anaesthetic medication in DCM. Low doses of acepromazine (2–10 µg/kg) may be tolerated if additional sedation is required, but it is best avoided in case relative hypovolaemia results. Alpha-2 adrenoceptor agonists are contraindicated.

Pericardial effusion

The most frequently identified cause of pericardial effusion (PE) in dogs is neoplasia, most commonly haemangiosarcomas, heart base tumours and mesotheliomas. Idiopathic PE is also common. In cats, the cause of PE is almost invariably CHF, although neoplasia (lymphoma) and other causes have been reported. Effusions in the relatively rigid pericardium increase intra-pericardial pressure. If intra-pericardial pressure exceeds right atrial pressure, cardiac filling is inhibited and clinical signs of right heart failure develop (cardiac tamponade). More chronic PEs can accrue in greater volumes due to stretching of the pericardium. Smaller PEs causing cardiac tamponade are more likely to be acute and thus indicate haemorrhage. In these cases, cardiac haemangiosarcoma is often diagnosed.

Stabilization of dogs with PE before anaesthesia is most easily achieved by pericardiocentesis. However, echocardiography should be performed before drainage, as the hypoechoic effusion may assist in delineating soft-tissue density masses, especially on the right atrium or auricle.

Anaesthetic management

It is unusual for patients with significant PE to require anaesthesia; in most patients, the effusion will be drained before anaesthesia. However, more fractious patients may require sedation to facilitate drainage. Diuretic therapy in patients with cardiac tamponade is contraindicated, as they are in a relatively hypovolaemic state.

As these patients tend to have a fixed SV, maintenance of their CO relies heavily on HR. In addition to maintaining HR, it is vital that preload is maintained. Any reduction in venous return or SVR may lead to a critical situation of further decreased cardiac filling and thus decreased CO.

Opioids may provide adequate sedation for pericardiocentesis, although care should be taken that the patient does not become bradycardic. Provided the patient does not require further (surgical) intervention, butorphanol (0.1–0.3 mg/kg i.v. depending upon the degree of debilitation) is often sufficient. Acepromazine and alpha-2 adrenoceptor agonists should be avoided until the cardiac tamponade has been relieved because they can reduce SVR and HR, respectively, both of which will result in decreased CO. If mechanical ventilation is used during anaesthesia, low inspiratory pressures should be employed, to maintain venous return.

These patients may be anaemic, particularly those patients with a chronic PE associated with a bleeding tumour. Chronic anaemia is often well tolerated in patients requiring anaesthesia. However, if a patient has either a PCV <15% or a PCV <20% with alterations in HR or ABP once the PE has been drained, a transfusion may be indicated. Whole blood, packed red blood cells, or haemoglobin-based oxygen-carrying solutions such as Oxyglobin® can be considered in such cases. Caution should be exercised when transfusing normovolaemic anaemic patients, to avoid fluid overload.

Key points:
- Optimize CO by maintaining HR and preload
- Maintain sinus rhythm.

Key points:
- Maintain HR and prevent bradycardia
- Maintain preload through adequate venous return and SVR.

Pulmonary hypertension

Pulmonary arterial pressure is normally 25–30 mmHg in systole and 10–15 mmHg in diastole. Pressures in excess of 32 mmHg systolic or 20 mmHg diastolic are indicative of PHT. Afterload on the RV is increased, which causes a combination of eccentric (dilation) and concentric (thickening) hypertrophy. Changes in the geometry and pressure of the RV and pulmonary artery often lead to tricuspid and pulmonic valve insufficiency. Echocardiography can be used to estimate pulmonary pressures indirectly by measuring the velocity of tricuspid (systolic) and pulmonic (diastolic) regurgitant flow. Over time, changes in the pulmonary vasculature become progressive and irreversible.

In dogs, the most common cause of PHT is chronic left-sided cardiac disease. In this condition, chronic elevation in pulmonary vascular pressure leads to changes in the structure and function of the pulmonary vasculature, causing increased pulmonary arterial pressure. A common cause of PHT in dogs in the UK is the lungworm *Angiostrongylus vasorum*. In heartworm-endemic areas or in patients with a history of travel, infection with *Dirofilaria immitis* should be considered. Other causes of PHT include: chronic respiratory disease (hypoxia); left-to-right shunting cardiac disease (e.g. PDA); PTE; obstructive neoplasia; and, rarely, an idiopathic condition. In the case of PTE, in addition to PHT and prolonged pulmonary transit time, ventilation–perfusion mismatch will occur. In dogs with PHT, previously closed arteriovenous shunts may open (Matos *et al.*, 2012), contributing to systemic hypoxaemia.

Anaesthetic management

Careful management of anaesthesia is required to avoid worsening PHT, which will further increase RV work and possibly precipitate CHF. Preoxygenation is recommended because hypoxaemia can worsen PHT via hypoxic pulmonary vasoconstriction.

Arterial blood pressure should be closely monitored because if hypotension occurs, coronary perfusion and oxygen delivery to the hypertrophied RV may be compromised; the resulting ischaemia may cause arrhythmias. Hypotension should be managed with vasopressors that do not have beta-1 adrenoceptor agonist action (e.g. phenylephrine or noradrenaline). Dopamine is not recommended because it may further increase pulmonary vascular resistance (PVR). In addition, adequate analgesia for surgical procedures on patients with PHT is important to reduce the risk of catecholamine surges caused by surgical stimulation.

Increased PVR can also result from hypercapnia. If hypoventilation occurs, IPPV is recommended. Although some authors advocate mild hyperventilation, excessive inspiratory or positive-end expiratory pressures can increase PVR and should be avoided. Efforts should also be made to prevent hypothermia, as this is another cause of increased PVR.

Most anaesthetic agents are safe to use in patients with PHT, provided they are used as part of a balanced anaesthetic protocol. However, it is probably safest to avoid nitrous oxide and ketamine because they may increase PVR.

Key points:
- Avoid hypotension to maintain coronary perfusion
- Maintain venous return and rapidly replace any fluid loss
- Avoid hypoxaemia, hypothermia, hypercapnia, pain and acidaemia.

Hyperthyroidism

In cats, the effects of hyperthyroidism on the myocardium are controversial. While some authors have reported concentric hypertrophy, others have not detected this change. However, hyperthyroid cats may have some degree of myocardial injury, evidenced by increased serum cTnI (Connolly *et al.*, 2005). Excess thyroid hormone can contribute to increased circulating volume through RAAS activation. This volume can increase filling pressures in cats with concurrent cardiomyopathy, leading to a risk of CHF. Clinical signs of CHF may be easier to control once thyroid disease has been treated, especially by radioactive iodine therapy.

Hyperthyroid cats can be managed similarly to those with HCM (as described earlier). It should be noted that the increased metabolic rate of these patients may lead to increased consumption of oxygen and production of carbon dioxide.

Systemic hypertension

Patients with hypertension often have clinical signs referable to their primary disease, or signs of target organ damage. The most common clinical sign in cats is acute blindness due to either retinal detachment or hyphaema. More subtle hypertensive retinopathy, renal disease or persistent tachycardia are less obvious clinical signs. High perfusion pressure damages capillary beds and chronic hypertension may result in vascular remodelling, further increasing SVR. Increased arterial blood pressure (ABP) (persistently >160–170 mmHg) increases afterload on the LV, causing concentric hypertrophy and fibrosis. In severe cases, the myocardium can become ischaemic due to relative hypoxia. Despite this, CHF is rare in hypertensive patients.

Anaesthetic management

In humans, poorly controlled hypertension is associated with intraoperative events such as myocardial ischaemia and arrhythmias. Worsening hypertension or even hypotension may also occur. For hypertensive animals requiring anaesthesia, stress should be minimized to prevent excessive sympathetic stimulation. Hypotension can occur following administration of anaesthetic agents. Hypertension may occur upon endotracheal intubation, although topical lidocaine applied to the larynx may help to reduce this exaggerated response. During anaesthesia, alterations in ABP can be minimized by inhalational agent titration and use of agents such as opioids as part of a balanced anaesthetic protocol, although vasopressors and/or vasodilators may also be required.

Chronic hypertension alters renal and cerebral autoregulation, which occurs over a higher range of pressures. Therefore, a higher MAP is required to maintain adequate cerebral and renal perfusion (>70–80 mmHg). However, excessive increases in MAP are undesirable in patients with significant myocardial hypertrophy, as myocardial work is increased. It is generally recommended that blood pressure is maintained within 10–20% of preoperative values.

Most anaesthetic agents can be used in these patients, although ketamine is generally not recommended as its sympathomimetic effects may worsen hypertension and increase myocardial work.

Key points:
- Minimize increases in myocardial work by moderating HR and SV
- Maintain or slightly increase MAP.

Congenital cardiovascular disease

Congenital cardiac disease accounts for approximately 21% of all cardiovascular diseases diagnosed in small animal referral hospitals (Oliveira *et al.*, 2011) but it is less frequent in general practice. Cats and dogs with congenital heart disease often have heart murmurs detected during physical examination before neutering. Most age-related flow murmurs in young animals do not persist beyond 15–16 weeks of age. Determining the significance of a detected murmur in a juvenile animal before the patient undergoes anaesthesia should therefore be recommended to the owners. In Europe, the most common congenital heart disease diagnosed in dogs is PS, followed by aortic stenosis (AS) and PDA. In cats, ventricular septal defects (VSDs) are the most common congenital disease, but congenital cardiac disease overall is rare.

Pulmonic stenosis

Left untreated, dogs with severe PS may either die as a result of ventricular arrhythmias, or eventually develop RV failure due to chronic pressure overload (Figure 21.18). Valvular stenosis is the most common form of the disease, but some dogs are affected by a muscular stenosis of the RV outflow tract. Prognosis is based on the severity of the pressure gradient across the stenotic valve. Stenosis is considered mild at pressure gradients <50 mmHg, moderate at 50–80 mmHg and severe at >80 mmHg. Medical treatment with beta blockers (e.g. atenolol) or surgical intervention is recommended for dogs with severe stenosis or those showing clinical signs. In some breeds (especially Bulldogs) PS may be associated with coronary artery anomalies.

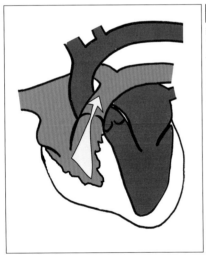

21.18 Schematic diagram illustrating major haemodynamic abnormalities in valvular pulmonic stenosis: pressure overload of the right ventricle due to valve leaflet fusion.

Anaesthetic management

Venous return and cardiac contractility should be maintained to prevent reduced SV. Maximum SV of the RV is fixed, which consequently limits LV output. As such, CO is heavily dependent upon HR and bradycardia should therefore be avoided. However, tachycardia reduces the time available for ventricular filling and is also undesirable.

As with PHT, factors that increase PVR should be avoided as this may further reduce RV output. Catecholamine surges should be avoided and care should be taken when providing IPPV.

Key points:
- Maintain preload/venous return
- Maintain myocardial contractility
- Maintain HR as near to pre-anaesthetic values as possible
- Avoid factors that may increase PVR.

Aortic stenosis

Aortic stenosis is classified according to lesion location, and most commonly occurs in the subaortic region. Here, fibrous tissue develops in the LV outflow tract (Figure 21.19). Severity of this pathology can range from small nodules with little clinical effect, to a fibrous ring or tunnel-like lesion. Although AS is often considered a congenital disease due to its young age of onset and familial nature, the development of subaortic stenosis lesions occurs gradually over the first year of life.

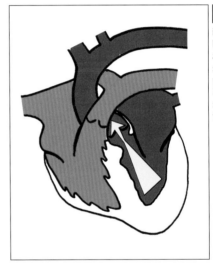

21.19 Schematic diagram illustrating major haemodynamic abnormalities in subaortic stenosis: pressure overload of the left ventricle due to a subaortic ridge of fibrous tissue.

Similarly to PS, prognosis is based on the severity of the pressure gradient across the valve. Stenosis is considered mild at gradients <50 mmHg, moderate at 50–80 mmHg and severe at >80 mmHg. Medical treatment with beta blockers (e.g. atenolol) may be implemented for dogs with severe stenosis or those with clinical signs. Both valvular and sub-valvular forms of the disease (the latter being more common) cause a fixed stenosis, limiting maximal SV and leading to LV pressure overload and concentric LV hypertrophy. Pressure in the LV leads to increased myocardial oxygen demand, relative ischaemia and fibrosis (acting as a substrate for arrhythmias); pressure may become so high that coronary blood flow reverses during systole (Pyle *et al.*, 1973). Eventually, untreated dogs with severe AS may die suddenly (presumably due to ventricular arrhythmias) or eventually develop LV failure and pulmonary oedema. Subvalvular and valvular AS has also been reported in cats.

Anaesthetic management

As patients with AS have a fixed SV, CO is dependent upon HR, and it is critically important to maintain HR close to pre-anaesthetic values. Bradycardia will result in CO reduction, while tachycardia will reduce ventricular filling time and predispose to myocardial ischaemia. Maintenance of sinus rhythm is essential to ensure appropriate ventricular filling, aided by atrial contraction. Loss of normally timed atrial contractions, as occurs in AF or ventricular arrhythmias, can lead to rapid reductions in CO. Electrocardiographic monitoring is therefore important and antiarrhythmic treatment should be instigated rapidly if necessary.

Diastolic dysfunction and reduced ventricular compliance resulting from LV hypertrophy also reduce SV. Patients with AS are therefore sensitive to rapid changes in intravascular volume, with hypovolaemia causing a rapid reduction in CO. Maintenance of circulating volume is also important to ensure adequate coronary perfusion. Hypotension rapidly causes reductions in coronary perfusion and myocardial oxygen delivery due to lower aortic diastolic pressure.

Although the use of opioids is appropriate, they may cause bradycardia. This should be controlled by the use of anticholinergic agents if necessary; glycopyrronium (5–10 µg/kg i.v.) may be preferable to atropine due to its reduced propensity to cause extreme tachycardia. Acepromazine is not suitable because it reduces SVR. Very small doses of an alpha-2 agonist (medetomidine or dexmedetomidine 1–3 µg/kg i.v or i.m) may be beneficial, as these agents maintain SVR and can be antiarrhythmic. Damage caused by high-velocity flow of blood against the aortic valve leaflets disrupts the epithelial lining and increases the risk of infective endocarditis. Prophylactic antibiotic cover should therefore be given when dogs with AS suffer wounds or are at risk of sepsis from surgical procedures.

> **Key points:**
> - Maintain HR close to pre-anaesthetic values
> - Maintain normal sinus rhythm
> - Maintain intravascular volume
> - Maintain normotension (avoid hypotension)
> - Avoid alterations in myocardial oxygen demand.

Patent ductus arteriosus

PDA occurs when the fetal ductus arteriosus fails to constrict as normal after birth, owing to an absence of smooth muscle in the vessel wall. Female dogs are three times as likely to be affected as males. Blood flows continuously through the PDA from the systemic circulation into the pulmonary vasculature because of persistently higher pressure in the descending aorta than in the pulmonary artery. This gives rise to the characteristic loud, continuous murmur associated with a PDA, located dorsally and cranially to the heart base (caudal to the triceps muscle). Pulse quality is often hyperkinetic, with reduced diastolic arterial pressure (DAP) caused by diastolic flow leaving the systemic circulation through the PDA. Over-circulation of the lungs leads to left sided heart overload (Figure 21.20). If PDA is untreated, left-sided heart failure often occurs, with a reported 50% mortality by 1 year of age. Large PDAs can be associated with severe PHT, causing balanced or right-to-left shunts (see below). Some dogs with small PDAs may remain asymptomatic, but occlusion of the PDA is almost always recommended due to the potential for effective prevention of clinical signs and good long-term prognosis.

Anaesthetic management

Patients may be anaesthetized for occlusion of their PDA, or for investigation or treatment of a concurrent disease.

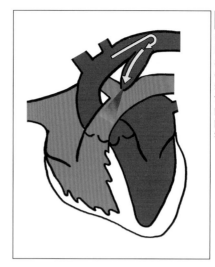

21.20 Schematic diagram illustrating major haemodynamic abnormalities in patent ductus arteriosus: systemic-to-pulmonary flow due to low pulmonary vascular pressure relative to systemic pressure.

These animals are usually young, and appropriate age-related anaesthetic considerations are important (see Chapter 30). Reduced DAP leads to reduced MAP, despite normal SAP. Hypotension is common during anaesthesia, particularly if SAP is reduced due to compromised myocardial function. Maintenance of CO is important in order to maintain adequate MAP.

The direction of shunt flow depends upon the balance between SVR and PVR. Sudden reductions in SVR, which can be produced by anaesthetic agents, may cause a left-to-right shunt to become right-to-left in patients with pre-existing PHT. Shunt reversal is considered unlikely in patients with normal pulmonary pressure before anaesthesia, as a large pressure change would be required to induce reversal. Where flow reversal does occur, arterial haemoglobin saturation with oxygen (S_pO_2) decreases in the caudal body and does not respond to oxygen therapy, and tissue hypoxia will result. Increases in PVR and decreases in SVR should be minimized in order to maintain left-to-right shunting.

Alpha-2 adrenoceptor agonists are contraindicated as they result in reductions in both HR and CO. Acepromazine is generally not recommended due to the resulting decreased SVR. However, very small doses of acepromazine (2–5 µg/kg i.v.) may be beneficial, as mild reductions in SVR can increase systemic blood flow.

At induction of anaesthesia, propofol, and to a lesser extent alfaxalone, can reduce SVR. Care should be taken to monitor the patient's perfusion status; ABP is often used as a surrogate measure of perfusion. The use of co-induction agents, such as potent opioids or benzodiazepines, may reduce the dose of induction agent required. Ketamine may also be used as it maintains or increases SVR, although its slower onset of action in comparison to other agents may make this choice less desirable. Similarly, attempts should be made to reduce the concentration of volatile agents, to limit their vasodilatory effects. Nitrous oxide has been reported to increase PVR and so its use may be best avoided.

Particular attention should be paid to HR once the PDA is occluded, as Branham's reflex may occur. With this reflex, increased DAP (and thus MAP) stimulates baroreceptors and causes bradycardia and vasodilation. This is most likely to occur within minutes of PDA occlusion but can occur postoperatively. Treatment with anticholinergics is not usually necessary, unless bradycardia is haemodynamically significant (see Figure 21.13).

Ventricular septal defects

Failure of the interventricular septum to fuse completely during cardiogenesis results in a VSD. Associated murmurs are located on the right hemithorax, often radiating cranioventrally from the right apex. Defects located in the membranous septum, just beneath the great vessels, are most common (Figure 21.21). They may be associated with other congenital malformations, including PS, AS or PDA. Muscular VSDs are rare but may be associated with complex or multiple congenital diseases. Small VSDs may resist flow (so-called 'resistive' defects) and allow maintenance of the normal interventricular pressure difference. Patients with this type of defect have a good long-term prognosis but a very loud murmur may be present. Smaller defects can be complicated if they lead to aortic valve prolapse and aortic insufficiency; this possibility should be considered before anaesthesia, as there may be a degree of ventricular dysfunction or a risk of volume overload. Larger defects are often associated with quieter murmurs because of a reduced interventricular pressure gradient, due to higher pulmonary artery and RV pressure. They are associated with a worse prognosis, as reversal of flow may occur (see below).

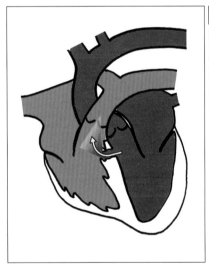

21.21 Schematic diagram illustrating major haemodynamic abnormalities in ventricular septal defect: left-to-right flow due to low pulmonary vascular resistance.

Anaesthetic management

In the absence of heart failure or significant PHT, most anaesthetic agents are relatively well tolerated. However, it is important to maintain left-to-right shunting through the VSD rather than induce flow reversal. Reduced SVR or increased PVR in a patient with a non-resistive VSD may lead to reversal. Clinically, shunt reversal is seen as reduced S_pO_2 that is unresponsive to oxygen therapy. Often, a reduction in the concentration of volatile anaesthetic agent will increase SVR and reduce desaturation. If volatile agent concentration is reduced, additional agents may be required to maintain anaesthetic depth; opioids are usually the first choice.

Right-to-left shunts

Animals with large defects such as a PDA or VSD may present with PHT and balanced (bidirectional, low-velocity) or reversed (right-to-left) shunt flow (Figure 21.22). Chronically increased pulmonary vascular flow can cause vasoconstriction (via shear stress) and increased PVR, leading to PHT. Eventually, irreversible changes in the pulmonary vasculature may result, due to medial hypertrophy, intimal fibrosis and reduced luminal diameter. An alternative hypothesis that has been suggested as the cause of right-to-left shunting is the persistence of high-resistance fetal vasculature in some individuals. Affected patients may develop right-to-left shunting during exercise or excitement (due to increased PVR and reduced SVR), leading to chronic hypoxaemia and a compensatory erythrocytosis. These patients may present with generalized (VSD) or differential caudal (PDA) cyanosis (Figure 21.23), or neurological signs related to hyperviscosity. The severity of PHT may be reduced by treatment with phosphodiesterase-V inhibitors, such as sildenafil. Treatment options for erythrocytosis are limited to phlebotomy, hirudotherapy (using medical-grade leeches) or chemotherapeutic suppression of the erythroid line. Sildenafil has been reported to reduce the severity of erythrocytosis in dogs with right-to-left PDA (Nakamura et al., 2011).

Tetralogy of Fallot is characterized by a large subaortic VSD, dextroposition of the aorta relative to the mitral annulus, PS and RV hypertrophy. In dogs with this condition, flow through the VSD is predominantly right-to-left due to the presence of PS, rather than PHT. Possible treatments for these patients are pulmonic balloon valvuloplasty or surgical bypass of the PS with a Blalock-Taussig procedure. Untreated dogs have a poor long-term prognosis.

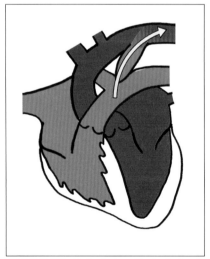

21.22 Schematic diagram illustrating major haemodynamic abnormalities in a right-to-left ('reverse') patent ductus arteriosus: pulmonary to systemic flow due to severe pulmonary hypertension causing high pulmonary vascular pressure relative to systemic arterial pressure. Note that admixture of blood occurs caudal to the brachycephalic trunk and left subclavian artery, leading to caudal hypoxia and cyanosis (see Figure 21.23).

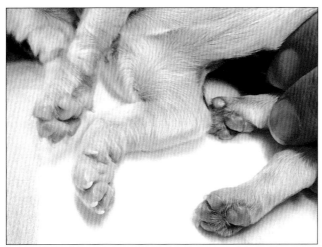

21.23 Caudal cyanosis, a typical clinical sign associated with right-to-left patent ductus arteriosus, in a puppy that suffered perinatal death. In this patient, the ductus arteriosus did not close and pulmonary vascular resistance remained high, mimicking a right-to-left PDA.

Anaesthetic management

With any intracardiac or vascular right-to-left shunt, the anaesthetist must ensure removal of all air bubbles before intravenous administration of fluids or drugs. If any bubbles remain, a systemic air embolus to the cerebral, renal or coronary arteries may be fatal.

Where flow reversal occurs during anaesthesia in a patient with a previously documented left-to-right shunt (more likely with PHT), adjustments to anaesthesia should be made as described above. In patients with pre-existing right-to-left or balanced shunts caused by a PDA or VSD, every effort to minimize right-to-left flow should be made by optimising SVR and PVR. Similar principles for the anaesthetic management of complex shunts should be employed.

In Tetralogy of Fallot, where fixed PS is more important than PVR in causing shunt direction, moderation of SVR is crucial. Intravascular volume and SVR should be maintained to minimize right-to-left flow. Factors that significantly increase PVR, such as excessive inspiratory pressures or acidosis, may worsen right-to-left shunting. However, these are less important than the presence of PS. Although most dogs with Tetralogy of Fallot are adapted to chronic hypoxaemia, if hypoxaemia worsens during anaesthesia a reduction in the volatile anaesthetic concentration may help. If this is not achievable even with the use of adjunctive agents, administration of a pure vasoconstrictor such as phenylephrine (5 µg/kg i.v. bolus or 1–3 µg/kg/min i.v. infusion) may be useful.

> **Key points:**
> - Prevent introduction of air emboli
> - Minimize right-to-left shunting:
>   - Maintain SVR – avoid decreases
>   - Maintain PVR – avoid increases
> - Maintain intravascular volume.

Mitral dysplasia

Mitral dysplasia is defined as a developmental abnormality of the mitral valve apparatus, causing insufficiency and/or stenosis. The pathophysiology of mitral regurgitation in association with dysplasia is similar to that of DMVD. In patients that also have mitral stenosis, the dependence of CO on preload can make management very challenging, as increased preload may risk pulmonary oedema. Mitral dysplasia is most common in the English Bull Terrier but has been reported in other breeds.

Anaesthetic management

Many of the considerations for mitral dysplasia are the same as those discussed for DMVD. It is important, however, to maintain preload without excessively increasing intravascular volume. With mitral stenosis, reduced SVR may not benefit the patient as greatly as if mitral regurgitation were the sole problem, because the stenosis represents a barrier to forward blood flow. Maintenance of preload will help to augment flow through the mitral valve and thus maintain CO. Patients with mitral stenosis are also prone to PHT, so increases in PVR should be avoided.

> **Key points:**
> - Avoid bradycardia and aim for a slight increase in HR above pre-anaesthetic values
> - Avoid increases in SVR and PVR
> - Maintain preload but avoid excessive volume expansion.

Tricuspid dysplasia

Tricuspid dysplasia is a developmental abnormality of the tricuspid valve apparatus, causing insufficiency and/or stenosis. It is a poorly defined condition, due to the wide variability of the normal canine tricuspid apparatus. Labradors and Golden Retrievers appear to be predisposed to the abnormality. Many cases may be subclinical. The most common clinical sign is right-sided CHF due to severely increased right atrial pressure. In dogs with severe right heart remodelling, such as severe PS or with PHT, the geometry of the tricuspid annulus may be abnormal; over time, abnormal flow may lead to myxomatous valvular degeneration. In this scenario, the presence of tricuspid dysplasia may be difficult to identify conclusively on echocardiography.

Anaesthetic management

Increases in PVR should be avoided in patients with tricuspid dysplasia, as this will result in an increased regurgitant fraction through the tricuspid valve. Factors influencing PVR are discussed earlier. Similar to DMVD, the aim is to maintain pre-anaesthetic HR, as bradycardia may worsen regurgitation through the valve.

Maintenance of preload will help to augment flow through the tricuspid valve and ultimately ensure that RV and LV CO is maintained. However, care should be taken to ensure that an excessive increase in intravascular volume is avoided, as this may precipitate or worsen right-sided CHF.

> **Key points:**
> - Maintain pre-anaesthetic HR and avoid bradycardia
> - Avoid increases in PVR
> - Maintain preload without excessive increases in intravascular volume.

Perioperative arrhythmias

The majority of arrhythmias encountered during anaesthesia of cats and dogs tend to be due either to the cardiovascular effects of drugs administered, or secondary to non-cardiac disease.

Arrhythmias encountered during the pre-anaesthetic period should be investigated and stabilized appropriately. This may require a period of several weeks to monitor the response of a patient to appropriate oral antiarrhythmic therapy, and serial Holter monitoring may often be needed. Where possible, anaesthesia should be postponed until the patient is more stable. For further details of treatment and monitoring, readers are referred to the *BSAVA Manual of Canine and Feline Cardiorespiratory Medicine*.

If an arrhythmia is detected in a patient where anaesthesia is unavoidable, intravenous treatment should be considered (Figure 21.24). Treatment should be given only in those patients where the arrhythmia is haemodynamically significant. In apparently stable patients, treatment should be prepared and ready to administer in case of acute worsening of arrhythmia or decompensation. Patients with arrhythmias causing clinical signs should be stabilized as a priority. Ventricular tachycardia or complex ventricular arrhythmias in dogs may be controlled with lidocaine (2 mg/kg i.v. bolus over 1–2 minutes, repeated after 10 minutes up to a total dose of 8 mg/kg, followed by an infusion given at 25–100 μg/kg/min i.v.). Supraventricular tachycardia (SVT) should be controlled with diltiazem (0.1–0.25 mg/kg i.v. bolus over 1–2 minutes, repeated after 5–10 minutes up to 0.75 mg/kg, followed by an infusion given at 0.1–0.3 mg/kg/h i.v.) or esmolol (50–500 μg/kg bolus over 5 minutes, followed by an infusion of 25–200 μg/kg/min i.v.). In animals with heart failure, beta blockers may cause severe negative inotropic effects, leading to potentially fatal pulmonary oedema. For this reason, it is sensible not to use esmolol where the presence or absence of structural heart disease is unknown.

It is important for the veterinary surgeon to identify arrhythmias early and decide whether to treat them immediately, or to delay treatment until there is further deterioration in haemodynamic status. The gold-standard method for identifying an arrhythmia is an ECG. If this method is unavailable, it may be possible to identify abnormalities in pulse quality on palpation, or by observation of the plethysmograph waveform on a pulse oximeter (if available), or the invasive ABP waveform. These modalities, however, do not allow definitive diagnosis of the arrhythmia, meaning that specific treatment is not possible.

Bradyarrhythmias

Bradyarrhythmias are defined as any slow rhythm, which may be regular or irregular. They may be precipitated or worsened by anaesthesia. A low HR may result in reduced CO and MAP, and thus requires treatment.

Sinus bradycardia and sinus arrhythmia

Sinus bradycardia is present when the HR is low and the ECG has consistent P waves and QRS–T complexes that are repeatably related. P waves and QRS complexes are upright in lead II, with narrow QRS complexes (see reference intervals, Figure 21.25). Sinus arrhythmia occurs when there is a patterned irregularity to the QRS complexes (they are 'regularly irregular'). There is a P for every QRS, and the morphology and measurements in lead II are normal. Wandering pacemaker (variable P

wave morphology) is often seen alongside sinus arrhythmia. Here, P waves are usually short where the preceding R–R interval is long, and taller when the preceding R–R interval is short.

Recent reports suggest that breed does not have a clinically significant influence on HR in dogs, although true differences between breeds do exist (Ferasin *et al.*, 2010; Hezzell *et al.*, 2013). However, species-specific reference intervals are important to consider, as is the athletic fitness of the patient. Physiologically fit dogs have a higher than average SV and are more likely to have a lower resting HR.

A number of underlying conditions can be associated with, or can precipitate, sinus bradycardia (see Figure 21.24). It is difficult to define specific cut-off values for treatment of bradycardia, as physiological bradycardia very rarely requires treatment. The treatment of sinus bradycardia depends upon its underlying cause, and the decision whether to treat is based upon the impact of bradycardia on perfusion status.

Sinus arrhythmia is normal at lower HRs in dogs. Clinically, sinus arrhythmia can be easily detected as shortening of the R–R interval during inspiration and lengthening of the R–R interval during expiration (see Figure 21.8a). It is associated with conditions causing high vagal tone, including anaesthesia. Sinus arrhythmia in dogs rarely requires treatment as it is a normal physiological finding. In the unlikely event that this arrhythmia is found in association with hypotension, it can be treated with anticholinergic agents (see Figure 21.24).

Sinus arrhythmia is uncommon in cats, and this finding should prompt investigation. Cats in the hospital environment have a predominance of sympathetic tone, which prevents the development of sinus arrhythmia. Therefore, if sinus arrhythmia is present it is often an indicator of underlying pathology, commonly upper respiratory tract obstruction.

Atrioventricular block

First-degree atrioventricular (AV) block is characterized by a prolonged P–Q interval. Second-degree AV block occurs where some P waves are non-conducted; this can be identified by a lack of QRS following the P wave (Figure 21.26). Type I second-degree AV block is defined as a progressively prolonged P–Q interval, followed by a non-conducted P wave. This arrhythmia tends to be cyclical and associated with high vagal tone. Type II second-degree AV block has no predictable prolongation of the P–Q interval, but is simply characterized by non-conducted P waves. This is less likely to be vagally mediated and may become more severe and progress to third-degree AV block. Second-degree AV block can also be described as high grade (frequent blocked P waves) or low grade. High-grade second-degree AV block may be an indication for pacemaker implantation if there are associated clinical signs.

Second-degree AV block is a common finding during anaesthesia. Opioids and alpha-2 agonists commonly induce second-degree AV block, particularly after rapid intravenous administration. The effect is usually transient and rarely requires treatment. Persistent AV block with concurrent severe bradycardia or hypotension may require treatment with anticholinergic agents. These drugs should be used with care when alpha-2 agonists have recently been administered; alpha-2 agonists cause bradycardia due to both central and peripheral effects from a reflex response to peripheral vasoconstriction. Administration of anticholinergics in this situation would cause HR to

Rhythm	Underlying cause	Treatment	Dose and dosing interval	Potential adverse effects
Bradyarrhythmias				
Sinus bradycardia	Anaesthetic drugs Anaesthetic overdose	Reduce or antagonize causative agent Consider treatment with anticholinergics	Atropine: 0.02–0.04 mg/kg i.v. Glycopyrronium: 0.005–0.01 mg/kg i.v. Repeat after 10–15 minutes if no response	Possibility that depth of anaesthesia will lighten Reduced efficacy with hypothermia Low doses may increase severity of bradycardia in the short term
	Hypertension (particularly sudden onset) Pain or noxious stimuli, vasoconstricting agents or phaeochromocytoma	Provide appropriate analgesia Administer vasodilators	Acepromazine: 0.005–0.01 mg/kg i.v. Phentolamine: 0.025–0.1 mg/kg i.v. Repeat phentolamine every 5–20 minutes if needed	Some analgesic agents (e.g. opioids, alpha-2 adrenoceptor agonists) may reduce heart rate further May reduce blood pressure without a concurrent increase in heart rate
	Hypothermia	Use external warming devices and consider warm lavage fluids to re-warm the patient	Continuous warming from anaesthetic induction is recommended. Minimize anaesthetic length to reduce degree of hypothermia	Avoid excessive heat to prevent burns and use equipment according to manufacturers' instructions
	Vagal reflex	Identify cause of stimulation and cease Consider treatment with anticholinergics	Atropine: 0.02–0.04 mg/kg i.v. Glycopyrronium: 0.005–0.01 mg/kg i.v. Repeat after 10–15 minutes if no response	Reduced efficacy with hypothermia Low doses may increase severity of bradycardia in the short term
	Hyperkalaemia	Calcium gluconate 10% Dextrose Dextrose ± insulin Sodium bicarbonate	Calcium gluconate: 50–100 mg/kg (0.5–1.0 ml/kg of 10% solution) i.v. over 10 minutes Dextrose: 0.5–1.0 g/kg i.v. over 5 minutes Regular insulin, 0.25–0.5 IU/kg i.v. with dextrose, 1–2 g per unit of insulin (2–4 ml of 50% dextrose, diluted into 8–16 ml of fluids, respectively, to make a 10% solution) Sodium bicarbonate: 1–2 mEq/kg i.v. over 15–30 minutes	Calcium may induce arrhythmias if administered rapidly Possible hypoglycaemia with insulin Electrolyte imbalances and volume overload with sodium bicarbonate
	Hypoglycaemia	Dextrose	0.5–1.0 g/kg i.v. over 5 minutes 2.5–5% dextrose i.v. infusion if prolonged hypoglycaemia is expected	Administration of concentrated (>10%) dextrose in peripheral veins can result in phlebitis
	Severe acidosis (pH <7.0)	Sodium bicarbonate	1–2 mEq/kg i.v. over 15–30 minutes	Electrolyte imbalances and volume overload with sodium bicarbonate
	Severe hypoxia	Increase inspired oxygen concentration and consider ventilation	Use 100% oxygen initially Reduce inspired concentration for long-term use	May not respond if severe right-to-left shunting is present. High inspiratory pressures may worsen haemodynamics
	Raised intracranial pressure	Mannitol Hypertonic saline (7.5%)	Mannitol: 0.2–2.0 g/kg i.v. over 30 minutes Hypertonic saline: 2–4 ml/kg i.v. over 20 minutes Repeat after 4–8 hours if required	Volume overload, electrolyte imbalances and acidosis
Second-degree AV block	High vagal tone	Anticholinergics	Atropine: 0.02–0.04 mg/kg i.v. Glycopyrronium: 0.005–0.01 mg/kg i.v. Repeat after 10–15 minutes if no response	Anticholinergics administered after alpha-2 adrenoceptor agonists can increase myocardial workload and oxygen consumption Reduced efficacy with hypothermia Low doses may increase severity of bradycardia in the short term
	Anaesthetic drugs: Opioids	Anticholinergics	Atropine: 0.02–0.04 mg/kg i.v. Glycopyrronium: 0.005–0.01 mg/kg i.v. Repeat after 10–15 minutes if no response	
	Alpha-2 adrenoceptor agonists	Antagonize alpha-2 agonists (atipamezole)	Atipamezole: use 0.25–0.5 the dose that would have been used to antagonize the administered dose of medetomidine i.m.	

21.24 Common causes and treatment options for the management of perioperative arrhythmias. AV = atrioventricular; DMVD = degenerative mitral valve disease; ECG = electrocardiogram; GSD = German Shepherd Dog; J = Joules; PCV =packed cell volume. (continues)

Rhythm	Underlying cause	Treatment	Dose and dosing interval	Potential adverse effects
Bradyarrhythmias continued				
Third-degree AV block	Inflammatory or degenerative AV nodal disease	Pacemaker	Pacemaker placement generally recommended for lifelong support	
Sick sinus syndrome	Unknown, although often associated with DMVD and sinus node fibrosis with vascular changes often seen	Anticholinergics Pacemaker	Atropine: 0.02–0.04 mg/kg i.v. Glycopyrronium: 0.005–0.01 mg/kg i.v. Pacemaker placement generally recommended	Reduced efficacy with hypothermia Low doses may increase severity of bradycardia in the short term
Asystole and pulseless electrical activity	Many possible causes, including those listed for sinus bradycardia	Initiate cardiopulmonary resuscitation immediately Attempt to identify and treat potential underlying causes	Perform basic life support continuously until there is a positive response or there has been no response for 10 minutes If possible, perform advanced life support once basic life support has been initiated	Treatment may not be successful Success rates of treating anaesthetic cardiac arrests are higher than for non-anaesthetic cardiac arrests if treatment is instigated rapidly
Tachyarrhythmias				
Sinus tachycardia	Inadequate anaesthesia or analgesia	Increase depth of anaesthesia Provide more analgesia	Depends on anaesthetic technique being employed Consider providing additional opioids or alternative analgesia	
	Hypovolaemia or hypotension	Volume resuscitation with i.v. crystalloid or colloid therapy Vasopressors or inotropes for hypotension without hypovolaemia	Volumes of intravenous fluid therapy required depend upon degree of hypovolaemia (see Chapter 18) For doses and dosing intervals of vasopressors and inotropes, see Figure 21.13	Take care to avoid volume overload in patients in cardiac failure
	Hypercapnia	Initiate or increase positive pressure ventilation Decrease depth of anaesthesia	Positive pressure ventilation may be required for the remainder of anaesthesia A decreased depth of anaesthesia may reduce the degree of hypoventilation	High inspiratory pressures may worsen haemodynamics
	Electrolyte disturbances: Hypokalaemia Hypercalcaemia Hypomagnesaemia	Assess plasma electrolytes and then supplement or instigate appropriate treatment to correct the disturbance	Hypokalaemia: potassium supplementation with fluid therapy, not to exceed 0.5 mEq/kg/h Hypercalcaemia: diuresis with 0.9% sodium chloride, salmon calcitonin 4–6 IU/kg s.c. q8–12 hours Hypomagnesaemia: magnesium supplementation at 0.15–0.3 mEq/kg i.v. over 5–15 minutes (equivalent to 19–37 mg/kg magnesium sulphate i.v. or 16–32 mg/kg magnesium chloride i.v.)	Care should be taken with the rate of K⁺ supplementation to avoid inadvertent hyperkalaemia Volume overload may occur with large volumes of i.v. fluid for diuresis in patients with cardiac disease
	Hypoxia or hypoxaemia	Increase inspired oxygen concentration and consider ventilation	Use 100% oxygen initially Reduce inspired concentration for long-term use	May not respond if severe right-to-left shunting is present. High inspiratory pressures may worsen haemodynamics
	Anaemia	Whole blood, packed red cells or Oxyglobin®	Chronic anaemia, if affecting haemodynamics, should be treated before anaesthesia to increase the PCV >20% Acute haemorrhage will primarily cause hypovolaemia, but support of oxygen-carrying capacity may be required secondarily Volumes of blood products or Oxyglobin® will depend upon the degree of anaemia and on the volume status of the patient	See Chapter 18 regarding potential adverse effects of blood products

21.24 (continued) Common causes and treatment options for the management of perioperative arrhythmias. AV = atrioventricular; DMVD = degenerative mitral valve disease; ECG = electrocardiogram; GSD = German Shepherd Dog; J = Joules; PCV = packed cell volume. (continues)

Tachyarrhythmias continued

Rhythm	Underlying cause	Treatment	Dose and dosing interval	Potential adverse effects
	Pre-existing disease, e.g. hyperthyroidism or phaeochromocytoma	Attempt to reduce catecholamine release (storms). Vagomimetics such as beta blockers or opioids may be useful	Beta blockers: see Figure 21.13. Short acting opioids: Fentanyl: 1–2 µg/kg i.v. Alfentanil: 1–2 µg/kg i.v. Remifentanil: 0.5–1.0 µg/kg i.v.	Bronchospasm may occur with propranolol
	Drug therapy, e.g. beta-1 adrenoceptor agonists	Cease causative drug therapy		
Idioventricular rhythm	Cardiac or extracardiac disease	Usually requires no specific treatment and usually self-resolves. Lidocaine may be administered, although this is rarely successful	Lidocaine i.v. bolus: 1–2 mg/kg (dogs), 0.5 mg/kg (cats). Lidocaine i.v. infusion: 25–100 µg/kg/min (dogs)	Lidocaine boluses may cause some cardiovascular depression, especially with repeated doses and any dose in cats. Maximum dose of 8 mg/kg (dogs) and 2 mg/kg (cats) over 10 minutes should be administered
Atrial fibrillation	Vagotonic in large or giant breeds (especially GSD). Atrial dilation – may be present in structurally normal hearts in giant-breed dogs	Usually requires no specific treatment in the peri-anaesthetic period unless newly developed due to anaesthesia; in this case, lidocaine should be used. Diltiazem or beta blockers may be useful to control heart rate in pre-existing atrial fibrillation. Electrical cardioversion may be performed	Lidocaine 2 mg/kg i.v. bolus, repeated every 10 minutes up to a total dose of 8 mg/kg. Beta blockers: see Figure 21.13. Diltiazem: 0.1–0.25 mg/kg i.v. bolus slowly over 1–2 minutes, repeat after 5–10 minutes up to 0.75 mg/kg. Diltiazem i.v. infusion: 0.1–0.3 mg/kg/h	Lidocaine boluses may cause some cardiovascular depression, especially with repeated doses and any dose in cats. Bronchospasm may occur with propranolol. Diltiazem may cause a mild reduction in systolic function
Ventricular tachycardia	Cardiac or extracardiac disease	Lidocaine. Magnesium may be attempted for refractory ventricular tachycardia	Lidocaine i.v. bolus: 1–2 mg/kg (dogs), 0.5 mg/kg (cats). Lidocaine i.v. infusion: 25–100 µg/kg/min (dogs). Magnesium i.v. bolus: 30 mg/kg over 10 minutes. Magnesium i.v. infusion: 0.5 mmol/kg/24 hours i.v. (equivalent to 5.2 mg/kg/h)	Lidocaine boluses may cause some cardiovascular depression, especially with repeated doses and any dose in cats. Maximum dose of lidocaine of 8 mg/kg (dogs) and 2 mg/kg (cats) over 10 minutes should be administered. Magnesium should be given slowly i.v. and an ECG is recommended for monitoring
Ventricular fibrillation	Many possible causes, including those listed for sinus tachycardia	Initiate cardiopulmonary resuscitation immediately. Attempt to identify and treat potential underlying causes. Instigate electrical defibrillation if available; otherwise attempt a precordial thump	Perform basic life support continuously until there is a positive response or there has been no response for 10 minutes. If possible, perform advanced life support once basic life support has been initiated. External electrical defibrillation: 4–6 J/kg. Internal electrical defibrillation: 0.5–1 J/kg	Treatment may not be successful. Success rates of treating anaesthetic cardiac arrests are higher than for non-anaesthetic cardiac arrests if treatment is instigated quickly

21.24 (continued) Common causes and treatment options for the management of perioperative arrhythmias. AV = atrioventricular; DMVD = degenerative mitral valve disease; ECG = electrocardiogram; GSD = German Shepherd Dog; J = Joules; PCV = packed cell volume.

Parameter	Dog	Cat
Heart rate (beats/min)	70–160	140–240
P wave duration (seconds)	<0.04	<0.04
P wave amplitude (mV)	<0.4	<0.2
P–Q interval (seconds)	0.06–0.13	0.05–0.09
QRS duration (seconds)	<0.06	<0.04
R wave amplitude (mV)	<2.5 (<3.0 in giant breeds)	<0.9
T wave character	<25% QRS complex height, can be negative in lead II	
Q–T interval (seconds)	0.15–0.25	0.12–0.18

21.25 Reference intervals for electrocardiographic measurements in the dog and the cat.

increase while the concurrent peripheral vasoconstriction persists. This can result in dramatically increased after-load, and thus increased myocardial work and oxygen demand. This may result in significant arrhythmias, most likely associated with myocardial hypoxia. For this reason, haemodynamically significant AV block caused by alpha-2 adrenoceptor agonist administration should be initially treated with atipamezole (see Chapter 13).

Third-degree AV block is an indication for pacemaker implantation. With this block, P waves are completely dissociated from QRS complexes, with the P wave rate usually greater than the QRS rate. QRS complexes are often wide and bizarre, representing a ventricular escape rhythm. Dogs often have an escape rate of 30–40 beats/min, and invariably have clinical signs associated with the arrhythmia. Cats can have an escape rate at 80–120 beats/min, so often do not exhibit clinical signs and the arrhythmia may be an incidental finding. In dogs, there is a risk of failure of the escape focus, but cats seem not to be at risk of sudden death. Third-degree AV block is very rarely vagally mediated and usually reflects damage to the AV node. Differential diagnoses include neoplastic or infiltrative disease, trauma or most commonly an idiopathic disease process. Some dogs with third-degree AV block have progressive myocardial dysfunction even if HR is normalized by pacemaker implantation. In these cases, third-degree AV block may represent an early stage of primary myocardial disease.

Sick sinus syndrome

Sinus node dysfunction, more commonly known as sick sinus syndrome (SSS), is an idiopathic disease of the sinus node. It is most commonly seen in West Highland White Terriers and Miniature Schnauzers. Other breeds are rarely affected. The ECG can appear chaotic, with periods of extreme tachycardia and bradycardia. Long pauses in the sinus rhythm (sinus arrest) are often followed by ventricular escape beats. The P wave morphology can vary, with first- and second-degree AV block often present (suggesting more diffuse conduction system disease in some patients). Long pauses in the rhythm can occur, sometimes for over 10 seconds. Pacemaker implantation is the treatment of choice for patients with clinical signs. Sick sinus syndrome can also be detected as an incidental finding; these patients should be monitored for the development of clinical signs.

If dogs with SSS are anaesthetized, pauses in the rhythm may become severely prolonged, which can lead to cardiac arrest. Although vagal tone may not be the sole cause, these patients should be treated with anticholinergic agents. Periods of tachycardia rarely require treatment, and the treatment of such tachycardia may exacerbate the sinus arrest.

Asystole and pulseless electrical activity

Asystole and pulseless electrical activity (PEA) are two of the three cardiac arrest rhythms. Emergency treatment is required if either of these is identified. Asystole is the absence of cardiac electrical activity on an ECG. Sometimes, PEA is identified. This rhythm often appears sinus in origin (P–QRS–T), but has a slow rate, prolonged P–Q interval and a wide QRS complex (Figure 21.27); T wave abnormalities may also be present. If asystole or PEA is identified, cardiopulmonary resuscitation should be immediately started (see Chapter 31).

Tachyarrhythmias

Tachyarrhythmias (rapid rhythms) may be regular or irregular, and can be intermittent in the case of VT or SVT. Severe tachyarrhythmias can reduce CO because SV is

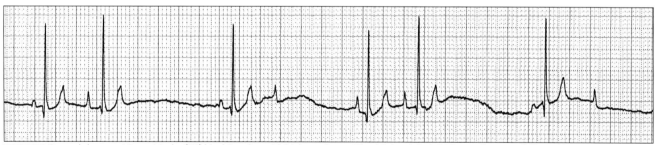

21.26 Second-degree atrioventricular (AV) block in a dog with high vagal tone. The third and sixth QRS complexes are followed by non-conducted P waves. Variable P–Q interval is present (Wenckebach phenomenon; easily seen when comparing the first and second complexes), typical of Type I second-degree AV block.

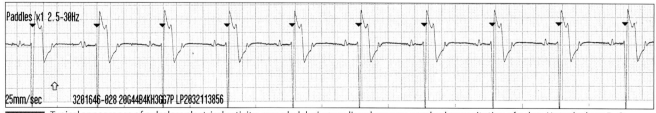

21.27 Typical appearance of pulseless electrical activity, recorded during cardiopulmonary–cerebral resuscitation of a dog. Note the long P–Q interval, wide QRS complex and right bundle branch block morphology.

decreased by a reduced diastolic filling time. The decision to treat tachyarrhythmias should be based on the severity of the haemodynamic effect. Some ventricular arrhythmias may be unstable and can lead to terminal arrhythmias.

Sinus tachycardia

A rhythm originating in the sinus node (positive P wave in lead II, with upright QRS complexes of normal duration in lead II), at a high HR for the species and context (see Figure 21.25), is defined as sinus tachycardia. This is a physiological response to sympathetic tone. Although this is a normal compensatory response in a patient with heart failure, there are a number of alternative reasons for sinus tachycardia, generally caused by sympathetic tone (see Figure 21.24).

The cut-off HR value between sinus rhythm and sinus tachycardia is somewhat arbitrary. Usual values are >160 beats/min in dogs and >220 beats/min in cats. In anaesthetized patients that develop sinus tachycardia, it is of paramount importance to identify the cause (e.g. lack of adequate analgesia/anaesthesia, hypovolaemia, hypotension).

Sinus tachycardia should be differentiated from SVT, if an overt cause of tachycardia cannot be identified. Regular rates of >300 beats/min are common with SVT, where identification of a discrete P wave is difficult due to overlap with the ST segment of the preceding complex. In dogs with SVT, a pathological process is usually responsible for the abnormal generation or propagation of electrical activity; this is not the case in sinus tachycardia.

Atrial fibrillation

Atrial fibrillation has no pattern to the arrhythmia (it is 'irregularly irregular'). QRS complexes are supraventricular in origin (i.e. traversing the AV node) but there are no discernible P waves. Often, fine undulations of the baseline (called F waves) are present (Figure 21.28). This can be differentiated from atrial flutter, which has larger, regular and repeatable undulations of the baseline that have a 'saw-toothed' appearance and often occur at a rate of approximately 400 beats/min. Atrial flutter is usually transient and rapidly converts to AF.

The most common cause of AF in small animals is severe atrial dilation caused by primary cardiac disease. Atrial fibrillation can also be identified in dogs without structural heart disease, most often in large or giant breeds. In some dogs, AF may be associated with hypothyroidism, and may also be an early sign of an underlying myocardial disease, such as DCM. After pericardiocentesis, AF can occur transiently; attempts at cardioversion should be considered if fibrillation persists for more than 12 hours.

Since atrial contraction contributes only approximately 20% to ventricular filling at rest, AF is unlikely to be life-threatening. This is especially the case during anaesthesia. Lack of atrial contraction has a greater impact during exercise or with higher HR. As patients with AF may have a high sympathetic tone due to CHF, HR can be high and CO will be further reduced by the development of AF.

Most patients with AF can be safely anaesthetized, and specific treatment for AF without underlying heart disease is rarely required during the perioperative period. Patients with AF and persistent tachycardia (best confirmed by Holter monitoring in the home environment), may require pre-anaesthetic stabilization with oral medication to control HR. In patients requiring immediate anaesthesia, beta blockers, diltiazem or vagomimetic agents (e.g. opioids) may be included in the anaesthetic protocol to provide control of HR. However, beta blockers should not be used in patients with LA dilation or CHF. In patients that are anaesthetized specifically for electrical cardioversion of AF, higher doses of vagomimetic drugs should be avoided as they may reduce the likelihood of successful conversion.

Anaesthesia itself may cause AF in some dogs. These patients are most likely to be large dogs receiving significant intravenous fluid therapy and treatment with lidocaine (as for VT) may be used in an attempt to restore sinus rhythm. If AF persists beyond the initial recovery period with bolus lidocaine treatment, either prolonged intravenous infusions of lidocaine can be used or electrical (DC) cardioversion may be indicated. In patients with post-anaesthesia AF, opioids may be antagonized and intravenous fluid rate reduced before attempting cardioversion. Care should be taken when antagonizing opioids in postsurgical patients, as this can make subsequent analgesia extremely challenging. If AF is not adversely affecting haemodynamics, it may be more appropriate to delay cardioversion until the patient no longer requires opioid treatment.

Isolated ventricular premature complexes

With this arrhythmia, the QRS complexes of ventricular origin appear wide and bizarre compared with supraventricular complexes (see Figure 21.8b). They have no repeatable preceding P waves and the T wave is opposite in polarity to the QRS. When a ventricular ectopic complex occurs before the next sinus complex would normally be

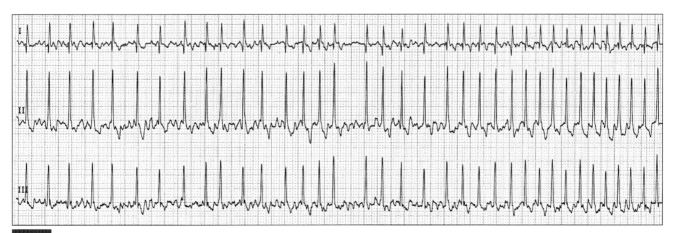

21.28 Atrial fibrillation, identified by a highly irregular arrhythmia with no P waves, an undulating baseline and supraventricular QRS complexes.

expected, it is defined as a VPC. Following a VPC, there is a pause in the background rhythm. Two VPCs in sequence are termed a couplet, three a triplet, and four or more a run of VT. In ventricular bigeminy, every other beat is a VPC. In ventricular trigeminy, every third beat is a VPC. In lead II with the patient in right lateral recumbency, negative complexes suggest a left ventricular origin, while positive complexes suggest a right ventricular origin.

Ventricular premature complexes may be associated with both cardiac and non-cardiac causes. In dogs, non-cardiac causes are probably more common. In the authors' experience, ventricular arrhythmias in cats are almost always associated with an underlying cardiomyopathy. It is normal for healthy dogs to have small numbers of VPCs (<50 per day).

During anaesthesia, VPCs rarely require specific treatment as they are unlikely to affect cardiovascular function, especially if they are isolated. However, if more complex ventricular arrhythmias are detected (couplets, triplets, VT), myocardial hypoxia or undetected cardiac disease should be considered.

Ventricular rhythms

When ventricular QRS complexes predominate for a period of time at a HR within the normal reference interval, the rhythm is known as an accelerated idioventricular rhythm. When the HR is significantly higher than the reference interval for sinus rhythm, it is called VT. The rate, complex morphology and patient haemodynamics should help guide the decision of when to treat.

Idioventricular rhythm is common during anaesthesia of dogs in American Society of Anesthesiologists (ASA) physical status categories grades 3–5, particularly when abdominal disease is present (e.g. GDV, sepsis, haemoabdomen). Where the arrhythmia has a non-cardiac cause, it usually resolves over a period of hours to days once the underlying disease has been treated (Figure 21.29). An idioventricular rhythm (cardiogenic or not) may also be intermittent during anaesthesia, due to alterations in autonomic tone. Idioventricular rhythms rarely require specific treatment because ventricular filling is not significantly compromised at normal HRs and so blood pressure is rarely affected. However, the arrhythmia may cause asynchronous ventricular contraction, which could reduce SV. If idioventricular rhythm is thought to be haemodynamically significant, lidocaine is the first-line drug for attempted cardioversion. However, its action is transient and cardioversion is not always successful. An infusion of lidocaine may also be beneficial as part of multimodal anaesthesia and analgesia for ASA category 3–5 patients.

In patients with continuous or paroxysmal VT, tachycardia (often >200–300 beats/min) increases the haemodynamic significance because of reduced diastolic filling time. In addition, higher ventricular rates lead to electrical

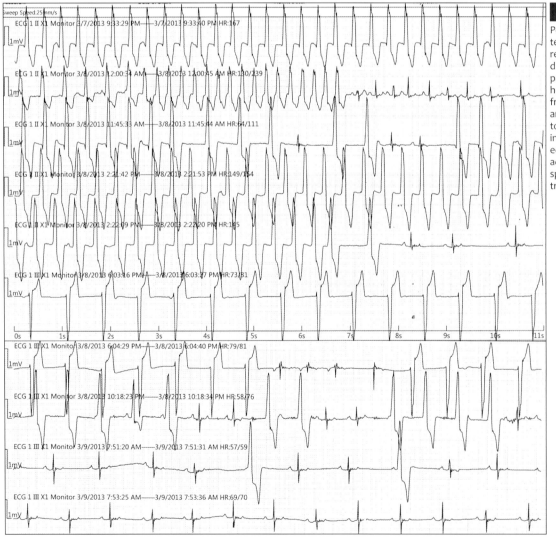

21.29

Postoperative telemetric ECG recording from a gastric dilatation–volvulus patient. Over the first 24 hours postoperatively, frequent ventricular arrhythmias converted to sinus rhythm with infrequent ventricular ectopy, without administration of any specific antiarrhythmic treatment.

instability in the myocardium and stimulation of cells during their refractory period. When combined with myocardial hypoxia due to reduced diastolic coronary perfusion, VT can deteriorate to VF. Differences in ventricular complex morphology (polymorphic VT) on the ECG suggest that the electrical rhythm is less stable and there may be a greater risk of deterioration; treatment should be instigated for these cases. In the peri-anaesthetic period, the first-line treatment is intravenous lidocaine. Underlying triggers of ventricular arrhythmias should be excluded (see Figure 21.24). For patients that do not respond to lidocaine, hypomagnesaemia and hypokalaemia should be excluded; if present, these electrolyte abnormalities should be corrected and conversion to sinus rhythm re-attempted.

Ventricular fibrillation is a cardiac arrest rhythm. It is identified by a chaotic, undulating line on the ECG. No defined QRS complexes are present. ECG lead disconnection, electrical interference and artefact can be misinterpreted as VF, so these must be quickly excluded if VF is suspected. Once VF is confirmed, cardiopulmonary resuscitation should be initiated and electrical defibrillation is indicated, either externally or internally (see Chapter 31).

Bundle branch blocks

Bundle branch blocks (BBBs) are seen when electrical activity within the ventricular myocardium is re-routed from rapid conducting fibres (the left and right bundle branches) and travels more slowly through myocardial cells. They can be intermittent or persistent. The ECG shows wide, bizarre QRS complexes, which may at first be presumed to represent ventricular complexes; however, BBBs can be differentiated from idioventricular rhythm by the identification of repeatable P waves preceding the QRS complexes in BBB. Occasionally, concurrent AF may be present. In this case, the rhythm can be differentiated from a ventricular arrhythmia by the complete lack of regularity and absence of any normal sinus complexes. Right BBB has wide negative QRS complexes in lead II. It is commonly associated with anaesthesia or is an incidental finding in dogs. It is also relatively common after pulmonic balloon valvuloplasty. Left BBB has wide positive QRS complexes in lead II. In the authors' experience, left BBB is more commonly identified in patients with cardiac disease. Occurrence of BBB during anaesthesia does not require specific treatment, although causes of myocardial hypoxia should be excluded.

Interventional cardiology

Pulmonic balloon valvuloplasty

Severe PS or moderate PS with clinical signs are typical indications for pulmonic balloon valvuloplasty. Approach is via the right jugular or femoral vein, using a percutaneous modified Seldinger method. The balloon catheter is passed into the vena cava, then the right atrium and through the tricuspid valve. From the RV, the RV outflow tract and pulmonary artery are catheterized. Balloon dilation of the stenotic pulmonary valve is accomplished by multiple forceful inflations of the balloon catheter under fluoroscopic guidance (Figure 21.30). Success is defined as a 50% or greater reduction in severity of the pressure gradient.

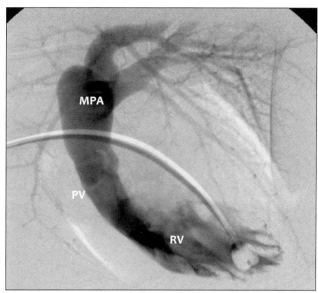

21.30 Angiogram (digital subtraction) from a 1-year-old entire male Miniature Pinscher with valvular pulmonic stenosis. A balloon-tipped catheter can be seen in the right ventricle (accessed from the jugular vein and cranial vena cava). Opacification of the right ventricular outflow tract, pulmonic valve and pulmonary artery shows abnormal, fused valve leaflets that are not fully open during systole. MPA = main pulmonary artery; PV = pulmonic valve; RV = right ventricle.

Common complications:

- Haemorrhage from the venous access site
- Ventricular arrhythmia during catheterization of the RV outflow tract and balloon dilation of the pulmonic valve
- Supraventricular arrhythmias during right atrial catheterization
- Damage to the tricuspid apparatus or pulmonary artery.

Anaesthetic management

With inflation of the balloon catheter, there is a temporary complete occlusion of the RV outflow tract. This reduces pulmonary perfusion and LV output and causes a pronounced reduction in SAP. Ventricular arrhythmias are very common during this procedure and can be treated with lidocaine boluses and/or infusion. The balloon may need to be deflated early if haemodynamics are critically affected. Time should be allowed for the cardiovascular system to recover before repeat balloon inflation is performed.

The authors routinely use infusions of lidocaine (30–50 μg/kg/min i.v.) and low-dose fentanyl (0.05–0.1 μg/kg/min i.v.) in combination with volatile agents; the infusions help to reduce volatile anaesthetic requirement and contribute to a balanced anaesthetic technique.

Device occlusion of a patent ductus arteriosus

Left-to-right flow through a PDA is the typical indication for occlusion of the ductus, even in the absence of clinical signs. Approach is via the femoral artery, using a vascular cut-down and modified Seldinger technique. The catheter is passed into the aorta, through the PDA and into the pulmonary artery. An Amplatz canine ductal occluder (ACDO) or thrombogenic coil can then be placed to occlude the flow. The arterial access site is then ligated or repaired, followed by surgical closure of the wound. A successful procedure leads to a significant reduction in shunt flow.

Common complications:

- Failure to occlude PDA flow
- Arterial haemorrhage at the vascular access site
- Device loss (catastrophic if in the aorta, causes iatrogenic PTE if in the pulmonary artery)
- Haemodynamically significant bradycardia after occlusion
- Damage to the pulmonary artery
- Rupture of the PDA
- Haemolysis caused by a thrombogenic coil.

Anaesthetic management

If guide wires or catheters are passed into the RV outflow tract during the procedure when attempting to place them in the main pulmonary artery, ventricular arrhythmias may occur, as with pulmonic balloon valvuloplasty (see above). Bradycardia after occlusion rarely requires treatment with anticholinergic agents, as previously discussed.

Pacemaker implantation

A permanent transvenous pacemaker is indicated for bradyarrhythmias associated with clinical signs, such as SSS, third-degree AV block, high-grade second-degree AV block or persistent atrial standstill. Approach is via the right jugular vein, using a surgical cut-down and vessel isolation. Temporary trans-thoracic or transvenous pacing can be performed at the beginning of anaesthesia to minimize the risk of bradycardia worsening after induction (see also Chapter 23). The pacemaker lead is inserted into the RV, via the cranial vena cava and right atrium (Figure 21.31). The lead tip is anchored either passively around the RV trabeculae or screwed into the endocardium of the RV (active fixation). Ligation of the venous access site is performed at the lead entry site. The wound is then closed surgically. Pacemaker implantation is rarely performed in cats; in this species pacemaker attachment is epicardial and is achieved via a transdiaphragmatic approach. Success is defined as the abolition of clinical signs associated with the bradyarrhythmia.

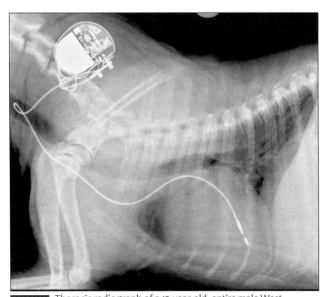

21.31 Thoracic radiograph of a 13-year-old, entire male West Highland White Terrier after pacemaker implantation (right lateral view). The pacemaker pulse generator can be seen in the prescapular region, with the pacemaker lead traversing the right jugular vein, cranial vena cava and right heart. The tip of the pacemaker lead is passively fixed in the apical right ventricle.

Common complications:

- Postoperative lead dislodgement or damage
- Ventricular arrhythmia during pacemaker lead insertion
- Damage to the tricuspid apparatus
- Ventricular perforation (with active fixation)
- Postoperative PTE.

Anaesthetic management

After administration of sedative or anaesthetic agents, there is a vulnerable period before permanent artificial pacing can be initiated. The risk is greatest where drugs with a negative effect on HR are used (e.g. opioids). Sedation with a combination of acepromazine and buprenorphine should have minimal effect on HR, although low doses of full mu opioid receptor agonists can be used successfully. When the patient is sedated, a temporary transvenous pacemaker lead can be inserted into the RV; this will reduce the risk of general anaesthesia. Patients requiring external pacing must be anaesthetized beforehand to avoid significant discomfort from the external electrical impulses. As external stimulation of skeletal muscles causes significant patient twitching, neuromuscular blockade (see Chapter 16) and artificial ventilation are necessary. Once temporary pacing has begun, anaesthesia usually proceeds with minimal complications.

References and further reading

Connolly DJ, Guitian J, Boswood A and Neiger R (2005) Serum troponin I levels in hyperthyroid cats before and after treatment with radioactive iodine. *Journal of Feline Medicine and Surgery* **7**, 289–300

Dugdale A (2010a) Some cardiac considerations. In: *Veterinary Anaesthesia Principles to Practice, 1st edn*, ed. A Dugdale, pp. 341–343. Wiley-Blackwell, Chichester

Dugdale A (2010b) Cardiopulmonary cerebral resuscitation (CPCR). In: *Veterinary Anaesthesia Principles to Practice, 1st edn*, ed. A Dugdale, pp. 359–370. Wiley-Blackwell, Chichester

Ferasin L, Crews L, Biller DS, Lamb KE and Borgarelli M (2013) Risk factors for coughing in dogs with naturally acquired myxomatous mitral valve disease. *Journal of Veterinary Internal Medicine* **27**, 286–292

Ferasin L, Ferasin H and Little CJ (2010) Lack of correlation between canine heart rate and body size in veterinary clinical practice. *Journal of Small Animal Practice* **51**, 412–418

Hezzell MJ, Humm K, Dennis SG, Agee L and Boswood A (2013) Relationship between heart rate and age, body weight and breed in 10,849 dogs. *Journal of Small Animal Practice* **54**, 318–324

Höllmer M, Willesen JL, Jensen AT and Koch J (2008) Aortic stenosis in the Dogue de Bordeaux. *Journal of Small Animal Practice* **49**, 432–437

Hopkins A, Giuffrida M and Larenza MP (2014) Midazolam, as a co-induction agent, has propofol sparing effects but also decreases systolic blood pressure in healthy dogs. *Veterinary Anaesthesia and Analgesia* **41**, 64–72

James TN, Robertson BT, Waldo AL and Branch CE (1975) De subitaneis mortibus. XV. Hereditary stenosis of the His bundle in Pug dogs. *Circulation* **52**, 1152–1160

Johns SM, Nelson OL and Gay JM (2012) Left atrial function in cats with left-sided cardiac disease and pleural effusion or pulmonary edema. *Journal of Veterinary Internal Medicine* **26**, 1134–1139

Kudnig ST and Mama K (2002) Perioperative fluid therapy. *Journal of the American Veterinary Medical Association* **221**, 1112–1121

Lamont LA, Bulmer BJ, Sisson DD, Grimm KA and Tranquilli WJ (2002) Doppler echocardiographic effects of medetomidine on dynamic left ventricular outflow tract obstruction in cats. *Journal of the American Veterinary Medical Association* **221**, 1276–1281

Levick JR (2010) Specialization in individual circulations. In: *An Introduction to Cardiovascular Physiology, 5th edn*, ed. JR Levick, pp. 116–146. Hodder Arnold, London

Luis Fuentes V, Johnson LR and Dennis SG (2010) *BSAVA Manual of Canine and Feline Cardiorespiratory Medicine, 2nd edn*. BSAVA Publications, Gloucester

Machen MC, Oyama MA, Gordon SG *et al.* (2014) Multi-centered investigation of a point-of-care NT-proBN ELISA assay to detect moderate to severe occult (pre-clinical) feline heart disease in cats referred for cardiac evaluation. *Journal of Veterinary Cardiology* **16**, 245–255

Martin MWS, Stafford Johnson MJ and Celona B (2009) Canine dilated cardiomyopathy: a retrospective study of signalment, presentation and clinical findings in 369 cases. *Journal of Small Animal Practice* **50**, 23–29

Matos JM, Schnyder M, Bektas R *et al.* (2012) Recruitment of arteriovenous pulmonary shunts may attenuate the development of pulmonary hypertension in dogs experimentally infected with *Angiostrongylus vasorum*. *Journal of Veterinary Cardiology* **14**, 313–322

McNally EM, Robertson SA and Pablo LS (2009) Comparison of time to desaturation between preoxygenated and nonpreoxygenated dogs following sedation with acepromazine maleate and morphine and induction of anesthesia with propofol. *American Journal of Veterinary Research* **70**, 1333–1338

Moïse NS, Pariaut R, Gelzer AR, Kraus MS and Jung SW (2005) Cardioversion with lidocaine of vagally associated atrial fibrillation in two dogs. *Journal of Veterinary Cardiology* **7**, 143–148

Nakamura K, Yamasaki M, Ohta H *et al.* (2011) Effects of sildenafil citrate on five dogs with Eisenmenger's syndrome. *Journal of Small Animal Practice* **52**, 595–598

Oliveira P, Domenech O, Silva J *et al.* (2011) Retrospective review of congenital heart disease in 976 dogs. *Journal of Veterinary Internal Medicine* **25**, 477–483

Pariaut R, Moïse NS, Koetie BD *et al.* (2008) Lidocaine converts acute vagally associated atrial fibrillation to sinus rhythm in German Shepherd dogs with inherited arrhythmias. *Journal of Veterinary Internal Medicine* **22**, 1274–1282

Pyle RL, Lowensohn HS, Khouri EM, Gregg DE and Patterson DF (1973) Left cirumflex coronary artery hemodynamics in conscious dogs with congenital subaortic stenosis. *Circulation Research* **33**, 34–38

Quintavalla C, Guazzetti S, Mavropoulou A and Bussadori C (2010) Aorto-septal angle in Boxer dogs with subaortic stenosis: an echocardiographic study. *Veterinary Journal* **3**, 332–337

Robinson RL and Borer-Weir K (2013) A dose titration study into the effects of diazepam or midazolam on the propofol dose requirements for induction of general anaesthesia in client owned dogs, premedicated with methadone and acepromazine. *Veterinary Anaesthesia and Analgesia* **40**, 455–463

Rodighiero V (1989) Effects of cardiovascular disease on pharmacokinetics. *Cardiovascular Drugs and Therapy* **3**, 711–730

Summerfield NJ, Boswood A, O'Grady MR *et al.* (2012) Efficacy of pimobendan in the prevention of CHF or sudden death in Doberman Pinschers with preclinical dilated cardiomyopathy (The PROTECT Study). *Journal of Veterinary Internal Medicine* **26**, 1337–1349

Wagner T, Luis Fuentes V, Payne JR, McDermott N and Brodbelt D (2010) Comparison of auscultatory and echocardiographic findings in healthy adult cats. *Journal of Veterinary Cardiology* **12**, 171–182

Chapter 22

Respiratory compromise

Tamara Grubb

Causes of respiratory compromise can range from stenotic nares to severe alveolar collapse, and anaesthesia of patients with these conditions can exacerbate or even create further problems. The choice of anaesthetic agents will be mainly dictated by the overall health of the patient, but the chosen anaesthetic technique is often critical. Patient stabilization, monitoring and support should be directed towards normalizing and supporting respiratory function. Appropriate anaesthetic and analgesic management are the keys to success, regardless of the location of the airway disease or dysfunction.

General pathophysiology

Respiratory compromise can have varying impacts on gas exchange. Hypoventilation may be caused by, for example, central nervous system (CNS) depression or impaired thoracic and/or diaphragmatic movement, resulting in hypercapnia (arterial carbon dioxide tension (P_aCO_2) >45 mmHg (6 kPa)). If this occurs when the patient is breathing room air (inspired oxygen fraction (F_iO_2) 0.21), hypoxaemia (arterial oxygen tension (P_aO_2) <60 mmHg (8 kPa)) can also develop. Providing supplemental oxygen will improve oxygenation, but the definitive treatment is to improve alveolar ventilation. States that cause pulmonary atelectasis (e.g. dorsal recumbency, gastrointestinal distension, external thoracic compression) or lung consolidation (e.g. tumours, abscesses) can increase intrapulmonary shunting of blood, where blood passes through these areas of collapsed lung without taking part in gaseous exchange. This deoxygenated blood then enters the arterial circulation, lowering the overall oxygen content of the blood. Normal physiological shunt is approximately 3–5% of cardiac output; increased shunt can lead to hypoxaemia either with or without concurrent hypercapnia.

Alveolar dead space can increase with some respiratory diseases (emphysema) or vascular accidents (pulmonary thromboembolism), with the result that alveoli with little or no perfusion are ventilated. Normal lungs have little alveolar dead space, which means that end-tidal carbon dioxide ($P_E'CO_2$) measurements are very similar to P_aCO_2 and thus provide a non-invasive way of monitoring alveolar ventilation (see Chapter 7).

Alveolar ventilation is normally well matched to lung perfusion; however, the combined effects of increased alveolar dead space and intrapulmonary shunt lead to changes in alveolar ventilation (V_A)/perfusion (Q) ratios

(V_A/Q) within the lung. The normal V_A/Q ratio is approximately 1; ratios <1 indicate relatively increased intrapulmonary shunt, and ratios >1 indicate relatively increased alveolar dead-space ventilation. Oxygen supplementation will increase arterial oxygenation in cases of hypoventilation, but has minimal effect when intrapulmonary shunting is present (severe V_A/Q mismatch). Certain congenital heart defects can also cause blood to pass directly from the right side of the circulation into the systemic circulation (anatomical shunt), which results in hypoxaemia with normal or low P_aCO_2.

Hypoxaemia can also be caused by diffusion abnormalities (pulmonary oedema or fibrosis). In these patients, supplemental oxygen should improve arterial oxygenation; however, where possible, the underlying cause should be treated before the patient undergoes anaesthesia.

Work of breathing (WOB) represents the energy required for inhalation and exhalation. Increased WOB due to respiratory compromise will increase the total oxygen demand; in this situation, the patient may become too exhausted to meet these energy and oxygen requirements. Myocardial workload can also increase during periods of increased WOB because of the extra oxygen demand from the respiratory system and the pulmonary hypertension that results from hypoxic pulmonary vasoconstriction. Hypoxic pulmonary vasoconstriction is normally a protective reflex that shunts blood away from areas of lung with poor gas exchange to areas that are better ventilated. However, in the situation of globally low alveolar PO_2, this vasoconstrictive response will result in pulmonary arterial hypertension and increased right ventricular work. These patients will benefit from oxygen supplementation; in addition, lung ventilation is sometimes needed to reduce the WOB and myocardial workload as much as possible.

General patient assessment

Patients may require anaesthesia for surgery of the respiratory system (e.g. arytenoid cartilage lateralization or removal of a consolidated lung lobe) or for unrelated procedures when concurrent respiratory problems exist (e.g. severe brachycephalic obstructive airway syndrome; removal of an intestinal foreign body when there is aspiration pneumonia). Every patient should be comprehensively evaluated before anaesthesia. Specific tests to assess respiratory function are described in Figure 22.1. During the evaluation the patient should be

Test	Comments
Pulmonary-specific tests	
Methodical auscultation of the thorax, trachea and larynx/pharynx	Identification of abnormalities in sounds (crackles, wheezes, absence of sound, etc.) may assist in disease differentiation and location
Cervical and thoracic radiographs	Specific abnormalities may be identified Thorax: pneumothorax, pulmonary masses, congestion or contusions; pleural effusions Cervical region: tracheal collapse, airway foreign bodies, masses
Pulse oximetry	Identifies abnormalities in saturation of haemoglobin with oxygen. Can be relatively easily assessed in conscious patients
Measurement of end-tidal carbon dioxide ($P_E'CO_2$)	Identifies hypo- or hyperventilation. Primarily performed only in intubated patients, although sidestream analysis can be done in conscious patients or from pre-placed nasal catheters
Arterial blood gas analysis	Gold standard pulmonary function test
Venous blood gas analysis (jugular blood samples are more representative of mixed venous blood compared to peripheral venous blood samples)	Provides information on tissue oxygen utilization; may provide information on oxygen delivery alongside clinical signs related to cardiac output and lung function. Venous blood is easier to obtain than arterial blood
Respiratory volumes and spirometry	Using a facemask or in intubated patients, a Wright's respirometer can measure tidal volume. A spirometer can also give flow–volume analysis
Other tests as needed	Many other tests require anaesthesia (e.g. bronchoscopy, bronchoalveolar lavage)
General tests	
Serum lactate concentration	Elevation indicates decreased tissue oxygen delivery due to any cause (decreased oxygen content, decreased tissue perfusion)
Serum chemistry	Decreased oxygen delivery can lead to hypoxia-induced damage in any organ system
Complete blood count	Significant findings include anaemia, polycythaemia due to hypoxaemia, increased white blood cell count with pneumonia

22.1 Tests that can be used to assess respiratory function.

handled gently to avoid increases in WOB resulting from stress or fear, and exacerbation of respiratory dysfunction. All patients with any degree of respiratory distress during handling should receive oxygen administered by using a face mask or 'flow-by' technique (Figure 22.2). Patients that are distressed or fractious may require sedation, and those showing signs of pain will require analgesia. If the patient begins to show signs of respiratory distress, the physical examination should be stopped immediately and the patient placed in an oxygen cage or quietly restrained and oxygen delivered using a facemask. The veterinary surgeon (veterinarian) should be prepared for emergency induction of anaesthesia by placing an intravenous catheter if possible and preparing items for endotracheal intubation to gain control of the airway and provide ventilation if required.

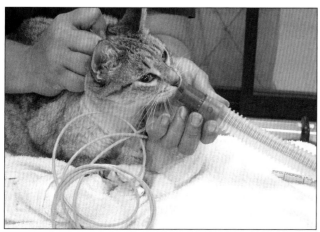

22.2 A cat receiving oxygen supplementation. 'Flow-by' or 'blow-by' oxygen can be delivered from an anaesthetic machine or other oxygen source. The tube delivering the oxygen should be held as close to the patient's nares or mouth as possible, otherwise the technique will be inefficient. This method of oxygen delivery may increase inspired oxygen from 21% (the proportion in room air) to 30–40%.

Observation of the patient's breathing can help to locate the respiratory lesion and to determine its extent and severity. Restrictive diseases such as pulmonary oedema, pneumonia, fibrosis or pleural effusion result in poor lung compliance and a rapid and shallow breathing pattern. Obstructive diseases such as laryngeal paralysis, tracheal collapse and small airway disease are characterized by a breathing pattern with a slower rate and increased respiratory effort. Differentiating between inspiratory dyspnoea (usually due to extrathoracic causes) and expiratory dyspnoea (intrathoracic and intra-airway causes) may also aid in locating the lesion. Observation of chest and diaphragm movements may help to differentiate a problem with neuromuscular function from a pulmonary lesion. A paradoxical breathing pattern will cause the thoracic wall to collapse during inspiration, the diaphragm to move caudally and the abdomen to expand. These changes can be associated with severe respiratory obstruction, paralysis of the intercostal muscles, or a CNS lesion that has altered the normal respiratory rhythm.

Assessment of mucous membrane colour may help to determine which further examinations should be made. Cyanosis indicates the presence of hypoxaemia; however, studies in humans have shown that clinicians cannot always visually detect cyanosis. The appearance of the mucous membranes may be affected by the quality or type of ambient light (particularly fluorescent lights); in addition, desaturated haemoglobin must be present at a concentration of at least 15 g/l before cyanosis can be detected accurately (Goss *et al.*, 1988). Nevertheless, when cyanosis is present, it indicates that immediate oxygen therapy is required. Pulse oximetry is therefore a useful tool for identifying abnormalities in haemoglobin oxygen saturation and monitoring any changes once oxygen therapy is initiated. Flushing of the mucous membranes may occur with hypercapnia, but (unlike cyanosis) this is not a pathognomonic sign.

Auscultation of the lungs and trachea is important to help identify the location and nature of the lesion. Although difficult to assess accurately in small animals, percussion of the lung fields may also detect areas of hypo-resonance associated with fluid/solid masses, or hyper-resonance associated with pneumothorax. Radiographic or ultrasonographic examinations can be useful to further define the lesion; when performing these, it is important to ensure that oxygen is available if needed. In a patient with pleural effusion, thoracocentesis should be performed to obtain a sample of fluid for further diagnostic investigations. When attempting thoracocentesis in an obese patient, it is especially important to confirm that the distal end of the needle/catheter has entered the pleural cavity before accepting that a negative result truly indicates absence of fluid. Preoperative measurement of respiratory volumes can be performed using a tight-fitting facemask and a Wright's respirometer, or spirometry loops can be obtained using an electronic spirometer (Rozanski and Hoffman, 1999). Measurement of P_aO_2 and P_aCO_2 by arterial blood gas analysis is the best way to assess changes in respiratory function. The results obtained will depend to some extent on the animal's behaviour during blood sampling. Hyperventilation caused by stress can mask the degree of hypoxaemia and may decrease P_aCO_2, and sampling should be abandoned if a dyspnoeic patient objects to restraint. Blood samples from the jugular vein can be analysed to obtain information on acid–base status, venous oxygen tension (P_vO_2) and venous carbon dioxide tension (P_vCO_2).

Choice of drugs for patients with respiratory compromise

Sedation may be necessary to calm a distressed or fractious patient and analgesia may be required to relieve pain-induced hyperventilation or hypoventilation; the latter might occur if the pain originates from the thorax or cranial abdomen. Although sedative drugs and some opioids may cause CNS depression and reduce respiratory function, in many cases the beneficial effects of a judiciously chosen small dose of these drugs will improve respiratory function.

Acepromazine

Acepromazine (0.01–0.03 mg/kg i.v. or i.m. in dogs; 0.03–0.05 mg/kg in cats i.v. or i.m.) causes minimal to no adverse effects on ventilatory function (Popovic et al., 1972) and is often used to calm anxious patients with airway disease or dysfunction. Acepromazine produces mild sedation but has no analgesic effect, and has a relatively long duration of action. If sedation is excessive, it may result in a recumbent patient that is unable to maintain a patent airway and cause some relaxation of the pharyngeal muscles, which might lead to further airway dysfunction.

Benzodiazepines

Use of benzodiazepines alone should be avoided, as they rarely provide adequate sedation in distressed dogs or cats and can even make them more excitable. Midazolam and diazepam (0.2–0.3 mg/kg i.v. for either drug) cause minimal to no respiratory depression but can result in some relaxation of the muscles of the upper airway. In some debilitated or calmer, older patients, benzodiazepines can be combined with an opioid to provide sedation.

Opioids

If the animal shows signs of moderate to severe pain, a full mu opioid receptor agonist (e.g. morphine or methadone) may be required to provide adequate analgesia. Animals appear to be more tolerant of opioid-mediated respiratory depression compared with humans; however, if excessive sedation is observed, the patient's respiratory function should also be assessed for any signs of compromise. If necessary, the effects of these drugs can be partially reversed with butorphanol or fully reversed with naloxone. Butorphanol (0.2–0.4 mg/kg slow i.v.) can be used to reverse the mu receptor-mediated effects while still providing some analgesia via kappa receptors. Buprenorphine may be useful; it produces minimal sedation or respiratory depression, has a long duration of analgesic effect and can be used in patients with mild to moderately painful conditions but the slow onset of action may limit its use for reversal. Opioids can cause panting due to an effect on the thermoregulatory system, but without compromising respiratory function in normal patients.

Drug combinations

Butorphanol (0.2 mg/kg i.v. or i.m.) or buprenorphine (0.02 mg/kg i.v. or i.m.) combined with acepromazine (0.02 mg/kg i.v. or i.m.) or midazolam (0.2-0.3 mg/kg slow i.v. or i.m.) are popular sedative and analgesic combinations for cats and dogs with respiratory compromise.

Alpha-2 adrenoceptor agonists

Alpha-2 agonists have potential to result in profound sedation, relaxation of the upper airway musculature, decreased respiratory rate and decreased central respiratory drive; they are thus not recommended for patients with moderate to severe respiratory compromise.

Non-steroidal anti-inflammatory drugs and local anaesthetic agents

Due to their reliable and long duration of action and absence of sedative and respiratory depressant effects, non-steroidal anti-inflammatory drugs (NSAIDs) should not be withheld unless contraindicated in the individual patient. Local anaesthetic agents do not cause sedation when used for nerve blocks; local anaesthesia techniques specific for rhinoscopy and the thorax are found in Chapters 11 and 23.

Anaesthesia for patients with respiratory compromise

A plan for anaesthesia, monitoring and support of the patient should be formulated and implemented before inducing anaesthesia, and continued well into the recovery period. Anaesthesia for intrathoracic surgery is discussed in Chapter 23. Patients with upper airway problems include those listed in Figure 22.3, and those with lower airway problems are listed in Figure 22.4. Both induction of, and recovery from, anaesthesia are high-risk phases for patients with upper airway disease or dysfunction. However, the maintenance phase of anaesthesia is often straightforward because during this period the airway is protected by an endotracheal tube (ETT) and the

Patients with upper airway disease or dysfunction include those with:

- Laryngeal paralysis or other laryngeal/pharyngeal abnormalities
- Tracheal collapse
- Upper airway foreign bodies
- Brachycephalic obstructive airway syndrome (BOAS). This syndrome includes the presence of an elongated soft palate, everted laryngeal saccules, hypoplastic trachea and stenotic nares. BOAS is common in brachycephalic dogs; brachycephalic cats can also suffer from the syndrome, although generally to a lesser degree than dogs
- External compression of the airway, e.g. due to enlarged pharyngeal lymph nodes or grossly enlarged thyroid glands
- Inability to open the mouth or to move air through the nares

22.3 Patients with upper airway disease or dysfunction.

Patients with lower airway disease or dysfunction include those with:

- Asthma
- Chronic obstructive pulmonary disease
- Pneumonia
- Pneumo-, haemo-, pyo- or chylothorax
- Intrathoracic masses
- Consolidated lung lobe(s) or torsion
- Diaphragmatic hernia
- Impaired thoracic movement, e.g. fractured ribs, muscle weakness or abdominal distension

22.4 Patients with lower airway disease or dysfunction.

patient is receiving supplemental oxygen. However, in anaesthetized patients requiring upper airway surgery or diagnostic procedures, the ETT may need to be removed, which in-creases the risk of a life-threatening respiratory emergency. Patients with lower airway dysfunction often have more severe systemic disturbances than those with upper respiratory disease but are not prone to sudden airway obstruction. However, patients with some lower airway diseases may be more prone to bronchoconstriction. Specific treatment of emergency patients with severe airway disease and anaesthesia for long-term ventilatory support are both covered in the *BSAVA Manual of Canine and Feline Emergency and Critical Care*.

Pre-anaesthetic preparation

Pain, excitement, fear and struggling will increase the patient's WOB and exacerbate negative pressure within the upper airway. This pronounced negative pressure promotes inward collapse of the airway, leading to further narrowing or even total obstruction of the airway. A small decrease in airway diameter can have a major impact on WOB: for every 50% reduction in airway diameter there is a 16-fold increase in airflow resistance. For mildly dyspnoeic patients, consider using low doses of sedative and/or analgesic drugs, which may allow the patient to breathe more slowly and deeply, resulting in reduced airflow turbulence and decreased WOB. It is also important to avoid the patient developing hyperthermia, or immediately start cooling processes (using fans, ice, etc.) if the patient is already hyperthermic, as hyperthermia-induced panting can exacerbate upper airway dysfunction. Excessive sedation may produce airway muscle relaxation, and these patients should therefore be observed at all times for signs of airway dysfunction. A patient that is struggling to breathe and in danger of immediate ventilatory failure may require immediate anaesthesia and rapid control of the airway without prior use of sedatives or opioids; these drugs can be administered after control of the airway and ventilation is achieved.

The use of anticholinergic agents in patients with airway problems is controversial. Anticholinergics can cause tachycardia, which increases myocardial work and oxygen demand with the risk of cardiac arrhythmias, especially in patients that are already hypoxaemic. The antisialogogue action of these agents causes the composition of secretions to change from a watery fluid to thick mucus, which may not be cleared by a compromised mucociliary system. If the secretions accumulate they can block small airways, promoting atelectasis, and they also provide a medium for bacterial growth. However, laryngeal manipulation can cause a vagally mediated bradycardia and so anticholinergics may be indicated for procedures involving the larynx, although their use may not guarantee protection from a strong vago-vagal reflex. The bronchodilating action of anticholinergics may be of benefit in individuals with reactive airways; the smooth muscle relaxation is most pronounced in large and medium-sized bronchi. Bronchodilation leads to reduced airway resistance and eases WOB, but also increases anatomical dead space, particularly in patients with asthma or chronic bronchitis. When considering using anticholinergics, the possible beneficial effects of bronchodilation should be weighed against the detrimental effects of tachycardia and inspissation of respiratory secretions.

The administration of a single dose of short-acting corticosteroids (0.2–2.0 mg/kg dexamethasone i.v.) is often recommended to alleviate acute swelling of the upper airway in patients with severe dyspnoea and/or those in which intubation was traumatic (Lodato and Hedlund, 2012). The decision to use corticosteroids is usually urgent, but where possible concurrent administration of NSAIDs should be avoided.

Induction and endotracheal intubation

The patient should be preoxygenated before induction of anaesthesia. Delivery of 100% oxygen for at least 3 minutes by means of a facemask can prevent desaturation (oxygen saturation of haemoglobin (S_pO_2) <90%) for up to 5 minutes after induction of anaesthesia (McNally *et al.*, 2009). If not already present, an intravenous catheter should be placed before induction. Anaesthesia should be induced rapidly and the trachea intubated immediately after induction. Propofol, thiopental and alfaxalone will produce rapid induction of anaesthesia in 30–60 seconds and can be titrated to effect. These agents can produce induction apnoea but this effect can be minimized by administering the drug over 30–60 seconds. However, if there is life-threatening airway dysfunction, the induction drug should be administered rapidly and an ETT placed immediately. Intermittent positive pressure ventilation (IPPV) can be used to overcome any induction apnoea. Ketamine–benzodiazepine or tiletamine–zolazepam combinations will induce anaesthesia in 30–90 seconds and are useful in patients with haemodynamic instability. Ketamine preserves laryngeal and pharyngeal reflexes, which may exacerbate laryngospasm during intubation, but its combination with a benzodiazepine decreases the likelihood of this occurrence. Both ketamine and propofol cause mild bronchodilation and may reduce bronchospasm in patients with asthma. Some clinicians advocate the use of a combination of propofol and ketamine, using a half dose of each mixed in the same syringe, to combine the advantageous effects of both drugs.

For short procedures, the impact of the induction drug on quality of recovery should also be considered, since any residual effects may cause problems such as excitement in the recovery period and interfere with oxygenation and ventilation. In an emergency during recovery, alfaxalone, thiopental or propofol can be used for induction of anaesthesia without pre-anaesthetic medication (higher doses will be required). Recovery excitement can be prevented with a low dose of acepromazine (0.01–0.02 mg/kg i.v.) given just before the animal recovers from anaesthesia. Tiletamine–zolazepam can cause prolonged and dysphoric recoveries, especially in dogs and for this reason may not be the best drug combination.

It is essential to be prepared for endotracheal intubation, because control of the airway must be gained as rapidly and smoothly as possible. Ensure that the patient is placed in the correct position for intubation (Figure 22.5). General guidelines for intubation are as follows:

- Ensure that several different diameter sizes and lengths of ETTs, a tube tie, a laryngoscope, lidocaine spray, a stylet (especially useful for intubation of cats) and a tracheotomy kit are all readily available (Figure 22.6)
- In cats, Xylocaine® spray should not be used for desensitizing the larynx as it may result in severe laryngeal oedema, excess respiratory secretions and possibly death due to upper airway obstruction. One of the carriers in this product and not the active agent, lidocaine, is suspected as the cause of these adverse

effects (Brearley, 2010; Fisher, 2010). Benzocaine spray should also not be used because it can increase circulating methaemoglobin concentration. Intubeaze® (20 mg/ml) can be used in cats, as can regular 20 mg/ml lidocaine
- The ETT should be pre-measured against the patient to ensure it is long enough to bypass any upper airway narrowing but not long enough for the distal tip to enter a bronchus
- In all patients, the larynx should be visualized and the ETT observed to pass between the arytenoids. Accidental oesophageal intubation will delay delivery of oxygen and anaesthetic gases to the patient, and may promote regurgitation
- Laryngeal structure and function should be assessed at intubation and a plan made if any abnormalities are found. Anaesthesia required for a laryngeal examination is discussed later
- Bronchoconstriction can occur in patients with reactive airways if the plane of anaesthesia is light, especially during intubation. Thus, it is important to achieve an adequate anaesthetic depth to eliminate laryngeal reflexes before attempting intubation.

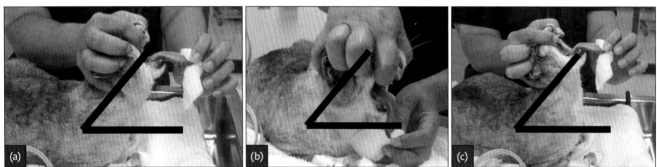

22.5 Positioning of the patient for endotracheal intubation. (a) The larynx is easiest to visualize if the head and neck are stretched out from the body at approximately a 45 degree angle with the tongue gently pulled forward. (b) Under-extension or (c) over-extension of the head and neck will make the larynx difficult to visualize.

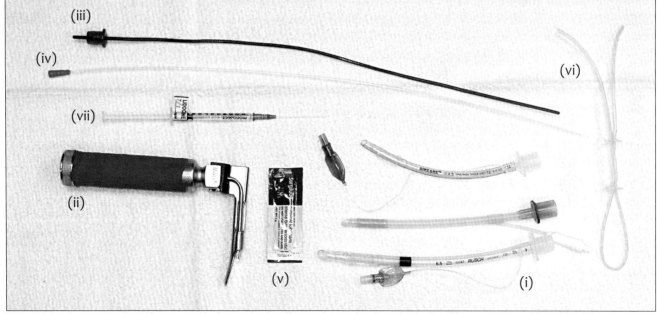

22.6 Equipment that should be prepared before intubation: (i) several sizes of endotracheal tubes; (ii) laryngoscope with working light source; (iii) rigid stylet; (iv) soft stylet; (v) sterile lubricant to lubricate the tube; (vi) a means of securing the tube (e.g. tubing); (vii) lidocaine in a syringe with a catheter attached.

Endotracheal tube management

In all patients, the ETT cuff should be carefully inflated only to the point at which leaks are prevented at a peak inspiratory pressure (PIP) of 20 cmH$_2$O (as measured by the circuit manometer) during delivery of a positive-pressure breath (ie, delivered by squeezing the reservoir bag in the breathing system or by initiating IPPV) (Figure 22.7). An overinflated cuff can cause damage to the tracheal mucosa, possibly resulting in scarring and constriction. To prevent the ETT and inflated cuff from damaging the trachea, the ETT should be disconnected from the breathing system when the patient is moved or repositioned and then reconnected afterwards. Tracheal rupture may occur if the patient is repositioned while still connected to the breathing circuit, as a result of twisting of the ETT, especially in cats (Hardie *et al.*, 1999; Mitchell *et al.*, 2000).

Intubation techniques

With all patients it is important to anticipate that intubation may be difficult. A checklist for steps to take with a difficult intubation is given in Figure 22.8.

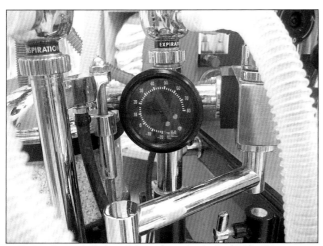

22.7 Proper inflation of the endotracheal tube (ETT) will just prevent a leak when the pressure relief (or 'pop-off') valve is closed and the system is pressurized to 20 cmH$_2$O as measured by the manometer. Pressurizing the system at pressures higher than 20 cmH$_2$O is not necessary and may result in overinflation of the ETT cuff and excessive pressure on the tracheal mucosa, which could damage the mucosa and lead to tracheal constriction.

If intubation is difficult:

- For best visualization of the larynx, the head should be gently extended (neither too flexed nor too extended) and the tongue carefully pulled forward (see Figure 22.5)
- If the larynx can be visualized but the endotracheal tube (ETT) cannot be placed into the trachea, place a soft stylet (e.g. a feeding tube) through the ETT and into the trachea, and use this as a guide for the ETT
- If the soft palate is obscuring visualization of the airway, the ETT or a more rigid stylet can be used gently to lift the soft palate out of the way
- Consider using an endoscope to aid intubation
- Laryngospasm: apply a few drops of lidocaine on the arytenoids and administer oxygen for 1–2 minutes before again attempting to intubate. Lidocaine should be routinely used for intubation of cats since they are prone to laryngospasm
- Small boluses of propofol (1–2 mg/kg i.v.) or alfaxalone (0.5–1.0 mg/kg i.v.) will improve laryngeal relaxation and facilitate intubation
- If endotracheal intubation is not possible, consider a tracheotomy
- If an ETT would interfere with the surgical approach, consider a tracheotomy or pharyngotomy

22.8 Checklist for performing a difficult intubation.

Intubation using an endoscope: If the upper airway cannot be visualized by standard methods, an endoscope can be passed through the oral cavity to the larynx. If the airway is large in comparison to the endoscope, the ETT can be placed over the endoscope (such that the endoscope serves as a 'stylet' for the tube); the endoscope can be manipulated into the trachea, and the ETT can then be passed off the endoscope into the airway. If the airway is small in comparison to the endoscope, the scope can be used to visualize the upper airway but cannot serve as a stylet to help place the ETT.

Emergency tracheotomy: Patients requiring an emergency tracheotomy can be in severe respiratory distress and panic, and may be difficult to restrain. These patients may require sedation, and oxygen should be continuously supplemented. A combination of acepromazine (0.02 mg/kg) with butorphanol (0.2 mg/kg) and local anaesthesia can provide suitable conditions for transcutaneous placement of a catheter or large-bore needle into the trachea to facilitate delivery of oxygen. Note that the trachea may be deeply situated within the neck when it is in a flexed position. It may be better to perform an emergency tracheotomy with the patient in dorsal recumbency and with the head and neck extended to bring the trachea just under the skin, but this may require a short-acting injectable anaesthetic (Figure 22.9).

Intubation using a pharyngotomy: Occasionally, the ETT may need to be placed in a position that enables the mouth to be closed in order to check the gape or bite. Injectable anaesthesia is used to place an ETT via a pharyngotomy; oxygen should be available during this procedure. The ETT can be passed through an incision made just caudal to the lower mandible (Figure 22.10) and turned

Preparation
- Obtain a tracheotomy kit (scalpel, suture material, sterile tracheotomy or endotracheal tube). Clip the hair from the surgical site and prepare the skin aseptically – preparation may be brief if the procedure is an emergency. The patient should receive supplemental oxygen during preparation

Sedation/anaesthesia
- Emergency tracheotomy is often done with no sedation (if the patient is syncopal), or under light sedation with acepromazine and butorphanol and local anaesthetic blockade of the incision site. Elective tracheotomy should be done under general anaesthesia with injectable anaesthetic drugs and supplemental oxygen

Landmarks
- Ventral surface of the trachea at the level of the second, third or fourth tracheal rings

Technique
- Make a midline incision at the site described above and retract the sternohyoideus muscles. Place stabilizing sutures around a tracheal ring on either side of the tracheal incision site. Make a transverse incision between the rings, of <65% of the tracheal circumference. Use the sutures to pull the incised portion of the trachea open and insert a tracheotomy tube or a sterile endotracheal tube for anaesthesia

Aftercare
- Leave the endotracheal tube in the airway during recovery from anaesthesia. Replace with a dedicated tracheotomy tube if longer-term airway care is required. Once the tube has been removed, the incision is generally allowed to heal by granulation. The incision could be closed, but this increases the risk of subcutaneous emphysema

22.9 Technique for a tracheotomy.

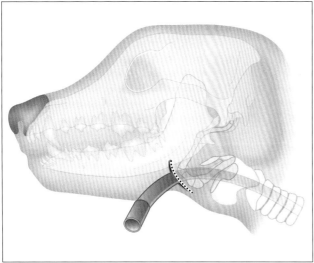

22.10 Placement of an endotracheal tube through a pharyngotomy site.

with forceps such that the distal end can be passed into the trachea. When inserted using this method, the ETT may be difficult to bend, and intubation can take some time to accomplish. Alternatively, the ETT can be placed into the trachea as normal and the proximal end can then be passed through the incision to the exterior, and connected to a breathing system. The latter method requires a larger incision to allow passage of the cuff inflation valve and tubing, which may be undesirable.

Maintenance of anaesthesia

If the procedure involves the airway itself so that the patient cannot be intubated, anaesthesia can be maintained with injectable anaesthetic agents. An intravenous infusion of propofol (0.1–0.4 mg/kg/min) or alfaxalone (0.05–0.2 mg/kg/min) with intermittent boluses of fentanyl (1–2 µg/kg i.v.) or an intravenous infusion of fentanyl (5–40 µg/kg/h) is an effective technique, but infusions of fentanyl given at the high end of the rate range should be decreased prior to recovery to avoid residual respiratory depression. Oxygen supplementation when using this technique is described later.

For procedures that will allow endotracheal intubation, once the trachea has been intubated and the ETT connected to a suitable breathing system, ventilation can be spontaneous as long as adequate gas exchange occurs. Sevoflurane and isoflurane have a bronchodilating effect: although this is unlikely to be significant in patients with normal airways, it may be beneficial in patients that have reactive and/or constricted airways (e.g. cats with asthma). The bronchodilating effect of these agents is also useful in patients undergoing bronchoalveolar lavage (BAL) or lung lobectomy. In addition, modern inhalant anaesthetics are rapidly eliminated, allowing the patient to recover from anaesthesia fully with a short transition time between extubation and complete consciousness, and without any 'hang-over' effect. However, these drugs (especially isoflurane) are potent respiratory depressants and produce a dose-dependent decrease in alveolar ventilation. This depression results in hypercapnia, and possibly hypoxaemia if pulmonary pathology is severe. Excessive anaesthetic depth must therefore be avoided. Administration of analgesics to decrease anaesthetic gas requirements (i.e. a balanced anaesthetic technique) and the ability to provide IPPV if needed are important.

Intermittent positive pressure ventilation and positive end-expiratory pressure

More information on mechanical ventilators and IPPV can be found in Chapters 6 and 23. IPPV is generally recommended to maximize alveolar function in these patients and is mandatory when there is an open thorax. Ventilation can be started using 10–15 breaths per minute, a tidal volume of 10–15 ml/kg and a PIP of 10–20 cmH$_2$O, delivered either by a mechanical ventilator or by a dedicated staff member squeezing the reservoir bag of the breathing circuit. The $P_E'CO_2$ should be maintained between 35 and 55 mmHg (4.7–7.3 kPa) and arterial blood gas analysis used, if possible, to confirm the accuracy of the capnogram. A decrease in P_aO_2 can occasionally occur with IPPV; this can be due to an increase in V_A/Q mismatch as blood flow redistributes from the ventilated to the non-ventilated alveoli because the positive pressure within the ventilated alveoli collapses alveolar blood vessels.

Positive end-expiratory pressure (PEEP) can be provided using special valves within the breathing system or ventilator and is occasionally necessary to improve gas exchange. It is useful to provide PEEP in combination with an alveolar recruitment manoeuvre, to reopen non-ventilated (collapsed) alveoli (see below for a description of the manoeuvre). In general, the application of IPPV and PEEP (3–5 cmH$_2$O) will improve arterial oxygenation in cats and dogs. However, aggressive use of IPPV and PEEP (>5 cmH$_2$O) can cause excessive airway pressures and may lead to collapse of the intrathoracic venae cavae, with a subsequent decrease in preload and decreased cardiac output, especially in hypovolaemic patients.

To perform the alveolar recruitment manoeuvre, close the pressure-relief valve on the breathing system and expand the lungs for 20 seconds to a PIP of 40 cmH$_2$O for dogs or 30 cmH$_2$O for cats. Blood pressure will decrease transiently during this time, and so it is important not to exceed 20 seconds duration. Recruitment manoeuvres should not be used if there is chance of creating a pneumothorax, or in severely hypovolaemic and hypotensive patients. Ideally, PEEP should be used to keep the alveoli open once they have been re-expanded.

Life support

Delivery of oxygen is still required during injectable anaesthesia and airway procedures that make placement of an ETT impossible. Provision of supplemental oxygen is imperative, and can be achieved using a small tube placed using an orotracheal approach or through a percutaneous catheter inserted into the trachea. A low insufflation rate of 30–50 ml/kg/min should be used, which requires a suitably calibrated flowmeter. This method will provide high inspired concentrations of oxygen but does not remove carbon dioxide from the lungs. The catheter must be securely attached to the oxygen tubing so that it cannot become dislodged into the trachea. It is important to observe the patient closely and ensure that the airway does not become occluded. If airway occlusion occurs, there is no route by which the insufflated oxygen may escape and airway pressure can rapidly increase, potentially causing pulmonary rupture (with subsequent pneumothorax) and possibly cardiovascular collapse.

A much less common technique is to use a high-frequency jet ventilator (HFJV). A catheter can be placed in the trachea and attached to the HFJV (Figure 22.11). This manually operated device can provide high concentrations of oxygen while also oscillating the gas in the airway,

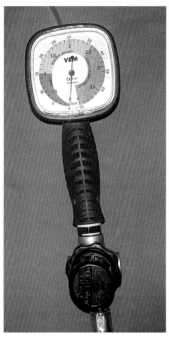

22.11 A manually operated high-frequency jet ventilator (Manujet; VBM). The insufflation tube (top of the image) is inserted into the airway. The unit is connected to a source of pressurized oxygen (400 kPa) and the black knob allows adjustment of delivered pressure in the range 50–350 kPa.
(Courtesy of Chris Seymour, Royal Veterinary College, London, UK)

enhancing the removal of carbon dioxide. The trigger on the HFJV is pressed as often as possible and can provide small tidal volume 'breaths' at a frequency of about 60 times per minute.

Oxygen delivery to the tissues is dependent on both arterial oxygen content and cardiac output, and tissue perfusion requires the mean arterial blood pressure to be maintained above 60 mmHg. To support cardiac output and tissue oxygen delivery:

- Intravenous fluid support should be used in all patients (see Chapter 18). Plasma and/or colloids should be considered in hypoproteinaemic patients to prevent the development of pulmonary oedema
- Blood products should be considered for any patient with anaemia, since low haemoglobin concentrations will contribute significantly to decreased oxygen delivery
- Positive inotropes and vasopressors should be used in patients that remain hypotensive despite an appropriate anaesthetic depth and adequate fluid support (see Chapter 17).

If hypoventilation is apparent, the cause should be identified and corrected if possible, and IPPV should be considered to support ventilation. Another potential treatment for some causes of hypoventilation is to change the position of the patient (if possible) to allow better thoracic and diaphragmatic excursion. 'Ties' used to maintain a patient's position on the table can also produce external thoracic compression, and removing these can help to improve ventilation (see Chapter 3). Hypoxaemia may also be caused by hypoventilation when the patient is breathing room air; this can be corrected by increasing ventilation and providing oxygen.

Both the duration of anaesthesia and the degree of pain are correlated with increased risk of respiratory dysfunction during the postoperative period. Analgesics should be administered to control pain and enable the patient to breathe as normally as possible. The degree of pain management should be based on the type of the procedure, and is covered in Chapters 9 and 10. Thoracotomy is particularly painful, and multimodal analgesia should be

used (see Chapter 23). Useful local anaesthetic techniques for these patients include intercostal nerve and interpleural blocks, and wound diffusion catheter implantation (see Chapters 11 and 23).

Monitoring

Arterial blood gas analysis is the most accurate method of diagnosing hypoxaemia and hypercapnia, but may not always be available or feasible. Pulse oximetry is a useful technique to measure oxygen saturation of haemoglobin (S_pO_2), and P_aO_2 can be derived from the oxygen–haemoglobin dissociation curve when the P_aO_2 is below 100 mmHg (13.3 kPa) (Figure 22.12; see also Chapter 7). However, the pulse oximeter is not a sensitive measure of ventilation and tissue oxygen delivery. Patients receiving supplemental oxygen may not ventilate adequately to maintain normocapnia, yet may have an acceptable S_pO_2 as measured by pulse oximetry. Similarly, patients with anaemia or abnormal haemoglobin may not have adequate tissue oxygen delivery, yet may have an acceptable S_pO_2.

In the absence of a profound V_A/Q mismatch, P_aCO_2 can be indirectly determined by measuring $P_E{'}CO_2$ using capnography or capnometry (Figure 22.13; see also Chapter 7). The P_aCO_2 is normally approximately 2–5 mmHg greater than $P_E{'}CO_2$. An increased P_aCO_2–$P_E{'}CO_2$ gradient indicates increased alveolar dead-space ventilation. Hypoventilation can also cause retention of carbon dioxide, but will not increase the gradient.

Since perfusion of the lungs is an important aspect of pulmonary function, arterial blood pressure and the electrocardiogram should also be monitored. Monitoring considerations and normal values for parameters are listed in Figure 22.14 and are covered in depth in Chapters 7 and 17.

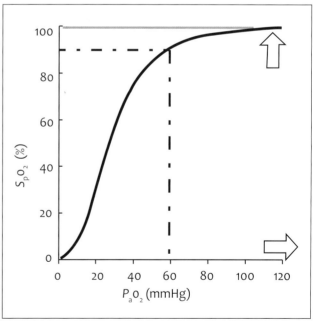

22.12 Oxygen–haemoglobin dissociation curve, with the partial pressure of oxygen in arterial blood (P_aO_2) on the horizontal axis and the percentage of haemoglobin saturated with oxygen (S_pO_2) on the vertical axis. Note that at values of S_pO_2 <90%, further decreases in P_aO_2 result in a rapid decline in oxygen saturation (dashed line). At this point, the saturation can be a sensitive indicator of ventilation because decreased ventilation will cause immediate desaturation. Once 100% saturation is reached, as will occur with supplemental oxygen therapy, the P_aO_2 can continue to increase but S_pO_2 cannot increase beyond 100% (open arrows). At this point, the S_pO_2 is a very insensitive indicator of ventilation because decreased ventilation can occur with no decrease in saturation.

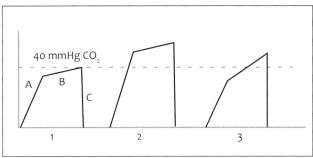

22.13 Capnographic waveforms can be used to diagnose some types of respiratory compromise. Waveform 1 is normal. Slope A represents the beginning of expiration when carbon dioxide (CO_2) in the exhaled breath increases rapidly. Slope B represents the slower rise as CO_2 is exhaled from the alveoli. Slope C results from the switch to inhalation, when the CO_2 drops back to zero. The intersection of slopes B and C is the point where end-tidal carbon dioxide ($P_E'CO_2$) is measured by the capnometer; this value should be approximately 40 mmHg (5.3 kPa), as indicated by the dotted line. Waveform 2 represents hypoventilation. The waveform shape is normal but $P_E'CO_2$ is elevated. Waveform 3 represents an obstructed airway, which is indicated by the longer, steeper slope B. The airway obstruction may be in either the upper airway (e.g. plugged or kinked endotracheal tube) or the lower airway (bronchoconstrictive disease, e.g. asthma) (see also Chapter 7).

Monitoring	Normal values and appearance	Comments
Pulse oximeters measure the S_pO_2	S_pO_2 should be >90% (ideally >95% with an F_iO_2 of 100%) Values <90% indicate hypoxaemia	Pulse oximeters are considered to be monitors of oxygenation, not monitors of ventilation Patients inhaling 100% oxygen may still hypoventilate and may develop a respiratory acidosis
End-tidal carbon dioxide monitors measure the partial pressure of carbon dioxide (P_aCO_2) in exhaled gases	Normal values in anaesthetized patients are 35–50 mmHg (4.7-6.7 kPa). Note: a mild degree of hypercapnia is acceptable under anaesthesia	Efficient monitors of ventilation and should be used in all patients with respiratory dysfunction Generally, the $P_E'CO_2$ will be close to the arterial values of P_aCO_2 Profound V_A/Q mismatch and increased alveolar dead space will cause increased $P_aCO_2 - P_E'CO_2$ gradient
P_aO_2, P_aCO_2 and arterial blood pH	Normal values for cats and dogs can be found in Chapter 7	Arterial blood gases are the gold standard for assessment of respiratory function Minor variations will occur between species and between laboratories
P_vO_2, P_vCO_2 and venous blood pH	Normal values for cats and dogs can be found in Chapter 7	Venous blood gases and pH provide some information on tissue oxygen delivery and utilization Minor variations will occur between species and between laboratories
Electrocardiogram	Sinus rhythm	Hypoxaemia, hypercapnia and acid–base imbalances can irritate the heart. The cause should be identified and corrected. Sinus tachycardia, sinus bradycardia and ventricular premature contractions are common anaesthesia-induced arrhythmias. See Chapters 21 and 31

22.14 Monitoring considerations for patients with respiratory compromise, and normal values of the key variables. F_iO_2 = inspired oxygen fraction; P_aCO_2 = arterial carbon dioxide tension; P_aO_2 = arterial oxygen tension; $P_E'CO_2$ = partial pressure of end-tidal carbon dioxide; P_vCO_2 = venous carbon dioxide tension; P_vO_2 = venous oxygen tension; S_pO_2 = percentage of haemoglobin saturated with oxygen; V_A/Q = alveolar ventilation/perfusion ratio.

Recovery from anaesthesia

For patients with respiratory compromise, a calm, stress-free recovery is essential and a rapid return to conscious-ness is desirable. Excitement and pain will promote airway narrowing and/or obstruction, increase WOB and myocar-dial work, and impair the ability to breathe. These patients may therefore require sedation and analgesia (acepro-mazine and opioids) during recovery, but excessive seda-tion should be avoided. The ETT should remain in place for as long as possible, depending on the species, breed and procedure. If a pharyngotomy or tracheotomy tube has been placed, it should remain in place for as long as there is a risk of upper airway obstruction. If the patient becomes dyspnoeic, the following steps should be attempted:

- Extend the head and neck to open the airway
- Position the patient in sternal recumbency to allow bilateral chest excursions
- Promote mouth-breathing by pulling the tongue rostrally, open the mouth (a suitably sized roll of adhesive tape may be used as a gag) and lift the lips if they are restricting movement of air
- Provide oxygen by facemask or flow-by
- Consider giving corticosteroids
- Prepare to re-anaesthetize the patient and re-intubate the trachea. Injectable anaesthetic agents, a laryngoscope and a variety of ETTs should be readily available during recovery. Another plan for recovery may be required, including emergency corrective surgery and/or tracheotomy

- Monitoring and support of respiratory and cardiovascular function should continue well into the recovery period (see Chapters 17 and 18)
- Management of chest drains is covered in the *BSAVA Manual of Canine and Feline Emergency and Critical Care*.

Methods of oxygen administration during recovery

Supplemental oxygen may be necessary during recovery, and can be provided by the following methods:

- 'Flow-by' oxygen can be provided by placing the tube of a breathing system or other oxygen source close to the nares of the patient (see Figure 22.2)
- A facemask can be placed over the muzzle and oxygen delivered using an anaesthetic machine or other oxygen source
- Nasal catheters (feeding tubes) can be placed in one or both nasal meatus and oxygen supplied (see Chapter 3)
- The patient can also be placed in an oxygen cage, which will provide some degree of freedom to move. The disadvantages of this option include high oxygen usage, loss/waste of oxygen when the cage door is open and lack of hands-on patient assessment when the door is closed
- Small patients can be placed in an incubator designed for use with human infants. However, the small volume of an incubator will render these patients prone to hyperthermia

Patients receiving supplemental oxygen should be monitored by pulse oximetry and arterial blood gas analysis (Figure 22.15). If possible, the F_iO_2 should be measured. If P_aO_2 remains low (P_aO_2 <50–60 mmHg (6.7–8 kPa)) with an F_iO_2 >0.6, or if P_aCO_2 markedly increases with oxygen therapy (suppression of hypoxaemic ventilatory drive), then anaesthesia, intubation and IPPV may be required.

Specific considerations

Rhinoscopy or removal of a nasal foreign body

Although cats and dogs can mouth-breathe, nasal problems may still affect respiratory function, especially in sedated animals. Cats appear reluctant to mouth-breathe when they are sedated, so anaesthetic drugs that are rapidly eliminated are useful to prevent any residual sedation during recovery. Anaesthesia itself is often straightforward for rhinoscopy or removal of a foreign body from the nasal passages, but close observation of the patient during the recovery phase is warranted to ensure a patent airway. It is also important to ensure that the nares are kept clean of secretions.

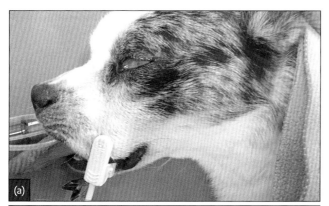
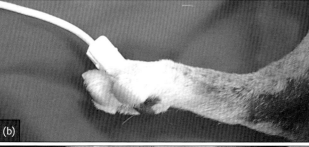
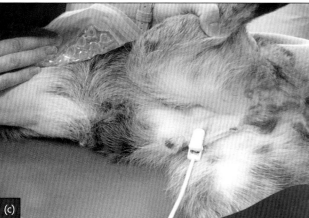

22.15 If the tongue is not available, the pulse oximeter probe can be placed on any relatively thin, non-pigmented skin. Sites that may be suitable include the (a) lip, (b) toe and (c) prepuce. Other suitable sites include the ear, vaginal fold and flank.

During the procedure, the ETT cuff should be fully (but not excessively) inflated, to prevent aspiration of blood and/or fluids. The patient may react to procedures within the nasal passages or nasopharynx by reflex sneezing and gagging even when the depth of anaesthesia is adequate. Providing appropriate analgesia, by blocking either the infraorbital or the maxillary nerve, can help prevent this response to manipulation. More information on these blocks is provided in Chapter 20. Alternatively, an intravenous bolus of fentanyl (2 µg/kg) can be used to provide 15–20 minutes of analgesia and reflex suppression. In extreme cases, neuromuscular blockade may be required (see Chapter 16); a means of providing IPPV is mandatory for these cases.

Laryngeal examination

Laryngeal function may need to be assessed either before surgery or as a stand-alone procedure. The examination requires a light plane of anaesthesia or deep sedation in order to open the patient's jaws and observe vocal cord movement. Excessive anaesthetic depth will impair laryngeal function and can produce false positive diagnoses. Acepromazine (0.02 mg/kg) or either midazolam or diazepam (0.2–0.3 mg/kg of either) followed by propofol or alfaxalone administered 'to effect' is an ideal combination. Some veterinary surgeons prefer not to use acepromazine, based on a report that it may interfere with the assessment of laryngeal function (Jackson et al., 2004). In another study, the time to observation of normal function after drug administration, and the occurrence of swallowing, laryngospasm, or breathing did not differ between drugs when using thiopental, propofol, or diazepam–ketamine for induction, but jaw tone was significantly less and exposure of the larynx greater with thiopental or propofol compared with diazepam–ketamine induction (Gross and Dodam, 2002).

The loss of the cough reflex is unlikely to affect the ability to assess laryngeal function adequately, but some veterinary surgeons also advocate the exclusion of opioids (cough suppressants) from the protocol. Opioids can be administered after the examination if they are considered necessary as part of the protocol for surgery. Administration of doxapram (0.5–1 mg/kg i.v.) causes deepening of breaths by briefly stimulating the respiratory centre, which may facilitate the assessment of laryngeal function (Tobias et al., 2004). Although adverse effects are rare at this dose, doxapram can cause tachycardia, hypertension and seizures, and should not be administered to patients with pre-existing problems that could be exacerbated.

Arytenoid cartilage lateralization ('tie-back' surgery)

It may be necessary to extubate the trachea during this procedure to prevent accidental damage to the ETT or to evaluate airway diameter following lateralization. Increments of injectable anaesthetic drugs (alfaxalone or propofol) can be used to maintain anaesthesia. A laryngoscope, a range of ETT sizes and a stylet must be readily available for re-intubation if required.

Brachycephalic breeds

Brachycephalic breeds of dogs and cats are predisposed to upper airway dysfunction, but many individuals (especially cats) can have fairly normal upper airway function.

With these patients, careful assessment is important to determine the degree of airway compromise. These animals require light sedation, rapid induction of anaesthesia and the use of anaesthetic agents that allow a rapid recovery. Recovery from anaesthesia is a critical period, but brachycephalic dog breeds are known to tolerate the ETT for a long period after they become completely conscious (Figure 22.16). The ETT should be removed once the patient is alert, able to maintain its airway and no longer tolerates the ETT. If dyspnoea occurs, the recommendations in the previous section on recovery should be followed; it is important to be prepared to re-anaesthetize and re-intubate the patient. Corrective surgery or temporary tracheotomy may be required. Treatment with corticosteroids should be considered if upper airway inflammation is moderate to severe. Brachycephalic cats usually have less severe problems compared with dogs, but should still be closely observed during recovery and can be extubated once they are swallowing.

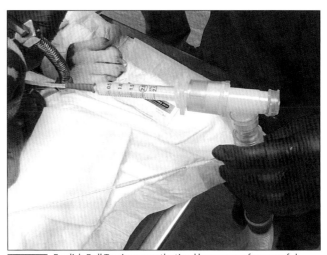

22.17 English Bull Terrier anaesthetized by means of a propofol infusion for removal of a bronchial foreign body. Oxygen supplementation is being provided by a urinary catheter placed in the trachea and connected via a 2.5 ml syringe to the anaesthetic breathing system.
(Courtesy of Marieke de Vries, Davies Veterinary Specialists, Higham Gobion, UK)

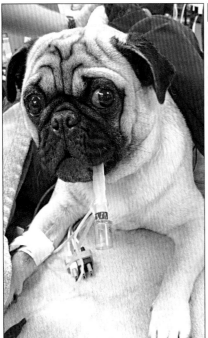

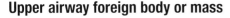

22.16 Brachycephalic breeds, like this Pug, generally tolerate an endotracheal tube in the trachea until they are completely conscious.

be placed in an oxygen cage. Conversely, in some patients only the typical 'honking' sound may be heard. If the tracheal collapse is confined to the cervical region, breathing will be normal once an ETT is placed. If the collapse is lower cervical or intrathoracic, IPPV will be required to keep the airway open (Figure 22.18). Endotracheal intubation should be performed with the patient at a suitable depth of anaesthesia to eliminate the gag reflex; coughing and gagging may promote bronchoconstriction, especially in patients with reactive airways.

Bronchoconstriction can be identified by a sudden onset of dyspnoea, resistance being felt to lung expansion during manual ventilation, desaturation (S_pO_2 <90%) and a capnogram typical of airway constriction (see Figure 22.13, waveform 3). Deepening the plane of anaesthesia may be

Upper airway foreign body or mass

Injectable anaesthesia with supplemental oxygen is usually required in these cases. If the foreign body is not completely occluding the airway, a small-bore tube (e.g. a feeding tube or urinary catheter; Figure 22.17) can be passed beyond the foreign body for administration of oxygen. Use of an ETT may push a foreign body deeper into the airway. If there is a mass attached to the tracheal mucosa (e.g. a tumour), it may be possible to pass a smaller ETT beyond the mass. Care should be taken to ensure that the ETT is secure and does not slide cranial to the mass, otherwise an obstruction may occur; if the foreign body is completely occluding the trachea, emergency oxygenation, via a percutaneous tracheal catheter and/or a tracheotomy, will be required.

Tracheal collapse

Management of patients with tracheal collapse will depend on the severity and location of the collapse. If the patient is in respiratory distress, it should receive light sedation and

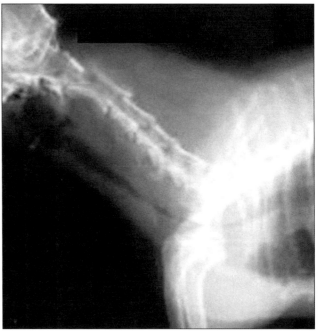

22.18 Tracheal collapse that extends beyond the location that can be reached by an endotracheal tube, as seen in this radiograph, may necessitate IPPV during the maintenance phase of anaesthesia.

sufficient to relax bronchoconstriction, otherwise specific bronchodilator drugs such as terbutaline or albuterol can be administered (see Chapter 31). Recovery from anaesthesia can present a greater risk for the patient with severe tracheal collapse when corrective surgery has not been performed. The ETT may need to be removed early so that a cough reflex, which may exacerbate the collapse, does not occur. Opioids provide good cough suppression, especially butorphanol. These patients should receive oxygen, sedation and analgesia as needed.

Tracheal stent: Tracheal collapse may be corrected by placing external or internal stents. An external stent may be sewn to the tracheal rings in order to hold them in a dilated position. Anaesthesia for this procedure is routine once the ETT has been placed. The main concerns involve damage to the laryngeal nerves during surgery (especially the recurrent laryngeal nerve) and laryngeal paralysis, which may complicate recovery.

Internal stenting with nitinol mesh is a less invasive procedure but requires specific management of the airway. In order to decide on the size and length of the stent, the ETT must be withdrawn until the cuff and distal end are positioned within the larynx, and the airway pressurized (using the reservoir bag) to a PIP of 15–20 cm H_2O, while a lateral radiograph is taken. Alternatively, special graduated markers can be used during fluoroscopy. If a ≥4 mm internal diameter ETT can be placed, the stent can be deployed through the ETT using adapters attached between the ETT and breathing system, similar to those described for bronchoscopy (see later), and anaesthesia maintained using an inhalant agent (see Figure 22.19). If only smaller ETT sizes can be placed, oxygen supplementation and total intravenous anaesthesia (TIVA) will be required for placement of the stent. Low-dose acepromazine and butorphanol are suitable for pre-anaesthetic medication, with propofol or alfaxalone infusion used for TIVA. These anaesthetic drugs provide a rapidly adjustable depth of anaesthesia with a smooth recovery. However, cats can have a delayed recovery after a propofol infusion if the maintenance rate is high or if the cat is anaesthetized for more than about 30 minutes (see Chapter 14).

Tracheal wash and bronchoalveolar lavage

The S_pO_2 should be closely monitored in patients undergoing tracheal wash or BAL because rapid desaturation is common during these procedures, especially when TIVA is used for anaesthesia without the use of supplemental oxygen. Supplemental oxygen should therefore be provided throughout, and the procedure should be stopped if desaturation occurs; in this situation, intubation and IPPV may be necessary. Several positive pressure breaths may be required to return S_pO_2 to normal, after which the procedure can be continued if necessary. Monitoring of saturation during recovery is also required because some BAL fluids can remain within the lung and can cause a decrease in S_pO_2. In patients with reactive airways, it is also important to monitor for signs of bronchoconstriction. Rarely, pneumothorax has been observed in cats undergoing these procedures.

Bronchoscopy

Most patients undergoing bronchoscopy are likely to have compromised pulmonary function, and oxygen supplementation is therefore important. In asthmatic cats, pre-treatment with inhaled or injected terbutaline can reduce the likelihood of acute bronchoconstriction occurring during the procedure. Where possible, a short ETT with >7.5 mm internal diameter should be selected and the cuff positioned just distal to the larynx; this will enable the greatest length of trachea to be examined.

A standard endoscope can pass through an adapter placed between the ETT and the anaesthetic breathing system (Figure 22.19). A double-diaphragm adapter arrangement is less likely to leak, reducing the likelihood that personnel are exposed to waste anaesthetic gases. With this arrangement, anaesthesia is maintained with an inhalant anaesthetic and oxygen; it is also possible to provide IPPV if required. In smaller patients, it may be feasible to use a human laryngeal mask airway (LMA; see Chapter 5); these devices have a large external tube and can accommodate an appropriate diameter endoscope. The same type of adapter can be used on the external end of the LMA so that an anaesthetic breathing system can be attached, as described above. The slight curve of the LMA may make it slightly more difficult to manipulate the endoscope, so the LMA tubing should be cut as short as possible. In a patient where an ETT or LMA cannot be used, anaesthesia must be maintained with an injectable technique. For short procedures, most of the injectable anaesthetics are probably suitable, but for longer procedures propofol or alfaxalone infusions are used. For these cases,

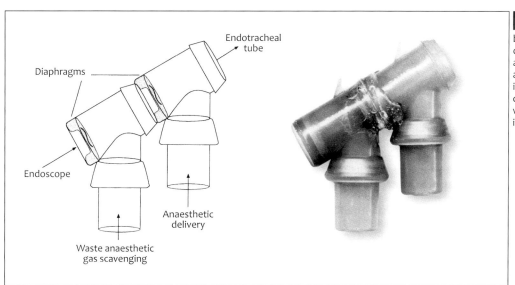

22.19 Diagram and picture of an adapter used for bronchoscopy. The double diaphragm used with this arrangement reduces the amount of anaesthetic spilling into the room while allowing the delivery of inhalant anaesthetics with positive pressure ventilation if needed.

Diaphragms

Endotracheal tube

Endoscope

Anaesthetic delivery

Waste anaesthetic gas scavenging

oxygen can be supplied using the methods described earlier, or by passing oxygen through one of the channels of the endoscope. This method can deliver oxygen deep into the lungs, but supply may be limited to one lung (if the distal end of the endoscope is in a bronchus) and may need to be discontinued if the channels are needed for equipment (e.g. suction or sampling). The flow rate should not be so high that excessive pressure develops; use 10–50 ml/kg/min. While this method will supply oxygen, carbon dioxide is not removed from the lungs and the procedure duration should be kept to a minimum.

A pulse oximeter is ideal for monitoring oxygenation, because desaturation often occurs when the endoscope blocks off various portions of the lung. The endoscope should be moved or completely removed if desaturation occurs. Biopsy may cause significant haemorrhage into the airway and compromise gas exchange. If this occurs, blood should be removed using the suction channel on the endoscope, if possible. Occasionally, a biopsy may result in a ruptured airway, or spontaneous rupture can occur if there is severe lung pathology present. Airway rupture manifests as rapid desaturation, an increase in respiratory rate and a change in pulmonary compliance. Immediate thoracocentesis is required to remove air from the pleural space, and a chest drain is placed for further air removal.

Use of spring-held mouth gags to allow passage of the endoscope can cause problems, especially in cats. When the gape is wide, the position of the mandible interferes with blood flow through the maxillary artery to the brain (Barton-Lamb *et al*., 2013). Electroretinograms and computed tomographic imaging have linked the use of mouth gags to cortical blindness, deafness and neurologic deficits in cats following endoscopy or dental procedures (Stiles *et al*., 2012).

Once endoscopy is finished, the trachea can be intubated and oxygen provided. Inhalational anaesthesia can be used if necessary, or oxygen given until extubation. It is essential to continue monitoring with pulse oximetry and oxygen supplementation into the recovery period.

Asthma

Cats with asthma should be stabilized before anaesthesia, although they are still liable to have an acute bronchoconstrictive response to anaesthesia and/or airway procedures (e.g. BAL). Asthmatic patients should be preoxygenated for at least 3 minutes and can be sedated with an acepromazine and opioid combination (doses given earlier in the section on choice of drugs). If more profound sedation is required, an alpha-2 adrenoceptor agonist can be used, if not contraindicated, or a combination of intramuscular ketamine or alfaxalone with midazolam and/or butorphanol (see Chapter 13 for doses). However, alfaxalone administered by the intramuscular route requires a large volume to produce sedation and should be used with caution in healthy cats, as it may create a hyper-reactive state (Grubb *et al*., 2013). The choice of anaesthetic induction agent is probably not as critical as achieving an appropriate depth of anaesthesia before rapid intubation (propofol or alfaxalone are suitable). Ketamine, combined with a benzodiazepine, is also a good choice because of its bronchodilatory effects. Mask induction with any inhalant agent is slow and not recommended for most patients with airway disease; in addition, mask induction with desflurane should not be used as it may cause airway hyper-reactivity. Laryngeal stimulation may cause bronchospasm, so it is important to ensure that the patient is at a suitable depth of anaesthesia that

prevents gag reflexes, and lidocaine should be applied to the arytenoids before endotracheal intubation. Terbutaline, with or without a corticosteroid, should immediately be administered (see Chapter 31) if bronchoconstriction occurs (signs of bronchoconstriction are described earlier, in the section on tracheal collapse). A 'puff' of albuterol from an inhaler may also be effective. To deliver this, a standard albuterol inhaler is connected to the end of the ETT, and one press on the inhaler activation tab delivers the drug into the ETT. The inhaler should then be immediately removed to prevent impaired ventilation. During recovery, asthmatic patients should be extubated before return of the gag reflex.

Pulmonary bullae

Pulmonary bullae (Figure 20.20) can occur with some forms of chronic respiratory disease in dogs (Lipscomb *et al*., 2003) and cats, although bullae are less common in the latter species (Milne *et al.*, 2010). These bullae can rupture spontaneously or can be ruptured with aggressive IPPV in anaesthetized patients. Anaesthetic protocols are the same as for those patients with other lower airway disease but IPPV should be used cautiously. A respiratory rate of 8–10 breaths per minute, with PIP not exceeding 10 cmH$_2$O is recommended. If possible, patients with pulmonary bullae should be allowed to breathe spontaneously.

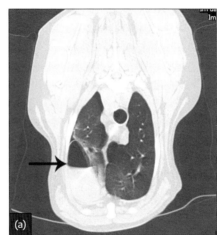
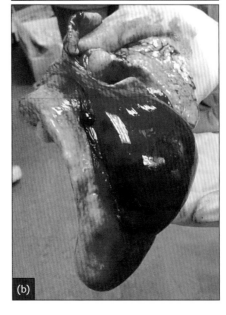

22.20 (a) Sagittal computed tomography image from a dog which had developed sudden onset of dyspnoea and spontaneous pneumothorax. Note the fluid-filled bulla (arrowed) in the left cranial lung lobe. (b) Appearance of the bulla after lung lobectomy.
(Courtesy of Chris Seymour, Royal Veterinary College, London, UK)

Pleural space disease

Air or fluid in the pleural space will reduce the ability of the alveoli to expand. Ventilation of the lungs can be more difficult if fluid is present because it is less compressible than air. Anaesthesia is usually straightforward in these cases, but removal of air and/or fluid may be required before induction of anaesthesia. A mild pneumothorax may not require treatment before anaesthesia, but may become more severe if overzealous IPPV ruptures friable tissues. To reduce the risk of this, low PIPs should be used, but not so low as to promote atelectasis (10–15 cmH$_2$O).

If the pneumothorax is causing respiratory distress, and especially if it is a tension pneumothorax (Figure 22.21), the air must be removed immediately, before induction of anaesthesia. Thoracocentesis can often be performed with no or only light sedation, with the puncture site desensitized by infiltration of a local anaesthetic agent. Drainage of air is generally performed with the patient either standing or in sternal or lateral recumbency, and with the puncture site at the seventh or eighth intercostal space at the junction of the mid- and dorsal third of the thorax. An over-the-needle catheter, hypodermic needle or butterfly needle can be used to penetrate the chest wall. A large syringe with tubing and a 3-way tap (stopcock) included is attached to the needle hub to remove air from the pleural cavity. A negative pressure of no greater than 2–5 ml on the syringe barrel markings should be applied. The needle can be directed so it lies against the inner chest wall but the bevel faces into the pleural cavity to avoid accidental lung puncture. Once no more air can be suctioned, the needle is removed. Supplemental oxygen should be given during the procedure. For pleural fluid, drainage is usually performed at the seventh or eighth costochondral junction, with the patient either in sternal recumbency or standing (Figure 22.22).

Pneumonia, pulmonary contusions and rib fractures

It is best to let pneumonia resolve before anaesthesia for elective procedures. Thoracic trauma can cause pneumothorax, pulmonary contusions and rib fractures, all of which can impair gas exchange. Pulmonary contusions will result in areas of V_A/Q mismatch, and rib fractures can

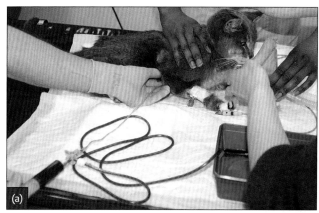

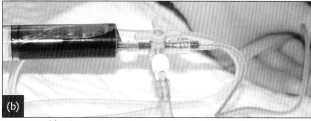

22.22 (a) Feline patient with pleural haemorrhagic effusion. After sedation with butorphanol and local infiltration with lidocaine, the chest is drained in a sterile manner by means of a butterfly needle with the cat in sternal recumbency. Extra oxygen is provided and an ECG is attached to monitor heart rate and rhythm. (b) Close up of the connection of the syringe, 3-way tap, butterfly needle and extension set. During aspiration, the 3-way tap blocks off the connection to the extension line. To empty the syringe, the 3-way tap is closed towards the butterfly needle to avoid injecting aspirate back into the chest.
(Courtesy of Marieke de Vries, Davies Veterinary Specialists, Higham Gobion, UK)

cause pain that leads to hypoventilation. This hypoventilation is further exacerbated if the ribs are isolated from their vertebral attachments, creating a 'flail chest'. A flail segment impairs the ability to create sufficient negative intrathoracic pressure for lung inflation, which will greatly increase WOB. Mild pulmonary contusions generally do not require treatment, but if possible, anaesthesia should be delayed until the patient's gas exchange is acceptable. Patients with moderate pulmonary contusions may require supplemental oxygen and those with severe contusions occasionally require judicious use of IPPV. Appropriate analgesia should be provided if the animal shows signs of pain; local anaesthetic block of the intercostal nerves can provide analgesia without the need for sedation. Opioids should also be considered if pain is limiting ventilation.

Summary

Respiratory disease encompasses a wide range of complications, but regardless of the location or type of disease, monitoring and support of the patient is generally more important for anaesthetic safety than the choice of anaesthetic agent.

References and further reading

Anagnostou TL, Pavlidou K, Savvas I et al. (2012) Anesthesia and perioperative management of a pneumonectomized dog. Journal of the American Animal Hospital Association **48**, 145–149

Barton-Lamb AL, Martin-Flores M, Scrivani PV et al. (2013) Evaluation of maxillary arterial blood flow in anesthetized cats with the mouth closed and open. Veterinary Journal **196**, 325–331

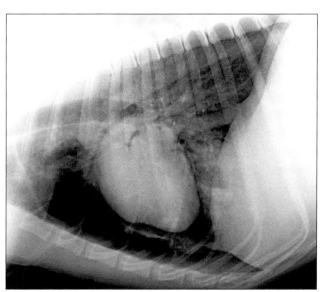

22.21 Pneumothorax and pulmonary contusions in a dog following blunt trauma. Patients with this presentation should have air removed from the thorax before anaesthesia.

Brearley JC (2010) Use of xylocaine spray in cats. *Veterinary Record* **167**, 627

Clutton E (2007) Respiratory disease. In: *BSAVA Manual of Canine and Feline Anaesthesia and Analgesia, 2nd edn*, ed. C Seymour and T Duke-Novakovski, pp. 194–200. BSAVA Publications, Gloucester

Cremer J, Sum SO, Braun C, Figueiredo J and Rodriguez-Guarin C (2013) Assessment of maxillary and infraorbital nerve blockade for rhinoscopy in sevoflurane anesthetized dogs. *Veterinary Anaesthesia and Analgesia* **40**, 432–439

De Monte V, Grasso S, De Marzo C, Crovace A and Staffieri F (2013) Effects of reduction of inspired oxygen fraction or application of positive end-expiratory pressure after an alveolar recruitment maneuver on respiratory mechanics, gas exchange, and lung aeration in dogs during anesthesia and neuromuscular blockade. *American Journal of Veterinary Research* **74**, 25–33

Duggan M and Kavanagh BP (2010) Perioperative modifications of respiratory function. Best Practice and Research. *Clinical Anaesthesiology* **24**, 145–155

Duke-Novakovski T (2007) Dental and oral surgery. In: *BSAVA Manual of Canine and Feline Anaesthesia and Analgesia, 2nd edn*, ed. C Seymour and T Duke-Novakovski, pp. 194–200. BSAVA Publications, Gloucester

Fisher J (2010) Use of Xylocaine spray in cats. *Veterinary Record* **167**, 500

Goss GA, Hayes JA and Burdon JG (1988) Deoxyhaemoglobin concentrations in the detection of central cyanosis. *Thorax* **43**, 212–213

Gross ME and Dodam J (2002) A comparison of thiopental, propofol, and diazepam-ketamine anesthesia for evaluation of laryngeal function in dogs premedicated with butorphanol-glycopyrrolate *Journal of the American Animal Hospital Association* **38**, 503–506

Grubb T (2010) Anesthesia for patients with respiratory disease and/or airway compromise. *Topics in Companion Animal Medicine* **25**, 120–132

Grubb TL, Greene SA and Perez TE (2013) Cardiovascular and respiratory effects, and quality of anesthesia produced by alfaxalone administered intramuscularly to cats sedated with dexmedetomidine and hydromorphone. *Journal of Feline Medicine and Surgery* **15**, 858–865

Hardie EM, Spodnick GJ, Gilson SD, Benson JA and Hawkins EC (1999) Tracheal rupture in cats: 16 cases (1983–1998). *Journal of the American Veterinary Medical Association* **214**, 508–512

Jackson AM, Tobias K, Long C, Bartges J and Harvey R (2004) Effects of various anesthetic agents on laryngeal motion during laryngoscopy in normal dogs. *Veterinary Surgery* **33**, 102–106

Johnson LR (2014) Canine and feline respiratory medicine. *Veterinary Clinics of North America: Small Animal Practice* **44**, 1–190

King LG and Boag A (2007) *BSAVA Manual of Canine and Feline Emergency and Critical Care, 2nd edn*. BSAVA Publications, Gloucester

Lipscomb VJ, Hardie RJ and Dubielzig RR (2003) Spontaneous pneumothorax caused by pulmonary blebs and bullae in 12 dogs. *Journal of the American Animal Hospital Association* **39**, 435–445

Lodato DL and Hedlund CS (2012) Brachycephalic airway syndrome: pathophysiology and diagnosis. *Compendium on Continuing Education for the Practicing Veterinarian* **34(7)**, E3

Lumb AB (2010) *Nunn's Applied Respiratory Physiology, 7th edn*. Churchill Livingstone Elsevier, London

McNally EM, Robertson SA and Pablo LS (2009) Comparison of time to desaturation between preoxygenated and nonpreoxygenated dogs following sedation with acepromazine maleate and morphine and induction of anesthesia with propofol. *American Journal of Veterinary Research* **70**, 1333–1338

Milne ME, McCowan C and Landon BP (2010) Spontaneous feline pneumothorax caused by ruptured pulmonary bullae associated with possible bronchopulmonary dysplasia. *Journal of the American Animal Hospital Association* **46**, 138–142

Mitchell SL, McCarthy R, Rudloff E and Pernell RT (2000) Tracheal rupture associated with intubation in cats: 20 cases (1996–1998). *Journal of the American Veterinary Medical Association* **216**, 1592–1595

Padrid P (2000) Feline asthma. Diagnosis and treatment. *Veterinary Clinics of North America: Small Animal Practice* **30**, 1279–1293

Pardali D, Adamama-Moraitou KK, Rallis TS, Raptopoulos D and Gioulekas D (2010) Tidal breathing flow-volume loop analysis for the diagnosis and staging of tracheal collapse in dogs. *Journal of Veterinary Internal Medicine* **24**, 832–842

Popovic NA, Mullane JF and Yhap EO (1972) Effects of acetylpromazine maleate on certain cardiorespiratory responses in dogs. *American Journal of Veterinary Research* **33**, 1819–1824

Rozanski EA and Hoffman AM (1999) Pulmonary function testing in small animals. *Clinical Techniques in Small Animal Practice* **14**, 237–241

Stiles J, Weil AB, Packer RA and Lantz GC (2012) Post-anesthetic cortical blindness in cats: twenty cases. *Veterinary Journal* **193**, 367–373

Sumner C and Rozanski E (2013) Management of respiratory emergencies in small animals. *Veterinary Clinics of North America: Small Animal Practice* **43**, 799–815

Tobias KM, Jackson AM and Harvey RC (2004) Effects of doxapram HCl on laryngeal function of normal dogs and dogs with naturally occurring laryngeal paralysis. *Veterinary Anaesthesia and Analgesia* **31**, 258–263

Trappler M and Moore K (2011a) Canine brachycephalic airway syndrome: pathophysiology, diagnosis, and nonsurgical management. *Compendium on Continuing Education for the Practicing Veterinarian* **33**, E1–5

Trappler M and Moore K (2011b) Canine brachycephalic airway syndrome: surgical management. *Compendium on Continuing Education for the Practicing Veterinarian* **33**, E1–8

West JB (2012) *Respiratory Physiology: The Essentials, 9th edn*. Lippincott Williams and Wilkins, Baltimore

West JB (2013) *Pulmonary Pathophysiology: The Essentials, 8th edn*. Lippincott Williams and Wilkins, Baltimore

Chapter 23

Intrathoracic surgery and interventions

Peter J. Pascoe

A thoracotomy is still required for many procedures but less invasive procedures are becoming more popular. These include thoracoscopic approaches to pericardiectomy, lung lobectomy, and the use of implantable coils to treat patent ductus arteriosus. These newer techniques may result in less surgical morbidity, but the veterinary surgeon (veterinarian) must fully understand the underlying pathophysiology of the condition and the planned procedure in order to devise a suitable and safe anaesthetic technique.

Preoperative evaluation

Whenever the thoracic wall is breached, there will be significant effects on the pulmonary system. It is therefore essential to perform a careful evaluation of the pulmonary system before embarking on thoracic surgery. Preoperative evaluation of the patient is also covered in Chapters 2 and 22, but is summarized here with emphasis on issues relevant to conditions of the pulmonary system. Cardiovascular system diseases are covered in Chapter 21.

History

Historical information about the patient is an important part of the evaluation of respiratory and cardiovascular disease, and contributes to the achievement of an accurate diagnosis. Chronic respiratory disease may produce a slowly changing condition with few clinical signs as a result of the physiological reserve, but may manifest as acute disease when the physiological reserve becomes exhausted (Figure 23.1). It is helpful to ask the owner about the patient's exercise tolerance; this can provide important information with regard to the inherent risks of anaesthetizing the animal. An animal with poor exercise tolerance (due to an intrathoracic lesion) has a greater risk of perioperative problems than an animal with normal tolerance. Another question that can provide useful information is whether the patient adopts any abnormal postures when it sleeps; for example, an animal with a bilateral pleural effusion may have learned to sleep in a relatively upright position while an animal with unilateral changes may always sleep on one side.

Clinical pathology

Before undertaking a major surgical intervention, it is appropriate to obtain a complete blood count and bio-chemical profile to rule out further unrecognized

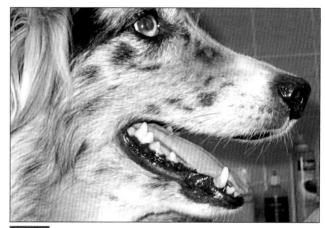

23.1 Cyanosis of the tongue in a dog with hypoxaemia.

intercurrent disease. An increased haematocrit may be evidence of chronic hypoxaemia, while a decreased haematocrit may represent chronic illness or blood loss. Anaemia may not be well tolerated in an animal with poor cardiac output, and it is important to take this into account when deciding whether to give a preoperative or intraoperative blood transfusion. Cats and dogs can tolerate a haematocrit of 0.15–0.2 l/l by increasing cardiac output so that oxygen delivery to the tissues is maintained. However, an animal with a relatively fixed cardiac output (e.g. aortic stenosis) may barely survive at a haematocrit of 0.3 l/l.

Preparation

Pulmonary system

Stabilization of the patient is important, and any conditions that can be treated before the animal undergoes anaesthesia should be addressed. An animal with pneumonia amenable to antibiotics and without risk of further infection should be treated if the surgery can be delayed. If there is air or fluid in the pleural space, or fluid in the pericardium or abdomen, this should be drained as much as possible before induction of anaesthesia.

Ascites

The presence of ascites can impair ventilation and produce significant hypotension if the patient is placed in dorsal recumbency. The fluid can usually be drained using a 14–16 G catheter, entering the abdomen 3–10 cm from the midline, midway between the ribs and the pelvic limb on the right side. If the left side is used, care must be taken to avoid penetrating the spleen. Catheters with extra fenestrations cut in them are best for this procedure because the omentum is less likely to plug all the holes at the same time. Fluid should be drained slowly to avoid rapid changes in abdominal pressure. An animal that has compensated for an increase in intra-abdominal pressure due to ascites may develop severe hypotension and cardiovascular collapse if the fluid is removed too quickly. Using a 14G catheter rather than a larger access will slow fluid removal and minimize the chance of rapid changes in abdominal pressure and associated sequelae.

Pleural drainage

Pleural drainage can be achieved with minimal restraint in most animals, but cats requiring this intervention are often extremely fractious and may need an analgesic before any attempt is made to carry out thoracic puncture. Opioids, such as methadone (0.1–0.2 mg/kg i.m.), hydromorphone (0.1 mg/kg i.m.) or butorphanol (0.2 mg/kg i.m.), provide analgesia and some sedation, which is beneficial in these cases. After the opioid has been administered, the animal should be placed in an oxygen-rich environment for 15–20 minutes before an attempt is made to drain the chest. A local anaesthetic agent should be used before tapping the chest or placing a chest drain. Lidocaine has a sufficient duration of effect for either of these procedures and can be infiltrated directly into the site of puncture and then forward along the track of the catheter or chest drain. If the site of puncture is in the ventral half of the thoracic wall, lidocaine can also be used to perform two to three intercostal nerve blocks (for the skin site and the site of penetration through the chest wall) (see Chapter 11). Generally, an animal with a pleural effusion can be tapped and drained several hours before thoracic surgery, with minimal chance of the fluid returning within that time frame. However, in animals with either a haemo- or pneumothorax, rapid recrudescence can occur; in such cases a chest drain and (continuous) controlled suction will be required (Lombardi et al., 2012). If it is not possible to maintain suction during transport to the operating room, an implanted chest drain should be clamped off or connected to a water trap or Heimlich valve so air cannot enter the pleural space.

Lung ventilation

With any surgery involving entry into the thoracic cavity, it is essential to provide intermittent positive pressure ventilation (IPPV). This can be achieved simply by having someone squeeze the reservoir bag of the breathing system intermittently, but this is labour intensive, so ventilation is usually achieved with the assistance of a mechanical ventilator (see Chapter 6). Before anaesthetizing the patient, it is important to ensure that the ventilator is functioning properly and that it is suitable for that particular animal. Some machines are not able to provide small enough tidal volumes for patients weighing <5 kg, while others cannot cope with giant breeds weighing 70–100 kg. The ability to apply positive end-expiratory pressure (PEEP) or continuous positive airway pressure (CPAP) to the airway once the thoracic cavity has been opened is helpful.

In normal circumstances, the tendency of the lung to collapse is balanced by the tendency of the thoracic wall to spring outwards. Once the chest has been opened the 'adhesion' between the chest wall and the lung is broken, and the lung collapses to a smaller volume. Once this has happened it is necessary either to increase the tidal volume or to add PEEP/CPAP in order to maintain adequate gas exchange. In the author's experience, the addition of PEEP/CPAP has been helpful in reducing the atelectasis often associated with intrathoracic procedures.

The effect of PEEP can be achieved by adding resistance to the expiratory limb of the breathing system. The simplest method is to pass the expiratory limb through a beaker of water. With this method, the depth of the hose under the water determines the amount of PEEP: if the hose is 7 cm under water then the PEEP should be 7 cmH$_2$O. The same outcome can be achieved by placing the scavenge hose from the ventilator under water, although this should be tested with the ventilator before using with a patient as some machines do not work properly when back pressure is exerted on the exhaust valve of the system. However, this approach is likely to be inconvenient because of difficulties in scavenging waste anaesthetic gases after they have bubbled through the water. PEEP valves are available commercially. These usually have preset values of 2.5, 5 or 10 cmH$_2$O; they can be used in sequence to provide 7.5 or 12.5 cmH$_2$O pressure (Figure 23.2). Some ventilators are equipped with a PEEP or CPAP setting and the value required is set on the machine. With any of these techniques, a manometer placed in the system, or the use of spirometry, allows measurement of the effect produced by the PEEP/CPAP manoeuvre. The author normally aims for a value of 3–7 cmH$_2$O, observes the effects on circulation, gas exchange and surgical access and then, if necessary, modifies accordingly.

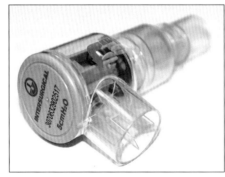

23.2 A positive end-expiratory (PEEP) valve for use in breathing systems. (Courtesy of Asher Allison, Animal Health Trust, Newmarket, UK)

Computed tomography

For patients requiring a computed tomography (CT) scan, it is best to induce and maintain anaesthesia with the patient in sternal recumbency until the scans are complete. Small areas of atelectasis rapidly form and these denser areas of tissue may hide lesions that would be visible if the lung was fully expanded. With modern CT technology it is usually possible to scan a thorax in under 60 seconds, so it is feasible to perform a breath-hold, or hyperventilate the lungs to produce apnoea, for this procedure. The airway pressure is typically held at 15–20 cmH$_2$O for this period. This pressure will significantly decrease venous return, so it is important that the animal has a normal circulating blood volume, and the blood pressure should be monitored during the scan (Akça et al., 1999). Another method to help reduce atelectasis is to use a reduced inspired fraction of oxygen (F$_i$O$_2$) to deliver the anaesthetic. This can be achieved by adding air to the mixture and it appears that reducing F$_i$O$_2$ to a value between 0.3 and 0.8 is effective.

Tracheal surgery

With some tracheal surgeries (e.g. tracheal resection), it may be necessary to place a tracheotomy tube during surgery and then continue anaesthetic delivery through this new tube (Figure 23.3). For these cases it is essential to have a range of sterile tracheotomy tubes or endo-tracheal tubes and a sterile breathing system available so they can be placed without risk of contaminating the surgical field. Before proceeding with the placement of a tracheotomy tube, check that all the connections between tubes are compatible to prevent delay in switching from one system to the other.

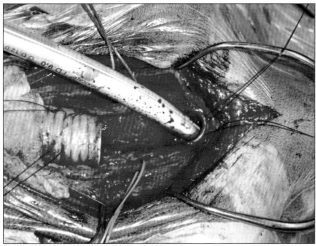

23.3 Insertion of a sterile endotracheal tube into the distal trachea of a dog to continue administration of oxygen and anaesthetic gases.
(Courtesy of Dan Brockman, Royal Veterinary College, London, UK)

Lung separation techniques

In a patient with a pulmonary mass (e.g. an abscess or tumour with a necrotic centre), a bronchial blocker can be used to prevent material from the lesion entering the healthy lung during surgery. Endotracheal tubes designed for humans (e.g. TCB Univent) can be used for this purpose in dogs of around 12–20 kg bodyweight (the maximum tube size has an internal diameter of 9.0 mm and the integral bronchial-occluding catheter is too short for larger dogs) (Figure 23.4). By using the curvature of the tube and catheter, it is possible to blindly direct the catheter into the left or right mainstem bronchus. However, this can be very difficult, so it may be easier to direct the catheter with the aid of an endoscope (Figure 23.5). Once the catheter is in place, the balloon on the catheter tip is inflated to seal the bronchus. The catheter also has an end-hole, which makes it is possible to slowly deflate or reinflate the lung beyond the balloon occlusion. The major disadvantage of these tubes is that the main tube has a 'D' shape (in cross-section), which means that a very small endoscope is needed in order to visualize placement of the catheter.

Another alternative is to use a Fogarty catheter; this can be placed in the airway before the endotracheal tube so that it passes between the endotracheal tube and tracheal wall. Once the animal is positioned for surgery, an endoscope can be used to guide the Fogarty catheter into the appropriate bronchus, and the balloon on the catheter tip can then be inflated to occlude that airway. The two main disadvantages of using a Fogarty catheter are that the catheter lacks an end-hole, and that the catheter and balloon can be easily dislodged back into the trachea. If this happens, an immediate total airway

occlusion develops, necessitating deflation of the balloon and repositioning of the catheter.

The Arndt bronchial blocker has some advantages over other types of bronchial blocker. It allows the catheter to be passed down the endotracheal tube with a guide loop placed over the endoscope (Figure 23.6). This system includes an adapter that allows connection of the breathing system while the endoscope is passed through one port and the bronchial blocker through another. By passing the endoscope into the required bronchus, the blocker can be directed appropriately. One version of this catheter has a pear-shaped balloon that makes it less likely to be dislodged from the airway. These catheters also have an end-hole to allow inflation or deflation of the blocked lung.

There are several other bronchial blockers available, each of which has its own advantages. The Cohen endo-bronchial blocker has a wheel on the proximal end that allows the operator to deflect the tip of the catheter in the desired direction (Figure 23.7a). The Coopdech bronchial blocker has a preformed angulation at the distal end; this catheter is relatively stiff, which enables the operator to rotate the end towards one lung or the other simply by rotating the proximal end (Figure 23.7b). The EZ blocker is a double-ended (Y-shaped) catheter with one balloon on

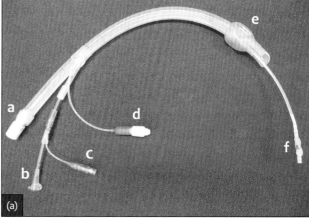

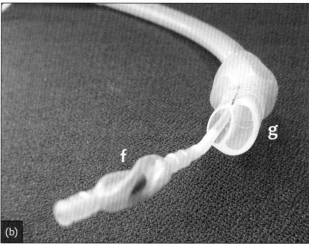

23.4 (a) A Univent endotracheal tube with bronchial blocker. a = breathing system end; b = tube to allow low-flow oxygen to be insufflated into collapsed lung or gently remove any air in alveoli and promote collapse; c = valve to inflate bronchial blocker cuff; d = valve to inflate main tube cuff; e = main tube cuff; f = bronchial blocker with cuff. (b) The distal end of the Univent tube. g = the D shaped main tube for ventilation and the channel for the bronchial blocker with cuff (f).
(Courtesy of Tanya Duke-Novakovski, Western College of Veterinary Medicine, University of Saskatchewan, Canada)

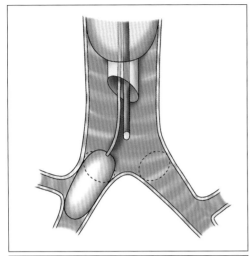

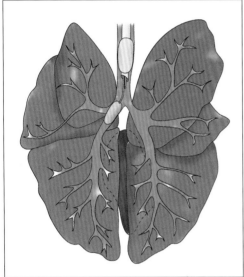

23.5 Insertion of a bronchial blocker into a bronchus using an endoscope.

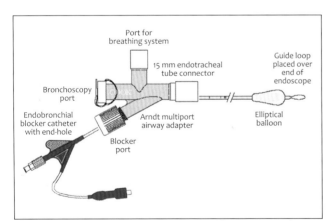

23.6 Diagram of the Arndt endobronchial blocker system. The adapter is connected to the endotracheal tube and the anaesthetic breathing system is attached to the right-angled port. The endoscope can then be put down the central port while the endobronchial blocking catheter is fed down the angled side port. The loop is slipped over the end of the bronchoscope and the catheter and endoscope can be advanced together. The balloon is shown inflated to illustrate its shape but it would not normally be inflated until placed into the airway. Once it is in place the endoscope is removed and the central port closed. The screw cap on the side port is tightened to fix the catheter in place. The blocked lung can be deflated, or positive end-expiratory pressure can be applied through the catheter.
(Drawing adapted from Cook Medical diagrams)

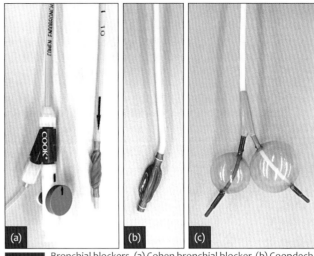

23.7 Bronchial blockers. (a) Cohen bronchial blocker. (b) Coopdech bronchial blocker. (c) EZ bronchial blocker.

each end. With this device, if the catheter is advanced until the division between the balloons reaches the carina, there should be one balloon in each bronchus and the anaesthetist can then choose which balloon to inflate (Figure 23.7c).

As an alternative to using a bronchial blocker, a double-lumen tube allows intubation of one mainstem bronchus and functional separation from the other lung. This technique has been described a number of times by various authors but has been difficult to apply clinically because of the anatomy of the canine respiratory tract (see section on thoracoscopy later in this chapter).

If none of these approaches is possible, the surgeon should clamp the bronchus of the lobe nearest to the lesion or, if that is not accessible, clamp the mainstem bronchus until the mass has been removed. Before the transected bronchus is closed, the airway should be suctioned to remove any material.

Cardiovascular system

Before anaesthetizing a patient with cardiovascular disease for intrathoracic surgery, it is important to optimize medical therapy to improve the patient's condition, if the procedure can be delayed to allow this. If vasodilators, inotropes, diuretics or antiarrhythmic drugs can improve the patient's cardiovascular system function, this treatment should be provided for long enough to have an effect. Cats with hyperthyroidism and associated cardiac changes should be given carbimazole or methimazole for at least one week before surgery, as the mortality rate in these patients is much higher without such treatment (see Chapter 27).

Pacemakers

For patients with bradycardia that is non-responsive to anticholinergic therapy, or those with sick sinus syndrome, it is advisable to place a temporary pacemaker until a permanent pacemaker can be implanted (Figure 23.8). Although many third-degree atrioventricular blocks are relatively stable in the conscious animal, they can become unstable once the patient is anaesthetized. Sick sinus syndrome is inherently unstable and may devolve into a fatal dysrhythmia at any time. In order to ensure that induction of anaesthesia is as safe as possible, it is best to employ a method to pace the animal temporarily during this period (see also Chapter 21).

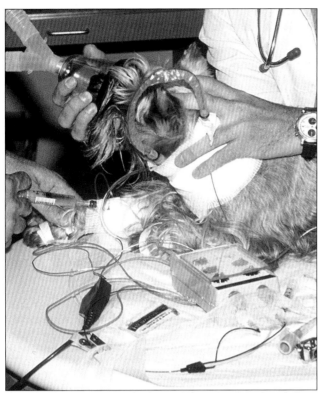

23.8 Temporary pacemaker inserted through an introducer in the jugular vein. The pacing generator can be seen in the foreground. The animal has had the pacemaker inserted under sedation and will have a constant regulated heart rate during the induction and maintenance of anaesthesia.

External pacing (transcutaneous pacing): Pacing can be achieved by attaching electrodes over the thorax between the fifth and seventh intercostal spaces, with the centre of the electrodes placed close to the intercostal junctions. After clipping and cleaning the skin in this area on both sides of the animal, the electrodes, usually adhesive pads, are placed. The negative electrode is generally placed on the left side of the chest as this requires the least current for capture. The electrodes should be about 20 cm^2 in area; electrodes smaller than 10 cm^2 have been reported to give a poor result (Lee *et al.*, 2010). The required size of the electrodes appears to be weakly correlated to body-weight, and therefore electrodes designed for paediatric use in humans are generally used for dogs.

The stimulus waveform is usually a square wave and is 20–40 milliseconds in duration. A wider waveform is reportedly more comfortable for the patient (Heller *et al.*, 1989). The ideal pacing system would be able to detect and display the electrocardiogram (ECG) without the need to place further electrodes, but some machines require a separate ECG recording. It is important that the pacemaker applies the pacing current at the appropriate time in the cardiac cycle, to avoid fibrillating the heart.

This technique is straightforward and quick to apply and is the method of choice for managing a life-threatening bradyarrhythmia. However, in the conscious patient, the skeletal muscle contractions that usually accompany the cardiac stimuli are often painful; therefore, once the electrodes are applied and connected to the pacing device, the patient can be anaesthetized before pacing begins (DeFrancesco *et al.*, 2003). Following induction of anaesthesia, the pacemaker is activated and the current adjusted until capture (electrical depolarization and myocardial contraction stimulated by the pacemaker) is achieved. Usually, the current is then increased by a factor of 1.5–3 to ensure that capture continues. In one study, the current required for external pacing in dogs ranged from 30–160 mA, although in 2 of 82 dogs capture failed (Noomanová *et al.*, 2010). In another retrospective study of 42 dogs, all dogs captured successfully (DeFrancesco *et al.*, 2003).

The major disadvantage of external pacing is movement of the patient each time the stimulus is applied, due to skeletal muscle contraction. Neuromuscular blocking agents may be used to prevent this muscle contraction, to provide better conditions for surgery. Another disadvantage is that the electrodes are placed close to the surgical site required for permanent pacemaker implantation. This may compromise the sterile surgical area, particularly in smaller patients.

Transoesophageal pacing: This method appears to be effective only for atrial pacing and is therefore unsuitable for patients with third-degree atrioventricular block. For atrial pacing, a bipolar electrode is passed down the oesophagus until the tip is located just beyond the level of the carina (Sanders *et al.*, 2010). The use of pacing currents in the range of 2.5–15 mA in dogs weighing 10.5–26 kg has been reported (Chapel and Sanders, 2012).

Transvenous pacing: This commonly used technique provides a reasonably secure pacing directed to the atria or the ventricles. Low currents can be used because this method provides direct contact with the endocardium. Placement of a temporary transvenous pacemaker (TTVP) is the author's preferred approach. The TTVP is placed after the animal has been given pre-anaesthetic medication but before induction of anaesthesia. Slightly deeper sedation than normal is needed to allow placement of an introducer sheath catheter and passage of the pacemaker wire. Either the left jugular vein or one of the lateral saphenous veins is catheterized for pacemaker placement; the latter are preferable, where possible, because the catheter can be manipulated without interfering with the surgical site or trying to find the access site beneath the animal. A 5 F introducer with a haemostasis valve is placed under aseptic conditions, sutured in place, bandaged and capped. The transvenous pacemaker wire is advanced into the heart under fluoroscopic guidance and positioned as desired for capture. The stimulator is attached and adjusted to an appropriate value for that patient, and the catheter is taped to the introducer and/or the animal to prevent it from backing out or accidentally being pulled out.

Whenever possible, the author's usual practice is to place a TTVP in each patient destined for a permanent pacemaker. In a study conducted at seven referral institutions, only 69 of 150 dogs received TTVP, and 9 of 154 dogs arrested during permanent pacemaker implantation (Oyama *et al.*, 2001). At the time of writing, among the most recent 113 cases of permanent pacemaker implantation performed with TTVP at the author's institution no cardiac arrests occurred during the procedure. In only two animals was the TTVP placed after induction of anaesthesia; one dog was too restless for TTVP placement under sedation, and the other patient had veins that were difficult to locate. Once the TTVP is pacing the heart, induction of anaesthesia should present few problems if there is no pre-existing myocardial failure. At the author's institution, fentanyl infusions are often used as part of a balanced anaesthetic protocol (~40% cases) and hypotension is treated with dopamine or dobutamine in many cases

(~30%). It is important that recovery from anaesthesia is smooth in these patients. Acepromazine may be useful in dogs that are either expected to have, or are having, a rough recovery, in order to reduce tension on the pacemaker lead.

Pericardial effusions

Patients with a pericardial effusion of sufficient magnitude to restrict myocardial function should have the fluid drained before surgery. In this procedure, a needle or catheter is used to drain enough fluid to release any pressure in the pericardial sac. The animal is usually positioned in left lateral recumbency and pericardiocentesis is performed through the right fourth to sixth intercostal spaces. Ideally, an over-the-needle catheter with multiple fenestrations should be used alongside ultrasonographic guidance, as this technique will minimize the risk of trauma to the heart.

Blood loss

The risk of surgical blood loss should be assessed before the procedure and, using the current haematocrit and cardiovascular status of the patient, a decision should be made as to whether blood is likely to be needed. If this is the case, the necessary arrangements should be made to obtain an adequate supply of compatible blood or packed red cells (see Chapter 18).

Surgical approach

Both lateral and sternal approaches to the chest involve some risk of damage to the underlying structures when the pleural membrane is incised. Controlled ventilation should be established before the thorax is opened, but it should be stopped for the brief period required to open the pleura, as this reduces the risk of accidental injury to the lung during entry into the chest. A lateral thoracotomy may involve a single intercostal space, or may entail the removal of one or more ribs. If surgery involves the heart, mediastinum or oesophagus, the surgeon may need to pack off the lung in the surgical field. Compression of the uppermost lung will reduce its compliance and promote more movement of gas to the lower lung. Packing off lungs should be done carefully so that the effect on the surface area for gas exchange is as small as possible, but a decrease in the arterial oxygen tension (P_aO_2) resulting from reduced exchange surface should be anticipated.

With a sternal approach, it is less likely that the lung fields will need to be compressed, but the alteration in the orientation of the heart can lead to a decrease in venous return. As a result, it may be necessary to increase fluid therapy in order to increase preload (see Chapter 18). During surgery, certain manipulations can cause a sudden and dramatic decrease in arterial blood pressure due to occlusion of large blood vessels. The surgeon and the anaesthetist should work together to define these deleterious events so that their effects can be minimized. It is more common to see cardiac arrhythmias with a sternal approach; the ECG should be monitored carefully for evidence of these, and therapy initiated if the arrhythmias appear to be detrimental to cardiovascular function.

Nitrous oxide is contraindicated during any thoracotomy because it rapidly accumulates in gas pockets in the interpleural space. Since the pleural space is well vascularized and is in direct contact with the lung containing nitrous oxide, the nitrous oxide diffuses down the concentration gradient and can double the volume of a closed pneumothorax in 10–15 minutes.

Analgesia

Analgesia for thoracotomy can be provided in a number of ways. A lateral thoracotomy appears to cause less pain than a sternotomy, and many dogs will show few signs of pain after a single intercostal incision if other muscle groups have not been transected. Epidural injection of an opioid such as morphine certainly provides some bilateral analgesia for a lateral or sternal thoracotomy, and can be administered before surgery to achieve a pre-emptive effect. Recent studies have shown that an opioid diluted to a total volume of 0.2 ml/kg provides sufficient volume for the drug to spread to the cranial thoracic region (Iseri et al., 2010; Son et al., 2011), and the author has used 0.3 ml/kg in many years of clinical practice. Local anaesthetic agents should not be used at volumes greater than 0.25 ml/kg because there is a risk that the intercostal and phrenic nerves (C4–5) may be blocked, causing respiratory muscle paralysis. If analgesia is required for longer periods, an epidural catheter can be placed via the lumbosacral space and its tip advanced up to the mid-thoracic region. This can be used to deliver morphine and/or small volumes of local anaesthetic (0.1–0.15 ml/kg would be acceptable) by intermittent boluses or by continuous infusion, and can be left in place for several days after surgery.

Intercostal nerve blocks will provide some analgesia for a lateral approach, but when applied before surgery they are unlikely to give complete analgesia over the dorsal half of the thorax. The lateral/ventral cutaneous branch of these nerves does not extend far dorsally in cats and dogs (in contrast to humans); in other words, the dorsal branches of the thoracic nerves supply the cutaneous structures of the dorsal half of the thoracic wall. The block will be more effective if injections are made from inside the thorax once the chest has been opened, aiming out towards the vertebrae where the nerves exit the intervertebral canal (Figure 23.9).

A paravertebral approach to the thoracic nerves is used in humans and gives excellent results. This block can be performed either as:

- A single injection with the needle approaching from a point lateral to the dorsal spinous processes
- A catheter introduced into the same site to facilitate repeated bolus injections or continuous infusion
- A catheter introduced into the subpleural space during surgery with visual confirmation of the location, and local anaesthetic agent then infused through the catheter.

An exploratory study using electrolocation and CT imaging of contrast agent injected into this area has been carried out in dogs, but there are no published data on the use of this technique in clinical pain management following thoracotomy in cats and dogs (Portela et al., 2012).

An interpleural block can be carried out via a preplaced chest drain after the chest has been closed; this technique has been reported to be effective (Conzemius et al., 1994; Thompson and Johnson, 1991). For a lateral thoracotomy, the animal is placed in dorsolateral recumbency (incision

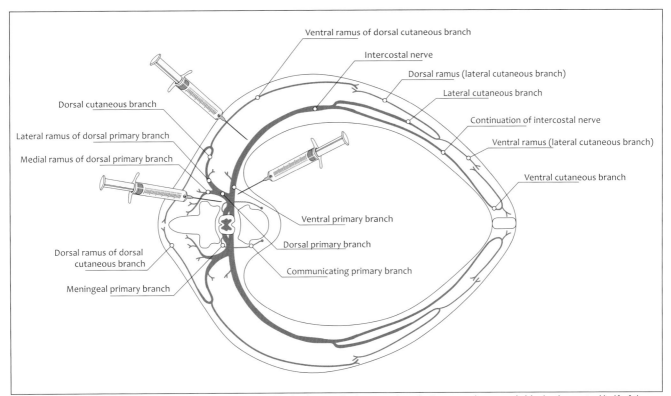

23.9 Diagram showing the sites for an intercostal nerve block. The standard approach to the intercostal nerve only blocks the ventral half of the thorax. Approaches dorsally close to midline or ventrally from inside the thorax can block the whole thoracic wall by reaching the thoracic nerve before it branches.

side down) and the local anaesthetic (usually 0.1–0.2% bupivacaine at 1–2 mg/kg) is injected through the chest drain. The anaesthetic agent gravitates to areas of the chest closest to the table and diffuses through the thoracic wall into the intercostal nerves. For a sternotomy, the local anaesthetic is injected through the chest drain with the animal in sternal recumbency or standing. In both instances the animal should be kept in that position for at least 10 minutes after injection so that the drug can be absorbed by the relevant tissues. Interpleural analgesia in cats has been documented in case reports but has not been assessed scientifically.

There is concern about the uptake of local anaesthetic agent into the blood, since the thoracic cavity is highly vascular and local anaesthetics are rapidly absorbed from this location, but doses of bupivacaine lower than 2 mg/kg do not appear to have toxic side effects. In an experimental study, uptake into the phrenic nerve was observed after bupivacaine was instilled directly over the mediastinum. However, this uptake is unlikely to occur with the techniques of administration described above (Kowalski et al., 1992). Uptake of bupivacaine into the heart is likely, particularly after a pericardiectomy, but seems to cause problems only at bupivacaine doses in excess of 2 mg/kg (Bernard et al., 2006).

Monitoring

Monitoring of an animal during a thoracotomy should allow the veterinary surgeon to assess the adequacy of ventilation and to diagnose arrhythmias, and should provide information on changes in cardiac function, which is especially important in a patient with cardiac disease. The open thorax does not move in a manner that allows tidal volume to be estimated; monitoring of ventilation therefore involves measuring airway pressure, minute volume, end-tidal carbon dioxide or arterial carbon dioxide tension (P_aCO_2); this list of monitoring techniques is ordered in increasing desirability.

Airway pressure indicates the force that is applied to the pulmonary system but does not give any information about gas exchange. Peak airway pressures in the range of 10–15 cmH$_2$O in the cat and 10–20 cmH$_2$O in the dog are considered to be normal. If higher pressures are required to achieve adequate inflation, this may be an indication of decreased chest wall and/or lung compliance.

Minute volume is an accurate representation of gas movement in and out of the lungs, but does not indicate whether there is adequate gas exchange. End-tidal carbon dioxide should reflect the value for P_aCO_2, but there is often an unknown discrepancy between the two values when the thorax is open. However, in the absence of lung pathology the two values are usually close enough to allow accurate estimation of whether lung ventilation is adequate. Continuous capnography will provide rapid feedback on changes in ventilation (see Chapter 7).

Blood gas analysis of arterial or free-flow lingual venous blood samples provides a definitive assessment of ventilation. Pulse oximetry is very helpful in cases where desaturation of haemoglobin may be expected (e.g. extensive pulmonary disease, right-to-left shunt) or where other techniques for measuring ventilation are not available. A pulse oximeter provides limited information in the early stages of ventilation/perfusion mismatching or alterations in shunt fraction, but if desaturation occurs it is likely that the monitor will sense this and provide a warning so that management can be instigated before it is too late.

The combination of capnography, arterial blood gas analysis and pulse oximetry is ideal for patients undergoing thoracotomy since the two non-invasive, continuous monitors can be verified intermittently by the measurement of blood gases, allowing more accurate interpretation of the values displayed. Electrocardiography is also essential to allow diagnosis of arrhythmias. Early diagnosis and management of arrhythmias may help prevent progression to ventricular fibrillation.

Haemodynamic monitoring should include measurement of arterial blood pressure. Direct (invasive) measurement via an arterial catheter is the preferred technique, and also allows sampling of blood for arterial blood gas analysis. In some conditions it may also be beneficial to monitor central venous pressure (CVP) (see Chapter 7) and/or pulmonary arterial pressure.

Individual conditions

Trauma

Immediate surgical intervention may be required for trauma such as a flail chest, puncture wounds to the thoracic cavity and intrathoracic bleeding. Delayed intervention is possible for fractured ribs, although these are rarely surgically repaired.

An animal with a flail chest may be unable to ventilate normally as the flail segment is pulled inwards during inhalation. As a result, ventilation is very inefficient and the animal may be hypoxaemic and hypercapnic. However, some cats and dogs seem to cope quite well with a three- or four-rib flail segment and may not become hypoxaemic. While preparing the patient for anaesthesia, oxygen should be supplemented and the animal should be positioned with the flail segment down; this position will minimize the movement and pathophysiological effects of the flail piece and improve ventilation. The anaesthetic technique should enable rapid control of the airway. This is best achieved using drugs with a rapid onset of action such as propofol, alfaxalone, thiopental or etomidate. Thiopental and alfaxalone provide the most rapid induction with peak effects occurring in 20–30 seconds. Propofol should be given over 60 seconds in order to minimize respiratory depression and possible hypotension. Ketamine- and tiletamine-based anaesthetics take effect in about 60 seconds. If using these agents, oxygen should be administered throughout the induction period until intubation is performed. When used for induction, opioids take at least 2 minutes to reach peak effect and, again, oxygen should be administered during this time. Once the trachea is intubated, the lungs should be ventilated until the flail segment has been stabilized. Since fractured ribs can damage the lungs, it is essential to monitor the patient carefully for signs of pneumothorax.

Diaphragmatic hernia

Diaphragmatic hernias may be traumatic or congenital. Traumatic hernias are usually caused by an excessive force applied to the abdomen, causing viscera to rupture through the diaphragm into the chest. Most patients with a traumatic diaphragmatic hernia are dyspnoeic and may be presented *in extremis* immediately following the trauma. However, some animals can be totally asymptomatic and the hernia may be discovered as an incidental finding on abdominal radiographs or ultrasonograms. The liver is the most common organ to herniate, and so ascites and hepatic dysfunction may be observed. The severity of dyspnoea usually relates to the loss of space in the chest,

which limits normal pulmonary function. It may be helpful to lift these animals on to their pelvic limbs so that their back is perpendicular to the ground, allowing emptying of the chest and alleviating compression of the lungs, and to lay them on a tilted board during preparation for surgery (Figure 23.10).

Many of these animals also have fractured limbs, pulmonary contusions and myocardial trauma, and these conditions need to be assessed before proceeding with repair of the diaphragmatic hernia. The timing of surgical repair is controversial: it is suggested that one should 'never let the sun go down' on a diaphragmatic hernia, even in cases where the diagnosis has been made months after the traumatic incident. The justification for immediate repair is that it is possible for more abdominal content to shift into the thoracic cavity and for the animal to become severely dyspnoeic, or even die, overnight; this author has encountered such incidents. The disadvantages of carrying out the repair on the same day may relate to scheduling conflicts and the inability to stabilize the patient before surgery if immediate repair is chosen. The author favours not delaying, since there is usually time to provide adequate restoration of circulating volume (after trauma); in addition, delaying the repair may allow decompensation, which can result in death in a matter of minutes. Cases of acute trauma need to receive adequate fluid therapy and should be preoxygenated before induction of anaesthesia.

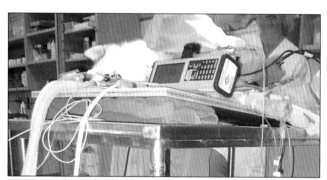

23.10 A dog with a diaphragmatic hernia being prepared for surgery. Note that the board provides a head-up position to alleviate lung compression.
(Courtesy of Tanya Duke-Novakovski, Western College of Veterinary Medicine, University of Saskatchewan, Canada)

Pre-anaesthetic medication with an opioid, at low doses, with or without an anticholinergic is appropriate. In recently traumatized (<5 days) or debilitated patients, acepromazine should be avoided as it may uncover occult volume depletion and exacerbate hypotension, and it can cause splenic enlargement. Preoxygenation should be carried out for five minutes, using a tight-fitting facemask to increase the inspired oxygen concentration to >95%. The facemask should be kept in place during induction until the animal is ready to be intubated. Induction with a benzodiazepine combined with a dissociative agent, propofol, alfaxalone or etomidate, is ideal; this allows rapid control of the airway so that the lungs can be ventilated immediately. Thiopental commonly causes splenic enlargement, which could lead to severe respiratory distress if the spleen is wholly or partially in the chest.

Once the trachea is intubated, IPPV should be initiated. It is important to re-expand a chronically atelectatic lung slowly, to avoid the development of pulmonary oedema. This can be achieved by using a higher respiratory frequency with lower peak airway pressures. Arterial blood oxygenation should be monitored carefully, as the author has found it difficult to avoid hypoxaemia if tidal volume is restricted excessively. As described above, the use of a lower F_iO_2 may provide a nitrogen splint to decrease the likelihood of further absorption atelectasis when using low tidal volumes. The pathophysiology of re-expansion pulmonary oedema is still unknown, but appears to be the result of the production of reactive oxygen species. The aim with these cases is to provide adequate lung ventilation to prevent hypoxaemia and excessive hypercapnia but not to re-expand the atelectatic lung. Once the hernia has been repaired, air should be evacuated from the chest slowly over the next 6–12 hours and the lung will expand gradually with normal, spontaneous breathing, hopefully sufficiently slowly to prevent acute lung injury.

The usual surgical approach for diaphragmatic hernia repair is via a midline laparotomy, with extension of the incision into the sternum if necessary. Some authors advocate a lateral thoracotomy and repair of the hernia from the cranial surface of the diaphragm; this approach is quite successful as long as the location of the hernia has been adequately defined (e.g. right lateral thoracotomy for a right-sided hernia). It may be helpful to place a chest drain so that air can be removed from the thoracic cavity and normal negative interpleural pressure restored, or air can be removed using a catheter inserted into the chest cavity through the diaphragm (Figure 23.11).

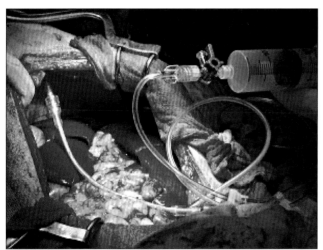

23.11 Evacuation of pleural air using a catheter inserted through the diaphragm and attached to a 3-way stopcock and syringe.
(Courtesy of Tanya Duke-Novakovski, Western College of Veterinary Medicine, University of Saskatchewan, Canada)

Space-occupying lesions not associated with the cardiopulmonary system: thymoma

The most common tumours found in the thoracic cavity that do not involve the heart or lungs are thymomas. These tumours can be large enough to interfere with pulmonary function by causing compression of the trachea, or to affect venous return by compressing the cranial vena cava, thus rendering the patient susceptible to postural hypotension (Johnson *et al.*, 1991). Myasthenia gravis is also associated with thymoma; in these patients, a megaoesophagus may be seen on thoracic radiographs (Shilo *et al.*, 2011). Regurgitation and aspiration pneumonia are possible complications of this condition (see Chapters 22 and 24). Patients with myasthenia gravis are normally treated with an anticholinesterase (pyridostigmine). This therapy should be given on the morning of surgery if the signs of myasthenia have been relatively severe. The presence of long-acting anticholinesterases may shorten

the duration of action of some opioids. The response to neuromuscular blocking agents is variable, but in general, these patients have an increased sensitivity to these agents. If it is necessary to use them, smaller than usual doses should be administered while the response is monitored (see Chapter 16).

The choice of pre-anaesthetic medication should be appropriate for the physical status of the patient (see Chapters 2 and 13). The patient should be preoxygenated before induction of anaesthesia, and suction apparatus should be immediately available if the animal has a megaoesophagus. An induction agent with rapid onset should be used in patients with a megaoesophagus, but if megaoesophagus is not present, the induction technique is not overly important. Maintenance with an inhalant anaesthetic agent would be typical. It is important to be prepared for sudden decreases in venous return during changes in patient position. A second intravenous catheter, or a central venous catheter, should be placed in case more than one infusion is necessary. Some thymomas wrap around the major blood vessels; significant blood loss is possible in these cases, and there should be blood available for transfusion. Postoperatively, the patient should be monitored carefully for signs of respiratory failure resulting from excessive airway secretions, laryngeal swelling or weakness of the respiratory musculature. The trachea should be reintubated if the patient is unable to maintain adequate gas exchange (Shilo *et al.*, 2011).

Oesophageal lesions including persistent right aortic arch

Congenital lesions, such as persistent right aortic arch (PRAA) or other aortic arch anomalies, may cause a restrictive lesion of the oesophagus. These animals are therefore prone to similar problems to those with megaoesophagus from other causes, and should be handled in a similar way. While PRAA is usually an avascular remnant, some other anomalies causing oesophageal stricture may involve patent blood vessels, and significant blood loss can occur during surgery. These patients should have two venous catheters, including a central venous catheter, placed, and blood for transfusion should be available. In cases of oesophageal tears or foreign bodies, the greatest risks are from infection, pneumothorax if a foreign object has damaged some lung as well as the oesophagus, and damage caused by the endoscope. Depending on the nature or position of a foreign body, a chest drain should be placed before IPPV is initiated.

Pulmonary lesions

Most patients with pulmonary lesions have some degree of respiratory compromise and will need 3–5 mins of preoxygenation via facemask before induction of anaesthesia. The mask should be kept in place during induction until the animal is ready to be intubated. If the mask is removed and the animal begins to breathe room air, any benefit of preoxygenation will be lost within a few breaths because there are no oxygen 'stores' in the body. If the animal will not tolerate a facemask, a plastic bag placed over the head and closed on to the neck with an oxygen inlet, may be better tolerated. If this technique is not feasible, it may be necessary to start the induction and place the facemask as soon as the animal begins to lose consciousness. Although it may take up to 5 mins to reach peak P_aO_2, the initial rise is steep and the animal will benefit from even a few breaths of 100% oxygen.

Pneumothorax is usually the result of damage to the lung or major airways. If the air leakage appears to be ongoing, a chest drain should be placed and the animal connected to a continuous suction device. If the amount of air in the thorax is minimal and there does not appear to be any ongoing leakage, thoracocentesis may be performed, but a chest drain with suction may not be necessary, as long as the time from induction to surgical opening of the thoracic cavity is short. The use of a total intravenous anaesthetic (TIVA) protocol should be considered in cases where there is likely to be significant ongoing air leakage from pulmonary tissue until the surgeon can oversew or remove the damage. The use of TIVA avoids leakage of volatile agent into the thoracic cavity so that surgeons and assistants do not breathe in anaesthetic gases. For TIVA, a propofol/opioid or alfaxalone/opioid infusion technique is ideal; combinations used at the author's institution are propofol (0.1–0.3 mg/kg/min) or alfaxalone (0.07–0.2 mg/kg/min) with an opioid such as fentanyl (18 to 60 μg/kg/h). In cats, the dose of fentanyl should not exceed 24 μg/kg/h since there appears to be limited benefit above this dose and there may be an increased risk of postoperative excitation.

Animals with pulmonary contusions need to be ventilated very carefully, because there is a risk that blood vessels that ruptured to cause the contusion can be opened up again if the lung is excessively stretched. Further haemorrhage into the lung may cause a significant loss of gas exchange area and lead to severe respiratory compromise. In these animals, ventilation should be with low tidal volumes and high frequencies (e.g. tidal volume 5–10 ml/kg, 20 breaths per minute).

Preoperatively, it is often difficult to differentiate between a pulmonary abscess and a tumour. If it is suspected that the lesion may be an abscess or a tumour with a necrotic centre, then the use of bronchial blockers should be considered (as described earlier in this chapter). It is also wise to have a suction device available in case the above measures fail to contain the pus. Any major drainage of pus into the lower lung carries a very poor prognosis for the patient.

Another concern with pulmonary lesions is that there may be adhesions between the lung and the parietal pleura, such that surgical entry through the pleura results in entry into the lesion. The anaesthetist should be prepared to manage the blood loss or air leakage that can occur in these circumstances.

Lung lobe torsion is usually treated by excision of the lobe. This is normally a relatively straightforward procedure, especially if advanced stapling techniques are used. Apart from the considerations described above (preoxygenation, ventilation, etc.) there are no major considerations for this type of surgery.

Chylothorax

Concerns with chylothorax and other pleural effusions relate to the amount of fluid in the chest and the possibility that adhesions to the parietal pleura may have formed, increasing the chance of pulmonary injury when the thoracic cavity is opened. If possible, the fluid should be drained from the chest before the patient is anaesthetized to improve intraoperative ventilation. Blood loss is minimal if the lymphatic duct is tied off or a drainage system is implanted into the diaphragm, but it can be substantial if pleurodesis is performed. It is now common to identify the

thoracic duct by injecting iohexol and/or methylene blue into the mesenteric lymph nodes using CT guidance and ultrasound imaging, and then use a thoracoscopic approach to visualize and ligate the duct. The magnification provided by thoracoscopy makes this technique much more precise than an open thoracotomy. Ligation of the thoracic duct is often accompanied by subtotal pericardiectomy to relieve any effect of pericardial thickening on diastolic filling.

Pericardiectomy

Pericardiectomy may be undertaken for a pericardial effusion or a pericardial constriction. Animals with cardiac tamponade (where intrapericardial pressure approaches right ventricular diastolic filling pressure) are at immediate risk of circulatory collapse. An intrapericardial pressure of 9 mmHg can cause a 60% reduction in cardiac output, although in some cases pressures as high as 12–13 mmHg may be tolerated. Drainage of fluid from the pericardium should be carried out to relieve these signs before the animal is anaesthetized. A sternotomy will give the best access to the pericardium, but a lateral approach may be used in some cases. Pericardiectomy may also be amenable to thoracoscopic approaches (see later).

If an animal with cardiac tamponade must be anaesthetized, it should be pretreated with fluids to ensure optimum venous return. An anaesthetic technique should be chosen that will not affect myocardial contractility and heart rate; in these patients, heart rate is usually elevated in an attempt to maintain cardiac output in the presence of a reduced stroke volume. Etomidate is the ideal induction drug, but an opioid-based induction could be used as long as care is taken to ensure that the heart rate does not decrease significantly (e.g. pre-administration of an anticholinergic). Once the patient is intubated, spontaneous ventilation should be maintained to minimize any further reduction in venous return. If IPPV is used before the thoracic cavity is opened, it is best to use a higher respiratory frequency to help limit peak airway pressure, and PEEP should be avoided. Dobutamine can be given to improve cardiac output; this drug also delays the onset of tissue hypoxia, compared with noradrenaline (norepinephrine) (Zhang *et al.*, 1994). Dopamine can also increase cardiac output and improve myocardial perfusion. Once the tamponade has been reduced, anaesthetic management of these patients during pericardiectomy is relatively straightforward. Ventricular arrhythmias are common during manipulation of the pericardium, and lidocaine should be readily available to use if arrhythmias begin to alter haemodynamic function. Haemorrhage may be marked if decortication of the epicardium is undertaken, and it is necessary to have adequate supplies of typed and cross-matched blood ready for transfusion in the event of severe blood loss.

Patent ductus arteriosus

Most animals anaesthetized for correction of a patent ductus arteriosus (PDA) (see Chapter 21) are young and usually in good health apart from the changes caused by the PDA. If the PDA is in the early stages, there are usually very few myocardial changes. However, if the ductus is large and/or the lesion has not been recognized early, there can be significant enlargement of the left ventricle and eventually cardiac failure due to volume overload.

If surgery is performed before significant changes have occurred, there are few concerns. Young patients have a lower arterial blood pressure than adults due to their stage of development. Coronary perfusion depends on maintaining diastolic pressure, which will be very low before ligation of the ductus because the ductus connects the systemic circulation to the low-resistance pulmonary system. Because of this, phenothiazines should be avoided for pre-anaesthetic medication because the alpha-1 adrenergic blockade decreases systemic vascular resistance (SVR), decreasing diastolic pressure even further. In these patients systolic pressure is usually normal to high but, because of the low diastolic pressure, mean arterial pressure is normal or reduced and is often in the 50–60 mmHg range during surgical approach to the ductus. Positive inotropes may increase systolic pressure and also increase mean pressure but should be used only if systolic pressure falls below 90 mmHg. Peripheral vasoconstrictors should not be used since an increased SVR will tend to increase the shunt through the ductus and may lead to pulmonary oedema.

If dissection of the ductus is difficult, massive haemorrhage may occur very quickly. A second intravenous catheter or central catheter should be placed so that fluids can be given rapidly if needed, although the outcome is rarely favourable if the ductus is ruptured. It may be advisable to give an anticholinergic agent before ligation because the sudden increase in diastolic (and hence mean) arterial blood pressure associated with ligation can elicit a strong baroreceptor reflex (Figure 23.12), which can even cause cardiac arrest. Anticholinergics block the vagal part of this reflex. The anticholinergic can be given either at the time of pre-anaesthetic medication, or closer to the time of ligation. Monitoring of direct arterial blood pressure will enable assessment of moment-to-moment changes and is also useful to confirm that the ductus has been fully ligated.

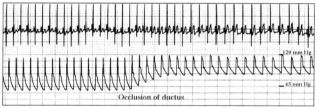

23.12 Arterial blood pressure and ECG tracing from a dog undergoing a patent ductus arteriosus occlusion. Note the increase in diastolic pressure with minimal change in systolic pressure. The heart rate decreases from 128 to 108 beats/minute in response to the increased pressure (baroreceptor response). The trace is at 6.25 mm/second.

Patients with signs of cardiac failure or pulmonary oedema should be treated with diuretics and positive inotropes (e.g. pimobendan) for 1–2 days before surgery. The anaesthetic technique chosen should aim to maintain myocardial function and perfusion as much as possible and not cause further decreases in SVR. Pre-anaesthetic medication with an opioid–anticholinergic combination is useful, and induction with an opioid–benzodiazepine technique, or etomidate with or without benzodiazepine, is preferred. Anaesthesia can be maintained in these patients with a standard inhalant agent, although if signs of myocardial failure are present, a balanced technique combining an opioid and/or a neuromuscular blocking agent with the inhalant would be advantageous.

Right-to-left shunts are rarely amenable to surgical correction, since closure of the duct often results in right heart failure due to pulmonary hypertension. The location of the ductus means that oxygenated blood is supplied to the coronary arteries and brachiocephalic trunk while the caudal end of the body receives the shunted blood. This leads to the caudal parts of the body becoming cyanotic relative to the thoracic limbs and head (see Figure 21.23).

In response to hypoxia, the kidneys release erythropoietin, resulting in polycythaemia. These animals can be managed medically by intermittent phlebotomy to control blood viscosity and may also be treated with hydroxyurea to reduce red cell production. Drugs such as sildenafil or tadalafil may decrease pulmonary vascular resistance and improve the patient's exercise tolerance, but are unlikely to reverse the shunt. With medical management, dogs with this condition may still live a long time. If these patients require anaesthesia for part of the diagnostic work-up or for other reasons, the regimen described for PDA with some degree of heart failure should be used. It is important to maintain or increase SVR while aiming to reduce (not increase) pulmonary vascular resistance.

Non-surgical repair of the PDA is achieved by the use of coils, plugs or occluders deployed into the ductus from a catheter introduced via the femoral artery or femoral vein, or rarely, the carotid artery. This procedure is relatively non-invasive and has a high success rate. The tip of the catheter is positioned at the entrance to the PDA and the coil or other device is released into the ductus. Coils that are 'dropped' and pass through the ductus into the lung rarely seem to cause problems; in contrast, coils that travel down the aorta can end up in critical vessels (e.g. mesenteric artery), with catastrophic results. The Amplatz canine ductal occluder (ACDO) deployed from the femoral artery appears to be the safest and most successful approach, but animals weighing 1–3 kg may require coils. In these smaller patients, passing the catheter through the right heart into the pulmonary artery, using the femoral vein for access, may be more successful because the vein can accommodate a larger catheter than the femoral artery. Significant haemorrhage from tearing of the femoral artery and percutaneous catheterization of either the artery or vein has been reported in a small number of cases (Singh *et al.*, 2012). Anaesthetic techniques for non-surgical PDA repair are similar to those described for the surgical approach except that a thoracotomy is not necessary; this obviates the requirement for IPPV and means that fewer postoperative analgesics will be required. With a transvenous approach, the catheter frequently elicits arrhythmias as it passes through the heart, and an intravenous lidocaine infusion is often included in the anaesthetic protocol.

Thoracoscopy

Thoracoscopy may be used for diagnostic purposes (e.g. biopsy of a mass) or for surgical approaches (e.g. pericardiectomy, PDA, PRAA, thoracic duct ligation or lung lobectomy). The basic procedure involves the introduction of a rigid or flexible fibreoptic endoscope into the thoracic cavity, and the use of air, carbon dioxide or another gas to create a pneumothorax, allowing visualization of intrathoracic structures. One or more ports on the endoscope allow the introduction of gas or instruments required for the surgical manipulation. The approach may be made laterally with the animal in lateral recumbency, or ventrally (subxiphoid) with the animal in dorsal recumbency. A lateral approach requires the upper lung to be collapsed, and in this situation selective one-lung ventilation (OLV) is useful.

One-lung ventilation

In the dog, the right lung is about 1.5 times the size of the left lung and receives almost 60% of the blood supply. It is possible to achieve adequate ventilation of the patient by ventilating only the right lung, although some desaturation can occur during the first few minutes. In cats it is difficult to achieve adequate oxygenation if the right lung is blocked off (Mayhew *et al.*, 2014).

Bronchial blockers can be used for OLV, in which case the blocker is placed in the lung to be collapsed (see Figure 23.5). Alternatively, a very long silicone endotracheal tube can be advanced down one bronchus; however, with this method the cuff and the piece beyond the cuff are long enough that they may block off the cranial lobe of the inflated lung. The preferred method is to use a double-lumen tube so each lung can be collapsed separately if a bilateral thoracoscopic procedure is undertaken. In dogs, the Robertshaw type of double-lumen tubes, which have a long and a short tube with two cuffs, have been used (see Figure 23.14). Carlens and Dr White double-lumen tubes have been evaluated and were not found to be useful in dogs (Mayhew *et al.*, 2012). The longer tube of the Robertshaw is placed in the bronchus while the shorter tube should remain in the trachea. Once the cuffs are inflated, the right and left lungs should be functionally isolated from each other. The tubes are supplied as right and left versions: the right tube has an orifice in the side of the cuff that, in humans, is placed at the entrance to the bronchus of the right upper lobe. This does not work well in dogs because of the different position of the right apical lobe bronchus, and it is difficult to place an endobronchial tube on the right side without losing ventilation to the right apical and cardiac (middle) lobes of the lung (Figure 23.13).

Because of this difference in anatomy, it is better to use a left-sided Robertshaw tube. The tube cuffs are bright blue to improve visualization and an endoscope is necessary to ensure correct placement of the tube. Studies in humans have reported that blind positioning of the tube results in a high (38–78%) incidence of malpositioning. The endoscope should be passed down both tubes to ensure that the ends of the tubes are not impacted against a bronchial wall and that the right tube has not slipped into the left main bronchus, and that the cuff is adequately inflated in the correct position. A 4.9 mm (outside diameter) endoscope will work for the larger sizes of tube (39 and 41 Fr), but an endoscope less than 4.2 mm is needed for the smaller tubes (28–37 Fr). For a midline thoracoscopy where both lungs can be seen, it is possible to pass the Robertshaw blindly with the angle of the longer tube aimed at the left mainstem bronchus. The distal cuff is then inflated and the veterinary surgeon evaluates which lung lobes are inflated with ventilation. The tube can then be slowly withdrawn until the complete left lung is ventilated. Robertshaw tubes are designed for humans and are too short to be used in dogs over approximately 30 kg. This means that their use is impractical in many canine patients. Endobronchial blockade or endobronchial intubation with a long single-lumen endotracheal tube are the most practical approaches for OLV in these larger dogs.

If a lateral approach is being used, then the dependent lung is ventilated while the upper non-dependent lung is collapsed. OLV appears to be adequate for the removal of carbon dioxide, but P_aO_2 decreases because of the loss of gas exchange area and shunting of blood through the non-ventilated lung. Studies examining OLV in healthy animals have shown that despite the decrease in P_aO_2, oxygen delivery to the periphery is unchanged because haemoglobin is still fully saturated and cardiac output is maintained. However, thoracoscopy is often performed on animals with abnormal lungs and so hypoxaemia is always a concern. Strategies to improve oxygen exchange include:

- Application of PEEP to the dependent lung. The combination of gravity, the weight of the heart and surgical manipulation all tend to induce collapse of the dependent lung. The application of PEEP will minimize these changes and keep the airways open. However, the ideal value of the PEEP is not easy to determine, since too low a value will produce no effect, and too high a value will increase pulmonary intravascular resistance. Increased pulmonary intravascular resistance decreases cardiac output and may also shunt blood into the upper (unventilated) lung. Nevertheless, in humans the application of 10 cmH$_2$O PEEP to the dependent lung has been reported to improve P_aO_2 in patients with a P_aO_2 <80 mmHg (<10.7 kPa). In normal dogs, 5 cmH$_2$O PEEP applied to the dependent lung does not significantly improve P_aO_2 or decrease cardiac output (Riquelme *et al.*, 2005b)
- Application of CPAP to the non-dependent lung using a double-lumen tube or through the catheter of a bronchial blocker with an end-hole. CPAP is applied to the upper lung before deflation or after a large tidal volume before lung collapse is allowed to occur. An adjustable, disposable CPAP valve can be used for this application (Broncho-Cath® with CPAP system; Figure 23.14). The CPAP valve is applied to the upper lung endotracheal tube and oxygen is administered at 5 l/min. This approach allows some mass diffusion of oxygen into the upper lung and improves oxygenation more than the application of PEEP to the dependent lung alone

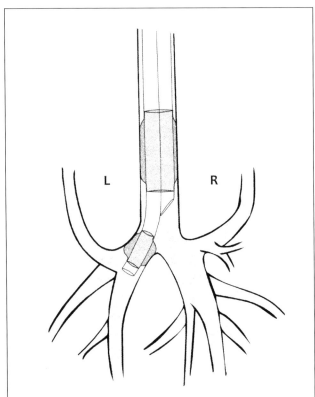

23.13 Diagram of the trachea and bronchi of the dog with a Robertshaw tube placed in the left mainstem bronchus. Note the proximity of the distal end of the tube to the bronchi in the left cranial lobe, showing the likelihood of occluding one or more of these bronchi.

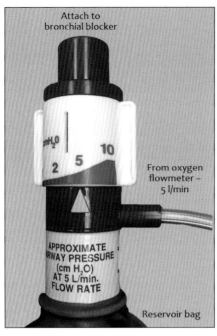

23.14 Disposable Broncho-Cath® CPAP system for use with bronchial blockers and double-lumen endotracheal tubes.

(figure labels: Attach to bronchial blocker; From oxygen flowmeter – 5 l/min; Reservoir bag; mmH₂O 2 5 10; APPROXIMATE AIRWAY PRESSURE (cm H₂O) AT 5 L/min. FLOW RATE)

- Application of high-frequency jet ventilation to the non-dependent lung. In humans, this technique reportedly gave comparable results to the application of CPAP in terms of P_aO_2 but interfered less with cardiac output, thus providing better oxygen delivery to the tissues (Nakatsuka et al., 1988). In this study, a high-frequency jet ventilator was used, set at a rate of 150 breaths per minute. The author has not had success with this technique in dogs.

If the other hemithorax also requires thoracoscopy, the use of a double-lumen tube enables the process to be reversed, so the collapsed lung can be re-expanded while the other lung is deflated.

When using the subxiphoid approach for thoracoscopy (e.g. for pericardiectomy), OLV may not be necessary, since both lungs may need to receive relatively low tidal volumes in order to improve visualization. It is essential during these procedures that the surgeon and anaesthetist coordinate their activities to achieve maximum visibility while maintaining adequate oxygenation. This often requires the use of manual ventilation to provide irregular ventilatory cycles between bouts of surgical activity. The use of a double-lumen tube may allow more flexibility in achieving the best ventilation with the least interference with surgery. Using PEEP/CPAP for this approach may also be beneficial in improving oxygenation.

Animals undergoing thoracoscopy should be monitored using pulse oximetry, so that any desaturation can be recognized and treated straight away. The addition of capnography, electrocardiography, direct arterial blood pressure and arterial blood gas analysis will improve the ability to recognize problems early and treat them immediately. CVP will be affected by the amount of air or carbon dioxide in the chest, so monitoring of CVP will make it easier to recognize excessive pneumothorax (>6 mmHg) (Daly et al., 2002). Low levels of intrathoracic pressure (2–3 mmHg) should be used, and these should still provide good visibility (Daly et al., 2002; Polis et al., 2002). Once the thoracoscopic procedure has been finished, air should be removed from the chest and a chest drain placed, so that any remaining air can be removed and any subsequent haemorrhage or air leaks recognized.

Postoperative care

Many animals undergoing thoracic procedures are at risk of postoperative hypoxaemia. This can be minimized by taking the following precautions:

- Take steps to ensure that the animal is normothermic in recovery. An animal that is shivering may increase its oxygen consumption by 300%. This extra demand may exacerbate any hypoxaemia caused by poor pulmonary function
- Ensure that the animal has received analgesics (if necessary), and monitor the recovery to ensure that the animal emerges calmly from the anaesthetic. It may be necessary to give a tranquillizer if the animal becomes agitated during recovery, to avoid the increased oxygen consumption that would occur during a rough recovery
- Place a chest drain and provide timely intermittent drainage or continuous suction if there is a risk of pneumo- or haemothorax. Remove the chest drain as soon as it is deemed safe to do so
- Provide an enriched supply of oxygen. If tolerated by the patient, a facemask can be used in the early postoperative period. Using a tight-fitting mask allows delivery of 100% oxygen but requires someone to be with the animal all the time, as most animals do not tolerate this technique for long. The delivery of approximately 75% oxygen can be achieved by placing bilateral nasal insufflation catheters before recovery and beginning oxygen insufflation as soon as the animal is extubated (Dunphy et al., 2002). This technique is less efficacious in larger dogs, but allows continuous delivery of oxygen while the animal is being examined or treated
- High concentrations of oxygen (40–100%) can be supplied by placing the patient in an oxygen cage. Inspired oxygen concentration can be adjusted according to the needs of the patient, but handling the animal involves losing the benefit of the increased oxygen
- If surgery has been carried out on the heart or lungs, the animal must be monitored carefully for signs of respiratory distress, cardiac arrhythmias, congestive heart failure or shock.

References and further reading

Akça O, Podolsky A, Eisenhuber E et al. (1999) Comparable postoperative pulmonary atelectasis in patients given 30% or 80% oxygen during and 2 hours after colon resection. Anesthesiology 91(4), 991–998.

Arndt GA, DeLessio ST, Kranner PW et al. (1999) One-lung ventilation when intubation is difficult – presentation of a new endobronchial blocker. Acta Anaesthesiologica Scandinavica 43, 356–358

Bailey CS, Kitchell RL, Haghighi SS and Johnson RD (1984) Cutaneous innervation of the thorax and abdomen of the dog. American Journal of Veterinary Research 45, 1689–1698

Baraff LJ (1993) Capillary refill: is it a useful clinical sign? Pediatrics 92, 723–724

Barnett HB, Holland JG and Josenhans WT (1982) When does central cyanosis become detectable? Clinical and Investigative Medicine 5, 39–43

Benumof J (1993) The position of a double-lumen tube should be routinely determined by fiberoptic bronchoscopy. Journal of Cardiothoracic and Vascular Anesthesia 7, 513–514

Bernard F, Kudnig ST and Monnet E (2006) Hemodynamic effects of interpleural lidocaine and bupivacaine combination in anesthetized dogs with and without an open pericardium. Veterinary Surgery 35, 252–258

Brasmer TH (1984) A is for airway. In: The Acutely Traumatized Small Animal Patient, pp. 55–95. WB Saunders, Philadelphia

Cantwell SL, Duke T, Walsh JP et al. (2000) One-lung versus two-lung ventilation in the anesthetized dog: a comparison of cardiopulmonary parameters. Veterinary Surgery 29, 365–373

Chapel EH and Sanders RA (2012) Efficacy of two commercially available cardiac pacing catheters for transesophageal atrial pacing in dogs. *Journal of Veterinary Cardiology* **14**, 409–414

Cohen E and Eisenkraft JB (1996) Positive end-expiratory pressure during one-lung ventilation improves oxygenation in patients with low arterial oxygen tensions. *Journal of Cardiovascular Anaesthesia* **10(5)**, 578–582

Cohen E, Eisenkraft JB, Thys D, Kirschner PA and Kaplan JA (1988) Oxygenation and hemodynamic changes during one-lung ventilation: effects of CPAP10, PEEP10, and CPAP10/PEEP10. *Journal of Cardiothoracic Anesthesia* **2**, 34–40

Cohen E, Thys DM, Eisenkraft JB and Kaplan JA (1985) PEEP during one lung anesthesia improves oxygenation in patients with low arterial P_aO_2. *Anesthesia and Analgesia* **64**, 201

Conzemius MG, Brockman DJ, King LG and Perkowski SZ (1994) Analgesia in dogs after intercostal thoracotomy: a clinical trial comparing intravenous buprenorphine and interpleural bupivacaine. *Veterinary Surgery* **23**, 291–298

Daly CM, Swaleo-Yobias K, Tobias AH and Ehrhart N (2002) Cardiopulmonary effects of intrathoracic insufflation in dogs. *Journal of the American Animal Hospital Association* **38**, 515–520

DeFrancesco TC, Hansen BD, Atkins CE, Sidley JA and Keene BW (2003) Noninvasive transthoracic temporary cardiac pacing in dogs. *Journal of Veterinary Internal Medicine* **17**, 663–667

Dunphy ED, Mann FA, Dodam JR et al. (2002) Comparison of unilateral versus bilateral nasal catheters for oxygen administration in dogs. *Journal of Veterinary Emergency and Critical Care* **12**, 245–251

Elliott AR, Steffey EP, Jarvis KA and Marshall BE (1991) Unilateral hypoxic pulmonary vasoconstriction in the dog, pony and miniature swine. *Respiration Physiology* **85**, 355–369

Fellows CG, Lerche P, King G and Tometzki A (1998) Treatment of patent ductus arteriosus by placement of two intravascular embolisation coils in a puppy. *Journal of Small Animal Practice* **39**, 196–199

Fordyce WE and Tenney SM (1984) Role of the carotid bodies in ventilatory acclimation to chronic hypoxia by the awake cat. *Respiration Physiology* **58**, 207–221

García F, Prandi D, Pena T et al. (1998) Examination of the thoracic cavity and lung lobectomy by means of thoracoscopy in dogs. *Canadian Veterinary Journal* **39**, 285–291

Gillespie DJ and Hyatt RE (1974) Respiratory mechanics in the unanesthetized dog. *Journal of Applied Physiology* **36**, 98–102

Grifka RG, Miller MW, Frischmeyer KJ and Mullins CE (1996) Transcatheter occlusion of a patent ductus arteriosus in a Newfoundland puppy using the Gianturco-Grifka vascular occlusion device. *Journal of Veterinary Internal Medicine* **10**, 42–44

Heller MB, Peterson J, Ilkahpamipour K, Kaplan R and Paris PM (1989) A comparative study of five transcutaneous pacing devices in unanesthetized human volunteers. *Prehospital and Disaster Medicine* **4**, 15–19

Ilkiw JE, Pascoe PJ, Haskins SC, Patz JD and Jaffe R (1993) The cardiovascular sparing effect of fentanyl and atropine, administered to enflurane anaesthetized dogs. *Canadian Journal of Veterinary Research* **57**, 248–253

Iseri T, Nishimura R, Nagahama S et al. (2010) Epidural spread of iohexol following the use of air or saline in the 'loss of resistance' test. *Veterinary Anaesthesia and Analgesia* **37**, 526–530

Johnson D, Hurst T, Cujec B and Mayers I (1991) Cardiopulmonary effects of an anterior mediastinal mass in dogs anesthetized with halothane. *Anesthesiology* **74**, 725–736

Kienle RD (1998a) Aortic stenosis. In: *Small Animal Cardiovascular Medicine, 1st edn*, ed. MD Kittleson and RD Kienle, pp. 260–272. Mosby, St. Louis

Kienle RD (1998b) Congenital pulmonic stenosis. In: *Small Animal Cardiovascular Medicine, 1st edn*, ed. MD Kittleson and RD Kienle, pp. 248–259. Mosby, St. Louis

Kitchell RL, Whalen LR, Bailey CS and Lohse CL (1980) Electrophysiologic studies of cutaneous nerves of the thoracic limb of the dog. *American Journal of Veterinary Research* **41**, 61–76

Koller ME, Smith B, Sjostrand U and Brevik H (1983) Effects of hypo-, normo-, and hypercarbia in dogs with acute cardiac tamponade. *Anesthesia and Analgesia* **62**, 181–185

Kowalski SE, Bradley BD, Greengrass RA, Freedman J and Younes MK (1992) Effects of interpleural bupivacaine (0.5%) on canine diaphragmatic function. *Anesthesia and Analgesia* **75**, 400–404

Lee S, Nam SJ and Hyun C (2010) The optimal size and placement of transdermal electrodes are critical for the efficacy of a transcutaneous pacemaker in dogs. *Veterinary Journal* **183**, 196–200

Lombardi R, Savino E and Waddell LS (2012) Pleural space drainage. In: *Advanced Monitoring and Procedures for Small Animal Emergency and Critical Care*, ed. JM Burkitt Creedon and H Davis, pp. 378–392. Wiley-Blackwell, Chichester

Martins JB, Manuel WJ, Marcus ML and Kerber RE (1980) Comparative effects of catecholamines in cardiac tamponade: experimental and clinical studies. *American Journal of Cardiology* **46**, 59–66

Mattila I, Takkunen O, Mattila P et al. (1984) Cardiac tamponade and different modes of artificial ventilation. *Acta Anaesthesiologica Scandinavica* **28**, 236–240

Mayhew PD, Culp WT, Pascoe PJ, Kass PH and Johnson LR (2012) Evaluation of blind thoracoscopic-assisted placement of three double-lumen endobronchial tube designs for one-lung ventilation in dogs. *Veterinary Surgery* **41**, 664–670

Mayhew PD, Pascoe PJ, Shilo-Benjamini Y, Kass PH and Johnson LR (2015) Effect of one-lung ventilation with or without low-pressure carbon dioxide insufflation on cardiorespiratory variables in cats undergoing thoracoscopy. *Veterinary Surgery* **44**, 15–22

Mure M, Domino KB, Robertson T, Hlastala MP and Glenny RW (1998) Pulmonary blood flow does not redistribute in dogs with reposition from supine to left lateral position. *Anesthesiology* **89**, 483–492

Nakatsuka M, Wetstein L and Keenan RL (1988) Unilateral high-frequency jet ventilation during one-lung ventilation for thoracotomy. *Annals of Thoracic Surgery* **46**, 654–660

Noomanová N, Perego M, Perini A and Santilli RA (2010) Use of transcutaneous external pacing during transvenous pacemaker implantation in dogs. *Veterinary Record* **167**, 241–244

Oyama MA, Sisson DD and Lehmkuhl LB (2001) Practices and outcome of artificial cardiac pacing in 154 dogs. *Journal of Veterinary Internal Medicine* **15**, 229–239

Pascoe PJ (1988) Oxygen and ventilatory support for the critical patient. *Seminars in Veterinary Medicine and Surgery (Small Animal)* **3**, 202–209

Pascoe PJ and Dyson DH (1993) Analgesia after lateral thoracotomy in dogs. Epidural morphine vs. intercostal bupivacaine. *Veterinary Surgery* **22**, 141–147

Polis I, Gasthuys F, Gielen I et al. (2002) The effects of intrathoracic pressure during continuous two-lung ventilation for thoracoscopy on the cardiorespiratory parameters in sevoflurane anaesthetized dogs. *Journal of Veterinary Medicine* **49**, 113–120

Popilskis S, Kohn D, Laurent L and Danilo P (1993) Efficacy of epidural morphine versus intravenous morphine for post-thoracotomy pain in dogs. *Journal of Veterinary Anaesthesia* **20**, 21–25

Popilskis S, Kohn D, Sanchez JA and Gorman P (1991) Epidural vs. intramuscular oxymorphone analgesia after thoracotomy in dogs. *Veterinary Surgery* **20**, 462–467

Portela DA, Otero PE, Sclocco M et al. (2012) Anatomical and radiological study of the thoracic paravertebral space in dogs: iohexol distribution pattern and use of the nerve stimulator. *Veterinary Anaesthesia and Analgesia* **39**, 398–408

Riegler FX, VadeBoncouer TR and Pelligrino DA (1989) Interpleural anesthetics in the dog: differential somatic neural blockade. *Anesthesiology* **71**, 744–750

Riquelme M, Monnet E, Kudnig ST et al. (2005a) Cardiopulmonary changes induced during one-lung ventilation in anesthetized dogs with a closed thoracic cavity. *American Journal of Veterinary Research* **66**, 973–977

Riquelme M, Monnet E, Kudnig ST et al. (2005b) Cardiopulmonary effects of positive end-expiratory pressure during one-lung ventilation in anesthetized dogs with a closed thoracic cavity. *American Journal of Veterinary Research* **66**, 978–983

Sanders RA, Green HW 3rd, Hogan DF, Trafney D and Batra AS (2010) Efficacy of transesophageal and transgastric cardiac pacing in the dog. *Journal of Veterinary Cardiology* **12**, 49–52

Saunders AB, Miller MW, Gordon SG and Bahr A (2004) Pulmonary embolization of vascular occlusion coils in dogs with patent ductus arteriosus. *Journal of Veterinary Internal Medicine* **18**, 663–666

Sawafuji M, Ishizaka A, Kohno M et al. (2005) Role of Rho-kinase in reexpansion pulmonary edema in rabbits. *American Journal of Physiology. Lung Cellular and Molecular Physiology* **289**, 946–953

Shilo Y, Pypendop BH, Barter LS and Epstein SE (2011) Thymoma removal in a cat with acquired myasthenia gravis: a case report and literature review of anesthetic techniques. *Veterinary Anaesthesia and Analgesia* **38**, 603–613

Singh MK, Kittleson MD, Kass PH and Griffiths LG (2012) Occlusion devices and approaches in canine patent ductus arteriosus: comparison of outcomes. *Journal of Veterinary Internal Medicine* **26**, 85–92

Son WG, Kim J, Seo JP et al. (2011) Cranial epidural spread of contrast medium and new methylene blue dye in sternally recumbent anaesthetized dogs. *Veterinary Anaesthesia and Analgesia* **38**, 510–515

Stokhof A (1986) Diagnosis and treatment of acquired diaphragmatic hernia by thoracotomy in 49 dogs and 72 cats. *Veterinary Quarterly* **8**, 177–183

Thompson SE and Johnson JM (1991) Analgesia in dogs after intercostal thoracotomy. A comparison of morphine, selective intercostal nerve block, and interpleural regional analgesia with bupivacaine. *Veterinary Surgery* **20**, 73–77

VadeBoncouer TR, Riegler FX and Pelligrino DA (1990) The effects of two different volumes of 0.5% bupivacaine in a canine model of interpleural analgesia. *Regional Anesthesia* **15**, 67–72

Wagner AE, Gaynor JS, Dunlop CI, Allen SL and Demme WC (1998) Monitoring adequacy of ventilation by capnometry during thoracotomy in dogs. *Journal of the American Veterinary Medical Association* **212**, 377–379

Wilson CW and Benumof J (2005) Anesthesia for thoracic surgery. In: *Miller's Anesthesia, 6th edn*, ed. RD Miller, pp. 1847–1940. Elsevier/Churchill Livingstone, Philadelphia

Wilson G and Hayes H (1986) Diaphragmatic hernia in the dog and cat: a 25-year overview. *Seminars in Veterinary Medicine and Surgery (Small Animal)* **1**, 318–326

Zhang H, Spapen H and Vincent JL (1994) Effects of dobutamine and norepinephrine on oxygen availability in tamponade-induced stagnant hypoxia: a prospective, randomized, controlled study. *Critical Care Medicine* **22**, 299–305

Chapter 24

Gastrointestinal, laparoscopic and liver procedures

Ian Self

The gastrointestinal (GI) system consists of all structures from the oral cavity to the rectum, including associated exocrine and endocrine glands. It supplies the body with water and nutrients and allows waste material to be excreted. Dysfunction of the system therefore results in inadequate nutrition and water balance, which can lead to a variety of metabolic changes that need to be considered and corrected before the patient is anaesthetized. Disorders of the GI system and liver are commonly encountered in veterinary practice and many patients require anaesthesia either for diagnostic procedures or management of these disorders; alternatively, patients may have incidental GI disease but require anaesthesia for unrelated conditions.

Anaesthesia for disorders of the oral cavity is covered in Chapter 20.

The oesophagus

Obstruction

Oesophageal obstruction may occur acutely as a result of ingestion of a foreign body (Figure 24.1ab), or chronically due to oesophagitis and stricture development. In addition, young patients with congenital vascular ring anomalies may have a sudden onset of regurgitation once they begin to ingest solid food. Patients with an oesophageal obstruction may require anaesthesia to enable imaging and endoscopy, removal of a foreign body, balloon dilation of an oesophageal stricture or, occasionally, thoracotomy to correct the cause of the obstruction.

Pre-anaesthetic considerations

Patients with oesophageal obstruction may be dehydrated and have electrolyte disturbances, which should be corrected before anaesthesia if possible. These patients are at risk of aspiration pneumonia and a thorough examination of the respiratory and cardiovascular systems is essential. Aspiration pneumonia reduces the functional capacity of the respiratory system and may lead to altered oxygen, carbon dioxide and inhalant anaesthetic exchange.

Anaesthetic management

Analgesia is an important consideration for these patients. Acute obstruction of the oesophagus is often painful. If the patient is likely to require a thoracotomy, a full mu opioid

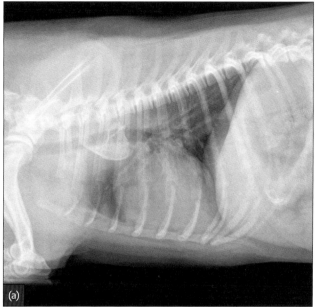

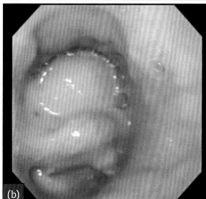

24.1 (a) Right lateral radiograph of a dog showing a radio-opaque oesophageal foreign body at the level of the heart base. (b) The same foreign body viewed on oesophagoscopy.
(Courtesy of Internal Medicine Service, Royal Veterinary College, London, UK)

receptor agonist should form part of the anaesthetic protocol; however, drugs that may cause vomiting or increase the incidence of regurgitation (such as morphine, hydromorphone or alpha-2 adrenoceptor agonists) should be avoided. Opioids such as pethidine (meperidine) (3–5 mg/kg i.m.) or methadone (0.1–0.3 mg/kg i.m. or i.v.) would be suitable choices. If a thoracotomy is deemed unlikely, then buprenorphine (20 μg/kg i.m. or i.v.) or butorphanol (0.2–0.4 mg/kg i.m. or i.v.) may be sufficient; butorphanol has antiemetic properties and is useful for straightforward cases. Balloon dilation of oesophageal strictures can be painful, and further analgesics such as fentanyl (2–5 μg/kg i.v.) may be required during the procedure. Acepromazine may be useful because of its antiemetic and sedative effects; however, the individual patient's hydration status must be considered when deciding whether to use this drug because it causes vasodilation, which can precipitate profound hypotension in hypovolaemic patients. Administration of low doses of acepromazine (0.005–0.01 mg/kg i.v.) following relief of the oesophageal obstruction can be useful to facilitate a smooth recovery from anaesthesia. It is essential to monitor the patient closely after giving pre-anaesthetic medication, because any fluid and/or food that has accumulated proximal to the obstruction is more likely to be aspirated in the sedated patient.

Before anaesthesia, the patient should be positioned in sternal recumbency and intravenous access should be secured. The head should be raised in order to minimize the risk of aspiration (Figure 24.2) until the airway is secured with a cuffed endotracheal tube (ETT). Either a surgical suction machine or a large syringe attached to a urinary catheter can be used to suction the oropharynx and remove secretions. In humans, the oesophagus may be temporarily occluded by compressing it between the larynx and the spinal column (Sellick's manoeuvre) when regurgitation/vomiting and aspiration are potential complications. There are only anecdotal reports of its use in animals.

Anaesthesia can be induced with propofol, alfaxalone or a ketamine/benzodiazepine combination, to allow rapid, atraumatic endotracheal intubation with a suitably sized and cuffed ETT. In these cases, the use of high-pressure, low-volume cuffs (silicone or red rubber) may provide a more secure barrier against leakage of oesophageal contents around the cuff. The cuff should be inflated until no leak is detected (see Chapter 5). In dogs, the oesophagus is composed of striated muscle throughout its length, but in cats only the proximal third is striated muscle. For this reason, neuromuscular blocking agents, such as vecuronium or atracurium, frequently improve the ability to remove a foreign object from the oesophagus in dogs; if these agents are administered, it is essential to have available a method of ventilating the lungs and of monitoring the block (see Chapter 16).

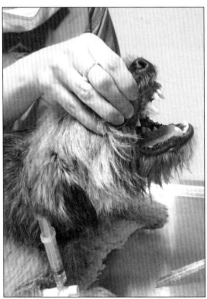

24.2 Correct positioning of a patient at risk of regurgitation before endotracheal intubation.

During the procedure, the oesophagus may develop full-thickness tears, leading to leakage of air and secretions into the thoracic cavity. Pneumothorax causes reduced oxygen saturation, exaggerated respiratory effort, increased resistance during intermittent positive pressure ventilation (IPPV) and decreased lung sounds on auscultation. If pneumothorax is suspected, anaesthesia and ventilation should be maintained, thoracocentesis used to confirm and remove pleural air, and oesophagoscopy performed to check for the presence of a tear that may require surgical repair. Patients with an oesophageal foreign body within the thoracic cavity that is considered to be too difficult to remove endoscopically, or is chronic in nature, should be referred to a veterinary specialist with expertise in thoracotomies, because of the increased risk of oesophageal tears in these cases. During the procedure, aspiration of oesophageal contents is still possible despite the presence of a cuffed ETT. To minimize the risk of aspiration, the oropharynx should be continually suctioned throughout the procedure. On recovery from anaesthesia, it is good practice to remove the ETT with the cuff still partially inflated to 'sweep' debris from the proximal trachea into the oral cavity, where it can be suctioned. Monitoring should continue into the recovery period, again paying close attention to the respiratory system.

The requirement for postoperative analgesia will depend on the severity of the obstruction and the procedure. Full mu opioid receptor agonists are recommended as they provide excellent analgesia. Due to the risk of GI ulceration and possibly altered fluid balance caused by the obstruction (and subsequent effects on renal blood flow), perioperative use of non-steroidal anti-inflammatory drugs (NSAIDs) is not usually recommended. Oesophageal protectants such as sucralfate may contribute to pain control, by minimizing further damage, along with proton pump inhibitors (omeprazole 0.5–1.5 mg/kg i.v. q24h) and a limited period of nil by mouth.

Megaoesophagus

Patients with megaoesophagus rarely require anaesthesia for the condition itself, but may require anaesthesia for unrelated conditions or for imaging of the oesophagus. Many patients with megaoesophagus have concurrent myasthenia gravis, hypoadrenocorticism or dysautonomia; there may also be an association with hypothyroidism, although this remains contentious. Megaoesophagus should be suspected in young animals with congenital vascular ring anomalies. Generalized myasthenia gravis leads to muscle weakness that can affect respiratory function, and is discussed in Chapter 28. Similarly, hypoadrenocorticism leads to generalized muscle weakness as well as electrolyte imbalance, which should be corrected before anaesthesia where possible (see Chapter 27). Anaesthetic management of patients with megaoesophagus is similar to that for animals with oesophageal obstruction, as the main risk is aspiration of oesophageal contents.

Oesophagitis

Oesophagitis is relatively rare in cats and dogs. Clinical signs include dysphagia, excessive salivation and reduced appetite. It can occur after ingestion of corrosive substances, after removal of an oesophageal foreign body (Figure 24.3), in association with chronic vomiting, and with gastro-oesophageal reflux (GOR), which is a particular concern during anaesthesia.

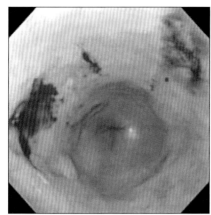

24.3 Marked oesophagitis and oesophageal trauma after endoscopically-guided removal of a foreign body.
(Courtesy of Internal Medicine Service, Royal Veterinary College, London, UK)

The incidence of regurgitation during anaesthesia is reported to be approximately 1% (Lamata *et al.*, 2012), but the incidence of subclinical oesophageal reflux may be as high as 55% (Wilson *et al.*, 2005). As a result, it is possible that many patients may have subclinical oesophagitis following anaesthesia. Treatment with opioids and anticholinergics, abdominal surgery and positioning in dorsal recumbency have all been associated with an increased risk of GOR (Galatos and Raptopoulos, 1995a, 1995b; Raptopoulos and Galatos, 1995). If GOR occurs during anaesthesia, it may be detected by identifying a decrease in distal oesophageal pH or by the appearance of reflux in the oral cavity or at the nostrils. If this occurs, the first step is to ensure that the ETT is correctly positioned and the cuff is properly inflated, followed by suctioning. The oesophagus can be lavaged with warm saline to increase the pH of the reflux fluid, followed by gentle suctioning, but this should be done only if a secure airway is guaranteed (Figure 24.4). Ignoring the presence of GOR may increase the likelihood of post-anaesthetic complications such as oesophageal stricture formation. Both metoclopramide and omeprazole can reduce the incidence of GOR when used perioperatively, although neither has been reported to eliminate its occurrence completely (Wilson *et al.*, 2006; Panti *et al.*, 2009). In cases where GOR is considered likely, these drugs may be included in the preanaesthetic medication.

Medical management of oesophagitis should include adequate control of pain and the use of antacids such as ranitidine and omeprazole (Han, 2003), and sucralfate.

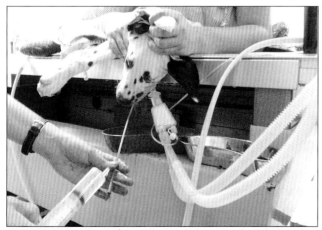

24.4 Management of regurgitation during anaesthesia by lavaging the oesophagus with warm saline followed by gentle suctioning using a syringe and urinary catheter. Note the head-down position of the patient.
(Courtesy of Marieke de Vries, Davies Veterinary Specialists, Higham Gobion, UK)

The stomach and intestines

A wide range of gastric and intestinal conditions is encountered in small animal practice, and patients with these conditions may require anaesthesia for treatment or diagnosis. These conditions include obstruction by intra- and extraluminal structures, GI haemorrhage, acute anatomical alterations such as gastric dilatation–volvulus (GDV) or intussusceptions, and chronic inflammatory and malabsorptive syndromes. Depending on the severity and chronicity of the underlying condition, patients can have a wide range of systemic disturbances and will often require stabilization before anaesthesia. Dehydration is a common finding and may occur as a result of excessive losses (diarrhoea and vomiting) or reduced food and water intake. Treatment should aim to correct both hypovolaemia and dehydration; the volume of fluids administered should be based on the underlying severity and the response to treatment (see Chapter 18).

In most cases, pre-anaesthetic haematology and biochemistry will provide information on the degree of metabolic disturbance. For example, chronic GI disease often results in hypokalaemia, which may lead to muscle weakness. Patients may have reduced plasma protein concentrations; for highly protein-bound drugs such as propofol, this may lead to an increase in the amount of unbound (and therefore active) drug, increasing the clinical effect. All patients with low plasma protein concentrations should have intravenous anaesthetic drugs carefully titrated to effect. Acid–base disturbances are also common, and if facilities allow, jugular venous or arterial blood gas analysis should be performed. Acute prepyloric vomiting will initially result in a hypochloraemic metabolic alkalosis, which can be corrected with an infusion of 0.9% sodium chloride. However, most cases of GI disease and chronic prepyloric vomiting will typically have a metabolic acidosis, which should be treated with an alkalizing fluid (e.g. Hartmann's solution) and whole body fluid deficits should be corrected.

Gastric dilatation–volvulus

This condition is most common in medium- to large-breed dogs and has an acute or hyperacute onset. In GDV, the presence of a large gas-filled viscus (the stomach) in the cranial abdomen compromises blood supply to the stomach wall and spleen, resulting in tissue necrosis of these organs. The dilated stomach also compresses the caudal vena cava, reducing venous return to the heart, with a consequent decrease in cardiac output (obstructive shock). Other features include 'splinting' of the diaphragm and impaired ventilation, sequestration of fluid and/or blood in the stomach ('third space' losses), release of endotoxins from the compromised stomach wall and spleen, acid–base and electrolyte disturbances and associated cardiac arrhythmias (ventricular premature contractions and ventricular tachycardia) (Tivers and Brockman, 2009ab).

Pre-anaesthetic considerations

The degree of pre-anaesthetic preparation will depend on the clinical state of the patient. An attempt should be made to decompress the stomach by passing a large-bore stomach tube, inserted via a tube gag (Figure 24.5). This procedure is unlikely to be successful in cases of volvulus, where passage of the tube through the lower oesophageal sphincter is not possible. In such cases, consideration should be given to placing a percutaneous trochar to relieve the pressure temporarily while the patient

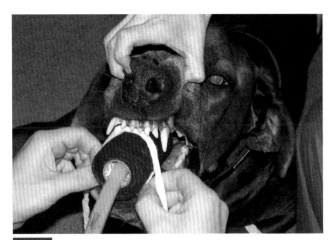

24.5 Attempted passage of a stomach tube using a tube gag.

is stabilized; however, this procedure carries the risk of causing stomach wall tears and subsequent peritonitis.

It is useful to obtain baseline measurements of packed cell volume and total protein (both are often elevated), electrolytes (potassium derangements are common) and lactate, in order to direct subsequent therapy. Trends in these variables should be monitored. Plasma lactate concentration at the time of hospital admission is a good predictor of gastric necrosis and outcome (Beer *et al.*, 2013). Patient stabilization involves the correction of hypovolaemia and acid–base and electrolyte disturbances. Hypovolaemia, the major problem, will require intravenous fluid therapy; this is covered in more detail in Chapter 18. Catheters should be placed in both cephalic veins to allow rapid correction of hypovolaemia. Crystalloids and/or colloids can be used, but colloids may restore circulating fluid volume more effectively. As an alternative, to aid rapid volume expansion, hypertonic (7.2%) saline can be given as a 2–4 ml/kg bolus provided the patient does not have pre-existing hypernatraemia (see Chapter 18).

Anaesthetic management

If the patient is in a very debilitated or collapsed state, it may require little or no pre-anaesthetic medication, although analgesia will be required for surgery. Drugs that induce vomiting or have marked negative effects on the cardiovascular system should be avoided. Pethidine (3–5 mg/kg i.m.) often provides good sedation and visceral analgesia without depressing cardiac output, but has only a short duration of action. Alternatively, methadone (0.1–0.3 mg/kg slow i.v.) or hydromorphone (0.05–0.1 mg/kg slow i.v.) can be used.

Before induction of anaesthesia, the patient should be preoxygenated for 3–5 minutes via a facemask unless this causes the animal distress. Patients with GDV commonly have cardiac arrhythmias and the electrocardiogram (ECG) should be monitored continuously. Ventricular arrhythmias are more common in these patients and boluses of lidocaine (1–2 mg/kg i.v.) should be prepared in advance so that they are immediately available if required. Suction should also be available to remove excess secretions in the oropharynx, which could complicate endotracheal intubation.

For induction of anaesthesia, a combination of agents suitable for an animal with unstable haemodynamics should be used. The author's preference is to use familiar agents such as propofol or alfaxalone alongside a benzodiazepine; for example, 1 mg/kg propofol i.v. followed by 0.1–0.3 mg/kg midazolam or diazepam i.v. The intravenous

catheter is then flushed with saline and a final dose of propofol (usually 1–2 mg/kg) given to effect until intubation with a cuffed ETT is possible. Alternatively, a similar approach can be used in which fentanyl or sufentanil (2–5 µg/kg i.v.) is either added to or substituted for the benzodiazepine (for further details see Chapter 14). Induction of anaesthesia with a volatile agent (isoflurane or sevoflurane) is not suitable for patients with GDV because the longer induction time with these agents increases the risks of impaired ventilation and regurgitation.

Anaesthesia is usually maintained with isoflurane or sevoflurane in oxygen. Nitrous oxide may increase gastric distension, further impeding venous return, and should be avoided at least until the stomach has been decompressed. An alternative technique, which utilizes intravenous infusions of sufentanil and midazolam, has been described (Hellebrekers and Sap, 1991). Patients should be handled carefully because there is a risk of rupture of the distended stomach. Monitoring should include heart and pulse rates, respiratory rate, pulse oximetry, ECG, capnography, and arterial blood pressure (ideally measured directly). Spirometry and arterial blood gas analysis also provide valuable information, if available. Ventilation should be controlled to prevent hypoventilation, but high peak respiratory airway pressures should be avoided as they may adversely affect cardiovascular function. Ventricular arrhythmias are common and should be managed with lidocaine (1–2 mg/kg i.v. bolus followed by infusion at 25–100 µg/kg/min). There is some evidence that early treatment with an intravenous lidocaine bolus, followed by an infusion of lidocaine at 50 µg/kg/min for 24 hours after admission, significantly decreases the occurrence of cardiac arrhythmias and acute kidney injury, and shortens hospitalization time in dogs with GDV (Bruchim *et al.*, 2012). Fluid therapy should be continued throughout surgery and appropriate analgesics provided, for example, methadone (0.1–0.3 mg/kg i.v. q3–4h), hydromorphone (0.05–0.1 mg/kg i.v. q2–3h), fentanyl boluses (2–5 µg/kg i.v. every 20 minutes) or fentanyl infusions (5–40 µg/kg/h i.v.).

Following surgery and recovery, the patient should be monitored for signs of continuing cardiovascular compromise. Ventricular arrhythmias can still develop during the first two days after surgery (Muir, 1982). Close attention should be paid to analgesia, fluid balance and nursing care in this period.

Upper gastrointestinal tract endoscopy

Endoscopic examination of the upper GI tract is commonly performed, as this minimally invasive procedure allows visualization and biopsy sampling of the GI mucosa.

Pre-anaesthetic considerations

Patients may have a variety of pre-existing conditions and clinical signs, including anorexia, vomiting, diarrhoea, weight loss, anaemia, and altered plasma protein and electrolyte concentrations. As endoscopy is usually an elective diagnostic procedure, any pre-existing abnormalities should be corrected as much as possible before anaesthesia.

Anaesthetic management

Endoscopy and biopsy sampling are not considered to be painful procedures; in humans, pinch biopsies of the upper GI tract do not elicit pain. However, in humans, the inflation of a hollow viscus with air causes a dull, cramping pain typical of non-specific, poorly localized GI discomfort (see later section on visceral pain); this is especially the case if there is pre-existing pathology. Although patients rarely require analgesic support following endoscopy, intra-operative analgesia provides a more stable plane of anaesthesia; pre-anaesthetic medication for these patients therefore usually includes an opioid receptor agonist. Acepromazine may also be used unless the patient is hypovolaemic or dehydrated. Pyloric sphincter tone may be increased by full mu opioid receptor agonists, which may create problems during endoscopy or foreign body removal. Some clinicians prefer to use butorphanol, or no opioid at all. One study in cats evaluated the ease of passage of the endoscope into the duodenum after administration of hydromorphone or butorphanol, and found no differences between these opioids (Smith et al., 2004). However, clinical experience suggests that there may be some hindrance to passage of the endoscope if mu opioid receptor agonists are used, which may cause problems in some situations. If such problems are observed, butorphanol can be used to antagonize these mu opioid effects during anaesthesia. Morphine and other opioids known to cause nausea and vomiting should be avoided in patients with pre-existing vomiting, and NSAIDs are contra-indicated because of their ulcerogenic potential.

For induction of anaesthesia, any familiar intravenous induction agent can be used. The patient's head should be kept raised until a cuffed ETT has been placed to avoid aspiration (see Figure 24.2). Anaesthesia should be maintained by using a volatile anaesthetic agent vaporized in oxygen. Nitrous oxide should be avoided as it can increase distension of a gas-filled viscus.

During the procedure, careful attention should be paid to the degree of GI distension caused by air inflation. Excessive distension can impede ventilation by applying pressure to the diaphragm, which may in turn reduce the depth of anaesthesia if alveolar delivery of volatile anaesthetic agent is inadequate. The degree of distension can be assessed by gently palpating the abdomen and the level of inflation reduced as necessary. If the patient reacts to the stimulation of endoscopy, IPPV should be started and a short-acting opioid such as fentanyl (2–5 μg/kg) given as an intravenous bolus; a higher dose of fentanyl may be required if butorphanol was used as part of pre-anaesthetic medication. If fentanyl is used, ventilation may need to be supported for a short period of time as it is a respiratory depressant. Fluids should be administered throughout.

Overdistension of the GI tract may also reduce venous return by compressing the caudal vena cava, and thus decrease cardiac output. A more serious (but uncommon) complication is sudden vagal stimulation, as the vagus nerve supplies the majority of the GI tract. If the GI tract becomes overdistended, stretch receptors within its walls may be activated and cause sudden, profound vagally-mediated bradycardia. In this event, the GI tract should immediately be deflated, and atropine 20–40 μg/kg administered intravenously. The degree of distension must be continually checked as described earlier, and ECG/peripheral pulses closely monitored for sudden changes in heart rate.

Lower gastrointestinal tract endoscopy

Similar anaesthetic considerations apply as for gastro-duodenoscopy. While inflation of the lower GI tract seems to cause less respiratory impairment than inflation of the upper GI tract, colonic distension is more painful and also more likely to induce episodes of vagally-mediated bradycardia. Close monitoring is necessary and atropine should always be available.

Percutaneous placement of feeding tubes

A variety of methods may be used to provide enteral nutrition if a patient is not voluntarily taking food, including gastrostomy and oesophagostomy feeding tubes. The placement of these tubes is a well tolerated procedure and anaesthesia follows the same guidelines as for gastro-duodenoscopy discussed earlier.

Gastric ulceration

Data sheets for veterinary-licensed NSAIDs commonly list 'GI ulceration' and 'GI disease' as contraindications and adverse effects. Certainly, NSAIDs can elicit vomiting and/or diarrhoea, with or without haematemesis/melaena, in susceptible patients (Monteiro-Steagall et al., 2013). These drugs act by inhibiting cyclo-oxygenase (COX) enzymes, which are partly responsible for maintenance of normal GI secretions, regulation of gastric pH and regulation of blood flow to the GI mucosa. The newer NSAIDs preferentially inhibit COX-2; COX-2 is thought to be the predominant isoform of the enzyme expressed in inflammatory states, although recent studies have clearly shown a role for COX-2 in mucosal healing and therefore even the newer, COX-2-selective NSAIDs can have adverse effects. The co-administration of corticosteroids and NSAIDs is contraindicated and has been reported to increase the risk of ulceration in the GI tract. In addition, there is a strong association between mast cell tumours and gastroduodenal ulceration because of the effects of histamine on GI blood flow and secretion of hydrochloric acid by gastric parietal cells. The use of NSAIDs in patients with mast cell tumours is therefore not recommended.

Further information on NSAIDs and recommendations for GI ulcer prevention and treatment can be found in Chapter 10.

Anaesthesia for laparoscopy

Laparoscopy carries a lower risk of postoperative abdominal wound dehiscence compared with more invasive procedures. A total of three ports, or 'keyholes', are created in the abdominal wall: one for carbon dioxide insufflation, one for a laparoscopic camera and the third for the surgical instruments. Carbon dioxide is used in laparoscopy because it is very soluble in blood and does not support combustion. During the procedure, carbon dioxide is insufflated into the abdominal cavity to an intra-abdominal pressure of 10–15 mmHg, to allow visualization of the abdominal viscera with the camera. The patient may be positioned 'head down' (Trendelenburg position) for neutering procedures, or in a 'head up' position for procedures such as liver biopsy (Perrin and Fletcher, 2004).

The underlying condition will dictate the course of anaesthesia and analgesia and its management, but there are some specific complications associated with laparoscopic procedures. Insufflation with carbon dioxide may lead to increased end-tidal carbon dioxide values, as the gas freely diffuses into the splanchnic circulation; an increase in minute volume will be required if end-tidal carbon dioxide becomes unacceptably high (Duke et al., 1996). If lung ventilation is inadequate, the patient may show signs of hypercapnia (see Chapter 31). Most haemodynamic changes occur in the first 15 minutes following insufflation and result mainly from carbon dioxide accumulation and/or abdominal distension. It is important to keep abdominal pressure as low as possible (≤15 mmHg) to avoid causing compression of the caudal vena cava and consequent reduced venous return. Healthy cats may be able to ventilate adequately if intra-abdominal pressure is kept to 12 mmHg (Beazley *et al.*, 2011). Pressure on abdominal viscera is probably minimal at the low intra-abdominal pressures used.

In humans, pain after laparoscopy is usually short-lived but can be intense, with 80% of patients requiring opioid analgesia at some stage postoperatively (Hayden and Cowman, 2011); it is likely that cats and dogs undergoing the procedure will have similar analgesic requirements. Referred pain in the shoulder is also common in humans, although this usually dissipates once all the carbon dioxide has been reabsorbed from the peritoneal cavity.

Risk of air embolism

A rare yet serious complication of laparoscopy is major gas embolism due to incorrect positioning of the insufflator or absorption of carbon dioxide via a ruptured blood vessel (Staffieri *et al.*, 2007). Microemboli pass through the right side of the heart and can be eliminated through the lungs; they may cause a decrease in end-tidal carbon dioxide or occasionally an increase as they diffuse across the alveolar membranes. However, large gas emboli have the potential to become lodged in the right atrium or ventricle, where they act as a 'gas lock', effectively stopping the passage of blood through the heart. Unless recognized early, these emboli are rapidly fatal. Various treatments for major gas emboli in humans include using a central venous catheter to remove the gas, and repositioning the patient in left lateral recumbency, which may help to 'unlock' the emboli from the right side of the heart and improve cardiac output. However, neither of these measures has been shown to be useful in cats or dogs.

The large intestines, rectum and perineum

Common conditions of the lower GI tract and perineum that require anaesthesia for management include constipation, anal sac disease and perineal herniation. It is advisable to carry out pre-anaesthetic haematological and biochemical examinations, as a significant proportion of patients undergoing these procedures are geriatric and may have diminished organ function (see Chapter 30). In animals where medical treatment of constipation has been unsuccessful, anaesthesia may be required for manual removal of faecoliths. The effect of the underlying condition must be considered before these patients undergo anaesthesia; patients will often be dehydrated and malnourished, and appropriate fluid therapy should be given during the peri-anaesthetic period to correct any imbalances revealed by biochemical examination. Subtotal colectomy is occasionally required for patients with idiopathic megacolon, a perforating foreign body or tumour. Some cases may require a pelvic split, which can result in significant blood loss; in these cases blood typing or cross-matching should be performed before anaesthesia is induced, and adequate supplies of compatible blood should be available. Anal gland carcinomas are commonly associated with hypercalcaemia (which may cause clinical signs of polyuria/polydipsia, muscle weakness and cardiac arrhythmias); this imbalance should be corrected before anaesthesia. In cases of perineal hernia, the contents of the hernia can include the bladder, which may cause post-renal azotaemia and electrolyte imbalances. In all cases, perioperative fluid therapy with a balanced electrolyte solution is essential (see Chapter 18).

The general approach to all these conditions is similar, with analgesia being a primary concern, especially for cases requiring major surgery. Epidural administration of preservative-free morphine (0.1 mg/kg; 10 mg/ml) with or without a local anaesthetic (e.g. lidocaine 1–2 mg/kg; 2% solution) is recommended, particularly for major surgery. Patients with long-standing discomfort commonly respond to surgical manipulation during anaesthesia and epidural analgesia will help to provide a more stable plane of anaesthesia in these cases. The effect of epidural morphine, although variable in onset (20–60 minutes), may last for up to 24 hours. A multimodal approach to analgesia, involving systemic administration of opioids and other adjunct drugs, is likely to be more effective. In dogs, infusions of lidocaine (1–2 mg/kg i.v. bolus followed by 50 µg/kg/min i.v.) are particularly useful because lidocaine also possesses anti-inflammatory and prokinetic properties and may help to reduce the unwanted constipating effects of opioids (Cassutto and Gfeller, 2003). If the surgery does not directly involve the GI tract (e.g. anal sac removal, perineal hernia repair) the use of NSAIDs is acceptable if these drugs are not otherwise contraindicated.

For anal sac removal/flushing and perineal herniorrhaphy, the patient should be placed in sternal recumbency, in a head-down (Trendelenburg) position, with the abdomen raised and the legs extended ventrally. In this position, the diaphragm is pushed cranially, which reduces functional residual capacity (FRC); ventilation should therefore be monitored continuously, ideally with capnography and spirometry, and IPPV provided if necessary. This position will also place stress on the joints and muscles and it is therefore important to use good padding and ensure that tie-downs are not excessively tight (Figure 24.6).

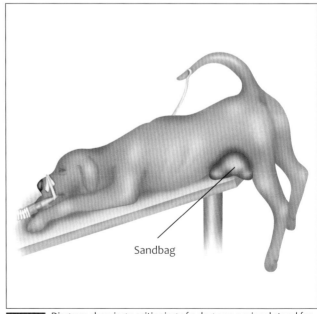

24.6 Diagram showing positioning of a dog on a perineal stand for perineal surgery. Note the sandbag under the pubis. This raises the abdomen a little, decreases intra-abdominal pressure and permits the diaphragm to move more easily. If used, care must be taken to avoid too much tension on the leg ties to prevent nerve and muscle damage.

The liver

General considerations for anaesthesia of patients with liver disease

The liver has many metabolic functions, which may have implications for the conduct of anaesthesia (Figure 24.7). To fuel these functions, the liver receives about 25% of the cardiac output, with blood flow being derived from both the hepatic artery (30%) and the portal vein (70%). Portal venous blood provides 50–60% of the oxygen supply to the liver. Unlike many other regional circulations (e.g. renal, cerebral, coronary), autoregulation of hepatic arterial and portal vein blood flow is poorly developed (Eipel et al., 2010). Arterial flow changes reciprocally with portal venous blood flow: this is known as the hepatic arterial buffer response and it may be impaired in disease states. Activation of the sympathetic nervous system causes constriction of the hepatic arteries and veins; in this way, approximately half the blood volume in the liver can be redistributed into the systemic circulation. Factors affecting hepatic blood flow are shown in Figure 24.8; a useful review of liver haemodynamics is provided by Furneaux (2011).

Some patients with mild hepatic dysfunction may require anaesthesia for unrelated conditions (e.g. dental treatment), but only patients anaesthetized for liver-specific procedures will be considered here.

Pre-anaesthetic evaluation should include an assessment of liver function. Clinical signs (e.g. hepatic encephalopathy (HE), vomiting, diarrhoea, anorexia, jaundice) are

Increased flow
- Hypercapnia
- Food intake
- Hepatitis
- Beta adrenoceptor agonists
- Enzyme-inducing drugs

Decreased flow
- Hypotension
- Hypocapnia
- Hypoxaemia
- IPPV
- Surgery (e.g. laparoscopy)
- Cirrhosis
- Alpha adrenoceptor agonists
- Histamine (H₂) receptor antagonists
- Vasopressin

24.8 Factors affecting hepatic blood flow. IPPV = intermittent positive pressure ventilation.

likely to be more pronounced in animals with severely impaired liver function. Animals with a congenital porto-systemic shunt (PSS) are likely to be thin and poorly developed for their age. Serum biochemistry may show hypoalbuminaemia, decreased urea, hypoglycaemia, decreased cholesterol, hyperammonaemia, increased bile acids and hypokalaemia; liver enzyme activity may be normal or increased. Haematology may reveal anaemia. There may also be coagulation abnormalities; one study in dogs with PSS found that they had lower platelet counts, lower activity of factors II, V, VII, and X, and increased factor VIII and activated partial thromboplastin

Liver function	Consequences of severe dysfunction
Metabolic	
• Carbohydrate: gluconeogenesis and glycogenolysis • Lipid metabolism • Protein metabolism • Synthesis of albumin • Synthesis of coagulation factors, anticoagulants (antithrombin III, Proteins C, S), fibrinolytic factors, clearance of activated factors • Synthesis of angiotensinogen All these processes involve exothermic reactions, thus generating heat	• Hypoglycaemia • Hypoproteinaemia: peripheral and lung oedema, altered drug–protein binding • Coagulopathies • Anaemia (e.g. from haemorrhage, folic acid/vitamin B12 deficiency) • Acid–base disturbances (Ahya et al., 2006) Hypothermia may be more common during anaesthesia when thermoregulation is impaired
Biotransformation of drugs	
• Phase I: transformation to more polar compounds, e.g. oxidation, reduction, demethylation • Phase II: conjugation with e.g. glucuronic acid, sulphate, glutathione	• Reduced drug metabolism – prolonged effects
Storage	
• Glycogen • Fat-soluble vitamins • Iron • Copper • Blood (approximately 15% of blood volume is normally accommodated in the liver)	• Hypoglycaemia • Malnutrition
Excretory	
• Synthesis of urea • Breaks down erythrocytes and metabolizes waste products (75% of bilirubin from haem; remainder from non-erythrocyte haem (enzymes))	• Jaundice, difficulty in assessing mucous membrane colour • Affects some biochemistry measurements • Bile acids are irritant to endothelium and may cause refractory hypotension • Reduced ability to deal with increased haem breakdown from a blood transfusion
Immunological functions	
• Synthesis of immunoglobulins • Kupffer cells remove bacteria, endotoxins, immune complexes	• Increased risk of perioperative infection and endotoxaemia

24.7 Functions of the liver and their relevance to anaesthesia.

time compared with healthy dogs. Surgical attenuation of the shunt resulted in more pronounced abnormalities in coagulation times and factors in the immediate postoperative period (Kummeling et al., 2006).

Adequate preparation before anaesthesia is vital. Animals with HE should be treated with antibiotics, lactulose and an appropriate diet. Pre-existing fluid imbalances should be corrected using intravenous fluids, guided by results of haematology and biochemistry, with particular attention paid to the presence of hypoproteinaemia, hypoglycaemia, hypokalaemia and anaemia. Fresh frozen plasma can be administered to replace deficient clotting factors, although some veterinary surgeons (veterinarians) prefer to administer vitamin K for 1–2 days, depending on the clotting abnormality.

Direct hepatotoxicity caused by exposure to modern anaesthetic agents is rare (Elliott and Strunin, 1993). In humans, halothane has been shown to cause hepatitis, usually after multiple exposures, and is fatal in 20–50% of cases. The toxicity was attributed to a metabolite of halothane, trifluoroacetic acid (TFA), which can bind covalently to liver microsomal proteins. The TFA–protein complex incited an immune response in rare cases, and repeated exposure could lead to hepatic necrosis. Reports of toxicity after exposure to isoflurane and desflurane have also been reported in humans, but they are infrequent, and there have been no similar reports in cats or dogs.

Administration of drugs that require extensive hepatic metabolism should be avoided in these patients if possible, or should be short acting or reversible. For pre-anaesthetic medication, acepromazine should be avoided as its duration of action may be prolonged and it can potentiate hypotension. Alpha-2 adrenoceptor agonists reduce hepatic blood flow but are reversible, and may be useful to provide sedation in patients that are difficult to handle. The use of benzodiazepines is controversial in patients with liver disease, as they may have unpredictable effects (see later in the section on PSS). Pre-anaesthetic medication with an opioid alone will frequently be sufficient. However, the disposition of opioids may be dramatically altered in these patients: in dogs for example, the absorption of pethidine is slower and the elimination half-life longer, which means that the interval between repeat doses of this drug may need to be extended (Waterman and Kalthum, 1990).

Anaesthesia is commonly induced with propofol or alfaxalone given intravenously and titrated to effect, and maintained with isoflurane or sevoflurane vaporized in oxygen. Propofol probably has some extrahepatic metabolism (its plasma clearance is greater than hepatic blood flow) and may be preferable as an induction agent. Isoflurane undergoes less hepatic biotransformation than sevoflurane, and liver blood flow is maintained well with isoflurane, but either volatile agent is suitable. A balanced anaesthesia protocol including a neuromuscular blocking agent is useful; atracurium is a good choice as it undergoes Hofmann elimination (which is independent of hepatic metabolism) but the block should always be monitored by using a peripheral nerve stimulator. In dogs with PSS, cis-atracurium may offer some advantages (Adams et al., 2006). Remifentanil is an ideal choice for intraoperative analgesia as its elimination is independent of liver metabolism (it is metabolized by plasma and erythrocyte esterases), but other short-acting opioids such as alfentanil or fentanyl are acceptable. Epidural analgesia with morphine is useful and will provide up to 24 hours of analgesia, but is contraindicated if the patient has a coagulopathy (where there is a risk of epidural haematoma).

Monitoring requirements during anaesthesia will depend upon the patient's condition and the procedure being performed. Refractory hypotension is common in patients with PSS and disease of the biliary tract; it may be mediated by excessive production of nitric oxide, especially after shunt ligation (Howe et al., 2000), although hypoalbuminaemia and hypothermia probably also play a role. Increased concentrations of bile acids in the blood are irritant to the endothelium and may also contribute to hypotension. Hypotension must be treated appropriately (crystalloids, colloids, positive inotropes, vasopressors). In young patients with congenital PSS, it is important to monitor body temperature, blood glucose and electrolytes.

Liver biopsy

Liver biopsy is a diagnostic procedure performed in patients with clinical and/or biochemical evidence of liver disease. It may be performed via transcutaneous fine needle aspiration or percutaneous Tru-cut needle biopsy, via laparoscopy or during an exploratory laparotomy. The anaesthetic protocol will depend on the approach taken for biopsy. The percutaneous approach is a quick procedure, for which relatively short-acting drugs can be used. Pre-anaesthetic medication is often provided with an opioid alone; in patients with stable haemodynamics, small doses of alpha-2 adrenoceptor agonists such as medetomidine (2–5 µg/kg i.v.) or dexmedetomidine (1–2.5 µg/kg i.v.) may also be included, as they can be antagonized with atipamezole. Following anaesthesia, the patient should be examined regularly for signs of haemorrhage (assessing mucous membrane colour, pulse rate and quality, and arterial blood pressure) and appropriate action taken if signs of haemorrhage are apparent.

Portosystemic shunts

In patients with PSSs, blood passes directly from the portal circulation into the systemic circulation without perfusing the liver. Blood leaving the GI tract contains nutrients, ammonia and false neurotransmitters, which are normally processed in the liver (as described earlier; see also Figure 24.7). In cases of PSS, this metabolic processing does not occur. Unless there is concurrent portal vein hypoplasia, the liver itself is healthy, but too small to perform all normal hepatic tasks. A PSS may be extrahepatic (congenital or acquired) or intrahepatic. The most common reason for surgery is a single extrahepatic shunt, which is more commonly seen in small-breed dogs. Intrahepatic shunts are more common in large-breed dogs and in these cases haemorrhage is a major concern.

Pre-anaesthetic considerations

Patients with PSS have a variety of clinical signs, including neurological dysfunction (HE), GI disease (vomiting/diarrhoea, pica and occasionally foreign body ingestion) and urolithiasis. They also tend to be small in stature and have poor body condition. These patients should be stabilized with medical management before undergoing surgery.

HE has traditionally been attributed to high plasma ammonia concentration resulting from bacterial breakdown of amino acids in the GI tract; this ammonia is normally removed from the portal blood by the liver. Ammonia contributes to HE by down-regulating N-methyl D-aspartate receptors within the central nervous system. It is now known that a number of other substances such as tryptophan, serotonin and glutamate also play an important role in HE (Holt *et al.*, 2002). In addition, increased concentrations of endogenous benzodiazepines (Baraldi *et al.*, 2009) and neurosteroids have been found in the portal circulation of dogs with PSS and, although their role is controversial, some anaesthetists avoid the use of benzodiazepines in patients with PSS. Treatment of HE before surgery consists of a low-protein diet, antibiotics to reduce the GI bacterial load and lactulose to trap ammonium ions in the gut lumen. If the patient has a history of seizures, appropriate anticonvulsant therapy should be administered and continued into the perioperative period (Fryer *et al.*, 2011). Levetiracetam therapy has been shown to reduce postoperative mortality after PSS ligation.

Fluid therapy should be planned to correct the patient's fluid deficits and acid–base/electrolyte abnormalities. Hypoalbuminaemia with few clinical signs is a consistent finding in these patients, and infusion of large volumes of crystalloids is best avoided. Synthetic colloids or plasma infusions can be provided to support plasma colloid osmotic pressure. Typed and cross-matched blood should be available for transfusion, as haemorrhage is possible during intrahepatic shunt surgery (see Chapter 18).

Anaesthetic management

Animals requiring surgery for PSS are often young and may be at great risk of developing hypoglycaemia; for this reason, food should be withheld for the shortest time possible before anaesthesia (4–6 hours). Blood glucose should be monitored regularly throughout the perioperative period and glucose added to intravenous fluids if necessary (addition of 25 ml of 50% glucose to 500 ml Hartmann's solution will produce a 2.5% solution of glucose). Once the patient has been stabilized, pre-anaesthetic medication with an opioid such as pethidine (3–5 mg/kg i.m.), methadone (0.1–0.2 mg/kg i.m. or i.v.) or hydromorphone (0.05–0.1 mg/kg i.m. or i.v.) is normally sufficient. Opioids should be continued during surgery. Acepromazine has a prolonged duration of effect in these patients and so should be either avoided or used at very low doses. Low doses of alpha-2 adrenoceptor agonists can also be used, as they will contribute to visceral analgesia; if profound cardiovascular effects occur, their action can be antagonized with atipamezole if necessary. However, alpha-2 adrenoceptor agonists may cause hyperglycaemia; when their effects are antagonized, hypoglycaemia may rapidly develop. For reasons mentioned above, benzodiazepines are often avoided.

These patients can become hypothermic very quickly as a result of their small body size and reduced metabolic heat generation by the small liver. Active warming should be started before induction of anaesthesia and body temperature should be continuously monitored throughout the procedure and recovery period. Arterial blood pressure is best measured invasively; if arterial cannulation is impossible, then Doppler or oscillometric methods should be used. Hypotension is common in PSS patients and may be mediated by excessive production of nitric oxide, especially after shunt ligation (Howe *et al.*, 2000); it should be treated using appropriate fluid therapy, anticholinergics (atropine 20 μg/kg or glycopyrronium 10 μg/kg i.v.) or vasopressors, depending on the cardiovascular status of the patient (see Chapter 17). Previously, Hartmann's solution was not recommended because of concerns that lactate would accumulate as a result of lack of hepatic metabolism. Such concerns are unwarranted and Hartmann's solution can be used for crystalloid therapy in these patients.

Analgesia can be provided into the recovery period with opioids administered at appropriate dosing intervals. Epidural preservative-free morphine (0.1 mg/kg) diluted in saline to 0.2 ml/kg (maximum volume 6 ml) can be used, except in patients with a coagulopathy or those that have also undergone cystotomy to remove ammonium biurate calculi because of the risk of urinary retention. Patient monitoring should continue into the postoperative period and recovery is often slow due to reduced drug elimination and hypothermia. Seizures may occur and are commonly managed with an intravenous infusion of propofol (Heldmann *et al.*, 1999). Patients should also be observed for signs of portal hypertension, which include abdominal discomfort, ascites, vomiting and diarrhoea.

Hepatic tumours

Hepatic tumours are more common in older patients. Clinical signs range from mild hepatitis to life-threatening abdominal haemorrhage. Pre-anaesthetic preparation should include assessment of the degree of hepatic insufficiency using haematological and biochemical examinations. The major challenges for anaesthesia and surgery in these cases include acute haemorrhage and alterations in venous return when the mass is manipulated. Two large-bore catheters, or a central venous catheter, should be placed and compatible blood should be available in case transfusion is required.

Feline hepatic lipidosis

This condition is treated medically but patients may require anaesthesia for feeding tube placement (as described earlier in this chapter). Short-acting drugs that can be antagonized are preferable in these cases, although buprenorphine is also useful. There are some theoretical concerns regarding the use of lipid emulsions of propofol in these cases, but practical experience suggests that it does not cause problems (Posner *et al.*, 2008). In some situations, induction with a volatile agent may be considered. The use of NSAIDs is contraindicated due to the hepatic impairment and the potential for GI ulceration.

Diseases of the biliary tract

Patients occasionally require exploratory laparotomy for bile stasis or cholecystitis. These animals often have other GI signs, such as vomiting (risk of aspiration) or diarrhoea (electrolyte and acid–base disturbances), and should have a comprehensive biochemical and haematological examination, including coagulation profile. It is essential to stabilize these patients before anaesthesia. There is considerable debate regarding the effect of morphine on the sphincter of Oddi in cats and dogs. In humans, morphine and fentanyl have been shown to increase the tone of the sphincter of Oddi, leading to increased bile duct pressure above pre-administration levels. Studies have shown a 99% increase in pressure with fentanyl, a 53% increase with morphine and a 61% increase in tone with pethidine (Radnay *et al.*, 1980). Other studies in humans found no effect of pethidine on the sphincter of Oddi, whereas morphine increased tone, and tramadol and buprenorphine had very little effect (Staritz *et al.*, 1986; Wu *et al.*, 2004) Remifentanil increased sphincter tone in humans, but the effect was short-lived (Fragen *et al.*, 1999). Shore *et al.* (1971) reported morphine caused sphincter of Oddi spasm between 3 and 77 minutes following clinical i.v doses, and higher than clinical doses of pethidine caused spasm for 1–21 minutes in dogs. It is not known how the effects on bile duct pressure relate to the pancreatic duct (Thompson, 2001), and the bile and pancreatic duct sphincters function independently of each other in dogs (Shore *et al*, 1971). The incidence, however, of clinical problems associated with increased bile duct pressure in humans is only 3% even with fentanyl, and an increase in sphincter tone may not correlate with detrimental clinical signs (Radnay *et al*., 1980). It is now considered inappropriate to withhold these analgesics for fear of increasing the risk of pancreatitis or cholangitis. Although there are no reports in animals that mu opioid receptor agonists aggravate pancreatitis, there are still published recommendations that morphine should be avoided and pethidine or buprenorphine used instead (Zoran, 2006). When treating severe pain caused by pancreatitis, however, opioids still have a beneficial effect and should not be withheld (Dyson, 2008).

Pancreatic disease

Pancreatitis

Anaesthesia is rarely required for patients with acute pancreatitis unless there is evidence of pancreatic abscessation or tumours requiring excision. A full assessment is necessary to identify comorbidities and acid–base and fluid imbalances. Dehydration, hypokalaemia, hypocalcaemia and acidosis are common findings that should be treated before anaesthesia.

A major problem with these patients is pain control: acute pancreatitis is very painful and a multimodal analgesic protocol is likely to be more effective than a monotherapy approach (see later section on visceral pain). Epidural analgesia is effective and placement of an epidural catheter for longer-term analgesia should definitely be considered. In humans, a coeliac plexus block is sometimes performed, although the efficacy of this block in animals has not been studied and it requires specialist imaging to perform satisfactorily. In humans, pancreatitis can occur after administration of propofol (Mirtallo *et al*., 2010), although there is no evidence for this in animals.

Peritonitis

Peritonitis may result from perforation or rupture of the GI tract (septic peritonitis) or leakage of bile/urine into the abdominal cavity (aseptic peritonitis). Septic peritonitis is an acute emergency. These patients may have abdominal pain, dehydration, anorexia, mental obtundation, vomiting, pale tacky mucous membranes and tachycardia (or bradycardia in cats). Development of distributive shock is frequently observed, characterized by tachycardia, hypotension and a decrease in systemic vascular resistance caused by a massive inflammatory response. Endotoxins produced by bacteria activate mononuclear cells and platelets, leading to a release of inflammatory cytokines and prostanoids; this contributes to vasomotor paralysis and capillary occlusion, with secondary leakage of fluid into the interstitium (Minneci *et al*., 2007). These patients require aggressive fluid resuscitation using crystalloids and/or colloids including plasma, and frequently also require haemodynamic support (see Chapters 17 and 18). Blood transfusions may also be necessary if analysis of peritoneal fluid samples indicates the presence of

haemorrhage. If a septic cause is suspected, broad-spectrum antibiotics should be given. Initial diagnostic examinations should include haematology and biochemistry, abdominocentesis and imaging to identify the source of the peritonitis and to aid surgical planning.

Following appropriate stabilization, pre-anaesthetic medication in these cases is usually an opioid alone. Patients should be preoxygenated as they are at risk of developing myocardial dysfunction due to the high cardiac output and increased myocardial oxygen demand that may be present in the early stages of sepsis. For induction of anaesthesia, drugs that cause minimal cardiovascular depression should be used (see Chapter 14). However, etomidate is not a good choice for these patients because it inhibits cortisol synthesis: a study from human medicine has reported that septic patients receiving etomidate had significantly higher 28-day mortality than other patients in the trial (Sprung *et al*., 2008). A balanced protocol for maintenance of anaesthesia will reduce the disadvantages of using large doses of any one drug and also offers a multidimensional approach to pain control. However, NSAIDs should be avoided until GI/renal/hepatic involvement has been excluded and normal circulating volume restored. The use of epidural analgesia is contraindicated in cases of septic peritonitis because of the risk of introducing bacteria into the epidural space.

Patients should be monitored intensively, as described above for PSS ligation: invasive measurement of arterial blood pressure is preferable because refractory hypotension is common and very often requires pharmacological management (see Chapter 17). Clinically significant arrhythmias may also develop during surgery and will require specific treatment (see Chapters 21 and 31). Plasma colloid osmotic pressure and glucose concentration should ideally be measured, because the septic process and use of high-volume fluid replacement may reduce both.

Visceral pain

Viscera contain fewer nociceptors compared to the integument, but mechanoreceptors in organ walls, responding to stimuli such as stretch, are common. These receptors fire in a graded fashion in response to the degree of stretch, typically giving rise to 'waves' of pain sensation. The afferent nerves from abdominal viscera enter the dorsal horn of the spinal cord, where they synapse on to neurons receiving inputs from many different nociceptors. This phenomenon is called somatosensory convergence, and gives rise to the typical, poorly localized pain of varying intensity described in human patients with GI conditions. In the dorsal horn, pain sensations can be modulated or can stimulate local reflex arcs, or are passed to higher centres where pain is perceived, leading to behavioural changes (Sikandar and Dickenson, 2012).

Pain assessment is challenging in these cases: often mild behavioural signs such as hunching, inappetence, vocalization or aggression are seen, but these signs are not pain specific. The adoption of a 'praying' position may be seen with cranial abdominal pain such as pancreatitis but is not a consistent finding (Figure 24.9). Validated pain-scoring systems, such as the short form of the Glasgow Composite Measure Pain Score, may be useful to monitor the progression of pain, but should not be relied on exclusively; if an animal is suspected to be in pain, analgesia should be provided and changes in the patient's demeanour assessed (see also Chapter 9).

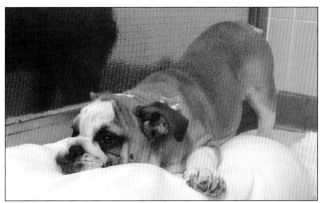

24.9 Dog in the 'praying' position typical of cranial abdominal pain. (Courtesy of Marieke de Vries, Davies Veterinary Specialists, Higham Gobion, UK)

Several agents are suitable for the relief of visceral pain and are shown in Figure 24.10. In general, intravenous infusions of analgesic agents are likely to be more effective than bolus dosing because plasma concentration can be maintained at a more constant level, and the total dose administered over a given period of time are likely to be reduced.

Obesity

Obesity typically results from excessive calorific intake over a prolonged period. Management of anaesthesia for obese animals presents a number of challenges (Love and Cline, 2015). It may be more difficult to auscultate the heart and lungs fully during pre-anaesthetic examination and so subtle cardiac or pulmonary changes may be missed. Identifying peripheral veins for catheterization and landmarks for local anaesthetic techniques may also be difficult in obese patients. Handling large, obese dogs may present challenges for staff, and adequate assistance and suitable equipment should be available in order to handle these animals safely.

Fat stores in the body have a relatively poor blood supply, which means that if drug doses are calculated based on total body mass, an exaggerated effect may result (Boveri et al., 2013). Therefore, doses of all drugs, especially rapidly acting anaesthetic induction agents, should be calculated using the ideal rather than actual body mass, to avoid potential overdose. Obese patients however, also have a relatively increased blood volume, which may minimize this effect. Theoretically, lipid-soluble drugs such as fentanyl and propofol redistribute preferentially to fat stores, especially when administered as an infusion, which may prolong recovery from anaesthesia; however, in humans, this has been reported to be dependent on the drug used, and recovery times may be relatively unaffected (De Baerdemaeker et al., 2004). Ideal maintenance agents include volatile agents with a low lipid solubility coefficient. Although isoflurane and sevoflurane are suitable, desflurane may offer advantages because it is significantly less fat soluble, and desflurane has been recommended for bariatric surgery in humans (Oggunaike et al., 2002).

Obesity has adverse effects on the respiratory system. Obese patients should be closely observed following administration of sedative drugs, because they may develop upper respiratory tract obstruction as the redundant pharyngeal tissue relaxes. During anaesthesia, obese patients tend to hypoventilate because thoracic wall excursion (owing to the presence of extra- and intrathoracic fat deposits) and diaphragmatic movement are reduced,

Drug	Loading dose (i.v. unless otherwise indicated)	Maintenance dose	Comment/adverse effects
Morphine	0.1–1.0 mg/kg slow	0.12–0.34 mg/kg/h	Usually only in dogs
Hydromorphone	0.05–0.1 mg/kg	0.05–0.1 mg/kg/h	Usually only in dogs
Fentanyl	0.002–0.005 mg/kg (2–5 µg/kg)	3–6 µg/kg/h i.v. in conscious patients 5–40 µg/kg/h intraoperative	IPPV required Bradycardia
Alfentanil	0.1 mg/kg	100 µg/kg bolus followed by 30–60 µg/kg/h i.v.	IPPV required Bradycardia
Sufentanil	0.003–0.005 mg/kg (3–5 µg/kg)	2.6–3.4 µg/kg/h i.v.	IPPV required Bradycardia
Remifentanil	Suggest using a loading dose of fentanyl at 0.003 mg/kg (3–5 µg/kg)	5–40 µg/kg/h i.v. Diluted to 0.1 mg/ml	IPPV required Bradycardia
Ketamine	0.2–1.0 mg/kg	2–10 µg/kg/min (commonly 5 µg/kg/min)	High infusion rates may cause dysphoria when used postoperatively although it is hard to see dysphoria under anaesthesia
Medetomidine	1–5 µg/kg i.v. or i.m. i.m. route preferred	1–5 µg/kg/h i.v.	Bradycardia
Dexmedetomidine	0.5–2.5 µg/kg i.v. or i.m. i.m. route preferred	0.5–2.5 µg/kg/h i.v.	Bradycardia
Lidocaine	Dog: 1–4 mg/kg	1–3 mg/kg/h	Haemodynamic depression (low blood pressures) in cats
MLK: Morphine Lidocaine Ketamine	Dog: 10 ml/kg; Cat: leave out lidocaine	0.2 mg/kg/h 3 mg/kg/h 0.6 mg/kg/h Infuse at 10 ml/kg/h during surgery Infuse at 2 ml/kg/h postoperatively	Add to 250 ml saline: 5 mg morphine 75 mg lidocaine 15 mg ketamine

24.10 Strategies for the treatment of visceral pain in cats and dogs. IPPV = intermittent positive pressure ventilation.

especially when in dorsal recumbency. The added weight of the abdominal contents will also press on the diaphragm, reducing FRC. It is advisable to preoxygenate such patients before induction, and IPPV may be necessary during anaesthesia, based on capnographic assessment of ventilation. Recovery may also present difficulties, as respiratory obstruction can occur following extubation; as a result, extubation should be delayed until the patient is capable of maintaining patency of its own airway.

Intravenous fluid therapy should be carefully monitored to avoid administration of excessive volumes for prolonged periods. Volumes of fluids should be based on estimated lean body mass (see Chapter 18). Although not normally a problem in temperate climates, it is possible that grossly obese patients may have an increased risk of developing hyperthermia during anaesthesia, and so body temperature should be continuously monitored.

References and further reading

Adams WA, Senior JM, Jones RS et al. (2006) cis-Atracurium in dogs with and without porto-systemic shunts. Veterinary Anaesthesia and Analgesia 33, 17–23

Ahya SN, Jose Soler M, Levitsky J and Batlle D (2006) Acid-base and potassium disorders in liver disease. Seminars in Nephrology 26, 466–470

Baraldi M, Avallone R, Corsi L et al. (2009) Natural endogenous ligands for benzodiazepine receptors in hepatic encephalopathy. Metabolic Brain Disease 24, 81–93

Beazley SG, Cosford K and Duke-Novakovski T (2011) Cardiopulmonary effects of using carbon dioxide for laparoscopic surgery in cats. Canadian Veterinary Journal 52, 973–978

Beer KA, Syring RS and Drobatz KJ (2013) Evaluation of plasma lactate concentration and base excess at the time of hospital admission as predictors of gastric necrosis and outcome and correlation between those variables in dogs with gastric dilatation–volvulus: 78 cases (2004–2009). Journal of the American Veterinary Medical Association 242, 54–58

Bexfield N and Watson P (2009a) Treatment of canine liver disease 1. Drugs and dietary management. In Practice 31, 130–135

Bexfield N and Watson P (2009b) Treatment of canine liver disease 2. Managing clinical signs and specific liver diseases. In Practice 31, 172–180

Boveri S, Brearley JC and Dugdale AHA (2013) The effect of body condition on propofol requirement in dogs. Veterinary Anaesthesia and Analgesia 40, 449–454

Bruchim Y, Itay S, Shira BH et al. (2012) Evaluation of lidocaine treatment on frequency of cardiac arrhythmias, acute kidney injury, and hospitalization time in dogs with gastric dilatation volvulus. Journal of Veterinary Emergency and Critical Care 22, 419–427

Buber T, Saragusty J, Ranen E et al. (2007) Evaluation of lidocaine treatment and risk factors for death associated with gastric dilatation and volvulus in dogs: 112 cases (1997–2005). Journal of the American Veterinary Medical Association 230, 1334–1339

Cassutto BH and Gfeller RW (2003) Use of intravenous lidocaine to prevent reperfusion injury and subsequent multiple organ dysfunction syndrome. Journal of Veterinary Emergency and Critical Care 13, 137–148

Center SA (2005) Feline hepatic lipidosis. Veterinary Clinics of North America: Small Animal Practice 35, 225–269

De Baerdemaeker LEC, Mortier EP and Struys MMRF (2004) Pharmacokinetics in obese patients. Continuing Education in Anaesthesia, Critical Care and Pain 4, 152–155

Dugdale A (2010) Veterinary Anaesthesia: Principles to Practice. Wiley-Blackwell, Oxford

Duke T, Steinacher SL and Remedios AM (1996) Cardiopulmonary effects of using carbon dioxide for laparoscopic surgery in dogs. Veterinary Surgery 25, 77–82

Dyson DH (2008) Analgesia and chemical restraint for the emergent veterinary patient. Veterinary Clinics of North America: Small Animal Practice 38, 1329–1352

Eipel C, Abshagen K and Vollmar B (2010) Regulation of hepatic blood flow: the hepatic arterial buffer response revisited. World Journal of Gastroenterology 16, 6046–6057

Elliott RH and Strunin L (1993) Hepatotoxicity of volatile anaesthetics. British Journal of Anaesthesia 70, 339–348

Fragen, RJ, Vilich, F, Spies, SM and Erwin WD (1999) The Effect of Remifentanil on Biliary Tract Drainage into the Duodenum. Anesthesia and Analgesia 89, 1561–1564

Fryer KJ, Levine JM, Peycke LE, Thompson JA and Cohen ND (2011) Incidence of postoperative seizures with and without levetiracetam pretreatment in dogs undergoing portosystemic shunt attenuation. Journal of Veterinary Internal Medicine 25, 1379–1384

Furneaux RW (2011) Liver haemodynamics as they relate to portosystemic shunts in the dog: A review. Research in Veterinary Science 91, 175–180

Galatos AD and Raptopoulos D (1995a) Gastro-oesophageal reflux during anaesthesia in the dog: the effect of preoperative fasting and premedication. Veterinary Record 137, 479–483

Galatos AD and Raptopoulos D (1995b) Gastro-oesophageal reflux during anaesthesia in the dog: the effect of age, positioning and type of surgical procedure. Veterinary Record 137, 513–516

Han E (2003) Diagnosis and management of reflux esophagitis. Clinical Techniques in Small Animal Practice 18, 231–238

Hayden P and Cowman S (2011) Anaesthesia for laparoscopic surgery. Continuing Education in Anaesthesia, Critical Care and Pain 11, 177–180

Heldmann E, Holt DE, Brockman DJ, Brown DC and Perkowski SZ (1999) Use of propofol to manage seizure activity after surgical treatment of portosystemic shunts. Journal of Small Animal Practice 40, 590–594

Hellebrekers LJ and Sap R (1991) Sufentanil-midazolam anaesthesia in the dog. Veterinary Anaesthesia and Analgesia 18, 191–193

Holt DE, Washabau RJ, Djali S et al. (2002) Cerebrospinal fluid glutamine, tryptophan, and tryptophan metabolite concentrations in dogs with portosystemic shunts. American Journal of Veterinary Research 63, 1167–1171

Howe LM, Boothe DM, Slater MR, Boothe HW and Wilkie S (2000) Nitric oxide generation in a rat model of acute portal hypertension. American Journal of Veterinary Research 61, 1173–1177

Kummeling A, Teske E, Rothuizen J and Van Sluijs FJ (2006) Coagulation profiles in dogs with congenital portosystemic shunts before and after surgical attenuation. Journal of Veterinary Internal Medicine 20, 1319–1326

Lamata C, Loughton V, Jones M et al. (2012) The risk of passive regurgitation during general anaesthesia in a population of referred dogs in the UK. Veterinary Anaesthesia and Analgesia 39, 266–274

Lamont LA (2008) Adjunctive analgesic therapy in veterinary medicine. Veterinary Clinics of North America: Small Animal Practice 38, 1187–1203

Love LJ and Cline MG (2015) Perioperative physiology and pharmacology in the obese small animal patient. Veterinary Anaesthesia and Analgesia 42, 119–132

Minneci PC, Deans KJ, Hansen B et al. (2007) A canine model of septic shock: balancing animal welfare and clinical relevance. American Journal of Physiology Heart and Circulatory Physiology 293, H2487–H2500

Mirtallo JM, Dasta JF, Kleinschmidt KC and Varon J (2010) State of the art review: Intravenous fat emulsions: Current applications, safety profile, and clinical implications. Annals of Pharmacotherapy 44, 688–700

Monteiro-Steagall BP, Steagall PVM and Lascelles BDX (2013) Systematic review of nonsteroidal anti-inflammatory drug-induced adverse effects in dogs. Journal of Veterinary Internal Medicine 27, 1011–1019

Muir WW (1982) Gastric dilatation-volvulus in the dog, with emphasis on cardiac arrhythmias. Journal of the American Veterinary Medical Association 180, 739–742

Ogunnaike BO, Jones SB, Jones DB, Provost D and Whitten CW (2002) Anesthetic considerations for bariatric surgery. Anesthesia and Analgesia 95, 1793–1805

Panti A, Bennett RC, Corletto F et al. (2009) The effect of omeprazole on oesophageal pH in dogs during anaesthesia. Journal of Small Animal Practice 50, 540–544

Perrin M and Fletcher A (2004) Laparoscopic abdominal surgery. Continuing Education in Anaesthesia, Critical Care and Pain 4, 107–110

Posner LP, Asakawa M and Erb HN (2008) Use of propofol for anesthesia in cats with primary hepatic lipidosis: 44 cases (1995–2004). Journal of the American Veterinary Medical Association 232, 1841–1843

Radnay PA, Brodman E, Mankikar D and Duncalf D (1980) The effect of equi-analgesic doses of fentanyl, morphine, meperidine and pentazocine on common bile duct pressure. Anaesthetist 29, 26–29

Raptopoulos D and Galatos AD (1995) Post anaesthetic reflux oesophagitis in dogs and cats. Veterinary Anaesthesia and Analgesia 22, 6–8

Robertson SA, Lascelles BDX, Taylor PM and Sear JW (2005) PK-PD modelling of buprenorphine in cats: intravenous and oral transmucosal administration. Journal of Veterinary Pharmacology and Therapeutics 28, 453–460

Savvas I, Rallis T and Raptopoulos D (2009) The effect of pre-anaesthetic fasting time and type of food on gastric content volume and acidity in dogs. Veterinary Anaesthesia and Analgesia 36, 539–546

Shore JM, Silverman A, Siegel M and Bakal M (1971) Direct observations of the canine sphincter of Oddi. Annals of Surgery 174, 264–273

Sikandar S and Dickenson AH (2012) Visceral pain: the ins and outs, the ups and downs. Current Opinion in Supportive and Palliative Care 6, 17–26

Smith AA, Posner LP, Goldstein RE et al. (2004) Evaluation of the effects of premedication on gastroduodenoscopy in cats. Journal of the American Veterinary Medical Association 225, 540–544

Sprung CL, Annane D, Keh D et al. (2008) Hydrocortisone therapy for patients with septic shock. New England Journal of Medicine 358, 111–124

Staffieri F, Lacitignola L, De Siena R and Crovace A (2007) A case of spontaneous venous embolism with carbon dioxide during laparoscopic surgery in a pig. Veterinary Anaesthesia and Analgesia 34, 63–66

Staritz M, Poralla T, Manns M and Meyer zum Buschenfelde K-H (1986) Effect of modern analgesic drugs (Tramadol, pentazocine, and buprenorphine) on the bile duct sphincter in man. Gut 27, 567–569

Thompson DR (2001) Narcotic analgesic effects on the sphincter of Oddi. A review of the data and therapeutic implications in treating pancreatitis. American Journal of Gastroenterology 96, 1266–1272

Thompson HC, Cortes Y, Gannon K, Bailey D and Freer S (2012) Esophageal foreign bodies in dogs: 34 cases (2004–2009). *Journal of Veterinary Emergency and Critical Care* **22**, 253–261

Tillson DM and Winkler JT (2002) Diagnosis and treatment of portosystemic shunts in the cat. *Veterinary Clinics of North America: Small Animal Practice* **32**, 881–899

Tivers M and Brockman D (2009a) Gastric dilation–volvulus syndrome in dogs 1. Pathophysiology, diagnosis and stabilisation. *In Practice* **31**, 66–69

Tivers M and Brockman D (2009b) Gastric dilation–volvulus syndrome in dogs 2. Surgical and postoperative management. *In Practice* **31**, 114–121

Trepanier LA (2013) Idiosyncratic drug toxicity affecting the liver, skin, and bone marrow in dogs and cats. *Veterinary Clinics of North America: Small Animal Practice* **43**, 1055–1066

Waterman AE and Kalthum W (1990) The effect of clinical hepatic disease on the distribution and elimination of pethidine administered post-operatively to dogs. *Journal of Veterinary Pharmacology and Therapeutics* **13**, 137–147

Watson PJ (2004) Chronic hepatitis in dogs: a review of current understanding of the aetiology, progression, and treatment. *Veterinary Journal* **167**, 228–241

Wilson DV, Evans AT and Mauer WA (2006) Influence of metoclopramide on gastroesophageal reflux in anesthetized dogs. *American Journal of Veterinary Research* **67**, 26–31

Wilson DV, Evans AT and Miller R (2005) Effect of preanesthetic administration of morphine on gastroesophageal reflux and regurgitation during anaesthesia in dogs. *American Journal of Veterinary Research* **66**, 386–390

Wilson DV and Walshaw R (2004) Postanesthetic esophageal dysfunction in 13 dogs. *Journal of the American Animal Hospital Association* **40**, 455–460

Wu SD, Zhang ZH, Jin JZ *et al.* (2004) Effects of narcotic analgesic drugs on human Oddi's sphincter motility. *World Journal of Gastroenterology* **10**, 2901–2904

Zoran DL (2006) Pancreatitis in cats: Diagnosis and management of a challenging disease. *Journal of the American Animal Hospital Association* **42**, 1–9

Chapter 25

Urogenital disease

Eva Rioja Garcia

Renal disease

Renal physiology

The kidneys accomplish their dual functions of excreting waste products and managing body fluid volume and composition by filtering large amounts of fluid and solutes from the blood, reabsorbing necessary components from the filtrate and secreting waste products into the tubular fluid. The kidneys receive approximately 20% of cardiac output (CO) and are able to filter 10% of this volume. More than 99% of the filtered fluid is reabsorbed into the circulation. This results in a urine output (UO) of 1–2 ml/kg/h in healthy animals. The processes of filtration and reabsorption can be influenced by changes induced by anaesthesia and surgery.

Renal blood flow (RBF) and glomerular filtration rate (GFR) are subject to autoregulation, which is effective over a range of mean arterial pressure (MAP) of 60–150 mmHg. Urine production itself is not subject to autoregulation, but there is an almost linear relationship between MAP >50 mmHg and UO (Figure 25.1). Renal medullary blood flow is low, constituting only 2% of total RBF; however, medullary blood flow is essential for concentration of the urine. The medullary thick ascending loop of Henle is metabolically very active and may be vulnerable to ischaemic injury during periods of decreased RBF, as can occur during anaesthesia.

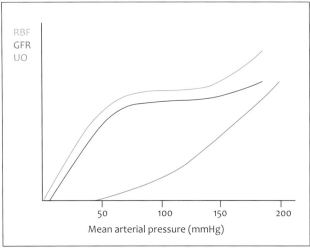

25.1 Relationship between mean arterial blood pressure and renal blood flow (RBF), glomerular filtration rate (GFR) and urine output (UO).

Pathophysiology of renal failure

Renal dysfunction can occur on a clinical continuum that ranges from compensatory (subclinical) dysfunction to renal failure. Patients with pre-existing renal dysfunction have limited ability to compensate during periods of stress, such as during anaesthesia and surgery, and are especially prone to postoperative acute renal failure (ARF).

The body responds to stress by activation of the sympathetic nervous system (SNS) and the renin–angiotensin–aldosterone system, and also by release of anti-diuretic hormone (ADH; also known as vasopressin). A modest activation of this stress response causes shifting of blood flow from the renal cortex to the medulla, avid reabsorption of sodium and water and decreased UO. A more intense stress response will lead to a decrease in RBF and GFR, which in extreme cases may lead to ischaemic damage to the kidney and ARF.

During stress states, renal ischaemia and hypotension, prostaglandins are produced in the kidneys by the enzymes phospholipase A_2 and cyclo-oxygenase (COX). Renal prostaglandins increase RBF by opposing the actions of ADH, noradrenaline (norepinephrine) and the renin–angiotensin–aldosterone system. They are therefore important in maintaining RBF and sodium and water excretion during periods of high physiological stress and poor renal perfusion.

Maintenance of adequate intravascular volume, CO, systemic arterial blood pressure and oxygenation is imperative to prevent renal hypoxia during anaesthesia. Renal hypoperfusion should be aggressively managed to prevent the development of ARF, especially in patients with pre-existing renal disease.

Preoperative assessment and stabilization

For detailed information on assessment of renal function in patients with acute kidney injury and chronic kidney disease (CKD), the reader is referred to reviews by Ross (2011) and Polzin (2011). Patients with ARF may have anuria or oliguria (UO <0.5 ml/kg/h), or polyuria (UO >2 ml/kg/h), with vomiting, diarrhoea and/or anorexia. These animals are commonly dehydrated. Signs related to the uraemic syndrome include halitosis, oral ulceration, tongue-tip necrosis, scleral injection, hypothermia, cutaneous bruising, uraemic gastritis or enteritis with diarrhoea and melaena. Uraemia induces a thrombocytopathy, which causes a prolongation of the buccal mucosal bleeding time despite a normal platelet count and coagulation profile. The urine is isosthenuric (urine specific gravity (USG) 1.007–1.015). In animals with acute tubular necrosis, a urine dipstick test may show glucosuria (without hyperglycaemia), proteinuria and haematuria. Metabolic acidosis, hyperphosphataemia and hyperkalaemia are also common in animals with ARF.

CKD is most common in older cats, although it can also be present in younger cats and in dogs. Animals that are asymptomatic may have only mild elevations of serum urea and creatinine concentrations. As CKD progresses, animals develop signs such as polyuria, polydipsia and weight loss. Decompensation of CKD will lead to dehydration and uraemic syndrome. Lack of erythropoietin synthesis by the kidneys leads to a non-regenerative anaemia, which may worsen if there is gastrointestinal blood loss caused by the uraemic syndrome. As in ARF, the uraemia induces a thrombocytopathy. Animals with CKD have low USG, and metabolic acidosis, hyperphosphataemia and hypokalaemia are commonly present, especially in more advanced stages. Hyperkalaemia is uncommon in cats with CKD, except in end-stage oliguric CKD. Systemic hypertension has been reported to occur in up to 61% of cats with CKD, with systolic arterial pressures of 146.6 ± 25.4 mmHg and diastolic arterial pressures of 96.6 ± 15.2 mmHg (Kobayashi et al., 1990). Dogs with CKD are more resistant to the development of hypertension, and pressures in this species may be relatively normal until renal function is severely compromised.

As part of pre-anaesthetic assessment, patients with renal disease should have a full haematological examination and serum urea, creatinine and electrolyte concentrations (sodium, potassium, chloride, ionized calcium, bicarbonate and inorganic phosphate) measured. Urinalysis and estimation of urine production are also recommended. It may be useful to place a urinary catheter before or during anaesthesia so that UO can be measured more accurately. Arterial blood pressure in CKD patients should also be measured preoperatively with a Doppler technique or by using oscillometry. Patients in ARF with hyperkalaemia and uraemic crisis should be stabilized over at least 24 hours before anaesthesia is considered. The choice of fluid type used for stabilization should be guided by the plasma sodium concentration, as the degree of free water loss relative to sodium loss can vary considerably. Rapid increases or decreases in plasma sodium concentration should be avoided as these may cause central nervous system dysfunction. In dehydrated patients, the amount of fluid necessary for rehydration should be calculated (% dehydration x bodyweight (kg) = fluid deficit (litres)) and administered over 12–24 hours (depending on the clinical signs).

The patient's fluid output should be estimated, including insensible losses (respiration, saliva), UO and any ongoing losses (vomiting, diarrhoea). Insensible losses are estimated to be approximately 20–70 ml/kg/day in dogs and 12–30 ml/kg/day in cats. If the patient is anuric, care should be taken to avoid overhydration.

Hyperkalaemic patients should receive intravenous fluids lacking potassium or alkalizing solutions with low potassium content (i.e. Hartmann's or lactated Ringer's) before anaesthesia. Specific treatment for hyperkalaemia includes the administration of insulin together with dextrose. Administration of sodium bicarbonate to correct metabolic acidosis results in an intracellular shift of potassium ions, but this treatment should be reserved for severely acidaemic animals and is contraindicated in patients with hypernatraemia and/or impaired respiratory function. In cases of life-threatening hyperkalaemia, 10%

calcium gluconate can be given intravenously in order to reduce cardiac membrane excitability and avoid the development of fatal arrhythmias; however, this therapy has no effect on plasma potassium concentration. (For more detail on the treatment of hyperkalaemia, see the section on urethral obstruction and uroabdomen later in this chapter.)

For animals that are anuric, diuretics may be administered to try to restore UO and control intravascular fluid volume, but there is no evidence that diuretics improve outcome in ARF. Mannitol (0.25–1 g/kg i.v. q4–6h) alone or combined with furosemide (0.5–4 mg/kg i.v., s.c., i.m. or orally q8–12h) may be used. Dopamine at low doses (0.5–3 μg/kg/min i.v.) promotes renal vasodilation and UO through stimulation of D_1-like receptors in dogs. Cats also possess D_1-like receptors in the kidneys, but they differ from those in dogs and are much less abundant. It seems that the dopamine-induced increase in UO in cats is mediated through alpha-adrenergic and not dopaminergic receptors, and higher doses of dopamine are needed to achieve this effect (>10 μg/kg/min). However, the so-called 'renal dose' of dopamine is generally no longer recommended because of the lack of a clear beneficial effect in management of renal failure in humans (Friedrich et al., 2005). If anuria persists in a uraemic patient, some form of dialysis may be the only effective treatment.

Patients with CKD should ideally be treated medically and stabilized before any elective procedure requiring anaesthesia. Dehydrated animals should have fluid deficits replaced over 12–24 hours; if there is haemodynamic instability or the patient is collapsed, the fluid deficit should be replaced more rapidly. In addition to replacement of fluid deficits, an empirical maintenance rate of 66 ml/kg/day is recommended in polyuric patients, although measurement of UO will give a more accurate idea of the individual patient's fluid requirements. If there are other fluid losses (e.g. through vomiting) the fluid rate should be adjusted accordingly.

Hypokalaemia is common in animals with CKD and most patients will need potassium supplementation in intravenous fluids (Figure 25.2). The rate of potassium supplementation should not exceed 0.5 mmol/kg/h. Signs of potassium overdose may be monitored with an electrocardiogram (ECG) (Figure 25.3).

Animals with CKD and concomitant hypertension should receive a calcium channel blocker such as amlodipine and/or an angiotensin converting enzyme (ACE) inhibitor such as enalapril or benazepril. Clinicians have differing opinions on whether or not these agents should be stopped before anaesthesia. Continued administration until the time of anaesthesia has the advantage of preventing hypertension and better preservation of remaining renal function. However, these drugs may promote

Serum potassium (mmol/l)	KCl to add to 250 ml of solution* (mmol)	KCl to add to 1 litre of solution* (mmol)	Maximum fluid infusion rate (ml/kg/h)
<2	20	80	6
2.1–2.5	15	60	8
2.6–3	10	40	12
3.1–3.5	7	28	18

25.2 Intravenous supplementation of potassium in hypokalaemic animals. KCl = potassium chloride. *Hartmann's solution contains 5 mmol/l of potassium and lactated Ringer's solution contains 4 mmol/l of potassium, which should be taken into account when adding KCl.
(Adapted from Greene and Scott, 1975)

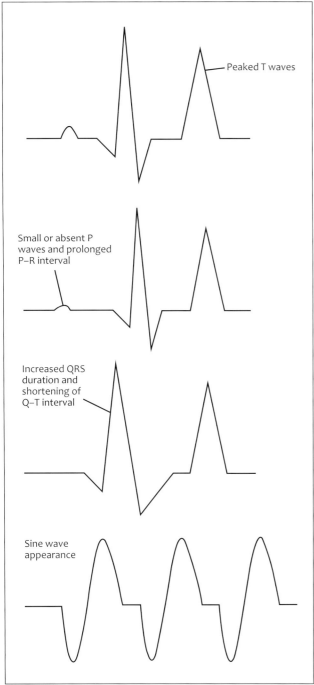

Peaked T waves

Small or absent P waves and prolonged P–R interval

Increased QRS duration and shortening of Q–T interval

Sine wave appearance

25.3 Progressive ECG changes associated with hyperkalaemia. These may be detectable only at potassium concentrations >7 mmol/l, and become progressively more obvious, particularly at concentrations >9 mmol/l. Bradycardia is a common feature.

hypotension during anaesthesia, which may be more difficult to treat and may require more aggressive fluid therapy and/or inotropic support.

Severely anaemic patients with clinical signs may need a blood transfusion (whole blood or packed red cells) before anaesthesia. In the absence of suitable blood products, Oxyglobin® (see Chapter 18 for administration rates) may be administered as a substitute to increase oxygen carrying capacity. Antagonists of histamine H_2 receptors, such as famotidine or ranitidine, or proton pump inhibitors, such as omeprazole, may be administered to animals with uraemic gastritis and vomiting to decrease gastric acid production. Lower than normal doses of these drugs should be given, as they are primarily eliminated by the kidneys. Sucralfate may be administered when gastric ulcers are suspected. Uraemia stimulates the chemo-receptor trigger zone, causing nausea and vomiting; centrally acting antiemetics, such as metoclopramide, maropitant or ondansetron, are sometimes necessary in patients that have intractable vomiting.

Anaesthetic management

Intravenous access is mandatory for patients in renal failure. Patients should receive intravenous fluids for some time before anaesthesia, with the volume and composition of fluids and the duration of infusion being tailored to their hydration, acid–base and electrolyte status, as discussed above. Monitoring of central venous pressure (CVP) will also aid perioperative fluid management, especially in patients with ARF and decompensated CKD; however, this technique is difficult in smaller patients. While the absolute value of CVP at any given time may be of limited clinical significance, especially in anaesthetized and mechanically ventilated patients, analysis of the trend in CVP will allow assessment of whether there is volume overload in oliguric/anuric patients, and inadequate volume replacement in polyuric patients. Urinary catheterization is also recommended for patients in renal failure to facilitate perioperative monitoring of UO. Normal UO should remain between 1 and 2 ml/kg/h, although a reduction is often observed during anaesthesia and in the post-anaesthetic period.

Invasive measurement of arterial blood pressure during anaesthesia is ideal, especially in patients with decompensated renal failure that are undergoing major procedures, although it may be difficult in very small animals. MAP should be maintained above 60–70 mmHg to ensure proper renal perfusion, especially because autoregulation of RBF is reduced in patients with renal disease. Non-invasive methods of blood pressure monitoring such as Doppler or oscillometric techniques may be more feasible, particularly in smaller patients. In chronically hypertensive animals, a slightly higher than normal MAP (>70–80 mmHg) should be targeted in order to preserve RBF and GFR.

Electrocardiography is also recommended, especially for hyperkalaemic patients (see Figure 25.3) and for animals with uraemia and acidaemia, which are also prone to the development of ventricular arrhythmias.

Capnography is very useful to determine the adequacy of ventilation and thus the requirement for mechanical ventilation. It is important to avoid hypercapnia, as it will lead to respiratory acidosis, and to potentially life-threatening acidaemia if metabolic acidosis is also present.

Pulse oximetry should also be used, especially during the recovery period, to ensure good haemoglobin oxygen saturation. In anaemic animals, who will have a low blood oxygen-carrying capacity, the haemoglobin oxygen saturation should be maintained above 96%, and oxygen supplementation should be provided to maintain saturation if necessary.

Animals with CKD might be very thin, rendering them prone to hypothermia. In these patients, efforts to maintain body temperature should be made using methods such as pre-anaesthetic heating in an incubator, active warming devices (forced warm air, warm water blanket, electric blanket), administration of warmed intravenous fluids, and heat and moisture exchangers. Further details of the effects and management of hypothermia can be found in Chapter 3.

A balanced anaesthetic protocol should be chosen to reduce the required dose of each individual agent and minimize the potential side effects. Drugs that are mainly eliminated unchanged by the kidneys or that have active metabolites that require renal elimination should be avoided, as their effects and duration will be unpredictable in patients with renal disease (e.g. ketamine in cats).

It is also important to note that protein binding of drugs may be reduced in animals with CKD; this will increase the free fraction (active fraction) of the drug, resulting in more pronounced drug effects. Therefore, lower doses of sedative and anaesthetic agents should be used and titrated carefully to the desired effect.

Pre-anaesthetic medication

The safest drugs to use for pre-anaesthetic medication of patients with renal failure include opioids and benzodiazepines, as they cause minimal cardiovascular depression, decrease requirements for other anaesthetic agents and can be antagonized if necessary. The choice of opioid should be based on the anticipated degree of pain for the procedure to be performed. Full mu opioid receptor agonists such as methadone or morphine (0.2–0.3 mg/kg i.m. or i.v.), pethidine (meperidine) (3–5 mg/kg i.m.), hydromorphone (0.05–0.1 mg/kg i.m. or i.v.) or fentanyl (3–5 µg/kg i.v.) are appropriate for procedures likely to cause moderate to severe pain. Control of mild pain may be achieved with butorphanol (0.2–0.3 mg/kg i.m. or i.v.) or buprenorphine (0.02 mg/kg, i.m., i.v. or (in cats) oral transmucosal). If only sedation is required, butorphanol may be useful. It is vital to control pain adequately, as untreated pain will stimulate the SNS stress response, which may lead to further renal hypoperfusion. Midazolam (0.2 mg/kg i.m. or i.v.) or diazepam (0.2 mg/kg i.v.) may cause disinhibition and excitement in healthy animals, especially following intravenous administration, but often cause sedation in sick animals.

Acepromazine maintains normal RBF and GFR in healthy cats and dogs during anaesthesia, despite causing hypotension (Boström et al., 2003). Therefore, acepromazine may be used at low doses (0.005–0.02 mg/kg i.m. or i.v.) in animals with compensated renal disease that are euvolaemic.

Alpha-2 adrenoceptor agonists such as medetomidine and dexmedetomidine cause initial peripheral vasoconstriction and a pronounced decrease in CO, resulting in redistribution of blood flow (decreased perfusion mainly to the skin but also to the kidneys). Because of this, these drugs are best avoided, especially in patients with decompensated CKD and ARF. In non-hypertensive patients with compensated CKD, alpha-2 agonists may be used at low doses (medetomidine ≤5 µg/kg i.m., or ≤3 µg/kg i.v.; dexmedetomidine ≤2.5 µg/kg i.m., or ≤1.5 µg/kg i.v.) if necessary.

In fractious cats, a moderate degree of sedation, sufficient to place an intravenous catheter, may be achieved by the intramuscular administration of an opioid (e.g. butorphanol 0.2–0.3 mg/kg), in combination with a low dose of an alpha-2 adrenoceptor agonist (e.g. medetomidine 2–5 µg/kg), and midazolam (0.2–0.3 mg/kg) or alfaxalone (1 mg/kg).

Induction of anaesthesia

Pre-oxygenation via a tight-fitting facemask for 3–5 minutes before induction of anaesthesia is recommended, especially in anaemic animals.

During induction, minimal cardiovascular depression is desirable; the use of a co-induction technique can be helpful in an attempt to preserve CO and RBF. Examples of suitable combinations include a benzodiazepine (midazolam or diazepam 0.2–0.5 mg/kg i.v.) or an opioid (e.g. fentanyl 3–5 µg/kg i.v.) administered before the agent chosen to induce anaesthesia. Induction of anaesthesia may be achieved by using propofol (1–4 mg/kg i.v.), alfaxalone (0.5–3 mg/kg i.v.) or etomidate (1–2 mg/kg i.v.), in each case titrated to effect. In uraemic animals, the permeability of the blood–brain barrier is increased, resulting in greater sensitivity to anaesthetic agents. As a result, lower doses, carefully titrated to effect, should be used in these patients. Thiopental should be avoided in animals with ARF and decompensated CKD because it may promote cardiac arrhythmias.

In fractious cats, sometimes the only option to induce anaesthesia might be with a volatile anaesthetic, using an induction chamber. Sevoflurane, which is less soluble in blood and less pungent than isoflurane, provides slightly faster and smoother inductions. However, isoflurane is an acceptable choice. The advantages of this technique are that it requires minimal restraint of the animal and oxygen is co-administered with the anaesthetic agent; both of these factors are of benefit in anaemic animals. The disadvantage is the lack of intravenous access before the cat is anaesthetized. Also, cats with hypovolaemia and uraemia may become rapidly anaesthetized with this technique and therefore careful attention needs to be paid to the depth of anaesthesia, and cats should be removed from the chamber as soon as they become unconscious.

Maintenance of anaesthesia

Volatile anaesthetics, including isoflurane, sevoflurane and desflurane, may be used for maintenance of anaesthesia, but they all cause dose-dependent vasodilation and hypotension. Animals with CKD that are being treated with calcium channel blockers and/or ACE inhibitors may develop excessive hypotension when volatile agents are administered. Therefore, balanced anaesthetic techniques that allow the delivery of lower volatile agent concentrations should be used, for example, intravenous infusion of fentanyl (5–40 µg/kg/h).

The reaction of sevoflurane with carbon dioxide absorbents such as soda lime produces a vinyl halide called Compound A, which has been shown to be nephrotoxic in rats. This compound is mainly produced when high concentrations of sevoflurane and low fresh gas flows (<10 ml/kg/min) are used; it may reach toxic levels during prolonged anaesthesia. Even though there have been no reports of nephrotoxicity in cats and dogs, it is advisable to use higher fresh gas flows (>20 ml/kg/min) when using sevoflurane in animals with renal failure. Compound A is not produced when non-rebreathing (Mapleson) systems are used.

Co-administration of nitrous oxide allows a reduction in the delivered concentrations of volatile anaesthetic and also provides some analgesia. Nitrous oxide also results in SNS stimulation and consequent vasoconstriction, which may counteract the vasodilation and hypotension caused by the volatile anaesthetic; however, if vasoconstriction is too pronounced it may decrease RBF.

Total intravenous anaesthesia (TIVA) techniques are an alternative to volatile agents. Propofol (0.2–0.4 mg/kg/min) or alfaxalone (0.07–0.11 mg/kg/min) infusions may be titrated to achieve an appropriate plane of anaesthesia. These agents may be combined with an opioid and/or a benzodiazepine to produce analgesia (opioids) and decrease anaesthetic requirements (opioids and benzodiazepines). Ideally, propofol infusions should not be used in cats, or only used for very short procedures, as they can lead to Heinz body formation and prolonged recovery. See Chapter 14 for further discussion of TIVA.

Local anaesthetic techniques should be used whenever possible. These have a number of benefits: they produce excellent analgesia, they decrease the requirements for general anaesthetic agents and therefore minimize cardiorespiratory depression, and they diminish the stress response to surgical stimulation. Neuraxial (epidural and intrathecal) administration of morphine provides excellent analgesia for up to 12–24 hours. Neuraxial administration of local anaesthetic agents may result in sympathetic blockade and vasodilation with subsequent hypotension, especially in hypovolaemic animals. However, vasodilation of the renal arteries increases RBF and has been reported not to worsen preoperative renal dysfunction in humans (Sharrock et al., 2006). Local anaesthetic agents may therefore be used, provided that the patient's blood pressure is monitored and hypotension is properly managed. However, the neuraxial administration of drugs is contraindicated in uraemic animals as they may suffer from a thrombocytopathy, making them prone to bleeding and possible epidural haematoma formation.

Intravenous fluids should be administered throughout the anaesthetic period to prevent or treat hypovolaemia and kidney hypoperfusion, with the aim of avoiding further kidney damage. The choice of fluid type will depend on the concentrations of serum electrolytes and plasma proteins. An isotonic crystalloid such as Hartmann's or lactated Ringer's solution should be administered intraoperatively at a rate that aims to match ongoing losses (respiratory, gastrointestinal, blood, urine). Measurement of UO and CVP may be used to guide fluid therapy, although they are not very sensitive indicators of fluid balance and renal perfusion. The rate of crystalloid fluid administration during surgery can be calculated as follows:

Maintenance rate for insensible losses (i.e. 1 ml/kg/h) + any pre-existing deficit (e.g. to correct 5% dehydration, 50 ml/kg over 12–24 hours is needed) + UO + 3–4 times the amount of blood loss (e.g. if blood loss is 50 ml the volume required is 150–200 ml) + other losses (e.g. diarrhoea, vomiting) (Figure 25.4).

If UO is not measured, an estimated value should be used. It is estimated that polyuric animals will need at least 3–4 times the maintenance rate of fluids (i.e. 6–8 ml/kg/h; Figure 25.4). Measurement of the patient's bodyweight before and after surgery will also give an idea of fluid balance (positive or negative). Infusion of an artificial colloid (e.g. gelatins) or fresh frozen plasma may be necessary in hypoproteinaemic animals. In severely anaemic animals, whole blood, packed red cells or Oxyglobin® may be necessary (see also Chapter 18).

For management of intraoperative hypotension (MAP <60 mmHg), efforts should be made to decrease the administered volatile agent concentration. If hypotension is associated with bradycardia, causing a low CO, an anticholinergic such as glycopyrronium (0.005-0.01 mg/kg i.v.) or atropine (0.02-0.04 mg/kg i.v.) may be administered. If hypotension persists or is not associated with bradycardia, a crystalloid fluid bolus may be administered in non-anaemic animals (10–20 ml/kg in dogs, 5–10 ml/kg in cats, over 10 minutes). If this does not correct hypotension, a bolus of a colloid solution (3–5 ml/kg in dogs, 2–3 ml/kg in cats, over 10 minutes) may be used. This may also help to restore UO in anuric/oliguric animals with undetected hypovolaemia or dehydration. Smaller boluses should be administered to animals with heart disease, starting at 25–33% of the fluid bolus (e.g. 5 ml/kg in dogs and 2.5 ml/kg in cats if a crystalloid solution is used).

If hypotension persists after more than adequate fluid resuscitation has been provided, positive inotropic drugs,

Sources of water loss	Estimated fluid rate*
(A) Insensible (respiratory, skin and saliva) Dog: 20–70 ml/kg/day Cat: 12–30 ml/kg/day	1 ml/kg/h
(B) Urine output Normal: 1–2 ml/kg/h Polyuria: >2 ml/kg/h	Normal: 1–2 ml/kg/h Polyuria: 6–8 ml/kg/h
(C) Blood loss	3 x amount of blood lost Example: Estimated blood loss 10% of blood volume Dog's blood volume is 80 ml/kg: 10% blood loss is 8 ml/kg Cat's blood volume is 60 ml/kg: 10% blood loss is 6 ml/kg Amount of fluid needed to replace losses is 8 x 3 = 24 ml/kg in a dog and 6 x 3 = 18 ml/kg in a cat If surgery lasts 2 hours, fluid rate should be 12 ml/kg/h in a dog and 9 ml/kg/h in a cat Note: Rate will depend on time course of blood loss. Ideally, administration rate should match rate of blood loss
(D) Pre-existing dehydration	Dehydration (%) x bodyweight = litres of fluid to administer over 12–24 hours For 5% dehydration = 50 ml/kg over 24–12 hours or 2–4 ml/kg/h For 7% dehydration = 70 ml/kg over 24–12 hours or 3–6 ml/kg/h For 10% dehydration = 100 ml/kg over 24–12 hours or 4–8 ml/kg/h Note: For dehydration ≥8%, hypovolaemia may also occur. Fluid boluses should be initially administered to stabilize the patient
(E) Other losses Diarrhoea Vomiting/regurgitation	Depending on estimated losses
Total fluid rate: A + B + C + D + E Example: Total fluid requirement in a polyuric cat with chronic kidney disease, undergoing a dental procedure (estimated blood loss of 2%) with 5% pre-existing dehydration: A (1 ml/kg/h) + B (6–8 ml/kg/h) + C (1.2 x 3 = 3.6 ml/kg/h) + D (2–4 ml/kg/h) + E (none) = 12.6–16.6 ml/kg/h	

25.4 Calculation of intraoperative intravenous fluid administration rate to maintain zero water balance. *Using a balanced crystalloid solution such as Hartmann's or lactated Ringer's.

such as dopamine (3–7 μg/kg/min i.v.) or ephedrine 0.02–0.05 mg/kg bolus i.v.) may be considered. Dopamine has no direct effect on renal function but it improves CO and blood pressure, thus helping to maintain renal perfusion and avoid further ischaemic damage to the kidney during anaesthesia-induced hypotension. Higher doses of dopamine may cause excessive peripheral vasoconstriction and promote arrhythmias. Ephedrine is a synthetic non-catecholamine agent that has intrinsic adrenergic effects and also promotes release of endogenous noradrenaline. This results in increases in CO, arterial blood pressure, arterial oxygen content and delivery, while the heart rate initially increases and then decreases (baroreceptor reflex response). Dobutamine, a beta-1 and beta-2 adrenoceptor agonist with minor alpha-1 adrenergic effects (seen only at high doses), may also be used (2–10 μg/kg/min i.v.) to improve CO and oxygen delivery to the tissues. However, even though dobutamine increases CO, blood pressure often does not change in cats and dogs, making it difficult to assess the clinical response. Pure alpha adrenoceptor agonists such as phenylephrine are contraindicated as they may decrease RBF. Noradrenaline is a potent vasoconstrictor with some positive inotropic effects. It is not recommended as initial therapy; however, it can be considered in cases where dopamine, ephedrine and dobutamine have failed, especially in septic animals (initial noradrenaline dose 0.1 μg/kg/min i.v., increasing slowly to effect up to a maximum of 1.0 μg/kg/min).

Mechanical ventilation may be required if the animal is hypoventilating (end-tidal or arterial carbon dioxide tension >45 mmHg (>6 kPa)) and especially if metabolic acidosis is present, as concomitant respiratory and metabolic acidosis may dangerously decrease the pH. Mechanical ventilation may however decrease venous return, CO and arterial blood pressure; therefore, adequate fluid resuscitation is needed before initiating lung ventilation. Prolonged positive pressure ventilation will promote fluid retention and decrease UO, although this is unlikely to be a problem during anaesthesia.

Non-depolarizing neuromuscular blocking agents such as atracurium and cisatracurium are suitable and have been reported to have a predictable onset and duration of action in human patients with CKD. Laudanosine, a metabolite of atracurium and cisatracurium, may accumulate during prolonged administration in patients with renal failure and may cause seizures, but this is unlikely after administration of clinically recommended doses for a short period of time. If neuromuscular blockade is used, it is mandatory to monitor neuromuscular function to detect possible prolonged blockade.

Non-steroidal anti-inflammatory drugs and renal failure

The use of non-steroidal anti-inflammatory drugs (NSAIDs) in patients with renal disease is controversial. These drugs inhibit renal production of prostaglandins, which regulate renal vasodilation, RBF and UO. In healthy animals that became hypotensive during anaesthesia, administration of meloxicam or carprofen (both preferential COX-2 inhibitors) before anaesthesia did not impair renal function or decrease RBF or GFR (Boström et al., 2002; Boström et al., 2006). However, another study found that administration of carprofen or etodolac to dogs with hypovolaemia or receiving concurrent furosemide treatment resulted in decreased renal function and GFR (Surdyk et al., 2012). Therefore, use of NSAIDs in animals with decompensated

CKD or ARF, or patients that are being treated with a diuretic, may be detrimental and is not recommended.

A retrospective study of 47 geriatric cats with osteoarthritis and clinically stable CKD (no elevation in urinary protein:creatinine ratio at the start of the treatment) found that long-term treatment with meloxicam at a median daily dose of 0.02 mg/kg (range 0.01–0.05 mg/kg) did not result in detrimental renal effects, faster progression of the disease or decreased life span (Gowan et al., 2012). In fact, less progression of renal disease was observed than in age- and CKD stage-matched cats not given meloxicam. Long-term use of the lowest effective dose of meloxicam for treatment of osteoarthritis may therefore be used in cats with clinically stable CKD, although these patients should be monitored regularly for any decline in renal function.

In dogs with stable CKD, tepoxalin has been used for long-term treatment of osteoarthritis-related pain. Renal function became worse in 1 of 16 dogs and improved after tepoxalin was discontinued (Lomas et al., 2013). The results of this study suggest that tepoxalin may be used with appropriate monitoring in dogs with stable CKD and osteoarthritis.

Postoperative care

Analgesia should be continued into the postoperative period, both to increase patient comfort and to decrease the stress response (which can lead to further renal hypoperfusion). Opioids can be administered intravenously if intravenous access has been established, or they can be injected via the intramuscular route. Full mu opioid receptor agonists such as methadone or morphine (0.2–0.3 mg/kg i.v. or i.m. q4h), hydromorphone (0.05–0.1 mg/kg i.v. or i.m. q4h) or fentanyl (3–6 μg/kg/h i.v. infusion) should be administered if the animal shows signs of moderate to severe pain. Buprenorphine (0.02 mg/kg i.v., i.m. or (in cats) oral transmucosal, q6–8h) may be administered for mild pain; it has the advantage of a long duration of effect. Buprenorphine administered by the oral transmucosal route in cats has excellent bioavailability.

During the postoperative period, the patient should be monitored continuously. Measurement of UO and serial blood and urine analyses, especially for creatinine and USG measurements, respectively, should be performed to assess the progression of the disease.

Fluids should be administered in the postoperative period to continue fluid resuscitation and rehydration until the animal is able to maintain fluid balance with oral fluid intake. Once fluid resuscitation and rehydration have been completed, the type of fluid administered for maintenance will depend on serum electrolytes. A solution with lower than normal sodium content such as 0.45% sodium chloride or half-strength Hartmann's solution (diluted 1:1 with sterile water) is more appropriate for these patients, as the damaged kidneys may not be able to excrete a high sodium load. Hypokalaemia may occur in animals that are receiving diuretics and in cases of polyuria; potassium supplementation will be necessary in these cases (see Figure 25.2).

Antibiotics should be administered perioperatively if urinalysis indicates the presence of infection (pyelonephritis could be the cause of ARF). Ideally, antibiotic therapy will be based on the results of culture and antibiogram. While antibiogram results are pending, or in cases of negative culture but the patient has undergone major surgery, a broad-spectrum antibiotic (e.g. cefazolin, cefalexin or co-amoxiclav) should be administered.

Urethral obstruction and uroabdomen

Pathophysiology

Urethral obstruction is more commonly anatomical (e.g. urolithiasis, neoplasia, post-surgery, post-trauma) but it can also be functional (e.g. reflex dyssynergia). It occurs more often in males than females. Uroabdomen due to bladder rupture is also quite common, and is most notably related to trauma. Both urethral obstruction and uroabdomen will lead to post-renal azotaemia and life-threatening hyperkalaemia and metabolic acidosis if they are not rapidly corrected. The clinical condition of the patient and severity of associated serum abnormalities will depend on the duration of the obstruction/uroabdomen and whether obstruction is partial or total. Animals with total urethral obstruction lasting for >36–48 hours will present with signs of shock; rapid treatment of these patients is vital. Anaesthesia will be required for either medical (urethral catheterization) and/or surgical correction of these conditions.

Preoperative assessment and stabilization

The animal should be stabilized with initial fluid therapy, and hyperkalaemia addressed before anaesthesia. Initial assessment should focus on the cardiorespiratory systems, and serum electrolyte concentrations (especially potassium) and acid–base balance should be evaluated. Measurement of haematocrit, urea and creatinine is useful to gain baseline values and facilitate monitoring of changes in these variables during treatment. Mixed acid–base disorders are usually observed, with concomitant metabolic acidosis (uraemic and lactic acidosis) and respiratory acidosis or alkalosis (depending on factors such as the condition of the respiratory system, degree of pain, level of central nervous system depression, etc). To establish the severity of the metabolic disturbance and aid in selecting appropriate therapy, it is important to interpret the pH together with the carbon dioxide tension, base excess and bicarbonate concentration measured in a central venous (or jugular) blood sample. Ionized calcium concentration should also be measured, as this can be extremely low in critically ill animals, predisposing them to cardiac arrhythmias. Note that ionized calcium may further decrease when acidosis is corrected.

Hyperkalaemia causes cardiac rhythm abnormalities and if severe (>9–10 mmol/l) will lead to cardiac arrest. Therefore, the initial priority is to correct abnormalities in serum potassium. In general, anaesthesia should not be induced until serum potassium concentration is <6 mmol/l. An ECG is useful to assess the presence of some arrhythmias associated with hyperkalaemia (see Figure 25.3). However, ECG changes do not normally occur until the potassium concentration is >7 mmol/l, and these patients may have no ECG abnormalities. If serum potassium cannot be measured, hyperkalaemia should be suspected if the animal has a normal to low heart rate in the presence of signs of pain and dehydration. In early acute hyperkalaemia, sinus tachycardia may be present; wide-complex tachycardia and ventricular tachycardia may also be seen. Lidocaine must not be used to treat these cardiac abnormalities as ventricular fibrillation or asystole may result.

Treatment of hyperkalaemia includes administration of fluids without potassium (e.g. 0.9% sodium chloride) or alkalizing crystalloid solutions (e.g. Hartmann's or lactated Ringer's), administration of dextrose ± insulin, and sodium bicarbonate (Figure 25.5). These treatments aim to reduce serum potassium concentration either by dilution (0.9% sodium chloride, but this solution will cause hyperchloraemic acidosis) or by driving potassium from the circulation into the cells (dextrose and insulin). Use of alkalizing solutions is preferable in acidaemic animals because they will facilitate translocation of potassium into the cells as the pH is restored. Hartmann's and lactated Ringer's solutions contain some potassium (5 and 4 mmol/l, respectively) but their infusion will still have a dilutional effect on plasma potassium concentration. Administration of dextrose ± insulin is preferable to sodium bicarbonate for treating hyperkalaemia without acidaemia. Plasma glucose concentration should be closely monitored when insulin is administered to avoid hypoglycaemia. Sodium bicarbonate should be administered only to animals with intact respiratory function (which is necessary to eliminate the carbon dioxide generated by the infusion). In general, it should be used only for severe metabolic acidosis because it may be associated with side effects such as paradoxical intracellular acidosis, a decrease in ionized calcium concentration and a decrease in blood pressure and CO.

Calcium gluconate is indicated in severe hyperkalaemia when ECG abnormalities are observed, while

Treatment	Dose	Comments
Alkalizing fluids (Hartmann's or lactated Ringer's solution)	5–10 ml/kg i.v. over 5–10 minutes Repeat as needed to restore circulation and pH	Caution with full bladder; perform cystocentesis as soon as possible
Regular insulin	0.25–0.5 IU/kg i.v.	Always administer dextrose concomitantly Monitor blood glucose
Dextrose	1–2 g dextrose per unit of insulin (2–4 ml of 50% dextrose, diluted with 8–16 ml of fluids, to make a 10% solution)	Do not administer >10% dextrose solution into a peripheral vein For a 5% dextrose solution, add 100 ml of 50% dextrose to 900 ml of fluids
Sodium bicarbonate	Total dose (mmol) to administer = BE x 0.3 x bodyweight (kg) (start with one-third and reassess) or 0.5–2 mmol/kg i.v. and reassess	Use only for severe metabolic acidosis, if pH <7.1, BE <-12 mmol/l or bicarbonate <12 mmol/l Administer slowly over 20 minutes and reassess acid–base Do not administer through the same line with calcium-containing fluids
Drain peritoneal urine and perform peritoneal dialysis	Irrigate peritoneum with a warm, potassium-free solution (0.9% sodium chloride)	In uroabdomen

25.5 Treatment options for hyperkalaemia. BE = base excess.

other therapies are being instituted to reduce serum potassium concentration. A bolus of 10% calcium gluconate (50–100 mg/kg; 0.5–1 ml/kg i.v. over 2–5 minutes) is administered and the ECG should be continuously monitored. This dose will decrease the membrane threshold potential for approximately 20 minutes, avoiding the development of fatal arrhythmias.

Anaesthetic management

In general, the same principles apply to these cases as to patients with renal disease. It is important to pre-oxygenate the patient before anaesthesia and to use a balanced anaesthetic protocol to avoid excessive cardiovascular depression associated with high doses of induction agents. Opioids and benzodiazepines are suitable options for pre-anaesthetic medication: the pain relief provided by opioids and the muscle relaxation by benzodiazepines may facilitate urinary catheterization. Some opioids, such as pethidine and fentanyl, also have some intrinsic spasmolytic effects. Alpha-2 adrenoceptor agonists are contraindicated due to their cardiovascular side effects and also because they increase diuresis and inhibit insulin release, which may interfere with the treatment the patient is receiving for hyperkalaemia. Phenothiazines should also be avoided in animals with fluid deficits.

For induction of anaesthesia, propofol, alfaxalone or etomidate may be used as described in the section on renal disease. A suitable alternative is ketamine (2–5 mg/kg i.v.) combined with a benzodiazepine (midazolam or diazepam 0.2–0.3 mg/kg i.v.), as this combination will cause some degree of cardiovascular stimulation via activation of the SNS. However, ketamine should not be administered to cats with suspected renal damage (e.g. cases with obstruction of long duration), as it is mainly eliminated unchanged by the kidneys in this species, or to animals with decompensated shock, as it may cause direct myocardial depression.

During anaesthesia of acidaemic animals, mechanical ventilation should be provided to avoid respiratory acidosis, which will worsen the acidaemia.

Rapid drainage of large volumes of urine from the abdomen can result in haemodynamic instability, with redistribution of blood causing sudden hypotension. In addition, the sudden loss of severe visceral nociceptive input that occurs when the distended bladder is emptied could markedly reduce plasma catecholamine concentrations, leading to cardiovascular collapse. In these instances, a fluid bolus (10–20 ml/kg crystalloid or 2.5–5 ml/kg colloid) and, if necessary, a positive inotrope (dopamine, dobutamine or ephedrine) should be administered immediately.

Epidural administration of local anaesthetic agents into either the lumbosacral or sacrococcygeal space will provide excellent pain relief, reduce anaesthetic requirements and relax the urethra, facilitating catheterization. Epidurally administered morphine may inhibit the micturition reflex, which is not desirable after urinary obstruction or bladder surgery. However, morphine may be administered epidurally if a urinary catheter is left in place postoperatively.

Administration of NSAIDs is recommended only for animals with no renal damage and stable haemodynamics following adequate fluid resuscitation. Their use is best withheld until the postoperative period, when the animal is sufficiently stabilized and renal function can be evaluated.

Postoperative care

The urinary catheter should be left in place for at least 24 hours or even a few days after relief of an obstruction, so that urine production can be assessed and also to avoid re-obstruction of the urethra due to inflammation (Figure 25.6ab). It is common to observe post-obstructive diuresis (UO >2 ml/kg/h) resulting from impaired tubular reabsorption of glomerular filtrate, which can lead to hypokalaemia (plasma concentration <3.5 mmol/l) and excessive fluid losses. Post-obstructive diuresis has been reported to occur in 50% of cats within 6 hours of relieving urethral obstruction, but in some cats it may not appear until 18–30 hours post-relief, and it may be present for up to 84 hours (Francis et al., 2010). Cats with acidaemia on admission seem to be at higher risk of post-obstructive diuresis. Close monitoring of fluid balance and serum electrolytes (especially potassium) is therefore necessary and should continue until the polyuria is resolved. Potassium should be added to balanced crystalloid solutions to prevent or treat hypokalaemia (see Figure 25.2); the rate of potassium supplementation should not exceed 0.5 mmol/kg/h.

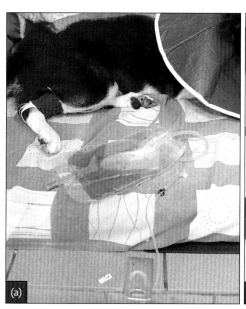
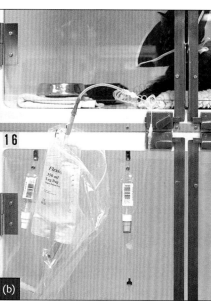

25.6 (a) Recumbent dog after spinal surgery with an indwelling urinary catheter and a closed urine collection system. The urine colour indicates that the urine is concentrated. (b) Cat with a urinary catheter and a closed urine collection system. The urine is very dilute because of post-obstruction diuresis.
(Courtesy of Marieke de Vries, Davies Veterinary Specialists, Higham Gobion, UK)

Pyometra

Pathophysiology

When inflammatory cells, bacteria and secretions accumulate within the uterus, endotoxaemia results, and eventually septic peritonitis and shock if uterine rupture occurs. The risk of uterine rupture is greater in closed (i.e. no vaginal discharge) than in open (with vaginal discharge) pyometra. The clinical signs of pyometra range from mild (e.g. polydipsia, polyuria) to severe with septic shock or peritonitis (e.g. lethargy, anorexia, fever, dehydration, tachycardia, tachypnoea, pale or hyperaemic mucous membranes). Endotoxins from *Escherichia coli* cause insensitivity to ADH, which results in impaired urine concentrating ability and increased diuresis. This can normally be reversed, but in some severe cases more permanent renal tubular damage occurs. Some animals may also have progesterone-induced diabetes mellitus (caused by insulin resistance), which may resolve after ovariohysterectomy.

Preoperative assessment and stabilization

It is helpful to obtain full haematological and biochemical panels. Neutrophilia with a high percentage of band neutrophils and anaemia of chronic disease may be present. Alterations in albumin (decreased), globulins (increased), urea and creatinine (increased), hepatic enzymes (increased), glucose (decreased in sepsis, increased in diabetes), electrolytes (hypochloraemia may occur when the animal has been vomiting) and blood gases (mixed disturbance of lactic acidosis due to hypovolaemia and hypochloraemic alkalosis due to vomiting) are common.

Animals in shock must be stabilized before anaesthesia. Intravenous fluid therapy with crystalloids and/or colloids should be provided to restore circulating volume and to correct any specific abnormalities (e.g. hypo- or hyperglycaemia, acidaemia). Severely anaemic patients should receive a transfusion of whole blood, packed red blood cells or Oxyglobin®. Broad-spectrum antibiotics should also be started. Animals with hyperglycaemia and suspected diabetes mellitus should be treated with insulin to prevent ketoacidosis.

A patient with a ruptured uterus will have septicaemia and frequently severe hypotension, which may be unresponsive to fluid therapy. In these cases, positive inotropes and/or vasoconstrictors may be required. Initially, ephedrine (0.02–0.05 mg/kg i.v. bolus) or dopamine (start with an infusion of 5 μg/kg/min i.v. and increase by 1 μg/kg/min every 2–3 minutes up to a maximum of 15 μg/kg/min) may be administered. Ephedrine will have little effect in animals with decompensated shock, because part of its effect is indirectly mediated via release of endogenous catecholamines. When administering dopamine, if the heart rate increases but there is no effect on blood pressure, noradrenaline may be administered instead (starting at 0.1 μg/kg/min i.v., increasing to effect up to a maximum of 1.0 μg/kg/min). Alternatively, dobutamine (2–10 μg/kg/min i.v.) in combination with phenylephrine (1–3 μg/kg/min i.v.) can be administered.

Anaesthetic management

The choice of anaesthetic agents will depend on the severity of the patient's systemic condition. In mildly affected animals, a protocol similar to that used for an elective ovariohysterectomy can be used, although greater caution should be exercised with cardiovascular depressant drugs.

Sicker patients are unlikely to need a sedative for pre-anaesthetic medication, but an opioid should always be administered to provide intraoperative analgesia. Alpha-2 adrenoceptor agonists and phenothiazines should, ideally, be avoided. Co-induction with a benzodiazepine or fentanyl may allow use of a lower dose of induction agent, resulting in less cardiovascular depression. Pre-oxygenation via a tight-fitting facemask for 3–5 minutes before induction is recommended.

In severely compromised animals, induction of anaesthesia can be achieved with an opioid (methadone 0.3–0.5 mg/kg, hydromorphone 0.05–0.1 mg/kg or fentanyl 5–10 μg/kg, all i.v.) in combination with a benzodiazepine (midazolam or diazepam 0.2–0.5 mg/kg i.v.). No pre-anaesthetic medication is necessary in these cases. If endotracheal intubation is not possible with this combination, a small dose of an intravenous anaesthetic agent (propofol 0.5–1 mg/kg, alfaxalone 0.25–0.5 mg/kg or ketamine 0.5–1 mg/kg) may be administered.

For maintenance, intravenous infusions of an opioid (fentanyl or remifentanil 10–40 μg/kg/h), a benzodiazepine (midazolam 0.1–0.2 mg/kg/h), ketamine (5–10 μg/kg/min) and/or lidocaine (only in dogs, 2 mg/kg bolus followed by 16.6–50 μg/kg/min) may be used to decrease the requirements for general anaesthetic agents. If a high dose of a longer-acting opioid such as methadone or hydromorphone has already been administered, the analgesia provided may last for the duration of surgery. High doses of opioids are more likely to cause respiratory depression; mechanical ventilation may therefore be necessary to avoid hypercapnia and exacerbation of acidaemia.

Intensive monitoring of the respiratory and cardiovascular systems is necessary during anaesthesia; monitoring should include capnography, pulse oximetry, arterial blood pressure (ideally by invasive measurement in critical cases) and ECG.

Animals with pyometra are prone to hypotension when positioned in dorsal recumbency as a result of compression of the vena cava by the full uterus, which causes a decrease in venous return and CO. Hypotension in these patients should be treated with aggressive intravenous fluid therapy and positive inotropes as previously described. For non-responsive hypotension in septicaemic animals, a vasoconstrictor such as noradrenaline or phenylephrine may be necessary (see preoperative stabilization, above). A possible complication during exteriorization of the uterus is the initiation of a vago-vagal reflex, which will cause a sudden drop in heart rate; if this occurs, atropine (0.04 mg/kg i.v.) or glycopyrronium (0.005–0.01 mg/kg i.v.) should be administered.

Postoperative care

Fluid therapy should continue into the postoperative period, until patients can maintain their fluid balance with oral intake. Patients that are anorexic may require placement of an oesophagostomy feeding tube. Blood should be sampled and analysed periodically to evaluate the progression of abnormal parameters and to guide interventions. Renal damage should be evaluated by urinalysis and measurement of UO, as well as serum urea and creatinine concentrations.

Postoperative analgesia should be provided using opioids (e.g. a full mu opioid receptor agonist for the first 24 hours, followed by a partial agonist such as buprenorphine for the next 2–3 days). NSAIDs are reserved for animals with no renal damage after adequate fluid resuscitation, and should only be administered postoperatively.

Other genital conditions

Several other genital conditions may necessitate anaesthesia and surgery. Some, for example ruptured prostatic abscess, may have a similar clinical presentation to a pyometra, and can be approached in a similar way. Others, such as paraprostatic cysts and testicular tumours, usually have a more stable clinical presentation. Testicular torsion is rare, but is associated with severe pain, and requires aggressive preoperative analgesic management, followed by prompt surgery.

References and further reading

Boström IM, Nyman GC, Hoppe A and Lord P (2006) Effects of meloxicam on renal function in dogs with hypotension during anaesthesia. *Veterinary Anaesthesia and Analgesia* **33**, 62–69

Boström M, Nyman GC, Kampa N, Häggström J and Lord P (2003) Effects of acepromazine on renal function in anesthetized dogs. *American Journal of Veterinary Research* **64**, 590–598

Boström IM, Nyman GC, Lord P *et al.* (2002) Effects of carprofen on renal function and results of serum biochemical and hematologic analyses in anesthetized dogs that had low blood pressure during anesthesia. *American Journal of Veterinary Research* **63**, 712–721

Clark KL, Robertson MJ and Drew GM (1991) Do renal tubular dopamine receptors mediate dopamine-induced diuresis in the anesthetized cat? *Journal of Cardiovascular Pharmacology* **17**, 267–276

Duke T, Caulkett NA and Tataryn JM (2006) The effect of nitrous oxide on halothane, isoflurane and sevoflurane requirements in ventilated dogs undergoing ovariohysterectomy. *Veterinary Anaesthesia and Analgesia* **33**, 343–350

Dyson D (1992) Anesthesia for patients with stable end-stage renal disease. *Veterinary Clinics of North America: Small Animal Practice* **22**, 469–471

Francis BJ, Wells RJ, Rao S and Hackett TB (2010) Retrospective study to characterize post-obstructive diuresis in cats with urethral obstruction. *Journal of Feline Medicine and Surgery* **12**, 606–608

Friedrich JO, Adhikari N, Herridge MS and Beyene J (2005) Meta-analysis: low-dose dopamine increases urine output but does not prevent renal dysfunction or death. *Annals of Internal Medicine* **142**, 510–524

Gowan RA, Baral RM, Lingard AE *et al.* (2012) A retrospective analysis of the effects of meloxicam on the longevity of aged cats with and without overt chronic kidney disease. *Journal of Feline Medicine and Surgery* **14**, 876–881

Gowan RA, Lingard AE, Johnston L *et al.* (2011) Retrospective case-control study of the effects of long-term dosing with meloxicam on renal function in aged cats with degenerative joint disease. *Journal of Feline Medicine and Surgery* **13**, 752–761

Greene RW and Scott RC (1975) Lower urinary tract disease. In: *Textbook of Veterinary Internal Medicine*, ed. SJ Ettinger, pp. 1572. Saunders, Philadelphia

Kobayashi DL, Peterson ME, Graves TK, Lesser M and Nichols CE (1990) Hypertension in cats with chronic renal failure or hyperthyroidism. *Journal of Veterinary Internal Medicine* **4**, 58–62

Lomas AL, Lyon SD, Sanderson MW and Grauer GF (2013) Acute and chronic effects of tepoxalin on kidney function in dogs with chronic kidney disease and osteoarthritis. *American Journal of Veterinary Research* **74**, 939–944

Machado CG, Dyson DH and Mathews KA (2005) Evaluation of induction by use of a combination of oxymorphone and diazepam or hydromorphone and diazepam and maintenance of anesthesia by use of isoflurane in dogs with experimentally induced hypovolemia. *American Journal of Veterinary Research* **66**, 1227–1237

O'Hearn AK and Wright BD (2011) Coccygeal epidural with local anesthetic for catheterization and pain management in the treatment of feline urethral obstruction. *Journal of Veterinary Emergency and Critical Care* **21**, 50–52

Pertek JP and Haberer JP (1995) Effects of anesthesia on postoperative micturition and urinary retention. *Annales Françaises d'Anesthésie et de Réanimation* **14**, 340–351

Polzin DJ (2011) Chronic kidney disease in small animals. *Veterinary Clinics of North America: Small Animal Practice* **41**, 15–30

Psatha E, Alibhai HI, Jimenez-Lozano A, Armitage-Chan E and Brodbelt DC (2011) Clinical efficacy and cardiorespiratory effects of alfaxalone, or diazepam/fentanyl for induction of anaesthesia in dogs that are a poor anaesthetic risk. *Veterinary Anaesthesia and Analgesia* **38**, 24–36

Ross L (2011) Acute kidney injury in dogs and cats. *Veterinary Clinics of North America: Small Animal Practice* **41**, 1–14

Sharrock NE, Beksac B, Flynn E, Go G and Della Valle AG (2006) Hypotensive epidural anaesthesia in patients with preoperative renal dysfunction, undergoing total hip replacement. *British Journal of Anaesthesia* **96**, 207–212

Sun L, Suzuki Y, Takata M and Miyasaka K (1997) Repeated low-flow sevoflurane anesthesia: effects on hepatic and renal function in beagles. *Masui* **46**, 351–357

Surdyk KK, Sloan DL and Brown SA (2012) Renal effects of carprofen and etodolac in euvolemic and volume-depleted dogs. *American Journal of Veterinary Research* **73**, 1485–1490

Chapter 26

Anaesthesia for Caesarean section and for the pregnant patient

Andy Claude and Robert E. Meyer

Case-based data are available to support or recommend best practice for anaesthesia for Caesarean section in cats and dogs. This chapter reviews the available literature, the relevant pharmacological and physiological changes that occur in the parturient small animal patient and, where possible, makes best-practice recommendations for maternal and neonatal patient care.

Pre-anaesthetic considerations

Overall, the rate of dystocia is approximately 5% in the dam and 3–6% in the queen (Smith, 2012). Risk factors for dystocia in the dam are breed (miniature breeds and Bulldogs are over-represented), age and parity (primiparous animals >6 years of age have significantly greater risk), larger litter size and smaller body size. The diagnosis of dystocia depends on multiple presenting clinical signs rather than one particular condition. The dam or queen may delay parturition when nervous or in unfamiliar surroundings but this is not necessarily dystocia. Criteria for the diagnosis of dystocia in the dog include pregnancy duration >70 days (>71 days in the queen); continuous straining for 1 hour without delivery of the first puppy; green or black discharge before delivery of the first puppy; 3 hours or more between puppies; the dam is ill or depressed; and the puppy is stuck or malpresented in the birth canal (Evans and Adams, 2010).

Ultrasonography can help to assess the condition of the uterus and viability of the fetuses. Generally speaking, fetal heart rates of <180 beats/min indicate fetal distress, while heart rates <160 beats/min warrant emergency intervention (Smith, 2012). Urgent patient stabilization and surgery can reduce fetal mortality from 9 to 3%; however, assessment of the dam/queen, progression of labour and fetal heart rate are used to indicate whether surgery is needed (Traas, 2008). The decision on which actions are appropriate should be based on physical examination and objective data (blood analysis, diagnostic imaging), and on the need for maternal stabilization. If the Caesarean is non-elective, the dam/queen may have biochemical and haematological abnormalities, electrolyte imbalances and absolute or relative volume losses. In an ideal situation, full bloodwork should be undertaken, but packed cell volume, total solids/total protein, blood glucose and blood urea nitrogen measurements are useful as a minimum database. The dam/queen may have eaten within the 6 hours before anaesthesia, making vomiting and/or regurgitation a strong possibility, and therefore it is essential to ensure a protected airway as soon as possible after induction of anaesthesia.

Review of outcome studies in small animals

Dogs

Puppy mortality rates are slightly higher for Caesarean section accompanying dystocia than for normal birth. In problem-free vaginal deliveries, the normal proportion of stillborn puppies and puppies that die in the immediate neonatal period is reported to be between 2.2 and 4.6%. The higher rates with Caesarean section probably result from a combination of physiological states that can occur during prolonged labour (maternal dehydration, hypovolaemia, sepsis, stress, exhaustion, hypocalcaemia), which can lead to fetal hypoxia, acidosis, hypercapnia, and distress *in utero* before anaesthesia. Additionally, puppies delivered by Caesarean section do not receive physical stimulation from passage through the birth canal, as would occur during vaginal birth.

When dystocia is not followed by Caesarean section, 15.6% of puppies are stillborn and 7.9% of live puppies may die soon after birth (Funkquist *et al.*, 1997). In puppies not born by Caesarean section, umbilical blood lactate concentration is an objective indicator of fetal distress and a valid predictor of neonatal survival (Groppetti *et al.*, 2010). In this study, fetal umbilical lactate concentration <5 mmol/l, an Apgar score >9 and effective uterine contractions were considered to be good prognostic indicators for survival.

In a multicentre prospective case series study, Moon *et al.* (1998) investigated mortality rates for 808 dams undergoing Caesarean section and for the 3410 puppies delivered. Neonatal survival rates were 92% immediately following delivery, 87% at 2 hours and 80% at 7 days. In 76% of the litters, all puppies delivered by Caesarean section were born alive. By comparison, the survival rates for 498 puppies born naturally during the study were 86% immediately following delivery, 83% at 2 hours and 75% at 7 days. Maternal mortality rate was reported to be 1% (9/808), and five of these deaths were attributed to pneumonia, possibly due to aspiration. Emergency surgery was required for 58% of the cases, most commonly in the Bulldog, Labrador Retriever, Boxer, Corgi and Chihuahua breeds. Breeds most commonly associated with elective surgery were the Bulldog, Labrador Retriever, Mastiff, Golden Retriever, and Yorkshire Terrier. The most commonly used anaesthetic protocols were isoflurane for induction and maintenance (34%), and propofol for induction followed by isoflurane for maintenance (30%).

A later analysis of the same data (Moon *et al.*, 2000) found that the following factors increased the likelihood of all puppies being alive following delivery:

- Surgery was not an emergency
- The dam was not a brachycephalic breed
- There were four puppies or fewer in the litter
- There were no naturally delivered or deformed puppies
- All puppies breathed spontaneously at birth
- At least one puppy vocalized at birth
- Neither methoxyflurane nor xylazine were used in the anaesthetic protocol.

However, 13 of the 23 litters exposed to xylazine also received ketamine, and this may indicate that the combination of xylazine with ketamine is detrimental. No other anaesthetic drugs were associated either positively or negatively with puppy survival at time of birth, and neonatal survival at 2 hours after delivery indicated no differences in residual anaesthetic effects at this time.

Using the same data set, Moon-Massat and Erb (2002) reported factors affecting puppy 'vigour', defined as spontaneous breathing and vocalizing within 2 minutes of delivery. This analysis indicated that the use of inhalant anaesthetics reduces the likelihood of any of the puppies in a litter breathing spontaneously or moving at delivery, emphasizing the need to minimize delivered concentrations of inhalant agents. The use of ketamine increased the odds that all puppies in a litter would require help to start breathing at delivery. Use of thiobarbiturates was associated with litters in which no puppies spontaneously moved at birth. Although the use of inhalant anaesthetics, ketamine and thiobarbiturates reduced puppy vigour at delivery, these drugs did not influence neonatal mortality.

In a prospective clinical study, Funkquist *et al.* (1997) studied neonatal survival rates after emergency Caesarean section in 141 dams. Anaesthesia was induced with propofol (6.5 mg/kg i.v.) and maintained with isoflurane (vaporizer setting 0.5–2.0%) and 65% nitrous oxide. An intentional 20-minute period was allowed to elapse between induction and delivery of puppies to allow time for propofol clearance. Of 412 puppies delivered, 71% survived, 3% were born alive but died within 20 minutes of delivery, and 26% were stillborn. Puppies were described as initially lethargic, but became lively and remained so after massaging and stimulation. Funkquist *et al.* (1997) compared these data with their own previous work, where Caesarean section was performed using either epidural lidocaine anaesthesia (118 dogs) or intravenous thiopental administered to effect followed by immediate delivery of puppies (48 dogs). The details are presented in Figure 26.1. The puppy mortality rate during the first 24 hours was highest with thiopental (20%), lower with propofol-isoflurane (6%) and lowest with epidural anaesthesia with lidocaine (4%). Specific consideration was not given to the duration of time that the dam had been in labour before Caesarean section, but this was mitigated somewhat by group classification based on the number of live and dead puppies born before the surgery. The puppy survival rate reported in this study for the Group 1 puppies using propofol–isoflurane anaesthesia (89%) is similar to the overall survival rate (92%) reported by Moon *et al.* (1998).

In another prospective clinical study, Luna *et al.* (2004) examined the effect of four different anaesthetic combinations on neurological and cardiorespiratory activity in puppies at birth. Chlorpromazine (0.5 mg/kg i.v.) was administered to 24 at-term dams, which were randomly assigned to groups of six to be anaesthetized as follows:

- Group 1: Thiopental (8 mg/kg i.v.) followed by enflurane maintenance
- Group 2: Midazolam (0.5 mg/kg i.v.) with ketamine (2.0 mg/kg i.v.) followed by enflurane
- Group 3: Propofol (5 mg/kg i.v.) followed by enflurane
- Group 4: Epidural anaesthesia with lidocaine (2.5 mg/kg; 2% solution) and bupivacaine (0.625 mg/kg; 0.5% solution) with adrenaline.

Puppy neurological reflexes were reported to be least depressed by epidural anaesthesia, followed by propofol–enflurane, thiopental–enflurane, and midazolam–ketamine–enflurane. There was no difference in puppy heart rate at delivery between the groups, although respiratory rate was highest in puppies delivered after epidural anaesthesia and lowest in the propofol–enflurane and midazolam–ketamine–enflurane groups. Two of 21 puppies from dams that received midazolam–ketamine–enflurane died within the first 24 hours after surgery, and one of the 24 puppies from dams receiving propofol–enflurane died 1 hour after anaesthesia. The authors concluded that differences in mortality between groups cannot be attributed solely to the anaesthetic induction agents because they did not control for other factors, such as duration of labour and puppy condition.

Prolonged anaesthesia time or a long surgical delivery time are both thought to be associated with increased neonatal mortality due to fetal exposure to anaesthetic agents, as well as reduction in uterine perfusion associated with anaesthesia and surgical manipulation. Different studies have used various strategies to limit fetal exposure to drugs (immediate delivery following induction) or to provide adequate time for drug clearance before delivery (20 minute delay after induction). There is no evidence that a very short time between induction of anaesthesia and delivery is advantageous, and puppy survival was not affected by either a long anaesthesia time (defined as >45 minutes) or a long delivery time (>10 minutes) (Moon-Massat and Erb, 2002).

Group	Percentage of puppies alive at delivery		
	Epidural lidocaine: n = 372 pups	Thiopental: immediate surgical removal after induction n = 121 pups	Propofol–isoflurane/N₂O: 20 minute delay after induction n = 380 pups
Group 1 (no puppies born prior to Caesarean section)	83% (229/277)	56% (32/57)	89% (197/221)
Group 2 (only live puppies born prior to Caesarean section)	72% (46/64)	34% (12/35)	70% (55/79)
Groups 3 (both live and dead puppies born prior to Caesarean section) and 4 (only dead puppies born prior to Caesarean section)	71% (22/31)	7% (2/29)	68% (54/80)

26.1 Results of the study by Funkquist *et al.* (1997) comparing puppy survival rates with three different anaesthetic protocols for Caesarean section.

Cats

In contrast to the dog, very few outcome data are available for Caesarean section in the cat. In one study of feline dystocia, 123 Caesarean sections were performed but no outcome data were given for either maternal or fetal survival (Ekstrand and Linde-Forsberg, 1994). In another study, 26 queens underwent Caesarean section accompanied by en bloc resection of the ovaries and uterus (Robbins and Mullen, 1994). A 58% incidence of stillborn kittens was reported in this group of cats; of kittens born alive, 10% died during the first week after delivery. One queen died nine days after surgery as a result of an ongoing coagulopathy.

Without adequate scientific data to support a best-practice approach, anaesthetic choice for feline Caesarean section will continue to depend largely on the drugs and facilities available, together with the veterinary surgeon's (veterinarian's) understanding of the physiological and pharmacological changes that accompany pregnancy. Until more data for injectable drugs are available, an inhalant anaesthetic is probably the best choice in cats.

Applied physiology of pregnancy

A number of physiological changes are present in the parturient patient that will significantly affect anaesthetic management. These changes are detailed below and summarized in Figure 26.2.

Oxygen consumption is increased by 20% in the parturient animal. To meet this increased oxygen demand, tidal volume is increased by 40% and respiratory frequency by 10%, together resulting in a 50% increase in alveolar ventilation. At the same time, cranial displacement of the diaphragm by the gravid uterus reduces total lung volume and functional residual capacity by 20%. The sum of these respiratory changes means:

- Without supplemental oxygen, the parturient patient will quickly become hypoxaemic should apnoea occur
- Induction with inhalant agents, and subsequent changes in anaesthetic depth, will occur much more rapidly than in a non-parturient patient.

Maternal plasma volume increases more than red blood cell volume, leading to the 'relative anaemia' of pregnancy. Anaemia becomes more pronounced as the number of fetuses increases. Cardiac output increases by 40%, with increased stroke volume accounting for two-thirds of the increase and heart rate for the remainder. Autoregulation of fetal blood flow does not occur and uteroplacental perfusion is pressure dependent. Compensatory cardiovascular reflexes to blood loss and hypovolaemia may be delayed, and the parturient patient may be less responsive to treatment with vasopressors, anticholinergics or inotropes. Colloids may be more effective in treating hypotension than crystalloids for intravenous fluid loading (Pascoe and Moon, 2001). Use of ephedrine to treat hypotension in the

Physiological changes	Potential effect	Potential complications	Preventative action
Respiratory			
Decrease in FRC, TLV	Lung volume closer to alveolar closing capacity	Atelectasis	Alveolar recruitment manoeuvre
Higher oxygen requirements and an increase in V_A	Hypoxaemia if hypoventilation or apnoea occurs	Hypoxaemia occurs quickly	3–5 minutes of pre-oxygenation with tight-fitting facemask at a rate of 5–6 l/min; oxygen supplementation during surgery
Decreased FRC and increased V_A	Uptake of inhalant anaesthetics is more rapidly achieved	Inhalational overdose possible	Vigilant attention to anaesthetic depth
Cardiovascular			
Increases in cardiac output and blood volume	If not maintained, hypotension occurs	Decreased blood flow to the fetus	Blood pressure monitoring; intravenous fluid therapy
Delay in compensatory cardiovascular reflexes to blood loss and hypovolaemia	Less responsive to therapeutic measures	Continued hypoperfusion despite standard treatment; anaemia as a result of amount of volume loading	Prophylactic therapy; immediate aggressive treatment
Neurological			
Sedative effects of progesterone; oestrogen- and progesterone-activated antinociception	Anaesthetic requirements and drug clearance decreased	Apparent sensitivity to anaesthetics; overdose with injectables or inhalants possible	Vigilant attention to anaesthetic depth
Gastrointestinal			
Delayed gastric emptying	Increased likelihood of ingesta in stomach		Rapid induction technique and protection of the airway
Decreased oesophageal sphincter tone	Increased incidence of regurgitation	Regurgitation and aspiration on induction or recovery causing aspiration pneumonia with pulmonary damage	Extubate when laryngeal reflexes present
Increased gastrin levels	Low pH of gastric fluid	Increased risk of regurgitation	Omeprazole
Mechanical			
Enlarged abdomen	Diaphragm pushed cranially	Hypoventilation, hypotension	Assist ventilation; give oxygen and intravenous fluids; care with positioning of patient

26.2 Physiological changes that occur during pregnancy and can affect the anaesthetic management of the patient. FRC = functional residual capacity; TLV = total lung volume; V_A = alveolar ventilation.

(Adapted from Pascoe and Moon, 2001)

parturient patient is controversial. In women undergoing Caesarean section, use of ephedrine during spinal anaesthesia resulted in fetal acidaemia and lower umbilical artery pH (Reynolds and Seed, 2005). Although dorsal recumbency leads to aortocaval depression and reduced uterine perfusion in humans, anatomical differences and greater collateral circulation tend to preserve uterine perfusion in small animals. Because of these circulatory changes:

- Maternal blood pressure should always be monitored during Caesarean section
- If maternal hypotension occurs, fetal perfusion will be reduced
- Intravenous fluid loading with a colloid is the first choice for treating maternal hypotension.

Anaesthetic requirement is reduced by 25–40% during pregnancy. This is due to a combination of increased concentrations of progesterone and its metabolites, which are potent positive allosteric modulators of gamma-aminobutyric acid A receptors (Erden *et al.*, 2005), and increased hormonal antinociception activated by oestrogen and progesterone during pregnancy (Gintzler and Liu, 2001). Epidural veins are engorged due to increased collateral blood flow, which decreases the epidural and cerebrospinal fluid spaces by 30–50%. As a result:

- Anaesthetic overdose is more likely unless inhalant or injectable anaesthetic doses are appropriately reduced
- A smaller volume is required for lumbosacral epidural or spinal anaesthesia to spread cranially to a specific dermatome.

Increased progesterone concentration during pregnancy also leads to delayed gastric emptying, increased gastric volume and reduced gastro-oesophageal sphincter tone. The increasing physical size of the uterus causes displacement of the pylorus, and increased gastrin level results in lowered gastric pH. These gastrointestinal changes can result in:

- Reduced lung volume
- Increased risk of regurgitation and aspiration during induction of or recovery from anaesthesia
- Increased pulmonary damage following accidental aspiration.

Pharmacological considerations

Placental transfer occurs with all anaesthetic agents, whether injectable or inhalant. The endotheliocortical placenta of dogs and cats allows rapid transfer of drugs from the mother to the fetus. Puppies and kittens delivered by Caesarean section will therefore be exposed to whatever anaesthetic agents have been administered to their mother. The amount of drug delivered to the placenta depends on placental blood flow and protein binding of the drug in the mother's blood, and the amount of drug available to the fetus depends on placental uptake and fetal metabolism and clearance.

Drugs cross biological membranes by simple diffusion. Most anaesthetic agents have relatively small molecular weights, which permit unimpeded transfer, and are also highly lipid-soluble. Non-ionized forms of drugs are more lipophilic than their ionized forms, and thus cross membranes more readily. Opioids and local anaesthetic agents are weak bases, with relatively low ionization at physiological pH and considerable lipid solubility. This means that, for these agents, the maternal-to-fetal concentration gradient is important as only 'free', non-protein-bound drug is available for transfer. At equilibrium, the concentrations of non-ionized drug in the fetal and maternal circulations will be similar. In an acidotic fetus, however, a weak base will tend to exist in the ionized form, which cannot diffuse back across the placenta into the maternal plasma. This phenomenon, known as 'ion trapping', can cause accumulation of opioids or local anaesthetics within fetal tissues and plasma, especially if the mother receives high or repeated doses.

Antacids and/or gastric protectants are recommended, especially in pregnant hospitalized patients. Examples of these drugs include H_2 receptor antagonists (cimetidine, famotidine, ranitidine), proton pump inhibitors (omeprazole) and antacids (calcium carbonate). However, there is little evidence regarding the prophylactic effects of antacids in pregnant veterinary patients and their offspring. In pregnant women, regurgitation or gastro-oesophageal reflux disease and resulting aspiration pneumonitis (Mendelson's syndrome) are always considered serious (Malfertheiner *et al.*, 2012).

Historically, chemically induced pneumonitis has been treated prophylactically by neutralization of gastric fluid with H_2 blockers and/or oral sodium citrate. In women scheduled to undergo Caesarean section, 30 ml of 0.3 M sodium citrate given orally within the 60 minutes before induction of general anaesthesia raised gastric pH, although the timing of administration had a critical effect on the results, and statistical analysis indicated that overall outcome was not improved (Dewan *et al.*, 1985). In another study, sodium citrate was shown to worsen nausea in women undergoing elective Caesarean deliveries (Kjaer *et al.*, 2006).

Emulsified antacids given to pregnant women caused significant pulmonary haemorrhage, exudation and oedema when aspirated into the lungs, compared with aspirated normal saline, alkalinized saline (Gibbs *et al.*, 1979) or sodium citrate (Kjaer *et al.*, 2006). Use of certain anti-nausea drugs (antacids and proton pump inhibitors) in the first trimester has been associated with infrequent development of cleft lip, cleft palate and neural tube defects in humans (Anderka *et al.*, 2012). Overall, these drugs appear to be safe when used after the first trimester.

To date, there are no reports on the efficacy of treatment in preventing aspiration pneumonitis, or on adverse and/or teratogenic effects of anti-nausea drugs or gastric protectants in veterinary obstetric patients.

Anaesthetic recommendations

In general, when planning an elective or emergency Caesarean section in a cat or dog, the veterinary surgeon should:

- Choose drugs with a short duration of action or drugs for which specific antagonists are available, to promote rapid recovery (Figure 26.3)
- Use the lowest possible dose of injectable or inhalant anaesthetics, bearing in mind that the pregnant patient has substantially lower anaesthetic requirements (see above). A general rule of thumb is to reduce the anaesthetic dose by 30–60%
- Use local anaesthetic techniques when possible and appropriate

Elective	Emergency patient in good health	Emergency patient in poor health	Precautions/concerns
Local anaesthetic techniques			
Opioid pre-anaesthetic medication plus epidural lidocaine	Opioid pre-anaesthetic medication plus epidural lidocaine	± Opioid pre-anaesthetic medication plus epidural lidocaine	May induce hypotension – measure blood pressure and be prepared to treat
	Opioid pre-anaesthetic medication plus local infiltration of the abdominal wall	Local infiltration of the abdominal wall	May not provide adequate analgesia – be prepared to induce general anaesthesia
General anaesthetic techniques			
Mask induction and maintenance	Mask induction and maintenance	Mask induction and maintenance	Be aware of regurgitation/aspiration risk and only use if risk is low
Opioid pre-anaesthetic medication plus propofol or alfaxalone inhalant	Opioid pre-anaesthetic medication plus propofol or alfaxalone inhalant	Propofol or alfaxalone inhalant	Propofol may cause significant hypotension in patient in poor health
Opioid pre-anaesthetic plus etomidate or alfaxalone inhalant	Opioid pre-anaesthetic plus etomidate or alfaxalone inhalant	± Opioid pre-anaesthetic medication plus etomidate or alfaxalone inhalant	May see myoclonus with etomidate – add low dose diazepam (0.05–0.1 mg/kg) or fentanyl (2–5 μg/kg) intravenously Flumazenil may be required in the neonate if diazepam is used in the mother

26.3 Anaesthetic agents that promote rapid recovery of the mother will allow her to care for her offspring as soon as possible.

- Monitor blood pressure and provide intravenous fluid support
- Provide supplemental oxygen to all patients
- Place an endotracheal tube if general anaesthesia is used.

In an emergency situation, it may be preferable to use a familiar technique rather than one that has not been used before, even if the familiar technique is less than ideal for Caesarean section (Pascoe and Moon, 2001). For Caesarean section in dogs, induction of anaesthesia with either an inhalant (via facemask) or injectable agent followed by maintenance with an inhalant is the usual technique. With general anaesthesia, the airway should be secured as quickly as possible to prevent aspiration. Mask induction is a simple technique that is familiar to most veterinary surgeons. With this technique, fetal depression is rapidly reversed after delivery with the onset of spontaneous breathing. The disadvantages are that maternal aspiration is a possibility before endotracheal intubation, and personnel will be exposed to waste anaesthetic gases. The authors' personal and recommended choice is mask induction for queens and very small dams, and induction with an injectable anaesthetic followed by maintenance with an inhalant agent for larger dogs. Ventilation of the lungs may be required to prevent hypoventilation once the patient is in dorsal recumbency (Figure 26.4), but it is important to avoid hyperventilation as this can reduce uterine perfusion.

The use of pre-anaesthetic medication will depend on the situation. Low doses of pre-anaesthetic drugs (see below for recommendations on the choice of drugs) can relieve maternal anxiety and distress, which will help to maintain uterine perfusion. They also reduce the required dose of induction and maintenance agents, thus helping to reduce fetal drug exposure. A healthy animal requiring an elective Caesarean section will probably need pre-anaesthetic medication; while a depressed, toxic animal requiring an emergency surgery will need much less, if any.

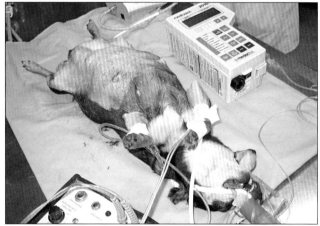

26.4 A heavily pregnant patient will have an enlarged abdomen, which could promote hypoventilation and atelectasis. Endotracheal intubation and ventilation of the lungs may therefore be necessary.
(Courtesy of Tanya Duke-Novakovski, Western College of Veterinary Medicine, University of Saskatchewan, Canada)

analgesia while producing minimal cardiovascular effects. Disadvantages include maternal respiratory depression requiring assisted ventilation, and possible bradycardia. If repeated or intraoperative re-dosing is considered likely, fentanyl (1–5 μg/kg i.v.) is preferred, as it is less likely to accumulate in an acidotic fetus than longer-acting opioids. If maternal bradycardia occurs it can be treated with atropine or glycopyrronium. Unlike glycopyrronium, atropine crosses the placenta, but it is unlikely to have an effect on fetal heart rate because of incomplete cardiac autonomic development in the fetus. It is important to be aware that bradycardia in the neonate is not vagally mediated and may be indicative of hypoxaemia. The opioid antagonist naloxone (0.01–0.02 mg/kg) can be administered to the neonate sublingually, intramuscularly or into the umbilical vein, to reverse opioid depression following delivery.

Mu opioid receptor agonists

The mu opioid receptor agonists (e.g., morphine, pethidine (meperidine), methadone, hydromorphone, fentanyl) can provide preoperative sedation and supplemental intraoperative

Phenothiazines

Phenothiazines (e.g. acepromazine, chlorpromazine) are not ideal choices for pre-anaesthetic medication before Caesarean section. The neonatal liver has limited ability to metabolize most drugs. In addition, phenothiazines may produce prolonged sedation, alpha-1 adrenoceptor-mediated vasodilation and hypotension, and disruption of thermoregulation in both the mother and neonate; these effects are undesirable. Nonetheless, these agents do not seem to be associated with increased maternal or neonatal mortality and, if judged necessary, can be effectively used at low doses (Moon *et al.*, 2000; Moon-Massat and Erb, 2002; Luna *et al.*, 2004).

Propofol

Propofol induction is associated with better neonatal outcome, similar to the outcome with epidural anaesthesia of the dam. Propofol crosses the placenta and reaches the fetus within two minutes of administration. Maternal blood concentration of propofol is three times higher than the concentration in the fetus following a single intravenous bolus, and six to nine times higher following one hour of continuous infusion; this indicates that there is a placental barrier effect. Mean residence times (the time that a drug is present in the body) are similar for the mother and fetus following a single intravenous bolus, but increased in the fetus with continuous infusion. Fetal elimination of propofol is prolonged following a single bolus or continuous infusion, with a half-life more than twice those observed for the dam. Plasma protein binding of propofol is higher in the dam than the fetus; this limits placental transfer because only unbound drug can pass (Gin *et al.*, 1991). However, because plasma protein binding is lower in the fetus, the free, pharmacologically active fraction of propofol may be higher in the fetus (Andaluz *et al.*, 2003). Based on the above, the use of continuous infusion or multiple boluses of propofol to maintain anaesthesia for Caesarean section is not recommended.

Thiobarbiturates

Outcome studies have shown reduced puppy vigour and increased mortality following thiobarbiturate administration to the mother (as described earlier in this chapter). Thiopental, an ultra-short-acting thiobarbiturate, is very lipid soluble and readily crosses the placenta following intravenous administration. In human infants, however, ultra-short-acting barbiturates are associated with higher Apgar scores (see later) and less neonatal depression at birth compared to either midazolam or propofol; this is due to a rapid decline in fetal blood concentration if delivery is delayed for at least 10 minutes after induction (Littleford, 2004). In the retrospective analysis of Moon *et al.* (2000) discussed earlier, it is not possible to determine the time between induction and delivery after thiobarbiturates were administered. In light of the data from human obstetrics, it is possible that in the study of Funkquist *et al.* (1997) puppy outcome may have improved in the thiopental group if more time had been allowed to elapse before delivery.

Alfaxalone

When used as induction agent in dams undergoing Caesarean section, alfaxalone has been found to have similar or better post-anaesthetic outcomes for both the mother and the puppies compared to propofol. A recent study, in which a modified Apgar scoring system was used to describe neonatal vitality, found that alfaxalone resulted in significantly better puppy vitality within the first 60 minutes after delivery, compared to propofol. However,

both induction agents were associated with similar puppy survival rates up to 3 months after delivery (Doebeli *et al.*, 2013a). A study by the same group reported significantly shorter maternal recoveries when alfaxalone was used as induction agent for emergency Caesarean sections, compared to propofol, but similar post-anaesthetic puppy survival rates were found for both agents (Doebeli *et al.*, 2013b).

Benzodiazepines

Benzodiazepines should be used cautiously, if at all, in cats and dogs requiring Caesarean section. Benzodiazepines are lipophilic, undissociated agents that readily penetrate membranes. Rapid placental transfer with significant fetal uptake occurs with these agents, and elimination from the neonate is quite slow. In human obstetric practice, benzodiazepine administration to the mother during labour is associated with lower Apgar and neurobehavioural scores and 'floppy infant syndrome', with symptoms such as mild sedation, hypotonia, reluctance to suck, apnoeic spells, cyanosis, and impaired metabolic responses to cold stress (Celleno, 1993; McElhatton, 1994). Similar depression of neurological reflexes has been observed in neonatal puppies following midazolam–ketamine–enflurane anaesthesia of the dam (Luna *et al.*, 2004). It is unknown whether benzodiazepine-associated neurological depression also occurs in neonatal kittens, but it seems likely. The antagonist flumazenil (0.01–0.03 mg/kg i.v.) can be tried in both cats and dogs, although it does not seem to be effective in cats (Ilkiw *et al.*, 2002).

Ketamine

Ketamine provides better maternal cardiovascular stability, especially in sick or depressed animals. However, it produces more profound fetal depression, necessitating intensive resuscitation (Pascoe and Moon, 2001). Although ketamine does not affect puppy survival, it reduces both spontaneous breathing at birth and neurological reflexes in puppies delivered by Caesarean section (Moon-Massat and Erb, 2002; Luna *et al.*, 2004). Because ketamine and the chemically similar agent tiletamine require concurrent benzodiazepine administration, these drugs should be used with caution.

Alpha-2 adrenoceptor agonists

Xylazine, an alpha-2 adrenoceptor agonist, significantly increases puppy mortality, probably by reducing uterine perfusion (Moon *et al.*, 2000). In an experimental study, bradycardia, hypertension and hypoxaemia lasting 20 minutes occurred in fetal lambs when xylazine was administered to conscious pregnant ewes (Perez *et al.*, 1991). Goats receiving 40 µg/kg of medetomidine intramuscularly demonstrated a 50% reduction in uterine blood flow, which resulted in fetal hypoxaemia and acidosis (Sakamoto *et al.*, 1997). Based on this evidence, the alpha-2 agonists should be avoided in Caesarean section in cats and dogs.

Injectable agents in critically ill dogs

Propofol, thiopental and alfaxalone can have significant adverse cardiovascular effects when administered rapidly and at high doses. These drugs should be used cautiously in depressed or critically ill patients to avoid causing reductions in cardiac output, arterial blood pressure and uterine perfusion. In critically depressed dams, a small dose of fentanyl can be given intravenously before induction. A reasonable alternative would be to use a low dose of propofol (1.0–2.0 mg/kg i.v.), thiopental (2.0–5.0 mg/kg i.v.) or alfaxalone (0.5–1.0 mg/kg i.v.) together with lidocaine (0.25–1.0 mg/kg i.v.) to facilitate endotracheal intubation. After intubation, start administration of isoflurane or sevoflurane, and wait at least 10 minutes before surgical delivery, to allow time for fetal concentrations of injectable agents to decline.

Local anaesthetics

Local anaesthetic techniques are generally considered to be the 'gold standard' in terms of optimal fetal and maternal viability, although Funkquist et al. (1997) reported similar neonatal puppy survival rates with either epidural lidocaine or propofol–isoflurane anaesthesia. Use of a local anaesthetic technique may require more time and skill, and adjunctive sedative or tranquillizer drugs may be needed to obtain maternal cooperation. On the other hand, local blocks can effectively augment analgesia and, when used as part of a balanced anaesthetic technique, can reduce the required concentrations of more depressant inhalant agents.

Caesarean section can be performed using a simple infiltrative line block (up to 3 mg/kg lidocaine diluted to the volume required to infiltrate the incision site). Once the puppies or kittens have been delivered, an inhalant anaesthetic agent and analgesics can be administered if needed for surgical wound closure, but this may prove impractical if the trachea is not already intubated: mask inhalant can be used at this point but is not considered to be the best method.

Lidocaine (2–3 mg/kg; of a 2% solution, 6 ml maximum volume) is the preferred agent for epidural anaesthesia for Caesarean section due to its rapid onset and relatively short duration of action. Adrenaline (epinephrine) (5 μg/ml) may be added to prolong analgesia and reduce systemic uptake of the lidocaine (Jones, 2001). If the dura mater is penetrated by the needle and cerebrospinal fluid observed in the hub of the needle (more likely in cats and small dogs), an attempt can be made to reposition the needle into the epidural space. Alternatively, 25–30% of the calculated volume can be injected into the subarachnoid space. If the needle strikes the floor of the spinal canal it may penetrate the distended epidural veins (see Chapter 11). Hypotension secondary to temporary spinal sympathetic nerve blockade may occur, and respiratory compromise or arrest can occur if the block spreads cranially to the cervical region. Hypotension associated with spinal anaesthesia can reduce uterine blood flow and umbilical cord pH more than either epidural or general anaesthesia (Reynolds and Seed, 2005).

Local anaesthetics can cause fetal depression if they accumulate within an acidotic fetus, but this problem usually occurs only when very high or repeated doses are administered. Morphine can also be included in the epidural for Caesarean section (see Chapter 11).

Postoperative analgesia

Unfortunately, at the time of writing there have been no reports of clinical studies investigating the safety of any analgesic drug in the pregnant cat or dog. Consequently, analgesics are often avoided or administered at doses too low to be effective because of concern regarding drug effects on the developing fetus or neonate. The canine fetal liver has limited drug-metabolizing capability, and therefore elimination of drugs is via immature renal mechanisms and/or passive diffusion through the placenta into the maternal circulation (Mathews, 2008).

An opioid can be used to provide maternal analgesia for Caesarean section. After delivery, a drop of naloxone administered sublingually can be used to antagonize the opioid in the neonates (see also below). Alternatively, administration of opioid to the dam/queen can be delayed until after the fetuses have been removed from the uterus; pethidine, butorphanol or buprenorphine will provide analgesia but not overly sedate the mother. In humans, methadone and buprenorphine have been shown to be fairly safe for the treatment of pain during pregnancy (Mathews, 2008).

Caesarean section (with or without concurrent ovariohysterectomy) does not in itself decrease milk production. However, studies in dogs have shown that inadequate pain control and/or poor surgical recovery is more likely to decrease milk production (Traas, 2008).

The non-steroidal anti-inflammatory drugs (NSAIDs) are particularly useful for controlling maternal pain after Caesarean section because they do not produce maternal depression, which was identified by Moon et al. (2000) as a cause of reduced neonatal survival. Although NSAIDs should ideally be administered to the dam before surgery to produce optimal postoperative analgesia, it may be safest to give them after removal of the neonates (Lascelles et al., 1998). Bleeding times are not increased following administration of meloxicam or carprofen in dogs (Deneuche et al., 2004; Fresno et al., 2005). Both NSAIDs and opioids (except hydromorphone) will partition into the mother's milk; however, the amounts are very low (1–2% of the maternal dose), such that use of these drugs for maternal pain control is considered safe for breast-feeding human infants (Spigset and Hagg, 2000). There have been no canine/feline studies measuring partitioning of tramadol into milk, but a study of human infants demonstrated that they receive approximately 2–3% of the total maternal dose via breast milk, with no clinical effects (Bloor et al., 2012). Due to their potential adverse effects on the developing fetal/neonatal kidneys, it is recommended that COX-2 inhibitors, such as carprofen or meloxicam, are administered only once in the nursing dam/queen (Mathews, 2008) (see Chapter 10).

Neonatal resuscitation

A warm, dry box should be prepared ahead of time to receive the neonates. Immediately following delivery, each neonate should be placed on a clean, dry, warm towel, and any membranes and fluid removed from the nose and mouth. Suction equipment can be useful, but cotton-tipped swabs and a bulb syringe are also effective. Bulb syringes have been reported to be effective for clearing fluids and mucus from the upper respiratory tract of newborn puppies following Caesarean section, and caused less trauma compared to a medical syringe attached to a small cannula (Goericke-Pesch and Wehrend, 2012). Vigorous body rubbing is used to dry the neonate and stimulate spontaneous breathing. Swinging the neonate to clear fluids is ineffective and may even be harmful (Seymour, 1999). Mouth-to-mouth/nose resuscitation using gentle pressure while monitoring thoracic movement can be used if the neonate makes no spontaneous breathing attempts; or the trachea can be gently intubated with a cannula or small-diameter tube to permit manual positive pressure ventilation.

Another option for neonatal ventilatory support is mechanical intermittent positive pressure ventilation. The McCulloch Medical™ Aspirator/Resuscitator device has been shown to be effective in clearing the respiratory tract of puppies and kittens, at the same time stimulating ventilation by gently pumping a controlled and repeatable volume of air into their lungs (Smith, 2012).

A slow heart rate, as determined by auscultation, palpation, or Doppler ultrasonography, may indicate neonatal hypoxia. Neonatal oxygen therapy has the potential to raise arterial oxygen tension significantly. Oxygen should therefore be available during resuscitation, especially for compromised neonates (Figure 26.5).

Naloxone (0.01–0.02 mg/kg diluted to an appropriate volume) can be administered intramuscularly, into the neonatal umbilical vein, or dripped sublingually to antagonize opioid-induced depression, if necessary. Doxapram is rarely used in resuscitation of human infants, is not effective during hypoxaemia and is unlikely to result in a positive response when administered to a neonate that is hypoxaemic due to hypoventilation; however, there are anecdotal reports that it can trigger a breath, which may be very effective if oxygen is also available (Pascoe and Moon, 2001).

Acupuncture stimulation of the Governing Vessel 26 point (GV 26) has been successfully used to resuscitate neonatal kittens following Caesarean section (Skarda, 1999). A 25 G, 1.6 cm needle can be used instead of a traditional acupuncture needle. The needle is inserted in the midline of the most dorsal aspect of the area between the upper lip and the nose (philtrum). The needle hub is held between the thumb and index finger and pressed 2–4 mm into the skin and subcutaneous tissue. Vigorous needle stimulation is continued until signs of arousal are observed. Acupuncture treatment of GV 26 may stimulate the sympathetic nervous system, as well as the respiratory and cardiovascular systems.

Apgar scoring, originally developed for assessing the condition of human infants at birth, can be used to examine neonatal survival following Caesarean section in small animals (Seymour, 1999). Each of five physical signs – heart rate, respiratory effort, muscle tone, reflexes, and colour – is scored at 1, 5, and 10 minutes following birth. The scores

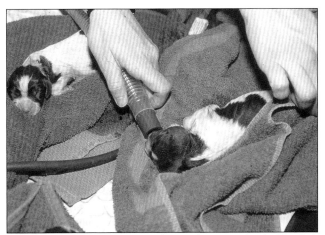

26.5 Puppies may require supplemental oxygen using the 'flow-by' technique. This technique will provide inspired levels of 40% oxygen.
(Courtesy of Tanya Duke-Novakovski, Western College of Veterinary Medicine, University of Saskatchewan, Canada)

provide a 'snapshot' of the newborn's status and the effectiveness of resuscitation (if applied) over time. In humans, the Apgar score is sufficiently sensitive to detect differences between newborns whose mothers received spinal anaesthesia *versus* general anaesthesia for Caesarean section, but it is not specific for the effects of anaesthesia on neonates (Littleford, 2004). Although it would be impractical to perform a complete Apgar score for each puppy in a litter, Luna *et al.* (2004) used an Apgar-like system (assessing heart and respiratory rates; ability to suckle; and withdrawal, anogenital and flexion reflexes) to evaluate neonatal depression following elective Caesarean section. Another study used a modified Apgar scoring system (heart rate, respiratory effort, reflexes, movement and mucous membrane colour) to evaluate puppies, within 5 minutes after birth, for viability and survival prognosis (Veronesi *et al.*, 2009). Puppies with a score of 6 or lower were more likely to die within 2 hours postpartum compared with those scoring 7–10. Delivery method did not affect puppy survival. Apgar scoring has also been combined with umbilical blood lactate concentrations to estimate newborn puppy distress (Groppetti *et al.*, 2010).

Fetal consciousness, sentience and welfare considerations during termination of pregnancy

In veterinary medicine, termination of pregnancy using an elective or emergency ovariohysterectomy is considered an acceptable practice, despite some aesthetic and ethical concerns. Advances in the understanding of mammalian fetal neurodevelopment have suggested that the most humane option for termination of unwanted canine and feline pregnancies is surgical removal of the gravid uterus (White, 2012).

According to recent guidelines on euthanasia produced by the American Veterinary Medical Association (AVMA), fetuses and embryos cannot consciously experience stressful events such as breathlessness or pain, and therefore they cannot 'suffer' while dying *in utero*, regardless of the cause (AVMA, 2013). Although fetal activity (respiratory and body movements) *in utero* is common, it does not indicate fetal consciousness or sentience. Fetal neurodevelopment occurs in a predictable sequence in all mammalian species, but species-specific neurodevelopment can vary following birth (White, 2012). Fetal brain electrical activity on an electroencephalogram (EEG) parallels neurological and behavioural development, and the differentiation of rapid eye movement (REM) from non-REM sleep correlates with the development of capacity for conscious awareness (Mellor, 2010; White, 2012). Mammalian fetuses have three primary degrees of neurodevelopment near the time of birth: exceptionally immature (marsupials), moderately immature (puppies, kittens, rodents, rabbits) and mature (humans, cattle, horses, pigs) (Mellor, 2010). In addition, even at full neurophysiological maturity, the fetal EEG remains quiescent and there is little differentiation between REM and non-REM sleep patterns *in utero* (White, 2012). Fetal EEG inactivity is related to the presence of adenosine, allopregnanolone and pregnenolone, prostaglandin D_2 and placental peptide neuroinhibitor; together, these prevent fetal awareness (Mellor *et al.*, 2010). Lacking consciousness, sentience and awareness, the fetus cannot perceive pain or suffering *in utero*.

Other factors that should be considered when planning an ovariohysterectomy to terminate pregnancy are the choice of anaesthetic agents, and fetal hypoxaemia. Anaesthetic agents administered to the dam will cross the placental barrier and anaesthetize or sedate the fetus, further inhibiting fetal brain activity. During periods of extremely low fetal arterial oxygen tension, for example, during birth or termination of pregnancy, fetal brain activity will become isoelectric, but this does not indicate fetal brain death (White, 2012). An isoelectric fetal brain EEG is a protective mechanism and provides further indication there is no fetal consciousness or sentience during surgical removal of the gravid uterus. After surgical removal, the uterus should not be opened or fetuses removed; exposure of the fetuses to an oxygen-rich environment may stimulate consciousness, necessitating other methods of euthanasia (White, 2012). The appropriate procedures for termination of pregnancy during an ovariohysterectomy are summarized in Figure 26.6.

- After exteriorizing the uterus, retain the fetuses within the placenta and leave alone for 1 hour. Do not open the placenta, otherwise there is a risk of fetal awareness/breathing occurring with exposure to an oxygen-rich environment
- Euthanasia via injection is unnecessary because the fetuses cannot appreciate pain/suffering, due to lack of consciousness, sentience or awareness
- Injecting euthanasia solution into the surgically removed uterine vasculature/umbilical vessels will not aid fetal death due to the lack of maternal placental circulation
- Injecting euthanasia solution into the placental vessels while the uterus is still attached to the dam is NOT recommended, due to inherent risks for the mother
- In the case of Caesarean section, intraperitoneal injection of pentobarbital is recommended for fetuses that have been removed from the uterus, regardless of breathing status (AVMA, 2013)

26.6 Appropriate procedures for termination of pregnancy during ovariohysterectomy in dams and queens (White, 2012).

Anaesthesia of pregnant patients not undergoing Caesarean section

Generally speaking, most elective procedures (e.g. prophylactic dental care, ear cleaning, skin mass removal) for the mother should be postponed until after the puppies/kittens have been weaned.

In cases where emergency surgery of a pregnant patient is necessary, the patient must be stabilized before anaesthesia. Most information regarding anaesthesia for pregnant veterinary patients is derived from human medical studies (Snegovskikh and Braveman, 2012). The main objectives of anaesthetic management in pregnant patients undergoing non-Caesarean procedures are preservation of maternal and fetal safety and prevention of premature labour, related to surgical manipulation and/or drug effects. Induction of, and recovery from, inhalant anaesthesia will be more rapid due to an increase in minute volume and decreased functional residual capacity. Reduced doses (by 25–30%) of local and general anaesthetic agents should be used due to increased sensitivity to these drugs during pregnancy (see also earlier in this chapter).

Teratogenicity (the production of fetal malformation) may occur at any stage during gestation, although the first trimester is the highest-risk period as it is the most critical period for organogenesis. At high doses, many anaesthetic or analgesic drugs have teratogenic effects, but no studies have provided evidence of similar effects with clinical doses. In human medicine, all drugs are classified on the basis of their potential risk in pregnancy. The classification places each drug in category A, B, C, D or X: category A indicates no risk to the fetus (this category contains no anaesthetic/analgesic drugs), while a drug in category X is contraindicated in women who are, or may become, pregnant (Mathews, 2008). Nitrous oxide has been shown to have teratogenic effects in animals, but only with prolonged (1–2 days) direct administration. Enato et al. (2011) reported a two-fold increase in fetal oral cleft malformation associated with benzodiazepine administration in women during early pregnancy. No recent studies have demonstrated teratogenic effects of benzodiazepines in pregnant dams/queens.

The same considerations regarding anaesthesia for Caesarean section can be applied to anaesthesia for non-obstetric procedures in pregnant patients; it is essential to ensure adequate maternal ventilation/oxygenation, blood pressure and maintenance of uterine perfusion in order to maintain fetal oxygenation. The risk of preterm labour should always be considered, especially when abdominal procedures are performed (Snegovskikh and Braveman, 2012).

Local and regional anaesthetic techniques can be considered in order to reduce excessive fetal exposure to anaesthetic/analgesic agents. Opioids are considered to be the analgesics of choice in pregnant animals (Mathews 2008). Studies in pregnant women using opioids for prolonged (weeks) periods have indicated that the fetus can be adversely affected. However, short-term opioid therapy in the pregnant dam/queen should not be withheld; studies in women have shown that methadone is safe at clinical dosages during pregnancy, and buprenorphine has a low transplacental transfer after a single dose. With repeated administrations, however, buprenorphine can accumulate within the placenta, which can result in continuous release into the fetal circulation. In pregnant women, fentanyl rapidly crosses the placental barrier and is detectable in the fetal brain after it has cleared from maternal blood. Fentanyl has also been associated with lower neuro-behavioural test scores at 24 hours after delivery in human infants. However, fentanyl is considered acceptable when combined with epidural bupivacaine during pregnancy. Morphine and its synthetic derivatives (hydromorphone, oxymorphone) can be used safely in pregnant dams/queens, although, as for other opioids, long-term use should be avoided (Mathews, 2008).

Although NSAIDs can be used to provide analgesia after Caesarean section, it is advisable not to administer them to pregnant dams/queens. Reported fetal adverse effects associated with NSAIDs are pulmonary hypertension, nephrotoxicity and renal insufficiency. Teratogenic effects (orofacial clefts and renal embryopathy syndrome) of certain NSAIDs have been reported in human infants (Mathews, 2008). Ideally, NSAIDs should be avoided completely in pregnant patients.

References and further reading

American Veterinary Medical Association (AVMA) (2013) AVMA guidelines for the euthanasia of animals: 2013 edition. Available at www.avma.org/KB/Policies/Documents/euthanasia.pdf.

Andaluz A, Tusell J, Trasserres O et al. (2003) Transplacental transfer of propofol in pregnant ewes. Veterinary Journal 166, 198–204

Anderka M, Mitchell A, Louik C et al. (2012) Medications used to treat nausea and vomiting of pregnancy and the risk of selected birth defects. Birth Defects Research. Part A: Clinical and Molecular Teratology 94, 22–30

Andersen AC (1957) Puppy production to the weaning age. *Journal of the American Veterinary Medical Association* **130**, 151–158

Bloor M, Paech MJ and Kaye R (2012) Tramadol in pregnancy and lactation. *International Journal of Obstetric Anesthesia* **21**, 163–167

Brock N (1996) Anesthesia for canine cesarean section. *Canadian Veterinary Journal* **37**, 117–118

Celleno D, Capogna G, Emanuelli M *et al.* (1993) Which induction drug for cesarean section? A comparison of thiopental sodium, propofol, and midazolam. *Journal of Clinical Anesthesia* **5**, 284–288

D'Alessio JG and Ramanathan J (1998) Effects of maternal anesthesia in the neonate. *Seminars in Perinatology* **22**, 350–362

Deneuche AJ, Dufayet C, Goby L, Fayolle P and Desbois C (2004) Analgesic comparison of meloxicam or ketoprofen for orthopedic surgery in dogs. *Veterinary Surgery* **33**, 650–660

Dewan DM, Floyd HM, Thistlewood JM, Bogard TD and Spielman FJ (1985) Sodium citrate pretreatment in elective cesarean section patients. *Anesthesia and Analgesia* **64**, 34–37

Doebeli A, Michel E, Bettschart R, Hartnack S and Reichler IM (2013a) Apgar score after induction of anesthesia for canine cesarean section with alfaxalone *versus* propofol. *Theriogenology* **80**, 850–854

Doebeli A, Michel E and Reichler I (2013b) Induction of anaesthesia for canine caesarean section with alfaxalone. *Reproductive Biology* **13**, 58 [Abstract]

Ekstrand C and Linde-Forsberg C (1994) Dystocia in the cat: a retrospective study of 155 cases. *Journal of Small Animal Practice* **35**, 459–464

Enato E, Moretti M and Koren G (2011) The fetal safety of benzodiazepines: an updated meta-analysis. *Journal of Obstetrics and Gynaecology Canada* **33**, 46–48

Erden V, Yangin Z, Erkalp K *et al.* (2005) Increased progesterone production during the luteal phase of menstruation may decrease anesthetic requirement. *Anesthesia and Analgesia* **101**, 1007–1011

Evans KM and Adams VJ (2010) Proportion of litters of purebred dogs born by caesarean section. *Journal of Small Animal Practice* **51**, 113–118

Fox MW (1966) Developmental physiology and behavior. In: *Canine Pediatrics*, ed. MW Fox and WA Himwich, pp. 22–25. Charles C. Thomas, Springfield

Fresno L, Moll J, Penalba B *et al.* (2005) Effects of preoperative administration of meloxicam on whole blood platelet aggregation, buccal mucosal bleeding time, and haematological indices in dogs undergoing elective ovariohysterectomy. *Veterinary Journal* **170**, 138–140

Funkquist PME, Nyman GC, Lofgren A-MJ and Fahlbrink EM (1997) Use of propofol–isoflurane as an anesthetic regimen for cesarean section in dogs. *Journal of the American Veterinary Medical Association* **211**, 313–317

Gibbs C, Schwartz D, Wynne J, Hodd CI and Kuck EJ (1979) Antacid pulmonary aspiration in the dog. *Anesthesiology* **51**, 380–385

Gin T, Yau G, Jong W *et al.* (1991) Disposition of propofol at caesarean section and in the postpartum period. *British Journal of Anaesthesia* **67**, 49–53

Gintzler AR and Liu NJ (2001) The maternal spinal cord: biochemical and physiological correlates of steroid-activated antinociceptive processes. *Progress in Brain Research* **133**, 83–97

Goericke-Pesch S and Wehrend A (2012) New method for removing mucus from the upper respiratory tract of newborn puppies following caesarean section. *Veterinary Record* **170**, 289

Groppetti D, Pecile A, Del Carro AP *et al.* (2010) Evaluation of newborn canine viability by means of umbilical vein lactate measurement, Apgar score and uterine tocodynamometry. *Theriogenology* **15**, 1187–1196

Hale TW, McDonald R and Boger J (2004) Transfer of celecoxib into human milk. *Journal of Human Lactation* **20**, 397–403

Herman NL, Li AT, Van Decar TK *et al.* (2000) Transfer of methohexital across the perfused human placenta. *Journal of Clinical Anesthesia* **12**, 25–30

Ilkiw JE, Farver TB, Suter C, McNeal D and Steffey EP (2002) The effect of intravenous administration of variable-dose flumazenil after fixed-dose ketamine and midazolam in healthy cats. *Journal of Veterinary Pharmacology and Therapeutics* **25**, 181–188

Johnston SD and Raksil S (1987) Fetal loss in the dog and cat. *Veterinary Clinics of North America: Small Animal Practice* **17**, 535–554

Jones RS (2001) Epidural analgesia in the dog and cat. *Veterinary Journal* **161**, 123–131

Kjaer K, Comerford M, Kondilis L *et al.* (2006) Oral sodium citrate increases nausea amongst elective Cesarean delivery patients. *Canadian Journal of Anesthesia* **53**, 776–780

Lascelles BD, Cripps PJ, Jones A and Waterman-Pearson AE (1998) Efficacy and kinetics of carprofen, administered preoperatively or postoperatively, for the prevention of pain in dogs undergoing ovariohysterectomy. *Veterinary Surgery* **27**, 568–582

Littleford J (2004) Effects on the fetus and newborn of maternal analgesia and anesthesia: a review. *Canadian Journal of Anesthesia* **51**, 586–609

Luna SPL, Cassu RN, Castro GB *et al.* (2004) Effects of four anaesthetic protocols on the neurological and cardiorespiratory variables of puppies born by caesarean section. *Veterinary Record* **154**, 387–389

Mace SE and Levy MN (1983) Neural control of heart rate: a comparison between puppies and adult animals. *Pediatric Research* **17**, 491–495

Malfertheiner SF, Malfertheiner MV, Kropf S, Costa S-D and Malfertheiner P (2012) A prospective longitudinal cohort study: evolution of GERD symptoms during the course of pregnancy. *BMC Gastroenterology* **12**, 131

Mathews KA (2008) Pain management for the pregnant, lactating, and neonatal to pediatric cat and dog. *Veterinary Clinics of North America: Small Animal Practice* **38**, 1291–1308

McElhatton PR (1994) The effects of benzodiazepine use during pregnancy and lactation. *Reproductive Toxicology* **8**, 461–475

Mellor DJ (2010) Galloping colts, fetal feelings, and reassuring regulations: putting animal-welfare science into practice. *Journal of Veterinary Medical Education* **37**, 94–100

Mellor DJ, Diesch TJ and Johnson CB (2010) When do mammalian young become sentient? *ALTEX—Proceedings of the 7th World Congress on Alternatives and Animal Use in the Life Sciences* **27**, 281–286

Meyer RE (1999) Anesthesia hazards to animal workers. *Occupational Medicine* **14**, 225–234

Moon PF, Erb HN, Ludders JW, Gleed RD and Pascoe PJ (1998) Perioperative management and mortality rates of dogs undergoing cesarean section in the United States and Canada. *Journal of the American Veterinary Medical Association* **213**, 365–369

Moon PF, Erb HN, Ludders JW, Gleed RD and Pascoe PJ (2000) Perioperative risk factors for puppies delivered by cesarean section in the United States and Canada. *Journal of the American Animal Hospital Association* **36**, 359–368

Moon-Massat PF and Erb HN (2002) Perioperative factors associated with puppy vigor after delivery by cesarean section. *Journal of the American Animal Hospital Association* **38**, 90–96

Pascoe PJ and Moon PF (2001) Periparturient and neonatal anesthesia. *Veterinary Clinics of North America: Small Animal Practice* **31**, 315–341

Perez R, Sepulveda L and SantaMaria A (1991) Xylazine administration to pregnant sheep: effects on maternal and fetal cardiovascular function, pH, and blood gases. *Acta Veterinaria Scandinavica. Supplementum* **87**, 181–183

Reynolds F and Seed P (2005) Anaesthesia for Caesarean section and neonatal acid–base status: a meta-analysis. *Anaesthesia* **60**, 636–653

Robbins MA and Mullen HS (1994) *En bloc* ovariohysterectomy as a treatment for dystocia in dogs and cats. *Veterinary Surgery* **23**, 48–52

Sakamoto H, Kirihara H, Fujiki M, Miura M and Misumi K (1997) The effects of medetomidine on maternal and fetal cardiovascular and pulmonary function, intrauterine pressure and uterine blood flow in pregnant goats. *Experimental Animals* **46**, 67–73

Seymour C (1999) Caesarean section. In: *Manual of Small Animal Anaesthesia and Analgesia*, ed. C Seymour and R Gleed, pp. 217–222. BSAVA Publications, Gloucester

Skarda RT (1999) Anesthesia case of the month: Dystocia, cesarean section and acupuncture resuscitation of newborn kittens. *Journal of the American Veterinary Medical Association* **214**, 37–39

Smith FO (2012) Guide to emergency interception during the parturition in the dog and cat. *Veterinary Clinics of North America: Small Animal Practice* **42**, 489–499

Snegovskikh D and Braveman FR (2012) Pregnancy-associated diseases. In: *Stoelting's Anesthesia and Co-Existing Disease, 6th edn*, pp. 558-582. Saunders-Elsevier, Philadelphia

Spigset O and Hagg S (2000) Analgesics and breast-feeding: safety considerations. *Paediatric Drugs* **2**, 223–238

Tan A, Schulze A, O'Donnell CP and Davis PG (2005) Air *versus* oxygen for resuscitation of infants at birth. *Cochrane Database of Systematic Reviews* **18**, CD002273

Traas AM (2008) Surgical management of canine and feline dystocia. *Theriogenology* **70**, 337–342

Veronesi MC, Panzani S, Faustini M and Rota A (2009) An Apgar scoring system for routine assessment of newborn puppy viability and short-term survival prognosis. *Theriogenology* **72**, 401–407

White SC (2012) Commentary: Prevention of fetal suffering during ovariohysterectomy of pregnant animals. *Journal of the American Veterinary Medical Association* **240**, 1160–1163

Chapter 27

Endocrine diseases

Kata O. Veres-Nyéki

Both general anaesthesia and surgery result in endocrine, immunological and haematological responses; together, these changes lead to a physiological stress response. Noxious stimuli – from surgical manipulation, starvation, dehydration, hypovolaemia, hypothermia, infection, immobilization and hypoxia – contribute to the afferent arm of the stress response. After central processing, this results in activation of the hypothalamic–pituitary–adrenal axis (HTP-AA) (Figures 27.1 and 27.2). Locally, these stimuli provoke release of cytokines, mainly interleukin (IL)-6, tumour necrosis factor-alpha and IL-1, which are responsible for initiating the acute phase response, the early systemic defence mechanism aiming to restore homeostasis through a group of inflammatory and physiological processes that are involved in the innate immune responses to infection, tissue trauma, stress, neoplasia and inflammation (Cray *et al.*, 2009). The magnitude and duration of the endocrine, immunological and metabolic changes are proportional to the invasiveness and duration of the procedure. However, provision of local and systemic analgesia can modify the afferent arm of the stress

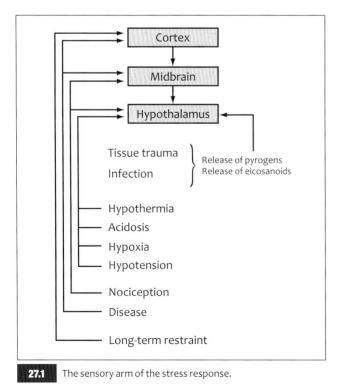

27.1 The sensory arm of the stress response.

response and mitigate the negative responses arising from tissue trauma and noxious stimulation.

Activation of the HTP-AA leads to increased secretion of pituitary hormones and ultimately, increased release of cortisol. In addition, endogenous catecholamines are released from the adrenal glands, resulting in tachycardia, hypertension and increased systemic vascular resistance. These hormones facilitate catabolic processes by increasing the metabolic rate and oxygen consumption. They also cause other metabolic changes such as hyperglycaemia, possibly through inhibition of alpha adrenoceptors and consequent reduced insulin release. Increased protein catabolism provides substrates for the liver to produce acute phase proteins and for gluconeogenesis. The release of antidiuretic hormone (ADH; also known as arginine vasopressin) from the posterior pituitary gland stimulates water retention to increase the circulating blood volume.

Cytokines are produced by white blood cells, fibroblasts and endothelial cells. They act on the receptors of many target cells and have a wide range of functions. As well as triggering the production of acute phase proteins in

27.2 The effector arm of the stress response.
ACTH = adrenocorticotropic hormone; CNS = central nervous system; CRH = corticotropin-releasing hormone.

the liver, they induce fever and stimulate the production and maturation of B and T lymphocytes and haemopoietic cells, and interact with the neuroendocrine system.

The function of the stress response is to preserve or restore homeostasis. However, a severe alteration in endocrine function will jeopardize the patient's ability to maintain homeostasis and may increase the likelihood of peri-anaesthetic complications.

This chapter describes the endocrine disorders of cats and dogs that may have an impact on anaesthetic management. Important physiological and pathophysiological considerations are highlighted. For each disease, the breed, age and sex predispositions, typical clinical signs and abnormalities in laboratory parameters are presented in Figures 27.3, 27.4 and 27.5.

Condition	Age/sex predisposition	Predisposed breeds
Feline hypersomatotropism	Middle-aged or older neutered males	None
Hyperadrenocorticism	Rare	None
Hypoadrenocorticism	Extremely rare	None
Feline hyperaldosteronism	Middle-aged or older	None
Hyperthyroidism	Middle-aged or older, no sex predisposition	None
Diabetes mellitus	None	In the UK: Burmese, Domestic Shorthair In the USA: Domestic Longhair, Maine Coon, Russian Blue, Siamese
Insulinoma	Very rare (only four reported cases)	Three were Siamese

27.3 Reported age, sex and breed predispositions of endocrine diseases in cats.

Condition	Age/sex predisposition	Predisposed breeds
Diabetes insipidus	None	German Shepherd, Husky, Miniature Poodle
Syndrome of inappropriate ADH secretion	Extremely rare	None
Hyperadrenocorticism	Middle-aged or older	Beagle, Boston Terrier, Boxer, Dachshund, Jack Russell Terrier, Miniature Poodle, Staffordshire Bull Terrier, Yorkshire Terrier
Hypoadrenocorticism	Young or middle-aged bitches	Bearded Collie, Great Dane, Leonberger, Nova Scotia Duck Tolling Retriever, Portuguese Water Spaniel, Rottweiler, Standard Poodle, Wheaten Terrier
Hyperparathyroidism	Older, no sex predisposition	Primary hyperparathyroidism is inherited in Keeshonds
Hypoparathyroidism	Uncommon	None
Hypothyroidism	None	Afghan Hound, Airedale Terrier, Borzoi, Boxer, Chow-Chow, Cocker Spaniel, Dachshund, Dobermann, English Bulldog, Giant Schnauzer, Golden Retriever, Great Dane, Irish Setter, Irish Wolfhound, Miniature Poodle, Miniature Schnauzer, Newfoundland, Rhodesian Ridgeback, Rottweiler, Scottish Deerhound, Shetland Sheepdog
Diabetes mellitus	Intact female dogs in dioestrus	In the UK: Cairn Terrier, Cavalier King Charles Spaniel, Border Collie, Labrador Retriever, Samoyed, Tibetan Terrier, Yorkshire Terrier, crossbreeds In the USA: Miniature Schnauzer, Miniature Poodle, Samoyed
Insulinoma	None	Boxer, Border Collie, Fox Terrier, German Shepherd, Irish Setter, Standard Poodle

27.4 Reported age, sex and breed predispositions of endocrine diseases in dogs. ADH = antidiuretic hormone.

Condition	Clinical signs	Typical laboratory findings
Diabetes insipidus	• PU/PD (up to 20 times greater water consumption and excretion than normal) • Anorexia • Weakness, ataxia • Seizures, stupor (hyperosmotic dehydration)	• Decreased urea concentration (washout) • Hyposthenuric (as low as 1.000 mOsm/l) or • isosthenuric urine • Increased PCV (if restricted access to water) • Hyperproteinaemia • Hypernatraemia (>170 mmol/l) • Serum hyperosmolarity (>375 mOsm/l) • Relative and absolute hypovolaemia • Prerenal azotaemia
Syndrome of inappropriate ADH secretion (Schwartz-Bartter syndrome)	• PU/PD • Weakness, lethargy • Nausea, vomiting • Tremor • Anorexia • Irritable behaviour, confusion • Cardiac arrhythmias • Head pressing • Seizures and coma	• Hyponatraemia • Hypokalaemia • Hypochloraemia and consequent metabolic alkalosis • Decreased urea concentration • High urine sodium (>20 mmol/l) despite hyponatraemia • High urine osmolarity (>150 mOsm/l) • Low plasma osmolarity (<280 mOsm/l)

27.5 Typical clinical signs and laboratory findings of endocrine diseases in cats and dogs. ADH = antidiuretic hormone; CK = creatine kinase; PCV = packed cell volume; PU/PD = polyuria/polydipsia. (continues)

Condition	Clinical signs	Typical laboratory findings
Feline hypersomatotropism	• Organomegaly (renomegaly, hepatomegaly and enlargement of endocrine organs) • Enlargement of extremities • Increased muscle mass • Cardiomegaly and consequent systolic murmur • Congestive heart failure • Azotaemia • Peripheral neuropathy	• Hyperglycaemia • Hypercholesterolaemia • Elevated liver enzymes • Hyperphosphataemia • Proteinuria • Glucosuria
Hyperadrenocorticism (Cushing's syndrome)	• PU/PD • Polyphagia, obesity • Heat intolerance • Lethargy • Hepatomegaly • Abdominal distension • Panting • Muscle weakness • Recurrent urinary tract infections • Dermatological problems • Slow tissue healing • Hypertension • Hypercoagulability and thromboembolism • Polyneuropathy and polymyopathy • Corneal ulceration	• Elevated liver enzymes • Increased bile acids • Hypercholesterolaemia • Hyperglycaemia • Decreased urea concentration • Low urine specific gravity with proteinuria • Stress leucogram • Erythrocytosis • Thrombocytosis
Hypoadrenocorticism (Addison's disease)	• Waxing and waning symptoms • Hypovolaemia, hypotension • Lethargy • Nausea, intermittent vomiting and diarrhoea • Impaired renal perfusion • Muscle weakness • Decreased cardiac conduction and bradycardia • Excitability • Anorexia	• Hyponatraemia (<135 mmol/l) • Hyperkalaemia (>5.5 mmol/l) • Sodium:potassium ratio of <25:1 • Hypochloraemia (<100 mmol/l) • Hyperphosphataemia • Azotaemia (prerenal or renal) • Metabolic acidosis • Increased PCV (dehydration) • Eosinophilia • Lymphocytosis • Low urine specific gravity (medullary washout)
Feline hyperaldosteronism (Conn's syndrome)	• Hypertension • Muscle dysfunction, weakness • Acute onset of blindness and other neurological signs • Left ventricular hypertrophy • Systolic heart murmur • Tachycardia • Gallop rhythm • Concomitant diseases: chronic kidney disease and hyperthyroidism	• Hypokalaemia • Metabolic alkalosis due to increased potassium and hydrogen ion excretion • Elevated CK concentrations if myopathy is present
Phaeochromocytoma	• Generalized weakness and episodic collapse • Tachycardia • Systemic hypertension • Excessive panting, tachypnoea • Arrhythmias • Retinal haemorrhage or detachment (hypertension)	• Increased PCV • Leucocytosis or stress leucogram • Catecholamine measurement from the urine can support the diagnosis
Hyperparathyroidism	• PU/PD (calcium acts as ADH antagonist) • Stranguria, pollakiuria, urolithiasis • Lethargy • Exercise intolerance • Shivering • Facial pain, discomfort when eating, inappetence • Vomiting • Constipation • Stiff gait and lameness	• Hypercalcaemia • Low serum phosphate concentration • If renal insufficiency is present: increased urea, creatinine and phosphate concentrations
Hypoparathyroidism	• Anorexia • Hyperventilation • Paraesthesia • Facial rubbing • Restlessness • Stiff, stilted gait • Generalized tetany and seizures	• Hypocalcaemia • Hyperphosphataemia
Feline hyperthyroidism	• Weight loss despite polyphagia • PU/PD • Hyperactive and difficult to handle • Hypertrophic cardiomyopathy	• Erythrocytosis • Stress leucogram • Increased urea concentration (increased catabolism) • Normal creatinine

27.5 (continued) Typical clinical signs and laboratory findings of endocrine diseases in cats and dogs. ADH = antidiuretic hormone; CK = creatine kinase; PCV = packed cell volume; PU/PD = polyuria/polydipsia. (continues)

Condition	Clinical signs	Typical laboratory findings
Feline hyperthyroidism (continued)	• Hypertension • Tachyarrhythmias	• Elevated liver enzymes • Decreased serum cholesterol • Mild hyperglycaemia • Hyperphosphataemia • Decreased serum total calcium • Hypokalaemia • Increased glomerular filtration and decreased urine specific gravity
Canine hypothyroidism	• Obesity • Lethargy, intolerance to cold • Bradycardia • Decreased cardiac contractility • Low-voltage R waves • Atherosclerosis • Neurological signs (facial nerve paralysis, vestibular disease, lower motor neuron disorders, myxoedema coma) • Dermatological signs (alopecia, thickened skin, dry coat, poor hair regrowth and retention of puppy hair) • Constipation, slow gastric emptying • Joint pain • Periorbital oedema • Reduced drug metabolism	• Anaemia • Hypercholesterolaemia (decreased conversion of lipids to bile acids) • Elevated liver enzymes and CK • Hyponatraemia (due to water retention)
Diabetes mellitus	• PU/PD • Dramatic, rapid weight loss with good appetite or anorexia • Weakness • Lethargy • Dehydration • Vomiting and diarrhoea • Unkempt hair coat • Enlarged liver • Strong acetone odour in breath • Cataracts (dogs), abnormal pupillary light reflexes or other cranial nerve abnormalities • Muscle twitching or seizure activity (severe hyperglycaemia) • Diabetic neuropathy (cats)	• Hyperglycaemia (up to >25 mmol/l), especially if severe dehydration is present • Elevated liver enzymes • Hypercholesterolaemia • Increased triglycerides • Increased urea and creatinine concentrations (due to dehydration)
Insulinoma	• Very weak, collapse possible • Neurological signs (altered mentation, dullness, recumbency, ataxia, blindness, altered vision, seizures, coma) • Tachycardia and arrhythmia (adrenergic activation by hypoglycaemia or electrolyte imbalances)	• Severe hypoglycaemia with high/normal insulin

27.5 (continued) Typical clinical signs and laboratory findings of endocrine diseases in cats and dogs. ADH = antidiuretic hormone; CK = creatine kinase; PCV = packed cell volume; PU/PD = polyuria/polydipsia.

Hypothalamus and hypophysis

The hypothalamus regulates body temperature, sleep, hunger, thirst, fear and aggression. It also provides neuroendocrine control of many organs via secretion of corticotropin-releasing hormone, thyrotropin-releasing hormone and gonadotropin-releasing hormone, all of which are involved in regulating the release of hormones from the anterior hypophysis (adenohypophysis) (Figure 27.6).

Adrenocorticotropic hormone

The anterior hypophysis releases adrenocorticotropic hormone (ACTH), which is primarily responsible for regulating the secretion of hormones from the adrenal cortex, especially cortisol. Release of cortisol has a diurnal rhythm, and also increases during periods of stress. Chronic glucocorticoid administration leads to functional atrophy of the HTP-AA, which may take several months to recover. Patients on long-term treatment with glucocorticoids often require corticosteroid supplementation during anaesthesia to prevent refractory hypotension.

Antidiuretic hormone

Direct activation of hypothalamic osmoreceptors results in synthesis of ADH, which is secreted from the posterior hypophysis (neurohypophysis). ADH synthesis can also be indirectly stimulated when cardiac stretch receptors and baroreceptors are stimulated by hypovolaemia, abolishing vagal inhibition of the osmoreceptors. The main role of ADH is to conserve water and to regulate the osmolarity of body fluids by activating aquaporin channels in the distal convoluted renal tubules and collecting ducts, which facilitates reabsorption of free water. Aquaporin channels are activated by stimulation of non-catecholamine transmembrane cell-signalling type V_2 receptors. If ADH is produced and released in excess, oxygen delivery to the tissues may become compromised because ADH also has powerful vasoconstrictive properties, which are mediated by stimulation of V_1 receptors. In contrast, production of insufficient ADH will lead to hypotension.

ADH release is provoked by a range of factors, such as exercise, nausea, stress, haemorrhage, pain, anaesthesia and certain drugs (opioids, apomorphine, beta adrenergic

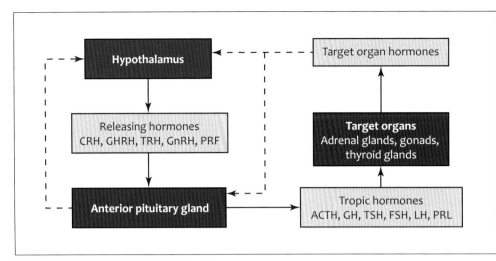

27.6 Feedback mechanisms in the hormone secretions of the hypothalamo-pituitary-adrenal axis. Solid line = stimulation of secretion; dashed line = negative feedback. ACTH = adrenocorticotropic hormone; CRH = corticotropin-releasing hormone; FSH = follicle-stimulating hormone; GH = growth hormone; GHRH = growth hormone-releasing hormone; GnRH = gonadotropin-releasing hormone; LH = luteinizing hormone; PRF = prolactin-releasing factor; PRL = prolactin; TRH = thyrotropin-releasing hormone; TSH = thyroid-stimulating hormone.

drugs, insulin, metoclopramide). Intermittent positive pressure ventilation (IPPV) decreases cardiac filling pressures, which also leads to increased release of ADH and consequent fluid retention. Conversely, water intake and certain drugs (glucocorticoids, all alpha adrenoceptor agonists, phenytoin, tetracyclines) may inhibit ADH release. As body water regulation is strictly controlled, both the lack of ADH (diabetes insipidus; see below) and its overproduction will severely affect this delicate balance.

Diabetes insipidus

There are two forms of diabetes insipidus (DI). Central DI is the result of insufficient ADH production, while in nephrogenic DI, renal receptors are unresponsive to ADH. The most common causes of central DI are brain tumours, infiltrative brain disease or head trauma. Pituitary surgery has also been reported to result in transient or permanent central DI in dogs (Teshima *et al.*, 2011). Hypokalaemia, hypercalcaemia, certain drugs (glucocorticoids, barbiturates, all alpha adrenoceptor agonists), cortisol, fluoride, lithium, pyelonephritis, pyometra, Gram-negative sepsis, portosystemic shunts, liver insufficiency, hypoadrenocorticism (in dogs) and hyperthyroidism (in cats) can all decrease renal responsiveness to ADH, thus provoking nephrogenic DI.

Complete central DI is the more common form in cats and dogs; partial central DI can also occur, although it is difficult to distinguish between the two types. Water deprivation before anaesthesia is contraindicated for patients with DI because severe dehydration, hypovolaemia and possible hyperosmotic encephalopathy may develop as the kidneys continue to excrete dilute urine, despite reduced or absent water intake. If the patient has hyperosmotic dehydration with hypernatraemia, slow correction with intravenous infusion of either 5% dextrose in water, or 0.45% saline with 2.5% dextrose, is recommended; it is important to avoid a decrease in plasma sodium concentration of >0.5 mmol/l/h, and the aim should be to correct dehydration completely over 72 hours. Providing the patient with sudden unrestricted access to water may lead to cerebral oedema.

Restoration of intravascular volume is a necessary part of pre-anaesthetic preparation. For patients with central DI, treatment with the synthetic ADH analogue desmopressin, administered nasally, may also be indicated. For those patients previously diagnosed and treated for DI, the patient's usual dose of desmopressin should be given

before anaesthesia. Isotonic fluid therapy should be administered to avoid development of water depletion and hypernatraemia (>160 mmol/l). If plasma osmolarity is increased, hypotonic fluids should be administered. Desmopressin has no action on V_1 receptors and so does not cause excessive vasoconstriction and hypertension. Stress and surgical stimulation can also increase endogenous ADH release in patients with central DI.

For patients with nephrogenic DI, a low-sodium and low-protein diet may help with pre-anaesthetic stabilization. In humans, chlorpropamide (5–40 mg/kg orally q24h) increases renal responsiveness to ADH, but has some additional diuretic effect in the loop of Henle and also provokes hypoglycaemia. The patient's blood glucose should therefore be monitored if chlorpropamide is administered. Hydrochlorothiazide (2.5–5.0 mg/kg orally q12h) has been used in cats and dogs to reduce hypernatraemia, but additional fluid therapy is essential to prevent further dehydration.

Syndrome of inappropriate ADH secretion (Schwartz–Bartter syndrome)

Either increased ADH release or increased renal response to ADH causes the syndrome of inappropriate ADH secretion (SIADH), which is extremely rare in cats and dogs (<10 reported cases). The transient nature of this syndrome may be partially responsible for the low incidence of diagnosis.

In humans, ectopic ADH production, altered control of ADH release or mutation of the V_2 receptor are known causes of the syndrome. The condition has been associated with pulmonary disease, neoplasia, central nervous system (CNS) disorders, bilateral head and neck surgery, adverse drug reactions (to antidepressants, neuroleptics, antineoplastic agents, non-steroidal anti-inflammatory drugs (NSAIDS), opioids), acquired immunodeficiency syndrome, prolonged strenuous exercise and senile atrophy. In dogs, dirofilariasis, granulomatous amoebic meningoencephalitis, hydrocephalus, meningeal sarcoma and trans-sphenoidal hypophysectomy have been reported as possible causes of SIADH (Chastain, 2009; Shiel, 2012).

Persistent ADH production despite decreased plasma osmolarity will lead to normovolaemic hyponatraemia (<120 mmol/l). The reabsorption of free water by the kidney results in extracellular volume expansion and the consequent natriuresis makes the hyponatraemia even worse.

Sedated or anaesthetized patients with SIADH that are receiving fluid therapy cannot compensate for the increased fluid load and therefore fluid restriction is recommended. In patients with severe hyponatraemia, hypertonic saline can be administered slowly (to achieve a maximum rate of increase in plasma sodium concentration of 0.5 mmol/l/h). Plasma potassium concentration should also be corrected. In addition, furosemide can be administered to facilitate excretion of excess free water. The successful use of a V_2 receptor antagonist OPC-31260 (3 mg/kg orally q12h) has been described for treatment of a dog with SIADH (Fleeman *et al.*, 2000). During the perianaesthetic period, the volume status of the patient should be monitored by using central venous pressure (CVP) measurements (see Chapters 7 and 18). Plasma sodium concentration, and if possible, plasma and urine osmolarity, should be monitored and tightly regulated.

Post-traumatic hypopituitarism and HTP-AA dysfunction

Brain trauma may cause suppression of hormone release from the anterior pituitary gland and decreased ADH secretion from the posterior pituitary gland. Trauma can therefore lead to central DI, hypoadrenocorticism, hypothyroidism and deficiencies in growth hormone (GH) and sex hormones, although these changes are usually transient. Patients with post-traumatic decreases in pituitary hormone release can be obtunded, anorexic and hypothermic, with hypernatraemia, hyperkalaemia, hypoglycaemia, hypotension and hyposthenuria.

Radiation therapy and hypophysectomy (see below) can also lead to temporary or long-term HTP-AA dysfunction.

Feline hypersomatotropism and canine pituitary-dependent hyperadrenocorticism

Excess GH secretion from a slowly growing pituitary somatotroph adenoma, after epiphyseal closure, is relatively common in cats, and results in acromegaly. Because GH is a potent modulator of cellular sensitivity to insulin, these patients often have uncontrolled insulin-resistant diabetes mellitus (DM), polyuria/polydipsia (PU/PD) and polyphagia, as well as weight gain. Over 25% of cats with insulin-resistant DM also have acromegaly (Figure 27.7). The facial soft tissue swelling, subglottic stenosis and enlarged tongue associated with acromegaly can make endotracheal intubation difficult in these patients. In addition, enlargement of abdominal viscera results in increased pressure on the diaphragm and can contribute to hypoventilation.

Hypophysectomy is a promising treatment for feline hypersomatotropism and also for canine pituitary-dependent hyperadrenocorticism (Cushing's disease; see later in this chapter). For the procedure, the animal must be placed in sternal recumbency with the mouth widely opened (Figure 27.8). In cats, extreme opening of the mouth may cause compression of the maxillary artery, which reduces cerebral blood flow and may result in postoperative blindness (Stiles *et al.*, 2012; Barton-Lamb *et al.*, 2013). During anaesthesia, access to the head is limited and use of an armoured endotracheal tube is recommended. Additional venous access and compatible blood should be available in the event that transfusion is required. Regular measurement of packed cell volume (PCV) (every hour), electrolytes (every hour) and glucose (every 30 minutes) is recommended. Close monitoring for any signs of increased intracranial pressure (ICP) is necessary, with appropriate treatment (mannitol,

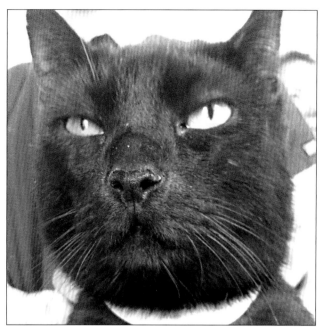

27.7 Acromegaly in a cat due to feline hypersomatotropism.
(Courtesy of Kieran Borgeat, Royal Veterinary College, London, UK)

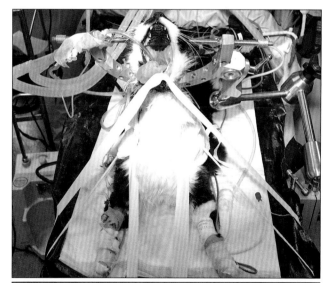

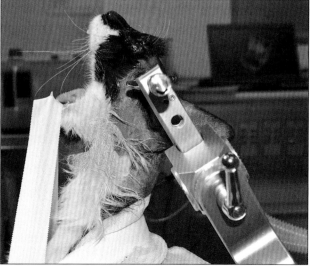

27.8 Postioning of a cat for hypophysectomy.

maintenance of normocapnia or even moderate hypocapnia; see Chapter 28) administered. To avoid detrimental increases in ICP, a central venous catheter should be placed postoperatively and not beforehand.

The pituitary gland is partially or completely resected via a trans-sphenoidal approach. After hypophysectomy, the patient will need transient (5 days to 2 weeks) or permanent hormone replacement therapy for hypoadrenocorticism, hypothyroidism and central DI. Hydrocortisone substitution (0.5 mg/kg/h i.v.) should be started and maintained until the animal can take oral medications. ADH replacement can be managed by the application of desmopressin eye drops. Replacement of sex hormones and GH is necessary only if the patient shows clinical signs. Hormone substitution therapy for cats and dogs is described in Figure 27.9. Postoperative alterations may occur in blood glucose and plasma sodium concentrations and in arterial blood pressure (ABP). Continuous monitoring of CVP and ABP and regular measurement (every 3–4 hours) of electrolytes, PCV, total solids and blood glucose is therefore recommended. If there is mild hypernatraemia, infusion of half-strength normal saline (0.45%) or 2.5% glucose, with potassium supplementation, is necessary. For severe hypernatraemia, 5% glucose with potassium supplementation can be administered. As these patients are often obtunded after the surgery, the eyes should be lubricated and attention paid to other areas of nursing care (see Chapters 3 and 28).

Radiation treatment can also be used for cats and dogs with hypersomatotropism or pituitary-dependent hyperadrenocorticism with concurrent neurological signs. This treatment option requires frequent anaesthetics for each dose of radiation, but the anaesthetist cannot be in the room during irradiation (Figure 27.10). See Chapter 29 for discussion of remote anaesthesia and Chapter 28 for anaesthetic considerations for patients with neurological disease.

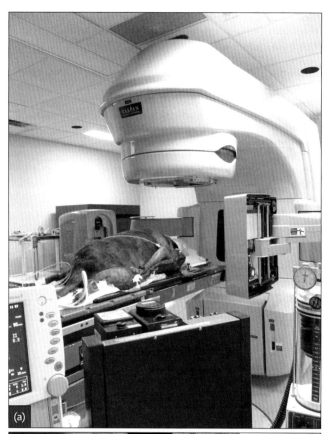

(a)

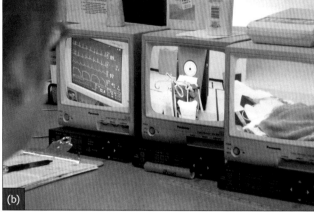

(b)

27.10 (a) Dog undergoing radiation treatment using a linear accelerator. (b) Closed circuit television is being used to observe the dog and anaesthetic monitors during anaesthesia while irradiation is underway.
(a, Courtesy of Vivian Fan, Western College of Veterinary Medicine, University of Saskatchewan, Canada; b, Courtesy of Michael Raine, Western College of Veterinary Medicine, University of Saskatchewan, Canada)

Cats[a]	
Drug	**Dose**
Hydrocortisone	0.5 mg/kg/h i.v. infusion until oral medication is possible
Desmopressin	1 drop (~5 µg) q8h topically on conjunctiva (alternating eyes)
As soon as the cat is drinking and eating: oral substitution therapy	
Hydrocortisone	2.5 mg orally q12h (reduced to q24h in second week)
Levothyroxine	15 µg/kg orally q12h (reduced to q24h in second week)
Desmopressin	1 drop (~5 µg) q8h (reduced over a period of 1–2 months)
Dogs[b]	
Drug	**Dose**
Prednisolone	0.05–0.2 mg/kg orally every other day
Desmopressin	3–5 µg/per eye topically on conjunctiva q12–24h
Levothyroxine	15–30 µg/kg orally q12–24h
Fludrocortisone acetate	If hyperkalaemia is present: 0.0025–0.01 mg/kg q12h

27.9 Postoperative hormone substitution therapy after hypophysectomy in cats and dogs.
([a] Protocol by Stijn Niessen, Royal Veterinary College, University of London, UK. [b] Data from Hara et al., 2003)

Adrenal glands

The adrenal cortex produces more than 30 different corticosteroids and sex hormones, while the adrenal medulla secretes adrenaline (epinephrine) and noradrenaline (norepinephrine). There are two major classes of corticosteroids: mineralocorticoids and glucocorticoids. Mineralocorticoids, of which aldosterone is the most important, regulate plasma sodium and potassium concentrations. Glucocorticoids, of which cortisol is the most important, regulate carbohydrate, fat and protein metabolism and also have anti-inflammatory effects. Release of mineralocorticoids is controlled by renin, which is produced by the kidney in response to decreased ABP or plasma sodium concentration. Renin transforms angiotensinogen (produced by the liver) to angiotensin I, which is then converted to angiotensin II by angiotensin converting enzyme (ACE). Angiotensin II stimulates the cortical zona glomerulosa to produce aldosterone and also causes vasoconstriction. Increased plasma potassium concentrations will also stimulate the zona glomerulosa to release aldosterone independently from the renin–angiotensin system. Aldosterone simultaneously stimulates sodium absorption and potassium secretion in the renal distal convoluted tubules and collecting ducts. Because water follows sodium, the action of aldosterone increases extracellular fluid volume, cardiac output and ABP.

Cortisol has mainly glucocorticoid activity; it improves cardiac function by increasing the number and/or responsiveness of beta adrenoceptors in the myocardium and permits normal responsiveness of arterioles to the vasoconstrictive action of catecholamines. Cortisol inhibits bone formation and produces skeletal muscle weakness by mobilizing amino acids from extrahepatic sites (except the heart and brain) to the liver for gluconeogenesis. It also increases the rate of lipolysis and redistributes fat into the liver and abdomen. In general, glucocorticoids inhibit the effect of ADH at the renal distal tubule.

The anti-inflammatory effects of cortisol include stabilization of lysosomal membranes and decreases in leucocyte migration, capillary permeability, numbers of circulating eosinophils and leucocytes, and antibody production. Because of these effects, corticosteroids are useful for the treatment of allergic reactions, although they do not alter histamine release. The basal output of cortisol strongly increases during the stress response and usually returns to normal after 24 hours (Church et al., 1994).

Opioids and locoregional anaesthesia both reduce the release of cortisol induced by surgical stimulation, although there is a marked increase in circulating cortisol concentration when the effects of the local nerve blockade wear off. Volatile anaesthetic agents also produce some suppression of cortisol release, and etomidate inhibits cortisol synthesis. Chronic administration of corticosteroids also reduces the ability of the adrenal glands to release endogenous cortisol in stressful situations.

The cells of the adrenal medulla are equivalent to postganglionic cells of the sympathetic nervous system (SNS) and release mainly adrenaline with some noradrenaline. Stress and hypoglycaemia are the main stimuli for catecholamine release. Adrenaline causes increases in blood glucose concentration via stimulation of hepatic glycogenolysis and gluconeogenesis, inhibition of insulin secretion via alpha-2 adrenoceptors and stimulation of glucagon secretion. Adrenaline also promotes lipolysis, which is potentiated by glucocorticoids. Activation of myocardial beta-1 adrenoceptors results in an increase in both the force and rate of contraction, with a shortening of de-polarization time. Both adrenaline and noradrenaline cause arteriolar vasoconstriction, but within the skeletal muscles and heart, adrenaline produces a beta-2-mediated vasodilation; as a result, total peripheral resistance and diastolic arterial blood pressure decrease while cardiac output increases. By acting on beta-2 adrenoceptors, adrenaline also causes relaxation of bronchial and gastro-intestinal smooth muscle. Both adrenaline and noradrenaline have an excitatory action on the CNS. They promote mydriasis and ciliary body relaxation, and they cause contraction of the urinary bladder neck and relaxation of the bladder body, which leads to urinary retention. The catecholamines also potentiate sweating and piloerection in some species.

Hyperadrenocorticism (Cushing's syndrome)

Hyperadrenocorticism is one of the most commonly diagnosed endocrinopathies in dogs. In 85% of cases, a pituitary tumour is responsible, but adrenal neoplasia or hyperplasia can also lead to hyperadrenocorticism, especially in large-breed female dogs. In cats, hyperadrenocorticism is rare and usually originates from pituitary dysfunction. Cushing's syndrome is usually managed medically, but patients with the disease may require anaesthesia for other reasons.

The increased cortisol production in hyperadrenocorticism stimulates gluconeogenesis and protein and fat catabolism, and leads to the redistribution of adipose tissue both dorsally and within the abdomen (Figure 27.11). Both the release and action of ADH are inhibited, resulting in polyuria, which necessitates adequate peri-anaesthetic fluid therapy to prevent dehydration.

As a result of the abdominal distension, respiratory muscle weakness, pulmonary mineralization and possible pulmonary thromboembolism that characterize this disease, these patients have poor respiratory function and are prone to hypoxaemia and hypercapnia. Ventilatory support is therefore recommended. These patients are usually hypertensive because of increased activation of the renin–angiotensin system, increased responsiveness to catecholamines and decreased release of vasodilatory prostaglandins. Decreased hepatic function, hypercoagulability (due to increased production of factors II, VII, IX and X), fragile skin that is prone to bruising and delayed primary wound healing may also be observed and should be taken into account.

Patients with hyperadrenocorticism can be stabilized by decreasing cortisol production. Trilostane blocks adrenal synthesis of glucocorticoids, mineralocorticoids and sex steroids, but may result in adrenal necrosis, with subsequent hypoadrenocorticism, vomiting and diarrhoea. Ketoconazole, which has a similar mode of action to trilostane, has also been used in the past. Mitotane, an adrenocorticolytic drug, selectively destroys the zonae fasciculata and reticularis of the adrenal cortex. Side effects of mitotane treatment are hypoadrenocorticism, anorexia, vomiting and diarrhoea. Selegiline, a monoamine oxidase (MAO) inhibitor, inhibits ACTH secretion from the pituitary gland by increasing dopaminergic tone, although its efficacy is reported to be poor. Co-administration of selegiline with pethidine (meperidine) and tramadol, other

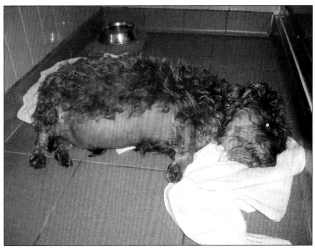

27.11 Dog with hyperadrenocorticism, with a typical pot-bellied appearance.
(Courtesy of Marieke de Vries, Davies Veterinary Specialists, Higham Gobion, UK)

MAO inhibitors and tricyclic antidepressants is contra-indicated because this may result in increased noradrenaline and serotonin concentrations, causing adverse effects (see Chapter 2).

In patients with a pituitary tumour, hypophysectomy may be considered (see above). Anaesthesia for adrenalectomy carries a high risk of complications, and the perioperative mortality rate can be as high as 26% (Barrera *et al.*, 2013). Preoperative staging with thoracic radiographs, computed tomography and abdominal ultrasonography provide a more detailed assessment of the patient's condition. The hypertrophied adrenal gland or adrenal tumour is usually fragile and there is a risk of haemorrhage during surgery. Compatible blood should be readily available during the procedure, and adequate venous access should be secured for rapid transfusion or for administration of emergency medications. Close monitoring of ABP is mandatory and the mean arterial blood pressure should be maintained within the range 70–90 mmHg in patients with pre-existing hypertension. In humans, perioperative use of angiotensin-converting enzyme (ACE) inhibitors reduces peripheral vascular tone and aldosterone secretion, but may result in refractory hypotension after adrenal tumour removal. In patients that have a unilateral adrenal tumour, the contralateral adrenal gland is often atrophied and glucocorticoid supplementation may be required (Figure 27.12). If the post-ACTH stimulation cortisol concentration remains within the range 30–100 µg/l, adrenocortical function is preserved; if not, supplementation will be needed. In cases of bilateral adrenalectomy, lifelong replacement therapy will be required.

Drug	Dose and comments
Dexamethasone	0.05–0.1 mg/kg i.v. total dose once tumour is removed 0.03–0.07 mg/kg i.v. q24h until oral prednisolone can be given
Prednisolone	0.2–0.5 mg/kg orally q24h for 3–4 months
If plasma serum sodium concentration <135 mmol/l or potassium >6.5 mmol/l:	
Desoxycorticosterone pivalate	2.2 mg/kg i.m. or s.c. Check sodium and potassium concentrations after 25 days: 1. If normal, re-evaluate after 7–10 days; if still normal, no further mineralocorticoid treatment needed 2. If hyponatraemia or hyperkalaemia is still present, 1.1 mg/kg s.c. and re-evaluate after 25 days

27.12 Protocol for postoperative corticosteroid substitution after adrenal tumour removal.
(Taken from recommendations by Galvao and Chew, 2011)

The hypercoagulable state of these patients means that pulmonary thromboembolism is a potential complication during the first 72 hours after surgery. To prevent this, routine anticoagulant therapy should be administered: heparinized plasma (35 IU/kg heparin to 10 ml/kg canine plasma) intraoperatively followed postoperatively by subcutaneous heparin (35 IU/kg s.c.) twice at an 8-hour interval and then tapered doses for 2–3 days (day 2: 25 IU/kg q8h; day 3: 15 IU/kg q8h). Postoperatively, frequent short walks will promote blood flow and minimize clot formation. Opioid medication for postoperative pain will help to allow the patient to exercise and also ensure better lung ventilation. NSAIDs should be avoided, as they can have severe side effects if the endogenous corticosteroid concentration is high.

Hypoadrenocorticism (Addison's disease)

Addison's disease results from deficient aldosterone and/or glucocorticoid production by the adrenal cortex. Primary idiopathic hypoadrenocorticism is the most common form in dogs, and is probably immune mediated. Its development is often precipitated by systemic mycosis, metastatic tumours, haemorrhagic infarction, cortical amyloidosis or canine distemper. Secondary hypoadrenocorticism is caused by decreased ACTH secretion (due to a pituitary tumour, hypothalamic lesion or prolonged negative feedback from exogenous corticosteroid therapy); this leads to glucocorticoid, but not mineralocorticoid, deficiency. Glucocorticoid deficiency impairs renal excretion of water, decreases carbohydrate, protein and fat metabolism and decreases stress tolerance, but rarely produces electrolyte imbalances. An ACTH stimulation test can help to guide diagnosis, and can reveal hypocortisolaemia and hypoaldosteronaemia; however, corticosteroid supplementation will interfere with the test because of cross-reaction in the cortisol assays (except dexamethasone).

These patients will require pre-anaesthetic stabilization: dehydration, electrolyte and acid–base disturbances should be corrected and corticosteroids administered. A dramatic improvement is usually seen following fluid therapy. Several treatment options have been described for administration of supplemental corticosteroids during critical hypoadrenocorticism (Figure 27.13). The crystalloid fluid of choice for intravenous therapy is 0.9% saline, but rapid correction of hyponatraemia should be avoided. During an Addisonian crisis, 10–30 ml/kg/h of 0.9% saline should be administered (depending on the condition of the patient) during the first 2–3 hours, followed by 5–7.5 ml/kg/h, and plasma sodium and potassium concentrations should be measured hourly.

Drug(s)	Dose and comments
Hydrocortisone sodium succinate	Equipotent glucocorticoid and mineralocorticoid activity Adheres to plastic and glass Incompatible with ampicillin sodium Minimum concentration is 1 mg/ml – needs to be diluted with saline 0.5 mg/kg/h i.v. infusion or bolus 4–10 mg/kg q6h
Prednisolone sodium succinate[a] and dexamethasone sodium phosphate[b]	[a] 4–20 mg/kg as bolus followed by [b] 0.05–0.1 mg/kg in fluid therapy, infused over 12 hours
Dexamethasone sodium phosphate	0.1–2.0 mg/kg i.v. bolus followed by i.v. infusion (0.05–0.1 mg/kg in fluid therapy, infused over 12 hours)

27.13 Options for corticosteroid substitution in Addisonian crisis.
(Taken from recommendations by Church, 2012)

Patients with hypoadrenocorticism have decreased stress tolerance; therefore, enough fluid should be provided during anaesthesia to counteract hypotension and hypovolaemic shock. Placement of a jugular catheter is recommended to facilitate fluid therapy. Animals with normal gastrointestinal and renal function should start on oral corticosteroid supplementation as soon as possible. Long-term hormone replacement therapy can be provided by using either the semi-selective mineralocorticoid fludrocortisone, or the selective mineralocorticoid desoxycorticosterone pivalate (DOCP) combined with the semi-selective glucocorticoid prednisolone.

Feline hyperaldosteronism (Conn's syndrome)

Hyperaldosteronism is increasingly being recognized as a cause of hypokalaemia and hypertension in cats. It usually originates from a unilateral adrenal neoplasm. In these patients, hypokalaemia and hypertension should be controlled before anaesthesia; amlodipine besylate is used to treat hypertension (0.625–1.25 mg/cat orally q24h), and the competitive aldosterone antagonist spironolactone (2–4 mg/kg orally q24h) can control both hypokalaemia and hypertension.

Surgical treatment usually consists of unilateral adrenalectomy, but has a very high mortality rate (33%). Expected complications are severe haemorrhage from the caudal vena cava, and the presence of a caval thrombus can make surgical resection more complicated. The chronic hypertension could cause retinal detachment and consequent blindness. Wound healing problems may also occur if the patient has concurrent hypercortisolism.

Phaeochromocytoma

Phaeochromocytomas are adrenal tumours characterized primarily by the secretion of noradrenaline, *not* adrenaline. The innervation of the tumour is different from that of the normal adrenal gland, and the circumstances that might provoke catecholamine secretion are not yet clear. At the time of diagnosis, one-third of dogs already have metastases. Neoplastic invasion of the vena cava is common and the eroded vena cava may rupture, resulting in haemoperitoneum or haemoretroperitoneum. Neurological signs may develop as a result of tumour metastasis or thromboembolism in the spinal cord. Unlike hyperadrenocorticism, a phaeochromocytoma does not cause atrophy of the contralateral adrenal gland. Abdominal ultrasonography and/or other diagnostic imaging techniques are used to assess tumour size and the presence of caval invasion or thrombus. An ophthalmic (fundic) examination should also be made to assess whether there is any retinal detachment. ABP measurement, haematology and biochemistry profiles, and blood typing or cross-matching are all recommended before surgery. The patient should be stabilized before surgery because of the potential for life-threatening haemodynamic instability, which is particularly likely to occur during induction of anaesthesia and during surgical manipulation of the mass.

Pre-anaesthetic treatment with the non-specific alpha adrenoceptor blocker phenoxybenzamine has been shown to reduce perioperative mortality in dogs with a phaeochromocytoma (Herrera *et al.*, 2008). The drug is administered in the 2–3 weeks before surgery at an initial dose of 0.5 mg/kg q12h, which is gradually increased every few days until either clinical signs of hypotension (lethargy, weakness, syncope) or vomiting occur, or to a maximum dose of 2.5 mg/kg q12h. Treatment is continued at the highest chosen dose and surgery scheduled for 1–2 weeks later. Prazosin is used in humans, but has been shown to provoke a significant decrease in blood pressure in Beagles (Fischer *et al.*, 2003); its use as a pre-treatment in dogs with phaeochromocytoma therefore requires further evaluation. Treatment with a beta adrenoceptor antagonist such as propranolol (0.2–1 mg/kg orally q8h) or atenolol (0.2–1 mg/kg q12–24h orally) should be started if severe, persistent tachycardia is also present. It is essential to ensure that alpha adrenergic blockade is established first before beta adrenergic blockers are administered, otherwise severe hypertension may occur

because of the patient's inability to produce beta-2 receptor-mediated vasodilation.

Arrhythmogenic (e.g. xylazine, thiopental) and anticholinergic drugs should be avoided in these patients. Neuromuscular blocking agents are relatively contraindicated because their effects may require reversal using anticholinergic drugs with neostigmine or edrophonium (see Chapter 16). Administration of metoclopramide should be avoided, as it blocks dopamine receptors and can increase catecholamine concentrations through this action. Continuous monitoring of the patient's electrocardiogram (ECG) is recommended before induction or even before pre-anaesthetic medication, as ventricular tachycardia, arrhythmias or cardiac arrest can occur as a result of noradrenaline release. The author prefers pre-anaesthetic medication with opioids alone, but the addition of a low dose of acepromazine can be considered, especially in nervous dogs, to provide anxiolysis and decrease SNS tone. However, acepromazine-induced blockade of alpha-1 adrenoceptors is long lasting, and the drug may have additive hypotensive effects when used with other alpha-1 antagonists. Ketamine increases SNS tone and etomidate depresses adrenocortical activity, so neither drug is recommended for induction.

Balanced anaesthetic techniques incorporating isoflurane or sevoflurane and an opioid infusion are recommended for maintenance. Nitrous oxide and desflurane should be avoided, as both increase SNS tone and may promote hypertension and/or cardiac arrhythmias. Epidural analgesia with opioids can provide good perioperative analgesia, but the use of epidural local anaesthetics, which can induce profound hypotension via sympathetic blockade, should be avoided. NSAIDs can be given at the end of the surgery (or anaesthesia), once the blood pressure is stable and within normal limits. Tumour removal will cause an acute decline in circulating catecholamine concentrations, and severe haemodynamic instability may result. If cardiovascular collapse occurs after tumour removal, intravenous administration of phenylephrine (1–3 µg/kg/min), noradrenaline (0.1–1 µg/kg/min) or, if catecholamine sensitivity is decreased, vasopressin (0.2–0.8 IU/kg bolus and/or 0.002–0.006 IU/kg/min infusion) can help to restore normal cardiovascular function. Higher infusion rates of fluids and vasopressors are often required in these patients compared to other patients.

Severe sinus tachycardia without hypotension can be treated by intravenous administration of esmolol (0.05–0.5 mg/kg bolus followed by 25–200 µg/kg/min). Pathological ventricular arrhythmias with polymorphic complexes and the R-on-T phenomenon will necessitate treatment with intravenous lidocaine (boluses of 2–4 mg/kg i.v.). Severe intraoperative hypertension can be treated by intravenous administration of the short-acting alpha adrenoceptor antagonist phentolamine (0.1 mg/kg loading dose followed by 1–2 µg/kg/min infusion) or the direct vasodilator sodium nitroprusside (0.1–10 µg/kg/min). Phentolamine should be readily available if phenoxybenzamine was not used before surgery. In humans, magnesium sulphate is sometimes used to provide intraoperative vasodilation (30 mg/kg infused over 10 minutes).

Adrenalectomy in these cases can cause severe intraoperative haemorrhage, especially if the right adrenal gland is affected and the caudal vena cava is involved. Clamping of the vena cava (to enable tumour removal) will reduce venous return and cardiac output, with severe haemodynamic consequences, such as reflex tachycardia or bradycardia due to suddenly reduced venous return (Bezold–Jarisch reflex). Temporary or permanent occlusion of the suprarenal vena cava may also lead to renal injury. If a collateral circulation has developed due to chronic partial obstruction of the vena cava, resection will be easier. The use of controlled intraoperative hypothermia will decrease oxygen consumption and may mitigate the effect of vessel occlusion, but will prolong coagulation times.

Invasive blood pressures (CVP and ABP) and ECG should be continuously monitored during anaesthesia and closely monitored in the first 24 hours postoperatively. Urinary output should be measured for at least 24 hours postoperatively. Ventricular tachyarrhythmias, dyspnoea, disseminated intravascular coagulopathy, acute pancreatitis, oliguric renal failure, abdominal incisional dehiscence, internal haemorrhage and vomiting are the most common postoperative complications (Brainard and Mandell 2009; Galvao and Chew, 2011).

Parathyroid glands

Hyperparathyroidism

Parathyroid hormone (PTH) is continuously secreted by chief cells, which are located in the four parathyroid glands. Its release is primarily stimulated by low plasma calcium concentrations. PTH release is also stimulated by adrenaline and high plasma phosphate concentrations, via stimulation of beta receptors located on the chief cells. High plasma magnesium and vitamin D concentrations decrease its secretion.

The main roles of PTH are to increase plasma calcium concentration and decrease plasma phosphate concentration; both directly, by acting on the kidneys and bone, and indirectly, by promoting vitamin D synthesis. Calcium has an essential role in coagulation, neuromuscular function and muscle contraction; it acts as a neurotransmitter, intracellular messenger and enzyme activator, and therefore its plasma concentration must be strictly controlled.

Primary hyperparathyroidism is rare, but is still the third most common cause of ionized hypercalcaemia in dogs. It is caused by either an adenoma, a carcinoma or adenomatous hyperplasia of a parathyroid gland. Secondary hyperparathyroidism may arise as a result of an underlying problem, such as chronic renal failure or hyperadrenocorticism; and, usually more parathyroid glands are involved in these cases.

If the patient has no signs of renal or cardiovascular dysfunction, hypercalcaemia usually does not require any special treatment before anaesthesia. However, dehydration should be corrected and the ionized calcium concentration should be normalized as much as possible; 0.9% saline should be administered at an appropriate rate to increase glomerular filtration and calcium loss by providing extra sodium ions to compete with calcium ions for reuptake. After adequate rehydration, furosemide (1–2 mg/kg i.v. or s.c., followed by an infusion of 0.2–1 mg/kg/h i.v. in a hypercalcaemic crisis; or 1–2 mg/kg orally q12h) can be given; this drug may also decrease tubular reuptake of calcium and thus facilitate calcium loss. Glucocorticoids increase renal calcium loss and decrease intestinal calcium uptake and bone resorption, and therefore they can be administered when fluid therapy and furosemide are insufficient. Bisphosphonates (inhibitors of bone resorption), calcitonin (4 IU/kg i.v. in emergency), plicamycin or dialysis may also be alternative therapeutic options. However, despite all treatments, the ionized calcium concentration may remain elevated.

The binding of calcium to albumin is decreased at lower plasma pH and ionized calcium increases; because of this, respiratory or metabolic acidosis can worsen hypercalcaemia. Intraoperative ECG monitoring is mandatory to detect S–T segment elevation, shortened P–R or Q–T intervals, arrhythmias or bradycardia caused by hypercalcaemia.

Administration of vitamin D 24–36 hours before surgery can prevent dramatic postoperative hypocalcaemia after parathyroid gland removal in hypercalcaemic patients. Up to three parathyroid glands can be removed during surgery, but at least one gland must remain in order to maintain calcium homeostasis. The remaining gland(s) may be atrophied, and therefore calcium homeostasis should be assessed by measuring ionized calcium concentration every 12 hours during the first 48 hours after surgery and once daily thereafter until the fifth postoperative day. If clinical signs of hypocalcaemia occur (muscle fasciculations or tremors, face rubbing, hypersensitivity to external stimuli, stiff and stilted gait, tetanic seizures, respiratory arrest, agitation, anxiety, vocalization, aggression, panting, pyrexia), calcium supplementation should be started. In an emergency situation, 10% calcium gluconate (0.5–1.0 ml/kg) should be administered slowly by the intravenous route over 20–30 minutes until the clinical signs resolve. Continuous ECG monitoring is necessary during calcium administration, and if S–T segment elevation, shortened P–R or Q–T intervals, arrhythmias or bradycardia are detected, administration should be stopped. After the first bolus, a further 10–15 ml/kg can be administered as an infusion over 24 hours if necessary. Calcium supplements must not be administered together with bicarbonate-containing fluids in the same intravenous line because precipitation of calcium salts will occur. Subcutaneous administration of calcium-containing solutions is contraindicated as this can result in sterile abscess formation or skin sloughing.

Hypoparathyroidism

In primary hypoparathyroidism, the low plasma PTH concentration causes hypocalcaemia and hyperphosphataemia. Other potential causes of hypocalcaemia include hypoalbuminaemia, hypomagnesaemia, hypovitaminosis D, citrate infusion or anticonvulsant therapy. Myocardial contractility is reduced and hypotension is common, and a prolonged Q–T interval may result in atrioventricular blocks. If the patient has any clinical signs of hypocalcaemia (usually apparent at ionized calcium concentrations <1.0 mmol/l), the ionized calcium concentration should be normalized before anaesthesia by administering calcium gluconate (see above). Seizures caused by hypocalcaemia do not respond to standard anticonvulsant therapy. Hyperventilation should be avoided because alkalosis will decrease the ionized calcium concentration and promote hypocalcaemia.

Thyroid glands

Feline hyperthyroidism

Hyperthyroidism is the most common endocrinopathy in cats caused by adenomatous hyperplasia, thyroid adenoma or adenocarcinoma. Patients with hyperthyroidism will require pre-anaesthetic stabilization of thyroid hormone concentration. Antithyroid medications for cats include methimazole (10–15 mg/cat divided in 2–3 oral doses/day or 5 mg applied to internal ear pinna every 12 hours in a transdermal gel form) or carbimazole (5 mg/cat orally q8h). Another option for treatment is therapy with radioactive iodine.

The increased concentration of thyroid hormone indirectly increases SNS tone to allow cardiac output to increase and meet the increased metabolic requirements associated with the disease. Over the longer term this will result in the development of hypertrophic cardiomyopathy or, very rarely, dilated cardiomyopathy. These changes may be reversible if the cat regains euthyroid status during the early stages. Hyperthyroid cats often have tachycardia (>240 beats/min), a 'gallop' rhythm and a systolic heart murmur, which usually originates from a dynamic right and left ventricular outflow obstruction. The high cardiac output can also mask underlying renal failure, and after successful treatment of hyperthyroidism deteriorating renal function and/or chronic renal failure may be observed. A sudden, rapid increase in circulating thyroid hormone may provoke a 'thyroid storm', which can manifest as hyperthermia, hypertension, CNS disturbances, severe vomiting and diarrhoea, abdominal pain, icterus, cardiac murmurs (with or without arrhythmias), atrial fibrillation, ventricular tachycardia, congestive heart failure, tachypnoea, pleural effusion, pulmonary oedema, retinopathies, extreme muscle weakness, cervical ventroflexion, thromboembolic disease or sudden death. Emergency treatment consists of beta blockers (esmolol) to manage ventricular tachycardia, and furosemide, ACE inhibitors (enalapril, benazepril), isosorbitol dinitrate, topical nitroglycerine and hydralazine for congestive heart failure. These drugs must be administered with care if the patient's renal function is compromised. Hyperthermia can be mitigated by the use of fans and fluid therapy with cool fluids. Other treatments may include potassium, dextrose and vitamin B supplementation (to prevent thiamine deficiency).

Hyperthyroid cats have an increased metabolic rate, which may make them more prone to tissue hypoxia if the higher oxygen demand is not met. Hyperthyroidism also results in a higher glucose demand and greater carbon dioxide production, and more rapid metabolism of drugs. Preoperative hypertension is usually treated with beta blockers or a calcium channel blocker such as amlodipine (0.625–1.25 mg/kg orally or rectally q12–24h).

Pre-anaesthetic medication should aim to decrease stress and catecholamine release, and reduce myocardial irritability. The combination of an opioid with a benzodiazepine is a good option; in addition, low doses of acepromazine may protect the heart from catecholamine-induced arrhythmias. A low dose of an alpha-2 adrenoceptor agonist (Lamont et al., 2002), combined with an opioid, can decrease heart rate and therefore myocardial oxygen demand. Nonetheless, preoxygenation before induction of anaesthesia is recommended. Alfaxalone (3 mg/kg s.c.) combined with butorphanol (0.2 mg/kg s.c.) has been reported to provide adequate sedation with cardiovascular stability in hyperthyroid cats; however, 24% of the cats had tremors during recovery (Ramoo et al., 2013).

Induction of anaesthesia can be performed by intravenous administration of propofol, alfaxalone or etomidate, or facemask induction with isoflurane or sevoflurane can be used in well-sedated cats. It is important to minimize stress to the patient, as stress can provoke a thyroid storm in hyperthyroid cats. Vigilant monitoring of the cardiovascular and respiratory systems is essential. To meet the increased glucose requirement, solutions containing 2.5–5% dextrose can be used for fluid therapy if required.

Supraventricular or ventricular tachycardia, ectopic atrial or ventricular arrhythmias or atrial fibrillation can be seen in uncontrolled hyperthyroid patients. Atrial fibrillation will potentiate the development of thromboembolic disease. To prevent thrombi formation, low-dose aspirin (5 mg/cat q72h orally) and heparin (200–400 IU/kg s.c. q6–8h until a markedly prolonged activated partial thromboplastin time is achieved) can be administered. Ventricular tachycardia can be treated with beta blockers. Acute hypertensive crises during anaesthesia can be treated with an intravenous infusion of either sodium nitroprusside (0.5-5.0 µg/kg/min) or nicardipine (0.5–5 µg/kg/min), although these drugs are unlikely to be available in first-opinion practices. If anticholinergic drugs are necessary, glycopyrronium is preferred over atropine to prevent excessive myocardial oxygen demand.

The thyroid mass may compress the trachea, which can compromise airflow and cause difficulties during intubation. After tumour removal, tracheomalacia and collapse can occur, and swelling at the surgical site can also lead to respiratory obstruction and dysphagia. Therefore, it is important to be prepared to reintubate the patient rapidly during the postoperative period in case of emergency.

The tumour may also compress other structures, causing dysphagia by pressing on the oesophagus, laryngeal nerve dysfunction or Horner's syndrome by the compression of the sympathetic trunk. Thyroid tumours are very vascular and their removal may cause severe haemorrhage; a transfusion may therefore be required. Inadequate perioperative perfusion of the parathyroid glands may provoke hypocalcaemia, and therefore the calcium concentration should be checked postoperatively, similar to following parathyroidectomy (see above). After bilateral thyroidectomy, patients will often need life-long thyroid hormone supplementation.

Further details on the anaesthetic management of hyperthyroidism may be found in Chapter 21.

Canine hypothyroidism

Dogs with clinical hypothyroidism tend to be overweight and have a decreased ventilatory response to hypoxaemia and hypercapnia, reduced functional residual capacity, decreased myocardial contractility, hypotension, impaired clearance of free water (leading to hyponatraemia), hypoglycaemia and possibly decreased anaesthetic requirements. Hypothyroidism should ideally be corrected before anaesthesia and thyroid hormone replacement medication given on the morning of anaesthesia. Untreated patients undergoing anaesthesia often require treatment with positive inotropes, vasopressors, aggressive fluid therapy and mechanical ventilatory support. Chronic hyponatraemia should be corrected slowly (see earlier). Due to a decreased metabolic rate, prolonged recovery is common, and these patients are also prone to hypothermia.

Drugs such as phenobarbital, diazepam, trimethoprim/sulphonamide, quinidine, NSAIDs and glucocorticoids decrease the plasma concentration of thyroid hormones and can potentiate a hypothyroid crisis. During a severe crisis (myxoedema coma), levothyroxine (5 µg/kg i.v. and later orally q12h) can be administered, and significant improvement is usually apparent within 24–30 hours (Pullen and Hess, 2006). Thyroid tumours may also cause problems for venous drainage from the head and may potentially produce an oedematous airway (Figure 27.14).

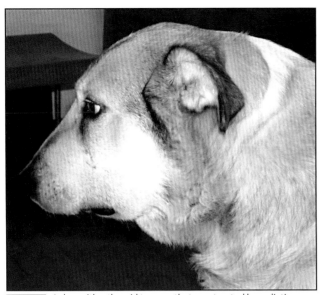

27.14 A dog with a thyroid tumour that was treated by radiation therapy in order to improve venous drainage from the head. Endotracheal intubation during treatment is essential to protect the airway.
(Courtesy of Dr Monique Mayer, Western College of Veterinary Medicine, University of Saskatchewan, Canada)

Pancreas

The islets of Langerhans in the pancreas release four main hormones: insulin (secreted by the beta cells), glucagon (alpha cells), somatostatin (delta cells) and pancreatic polypeptide (gamma cells). Insulin is an anabolic hormone with a short elimination half-life of 5 minutes. It promotes storage of glucose, fatty acids and amino acids, and causes glucose and potassium to move into cells where glucose is phosphorylated. Glucose transport into the brain, liver and red and white blood cells is, however, not insulin dependent.

Insulin secretion is regulated by a negative feedback mechanism, and is diminished at blood glucose concentrations <2.8 mmol/l. Peak insulin release occurs at glucose concentrations >16 mmol/l. Beta cells have a rich adrenergic innervation: beta adrenergic stimulation or the release of acetylcholine facilitates insulin release, while alpha adrenergic stimulation or beta blockade inhibits insulin release. Glucagon, GH and corticosteroids potentiate glucose-induced insulin secretion, but prolonged use of corticosteroids will lead to beta cell exhaustion and DM. Conversely, somatostatins, diazoxide, thiazide diuretics, volatile anaesthetic agents and (due to negative feedback) insulin itself all inhibit insulin secretion. Due to a particular gastrointestinal signalling mechanism, oral glucose intake provokes greater release of insulin compared to intravenous administration of glucose. Insulin facilitates the use of glucose for energy production, promotes glycogen production in the liver and skeletal muscle, and inhibits gluconeogenesis from amino acids. Cats are obligate carnivores and are not metabolically adapted to deal with excessive carbohydrate intake; as a result, their insulin response to dietary carbohydrates is unique, as amino acids are the main signal for insulin release. Cats can use gluconeogenic precursors such as amino acids to maintain a physiological glucose concentration for up to 72 hours of food deprivation. Feline insulin is most similar to bovine insulin, and canine insulin is identical to porcine insulin.

Glucagon is a catabolic hormone with an elimination half-life of 3–6 minutes, which mobilizes glucose, fatty acids and amino acids into the systemic circulation. Secretion of glucagon is stimulated by hypoglycaemia. Glucagon promotes hepatic gluconeogenesis and glycogenolysis in a similar way to adrenaline, and also enhances myocardial contractility. Somatostatin, which is identical to the GH-release inhibitory hormone secreted by the hypothalamus, regulates hormone secretion from the islet cells by inhibiting insulin and glucagon release.

Diabetes mellitus

Diabetes mellitus occurs with either an absolute insulin deficiency (type 1 DM; more common in dogs) or resistance to the effects of insulin (type 2 DM; more common in cats). The prevalence of DM in dogs in the UK is 0.32% (Davison et al., 2005). In female dogs, both progesterone produced in dioestrus and GH released from the mammary glands counteract the effect of insulin, and can thus provoke DM by hormonal antagonism. The insulin-resistant type of DM caused by progesterone can be prevented by early ovariohysterectomy.

Both type 1 and type 2 DM result in chronic hyperglycaemia, which leads to damage and dysfunction of the kidney, eye, autonomic nervous system, heart and vasculature, including the microcirculation. Damage to these tissues increases the overall anaesthetic risk. The renal threshold for glucose is 12–14 mmol/l; at higher concentrations, glucose cannot be reabsorbed any faster from the urine. This leads to an osmotic diuresis and consequent progressive dehydration and hyperosmolarity (>350 mOsm/l). Reduced glomerular filtration and concurrent renal failure may worsen the hyperglycaemia and hyperosmolarity. To compensate for the hyperosmolarity, increased natriuresis occurs, with subsequent hyponatraemia. Potassium and phosphorus are also lost as a result of diuresis. The plasma free fatty acid concentration increases as insulin-induced inhibition of lipase is removed. The liver produces ketones from free fatty acids to provide an energy source for skeletal and cardiac muscles; this increased ketone production usually leads to ketoacidosis, and urinary excretion of ketones results in further depletion of electrolytes, mainly potassium. However, hypokalaemia may not be observed, as intracellular potassium ions are exchanged for extracellular protons to mitigate extracellular acidosis, and oliguric patients can become hyperkalaemic. If some insulin secretion is maintained, it can block lipolysis and prevent ketoacidosis. Increased release of stress hormones will further worsen the metabolic acidosis and hyperglycaemia. This promotes osmotic diuresis and facilitates hyperviscosity, leading to thromboembolism, and exacerbates renal failure; all these factors can have fatal consequences. Approximately 50% of ketoacidotic dogs have a non-regenerative anaemia, left shift neutrophilia and thrombocytosis. In cats, increased plasma beta-hydroxybutyrate concentration and hypophosphataemia potentiate Heinz body formation and anaemia. Diabetic patients have compromised immune function, and concurrent diseases are also common. In dogs with DM, pancreatitis, urinary tract infection and hyperadrenocorticism are often seen, while in cats, hepatic lipidosis, chronic renal failure, acute pancreatitis, bacterial or viral infections and neoplasia are common. Diabetic patients may also suffer from autonomic neuropathy.

Stress can increase blood glucose concentration, especially in cats, to up to 10–15 mmol/l for at least 3–4 hours (Davison, 2012; Rand, 2012). As a result, blood glucose measurements made in the peri-anaesthetic period may increase above the reference range. To aid diagnosis, the concentration of glycosylated blood proteins (such as fructosamine) in the blood can be measured. The fructosamine concentration will reflect the average blood glucose concentration over the previous 1–2 weeks (depending on the protein turnover of the patient) and it therefore represents a more reliable monitor of glycaemic control in dogs. Unfortunately, in cats, fructosamine concentrations are unchanged until the blood glucose concentration constantly exceeds 20 mmol/l.

If a diabetic patient requiring an elective procedure has ketoacidosis, preoperative stabilization is highly recommended (Figure 27.15). Acidosis decreases myocardial contractility and causes peripheral vasodilation, and the patient may also become mentally obtunded. Fluid deficits should be replaced; this can effectively decrease the glucose concentration and alleviate acidosis, but may uncover severe hypokalaemia, which will require aggressive replacement therapy. Bicarbonate should be administered only if there is severe acidosis (pH <7.1 or bicarbonate <12 mmol/l). Fluid therapy should aim to decrease the glucose concentration slowly, to prevent rapid alteration in intracranial osmolarity and subsequent cerebral oedema. The main aims are to restore fasting glucose concentration, normalize plasma fructosamine concentration and reverse any complications.

For elective procedures, patients with DM should be fasted from midnight and scheduled to be anaesthetized in the morning, to allow full recovery and return to their normal schedule of feeding and insulin administration as soon as possible (see Figure 27.15 for insulin recommendations). It is advisable to measure plasma electrolytes, as unexpected abnormalities are sometimes found in these patients. If in doubt, urinalysis for the presence of ketones should be performed, and if ketonuria is present, the patient should be started on intravenous fluid therapy preoperatively. Unfortunately, commercially

available urinalysis sticks are not sensitive to beta-hydroxybutyrate, which is the main ketone in cats, and so this simple method is effective only in dogs. Stable diabetic patients can easily destabilize when a simple comorbidity, such as a urinary tract infection, is present; a good history and thorough pre-anaesthetic clinical examination are therefore very important (see Chapter 2). Ideally, drugs that can be antagonized (opioids, benzodiazepines) or that are rapidly eliminated (propofol, etomidate, alfaxalone, inhalant anaesthetics) without causing significant 'hang-over' should be used. Alpha-2 adrenoceptor agonist drugs exacerbate hyperglycaemia by inhibiting the release of insulin; therefore, they should be avoided. Neuromuscular blocking agents are commonly used in ocular surgeries and present no problems for DM patients. The use of local anaesthetic techniques is recommended, but in diabetic human patients the risk of nerve injury is higher and local anaesthetic requirements are lower because of neuropathy.

In humans, rigorous control of blood glucose concentration has been shown to improve wound healing and neurological outcome after CNS ischaemic insult, and to reduce risk of perioperative infections. However, owing to the stress related to anaesthesia and surgery, and to hospitalization in general, glucose concentrations are often increased in animals, and values >20 mmol/l are not unusual in normally treated diabetic patients. The frequency of glucose measurements will depend on the actual glucose concentration and its trend, but measurement every 30–60 minutes during anaesthesia is recommended. After recovery from anaesthesia, the patient should be fed a small amount of food as soon as possible, blood glucose measured and routine insulin treatment continued. Those patients injected with long-acting insulin once daily should return to their normal routine the next day, and patients on a twice-daily regimen should have their evening insulin dose on the day of surgery.

Unfortunately, hand-held glucometers developed for medical use are inaccurate at the low end of their scale, and can indicate a value 20–40% or 1–2 mmol/l lower than the actual glucose concentration. A veterinary-specific glucometer (AlphaTRAK©; www.alphatrakmeter.co.uk) is more reliable, requires only 0.3–0.6 μl of blood and is calibrated for both feline and canine blood (Figure 27.16). Whichever type of glucometer is used, always ensure that the same glucometer is used for measurements on an individual patient, to allow for inherent analyser error. In patients with severe hyperglycaemia, glucose can also be measured in the urine using a urinalysis stick.

Insulinoma

Insulinomas are insulin-secreting malignant tumours of the pancreatic beta cells. They are most commonly seen in middle-aged or older dogs; unfortunately, 50% of these patients will already have metastases at the time of diagnosis.

Pre-anaesthetic stabilization consists of feeding small, frequent meals that contain low amounts of simple sugars to prevent sudden insulin release and consequent severe hypoglycaemia. Glucocorticoids (prednisolone 0.5–1.0 mg/kg/day orally, divided into two doses), diazoxide (10 mg/kg/day up to 60 mg/kg/day orally, divided into two doses) or somatostatin analogues (octreotide 10–40 μg/kg s.c. q8–12h) can inhibit pancreatic insulin secretion and improve pre-anaesthetic stabilization. Streptozotocin selectively destroys pancreatic beta cells

Insulin administration on the morning of surgery	
Blood glucose	
<8 mmol/l	No insulin required
8–15 mmol/l	Give half of the regular dose of insulin
>15 mmol/l	Give full insulin dose
Blood glucose monitoring	
Depending on glucose values; at least every 30–60 minutes	
Management of severe alterations	
Hypoglycaemia (<3 mmol/l)	0.25–0.5 g/kg diluted glucose as slow intravenous bolus
Hyperglycaemia (>30 mmol/l)	Give normal insulin protocol and start intravenous fluid therapy
Intravenous administration of insulin for dogs with diabetic ketoacidosis	
2.2 IU/kg regular crystalline insulin added to 250 ml of 0.9% saline (flush set with 50 ml of the solution before administration)	
Blood glucose	
>14 mmol/l	0.9% saline 10 ml/h
11–14 mmol/l	0.9% saline with 2.5% dextrose 7 ml/h
8–11 mmol/l	0.9% saline with 2.5% dextrose 5 ml/h
5.5–8 mmol/l	0.9% saline with 5% dextrose 5 ml/h
<5.5 mmol/l	0.9% saline with 5% dextrose *without insulin*

27.15 Perioperative management of blood glucose in diabetic patients. Based on recommendations by Hess (2015).

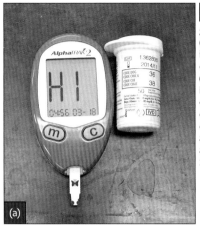

27.16 A veterinary-specific glucometer showing (a) high blood glucose level in an insulin-resistant diabetic cat and (b) glucose concentration in a dog with diabetic cataract, indicating that only half the regular dose of insulin is to be administered before anaesthesia (see Figure 27.15).

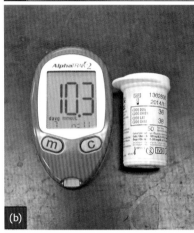

the effect of the medetomidine. Ketamine and propofol, with or without benzodiazepines, are commonly used for induction of anaesthesia. Pancreatitis has been reported following propofol administration in humans, albeit very rarely. Epidural anaesthesia and/or fentanyl infusions will usually provide adequate perioperative analgesia. It is recommended to obtain a second venous access to enable appropriate fluid therapy. Maintenance of adequate blood pressure is crucial to maintain good splanchnic perfusion and reduce the chance of postoperative pancreatitis.

Postoperatively, the blood glucose concentration should be measured every hour during the first 4–6 hours and then every 2–4 hours. Postoperative hyperglycaemia occurs in approximately one-third of these dogs, but only a few will require insulin therapy. If the patient is hyperglycaemic but blood glucose concentration is <20 mmol/l, stopping the administration of glucose-containing fluids is usually sufficient treatment. With more severe hyperglycaemia, a low dose of neutral protamine Hagedorn insulin (0.25 IU/kg s.c. q12h) can be given. Hyperglycaemia usually resolves within 1 month.

The risk of postoperative pancreatitis is high in these patients, and this condition may cause fatal sepsis. To prevent pancreatitis, postoperative fluid therapy at 60–110 ml/kg/day (Galvao and Chew, 2011) and feeding of small, frequent meals, low in fat and simple carbohydrate and high in fibre content, is recommended.

References and further reading

Barrera JS, Bernard F, Ehrhart EJ, Withrow SJ and Monnet E (2013) Evaluation of risk factors for outcome associated with adrenal gland tumors with or without invasion of the caudal vena cava and treated via adrenalectomy in dogs: 86 cases (1993-2009). *Journal of the American Veterinary Medical Association* **242**, 1715–1721

Barton-Lamb AL, Martin-Flores M, Scrivani PV *et al.* (2013) Evaluation of maxillary arterial blood flow in anesthetized cats with the mouth closed and open. *Veterinary Journal* **196**, 325–331

Brainard BM and Mandell DC (2009) Pheochromocytoma. In: *Small Animal Critical Care Medicine, 1st edn*, ed. D Silverstein and K Hopper, pp. 314–317. Saunders, Elsevier, Philadelphia

Brown AL, Beatty JA, Lindsay SA and Barrs VR (2012) Severe systemic hypertension in a cat with pituitary-dependent hyperadrenocorticism. *Journal of Small Animal Practice* **53**, 132–135

Calsyn JDR, Green RA, Davis GJ and Reilly CM (2010) Adrenal pheochromocytoma with contralateral adrenocortical adenoma in a cat. *Journal of the American Animal Hospital Association* **46**, 36–42

Chastain CB (2009) Syndrome of inappropriate antidiuretic hormone. In: *Small Animal Critical Care Medicine, 1st edn* ed. D Silverstein and K Hopper, pp. 304–306. Saunders Elsevier, Philadelphia

Church DB (2012) Canine hypoadrenocorticism In: *BSAVA Manual of Canine and Feline Endocrinology, 4th edn*, ed. C Mooney and M Peterson, pp. 156–166. BSAVA Publications, Gloucester

Church DB, Nicholson IA, Ilkiw JE and Emslie DR (1994) Effect of non-adrenal illness, anaesthesia and surgery on plasma cortisol concentrations in dogs. *Research in Veterinary Science* **56**, 129–131

Cray C, Zaias J and Altman NH (2009) Acute Phase Response in Animals: A Review. *Comparative Medicine.* **59(6)**, 517–526

Cunningham JG and Klein BG (2007) The endocrine system. In: *Textbook of Veterinary Physiology, 4th edn*, ed. JG Cunningham and BG Klein, pp. 410–427. Saunders Elsevier, Philadelphia

Cunningham JG and Klein BG (2007) Endocrine glands and their function. In: *Textbook of Veterinary Physiology, 4th edn*, ed. JG Cunningham and BG Klein, pp. 428–464. Saunders Elsevier, Philadelphia

Davison LJ (2012) Canine diabetes mellitus. In: *BSAVA Manual of Canine and Feline Endocrinology, 4th edn*, ed. C Mooney and M Peterson, pp. 116–132. BSAVA Publications, Gloucester

Davison LJ, Herrtage, ME and Catchpole B (2005) Study of 253 dogs in the United Kingdom with diabetes mellitus. *Veterinary Record* **156**, 467–471

Desborough JP (2006) Physiologic responses to surgery and trauma. In: *Foundations of Anesthesia: Basic Science for Clinical Practice, 2nd edn*, ed. HC Hemmings and PM Hopkins, pp. 867–873. Mosby Elsevier, London

Dugdale A (2010) Some endocrine considerations. In: *Veterinary Anaesthesia Principles to Practice, 1st edn*, ed. A Dugdale, pp. 333–336. Wiley-Blackwell, Oxford

and subsequently insulin production, but treatment with this drug necessitates aggressive fluid therapy to prevent renal failure (Kintzer, 2012).

Patients should not be fasted for longer than 6 hours to prevent hypoglycaemic seizures. Glucose administration should be avoided unless there are clinical signs of hypoglycaemia (behavioural changes, tachycardia, muscle weakness, tremor, seizures), as it can provoke insulin release, which may lead to severe hypoglycaemia. The aims are to maintain blood glucose concentration at above 2.5 mmol/l but not necessarily within normal limits, as the body will adapt to a lower concentration, and to avoid sudden changes in blood glucose concentration intraoperatively. In hypoglycaemic crisis, 1 ml/kg 50% dextrose can be diluted 1:4 with 0.9% saline and given intravenously over 5 minutes, followed by an intravenous infusion of 2.5–5.0% dextrose-supplemented isotonic solution. Glucagon (50 ng/kg bolus followed by 5–40 ng/kg/min i.v. infusion) can also be used but is expensive. Blood glucose concentration and electrolytes (especially potassium) should be measured before anaesthesia and every 30–60 minutes during anaesthesia.

Opioids can be used as required, as their effect on the sphincter of Oddi is considered to be clinically minimal (see Chapters 10 and 24). Medetomidine significantly decreases the insulin concentration in patients with insulinoma by acting on the neoplastic cells, and therefore its judicious use (5 μg/kg i.m. or 1 μg/kg i.v.) can be recommended (Guedes and Rude, 2013); as well as improving plasma glucose homeostasis, medetomidine (or dexmedetomidine) has an anaesthetic-sparing effect. If the patient is hyperglycaemic at the end of anaesthesia low doses of atipamezole can be administered to antagonize

Fischer JR, Lane IF and Cribb AE (2003) Urethral pressure profile and hemodynamic effects of phenoxybenzamine and prazosin in non-sedated male beagle dogs. *Canadian Journal of Veterinary Research* **67**, 30–38

Fleeman LM, Irwin PJ, Phillips PA and West J (2000) Effects of an oral vasopressin receptor antagonist (OPC-31260) in a dog with syndrome of inappropriate secretion of antidiuretic hormone. *Australian Veterinary Journal* **78**, 825–830

Foley C, Bracker K and Drellich S (2009) Hypothalamic-pituitary axis deficiency following traumatic brain injury. *Journal of Veterinary Emergency and Critical Care* **19**, 269–274

Galvao JFB and Chew DJ (2011) Metabolic complications of endocrine surgery in companion animals. *Veterinary Clinics of North America: Small Animal Practice* **41**, 847–868

Greco DS (2012) Endocrine causes of calcium disorders. *Topics in Companion Animal Medicine* **27**, 150–155

Guedes AGP and Rude EP (2013) Effects of pre-operative administration of medetomidine on plasma insulin and glucose concentrations in healthy dogs and dogs with insulinoma. *Veterinary Anaesthesia and Analgesia* **40**, 472–481

Hara, Y, Tagawa M, Masuda H *et al.* (2003) Transsphenoidal hypophysectomy for four dogs with pituitary ACTH-producing adenoma. *Journal of Veterinary Medical Science* **65**, 801–804

Harvey RC and Schaer M (2007) Endocrine disease. In: *Lumb and Jones' Veterinary Anaesthesia and Analgesia, 4th edn*, ed. WJ Tranquilli, JC Thurmon and KA Grimm, pp. 933–936. Blackwell Publishing Professional, Ames

Herrera MA, Mehl ML, Kass PH *et al.* (2008) Predictive factors and the effect of phenoxybenzamine on outcome in dogs undergoing adrenalectomy for pheochromocytoma. *Journal of Veterinary Internal Medicine* **22**, 1333–1339

Hess RS (2015) Diabetic ketoacidosis. In: *Small Animal Clinical Care Medicine, 2nd edn*, ed. D Silverstein and K Hopper, pp. 343–346. Saunders, Elsevier, Philadelphia

Johnson C and Norman EJ (2007) Endocrine disease. In: *BSAVA Manual of Canine and Feline Anaesthesia and Analgesia, 2nd edn*, ed. C Seymour and T Duke-Novakovski, pp. 274–283. BSAVA Publications, Gloucester

Kintzer PP (2012) Insulinoma and other gastrointestinal tract tumours. In: *BSAVA Manual of Canine and Feline Endocrinology, 4th edn*, ed. C Mooney and M Peterson, pp. 148–155. BSAVA Publications, Gloucester

Lamont LA, Bulmer BJ, Sisson DD, Grimm KA and Tranquilli WJ (2002) Doppler echocardiographic effects of medetomidine on dynamic left ventricular outflow tract obstruction in cats. *Journal of the American Veterinary Medical Association* **221**, 1276–1281

Lang JM, Schertel E, Kennedy S *et al.* (2011) Elective and emergency surgical management of adrenal gland tumors: 60 cases (1999–2006). *Journal of the American Animal Hospital Association* **47**, 428–435

Massari F, Nicoli S, Romanelli G, Buracco P and Zini E (2011) Adrenalectomy in dogs with adrenal gland tumors: 52 cases (2002–2008). *Journal of the American Veterinary Medical Association* **239**, 216–221

Meij BP, Auriemma E, Grinwis G, Buijtels JJ and Kooistra HS (2010) Successful treatment of acromegaly in a diabetic cat with transsphenoidal hypophysectomy. *Journal of Feline Medicine and Surgery* **12**, 406–410

Milovancev M and Schmiedt CW (2013) Preoperative factors associated with postoperative hypocalcemia in dogs with primary hyperparathyroidism that underwent parathyroidectomy: 62 cases (2004–2009). *Journal of the American Veterinary Medical Association* **242**, 507–515

Mooney CT and Peterson ME (2012) *BSAVA Manual of Canine and Feline Endocrinology, 4th edn*. BSAVA Publications, Gloucester

Niessen SJM (2010) Feline acromegaly: an essential differential diagnosis for the difficult diabetic. *Journal of Feline Medicine and Surgery* **12**, 15–23

Pullen WH and Hess RS (2006) Hypothyroid dogs treated with intravenous levothyroxine. *Journal of Veterinary Internal Medicine* **20**, 32–37

Ramoo S, Bradbury LA, Anderson GA and Abraham LA (2013) Sedation of hyperthyroid cats with subcutaneous administration of a combination of alfaxalone and butorphanol. *Australian Veterinary Journal* **91**, 131–136

Rand J (2012) Feline diabetes mellitus. In: *BSAVA Manual of Canine and Feline Endocrinology, 4th edn*, ed. C Mooney and M Peterson, pp. 133–147. BSAVA Publications, Gloucester

Roizen MF and Fleischer LA (2009) Anesthetic implications of concurrent diseases. In: *Miller's Anesthesia, 7th edn*, ed. RD Miller, pp. 1067–1150. Churchill Livingstone Elsevier, New York

Rose L, Dunn ME and Bédard C (2013) Effect of canine hyperadrenocorticism on coagulation parameters. *Journal of Veterinary Internal Medicine* **27**, 207–211

Rysnik M and Dugdale A (2011) Inadequate stress response to anaesthesia and surgery due to suspected glucocorticoid deficiency in a dog undergoing exploratory laparotomy with known Addison's disease. *Veterinary Anaesthesia and Analgesia* **39**, 315–316

Shiel RE (2012) Disorders of vasopressin production. In: *BSAVA Manual of Canine and Feline Endocrinology, 4th edn*, ed. C Mooney and M Peterson, pp. 15–27. BSAVA Publications, Gloucester

Sicken J and Neiger R (2013) Addisonian crisis and severe acidosis in a cat: a case of feline hypoadrenocorticism. *Journal of Feline Medicine and Surgery* **15**, 941–944

Silverstein D and Hopper K (2009) *Small Animal Critical Care Medicine, 1st edn*. Saunders, Elsevier, Philadelphia

Stiles J, Weil AB, Packer RA *et al.* (2012) Post-anesthetic cortical blindness in cats: twenty cases. *Veterinary Journal* **193**, 367–373

Stoelting RK and Hillier SC (2006) Endocrine system. In: *Pharmacology and Physiology in Anesthetic Practice, 4th edn*, ed. RK Stoelting and SC Hillier, pp. 803–816. Lippincott Williams and Wilkins, Philadelphia

Teshima T, Hara Y, Taoda T, Teramoto A and Tagawa M (2011) Central diabetes insipidus after transsphenoidal surgery in dogs with Cushing's disease. *Journal of Veterinary Medical Science* **73**, 33–39

Chapter 28

Neurological disease

Elizabeth A. Leece

Neurological disease may be caused by intracranial, spinal or neuromuscular pathology. Anaesthesia may be required for diagnostic investigation, surgical intervention or supportive management of neurological disease. Other patients with neurological problems may require anaesthesia for unrelated conditions. As always, a thorough understanding of pathophysiology and the effects of anaesthesia in each situation is important when formulating an appropriate anaesthetic protocol. Before anaesthesia, special consideration should be given to the following:

- Pain management: including not only management of acute postoperative pain, but also of those patients with pre-existing chronic pain states as a result of intervertebral disc protrusion or intracranial space-occupying lesions
- Maintenance of an adequate perfusion pressure to the central nervous system by maintaining cardiac output and arterial blood pressure (ABP)
- Maintenance of autoregulation
- Provision of neuroprotection
- Complications of surgical technique:
  - Positioning
  - Duration of anaesthesia and hypothermia
  - Haemorrhage
  - Seizures or worsening of neurological dysfunction
- Access to the patient
- Postoperative assessment of neurological function.

In the field of medical neuroanaesthesia, the controversies regarding best clinical practice in humans have still to be fully explored (Dinsmore, 2007), yet many of the recommendations for veterinary patients come from the medical field.

Occasionally, a non-neurological problem may present with neurological signs. It is vital to be able to differentiate these conditions (e.g. *Angiostrongylus* infestation or an Addisonian crisis) from those with a neurological aetiology.

Intracranial disease

The most common intracranial disease in veterinary patients is epilepsy, although other conditions, such as head trauma and intracranial neoplasia, may occur and require diagnosis and treatment. A good understanding of neuroanatomy and neurophysiology will allow appropriate anaesthetic management of these cases.

Pathophysiology

The function of the brain is dependent on maintenance of cerebral circulation within the restricted space of the cranium. Intracranial disease or injury interferes with the control of cerebral circulation, predisposing to further ischaemic damage. Anaesthesia should ideally maintain normal neurophysiology while limiting the extent of secondary damage. There are four intracranial components:

- Brain
- Cerebrospinal fluid (CSF)
- Arterial blood
- Venous blood.

These components are essentially non-compressible, although CSF and venous blood are connected to low-pressure systems outside the cranium and can be displaced if intracranial pressure (ICP) increases (Figure 28.1). The *Monro-Kellie doctrine* states that any increase in the volume of one of the intracranial components (brain, CSF or blood) will elevate the ICP. Increased ICP may occur because of trauma, haematoma, inflammation, oedema or a space-occupying lesion (SOL). Initially, displacement of CSF and blood allows good compensation so that ICP remains relatively stable with increasing volume. However, once these

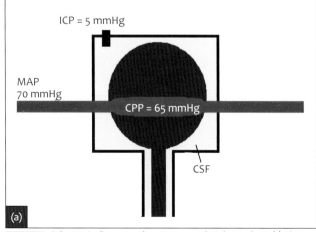

28.1 Schematic diagrams showing normal and raised ICP. (a) The normal intracranial compartment, consisting of the brain (80%), CSF (10%) and blood (10%) and their communication with the low-pressure systems. CPP = cerebral perfusion pressure; CSF = cerebrospinal fluid; ICP = intracranial pressure; MAP = mean arterial pressure. (continues) ▶

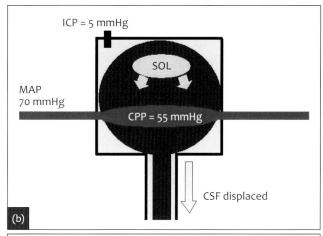

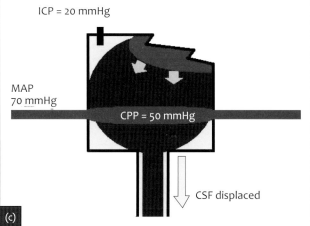

28.1 (continued) Schematic diagrams showing normal and raised ICP. As the brain is displaced by either (b) a space-occupying lesion or (c) trauma and haematoma, the CSF volume is reduced. As ICP increases, it opposes the driving pressure from the mean arterial pressure (MAP), which remains at 70 mmHg, and cerebral perfusion pressure (CPP) falls. CPP = cerebral perfusion pressure; CSF = cerebrospinal fluid; ICP = intracranial pressure; MAP = mean arterial pressure; SOL = space occupying lesion.

compensatory mechanisms are exhausted, ICP will increase rapidly (Figure 28.2). Since space is limited within the posterior fossa, ICP will increase relatively early in the case of SOLs in this area, and secondary hydrocephalus may occur if CSF outflow obstruction develops. Tentorial and tonsillar herniation of the brain (see later) may occur at the upper limit of ICP or if sudden increases in ICP occur.

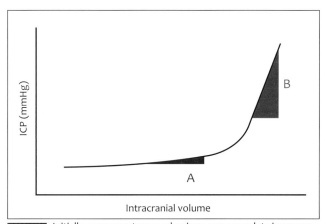

28.2 Initially, compensatory mechanisms accommodate increases in intracranial volume, and ICP remains relatively stable (A). Once these mechanisms are exhausted, ICP rises dramatically with only small increases in intracranial volume (B). ICP = intracranial pressure.

The aim of neuroanaesthesia is to optimize physiology. Specific aims include:

- Maintenance of cerebral perfusion pressure (CPP)
- Reduction of ICP
- Maintenance of autoregulation
- Maintenance of flow–metabolism coupling
- Maintenance of vascular carbon dioxide reactivity
- Avoidance of sudden increases in ICP
- Cerebral protection to minimize primary and secondary damage.

Cerebral blood flow

The primary goal of anaesthesia is to maintain cerebral blood flow (CBF), which is related to CPP and cerebral vascular resistance (CVR):

$$CBF = \frac{CPP}{CVR}$$

Many factors affecting these variables can be manipulated by the veterinary surgeon (veterinarian).

Cerebral perfusion pressure

CPP is determined by the mean arterial pressure (MAP), which is opposed by the ICP:

$$CPP = MAP - ICP$$

Perfusion is directly dependent on MAP and therefore the anaesthetist should pay particular attention to blood pressure monitoring and maintenance of cardiac output and systemic vascular resistance. Cardiovascular depression should be minimized. Fluid therapy is important in maintaining venous return and blood volume. It is advisable to maintain CPP above 70 mmHg in patients with intracranial pathology, which correlates to a MAP of 70–80 mmHg. This is important in the preoperative management of head trauma as well as management during anaesthesia. The patient's head should not be elevated by more than 30 degrees, otherwise a higher MAP would be required.

Cerebral vascular resistance

Autoregulation: In the normal brain, blood flow is maintained at a constant level over a wide range of perfusion pressures (50–150 mmHg). Outside this range, blood flow is dependent on MAP (Figure 28.3). Autoregulation of blood flow may be impaired in the injured brain and so sudden changes in blood pressure, such as increases in response to surgery, should be avoided. The use of agents that do not interfere with autoregulation, such as propofol and sevoflurane, may be beneficial.

Flow–metabolism coupling: CBF is normally well matched to metabolic requirements and this should be maintained during anaesthesia as far as possible.

Chemical factors: Hypoxaemia results in vasodilation of the cerebral vasculature, and should be avoided where possible and treated if it occurs.

As arterial carbon dioxide tension (P_aCO_2) increases, cerebral vasodilation occurs in a linearly proportional fashion (Figure 28.4). Conversely, with extreme hypocapnia, maximal cerebral vasoconstriction occurs, which can reduce cerebral oxygen delivery. Prolonged, severe hyperventilation leading to hypocapnia (P_aCO_2 <26 mmHg (<3.5 kPa)) has been shown to be detrimental in human

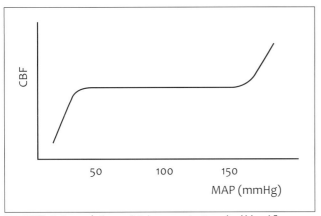

28.3 Autoregulation maintains a constant cerebral blood flow over a wide range of perfusion pressures (CPP or MAP) in the healthy brain. Outside this range, or in an injured brain where autoregulatory mechanisms are lost, CBF is directly related to the perfusion pressure. CBF = cerebral blood flow; CPP = cerebral perfusion pressure; MAP = mean arterial pressure.

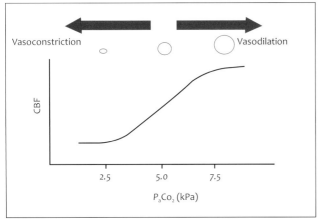

28.4 Cerebral blood flow is linearly related to P_aCO_2 except at extreme hypo- or hypercapnia, when maximum vasoconstriction or vasodilation occurs. Maintaining P_aCO_2 at the low end of the normal range is useful in reducing intracranial blood volume without the risk of excessive vasoconstriction and ischaemia. CBF = cerebral blood flow.

head trauma patients, although short periods of hyperventilation (P_aCO_2 26–30 mmHg (3.5–4.0 kPa)) as an emergency intervention may be beneficial in deteriorating patients while other therapy is instigated. In general, P_aCO_2 should be maintained at 30–33 mmHg (4.0–4.4 kPa) by using intermittent positive pressure ventilation (IPPV).

Some anaesthetic drugs alter vascular tone. Inhalant agents cause a dose-dependent vasodilation, although carbon dioxide reactivity is maintained with both sevoflurane and isoflurane to a similar degree, with maintenance of normocapnia counteracting the vasodilation. In humans, sevoflurane results in the least vasodilation at less than one minimum alveolar concentration (MAC) compared to the other inhalant agents when normocapnia is maintained, while maintaining intact autoregulation (Gupta *et al.*, 1997; Summons *et al.*, 1999). Therefore, sevoflurane appears to be the most suitable volatile agent for neuroanaesthesia. Propofol has the theoretical advantage of causing cerebral vasoconstriction, reducing cerebral blood volume and ICP while maintaining autoregulation and vasoreactivity. Propofol is therefore recommended in neuroanaesthesia, although its beneficial effects have not been demonstrated consistently in the clinical setting (Dagal and Lam, 2009).

Neuroprotection

A number of neuroprotective measures have been suggested to prevent or minimize pathophysiological processes. One such measure is to induce hypothermia, although its actual clinical benefit is controversial in human medicine. Some anaesthetic agents may possess neuroprotective properties through a variety of mechanisms, including reduced synaptic transmission, reduced calcium influx, membrane stabilization, improved regional CBF and improved glutamate uptake. Barbiturates, propofol and inhalant agents are the main anaesthetic agents thought to provide neuroprotection, but others, such as ketamine, may also have some effect (Doyle and Gupta, 2000).

Intracranial pressure

Normal ICP is 0–10 mmHg. Clinical signs of elevated ICP include depression, pupillary changes, alterations in respiratory pattern and cardiovascular abnormalities. ICP is rarely monitored in veterinary patients, although when magnetic resonance imaging (MRI) is available, the findings may be suggestive of raised ICP (Figure 28.5).

With severely raised ICP, vital medullary centres may be compressed, resulting in the *Cushing's triad*: hypertension, bradycardia and respiratory disturbances. The hypoxia caused by compression of the vasomotor centre

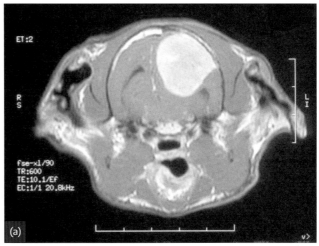

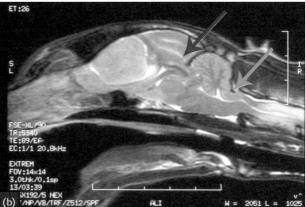

28.5 MRI findings may be suggestive of increased ICP. Reduced ventricular size, loss of normal gyral architecture and midline shift are good indicators of increased ICP on (a) a transverse scan, while (b) a sagittal scan is important to rule out subtentorial (red arrow) or tonsillar (blue arrow) herniation. The degree of oedema may also be assessed as a guide for treatment before recovering the patient from anaesthesia.

increases sympathetic outflow and increases ABP, with a concomitant bradycardia mediated via baroreceptors (Figure 28.6). Ventricular arrhythmias sometimes occur in dogs. Treatment must be instituted immediately to decrease ICP and maintain CPP, rather than simply treating the secondary cardiovascular effects.

Maintaining adequate CPP is vital, but a number of methods can be used to decrease ICP:

- Positioning: head slightly elevated (no more than 30 degrees)
- Avoid increases in central venous pressure (CVP): avoid jugular occlusion, provide pelvic support to reduce intra-abdominal pressure, minimize mean intrathoracic pressure during IPPV by altering peak inspiratory pressure and inspiratory time, and use a smooth intubation technique to avoid coughing
- Mannitol (0.2–1.0 g/kg i.v. over 10–20 minutes)
- Hypertonic (4.5–7.2%) saline (1–4 ml/kg i.v.)
- Furosemide (0.5–1.0 mg/kg i.v. bolus; constant rate infusion 1.0 mg/kg/h)
- IPPV to maintain P_aCO_2 at 30–33 mmHg (4.0–4.4 kPa).

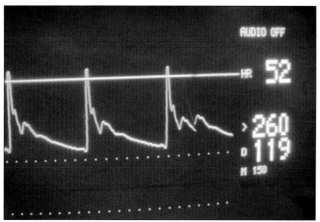

28.6 Invasive blood pressure monitoring showing the Cushing's reflex during brain herniation following craniotomy. Arterial blood pressure (ABP) is severely elevated, while the heart rate has decreased. Invasive ABP monitoring is important in this situation, as non-invasive measurements may fail. Treatment should be instituted immediately.

Traditionally, diuretics are used to reduce raised ICP. If using diuretics, it is important to maintain hydration with appropriate fluid therapy. Mannitol, an osmotic diuretic, decreases blood viscosity by increasing blood volume. The improved rheology (improved flow resulting from reduced viscosity) increases oxygen delivery to the brain, resulting in cerebral vasoconstriction and a rapid reduction in ICP. After 15–30 minutes, fluid will move from the interstitial and intracellular compartments to the intravascular compartment down an osmotic gradient, resulting in reduced brain volume. Mannitol (0.2–1.0 g/kg i.v. over 10–20 minutes) may be used and repeated as required. Constant rate infusions of mannitol do not produce the same osmotic effect and bolus administration is preferred.

Hyperosmolar solutions such as mannitol or hypertonic saline are used in the management of raised ICP in humans to improve CPP. Since the intact blood–brain barrier is impermeable to sodium, the hyperosmolarity of hypertonic saline will cause movement of water from the brain into the intravascular space by osmosis. Hypertonic saline is at least equally effective as mannitol for controlling intracranial hypertension for up to 6 hours after administration. For both hypertonic saline and mannitol, it is

debatable whether repeated boluses are effective, due to the brain's adaptive response to a sustained hyperosmolar state and also to uptake in the abnormal brain if the blood–brain barrier is no longer intact (Diringer, 2013). A survey of human neurointensive care clinicians found no difference in the numbers favouring the use of either mannitol or hypertonic saline therapy for raised ICP (Hays et al., 2011). When equiosmolar doses of mannitol and hypertonic saline were used in adult human head trauma patients, the decrease in ICP and the duration of effect were similar (Sakellaridis et al., 2011). Other reports suggest that hypertonic saline is superior (Kamel et al., 2011), although this superiority may be of limited clinical significance. The best choice of hyperosmolar solutions in veterinary patients is open for debate but may be guided by the animal's cardiovascular status.

Loop diuretics reduce CSF production as well as brain oedema. Furosemide (0.5–1.0 mg/kg i.v.) has been used in conjunction with mannitol in patients with life-threatening increases in ICP; however, current practice is moving away from furosemide due to the resulting diuresis, and it should be reserved for patients with severe elevations in ICP.

Pre-anaesthetic considerations for patients with raised ICP

Before any treatment is started, a complete haematology and serum biochemistry profile should be obtained. These patients are often depressed and may be dehydrated as a result. Electrolyte abnormalities are common. Alterations in sodium should be corrected; the time period over which correction should be performed depends on the rapidity of onset. A baseline urine specific gravity measurement is useful to guide fluid therapy. If raised ICP is suspected, mannitol administration may be beneficial (see above).

Pre-anaesthetic medication will depend on the mental status of the patient. Opioids are useful and do not cause respiratory depression in these patients at low doses. However, morphine and hydromorphone should be avoided if possible, as they may result in vomiting and consequently cause a massive increase in ICP, although this side effect is less common in patients that are in pain. Occasionally, more profound sedation may be required, particularly in cats, which can become aggressive if there is raised ICP associated with a SOL. Low intramuscular doses of medetomidine or dexmedetomidine (Figure 28.7) have been used in such aggressive cats where sedation is preferable to restraining for catheter placement. The effects of the alpha-2 adrenoceptor agonists on the cerebral vasculature are not well documented and occasionally vomiting may occur in cats at the higher doses (Figure 28.7). Since pain appears to be a frequent feature in these cats, opioids may be extremely helpful.

Anaesthetic considerations for patients with raised ICP

Patients should be preoxygenated to minimize hypoxaemia during induction, as long as this can be done with minimal restraint and minimal stress to the patient. It is important that an adequate plane of anaesthesia is achieved before attempting to intubate the trachea. Coughing during intubation will cause a profound increase in ICP, and the cardiovascular changes associated with a poor intubation technique also need to be avoided. Lidocaine (1 mg/kg i.v.) in dogs given 1 minute before induction may be useful to minimize these responses (Raisis et al., 2007). Lidocaine

Drug	Effect on ICP	Effect on seizure threshold	Neurological effects	Suggested doses for patients with raised ICP
Acepromazine	–	–	• Clinically relevant doses do not appear to affect incidence of seizures	0.01–0.03 mg/kg i.m. or i.v.
Medetomidine/dexmedetomidine	↓	↓	• Cerebral vasoconstriction • Dose-dependent systemic cardiovascular effects decreasing CBF • Decreases flow–metabolism coupling • May cause vomiting	1–5 µg/kg i.m. or i.v. Use lower doses for dexmedetomidine
Opioids	–	–	• No direct effect on ICP (high doses may cause hypoventilation and ↑ P_aCO_2) • Avoid morphine and hydromorphone, which may cause vomiting • Bradycardia with bolus administration, therefore i.v. infusion is more suitable during maintenance (see Figure 28.9)	Methadone 0.1–0.2 mg/kg i.m. Butorphanol 0.2–0.5 mg/kg i.m. Buprenorphine 0.01–0.02 mg/kg i.m. or oral transmucosal (cats) Fentanyl 2–5 µg/kg i.m. or i.v.
Benzodiazepines	↓	↑	• Potentiate respiratory depression seen with induction agents	0.1–0.2 mg/kg i.v.

28.7 Summary of the neurological effects of commonly used drugs for pre-anaesthetic medication. ↑ = increase; ↓ = decrease; – = no change; CBF = cerebral blood flow; ICP = intracranial pressure; P_aCO_2 = arterial carbon dioxide tension.

has also been shown to decrease ICP. Topical application of lidocaine to the larynx (in cats), or intravenous fentanyl used as a co-induction agent, can also decrease the response to intubation, although ensuring an adequate depth of anaesthesia is the most important factor. Care should be taken when intubating patients with caudal fossa disease, since an abnormal head position may be detrimental. Propofol, alfaxalone and thiopental are all suitable induction agents (Figure 28.8). IPPV and capnography should be implemented immediately following intubation and used to maintain end-tidal carbon dioxide between 30 and 33 mmHg (4–4.4 kPa) throughout anaesthesia. The minimal peak inspiratory pressures required to maintain these optimal carbon dioxide levels should be used during IPPV to minimize increases in intrathoracic pressure and, therefore, CVP.

Total intravenous anaesthesia (TIVA) has been suggested as the preferred anaesthetic technique in both humans and dogs. Variable rate infusions of propofol (0.1–0.4 mg/kg/min) and alfentanil (0.5–2 µg/kg/min) provide good cardiovascular stability during craniectomy in dogs (Raisis et al., 2007). Remifentanil is well suited to neuroanaesthesia due to its rapid elimination and recovery of respiratory function. Alfaxalone infusions have also been used successfully for craniotomy in dogs and cats. Sevoflurane appears to be the most suitable inhalational anaesthetic for neuroanaesthesia in humans, and has also been used in cats and dogs in association with opioid infusions (Leece et al., 2004). Due to prolonged recoveries in cats following TIVA, the use of sevoflurane for maintenance of anaesthesia may be preferable. When using propofol for

prolonged TIVA procedures, care must be taken when using the preparation containing benzyl alcohol (see Chapter 14). Opioid infusions are useful to minimize the amount of anaesthetic required while obtunding abrupt changes in MAP in response to surgery. Nitrous oxide should be avoided. The alpha-2 agonist dexmedetomidine has been used as an adjunctive agent, administered as an intravenous infusion both intraoperatively and during the immediate postoperative period; low-dose infusions provide good cardiovascular stability, may offer a degree of neuroprotection, and maintain cerebral vasoreactivity while not producing respiratory depression. Recoveries using this technique are smooth. However, dexmedetomidine causes a dose-dependent reduction in CBF while cerebral metabolic rate and oxygen consumption are maintained. A summary of maintenance agents in neuroanaesthesia is given in Figure 28.9.

Extensive monitoring, including invasive ABP monitoring where possible, is vital, particularly during surgery, when abrupt changes in cardiovascular variables may indicate associated brainstem compromise. Measurement of CVP may be helpful to guide fluid replacement following haemorrhage; increased CVP must be avoided as it opposes jugular drainage. Jugular catheters may be used for CVP measurement and fluid administration, although occlusion of the jugular vein during catheter placement can be detrimental in critically affected patients. Alternatively, peripherally inserted central catheters (PICC) may be introduced into the thoracic caudal vena cava via the medial saphenous vein (Figure 28.10).

Drug	Effect on ICP	Effect on seizure threshold	Dose	Comments
Propofol	↓↓	↑	1–8 mg/kg i.v.	• Administer to effect over 60 seconds to avoid profound respiratory depression
Thiopental	↓↓	↑	5–10 mg/kg i.v.	• Not suitable for i.v. infusion
Alfaxalone	–	–	1–2 mg/kg i.v.	• Administer to effect over 60 seconds to avoid profound respiratory depression
Ketamine	↑	↓	2–5 mg/kg i.m. combined with benzodiazepine	• Larger doses may increase ICP due to muscle rigidity and increased sympathetic tone • Avoid in patients with seizures • Has been used in aggressive cats for pre-anaesthetic medication with midazolam at low doses

28.8 Summary of the neurological effects of induction agents. ↑ = increase; ↓ = decrease; ↓↓ = profound decrease; – = no change; ICP = intracranial pressure.

Drug	Effect on ICP	Effect on seizure threshold	Dose	Comments
Fentanyl	–	–	Bolus: 2–5 µg/kg i.v. Infusion: 5–40 µg/kg/h i.v.	• Good cardiovascular stability • May accumulate with prolonged infusion
Alfentanil	–	–	30–60 µg/kg/h i.v.	• Can be used for prolonged infusions • Provide analgesia before discontinuing infusion
Remifentanil	–	–	5–40 µg/kg/h	• Does not rely on liver metabolism and is therefore rapidly eliminated • Provide analgesia before discontinuing infusion
Propofol	↓	↑	0.1–0.4 mg/kg/min i.v.	• Cerebral vasoconstriction results in good operating conditions • Prolonged infusions should be avoided in cats
Alfaxalone	–	–	Cats: 0.05–0.1 mg/kg/min i.v. Dogs: 0.05–0.2 mg/kg/min i.v.	• Suitable for infusions
Sevoflurane	↓	↑	<2 x MAC	• Maintains autoregulation and flow–metabolism coupling • Superior cardiovascular characteristics and easily titratable to effect • Indicated for neuroanaesthesia
Isoflurane	↓	↑	<1.5 x MAC	• Similar to sevoflurane but less favourable characteristics for neuroanaesthesia
Halothane	↑	↑	Not recommended	• Interferes with flow–metabolism coupling • Vasodilation cannot be regulated by P_aCO_2 and should therefore not be used
Nitrous oxide	↑	–	Not recommended	• Increases cerebral metabolic demand and cerebral blood flow

28.9 Summary of the neurological effects of agents used for maintenance of anaesthesia. ↑ = increase; ↓ = decrease; – = no change; ICP = intracranial pressure; MAC = minimal alveolar concentration; P_aCO_2 = arterial carbon dioxide tension.

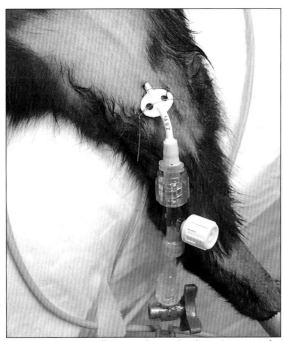

28.10 A peripherally inserted central catheter in a cat. Before placement, the catheter is measured to the correct length from the point of insertion in the medial saphenous vein to just caudal to the heart base. Central jugular catheters may also be used, but prolonged occlusion of the vein during placement may decrease venous return from the brain.

The use of neuromuscular blocking agents (NMBAs), such as atracurium, will help to decrease peak inspiratory pressure during IPPV while minimizing patient movement. Neuromuscular blockade must be monitored using a nerve stimulator to ensure full recovery necessary for adequate respiratory function postoperatively (see Chapter 16). Low heart rates are commonly seen during neuroanaesthesia, particularly with TIVA. Bradycardia should not be treated by administration of anticholinergic agents unless MAP is affected, because these drugs will mask changes in cardiovascular status associated with surgery or brainstem compression.

For intraoperative fluid therapy, normal (0.9%) saline may be preferable to lactated Ringer's or Hartmann's solution, Normosol® or Plasma-Lyte®, as these fluids are slightly hypotonic (see Chapter 18). However, hyperchloraemic acidosis may occur with prolonged infusions of normal saline. Hartmann's solution and lactated Ringer's solution contain calcium, which has been implicated in secondary brain injury. Currently, there is little evidence that the choice of fluid is likely to have marked clinical effects on the patient. Fluids are administered at rates of 5 ml/kg/h unless higher rates are required, for example, during haemorrhage. Hypotension and haemorrhage may be treated with infusions of colloids or hypertonic saline. The haemoglobin-based solution Oxyglobin® may be used in cases of severe haemorrhage although its effects on cerebral vasculature are poorly understood. Patients should be blood-typed and preferably cross-matched before surgery in case a blood transfusion is required.

The tongue should be protected using a moistened swab and positioned within the mouth, whenever possible, to avoid ischaemic damage and swelling. The endotracheal tube (ETT) should be connected securely to the breathing system to minimize the risk of disconnection; the use of elbow connectors can sometimes be beneficial. Secure intravenous access should be ensured and the use of extension lines and three-way tap (stopcock) connections is extremely useful. Care should be taken when administering drugs such as antibiotics if opioids are being infused upstream in the same intravenous line, because in smaller dogs and cats this can result in a serious opioid overdose.

Placement of an indwelling urinary catheter to facilitate measurement of urine output and improve patient comfort is recommended and should always be performed in obtunded patients.

Postoperative care

It is important to be able to monitor the patient's neurological status following anaesthesia in cases of elevated ICP, and often a rapid but smooth recovery is advocated to permit this monitoring. When performing prolonged procedures, sevoflurane has more favourable characteristics than isoflurane to allow earlier evaluation of neurological status.

However, prolonged anaesthesia and ventilation may be beneficial in patients where there has been marked surgical retraction, haemorrhage or severe brain trauma (Figure 28.11). If ventilation is to be continued, a mixture of air and oxygen should be used to minimize the risk of oxygen toxicity (King and Boag, 2007). Patients with severely raised ICP and those undergoing craniotomy under TIVA may also have prolonged recoveries. Warming of the patient should continue during the recovery period to prevent hypothermia and shivering. If body temperature is low then active rewarming should be attempted before recovery to minimize shivering. It is important to ensure good analgesia during the transition from anaesthesia to full consciousness, particularly when remifentanil has been used.

The risk of megaoesophagus and dysphagia occurring due to cranial nerve damage, particularly with caudal fossa surgery, makes it advisable to withhold food for 24 hours. Percutaneous endoscopic gastrostomy (PEG) tubes should be placed for nutritional support in cases of severe head trauma and caudal fossa surgery. Postoperative pneumonia is a potential complication if megaoesophagus and/or regurgitation are present (Fransson et al., 2001). Postoperative sedation should be used with caution in those patients at risk of developing megaoesophagus after surgery, but if sedation is required, then it may be advisable to reintubate the trachea and provide ventilation.

Dementia, apparent as inappropriate behaviour or circling, may be encountered following surgical trauma or haemorrhage, and must be differentiated from pain. Sedation is often required in these patients. Low doses of sedative agents have proved useful: acepromazine (5–10 µg/kg i.m. or i.v.), dexmedetomidine (0.5 µg/kg i.m. or i.v., or 0.5–1.0 µg/kg/h i.v.) or propofol (0.1–0.4 mg/kg/min i.v.). Many of these patients also have arterial hypertension, which may exacerbate haemorrhage. If MAP approaches 140 mmHg, it may be helpful to sedate the patient; alternatively, beta blockers such as esmolol (0.05–0.5 mg/kg i.v.

bolus or 25–200 µg/kg/min i.v.) or labetalol (0.1 mg/kg slow i.v. bolus repeated to effect, or 0.1 mg/kg/h i.v. titrated to effect) may be used.

Postoperative sedation with dexmedetomidine is becoming a popular choice after craniotomy. It provides analgesia, sedation and stable haemodynamics, although arterial hypertension may still be observed. Infusion at low rates can be continued for 12–48 hours postoperatively and neurological assessment can be performed if the infusion is stopped for a few minutes. Again, it is important not to over-sedate these animals as it increases the risk of regurgitation and aspiration.

Seizure activity should be controlled. Transfrontal approaches carry the risk of sneezing and aspiration, and pharyngeal packs should be placed preoperatively to reduce the risk of aspiration. Subcutaneous emphysema may develop. Tension pneumocephalus produces postoperative neurological deterioration with cervical pain, and requires prompt repeat surgery to repair the dural defect (Garosi et al., 2002; Cavanaugh et al., 2008). Constipation may be seen postoperatively, particularly in cats, and straining to defecate may severely elevate ICP. Constipation is more likely to occur if the patient is receiving opioids. Intravenous fluid therapy should be continued postoperatively and occasionally, warm saline enemas may be administered during anaesthesia in at risk patients.

Postoperative analgesia

Good analgesia is required during recovery to prevent the arterial hypertension that may occur secondary to nociception. The brain itself has no sensory or pain receptors, and it is a common misconception that patients undergoing craniotomy experience minimal postoperative pain. However, the skin, periosteum and meninges all have sensory innervation. People report headaches following craniotomy and it is not unreasonable to assume that similar pain is experienced by animals. Caudal fossa surgery is more painful than the supratentorial approach. Patients with increased ICP appear depressed, while cats with SOLs are often aggressive before craniotomy, which may suggest that they are experiencing pain.

Appropriate analgesia should therefore be provided; a multimodal approach is probably most effective. Opioids may be used, although intramuscular morphine should be avoided due to the likely side effect of vomiting. Care must be taken in severely obtunded patients; and the dose of opioids should be titrated to effect. Pupil size and responsiveness to light may be affected by opioids, particularly in cats, and may interfere with neurological assessment. An opioid should be administered at least 30 minutes before discontinuing a remifentanil infusion, particularly as remifentanil may cause an increase in postoperative opioid requirements and postoperative hyperalgesia (Guignard et al., 2000). Non-steroidal anti-inflammatory drugs (NSAIDs) may be used if the patient is not receiving corticosteroids; paracetamol (acetaminophen) is a useful alternative agent for neurological pain in dogs in these circumstances, and is used either intravenously or orally (note that paracetamol must not be used in cats). Local anaesthetic scalp blockade is commonly performed in human neuroanaesthesia and may be applicable to cats and dogs. Lidocaine patches applied close to the surgical site may also offer some benefit as there is limited systemic absorption. Intravenous lidocaine infusions may also be useful for analgesia because they can reduce ICP and are commonly employed for head trauma patients.

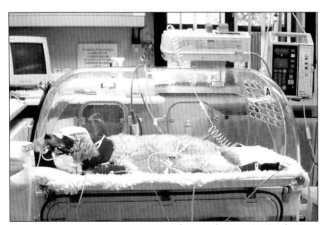

28.11 A patient in intensive care with anaesthesia maintained using TIVA. Patients may be recovered in either sternal or lateral recumbency. Sternal recumbency may allow better spontaneous ventilatory function, although care must be taken in arthritic patients and jugular occlusion should be avoided. Extubation should be performed as soon as possible to prevent coughing.

Anaesthetic considerations for specific conditions

Head trauma

The first 48 hours following head trauma are critical, with delayed deterioration occurring due to secondary injury, ongoing haemorrhage and inflammation or oedema. Anaesthesia may be required for management of the patient, diagnostic imaging or treatment of other injuries. Thorough systematic assessment is essential (Figure 28.12). Rapid fluid resuscitation is vital to maintain adequate cerebral perfusion to meet metabolic requirements. Analgesia is also required, and may aid patient assessment. Arterial hypotension and hypoxaemia are both associated with a poor outcome in human head trauma patients, so close monitoring of ABP and oxygenation (by pulse oximetry or arterial blood gas analysis) and aggressive therapy are required (see Chapter 17). Morbidity and mortality are significantly reduced if CPP is maintained at a value >70 mmHg. Fluid therapy should be administered to improve MAP and CVP and to normalize heart rate. Small volumes of hypertonic saline (1–4 ml/kg) or colloids are preferred for the initial phase of resuscitation, as they avoid the need for large volumes of relatively hypotonic crystalloids. Mild haemodilution (PCV 30–35%) is desirable because it improves cerebral oxygen delivery by reducing blood viscosity. Oxygen supplementation is beneficial during initial assessment and before anaesthesia.

Hyperventilation can be detrimental to the compromised brain because it causes cerebral vasoconstriction and a consequent reduction in oxygen delivery, although mild hyperventilation may be beneficial in the short term during patient stabilization.

Corticosteroids are contraindicated in head trauma and they may even be detrimental. In particular, they will cause hyperglycaemia. The severity of head trauma in veterinary patients correlates with the degree of hyperglycaemia (Syring *et al.*, 2001) and, since glucose is linked to increased brain injury, use of glucose-containing fluids should also be avoided. Occasionally, diabetes insipidus may result from head trauma, and so careful monitoring of urine output and specific gravity is helpful. This condition appears to be more common in cats.

Postoperatively, seizure activity may develop. This should be controlled to limit further injury. Nutritional support should be provided for comatose patients and those with facial fractures.

Mannitol is most commonly used to treat elevated ICP. However, during prolonged use, mannitol can cross the blood–brain barrier into the brain, where it might cause an increase in ICP. If active bleeding at the site of trauma is suspected, mannitol can still be used, although rapid management and control of bleeding is also necessary to ensure decompression. A recent review suggests that there is not only a reduced risk of mortality when using mannitol to control ICP, when compared with barbiturates but also that hypertonic saline may be superior to mannitol (Wakai *et al.*, 2013). Hypertonic saline (0.5–2.0 ml/kg of either 4.5 or 7.2% saline) has been successfully used to reduce elevated ICP in veterinary patients with acute traumatic brain injury, but clinical trials are needed before firm recommendations regarding this treatment can be made.

Space-occupying lesions

Corticosteroids are often used preoperatively to reduce oedema around a tumour. In this situation, they can dramatically improve clinical signs; their use should be continued perioperatively. Positioning of the patient for caudal fossa surgery involves flexion of the neck (Figure 28.13), and therefore, armoured ETTs (see Chapter 5) and elbow connectors to the breathing system are useful. Jugular obstruction should be avoided by careful positioning.

Relaxation of brain tissue is important to allow surgical access without excessive traction on the tissue. Mannitol can be administered before dural opening to facilitate this relaxation. In cases of meningioma, tumour removal can be associated with marked haemorrhage, particularly in cats; this can be minimized by avoiding increased CVP. Hypotension, haemorrhage and anaemia are the most commonly reported problems in cats undergoing craniotomy (Gordon *et al.*, 1994; Leece *et al.*, 2010).

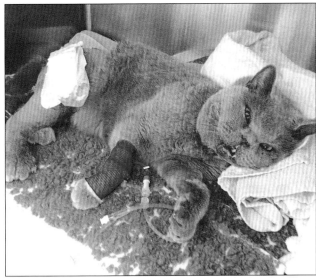

28.12 Patients may sustain head trauma as a result of road traffic accidents, falls, kicks or bites from dogs. Multiple other injuries may be sustained and so good assessment, fluid resuscitation and analgesia are vital.

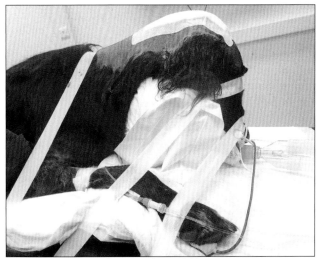

28.13 Positioning of a patient for caudal fossa surgery or suboccipital craniectomy involves flexion of the neck. An armoured endotracheal tube (ETT) avoids kinking of the tube and airway occlusion. If a normal ETT is used, it is important to monitor carefully for occlusion. ETT connections must be secure and elbow fittings can be useful. Capnography is very useful for early detection of kinking or disconnection from the breathing system. Jugular occlusion must also be prevented.

Hydrocephalus

Patients may require placement of a shunt to direct CSF from the ventricular system to the peritoneal cavity. Preoperative stabilization of these patients includes reducing CSF production, which may be achieved with carbonic anhydrase inhibitors, omeprazole and loop diuretics. Corticosteroids are also used to lower ICP, although their exact mechanism of action is unknown. Intraoperative use of opioids is advisable to avoid sympathetic stimulation from tunnelling of the catheter subcutaneously.

Epilepsy

Epilepsy should be differentiated from syncopal attacks and extracranial causes of seizure-like activity, such as hypoglycaemia or hepatic disease. Anti-epileptic drugs alter serum biochemistry values: phenobarbital may increase alkaline phosphatase and decrease calcium concentrations, while potassium bromide falsely elevates chloride concentrations. These drugs also cause polydipsia, and water should be available until pre-anaesthetic medication is given. Intravenous access should be secured and the patient observed, allowing prompt treatment of seizures. Anti-epileptic medications should *not* be discontinued during the peri-anaesthetic period.

Pre-anaesthetic medication should minimize stress and provide analgesia. Many commonly employed anaesthetic drugs affect neurotransmission and the use of some drugs in seizure patients is controversial. Manufacturers of acepromazine previously advised that the drug should not be used in patients with epilepsy, since high doses of a similar drug reportedly caused a reduction in seizure threshold in humans. However, acepromazine has been used at clinically relevant doses (0.005–0.07 mg/kg i.v. or i.m.) in dogs with epilepsy and does not alter the incidence of seizures (Tobias *et al.*, 2006). Opioids provide good sedation and analgesia without altering seizure activity, and low doses of alpha-2 adrenoceptor agonists will improve sedation in excitable patients. Benzodiazepines can cause dysphoria in non-seizuring patients and should not be used alone for pre-anaesthetic medication.

Propofol, alfaxalone and thiopental are suitable induction agents. Theoretically, ketamine should be avoided in patients with epilepsy, although infusions of ketamine at low doses may be administered to dogs with status epilepticus that is refractory to conventional therapy (see also later). Sevoflurane and isoflurane are the inhalant agents of choice. TIVA with propofol or alfaxalone is suitable for maintenance and is also used for longer-term control of status epilepticus, although care should be taken with prolonged infusions in cats, especially when using the propofol preparation containing benzyl alcohol as a preservative. Facemask induction of anaesthesia may result in excitement and is best avoided. Patients should be monitored carefully in a quiet recovery environment.

Perhaps the most important consideration when anaesthetizing patients with epilepsy is to monitor each patient carefully and be prepared to treat any seizure activity. Maintaining intravenous access is helpful for this, although rectal diazepam may also be used.

Seizure management

Control of prolonged seizure activity (status epilepticus or cluster seizures) is preferable to prevent further neurological damage and minimize hypoxaemia, hypoglycaemia and hyperthermia. Initially, diazepam (0.2–2.0 mg/kg i.v. or rectally) or midazolam (0.05–0.5 mg/kg i.v. or i.m.) can

be used while loading with other anti-epileptic drugs. Refractory seizure activity may require further sedation or anaesthesia. Propofol (4–8 mg/kg i.v. followed by 0.1–0.4 mg/kg/min infusion to provide continuing sedation) is useful, although respiratory monitoring will be required. Occasionally, muscle tremors may be seen during recovery from intravenous sedation. These are often localized to the head and neck. Patients should be monitored closely during this time for worsening of these tremors, which may indicate actual seizure activity. Experimental models have demonstrated the existence of reduced numbers of gamma-aminobutyric acid A ($GABA_A$) receptors with prolonged status epilepticus; this may explain why large doses of propofol are often required to manage seizures. Expression of *N*-methyl-D-aspartate (NMDA) receptors increases, and their stimulation by glutamate potentially propagates seizure activity. Ketamine has shown some promise as an adjunctive treatment for refractory status epilepticus in humans (Synowiec *et al.*, 2013) and has also been used in veterinary patients (Serrano *et al.*, 2006).

Body temperature and blood glucose concentration should be checked before weaning from the infusions. Heavily sedated patients will require a high level of supportive care, including:

* Airway management
* Respiratory monitoring
* Adequate bedding
* Turning every 4 hours
* Bladder care, preferably by placing an indwelling urinary catheter
* Eyes should be lubricated at least every 2 hours
* If intubated, oral hygiene should be addressed, including cuff deflation and repositioning, changing the ETT (tubes with low-pressure, high-volume cuffs are preferred) and moistening the mouth.

Vestibular disease

Anaesthesia of patients with vestibular disease often results in a degree of decompensation for 24–48 hours after anaesthesia, and owners should be warned of this possibility before the procedure. The use of short-acting agents is advisable. Low-dose medetomidine or dexmedetomidine will reduce the amount of intravenous induction agent required and help to expedite a smooth, rapid and complete recovery. Nausea may be seen following anaesthesia and can be treated with prochlorperazine (0.1–0.2 mg/kg i.v. or i.m. q6–8h) or maropitant (1 mg/kg s.c. or orally q24h).

Meningoencephalitis of unknown aetiology

Meningoencephalitis of unknown aetiology (MUA) is a common inflammatory disease in dogs, particularly small breeds. It is a multifocal disease that is normally acute in onset and progressive. MRI of the brain or spinal cord may be required and careful peri-anaesthetic monitoring and management is vital given the potential for rapid progression. The high mortality observed during anaesthesia depends on the areas affected, and patients demonstrating elevated ICP are at higher risk (Lowrie *et al.*, 2013). These patients also require close monitoring following diagnostic imaging, similar to patients with head trauma/SOLs, as well as management of raised ICP and seizures (as described above). Treatment should be initiated early due to the rapid progression in some cases.

Spinal disease

Spinal cord injury may occur as a result of intervertebral disc disease, fibrocartilaginous embolism, neoplasia, infection and/or inflammation, trauma or congenital instability. Anaesthesia may also be required for the diagnosis of discospondylitis or meningitis. Destabilization of the spinal column or surgical trauma may result in further deterioration of neurological signs. Patients will experience varying degrees of pain and may develop severe neuropathic pain, which can be extremely difficult to manage.

Anaesthesia for spinal surgery

Patients may exhibit signs of pain due to compression of neuronal tissue. Analgesia should be provided as part of pre-anaesthetic medication to allow placement of intravenous catheters with only minimal restraint. A multimodal analgesic protocol is likely to be more effective and usually includes opioids and NSAIDs, with additional drugs as required. Good analgesia is particularly important for patients with severe neck pain, especially during intubation. An accessible, wide-bore intravenous catheter should be placed for rapid fluid replacement in cases where haemorrhage is anticipated.

Careful patient positioning for the different procedures is important to minimize excessive venous pressure, which may exacerbate venous haemorrhage (see below). If the surgical site is positioned above the level of the heart (for example for some cervical procedures) there is the risk of air embolism. Pulse oximetry and capnography can help detect pulmonary air embolism. The surgical site should be 'flooded' with saline, patient positioning altered to prevent more air being entrained and nitrous oxide discontinued.

Judicious use of IPPV may be beneficial for control of P_aCO_2 because ventilation is often impaired by excessive surgical pressure; in addition, hypercapnia causes vasodilation, which may contribute to blood loss. IPPV will also maintain a consistent respiratory rhythm, thus helping the surgeon. Since patient responses to stimulation can be quite marked during manipulation of disc material, particularly if there is a chronic disc extrusion causing nerve entrapment, IPPV can also help to minimize excessive motion by reducing the respiratory component.

Analgesia may be supplemented intraoperatively with intravenous infusions of short-acting opioids such as fentanyl, alfentanil or remifentanil. Ketamine infusions have proved to be extremely useful during and after spinal surgery and may also provide neuroprotection (Figure 28.14); however, one retrospective study reported that ketamine did not reduce opioid requirements following spinal surgery (Klöppel et al., 2009). Intravenous lidocaine may also be useful for providing analgesia and neuroprotection, and reducing the MAC of inhalant agents. Occasionally, marked autonomic responses occur during drilling, when distortion of the vertebral column can cause dynamic compression at the site of intervertebral disc extrusion, and also during manipulation of disc material. These responses are more common in patients with chronic conditions with nerve root entrapment. The use of an intravenous bolus of opioid may be helpful in these circumstances.

Many drugs have neuroprotective properties, although in humans their use has not been shown to translate to clinical benefits. The only agent that has been shown to be of benefit in spinal trauma is high-dose methylprednisolone if given within 8 hours after injury. During this

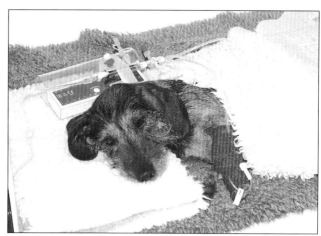

28.14 Ketamine infusions may be continued postoperatively for 12–24 hours and appear to substantially reduce opioid requirements. Lidocaine infusions may also be used.

specific time period, methylprednisolone probably acts as a free radical scavenger rather than via its anti-inflammatory properties (Bracken, 2012). Methylprednisolone should not be used in the presence of voluntary motor function, since in these circumstances, the prognosis is good without corticosteroid use. If given after 8 hours, corticosteroids may in fact be detrimental to the patient; many side effects have been reported, and there is no indication for their use at this time. Despite the documented side effects in animals, many spinal injury patients are treated with corticosteroids for their anti-inflammatory action; however, NSAIDs should be the primary choice. Suggested protocols for high-dose methylprednisolone are given in Figure 28.15.

Haemorrhage is commonly encountered during spinal surgery, and both MAP and the volume of blood lost should be monitored. Hypothermia will develop during prolonged procedures in smaller patients and should be minimized by the use of warming methods.

Analgesia for patients with spinal disease

Neuropathic pain is well recognized in human patients but may be difficult to identify in animals, although both cats and dogs can develop allodynia and hyperaesthesia. Neuropathic pain is very often difficult to treat with standard analgesic techniques such as opioids and NSAIDs, and a multimodal approach needs to be adopted. Neuropathic pain may result from a variety of causes, including

Time after injury	Methylprednisolone protocol
Up to 3 hours	30 mg/kg i.v. followed by 15 mg/kg i.v. at 2 and 6 hours after initial injection
	30 mg/kg i.v. followed by 5.4 mg/kg/h infusion for 24 hours
3–8 hours	30 mg/kg i.v. followed by 15 mg/kg i.v. at 2 and 6 hours after initial injection, then 2.5 mg/kg/h infusion for 42 hours
	30 mg/kg i.v. followed by 5.4 mg/kg/h infusion for 48 hours
Over 8 hours	Contraindicated

28.15 Suggested protocols for the use of high-dose methylprednisolone in patients with acute spinal cord trauma within the first 8 hours following injury (adapted from Bracken, 2012). Concomitant use of gastric protectants is recommended. NSAIDs may, however, be a more appropriate option than steroid use.

traumatic injury to nerves, nerve root entrapment, neoplasia (e.g. brachial plexus neoplasia), discospondylitis and meningitis. Animals show pain in several ways, such as depression, withdrawal from human interaction, anorexia, aggression or hyperaesthesia (see Chapter 9). Many analgesic protocols have been used for patients with neuropathic pain, including NMDA antagonists, systemic administration of local anaesthetic agents, alpha-2 adrenoceptor agonists, gabapentin and tricyclic antidepressants (Figure 28.16). If pain management is not satisfactory with high doses of opioids and NSAIDs, a combination of intravenous lidocaine and ketamine can be useful while the underlying cause is investigated and treated. Lidocaine infusions can be continued for several days in normovolaemic patients without liver disease, although they may develop tolerance. Once the underlying condition has been identified and treatment initiated, a gradual tapering of the dose of lidocaine and ketamine will allow re-evaluation of pain.

Pain associated with thoracolumbar spinal problems often benefits from the use of diazepam (0.3 mg/kg orally q8h). Its muscle relaxant properties are useful to reduce secondary pain and may be helpful pre- and postoperatively.

Preservative-free morphine (0.1 mg/kg) or hydromorphone (0.05 mg/kg) can be applied topically to the spinal cord before wound closure in thoracolumbar or lumbar surgery. The epidural application of preservative-free morphine has been reported to reduce postoperative opioid requirements in dogs (Wehrenberg et al., 2009; Aprea et al., 2012) and collagen implants can be soaked in morphine and left in situ prior to closure. Postoperatively, if prolonged opioid analgesia is anticipated, administration of transdermal fentanyl solution (see Chapter 10) may be worthwhile in dogs, and fentanyl patches are also useful (Bellei et al., 2011); however, lidocaine and/or ketamine should reduce the need for opioids.

Gabapentin has shown promise following spinal surgery. It binds to the presynaptic $\alpha_2\delta$ subunit of high-threshold voltage-dependent calcium channels in the dorsal root ganglion of the spinal cord and also acts on NMDA receptors. It is often suggested as the first-line treatment for neuropathic pain. However, in a recent study, gabapentin did not improve pain scores following hemilaminectomy in dogs concurrently treated with opioids (Aghighi et al., 2012). This may have been related to the dose used or to the fact that all dogs were treated simultaneously with opioids. It is also possible that the true analgesic effect of gabapentin may have become more obvious after the end of the study period. Gabapentin has proved to be a good adjunctive analgesic in feline trauma

Drug	Dose	Comments
Opioids	Methadone: 0.1–0.3 mg/kg i.v., i.m. (cats); 0.1–0.5 mg/kg i.v., i.m. (dogs) Morphine: 0.1–1.0 mg/kg i.m.; 0.05–0.1 mg/kg/h i.v. infusion (cats) 0.1–1.0 mg/kg i.m. or slow i.v.; 0.12–0.34 mg/kg/h i.v. infusion (dogs) Fentanyl: 2–40 µg/kg/h i.v. (cats); 5–40 µg/kg/h i.v. (dogs) Fentanyl patch: 4 µg/kg/h (cats); 2–5 µg/kg/h (dogs) Buprenorphine: 0.01–0.04 mg/kg i.v. or i.m. or oral transmucosally (cats) 0.01–0.03 mg/kg i.v. or i.m. (dogs) Hydromorphone: 0.05–0.1 mg/kg i.v., i.m. (cats) 0.05–0.2 mg/kg i.v., i.m.; 0.05–0.1 mg/kg/h i.v. infusion (dogs)	• Good for nociceptive pain but not very effective for neuropathic pain. High doses may be required • Methadone may have some NMDA antagonist effects and so may be indicated for use in neuropathic pain. May accumulate with repeated administration • Fentanyl patches have a long onset time and may not achieve significant plasma levels
NSAIDs	Carprofen 4 mg/kg orally, s.c., i.v. (dogs) Meloxicam: 0.2 mg/kg orally or s.c. on day 1 then 0.1 mg/kg orally q24h (dogs) 0.1 mg/kg orally or s.c. on day 1 then 0.05 mg/kg orally q24h for 4 days (cats) Robenacoxib 2 mg/kg s.c. then 1 mg/kg orally q24h (cats and dogs)	• Should be used in conjunction with other classes of analgesics
Paracetamol (acetaminophen)	10 mg/kg orally or i.v. q12h (dogs)	• May be useful for meningitis or pain caused by intracranial disease. May be used in conjunction with opioids. • **Do not use in cats**
Lidocaine	Loading dose 1 mg/kg i.v. followed by 25–50 µg/kg/min i.v. infusion (dogs only)	• Tolerance may develop during prolonged infusions • Lower doses should be used in hypovolaemic patients or those with liver disease
Ketamine	0.05–0.2 mg/kg i.m. or i.v. bolus followed by 5–10 µg/kg/min i.v. infusion	• NMDA antagonist
Medetomidine/ dexmedetomidine	2–5 µg/kg i.m. 0.5–1 µg/kg i.v. loading dose, followed by 0.5–2 µg/kg/h i.v. infusion	• Tolerance may develop during prolonged infusions and so dose may need to be adjusted. Infusions >48 hours may have decreased efficacy, although this is less of a problem with dexmedetomidine
Gabapentin	10 mg/kg orally q8h	• Side effect of mild sedation. Should not be discontinued abruptly
Amantadine	5 mg/kg orally q24h	• NMDA antagonist
Amitriptyline	1–2 mg/kg orally q12h (dogs) 0.25–1 mg/kg orally q24h (cats)	• Side effects include nausea and depression

28.16 Analgesic agents and doses used in acute and/or chronic neuropathic pain.

patients (Vettorato and Corletto, 2011). The author suggests using gabapentin at 10 mg/kg q8h following spinal surgery, unless side effects such as sedation are seen.

Lidocaine patches can be helpful in patients that still demonstrate allodynia and hyperaesthesia following surgery (Figure 28.17). Since there is minimal systemic absorption of lidocaine, any number of patches can be applied alongside the surgical wound to cover the area involved; patches may also be cut down to an appropriate size. No toxicity has been reported, but care must be taken if warming devices are used postoperatively.

Postoperative care

Movement of the patient should be restricted to minimize the risk of further haemorrhage, haematoma formation and resultant neurological deterioration. Some patients require sedation, which can be achieved by administration of opioids, alpha-2 adrenoceptor agonists or acepromazine. Recumbent patients should be turned every 4 hours to minimize positional atelectasis, and padded bedding should be provided to minimize bruising and the development of pressure sores. If prolonged recumbency or bladder dysfunction is expected, an indwelling urinary catheter should be placed.

A small percentage of patients with cervical spinal disorders will require postoperative ventilatory support (Figure 28.18). Patients undergoing surgery or suffering injury to the cervical spine should be assessed for adequate ventilatory function at the end of anaesthesia. Cyanosis may be seen if the patient is not receiving oxygen supplementation, although hypercapnia is a more reliable indicator of ventilatory dysfunction. Ideally, any patient demonstrating signs of paradoxical breathing should be closely monitored using pulse oximetry and

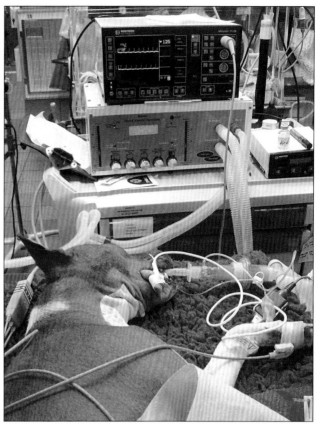

28.18 A patient requiring ventilatory support following ventral slot surgery at C2/C3. Respiratory function should be evaluated before extubation and, if possible, arterial catheters should be kept in place, as patients can deteriorate during the recovery period with ongoing inflammation affecting the phrenic nerve outflow.

analysis of arterial blood gases. Oxygen should be administered if oxygen saturation is low, but if P_aCO_2 increases, IPPV should be considered.

Anaesthetic considerations for specific spinal conditions or surgeries

Cervical spondylopathy

'Wobbler' surgery is often performed on Dobermanns. A buccal mucosal bleeding time should be measured before surgery, along with assessment of von Willebrand factor if possible. Dogs with von Willebrand's disease should be managed with desmopressin and plasma and cryoprecipitate transfusions where appropriate; drugs affecting platelet function, such as acepromazine and non-selective NSAIDs, should be avoided.

Dorsal approach to the spinal cord

Haemorrhage is a common complication of laminectomy. The anaesthetist can help to minimize blood loss by reducing venous pressures. Minimal peak inspiratory pressure should be used in ventilated patients, and excessive abdominal pressure should be avoided by appropriate patient positioning and emptying the bladder (Figure 28.19). Dachshunds often require hemilaminectomy; it has been shown that this breed has a tendency towards lower heart rates compared to similar-sized breeds when undergoing MRI (Harrison et al., 2012). It is therefore particularly important to avoid hypothermia in this breed as this could exacerbate the bradycardia.

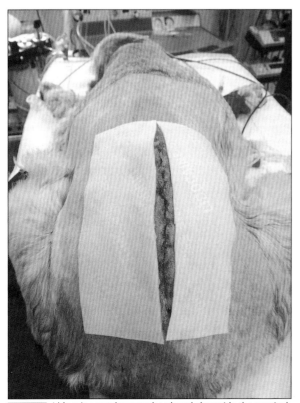

28.17 Lidocaine patches may be placed alongside the surgical wound, covering the dermatomes involved. This will help to manage allodynia and hyperaesthesia in some patients.

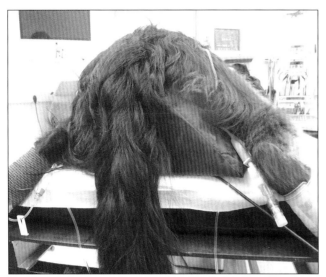

28.19 Abdominal pressure should be minimized in sternal recumbency by placing a support (sandbag or padding) underneath the pelvis to elevate it. The bladder should be expressed before surgery or a urinary catheter placed. Decreased intra-abdominal pressure will improve venous drainage from the vertebral canal, reducing the risk of haemorrhage during surgery.

Ventral slot surgery

During ventral slot surgery, the trachea and vagal trunk are retracted to allow surgical access. Use of NMBAs may improve surgical access. Excessive traction on the trachea may affect airway patency and alter ventilator setting requirements if a pressure-controlled ventilator is used. Iatrogenic damage to the recurrent laryngeal nerves will affect laryngeal function postoperatively; this may not always be immediately obvious in recovery. Vagal stimulation during surgery may cause bradycardia. If this occurs, retractors should be repositioned; anticholinergic drugs are rarely required. The patient is positioned with the neck fully extended (Figure 28.20) and care must be taken to place the head level with the body. If the head is lower than the body, this may exacerbate haemorrhage. Conversely, if the head is higher than the body, air embolism may occur during venous haemorrhage. Either invasive (direct) or non-invasive (indirect) ABP monitoring is advisable since haemorrhage is common with the ventral approach, due to the anatomy of the venous sinuses. Surgery at the level of the cervical vertebrae may result in respiratory compromise because of positioning; ventilation should therefore be monitored with capnography and pulse oximetry. Arterial blood gas analysis may also be helpful.

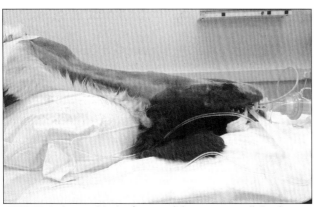

28.20 Patient positioning for ventral slot surgery usually involves extreme neck extension.

Atlantoaxial subluxation

Atlantoaxial subluxation is perhaps one of the most challenging spinal conditions for veterinary anaesthetists. It is typically a congenital or developmental condition affecting immature toy-breed dogs, and causes instability of the atlantoaxial joint with acute or chronic spinal cord compression. Damage at the atlantoaxial level can cause respiratory compromise or failure and so patients must be handled with great care, particularly at induction of anaesthesia. Adequate sedation will allow intravenous catheter placement with minimal restraint. It is particularly important to avoid struggling at this time, which could result in rapid deterioration. A rapid intravenous induction technique causing minimal respiratory depression is desirable; propofol, alfaxalone or thiopental are suitable choices. Benzodiazepines are best avoided, since they produce profound muscle relaxation, which may result in further destabilization of the joint. The patient should be preoxygenated before induction by using the 'flow-by' technique, if tolerated. The head and neck should be kept in the horizontal plane and the upper jaw supported, with the head remaining in a neutral position for intubation (Figure 28.21). Use of a laryngoscope is very helpful during intubation in this position.

Care must also be taken when positioning the patient for imaging. With smaller puppies, a supportive brace may be applied (Figure 28.22) to stabilize the neck while allowing growth until the patient is large enough for surgical intervention. However, the presence of a brace presents further problems for the anaesthetist during recovery and it should not be so tight as to compress the pharyngeal area. If the brace is too tight or poorly positioned, the patient may also experience difficulty in swallowing, increasing the risk of upper airway obstruction or aspiration pneumonia. The bandage supporting the brace should be cut before induction of anaesthesia in these patients, to allow rapid removal of the entire brace if intubation proves difficult. Suction should also be available.

Spinal trauma

Patients with spinal trauma should be stabilized on a board before being transported. Life-threatening conditions, such as a ruptured bladder, haemorrhage, lung or

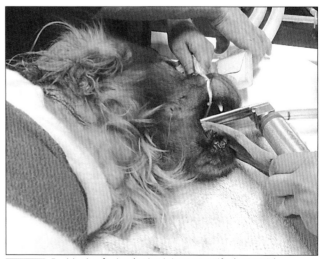

28.21 Positioning for intubation is important if atlantoaxial subluxation or cervical spinal fracture is suspected. The head and neck should be kept in a horizontal plane and in a neutral position. Preoxygenation is worthwhile, and the use of a laryngoscope will greatly aid intubation.

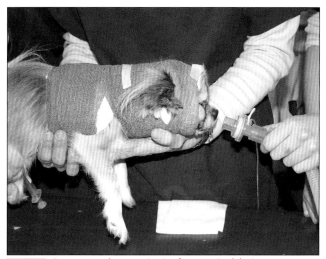

28.22 Oxygen supplementation is often required during recovery or before induction of anaesthesia in patients with a neck brace. If cyanosis develops, the brace should be loosened or reapplied. Before induction, the supporting bandage should be cut to allow rapid removal if difficulty arises at intubation.

myocardial contusions and pneumothorax, should be ruled out. Intravenous access should be secured, fluid therapy started and analgesics administered, ideally using intravenous opioids in the first instance. Cardiopulmonary variables should be stabilized before anaesthesia. If there is any possibility that the cervical spine is fractured, intubation should be performed with the patient in lateral recumbency (see Figure 28.21); once muscle tone is lost the support of the spinal column may be impaired.

Meningitis

Patients with meningitis may be extremely difficult to restrain due to severe pain and hyperaesthesia. Judicious use of low-dose medetomidine or dexmedetomidine administered intramuscularly in combination with an opioid should allow the patient to be handled for catheter placement. Intravenous agents such as lidocaine or ketamine may be used to provide analgesia, and low-dose medetomidine may be required in animals that have extreme pain. Usually, intravenous lidocaine infusions are sufficient while treatment for meningitis is started. Paracetamol may also be useful in dogs at a dose of 10 mg/kg i.v. or orally q12h.

Chiari malformation and syringomyelia

Patients with Chiari malformation often have chronic pain and so a multimodal analgesic protocol should always be used. The neuropathic pain syndrome may be correlated with the size and location of the syrinx and may be secondary to disordered sensory processing, which leads to spontaneous pain, allodynia and dysaesthesia. Patient handling may be difficult in the perioperative period if an analgesic is not provided as part of the anaesthetic plan. Sedation is also often required to avoid causing further stress during handling. Suboccipital craniectomy for foramen magnum decompression can be performed, although recurrence of syringomyelia is common. It is important to treat neuropathic pain aggressively at the time of surgery; suitable treatment choices are ketamine and lidocaine infusions intraoperatively and gabapentin perioperatively. Patient positioning for this procedure is similar to that for caudal fossa surgery and requires extreme neck flexion (see Figure 28.13).

Neuropathies and neuromuscular disease

Animals may have focal or generalized muscular weakness due to neuropathies or neuromuscular disease. Neuromuscular disease may also cause muscle rigidity, for example in tetanus, necessitating anaesthesia to provide supportive care such as ventilation, wound debridement and nutrition.

It is important to rule out treatable metabolic causes of muscular weakness before anaesthesia, such as electrolyte abnormalities. Myopathies may be associated with steroid use, as well as certain endocrinopathies such as hypothyroidism and hyperadrenocorticism (see Chapter 27).

Immune-mediated myasthenia gravis (MG) is among the most common neuromuscular diseases of dogs and cats. The disease may be focal or generalized. Some animals have signs of acute fulminating MG, which requires anaesthesia for management. In MG, a reduction in the number of functional postsynaptic acetylcholine receptors causes muscular weakness with sustained physical activity. Megaoesophagus and dysphagia are common findings in MG and both have important implications for anaesthesia. MG is associated with mediastinal thymoma and should be ruled out before surgical excision of a thymoma (see Chapter 23). Surgical stress may exacerbate MG, causing the patient's condition to deteriorate.

General anaesthesia is preferred to heavy sedation because it will allow proper airway control and ventilatory support. Benzodiazepines and alpha-2 adrenoceptor agonists exacerbate muscular weakness and should be avoided. Opioids with or without acepromazine will provide sedation, although morphine should be avoided in patients with suspected megaoesophagus (see Chapter 24). Radiographs to rule out megaoesophagus should be taken before induction of anaesthesia in patients with MG. The patient should be preoxygenated before induction. Use of a rapid intravenous induction technique using propofol, alfaxalone or thiopental will allow rapid airway control. The patient should be maintained in sternal recumbency with the head held in an elevated position until the ETT has been placed and the cuff inflated; this will help to prevent regurgitation and aspiration (Figure 28.23). Cricoid pressure (Sellick's manoeuvre) may be applied during intubation by applying upward pressure on either side of the trachea just below the larynx to minimize regurgitation. Suction should be available to clear any fluid or other material in the pharynx. In dysphagic patients, an excessive volume of saliva may be present in the oropharynx and dry swabs are helpful for tongue retraction, although suction or the use of sponge swabs may also be required.

Intraoperative monitoring of ventilation is important and IPPV will be required if hypoventilation occurs. The breathing system used should have minimal resistance to breathing. The use of inhalant agents allows rapid elimination of the agent and recovery, minimizing respiratory depression and improving airway protection. In patients with MG, the palpebral reflex may diminish with repeated stimulation and may not be a reliable indicator of depth of anaesthesia.

NMBAs may be used at low doses in patients with neuromuscular disease (see Chapter 16), but monitoring the extent of neuromuscular block with a nerve stimulator is mandatory.

In severely affected patients undergoing anaesthesia for diagnostic procedures, post-anaesthetic supportive care should be planned. In animals with megaoesophagus

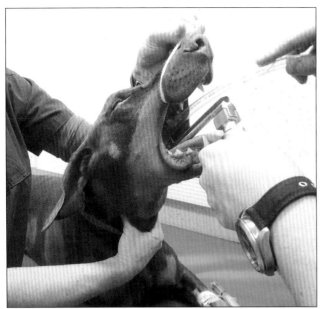

28.23 Patients with suspected megaoesophagus should be maintained in sternal recumbency with the head elevated for intubation to prevent aspiration. The cuff should be fully inflated before the head is lowered and suction should be available to clear pharyngeal fluid or other material.

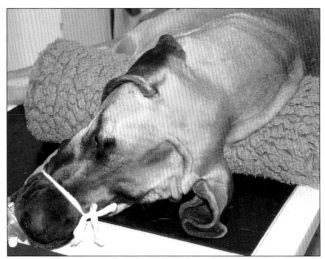

28.24 The pharynx should be raised above the level of the nose to allow fluid to drain from the oropharynx following extubation of patients with megaoesophagus or dysphagia.

or dysphagia, a PEG tube should be placed for nutritional support. Patients with severe ventilatory compromise may require tracheotomy to allow prolonged ventilatory support. Nasogastric and oesophagostomy tubes should be avoided in patients with oesophageal dysfunction. Baseline thoracic radiographs should be taken in case aspiration pneumonia develops.

For patients with tetanus, sedation with alpha-2 adrenoceptor agonists can often be extremely helpful. Anaesthesia for these patients requires the same general considerations as above. It is also important to provide a quiet, darkened recovery area to minimize stimulation. In severely affected patients, tracheotomy is advisable for both airway management and IPPV; nutrition can be managed with placement of a feeding tube. Acepromazine may also be used to provide sedation. Diazepam or midazolam infusions or bolus injections and also propofol or alfaxalone may also be administered to help aid relaxation of tetanic muscles.

Partial inflation of the ETT cuff during extubation will allow secretions to be drawn into the oropharynx from the airway. Following extubation, the pharynx should be supported higher than the nose to allow secretions or regurgitated fluid to drain through the mouth, minimizing the risk of aspiration (Figure 28.24). Adequate analgesia should always be provided because severely affected patients may not show normal signs of pain. Corticosteroids may be required for treatment in certain conditions, so NSAIDs should be avoided. Patients may be unable to generate heat by muscular activity (shivering) and hypothermia may result, so careful attention should be paid to monitoring and maintaining body temperature. Conversely, hyperthermia can be a severe complication in patients with progressive neuromuscular disease. This may result from a decreased ability to breathe and pant, and is more commonly seen in thick-coated breeds. Again, monitoring of body temperature is vital so hyperthermia can be treated early if it starts to develop.

Patients should be turned regularly to minimize atelectasis. Pulse oximetry is useful for monitoring ventilation in patients that are not receiving oxygen supplementation and may be used as a guide for oxygen therapy. Arterial blood gas analysis is an invaluable tool for detecting impending respiratory failure as P_aCO_2 increases and the results can be used as a guide for the implementation of IPPV.

Anaesthesia for neurological diagnostic procedures

Cerebrospinal fluid sampling

CSF may be sampled from the atlanto-occipital space or lumbar intervertebral spaces. Sampling from the cervical site carries an increased risk due to the possibility of spinal cord trauma and proximity to the brainstem. If elevated ICP is suspected, CSF sampling should be avoided, although if sampling is considered essential, the risk of tonsillar herniation can be minimized by judicious use of hyperventilation, sometimes in combination with osmotic diuretics. The patient should be adequately anaesthetized to prevent movement during collection of CSF. Ideally, an armoured ETT should be used (see Chapter 5) and 100% oxygen supplied during the procedure. Ventilatory effort and the capnograph should be observed for signs of respiratory tract obstruction, as older ETTs may 'kink' during flexion of the neck (Figure 28.25).

Electrodiagnostic tests

Electromyography is usually performed on patients with neuromuscular disease. There should be particular emphasis on ventilatory monitoring and support during the procedure. Electrical interference from monitoring equipment is common during electromyography, and ideally any monitors should be disconnected from the mains and run on battery power to limit this interference. If the plane of anaesthesia is too light this can also interfere with the testing. Nerve conduction testing can be extremely stimulatory and an adequate depth of anaesthesia must be provided to minimize patient interference. Hypothermia can affect brainstem auditory-evoked potentials. A 1°C decrease in limb temperature in dogs can decrease motor nerve conduction velocity by 1.7–1.8 m/s, and the amplitude of nerve and muscle potentials also increases in hypothermic patients.

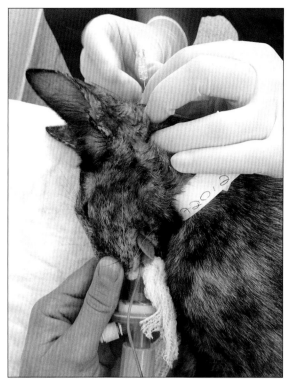

28.25 During CSF sampling, care must be taken to ensure that the endotracheal tube does not kink and that the patient does not move.

During electroencephalography, artefacts from patient movement can limit the value of testing. General anaesthetics can alter interpretation of the electroencephalogram and so sedation, usually with alpha-2 adrenoceptor agonists, is usually the best option to mimic sleep, and should not alter the recordings.

Myelography

Myelography is a relatively safe diagnostic tool for spinal cord disease. Intrathecal injection of contrast medium causes mild meningitis. The resultant meningeal irritation should be managed with anti-inflammatory agents or (in dogs) paracetamol. More serious side effects include seizures, apnoea, hyper- and hypotension, tachypnoea, tachycardia, bradycardia, arrhythmias and cardiac arrest.

Seizures may result from chemotoxicity and hyperosmolality; newer (second-generation) contrast media, such as iohexol, are theoretically less epileptogenic. Generalized seizures most commonly occur in the first hour of recovery, although they may be seen some hours later. Dogs over 20 kg have a higher incidence of seizures following myelography, possibly due to the relatively larger volume of contrast injected compared to CSF volume (Barone *et al.*, 2002; da Costa *et al.*, 2011). Cervical injection of contrast carries a higher risk than lumbar injection and the latter technique should be performed where possible. Rostral flow of contrast to the basal subarachnoid space and ventricular system can be minimized by slow injection over 1–2 minutes and maintaining the head in an elevated position afterwards. It is advisable to avoid the use of drugs that may lower the seizure threshold (see Figures 28.7 and 28.8). Seizures will normally be controlled successfully with intravenous or rectal diazepam; however, they can occur up to 24 hours following myelography (although the incidence with current contrast media may be reduced), and so maintenance of an intravenous catheter and close monitoring is advised.

Computed tomography

Accessibility is the major problem encountered during computed tomography (CT) scanning. Patients are often heavily sedated for this short procedure with drug combinations such as medetomidine and an opioid. Patients with suspected elevated ICP should be anaesthetized and IPPV provided. It is important to ensure intravenous access. Monitoring should be as standard. Some ETTs have radio-opaque markers that can interfere with CT scan quality.

Magnetic resonance imaging

The considerations specific to anaesthesia for MRI are covered in Chapter 29.

References and further reading

Aghighi SA, Tipold A, Piechotta M, Lewczuk P and Kästner SB (2012) Assessment of the effects of adjunctive gabapentin on postoperative pain after intervertebral disc surgery in dogs. *Veterinary Anaesthesia and Analgesia* **39**, 636–646

Aprea F, Cherubini GB, Palus V, Vettorato E and Corletto F (2012) Effect of extradurally administered morphine on postoperative analgesia in dogs undergoing surgery for thoracolumbar intervertebral disk extrusion. *Journal of the American Veterinary Medical Association* **241**, 754–759

Barone G, Ziemer LS, Shofer FS and Steinberg SA (2002) Risk factors associated with development of seizures after use of iohexol for myelography in dogs: 182 cases. *Journal of the American Veterinary Medical Association* **220**, 1499–1502

Bellei E, Roncada P, Pisoni L, Joechler M and Zaghini A (2011) The use of fentanyl-patch in dogs undergoing spinal surgery: plasma concentration and analgesic efficacy. *Journal of Veterinary Pharmacology and Therapeutics* **34**, 437–441

Bracken MB (2012) Steroids for acute spinal cord injury. *Cochrane Database of Systematic Reviews, CD001046*

Cavanaugh RP, Aiken SW and Schatzberg SJ (2008) Intraventricular tension pneumocephalus and cervical subarachnoid pneumorrhachis in a bull mastiff dog after craniotomy. *Journal of Small Animal Practice* **49**, 244–248

da Costa RC, Parent JM and Dobson H (2011) Incidence of and risk factors for seizures after myelography performed with iohexol in dogs: 503 cases (2002–2004). *Journal of the American Veterinary Medical Association* **238**, 1296–1300

Dagal A and Lam AM (2009) Cerebral autoregulation and anesthesia. *Current Opinion in Anaesthesiology* **22**, 547–552

Dinsmore J (2007) Anaesthesia for elective neurosurgery. *British Journal of Anaesthesia* **99**, 68–74

Diringer MN (2013) New trends in hyperosmolar therapy? *Current Opinion in Critical Care* **19**, 77–82

Doyle PW and Gupta AK (2000) Mechanisms of injury and cerebral protection. In: *Textbook of Neuroanaesthesia and Critical Care*, ed. BF Matta, DK Menon and JM Turner, pp. 42–43. Greenwich Medical Media, London

Fransson BA, Bagley RS, Gay JM et al. (2001) Pneumonia after intracranial surgery in dogs. *Veterinary Surgery* **30**, 432–439

Garosi LS, Penderis J, Brearley MJ et al. (2002) Intraventricular tension pneumocephalus as a complication of transfrontal craniectomy: a case report. *Veterinary Surgery* **31**, 226–231

Gordon LE, Thacher C, Matthiessen DT and Joseph RJ (1994) Results of craniotomy for the treatment of cerebral meningioma in 42 cats. *Veterinary Surgery* **23**, 94–100

Guignard B, Bossard AE, Coste C et al. (2000) Acute opioid tolerance: intraoperative remifentanil increases postoperative pain and morphine requirement. *Anesthesiology* **93**, 409–417

Gupta S, Heath K and Matta BF (1997) Effect of incremental doses of sevoflurane on cerebral perfusion pressure in humans. *British Journal of Anesthesia* **79**, 469–472

Harrison RL, Clark L and Corletto F (2012) Comparison of mean heart rate in anaesthetized dachshunds and other breeds of dog undergoing spinal magnetic resonance imaging. *Veterinary Anaesthesia and Analgesia* **39**, 230–235

Hays AN, Lazaridis C, Neyens R et al. (2011) Osmotherapy: use among neurointensivists. *Neurocritical Care* **14**, 222–228

Kamel H, Navi BB, Nakagawa K, Hemphill JC 3rd and Ko NU (2011) Hypertonic saline versus mannitol for the treatment of elevated intracranial pressure: a meta-analysis of randomized clinical trials. *Critical Care Medicine* **39**, 554–559

King LG and Boag A (2007) *BSAVA Manual of Canine and Feline Emergency and Critical Care, 2nd edn.* BSAVA Publications, Gloucester.

Klöppel H, Adams VJ, Brearley JC and Leece EA (2009) Opioid administration following spinal surgery in dogs receiving ketamine infusion compared to those not receiving ketamine: a retrospective study. *Veterinary Anesthesia and Analgesia* **36**, 6–7

Leece EA, Lujan Feliu-Pascual A and Joliffe C (2010) Perioperative complications in cats undergoing craniectomy: a retrospective study. *Veterinary Anaesthesia and Analgesia* **37**, 55–56

Leece EA, Raisis AL, Corletto F *et al.* (2004) Sevoflurane and intravenous alfentanil infusion for anaesthesia in cats with raised intracranial pressure. *Veterinary Anaesthesia and Analgesia* **31**, 5–6

Lowrie M, Smith PM and Garosi L (2013) Meningoencephalitis of unknown origin: investigation of prognostic factors and outcome using a standard treatment protocol. *Veterinary Record* **172**, 527. doi: 10.1136/vr.101431

Raisis AL, Leece EA, Platt SR *et al.* (2007) Evaluation of an anaesthetic technique used in dogs undergoing craniectomy for tumour resection. *Veterinary Anaesthesia and Analgesia* **34**, 171–180

Sakellaridis N, Pavlou E, Karatzas S *et al.* (2011) Comparison of mannitol and hypertonic saline in the treatment of severe brain injuries. *Journal of Neurosurgery* **114**, 545–548

Serrano S, Hughes D and Chandler K (2006) Use of ketamine for the management of refractory status epilepticus in a dog. *Journal of Veterinary Internal Medicine* **20**, 194–197

Simpson SA, Syring R and Otto CM (2009) Severe blunt trauma in dogs: 235 cases (1997–2003) *Journal of Veterinary Emergency and Critical Care* **19**, 588–602

Summons AC, Gupta AK and Matta BF (1999) Dynamic cerebral autoregulation during sevoflurane anaesthesia: a comparison with isoflurane. *Anesthesia and Analgesia* **88**, 341–345

Synowiec AS, Singh DS, Yenugadhati V *et al.* (2013) Ketamine use in the treatment of refractory status epilepticus. *Epilepsy Research* **105**, 83–88

Syring RS, Otto CM and Droatz KJ (2001) Hyperglycaemia in dogs and cats with head trauma: 122 cases (1997–1999) *Journal of the American Veterinary Medical Association* **218**, 1124–1129

Tobias KM, Marioni-Henry K and Wagner R (2006) A retrospective study on the use of acepromazine maleate in dogs with seizures. *Journal of the American Animal Hospital Association* **42**, 283–289

Vettorato E and Corletto F (2011) Gabapentin as part of multi-modal analgesia in two cats suffering multiple injuries. *Veterinary Anaesthesia and Analgesia* **38**, 518–520

Wakai A, McCabe A, Roberts I and Schierhout G (2013) Mannitol for acute traumatic brain injury. *Cochrane Database of Systematic Reviews, CD001049*

Wehrenberg A, Freeman L, Ko J, Payton M and Spivack R (2009) Evaluation of topical epidural morphine for postoperative analgesia following hemilaminectomy in dogs. *Veterinary Therapeutics* **10**, 1–12

Chapter 29

Magnetic resonance imaging: safety aspects for the anaesthetist

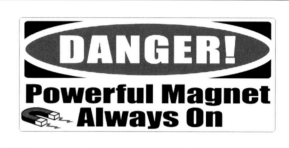

Julie A. Smith

Magnetic resonance imaging (MRI) is becoming more commonly available as a diagnostic tool in veterinary medicine. Although some MRI is performed using facilities designed for human use, the increased demand has driven the development and installation of dedicated veterinary imaging systems. Heavy sedation or general anaesthesia is necessary in cats and dogs to reduce patient response to machine noise and provide the immobilization necessary for obtaining optimal diagnostic images. In order to safely and effectively monitor vital signs during anaesthesia for MRI, it is essential to understand the unique environment and the dangers associated with this technology.

29.1 The strong magnetic field in an MRI system is always on, even when the system is not scanning.

How magnetic resonance images are obtained

The body is composed of many billions of atoms with randomly spinning protons, which act as small biological magnets. When exposed to the strong *magnetic* field that exists within the MRI machine, the atoms align themselves parallel to the applied field. Radio waves, tuned to a specific frequency, are pulsed into the tissue in short bursts to disrupt the alignment of the atoms. Following each burst, the atoms realign, or precess, with the applied field, and emit energy, called *resonance*. Receiver coils are used to capture and amplify this weak resonance signal, which is then digitally processed for magnetic resonance (MR) *image* formation. Each body tissue (e.g. bone, muscle, nerves) and any existing pathology displays different resonance characteristics, allowing the identification of different anatomical structures and any associated abnormalities.

Conditions and hazards in the MRI unit

The magnetic field

A powerful static magnetic field is the primary feature of the MRI system (Figure 29.1). The overall magnetic field strength is measured in Tesla (T) and the field is strongest at the centre of the magnet bore. Clinical MRI systems have magnetic fields ranging from 0.2–3.0 T. A 'fringe'

magnetic field extends beyond the bore of the magnet; this decreases in strength as distance from the magnet increases. The 'fringe' field strength is measured in Gauss (G) or milliTesla (mT). One mT equals 10 G (or 1 T equals 10,000 G). Within the 5 Gauss line (i.e. the area where the magnetic field exceeds 5 Gauss), there are safety restrictions (Figure 29.2) and appropriate warning signage must be displayed (Figure 29.3). The field strength increases rapidly within the 5 Gauss line and can cause accidents and medical device malfunction. The location of the 5 Gauss line varies with each MRI facility; a diagram of the fringe fields is provided by the device vendor, or can be obtained from the MR technologist (Figure 29.4).

No harmful biological effects have been associated with short-term exposure to strong magnetic fields in either patients or MR technologists. Often, however, the same personnel will provide the anaesthesia and monitoring required for all veterinary patients during MRI within a given clinic, and these personnel may have prolonged and repeated exposure to strong magnetic fields. Limited

- Non-compatible electronic medical devices (e.g. patient monitors, infusion pumps, ventilators, laryngoscopes)
- Metal instruments (e.g. haemostats, scissors, stethoscopes)
- Clipboards, pens, paperclips containing metal
- Hair clips, barrettes and bobby pins
- Analogue and digital watches, and jewellery
- Hearing aids
- Cards with a magnetic strip (e.g. ID badges, credit cards, hotel keys)
- Mobile cell phones and pagers
- Tablet computers
- Cameras
- Keys

29.2 Items that are restricted inside the 5 Gauss line (note that this is not a complete list).

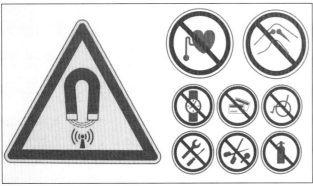

29.3 Example of a warning sign posted at the entrance to the MRI unit, outside the 5 Gauss line.

exposure to a strong magnetic field, not to exceed 0.2 T averaged over a given 8-hour period, is recommended until more is known about the long-term effects of exposure.

The 'missile' or 'projectile' effect is the most significant danger to personnel and patients when in the MRI unit. Any ferromagnetic objects, such as oxygen cylinders, patient trolleys, carts, mop buckets and floor cleaners, will be strongly attracted to the magnet, causing them to become projectiles, which will endanger the patient inside the magnet or anyone in the path of the projectile. The force of attraction may be very strong depending on the size and proximity of the object to the magnet and the magnetic field strength, and it will be difficult to stop the object moving toward the magnet once it has momentum. Large metal items are particularly difficult to remove due to the strong attraction, and removal may require a disruption of the magnetic field. As well as the risks to patients and personnel, this can result in significant costs due to equipment damage, costly restoration of the magnetic field and loss of revenue while the unit is out of action.

The safety of devices and equipment relative to a strong magnetic field are classified according to the ASTM International (formerly the American Society for Testing and Materials) classification system. Newly implemented classifications and their corresponding symbols are given in Figure 29.5. To protect against missile events, access to the magnet should be restricted to specific personnel, all equipment should be appropriately labelled as safe or unsafe (Figures 29.6 and 29.7) and, where indicated, metal detectors should be installed. It is wise to take a precautionary approach: *'When in doubt, keep it out!'*.

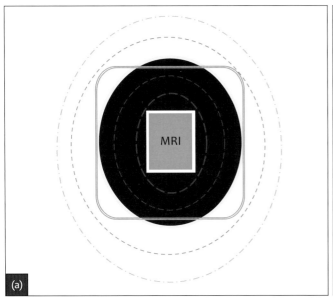

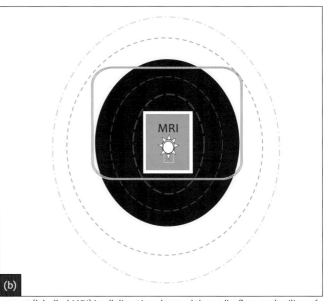

29.4 Illustration of the 'fringe' magnetic field that extends beyond the magnet (labelled MRI) in all directions beyond the walls, floor and ceiling of the MRI unit (orange double-lined box). The black area indicates the limited access area inside the 5 Gauss line (yellow line). The distance of the 5 Gauss line from the magnet will vary depending on the magnet strength and shielding. (a) View from above. (b) View from the front.

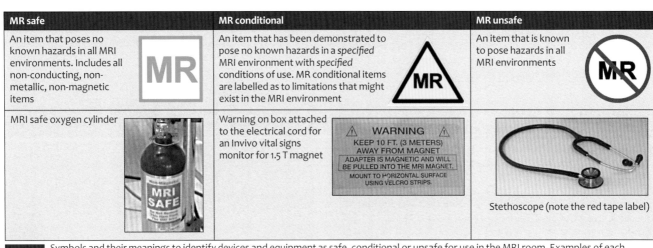

MR safe	MR conditional	MR unsafe
An item that poses no known hazards in all MRI environments. Includes all non-conducting, non-metallic, non-magnetic items	An item that has been demonstrated to pose no known hazards in a *specified* MRI environment with *specified* conditions of use. MR conditional items are labelled as to limitations that might exist in the MRI environment	An item that is known to pose hazards in all MRI environments
MRI safe oxygen cylinder	Warning on box attached to the electrical cord for an Invivo vital signs monitor for 1.5 T magnet	Stethoscope (note the red tape label)

29.5 Symbols and their meanings to identify devices and equipment as safe, conditional or unsafe for use in the MRI room. Examples of each classification are included.

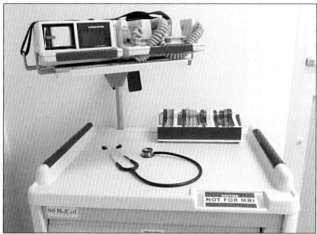

29.6 Crash cart and associated equipment labelled with red tape to alert users that it must not be taken into the MRI room. Crash carts and emergency equipment should be available outside the MRI room in case of emergency.

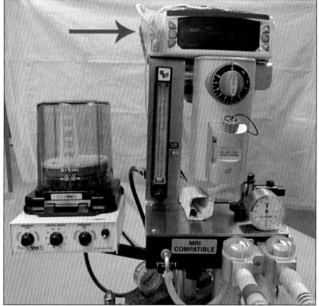

29.7 Carefully inspect any equipment before taking it into the MRI room. This MRI-compatible anaesthetic machine has a non-compatible capnograph on top of it (red arrow) that must be removed before the machine can safely be taken into the MRI room.

Rotational force, or torque, is an additional concern within the bore of the magnet where the field is strongest. Implanted, non-spherical metallic objects, such as aneurysm clips, will attempt to align with the magnetic field and may dislodge and tear vital structures. Once scarring has occurred, however, implanted microchips, vascular clamps, intravascular coils and stents are stable.

Radiofrequency fields

The energy generated by the radiofrequency (RF) pulses is transformed into heat in the tissues of the patient. This can increase body temperature, especially in large dogs and with prolonged imaging times. Elevated temperatures are observed after imaging with 3.0 T systems as the RF input is greatest with the stronger magnet. RF pulses also generate electrical currents that can overheat any conductive substance, such as wire cables from non-compatible electrocardiography or pulse oximetry equipment, within the magnetic field.

The RF transmitter/receiver used to deliver energy into the tissues and/or to capture the resonance energy produced as the atoms precess back into alignment with the magnetic field is called an RF coil. There are two main types of RF coils: body coils and surface coils. Surface coils are wrapped around or placed over the body part to be imaged (Figure 29.8), while body coils are built into the table or the main MR component.

There may be many extraneous sources of RF near the MRI room, which could affect image acquisition and quality. To prevent these radio waves from affecting the images, MRI units are lined with copper sheeting (Figure 29.9) or the magnet systems are encased in a metal Faraday cage (Figure 29.10). Many electronic devices, such as monitors and fluid pumps, emit RF that will affect image quality; unless marked as MR compatible, these devices should be kept outside the 5 Gauss line (see Figure 29.3).

Gradient magnetic fields

The 'clanging' noise heard during MRI is caused by gradient magnetic fields (gradients) generated by smaller magnets within the primary magnet, which enable the production of MR image slices. The level of acoustic noise

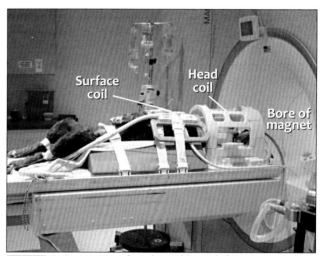

29.8 Patient positioned on a long table, inside foam positioning devices, surrounded with radiofrequency coils. Next, the patient will be covered with insulating blankets and moved into the middle of the narrow bore of the MRI unit, which will compromise patient access and visualization throughout the imaging procedure.

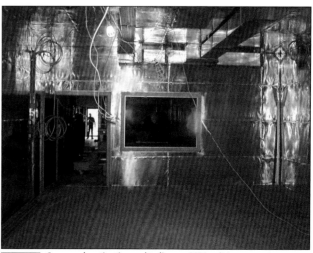

29.9 Copper sheeting is used to line an MRI unit to prevent radiofrequency (RF) interference from outside the room.

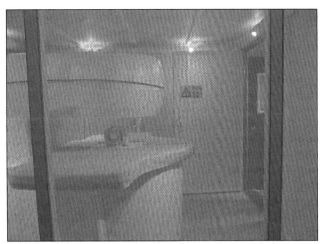

29.10 This photograph of an MRI unit was taken outside the radiofrequency shielding (Faraday) cage built around it. Patients can be observed through the metal shielding during imaging. (Courtesy of The Veterinary Surgical Referral Practice of Northern Virginia, USA).

can reach 90–130 decibels (dB) or even greater, depending on the scan sequence and the magnet strength. Noise increases with magnet strength: 3.0 T magnets create twice as much noise as 1.5 T systems. Permissible sound levels are limited to 99 dB by the International Electrotechnical Commission (IEC) and the US Food and Drug Administration (FDA). A maximum noise exposure of 85 dB over an 8-hour period is recommended by the Occupational Safety and Health Administration (OSHA) in the USA.

Hearing protection should always be worn in the MRI room during scanning. Close-fitting ear muff-style protection with a noise reduction rating (NRR) of 20–30 dB is most effective. Disposable ear plugs with an NRR of 30–33 dB can be worn alone, or in combination with the ear muffs to provide improved protection (Figure 29.11).

Cryogens

A great deal of energy and heat is generated by superconducting magnets (1.5 T and 3.0 T). As a consequence, they must be encased in cryogens (liquefied gases at very low temperatures), most commonly supercooled (4.22°K (−268.93°C)) liquid helium. If the system fails and heats up, the helium will vaporize and boil off very rapidly (5–15

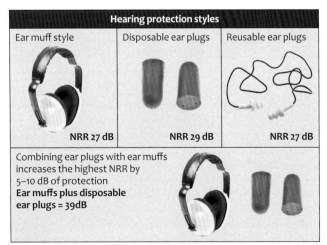

29.11 Hearing protection styles for wear during MRI scanning. The noise reduction rating (NRR) indicates the extent to which the noise will be reduced when wearing the hearing protection.

seconds) in an explosive event termed a 'quench'. Large vent pipes are installed in MRI rooms for evacuation of the helium vapour if a quench should occur. However, in the event that the vent pipe fails, the helium vapour will enter the MRI room. This extremely cold vapour will displace the oxygen in the room air, and any occupants will be at risk for asphyxiation and frostbite. A quench may occur if the cryogen system malfunctions, or it can be manually triggered in the event of a life-threatening situation, such as a fire in the MRI room or a person trapped against the magnet by a large ferromagnetic object, necessitating the termination of the magnetic field. In this situation, emergency and rescue personnel should be prevented from entering the magnet room until the magnetic field and helium cloud have had time to dissipate (this will take a few minutes). The anaesthetist should be familiar with the facility's procedure in the event of a quench (Figure 29.12).

- Evacuate the room immediately
- Stay close to the floor as the helium cloud will rise higher in the room
- Do not touch the magnet as it could have a high-voltage electrical charge
- Do not attempt to move the patient
- Break window or door if necessary to exit the room. Increased pressure in the room may make inward-opening doors difficult to open
- Prevent emergency personnel from running into the room. It will take a few minutes for the magnetic field to dissipate

29.12 Suggested procedure for a quench with vent failure. Make sure to familiarize yourself with the quench procedure for the facility where you are providing anaesthesia support, as it may vary from these guidelines.

Considerations for anaesthetic management

As patient access and visualization is limited in the MRI unit (see Figure 29.8), comprehensive monitoring of vital signs is critical for patient assessment during an MRI study. The capability and standards of monitoring should be the same in the MRI unit as in the operating theatre or any other area of the facility where general anaesthesia is administered. As part of patient preparation, intravenous catheters should be placed in the limb that will be the most accessible during the scan to ensure access for the administration of fluids, contrast agent and any other medications necessary during the procedure (Figure 29.13).

MR images are generated in series, repeated using different sequences (patterns of RF pulses and magnetic gradients), and then compared. Any motion, even from respiratory effort, can interfere with image quality; this will increase the scan time necessary to obtain good-quality images and, as a consequence, increase overall anaesthesia time. Controlled ventilation, achieved either manually or with an automatic ventilator, will keep respiratory motion consistent, allow for hyperventilation and maintain a more stable plane of anaesthesia. If a 'breath hold' scan is to be obtained, for which there must be no respiratory motion, the patient can be hyperventilated immediately before, to allow a short period of apnoea (20–40 seconds) for the scan to take place.

The anaesthetist should always be prepared for the possibility of longer than scheduled imaging times to enable additional sequences or imaging of further body

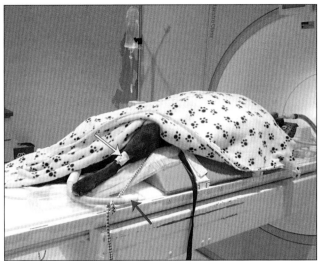

29.13 Patient placed on an absorbent pad to prevent urine or other fluids contaminating the table or leaking into components of the MRI system. Note the positioning of the intravenous catheter (yellow arrow) relative to the components of the magnet (red arrow indicates coil connection). Fluids from the intravenous infusion may damage coil connections.

- In an emergency, the patient should be removed from the MRI room to perform resuscitation procedures
- Inform and train support staff and emergency personnel about the hazards of the MRI room and *not* to run into the room in case of an emergency
- Construct *and practise* an emergency plan specific to the facility
- Identify an area close to the MRI room where emergency assessment and resuscitation procedures will be conducted
- Equip the designated area with an anaesthetic machine, vital signs monitors and a crash cart or box stocked with emergency drugs, additional intravenous catheters and fluids, endotracheal tubes, laryngoscope, suction and other supplies
- Make and display a flowsheet detailing the procedure to follow, similar to the following:
  • Signal or call for assistance
  • Discontinue inhalational or intravenous anaesthesia
  • Stop scanning
  • Move patient out of magnet bore
  • Assess patient
  • Begin cardiopulmonary resuscitation if no pulse
  • Remove from MRI unit to designated area for assessment and resuscitation
  • Notify clinician in charge
  • Transfer to intensive care unit/anaesthesia area

29.15 Guidelines for managing an anaesthetic emergency during MRI.

regions. Additional sedative and/or anaesthetic drugs, support fluids and other medications should be available in or close to the MRI unit. This is particularly important if the MRI facility is distant from the main anaesthesia area or in a trailer (mobile MRI unit) or other remote location.

A high proportion of patients scheduled to undergo MRI have spinal disease, are either weak or non-ambulatory and weigh >15 kg. An MR safe and compatible patient trolley or stretcher should be used to move these patients into and out of the MRI unit to keep the patient's spine stable and to prevent personnel sustaining lifting injuries (Figure 29.14). Some MRI systems have a detachable table that can be used to transport patients into and out of the MRI room.

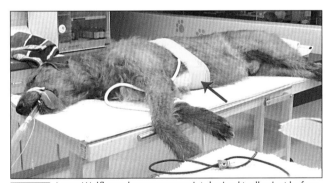

29.14 Large Wolfhound on an appropriately sized trolley just before transport into the MRI room. The red arrow indicates an ECG patch secured to the patient's chest with a light wrap.

Patients are virtually inaccessible during imaging. Because of this, in the event of cardiac arrest or other life-threatening changes occurring during imaging, it is best to remove the patient from the bore of the magnet and the MRI room for assessment and resuscitation. Guidelines for management of anaesthetic emergencies during MRI are provided in Figure 29.15.

Choice of sedation or general anaesthesia

Whether sedation or general anaesthesia is used for patient immobilization during MRI scanning, monitoring of vital signs should be thorough, and provision for intubation and respiratory support should always be part of the anaesthetic plan. Endotracheal tubes, equipment for manual ventilation (Ambu bag; see Chapter 31) and an oxygen source – either an anaesthetic machine or an MR safe portable aluminium oxygen cylinder equipped with an MR conditional regulator and flowmeter – are basic items that should be available.

Sedation, combined with the use of foam positioners and/or straps to insure immobility, may be preferred for obtunded but stable patients scheduled for short scans. However, sedated patients are more difficult to monitor, and the loud noise and vibration associated with MRI may cause unexpected patient arousal. The anaesthetist should maintain direct observation of the sedated patient by remaining in the MRI unit throughout the scan. If the patient becomes compromised, it will be necessary to interrupt the scan and move the patient in order to properly assess the patient and provide support. The anaesthetist must be prepared to intubate and to provide ventilatory support and/or to induce general anaesthesia in the event of respiratory depression or compromise, excessive patient movement, or when scanning time is prolonged.

General anaesthesia maintained using intravenous and/or inhalant agents provides a safe and manageable situation that allows easier and more accurate monitoring of vital signs. In addition, patients are intubated for delivery of oxygen and provision of respiratory monitoring and support. Total intravenous anaesthesia maintained by either infusion or repeated intravenous bolus injections may be indicated for particular patients or when an MR compatible anaesthesia machine and vaporizer are not available. It is important to inspect and secure the intravenous catheter and any connections before moving the patient into the bore of the magnet: disconnection or catheter problems may result in arousal, motion, and potential injury to the patient and damage to the magnet.

Maintenance of anaesthesia using an inhalant agent requires specialized equipment. Veterinary MR conditional machines are readily available and can also be used in the room next to the patient. However, it is important to be aware that an anaesthetic machine that is safe in a low-field or 1.5 T environment may not be safe in a 3.0 T field; MR conditional equipment will be labelled with details of such limitations (see Figure 29.5). Oxygen can be piped into the room or supplied using aluminium MR safe cylinders. Ensure that all cylinders that are safe to take into the room are labelled correctly, to prevent a projectile accident (see Figure 29.5). If a non-compatible machine is to be used inside the MRI unit, it must be located outside the 5 Gauss line and secured to prevent it moving towards the magnet. Alternatively, a non-compatible anaesthetic machine can be located outside the unit, with extra-long gas delivery hoses passed into the room through special wave guide portals that prevent the entrance of external radio waves into the unit (Figure 29.16). Delivery hoses need to be long enough to reach the patient when inside the bore of the magnet. Coaxial systems are commercially available in lengths up to 275 cm, and corrugated tubing can be purchased to connect to a Y-connector for customized systems. The risks associated with the use of long hoses include disconnection, obstruction, kinking or damage to the tubing. It is easier to make the necessary adjustments to delivery of inhalant agent when the patient can be assessed with the anaesthetic machine close to the patient. Intermittent positive pressure ventilation will provide respiratory support and control respiratory motion. Patients with brain disease in particular often have greater respiratory depression resulting from their disease process or when high doses of anticonvulsant medications are combined with sedation and/or general anaesthesia (see Chapter 28).

An active scavenging system for the removal of waste anaesthetic gases can be installed when the MRI unit is built, or a passive system can be used inside the unit (see Chapter 5).

Ideally, MR compatible anaesthetic machines should never leave the MRI room, in order to prevent potential risks from metal objects or non-compatible equipment being placed on the machine while it is outside the room and then inadvertently being brought into the MRI room (see Figure 29.6). Similarly, any equipment used in the MRI room (e.g. pumps, monitors, heat sources) should be left in place.

A second anaesthetic machine, labelled as MR unsafe to prevent it from inadvertently being brought into the MRI room, can be located outside the room for induction, recovery, transport and/or resuscitation procedures.

Monitoring of vital signs

A monitor that is compatible with a 1.5 T scanner may not be compatible with a 3.0 T scanner. Safe placement of monitoring equipment in the MRI room will differ with each facility, based on the fringe fields and manufacturer recommendations (Figure 29.17). It is important to check with the manufacturer about the compatibility of a monitor before using it with a different magnet.

Having a monitor inside the room next to the patient will facilitate assessment and adjustment of anaesthesia and support when the anaesthetist is close to the patient. If there is only one monitor, the anaesthetist will need to either stay in the room for the entire scan or observe the monitor through a window or door (Figure 29.18). A wireless connection to a remote monitor located outside the MRI unit, in the control room or induction/recovery area, will allow the anaesthetist to leave the room and monitor the patient remotely (Figure 29.19). Care is needed with equipment placement and connection, as long cables that cross the

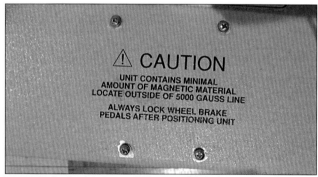

29.17 Caution label on an MRI compatible Invivo monitor. The 5000 Gauss line would be inside the bore of either a 1.5 or 3.0 T magnet, making this monitor safe for these systems.

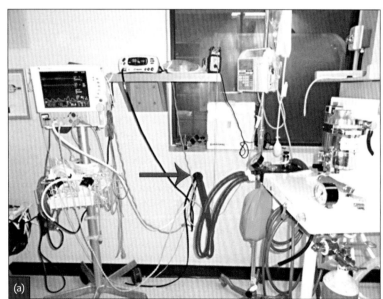
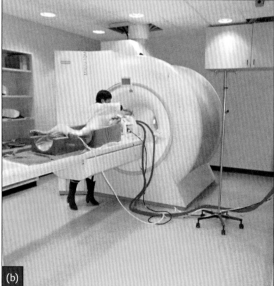

29.16 (a) Non-compatible anaesthetic machine, vital signs monitors, fluid pumps and other equipment located outside the MRI room (magnet can be seen through the window), with MRI compatible hoses, cables and fluid lines passed through an radiofrequency waveguide portal (red arrow) into the MRI room. (b) Hoses and cables inside the MRI room connected to the patient.
(Courtesy of Tanya Duke-Novakovski, Western College of Veterinary Medicine, University of Saskatchewan, Canada)

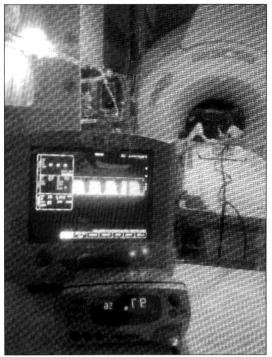

29.18 Multiple monitors located inside the magnet room of this MRI trailer can be seen through the RF-shielded glass window. From this position, the patient, anaesthetic machine and monitors can all be observed from outside the room during imaging.
(Courtesy of PetsDx Veterinary Imaging, USA)

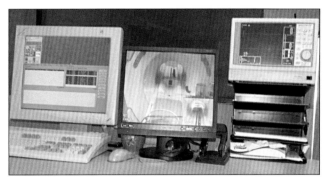

29.19 A remote vital signs monitor (on the far right) is located on the MR technologist's desk outside the MRI room. The monitor in the middle shows a video camera view into the bore of the magnet to enable optimal patient visualization during imaging.
(Courtesy of VCA Veterinary Referral Associates, USA)

work area may become damaged or disconnected, or be a trip hazard for personnel moving around the room. The noise of the gradients will make it difficult to hear any alarms in the MRI room, so it is ideal to choose monitors with large, easy-to-see displays and coloured flashing alarms.

Figure 29.20 lists guidelines for using monitoring and other equipment in an MRI environment.

Gadolinium-based contrast agents

Gadolinium-based contrast agents (GBCAs) are used for contrast studies during MRI. GBCAs are administered intravenously either by bolus injection or by using a rapid infusion system, depending on the study being made and the equipment available. They may also be administered intramuscularly if intravenous access is not available. GBCAs are excreted through the kidneys. The risk of nephrogenic systemic fibrosis, a rare debilitating or fatal condition, after GBCA administration is increased in

Do
• Use devices rated MR conditional for the strength of magnet in use
• Keep MR unsafe devices outside the magnet room (see Figure 29.16)
• Monitor S_pO_2 with fibreoptic technology designed for MRI
• Monitor ECG with insulated cables specifically designed for MRI
• Use carbon graphite ECG electrodes designed for MRI
• Use wireless technology for monitoring devices when available
• Run all cables parallel to the bore of the magnet (see Figure 29.25)
• Limit cable contact with the patient:
• Move cables off to the side of the patient as much as possible
• Insulate hairless or shaved areas where cables may have body contact
• Use sidestream capnography technology:
• Extra-long sampling lines are available
• Monitor indirect or direct blood pressure:
• Air- or fluid-filled lines are not hazardous
• Keep transducer outside the bore of the magnet
• Regulate the administration of intravenous fluids and other infusions:
• Use an MR compatible infusion pump
• If a compatible pump is not available, a non-compatible pump located outside the MRI room with tubing passed through a waveguide portal can be used (see Figure 29.16)
• In-line fluid regulators can be used safely in the MRI room, but are not very accurate, especially in small patients
• Support and monitor body temperature during imaging:
• MRI rooms are often very cold
• Turn off fan in bore of magnet
• Provide heat support in the form of warmed rice bags or 'snap' heat pads (see Figure 29.26). Properly insulate the patient to prevent burns from all heating devices
• Cover the patient with blankets, towels, bubble wrap or other insulating material to conserve body heat
• Monitor body temperature with a digital thermometer or fluoroptic thermometry (devices used to measure surface temperatures are unreliable in animals)
• Prolonged imaging in a 3 T magnet may cause hyperthermia

Do not
• Bring any device into the MRI room without first checking with the radiologist, MR technologist or magnet engineer to verify its safety and compatibility
• Use non-compatible devices inside the 5 Gauss line:
• Risk of device becoming a projectile
• Unreliable readings
• Image degradation and artefacts
• Use metal wires, cables or clips
• Overlap or loop cables in the bore of the magnet:
• Risk of thermal burns from voltages and currents generated during imaging
• Use a mainstream capnography sensor:
• Image artefacts
• Possible damage to the sensor
• Use hard-wired thermistor or thermocouple-based temperature sensors:
• Unreliable readings
• Image artefacts

29.20 Guidelines for using monitoring and other devices in an MRI environment. ECG = electrocardiogram; S_pO_2 = oxygen saturation of haemoglobin.

humans with compromised renal function due to acute or chronic renal disease. This condition has not been reported in animals, but the administration of contrast should be carefully considered in patients with impaired renal function.

Mild to severe anaphylactoid reactions following the intravenous administration of GBCAs have been reported in dogs, albeit rarely (Girard and Leece, 2010); dogs with a history of atopy may be more susceptible to an adverse reaction. Detection of an anaphylactoid reaction resulting from an injection of GBCA may be delayed due to anaesthesia and limited access to the patient during MRI. Following GBCA administration to a patient, the anaesthetist should remain in the MRI unit to monitor the patient closely for any sudden change in haemodynamic status or other signs of anaphylaxis.

Avoidance of imaging artefacts

Some common artefacts on MR images can be prevented by paying careful attention to the placement of objects such as intravenous lines and pilot balloons on endotracheal tubes, and preventing patient movement during imaging (Figures 29.21 and 29.22).

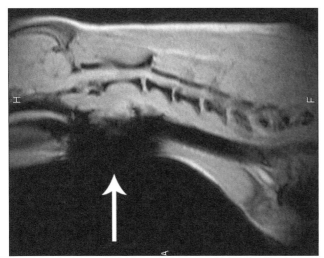

29.21 The large void (white arrow) seen on this MRI localizer image of a dog's neck is an artefact caused by the small amount of metal in the pilot balloon of the endotracheal tube, which was under the dog's neck. When positioning intubated patients, always ensure that the pilot balloon is moved away from the patient to avoid this artefact.

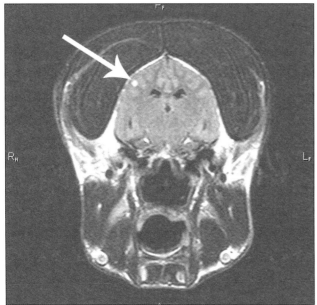

29.22 The small circular area (white arrow) seen on this brain scan was found to be an artefact from the fluid in the intravenous tubing that was running beside the head coil. Objects adjacent to radiofrequency coils can be inadvertently brought into the MR images. To avoid this artefact, ensure that fluid lines are kept away from the area being scanned.

Personnel considerations

Before providing anaesthetic support for a patient undergoing MRI, personnel should be screened and properly informed of the hazards and safety concerns for themselves and for the patient (Figures 29.23 to 29.26).

Anaesthetist

- Screen all anaesthesia personnel who will be working in the MRI unit for the presence of metal items in the body (aneurysm clip, ocular metal, pacemaker, hearing aid, cochlear implant, metal piercings, etc.)
- Make an MRI safety course mandatory for personnel and monitor compliance
- Provide routine reviews of formal safety and emergency procedures
- Restrict access: only individuals who have taken the safety course will be allowed to provide anaesthetic support to patients undergoing MRI
- Inform *all* personnel that the magnet is *always on*
- Be alert and constantly observe all personnel to ensure that no oxygen cylinders, clippers, stethoscopes, laryngoscopes, pens, scissors, haemostats, neurology hammers or other ferromagnetic objects are carried into the magnet room

Equipment

- Equipment not designated MR safe should *not* be taken into the room until it has been tested and labelled as MR safe or MR conditional by the magnet engineer, MR technologist and/or designated Safety Officer
- Conspicuously label all MR unsafe equipment located outside or in close proximity to the door of the MRI unit (see Figure 29.6)
- Be vigilant and recheck any equipment that leaves the MRI area and subsequently returns to ensure that it is MR safe
- When using equipment containing ferromagnetic components inside the MRI room, be sure to physically secure it at a safe distance from the magnet, outside the 5 Gauss line, using non-magnetic bolts, rope, plastic chains or weighted base assemblies as appropriate. Properly label the equipment and apply tape lines on the floor around it so it is easy to see where the equipment should be located

Patient screening

- Carefully screen patients before they enter the MRI unit for the presence of any metallic objects. Obtain a complete history of the presence of microchips, implants, pellets or shrapnel, ingested gravel or other metallic substances that may be a hazard or interfere with image acquisition
- Remove collars, harnesses, hair clips, etc.
- Remove transdermal patches if they are in the region that is to be scanned, as they may contain aluminium, which will heat up during imaging, causing skin irritation or burns
- *Always* remove blankets and other coverings before the patient enters the MRI room. Ferromagnetic items may be hidden under blankets and may become missiles upon entering the room
- Use a non-ferromagnetic gurney or stretcher to transport large patients into the MRI area
- Inspect any attached medical devices for metal parts or needles (urine bags (see Figure 29.24), triple-lumen catheters, infusion pumps, transdermal patches, etc.)

29.23 Personnel and patient safety guidelines for MRI.

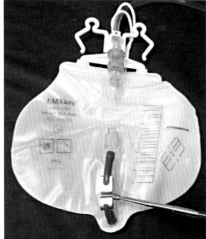

29.24 Urine bag attached to a patient scheduled for an MRI scan. The bag has a metal clamp which is attracted to the small hand-held magnet, demonstrating that it is ferromagnetic. For safety reasons, before this patient enters the MRI area, the clamp should be removed from the bag, or the bag can be temporarily removed from the urinary catheter for the duration of the scan.

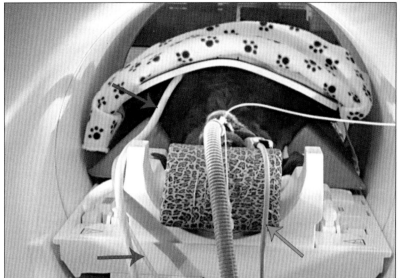

29.25 Dog in the bore of a 1.5 T magnet, with the monitoring cables placed parallel to the bore with limited contact with the body. Red arrow = insulated ECG cable; Green arrow = pulse oximeter fibreoptic cable; Blue arrow = air-filled blood pressure line.

The most common cause of accidents involving MRI scanners is human error. Communication and planning are vital to prevent accidents and ensure a safe and uneventful anaesthetic event for both the patient and the personnel involved.

References and further reading

American Society of Anesthesiologists Task Force on Anesthetic Care for Magnetic Resonance Imaging (2009) Practice advisory on anesthetic care for magnetic resonance imaging. *Anesthesiology* **110**, 459–479

Girard NM and Leece EA (2010) Suspected anaphylactoid reaction following intravenous administration of a gadolinium-based contrast agent in three dogs undergoing magnetic resonance imaging. *Veterinary Anaesthesia and Analgesia* **37**, 352–356

Kanal E, Barkovich AJ, Gilk T *et al.* (2007) ACR guidance document for safe MR practices: 2007. *American Journal of Roentgenology* **188**, 1447–1474

MHRA (2007) Device Bulletin: Safety guidelines for magnetic resonance imaging equipment in clinical use. DB2007(3). Available from http://webarchive. nationalarchives.gov.uk/20141205150130/http://www.mhra.gov.uk/Publications/ Safetyguidance/DeviceBulletins/CON2033018

Willis HRH (2009) Magnetic resonance imaging hazards and safety guidelines. *Willis Strategic Outcomes Practice Technical Advisory Bulletin.* www.willis.com/ Documents/Publications/Services/Claims_Management/MRI_Safety_ August_2009_V6.pdf

Useful websites

www.mrisafety.com

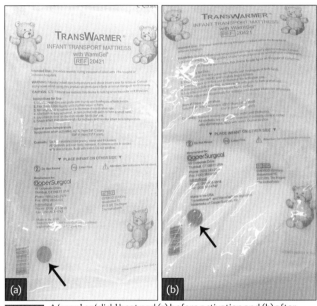

29.26 A 'snap' or 'click' heat pad (a) before activation and (b) after activation. Pads of this type are magnet safe, but the metal activation snap inside the pad (black arrows) will cause an image artefact if it is close to the region being imaged. Note that these pads become very hot upon activation and should not be placed in direct contact with a patient, otherwise serious burns may occur.

Chapter 30

Anaesthesia for paediatric and geriatric patients

Clara F. Rigotti and Jacqueline C. Brearley

Paediatric and geriatric patients will be discussed together in this chapter because the considerations for anaesthetic management are similar for patients at either extreme of the age spectrum. In the neonate, the body is still developing, and although organs may be capable of rapid repair they are also very vulnerable to damage, which may become evident only later in life. In the geriatric patient, the functioning of the various body systems becomes limited because of degeneration. A full understanding of the physiological differences in paediatric and geriatric patients compared to young adult animals is vital (Figure 30.1). The veterinary surgeon (veterinarian) must aim neither to cause any harm to a vulnerable and still developing paediatric patient, nor to accelerate the degenerative changes that will already be present in a geriatric patient. Old age *per se* is not a contraindication for anaesthesia, but some of the changes associated with age can be so.

For practical purposes, the term 'paediatric' refers to dogs and cats aged up to 6 months; these animals can be further classified as neonatal (0–2 weeks; Figure 30.2), infant (2–6 weeks), weanling (6–12 weeks) or juvenile (3–6 months). Animals older than 6 months of age are still growing but generally need doses of anaesthetic and analgesic drugs similar to those used in mature animals.

It is more difficult to define a 'geriatric' patient because individual animals age at different rates. One suggestion is that an animal can be regarded as geriatric when it has reached 75–80% of its normal expected lifespan for the species and breed; ultimately, however, each animal must be assessed and treated on an individual basis. Owners of geriatric patients should be informed that their animal may have some mental deterioration after anaesthesia. This is more evident in animals that already show signs of dementia.

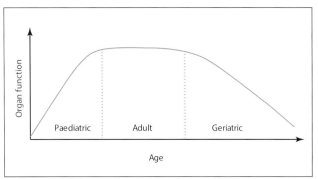

30.1 Graph showing the changes of an organ's function in relation to patient age.

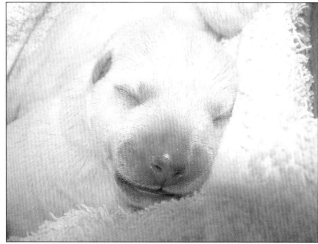

30.2 A neonatal puppy with closed eyes, a relatively large nose and the tip of a large tongue just visible.

Anatomy and physiology of paediatric and geriatric animals

Respiratory system

Paediatric patients

The tongue is relatively large in comparison to the oropharyngeal cavity, and this may result in upper airway obstruction when the muscles relax during sedation and anaesthesia. The tracheal lumen may be relatively narrow, and the very flexible tracheal cartilages may predispose to tracheal collapse. Endotracheal intubation is therefore recommended during general anaesthesia of paediatric patients; however, intubation can be challenging because of the small dimensions of the oropharynx and trachea. The chest wall is relatively flexible and compliant in young animals. The relatively small functional residual capacity of these patients predisposes them to lung atelectasis, which will decrease further their already limited respiratory reserves. Oxygen requirement in puppies <6 weeks of age is two times that of mature animals; this requirement results in a high basal respiratory rate that must be maintained during anaesthesia. The respiratory muscles fatigue easily because of the higher work of breathing; as a result, neonates cannot sustain an increase in minute volume in response to hypoxaemia for a long period of time. Hypoventilation and atelectasis can be corrected by using intermittent positive pressure ventilation (IPPV) during anaesthesia, but this must be applied carefully to avoid lung trauma.

Geriatric patients

Functional residual capacity increases with age, with an associated increase in closing volume, leading to small airway closure and a decrease in vital capacity (Robinson and Gillespie, 1973). Increased lung fibrosis ('old animal lungs') and reduced respiratory muscle function (i.e. muscle weakness) also contribute to these changes. The overall result is increased alveolar ventilation/perfusion mismatch and a decreased resting arterial oxygen tension. Ability to respond to hypercapnia and hypoxaemia is decreased. Furthermore, the laryngeal and pharyngeal protective reflexes are diminished, rendering geriatric patients more susceptible to aspiration. Endotracheal intubation is advisable to protect the airway against aspiration, allow efficient oxygen supplementation and allow IPPV if required.

Cardiovascular system

Paediatric patients

The paediatric heart is characterized by a less contractile myocardium and less compliant ventricles compared to the heart of mature animals. Stroke volume (SV) is limited and cardiac output (CO) is therefore dependent on heart rate (HR). Parasympathetic innervation of the heart is already mature and dominant at birth, whereas sympathetic innervation takes some time to develop; together, these factors make young animals more prone to bradycardia and hypotension in the presence of hypothermia, hypoglycaemia or certain drugs (e.g. opioids and alpha-2 adrenoceptor agonists). Systemic arterial blood pressure (ABP) in newborns is relatively low compared with blood pressure in older animals: an average systolic ABP of 54 mmHg, mean ABP of 40 mmHg and diastolic ABP of 30 mmHg are considered to be normal (Moon et al., 2001). Systemic vascular resistance, SV and ABP all increase to adult values during the first weeks of life, while HR, CO, plasma volume (per kg bodyweight) and venous pressure decrease. Because cardiac performance at rest is already high, the newborn has limited cardiac capacity to respond to stress. The immaturity of the baroreceptor reflex and sympathetic nervous system means that responses to acute changes in ABP normally seen in mature animals are not present. Haemorrhage is not well tolerated and even moderate blood loss of 5 ml/kg may result in severe hypotension and anaemia. The presence of a heart murmur during the neonatal period is not unusual, as functional closure of the foramen ovale occurs within 48 hours after birth in most animals and complete closure is usually achieved during the first 21 days of life (Oliveira et al., 1980).

At birth, 70–90% of total haemoglobin is still in the form of fetal haemoglobin (HbF). Over time, the proportion of HbF decreases and adult haemoglobin (HbA) comes to predominate. HbF binds oxygen more easily than HbA but releases oxygen to the peripheral tissues less readily because of low concentrations of erythrocyte 2,3-diphosphoglycerate (2,3-DPG), resulting in a left shift of the oxygen–haemoglobin dissociation curve. Haemoglobin concentration and packed cell volume (PCV) are lower

than in mature animals because of a shortened erythrocyte lifespan combined with a lower erythrocyte production rate. The haemopoietic system becomes more efficient at 2–3 months of age.

Geriatric patients

Maximum HR decreases with increasing age in adult animals, resulting in a decreased cardiac reserve. There is an increased incidence of valvular lesions, which increase myocardial work for a given CO. The consequent increase in myocardial oxygen demand makes the heart more sensitive to hypoxia. When leaky valves and regurgitation are present, effective SV decreases, but end-diastolic volume increases as forward flow is reduced. Other cardiovascular changes with age include decreased baroreceptor activity, decreased circulating blood volume and decreased vagal tone. Together these changes result in an increased resting HR and a decreased ability to respond to changes in blood pressure. Older animals have decreased vasoconstrictor and cardiac responses to reduced cardiac preload, but have an increased response to exogenous catecholamines. This suggests that the output of the autonomic nervous system may be reduced and that there is a consequent increase in receptor sensitivity or density. The conduction pathways in the heart also change in older patients, making them more prone to anaesthesia-induced arrhythmias. Overall, the changes within the circulatory system decrease the geriatric animal's ability to respond to circulatory changes or stress (Cheitlin, 2003).

Renal system

Paediatric patients

Nephrogenesis is complete at approximately 3 weeks of age, but renal excretion of drugs may be limited during the first 2 months of life until renal function is fully mature. Glomerular filtration rate (GFR) and tubular secretion are lower than in the mature animal due to high renal vascular resistance. Care must therefore be taken when large volumes of intravenous fluids are administered and when drugs dependent on renal excretion are used.

Geriatric patients

Unlike humans, hypertension is not associated with ageing in cats and dogs (Meurs et al., 2000), although hypertension secondary to, for instance, renal disease and hyperadrenocorticism, can occur in older animals (Brown et al., 2007). In cats, blood pressure increases with age and cats with chronic kidney disease are more likely to develop hypertension. In this species, creatinine concentration has been demonstrated to be an independent risk factor for the development of hypertension (Bijsmans et al., 2015). Renal reserve decreases with increasing age, as the kidney has no regenerative capacity. Cardiovascular changes can result in reduced renal blood flow and there is a decrease in the number of glomeruli and nephrons; together, these result in a decrease in GFR of up to approximately 50%. Tubular changes such as atrophy, decreased diameter and tubular disruption lead to a decreased ability to concentrate urine, which renders the patient more dependent on fluid intake and less tolerant of both fluid deficit and excess. In addition, with decreasing ability of the kidney to excrete hydrogen ions, acid–base balance is altered, resulting in changes in drug sensitivity, active drug forms and plasma protein binding. As a consequence, the effects of anaesthesia and surgery are exacerbated in geriatric patients, rendering them more susceptible to further renal damage. Decreased erythropoietin production by the kidney combined with decreased intestinal iron and vitamin B12 absorption (see below) may lead to chronic anaemia of old age.

Gastrointestinal system
Paediatric patients

The lower oesophageal sphincter is not fully developed until at least 5 weeks after birth (Spedale et al., 1982). Consequently, neonates have an increased incidence of regurgitation. This emphasizes the importance of endotracheal intubation during anaesthesia to protect the airway from aspiration.

Geriatric patients

There is a higher incidence of chronic intestinal problems in older cats and dogs. Lower oesophageal sphincter tone is reduced and gastric pH is lower, making these patients more prone to reflux and oesophagitis. Malabsorption and decreased uptake of essential nutrients can easily lead to nutritional deficiencies; in particular, decreased iron and vitamin B12 absorption may contribute to anaemia.

Hepatic function
Paediatric patients

The hepatic enzyme systems, such as cytochrome P450 hydroxylation and demethylation pathways, reach full capacity at approximately 5 months of age. At birth, oxidation is the most efficient metabolic pathway. All drugs that undergo metabolism in the liver may have a prolonged duration of action during the first months of life; consequently, it is recommended to use lower doses than would be administered to mature animals and to choose drugs with a short duration of action or those that can be antagonized. Hypoglycaemia is common, especially in the stressed and fasted neonate, because of these patients' small glycogen reserves.

Geriatric patients

The liver has the largest regenerative capacity of any internal organ but is prone to hepatopathy. Decreased immune function in the older patient may increase the risk of bacteraemia; synthesis of albumin and gluconeogenesis may also be reduced. Reductions in drug clearance and protein binding may increase effective drug concentrations. In addition to hypoproteinaemia, there may be decreased production of clotting factors.

Central and peripheral nervous systems
Paediatric patients

The central and peripheral nervous systems mature during the first 3 weeks of life. The blood–brain barrier is not mature in neonates and is more permeable than in adults (up to six times more permeable for certain drugs, e.g. morphine). However, cerebral autoregulation is immediately functional from birth.

Peripheral nerves are also immature in the neonate and require a lower dose of local anaesthetic agent to achieve conduction blockade. The minimum alveolar concentration of volatile agents is lower in the neonate but increases with age.

Geriatric patients

The increasing incidence of central nervous ischaemic episodes with age results in areas of cell death and dysfunction. This may be the mechanism behind post-anaesthetic cognitive dysfunction, which is well recognized in humans and becoming increasingly recognized in companion animals. These ischaemic episodes may also occur in younger animals, but the plasticity of their nervous system is able to accommodate the damage resulting from these insults. In older animals this neural reserve is not present and manifests as reduced brain weight. Manifestations of the post-anaesthetic syndrome can be severe (post-anaesthetic blindness or deafness) or milder (e.g. loss of learned behaviours).

Neuromuscular system
Paediatric patients

Reduced release of acetylcholine is evident in paediatric patients. This, rather than a lower number of postjunctional acetylcholine receptors, means that lower doses of non-depolarizing neuromuscular blocking agents (NMBAs) are required to produce neuromuscular blockade.

Geriatric patients

Although older animals are neither more resistant nor more sensitive to NMBAs, a longer onset time and duration of action of the steroidal NMBAs (e.g. vecuronium and pancuronium) can be observed in these patients. These agents are dependent on hepatic metabolism for termination of their action, unlike atracurium and cisatracurium (Arain et al., 2005). The variably increased duration of action of vecuronium, in combination with an inherent decrease in muscular function in geriatric patients, means that neuromuscular blockade with vecuronium should always be carefully monitored and antagonists given if deemed necessary. With atracurium-induced neuromuscular blockade, antagonism may be less commonly required, as spontaneous degradation of atracurium in plasma does not alter with age and so its duration of action is far more predictable in the normothermic geriatric patient. Geriatric patients receiving NMBAs should also be monitored closely in the recovery period, as a combination of residual blockade and decreased inherent muscle strength will rapidly result in hypoventilation and potential hypoxaemia.

Bones and joints
Paediatric patients

Care should be taken with positioning of young cats and dogs, as their ligaments are still lax and growth plates are still separated, increasing the risk of displacement when vigorous manipulations are carried out.

Geriatric patients

Osteoporosis and osteoarthritis in the geriatric animal will result in brittle bones and chronic pain, respectively. Signs of chronic pain may not be readily recognized by either the owner or the veterinary surgeon. Placing the animal in an abnormal position during anaesthesia and surgery may stimulate the sympathetic nervous system during the maintenance phase of anaesthesia and may worsen the chronic pain during the recovery period. Careful positioning and gentle handling are required to minimize this problem (Figure 30.3).

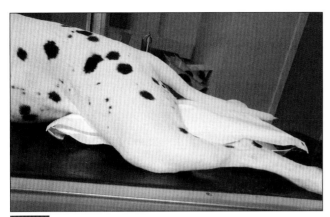

30.3 Careful positioning of the hip joints in an elderly Dalmatian.

Skin
Paediatric patients
Premature kittens and puppies may have a fragile skin; this is not generally a problem in the full-term neonatal or paediatric animal.

Geriatric patients
Geriatric animals exhibit slower healing in general, and particularly of the skin. The ability to form scar tissue is diminished and wounds take longer to heal. Concurrent corticosteroid administration to treat atopy or arthritis will exacerbate this delayed healing.

Thyroid function
Paediatric patients
Thyroid function, as determined by measurement of plasma concentrations of tri-iodothyronine (T3) and thyroxine (T4), is higher in neonates than in adults. This is reflected by the characteristically high metabolic rate of neonatal animals.

Geriatric patients
Thyroid function decreases as the animal ages. This appears to be secondary to an age-related reduction in metabolically active tissue mass in older animals, rather than an inherent decrease in the ability of the gland to respond to thyroid-stimulating hormone. Thermoregulation is impaired, in addition to other factors predisposing to hypothermia (see later). There may be thyroid-induced alterations in cognitive function, which may contribute to post-anaesthetic cognitive dysfunction.

Adrenal glands
Paediatric patients
The adrenal glands are still undergoing considerable changes around the time of birth and during the early neonatal period, which can result in a reduced response to stressors such as anaesthesia and surgery. However, there is little evidence that this causes clinical problems.

Geriatric patients
Age-related adrenal atrophy occurs, rendering the older animal less able to mount an adequate stress response to anaesthesia and surgery.

Senses
Paediatric patients
Both hearing and sight are usually well developed in kittens and puppies by the age of 4 weeks, with hearing maturing about a week before sight. Other senses, such as smell and touch, are also developing during this period. Hypoxic episodes during anaesthesia in this maturation phase may damage the sensory organs; it is therefore important to monitor oxygen saturation carefully and provide supplemental oxygen in very young patients.

Geriatric patients
Hearing is impaired in most geriatric animals. When at home, the animal may be able to accommodate this impairment, but in the hospital setting, with an unfamiliar environment and people, the animal may easily become confused and difficult to handle. Senile lenticular sclerosis and senile cataracts may impair vision in the older animal, resulting in the animal having difficulty in orientation to its new surroundings.

Temperature regulation
Paediatric patients
Neurological control of body temperature develops by 3 weeks of age; before this age the puppy or kitten will seek warmth but is unable to compensate for a cold environment. The large surface area:bodyweight ratio, minimal amount of subcutaneous fat and poorly developed shivering and vasoconstrictive mechanisms of young animals all predispose them to hypothermia. Non-shivering thermogenesis is responsible for 40% of total heat production and is mediated by the release of catecholamines and breakdown of brown fat. Great care must be taken to keep young patients in an environment warmer than that required by an adult patient (e.g. an incubator maintained at 38°C).

Geriatric patients
Temperature regulation is impaired in the geriatric patient. In conjunction with a decreased metabolic rate and changes in body composition (redistribution of fat stores), this renders the geriatric patient more susceptible to anaesthesia-induced hypothermia than a young adult animal (Mallet, 2002). This, in turn, may slow recovery from anaesthesia and potentially increase post-anaesthetic hypoxaemia if shivering occurs (see Chapter 3).

Body composition
Paediatric patients
At birth, water constitutes 84% of bodyweight, but this percentage decreases progressively with increasing age. Water distribution also changes: at birth, 62% of body water is in the extracellular fluid, but this amount slowly decreases until 6 months of age, when extracellular and intracellular fluid volumes are approximately equal. Despite their high water content, dehydration is poorly tolerated in

young animals. Neonates have a lower percentage of bodyweight as fat, and the amount of fat increases with age. Drugs may be better absorbed after subcutaneous injection in young animals unless peripheral vasoconstriction is present (e.g. as a result of hypothermia). Lipid-soluble drugs have a smaller volume of distribution in paediatric patients than in adults, and as a result, paediatric patients may be easily overdosed. In contrast, water-soluble drugs have a larger volume of distribution in paediatric patients and so the drug plasma concentration may be lower than expected. Albumin and plasma protein concentrations are lower in neonates. The albumin concentration reaches adult values at approximately 8 weeks of age, while it can take up to 6–12 months before total protein concentrations reach adult values (von Dehn, 2014). Neonates also have lower concentrations of alpha-1 acid glycoprotein, which is important for protein binding of certain drugs such as lidocaine, fentanyl, alfentanil and sufentanil. Drugs that are normally highly protein bound may show increased concentrations of the free, active form in the neonatal patient and may therefore exert greater therapeutic or toxic effects.

Geriatric patients

Decreased body fat content makes geriatric animals more susceptible to delayed recovery from injectable anaesthesia, as there is less tissue into which injectable anaesthetic agents can redistribute (see Chapter 14). Plasma concentrations are maintained at a higher level, which declines in proportion to inactivation of the agents; decreased muscle mass and strength may also contribute to delaying recovery to full muscular function. Hypothermia will further complicate recovery from anaesthesia. In comparison to the young adult and neonate, the geriatric patient tends to have lower body water content. This, in combination with reduced central thirst mechanisms and decreased renal water conservation, can lead to dehydration in the perioperative period.

Considerations for anaesthesia

Preoperative assessment

Paediatric patients

Preoperative assessment of the neonate can be challenging. Initial assessment should focus on the development of the puppy or kitten in comparison to its littermates or the breed standards; a smaller or weaker animal may require further diagnostic tests. A thorough physical examination with particular attention to the cardiopulmonary system should be performed. Thoracic auscultation can be difficult because of the small thoracic size and high heart and respiratory rates of very young patients. Furthermore, the presence of a heart murmur during the first 3 months of life is not unusual.

Measurement of blood glucose concentration is important to monitor for hypoglycaemia. When blood work is indicated, small blood samples can be taken by using capillary tubes. Bodyweight must be measured accurately to allow precise dosing of drugs, and either kitchen or analytical scales may be required to weigh very small patients.

Geriatric patients

An animal that looks and behaves 'old' rather than being chronologically 'old' may require further investigation.

Cardiopulmonary investigations, including an assessment of exercise tolerance, should be undertaken. If the animal's exercise tolerance is normal, then simple thoracic auscultation and pulse assessment is sufficient, whereas poor exercise tolerance warrants further investigation (e.g. electrocardiography, radiography or echocardiography). Assessment of renal function using measurement of blood urea nitrogen and creatinine concentrations will provide some indication of gross renal impairment, although approximately 75% of nephrons must be non-functional before measurable increases in these parameters occur. Other simple indicators of renal function should also be used, such as a history of polydipsia and polyuria, and measurement of urine specific gravity. Prerenal causes of any abnormalities should also be considered. Liver function tests (liver enzymes, total protein concentration, clotting profiles and pre- and postprandial bile acid concentrations) are a useful guide to the presence of liver damage and/or dysfunction. Liver enzyme concentrations remain constant with age, but an age-related decrease in liver mass reduces overall liver function. Prolonged exposure over time to environmental factors or toxins that are potentially damaging to the liver may be reflected in release of liver enzymes. Liver function is a reflection not just of metabolic capacity but also of hepatic blood flow (see Chapter 24); an age-related decrease in hepatic blood flow can result in decreased clearance and increased duration of action of drugs that undergo hepatic metabolism. Many older anaesthetic and sedative drugs are highly dependent on liver metabolism for deactivation (e.g. barbiturates), or actively cause liver damage (e.g. halothane and chloroform). However, with modern anaesthetics and sedatives that also undergo extrahepatic metabolism (propofol), or minimal metabolism (isoflurane), or for which antagonists are available (medetomidine/dexmedetomidine), the effect of hepatic function on recovery is a lesser consideration than was the case before their introduction. Of more importance is how anaesthesia and the associated hypotension may impair hepatic and renal blood flow, which carries a risk of causing further ischaemic damage.

Other investigations should be undertaken as indicated by the history and clinical examination. In a study investigating the influence of routine blood screening in 1537 dogs of all ages on the choice of anaesthetic subsequently delivered, there was little evidence to suggest that blood screening made any difference to outcome, unless potential problems had already been suggested by the history and thorough clinical examination (Alef et al., 2008). However, in a study in which 101 geriatric dogs (>7 years of age) underwent pre-anaesthetic screening, 30 animals were diagnosed with an abnormality on the basis of the screening and 13 did not undergo the proposed procedure under general anaesthesia (Joubert, 2007). Based on these findings, pre-anaesthetic screening in older patients (>7 years of age) is recommended, as 30–50% of animals in this age group have subclinical disease. The screen commonly includes measurement of PCV, total protein, urea, creatinine and glucose concentrations, and liver enzymes.

Anaesthetic preparation and pre-anaesthetic medication

Drug and dose recommendations for pre-anaesthetic medication and reversal agents in both paediatric and geriatric patients are provided in Figures 30.4 and 30.5.

Drug	Dose (mg/kg)	Route of administration
Diazepam	0.05–0.2	i.v.
Midazolam	0.05–0.2	i.v. or i.m.
Methadone	0.2–0.3 0.1–0.2	i.m. i.v.
Morphine	0.1–0.3 0.1–0.2	i.m. i.v.
Hydromorphone	0.05–0.1	i.v. or i.m.
Buprenorphine	0.005–0.02	i.v. or i.m. or OTM (cats)
Butorphanol	0.2–0.3 0.1–0.2	i.m. i.v.
Acepromazine	0.01–0.02 0.005–0.01	i.m. i.v.
Medetomidine	0.001 0.002–0.005	i.v. i.m.
Dexmedetomidine	Half the above dose of medetomidine	i.v. or i.m.

30.4 Suggested doses for sedation of paediatric and geriatric patients. OTM = oral transmucosal.

Drug	Dose (mg/kg)	Route of administration
Flumazenil	0.01–0.03	i.v.
Naloxone	0.004–0.04 0.01–0.1	i.v. i.m.
Atipamezole	Dogs: 5x previous medetomidine/dexmedetomidine dose (i.e. equal volume of solution to medetomidine or dexmedetomidine) Cats: 2.5x previous medetomidine/dexmedetomidine dose (i.e. half volume of solution to medetomidine or dexmedetomidine)	i.m.

30.5 Suggested doses for reversal agents in paediatric and geriatric patients.

Paediatric patients

Suckling animals should not be fasted before anaesthesia, and paediatric animals may require only 2 hours of fasting time. In these patients, hypoglycaemia caused by prolonged starvation is a greater risk than aspiration.

Depending on the patient's age and general condition, a sedative may not be necessary; use of sedatives should be minimized in neonatal patients. However, intravenous catheterization is often challenging in the non-sedated young animal (Figure 30.6). A small amount of topical anaesthetic

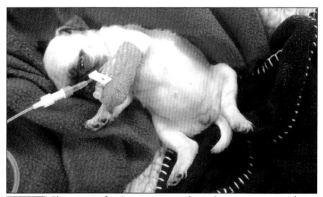

30.6 Placement of an intravenous catheter in a very young and small patient can be challenging.

cream (EMLA cream) can be applied to desensitize the skin before blood sampling or catheter placement, although care must be taken with the amount applied to minimize the risk of toxic side effects (e.g. oxidation of haemoglobin to methaemoglobin, seizures), especially considering that HbF oxidizes more rapidly than HbA.

A benzodiazepine combined with an opioid and administered intramuscularly is generally the authors' choice for sedating paediatric animals. Benzodiazepines provide effective sedation in young animals (unlike in adults), with minimal cardiovascular effects. If over-sedation with benzodiazepines occurs, it may be antagonized with flumazenil. Inclusion of an opioid will increase the sedative effect of the benzodiazepine and provide analgesia; however, administration of opioids can result in bradycardia, which may need treatment with an anticholinergic agent (e.g. atropine or glycopyrronium). Specific opioid antagonists can be used, such as naloxone, but these will also diminish the analgesic effects of the opioid.

Phenothiazines (e.g. acepromazine) have a long duration of action, and can cause profound sedation, vasodilation, possible cardiovascular collapse in the compromised patient and hypothermia. Acepromazine at low doses can be used in paediatric patients with stable haemodynamics, but is not recommended in neonates.

Alpha-2 adrenergic agonists (e.g. medetomidine, dexmedetomidine) are potent sedatives with additional analgesic properties. They also produce profound bradycardia, which results in a profound decrease in CO. They should be used only in relatively older and healthy paediatric patients, and their action should be antagonized by administering atipamezole at the end of the procedure if necessary.

Geriatric patients

Food should not be withheld for longer than necessary in the geriatric patient as hepatic glycogen reserves are often limited. Geriatric patients should be fasted for no more than 6 hours, but it is important to remember that even after this period they may still have a relatively full stomach and be prone to vomiting, regurgitation and aspiration. Water should be withheld either from the time of preanaesthetic medication or approximately 30 minutes before induction of anaesthesia. The animal should be handled carefully to minimize stress. Light sedation is often useful to facilitate handling, but the effects of any drugs given on the geriatric patient's organ systems should be taken into account, and minimal doses should be used. Although diazepam is often recommended in geriatric animals, even at moderate doses (0.2 mg/kg i.v.), it causes marked respiratory depression in elderly humans (Stewart, 1978); in the authors' experience, it has the same effect in dogs, particularly if used in combination with opioids. The respiratory depression produced by diazepam is characterized by decreases in both respiratory rate and tidal volume. If a benzodiazepine is to be used as a sedative/pre-anaesthetic medication it should be given at moderate doses, intramuscularly and close monitoring of respiratory function should be performed.

As with any anaesthetic procedure, venous access should be secured as early as possible in the preoperative period with minimal stress caused to the animal. It is important to appreciate that routine restraint may be painful to an animal with advanced arthritis, and in these cases, less conventional practices should be adopted, such as catheterization of the lateral saphenous vein in the standing animal.

Analgesia

Paediatric patients

Paediatric animals are known to perceive pain, and it has been shown that a painful insult in early life can influence their future nociception (Anand *et al.*, 1999; Lee, 2002).

In neonates, lower doses of full mu opioid receptor agonists are often required to provide analgesia, as very young patients are more sensitive to both their analgesic and side effects (Luks *et al.*, 1998). However, animals several weeks of age and older often require adult doses. It is best to start at the lower end of the dose range and increase the dose if necessary. Non-steroidal anti-inflammatory drugs (NSAIDs) are not recommended in animals less than 6 weeks of age because of the relatively late development of the hepatic and renal systems. NSAIDs inhibit the function of the enzyme cyclo-oxygenase–2, which is required for renal maturation and electrolyte balance. Their action also blocks the synthesis of various prostaglandins (see Chapter 10), which play a major role in closure of the ductus arteriosus after birth (see Chapter 26). In neonates, renal clearance of NSAIDs is lower and their terminal half-life is longer.

The application of locoregional blocks is encouraged. Local anaesthetic agents that can be used for this purpose include lidocaine, bupivacaine and ropivacaine. Lower doses than used in adults are recommended for paediatric patients, as their nerves are smaller and not yet completely myelinated. Furthermore, the metabolism of local anaesthetics of the amino-amide group may be reduced due to the still-immature metabolic pathways of the liver, which predisposes these patients to a higher risk of toxic effects (Yaster and Maxwell, 1989). Epidural analgesia is commonly performed in human paediatric patients (Patel, 2006); this procedure can also be performed in paediatric animals, although there are no published reports of its use. Care should be taken when administering an epidural block, as the spinal cord continues more caudally in the paediatric patient relative to the adult and the risks of entering the subarachnoid space and causing nerve trauma are therefore higher. For further reading on local anaesthetics, see Chapter 11.

Geriatric patients

Intraoperative analgesia may be required even for simple procedures such as radiography, because geriatric patients are likely to have muscle stiffness and joint pain. As in paediatric animals, the use of locoregional and other local anaesthesia techniques (e.g. line infiltration or splash blocks) will allow lower doses of anaesthetic agents to be used, and should be considered as an alternative or adjunct to general anaesthesia. Epidural blocks may be more difficult to perform successfully in older animals with ankylosis and new bone formation at the lumbosacral junction. If epidural analgesia is considered essential, it may be useful to refer to a spinal radiograph to help with needle placement. If the patient is already receiving a NSAID for arthritis or other chronically painful conditions, the medication should be continued, but particular attention should be paid to maintenance of ABP during anaesthesia.

The duration of action of anaesthetic and analgesic drugs in particular is age-related. For example, the elimination half-life of pethidine (meperidine) increases in dogs older than 10 years of age (146 minutes after intramuscular injection, compared to 51 minutes in younger patients) (Waterman and Kalthum, 1989, 1990). It is therefore important to observe the patient carefully and dose analgesics as required rather than at a set time interval.

Anaesthetic induction and maintenance

Paediatric patients

In most neonates it is easiest to induce anaesthesia with an inhalant anaesthetic delivered via facemask. Sevoflurane is the agent of choice for induction of anaesthesia because of its greater speed of onset and better tolerability compared with isoflurane (Figure 30.7). Because uptake is relatively fast in neonates and these patients are more sensitive to the effects of inhalant anaesthetics than older animals, a vaporizer setting of 3% is usually sufficient.

If venous access is available, injectable agents can be used, titrated to effect. If venous access cannot be obtained before induction of anaesthesia, it should be secured as soon as possible after induction.

Ketamine is commonly used in anaesthesia of human neonates because of its minimal cardiovascular depressant effects. Recovery from ketamine anaesthesia is dependent on renal excretion in cats and hepatic metabolism in dogs; recovery may therefore be prolonged in immature kittens or puppies whose renal and hepatic systems are not yet fully developed. Ketamine has been associated with neuronal cell death in rat pups, and so its use in the first 2–3 weeks of life should probably be avoided (Ikonomidou *et al.*, 1999).

Propofol and alfaxalone are suitable choices for use in young animals. These drugs are rapidly metabolized by the liver and propofol also undergoes some extrahepatic metabolism. Both agents cause dose-dependent cardiopulmonary depression; because of this it is important to administer the agent slowly over 45–60 seconds and titrate to effect. The use of alfaxalone in puppies and kittens <12 weeks of age has been reported (O'Hagan *et al.*, 2012ab). Dilution of both propofol and alfaxalone with saline has been shown to reduce dose

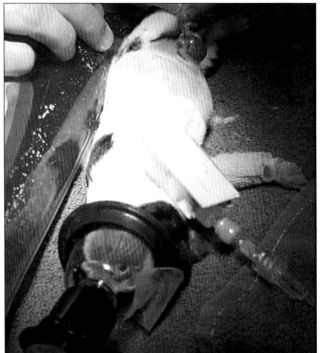

30.7 A 3-hour-old puppy requiring emergency umbilical hernia repair, anaesthetized with sevoflurane and N_2O delivered by facemask; hydromorphone was used to provide analgesia.
(Courtesy of Tanya Duke-Novakovski, Western College of Veterinary Medicine, University of Saskatchewan, Canada)

requirements and will also provide a larger volume, allowing more accurate administration in patients with low bodyweight (Zaki *et al.*, 2009).

Many young patients can be intubated with a small (2–3 mm) endotracheal tube (ETT). However, these narrow-bore tubes easily become obstructed by respiratory secretions, and the tube should be replaced if necessary. Extra care should be taken with intubation as laryngeal and tracheal trauma may easily occur, potentially resulting in oedema and upper airway obstruction. If tracheal intubation is impossible because of the size of the patient, a tight-fitting facemask should be used (see Figure 30.7). Use of a laryngeal mask airway device in kittens aged 12–15 weeks was found to be associated with an increased occurrence of gastro-oesophageal reflux compared to use of a conventional ETT (Sideri *et al.*, 2009). High resistance to breathing and increased apparatus dead space are two major concerns in paediatric anaesthesia. Both can be minimized by: using low-resistance non-rebreathing systems (T-piece, Bain or mini-Lack); choosing the appropriate length of ETT (distance from the nose to the point of the shoulder as a maximum length); and minimizing the space between the end of the breathing system and the ETT (Figure 30.8).

It is important to administer oxygen even if anaesthesia is being maintained with intravenous agents because of anaesthesia-induced hypoventilation and the higher oxygen consumption of paediatric patients compared to adults.

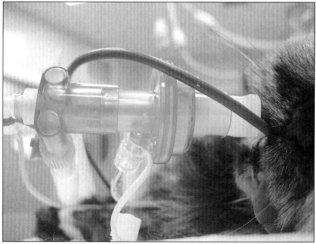

30.8 Care should be taken to minimize mechanical dead space in small patients. Although a paediatric heat and moisture exchanger is being used in this kitten, dead space is still considerable for a small patient.

Geriatric patients

Geriatric dogs and cats will probably benefit most from 5 minutes of preoxygenation delivered via a facemask, if they will tolerate it (Figure 30.9). Preoxygenation produces a greater alveolar oxygen reserve and helps to protect against hypoxaemia during induction of anaesthesia. Slow induction with propofol (administered intravenously over approximately 2 minutes) is probably the most suitable method, although it has the disadvantage that the airway is not secured quickly. The use of co-induction agents such as midazolam, diazepam or fentanyl can be considered but it is important to appreciate their respiratory depressant effects. Maintenance with isoflurane or sevoflurane is characterized by short recovery periods and fewer arrhythmias; these agents also require less metabolism than older

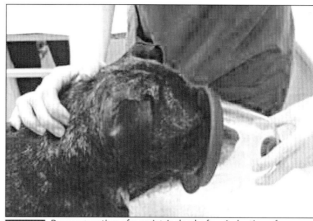

30.9 Preoxygenation of a geriatric dog before induction of anaesthesia.

volatile agents (e.g. halothane). Nitrous oxide may help to reduce oxygen-related atelectasis, but if using nitrous oxide as part of the gas mixture, care should be taken to maintain good oxygenation and avoid hypoxaemia.

Fluid therapy

Paediatric patients

Catheterization of superficial veins can be difficult in small patients. In very young patients, the intraosseous route can be a good alternative for fluid administration via a needle inserted into the medullary cavity of a bone, usually the femur, iliac crest or humerus (Beal and Hughes, 2000) (Figure 30.10).

Fluid therapy may help to correct hypotension during anaesthesia, but because of the decreased ventricular compliance in paediatric patients, CO will increase only minimally in response to volume loading.

Fluids containing 2.5–5% dextrose should be administered when hypoglycaemia is of concern, especially if the anaesthetic time is prolonged. Fluids should be titrated depending on the physical condition of the patient and the length and type of procedure. Fluid rate may be adjusted between 3 and 5 ml/kg/h and increased up to 10 ml/kg/h if necessary (Davis *et al.*, 2013). Accurate fluid pumps or burette administration sets should be used to avoid unintentional fluid overload. Gravity administration sets giving 50–60 drops/ml are also available, and will facilitate accurate administration (Figure 30.11). See Chapter 18 for further general guidelines on fluid therapy.

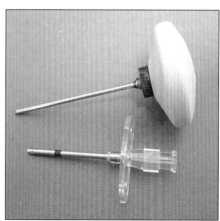

30.10 An intraosseous catheter.

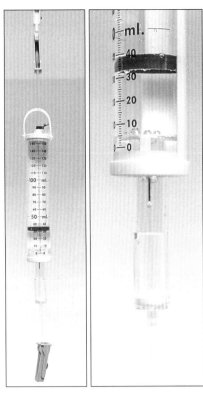

30.11 Intravenous administration set for small patients, giving a high number of drops/ml.
(Courtesy of Asher Allison, Animal Health Trust, Newmarket, UK)

Geriatric patients

Intravenous fluids should be provided during anaesthesia, as geriatric patients are less able to conserve fluid through resorption by the kidney and may therefore be more prone to dehydration than younger animals. A polyionic balanced crystalloid should be used, given at rates from maintenance (2 ml/kg/h) up to 10 ml/kg/h.

Monitoring

Paediatric patients

Monitoring small patients can be challenging, especially when they are covered by surgical drapes.

As stated earlier, CO is dependent on HR. For this reason it is particularly important to avoid bradycardia. Monitoring of HR by means of electrocardiography or an oesophageal stethoscope is highly recommended. ABP tends to be lower in young animals than in adults: a mean pressure of approximately 55 mmHg is acceptable in paediatric patients (Brierley *et al.*, 2009). Due to the small size of these patients, it can be difficult to monitor ABP as small enough blood pressure cuffs may not be available. Doppler ultrasonography is a very useful technique, as it provides an audible signal and gives information on changes in HR, heart rhythm and blood flow. In very small patients, the Doppler probe can be placed over the heart.

Body temperature should be closely monitored and hypothermia prevented or promptly corrected. Hypothermia can result in respiratory depression, acidosis, decreased CO and decreased drug metabolism and, hence, a prolonged recovery. To avoid hypothermia, the use of heating devices, insulating blankets, warmed surgical preparation solutions and infrared heat lamps is recommended. However, caution must be exercised when using heating devices, as they may cause burns to the patient (see Chapter 3).

Geriatric patients

The most comprehensive monitoring possible should be used if the planned procedure is expected to take longer than 20–30 minutes. Geriatric animals have little organ reserves, and any alteration in normal physiological variables should have the cause identified and immediately corrected.

Meticulous attention should be paid to the prevention of hypothermia in these patients, as they are less able than younger adults to maintain body temperature because of reduced central thermoregulatory mechanisms and altered body composition. In humans, infections resulting in sepsis are major contributors to accidental hypothermia (Mallet, 2002). Heat and moisture exchangers, warmed intravenous fluids and placing insulation or forced warm air blankets around the animal should all be considered, where possible, and body temperature should be monitored.

Recovery

During the recovery period, both paediatric and geriatric patients should be monitored closely until they have fully recovered their airway protective reflexes. Oxygen supplementation is particularly valuable in patients that have cardiopulmonary compromise or are shivering, as oxygen consumption can increase dramatically in these circumstances. If recovered in a cold environment, these patients can become rapidly hypothermic, may develop bradycardia that is unresponsive to anticholinergic drugs, and may quickly become apnoeic; it is therefore important to ensure that the recovery area is at an appropriate temperature. For small patients, a paediatric incubator is a very effective way to increase and maintain body temperature (Figure 30.12). Analgesia must be assessed regularly and continued into the postoperative period, especially in elderly patients that may experience pain if poorly positioned. As soon as the patient is conscious and able to eat, water and a small amount of food should be offered. Dextrose administration is often necessary in paediatric patients that have not had access to food for some time.

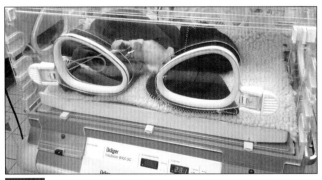

30.12 A paediatric patient recovering in an incubator.

Conclusion

While anaesthesia for paediatric and geriatric patients follows the same fundamental principles of good practice as for all patients, a good understanding of both developmental and ageing processes, and their consequences for anaesthesia, is imperative to ensure as good an anaesthetic outcome as possible.

References and further reading

Alef M, von Praun F and Oechtering G (2008) Is routine pre-anaesthetic haematological and biochemical screening justified in dogs? *Veterinary Anaesthesia and Analgesia* **35**, 132–140

Anand KJ, Coskun V, Thrivikraman KV, Nemeroff CB and Plotsky PM (1999) Long-term behavioural effects of repetitive pain in neonatal rat pups. *Physiology and Behaviour* **66**, 627–637

Arain SR, Kern S, Ficke DJ and Ebert T (2005) Variability of duration of action of neuromuscular-blocking drugs in elderly patients. *Acta Anaesthesiologica Scandinavica* **49**, 312–315

Baetge CL and Matthews NS (2012) Anesthesia and analgesia for geriatric veterinary patients. *Veterinary Clinics of North America: Small Animal Practice* **42**, 643–653

Beal MW and Hughes D (2000) Vascular access: theory and techniques in the small animal emergency patient. *Clinical Techniques in Small Animal Practice* **15**, 101–109

Bijsmans ES, Jepson RE, Chang YM, Syme HM and Elliott J (2015) Changes in systolic blood pressure over time in healthy cats and cats with chronic kidney disease. *Journal of Veterinary Internal Medicine* **29(3)**, 855–861

Brierley J, Carcillo JA, Choong K *et al.* (2009) Clinical practice parameters for hemodynamic support of pediatric and neonatal septic shock: 2007 update from the American College of Critical Care Medicine. *Critical Care Medicine* **37**, 666–688

Brown S, Atkins C, Bagley R, *et al.* (2007) Guidelines for the identification, evaluation, and management of systemic hypertension in dogs and cats. *Journal of Veterinary Internal Medicine* **21**, 542–558

Chang HY, Locker J, Lu R and Schuster VL (2010) Failure of postnatal ductus arteriosus closure in prostaglandin transporter-deficient mice. *Circulation* **121**, 529–536

Cheitlin MD (2003) Cardiovascular physiology—changes with aging. *American Journal of Geriatric Cardiology* **12**, 9–13

Davis H, Jensen T, Johnson A *et al.* (2013) 2013 AAHA/AAFP fluid therapy guidelines for dogs and cats. *Journal of the American Animal Hospital Association* **49**, 149–159

Grandy JL and Dunlop CI (1991) Anesthesia of pups and kittens. *Journal of the American Veterinary Medical Association* **198**, 1244–1249

Gregory GA, Wade JG, Beihl DR *et al.* (1983) Fetal anesthetic requirements (MAC) for halothane. *Anesthesia and Analgesia* **62**, 9–14

Harvey RC and Paddleford RR (1999) Management of geriatric patients: A common occurrence. *Veterinary Clinics of North America: Small Animal Practice* **29**, 683–701

Heavner JE and Racz GB (1990) Conduction block by lidocaine and bupivacaine: neonate versus adult. *Advances in Pain Research and Therapy* **15**, 181–187

Himms-Hagen J (1984) Thermogenesis in brown adipose tissue as an energy buffer. *New England Journal of Medicine* **311**, 1549–1558

Horster M, Kember B and Valtin H (1971) Intracortical distribution of number and volume of glomeruli during postnatal maturation in the dog. *Journal of Clinical Investigation* **50**, 796–800

Ikonomidou C, Bosch F, Miksa M *et al.* (1999) Blockade of NMDA receptors and apoptotic neurodegeneration in the developing brain. *Science* **283**, 70–74

Joubert KE (2007) Pre-anaesthetic screening of geriatric dogs. *Journal of the South African Veterinary Association* **78**, 31–35

Koehler RC, Traystman RJ and Jones MD Jr (1985) Regional blood flow and O$_2$ transport during hypoxic and CO hypoxia in neonatal and adult sheep. *American Journal of Physiology* **248**, 118–124

KuKanich B (2012) Geriatric veterinary pharmacology. *Veterinary Clinics of North America: Small Animal Practice* **42**, 631–642

Lee BH (2002) Managing pain in human neonates–applications for animals. *Journal of the American Veterinary Medical Association* **221**, 233–237

Luks AM, Zwass MS, Brown RC *et al.* (1998) Opioid-induced analgesia in neonatal dogs: pharmacodynamic differences between morphine and fentanyl. *Journal of Pharmacology and Experimental Therapeutics* **284**, 136–141

Mallet ML (2002) Pathophysiology of accidental hypothermia. *Quarterly Journal of Medicine* **95**, 775–785

Mathews KA (2008) Pain management for the pregnant, lactating, and neonatal to pediatric cat and dog. *Veterinary Clinics of North America: Small Animal Practice* **38**, 1291–1308

Meuldermans W, Woestenborghs R, Noorduin H *et al.* (1986) Protein binding of the analgesics alfentanil and sufentanil in maternal and neonatal plasma. *European Journal of Clinical Pharmacology* **30**, 217–219

Meurs KM, Miller MW, Slater MR and Glaze K (2000). Arterial blood pressure measurement in a population of healthy geriatric dogs. *Journal of the American Animal Hospital Association* **36**, 497–500

Meyer RE (1987) Anesthesia for neonatal and geriatric patients. In: *Principles and Practice of Veterinary Anaesthesia*, ed. C Short, pp. 330–337. Williams and Wilkins, Baltimore

Moon PF, Massat BJ and Pascoe PJ (2001) Neonatal critical care. Clinical theriogenology. *Veterinary Clinics of North America: Small Animal Practice* **31**, 343–367

O'Hagan B, Pasloske K, McKinnon C, Perkins N and Whittem T (2012a) Clinical evaluation of alfaxalone as an anaesthetic induction agent in dogs less than 12 weeks of age. *Australian Veterinary Journal* **90**, 346–350

O'Hagan BJ, Pasloske K, McKinnon C, Perkins NR and Whittem T (2012b) Clinical evaluation of alfaxalone as an anaesthetic induction agent in cats less than 12 weeks of age. *Australian Veterinary Journal* **90**, 395–401

Oliveira MC, Pinto e Silva P, Orsi AM, Mello Dias S and Define RM (1980) Observaciones anatómicas sobre el cierre del foramen oval en el perro (*Canis familiaris*). *Anatomica, Histologica, Embryologica* **9**, 321–324

Pascoe PJ and Moon PF (2001) Periparturient and neonatal anesthesia. Clinical theriogenology. *Veterinary Clinics of North America: Small Animal Practice* **31**, 315–341

Patel D (2006) Epidural analgesia for children. *Continuing Education in Anaesthesia, Critical Care and Pain* **6**, 63–66

Robinson NE and Gillespie JR (1973) Lung volumes in aging Beagle dogs. *Journal of Applied Physiology* **35**, 317–321

Sideri AI, Galatos AD, Kazakos GM and Gouletsou PG (2009) Gastro-oesophageal reflux during anaesthesia in the kitten: comparison between use of a laryngeal mask airway or an endotracheal tube. *Veterinary Anaesthesia and Analgesia* **36**, 547–554

Spedale SB, Weisbrodt NW and Morriss FH Jr (1982) Ontogenic studies of gastrointestinal function. II. Lower esophageal sphincter maturation in neonatal Beagle puppies. *Pediatric Research* **16**, 851–855

Stewart RC (1978) Respiratory depression with diazepam: potential complications and contraindications. *Anesthesia Progress* **25**, 117–118

von Dehn B (2014) Pediatric clinical pathology. *Veterinary Clinics of North America: Small Animal Practice* **44**, 205–219

Waterman AE and Kalthum W (1989) Pharmacokinetics of intramuscularly administered pethidine in dogs and the influence of anaesthesia and surgery. *Veterinary Record* **124**, 293–236

Waterman AE and Kalthum W (1990) Pharmacokinetics of pethidine administered intramuscularly and intravenously to dogs over 10 years old. *Research in Veterinary Science* **48**, 245–248

Webb JA, Kirby GM, Nykamp SG and Gauthier MJ (2012) Ultrasonographic and laboratory screening in clinically normal mature golden retriever dogs. *Canadian Veterinary Journal* **53**, 626–630

Yaster M and Maxwell LG (1989) Pediatric regional anesthesia. *Anesthesiology* **70**, 324–338

Zaki S, Ticehurst KE and Miyaki Y (2009) Clinical evaluation of Alfaxan-CD as an intravenous anaesthetic in young cats. *Australian Veterinary Journal* **87**, 82–87

Chapter 31

Anaesthetic complications, accidents and emergencies

Christine M. Egger

Most common anaesthetic complications are caused by central nervous system (CNS) and cardiopulmonary depressant effects of the drugs used in anaesthesia or by the procedure for which anaesthesia is required. Inhalational and injectable anaesthetic drugs often decrease heart rate, cardiac output (CO), arterial blood pressure (ABP), respiratory rate and tidal volume; they can also interfere with body temperature regulation. Surgical conditions may result in further depression of CO and ventilation (e.g. haemorrhage, pneumothorax, head-down positioning). However, human error remains the most frequent cause of problems encountered during anaesthesia, highlighting the importance of vigilance during the peri-anaesthetic period.

Lack of adequate pre-anaesthetic stabilization and peri-anaesthetic monitoring can lead to an increased incidence of complications. Most anaesthetic drugs have a narrow therapeutic index and therefore correct calculation of doses is critical to avoid an absolute overdose. Careful titration of drugs to achieve the desired effect in the individual patient, according to its physical status, is particularly important to avoid a relative overdose.

When complications do occur, appropriate evaluation, management and documentation are critical to minimize or eliminate negative outcomes. A planned course of action to deal with these events, should they occur, can result in improved patient outcome.

Anaesthetic complications

Respiratory complications

General effects of anaesthesia on the respiratory system

Respiratory centres located in the brainstem and central and peripheral chemoreceptors are depressed by general anaesthetic agents and potent mu opioid receptor agonists, resulting in reduced ventilatory drive. This, together with the peripheral depressant effects of anaesthetic drugs on the intercostal muscles and diaphragm, results in hypoventilation during anaesthesia, with consequent hypercapnia. Lung volume at the end of expiration (functional residual capacity (FRC)) is reduced during general anaesthesia, particularly when the patient is in dorsal recumbency. When the FRC is either close to, or less than, the point at which small airways start to close (closing volume of the lung), atelectasis develops when gas

trapped in the alveoli is absorbed into the circulation. The use of high inspired oxygen concentrations increases the rate at which this process occurs. Atelectasis may also develop as a result of lung compression and surfactant dysfunction. Blood flowing to atelectatic areas of lung does not take part in gas exchange; this results in right-to-left shunting of blood and possible hypoxaemia.

The ratio of alveolar ventilation (V_A) to pulmonary perfusion (Q) should be close to a value of 1 for optimal respiratory gas exchange. A V_A/Q mismatch is a common complication of general anaesthesia and may be caused by patient positioning, airway obstruction, accidental endobronchial intubation, bronchospasm, atelectasis, pneumonia, acute respiratory distress syndrome (ARDS) or pulmonary arterial hypotension. Mucosal ciliary paralysis, mucosal drying and depressed airway reflexes will further impair respiratory function during anaesthesia.

Respiratory complications, including hypoventilation, V_A/Q mismatch, atelectasis and airway obstruction will ultimately result in life-threatening hypoxaemia, hypercapnia or both, if not recognized and corrected.

Pathophysiological effects of hypoxaemia and hypercapnia

Effects of hypoxaemia on the cardiovascular system: The by-products of aerobic metabolism (oxidative phosphorylation) are carbon dioxide and water, which are normally easily excreted. Hypoxaemia results in cellular hypoxia; when mitochondrial oxygen concentration fall below a critical level, oxidative phosphorylation ceases. In these circumstances, anaerobic metabolism will still produce adenosine triphosphate (ATP), but much less efficiently than aerobic metabolism. The main waste metabolites of anaerobic metabolism are hydrogen and lactate ions; these are not easily excreted and accumulate in the circulation, resulting in metabolic acidosis and a base deficit. The clinical manifestations of hypoxaemia, tissue hypoxia and lactic acidosis are usually related to the most vulnerable organs: the brain, heart, spinal cord, kidneys and/or liver.

The cardiovascular response to hypoxaemia is a product of neural and humoral reflexes and direct effects. The neural reflexes occur first and result from stimulation of aortic and carotid chemoreceptors and from direct CNS stimulation. Humoral reflexes are mediated by catecholamines and the renin–angiotensin system. These reflexes together cause vasoconstriction. The direct local vascular effects of hypoxaemia are inhibitory and vasodilatory, and

BSAVA Manual of Canine and Feline Anaesthesia and Analgesia, third edition. Edited by Tanya Duke-Novakovski, Marieke de Vries and Chris Seymour. ©BSAVA 2016

occur later in the hypoxaemic period. Moderate hypoxaemia (oxygen saturation of haemoglobin (S_pO_2) 80–90%; arterial oxygen tension (P_aO_2) 50–60 mmHg (6.7–8.0 kPa)) causes general activation of the sympathetic nervous system (SNS) and release of catecholamines, resulting in increased heart rate, stroke volume, systemic vascular resistance, myocardial contractility and CO. With severe hypoxaemia (S_pO_2 <80%; P_aO_2 <50 mmHg (<6.7 kPa)), the local vasodilatory effects dominate and blood pressure rapidly falls. In sedated or anaesthetized patients, the early SNS reactivity to hypoxaemia may be reduced or unobserved, and hypoxaemia may manifest clinically as bradycardia, severe hypotension and cardiovascular collapse.

Hypoxaemia also promotes cardiac arrhythmias as a result of a decreased myocardial oxygen supply in relation to oxygen demand. Hypoxaemia directly decreases myocardial oxygen delivery, but catecholamines released in response to hypoxaemia cause tachycardia, which increases myocardial oxygen demand. Tachycardia also allows less time for ventricular filling during diastole and for coronary artery perfusion, further reducing myocardial oxygen delivery. Increased systemic vascular resistance during mild hypoxaemia causes increased left ventricular afterload, which also increases left ventricular oxygen demand. Systemic hypotension arising from severe hypoxaemia may decrease coronary perfusion pressure, further decreasing myocardial oxygen supply. If myocardial cells become hypoxic, ventricular premature complexes (VPCs), ventricular tachycardia (VT), and ventricular fibrillation (VF) can occur.

Effects of hypercapnia on the cardiovascular system: Hypercapnia, like hypoxaemia, can cause direct depression of both cardiac muscle and vascular smooth muscle, and at the same time cause reflex stimulation of the SNS. Mild hypercapnia (arterial carbon dioxide tension (P_aCO_2) 45–59 mmHg (6–7.9 kPa)) results in mild SNS stimulation, tachycardia and mild hypertension. With moderate to severe hypercapnia (P_aCO_2 60–90 mmHg (8–12 kPa)), SNS stimulation initially results in tachycardia and hypertension, which increases myocardial oxygen demand, and later results in decreased myocardial oxygen supply due to tachycardia and low diastolic blood pressure caused by global vasodilation. Significant hypercapnia causes direct depression of cardiac myocytes due to the extreme respiratory acidosis that also develops. With severe hypercapnia (P_aCO_2 >90 mmHg (>12 kPa)), severe CNS depression occurs as a result of extreme cellular acidosis, and this further depresses the cardiovascular system through depression of the vasomotor centre. Hypercapnia can also cause ventricular arrhythmias, including VF.

Effects of hypoxaemia and hypercapnia on the respiratory system: High alveolar carbon dioxide concentrations dilute alveolar oxygen, decreasing both alveolar and arterial oxygen concentrations. Hypercapnia causes a shift of the oxyhaemoglobin dissociation curve to the right, facilitating oxygen off-loading and tissue oxygenation but limiting oxygen binding to haemoglobin. At a P_aCO_2 of >100 mmHg (>13.3 kPa), ventilation eventually ceases due to brainstem depression. Severe hypoxaemia causes an inadequate supply of oxygen to the brainstem, resulting in depressed respiration, agonal gasping and eventual apnoea.

Recognition and causes of hypoxaemia

In conscious patients, the early clinical signs of hypoxaemia include restlessness and dysphoria, but these early signs will not manifest during general anaesthesia.

Following initial tachycardia and hypertension, signs of CNS depression, severe bradycardia, hypotension and ultimately cardiac arrest are observed. Cyanotic mucous membranes, another sign of hypoxaemia, may be difficult to see in anaemic patients or in poor lighting conditions. Using pulse oximetry, an S_pO_2 of <80% is equivalent to a P_aO_2 <50 mmHg (<6.7 kPa) and represents severe hypoxaemia. There are five main causes of hypoxaemia:

- Decreased inspired oxygen fraction (F_iO_2)
- Hypoventilation
- Impaired diffusion
- V_A/Q mismatch
- Right-to-left shunt.

Inadequate delivery of oxygen to the lungs will occur secondary to airway obstruction, bronchoconstriction or inhalation of a hypoxic gas mixture. Hypoventilation in a patient not receiving supplemental oxygen (i.e. on room air or 21% F_iO_2) may result in hypoxaemia even in the absence of lung disease. Apnoea can occur with a relative or absolute overdose of any anaesthetic agent, and can temporarily occur after the administration of thiopental, propofol, alfaxalone or ketamine. Pulmonary parenchymal disease such as oedema, pneumonia or parenchymal infiltrates will alter diffusion and cause V_A/Q mismatch. Increased intrapulmonary shunting due to atelectasis is a common cause of hypoxaemia both during and following general anaesthesia. Intrapulmonary shunting may also result from intrathoracic pathology such as pneumothorax and pleural effusion.

Tissue hypoxia results from hypoxaemia (low P_aO_2 and S_pO_2) and/or a significant decrease in CO (shock) or cardiac arrest. Severe anaemia produces inadequate blood oxygen-carrying capacity and also results in tissue hypoxia.

Prevention and treatment: Hypoxaemia during induction of anaesthesia can be prevented in many patients by pre-oxygenation with a tight-fitting facemask for 5 minutes before induction, providing the mask does not cause the patient distress. Preoxygenation is strongly recommended in patients with respiratory disease or where difficult endotracheal intubation is anticipated. The benefits of oxygen supplementation are lost after a few breaths of room air, therefore taking a patient from an oxygen cage to the induction area without continuing oxygen therapy will be inadequate (see Chapter 22). For treatment of hypoxaemia:

- Increase F_iO_2 by providing supplemental oxygen via nasal cannula, nasal prongs or facemask
- Intubate and provide oxygen and intermittent positive pressure ventilation (IPPV) for apnoeic patients and those in which oxygen supplementation alone is inadequate to maintain S_pO_2 >91%
- Check the anaesthetic machine, oxygen flowmeter, endotracheal tube (ETT) and breathing system to ensure they are functioning properly
- Use manual IPPV and auscultate both sides of the thorax to check for proper ETT placement; reposition the ETT as necessary
- Use manual IPPV to increase peak airway pressure (up to 40 cmH$_2$O) and hold for 20–30 seconds to re-expand atelectatic alveoli (alveolar recruitment manoeuvre). Consider the use of positive end-expiratory pressure (PEEP) to prevent recurrence of atelectasis
- Improve CO, ABP and pulmonary perfusion with intravenous fluid therapy, sympathomimetic drugs or cardiopulmonary resuscitation (CPR) if required

- Treat any underlying pathology: use thoracocentesis to remove pleural air or effusion, and consider diuretics, antibiotics and bronchodilators for pulmonary disease
- In significantly anaemic patients, increase oxygen-carrying capacity by transfusion of whole blood, packed red blood cells or oxygen-carrying solutions (Oxyglobin®) (see Chapter 18)
- In recovery, decrease oxygen consumption due to pain, shivering or fever (use analgesics, external warming devices, antipyretics) and continue oxygen supplementation
- Patients with relative shunting of blood through the lungs may benefit from oxygen supplementation, but those with an absolute shunt may not benefit.

Recognition and causes of hypoventilation

End-tidal carbon dioxide or P_aCO_2 >45 mmHg (>6 kPa) is indicative of hypoventilation. Hypoventilation is frequently encountered during anaesthesia because hypothermia, mu opioid receptor agonists, induction agents and volatile anaesthetics all directly depress the brainstem respiratory centres. Induction of anaesthesia and dorsal recumbency will significantly reduce minute volume and FRC because loss of normal end-expiratory diaphragmatic muscle tone allows the abdominal contents to press against the diaphragm, decreasing lung volume and reducing both thoracic and lung compliance. This results in alveolar hypoventilation, atelectasis and V_A/Q mismatch. Abdominal distension (ascites, uroabdomen, pregnancy, gastrointestinal obstruction, haemoabdomen) and a steep head-down position of greater than 30 degrees to horizontal will cause the abdominal contents to further impinge on the diaphragm, decreasing lung volume and compliance to a greater extent. Severe hypotension, resulting in inadequate perfusion of CNS respiratory centres, will cause hypoventilation and possibly a Cheyne–Stokes breathing pattern (repeated pattern of progressively increasing tidal volume, then progressively decreasing tidal volume followed by a long expiratory pause). Pain from upper abdominal disease (pancreatitis) or thoracic injury (fractured ribs, flail chest) frequently causes the patient to hypoventilate. Partial obstruction of the airway and increased work of breathing (WOB) (e.g. brachycephalic animals), obstruction of the ETT with secretions or blood or as a result of kinking, and placement of an inappropriately small ETT will also contribute to hypoventilation.

Prevention and treatment:

- Immediately provide supplemental oxygen delivered by facemask or nasal catheter to hypoventilating patients that have been breathing room air.
- Intubate patients with apnoea or severe hypoventilation and provide oxygen therapy and IPPV.
- Prevent and treat hypothermia by using warm intravenous and lavage fluids, circulating warm water blankets, and forced warm air blankets.
- Provide IPPV for patients placed in a steep head-down position.
- Provide IPPV for obese patients or those with abdominal distension.
- Improve CNS perfusion in patients with hypotension by decreasing the depth of anaesthesia, administering fluid therapy and sympathomimetic support.
- If there is chest trauma or abdominal disease, ensure appropriate analgesia.
- If there is significant CNS depression during recovery, consider antagonizing CNS depressant drugs where possible.

Tachypnoea

Tachypnoea can be a consequence of inadequate anaesthetic depth or a response to painful stimuli. It may also occur secondary to hypercapnia caused by exhausted carbon dioxide absorbent granules, or stuck or missing unidirectional valve(s) in a rebreathing system, improper connection of the breathing system, or insufficient fresh gas flow with a non-rebreathing system. Increased carbon dioxide production (hyperthermia and malignant hyperthermia) or administration (laparoscopy) can also cause tachypnoea. Hypoxic drive overrides the normal carbon dioxide-regulated control of breathing when P_aO_2 declines to values <60 mmHg (<8 kPa); therefore, hypoxaemia can also cause tachypnoea. Panting is sometimes seen after opioid administration to conscious animals, especially dogs.

Treatment:

- Rule out and treat hypercapnia or hypoxaemia.
- Rule out rebreathing of carbon dioxide by checking the breathing system, unidirectional valves (quickly remove, dry and replace; ensure correct size of valve or disc is used) and/or change absorbent granules if using a rebreathing system; increase fresh gas flow if using a non-rebreathing system.
- If the anaesthetic depth is inadequate, increase depth and/or administer additional analgesic drugs.
- If the patient is hyperthermic, turn off heating blankets, use cool intravenous fluids and wet the footpads with alcohol to promote evaporative heat loss.

Obstructive airway disease

Pathophysiology: During inspiration, work is performed against elastic and resistive forces in the lungs and chest wall (i.e. the WOB). Obstruction of the upper or lower airways can have a marked effect on the resistance and WOB. With obstructed airways, the animal will minimize the work needed to overcome the resistance forces by a combination of a reduced respiratory rate and increased tidal volume to maintain minute volume. The ability to compensate is reduced by the effects of many anaesthetic agents. In addition, many anaesthetics cause relaxation of the pharyngeal soft tissues, which results in further airway obstruction and increased resistance if an ETT is not in place. Airway obstruction can result in both hypercapnia and hypoxaemia.

Upper airway obstruction (inspiratory dyspnoea): Partial obstruction results in inspiratory stridor, with slow, deep breaths. The chest wall may be observed to move inwards during inspiration instead of outwards. Severe obstruction results in pronounced paradoxical breathing (abdomen expands and thorax moves inwards during inspiration) and hyperextension of the head and neck. If inspiratory efforts are profound, a dynamic inspiratory obstruction may occur because the marked pressure gradient in the upper airway causes airway soft tissues to collapse further (e.g. tracheal collapse). Prolonged obstruction and intense respiratory effort may lead to exhaustion and also to pulmonary oedema and acute lung injury.

Causes of upper airway obstruction include: soft palate entrapment (in heavily sedated, non-intubated patients); brachycephalic airway syndrome (breed predisposition); laryngospasm (common during a light plane of anaesthesia in non-intubated patients and can occur during intubation and after extubation); laryngeal paralysis (breed predisposition); laryngeal or pharyngeal inflammation or oedema (due to trauma during intubation, or prolonged pressure from the ETT); laryngeal or tracheal collapse (breed predisposition); laryngeal, pharyngeal, tracheal or nasal obstruction (blood, mucus, vomitus, saliva, tumour, foreign body); kinked or blocked ETT; excessively tight head and/or neck bandage (usually a problem after extubation); and insufficient fresh gas flow into the breathing system (reservoir bag will collapse during inspiration).

Prevention and treatment:

- Avoid stress and hyperthermia in brachycephalic breeds as it can result in panting and possibly laryngeal oedema.
- Avoid heavy sedation in brachycephalic breeds because relaxation of redundant pharyngeal tissue makes obstruction more likely.
- Establish i.v. access early in the peri-anesthetic period and maintain catheter until discharge home.
- Carefully intubate brachycephalic breeds and animals of breeds prone to laryngeal oedema/paralysis or laryngeal/tracheal collapse during general anaesthesia:
  - Brachycephalic animals will tolerate the ETT until fully conscious
  - Patients prone to laryngospasm or broncho-constriction may benefit from early extubation.
- IPPV may be required if the intrathoracic trachea or mainstem bronchi are collapsed.
- Administer corticosteroids and diuretics to reduce inflammation and oedema if there is significant airway swelling causing the obstruction.
- Ensure that head or neck bandages have not been applied too tightly.
- After extubation, maintain the patient in sternal recumbency with the head and neck extended, and the tongue pulled forward to reduce soft palate entrapment.
- Provide supplemental oxygen via a facemask or tracheal cannula (if upper airway obstruction).
- Re-intubation or emergency tracheotomy may be necessary if positioning does not relieve the obstruction.
- Light sedation is often helpful in the recovery period.

Lower airway obstruction (expiratory dyspnoea): Possible causes of lower airway obstruction include: bronchospasm, bronchitis, asthma, chronic obstructive pulmonary disease, and anaphylactic or anaphylactoid reactions.

Treatment:

- Provide supplemental oxygen (via nasal cannula, facemask or endotracheal intubation) as required.
- Consider a bronchodilator (adrenaline (epinephrine), albuterol, clenbuterol, terbutaline, aminophylline, theophylline). See Figure 31.1 for details.
- Consider corticosteroids (methylprednisolone, dexamethasone) and/or antihistamines (diphenhydramine, chlorphenamine).
- If an anaphylactic reaction is suspected, follow the treatment protocol given in Figure 31.2.

Restrictive pulmonary disease

Pathophysiology: Restrictive pulmonary diseases cause the lungs to collapse and become less compliant. Decreased lung compliance and increased lung elastance (tendency to collapse) can result from disease processes that are either intrinsic or extrinsic to the lungs. Decreased compliance results in increased WOB to overcome elastic forces and expand the lungs. To minimize WOB, a rapid shallow breathing pattern is adopted to reduce the need for lung expansion. Many anaesthetic agents decrease the patient's ability to compensate for the pathophysiology.

Intrinsic restrictive pulmonary disorders: These disorders reduce surfactant and bronchial mucus and increase lung water, reducing compliance. Causes include: ARDS, pulmonary oedema, pneumonia, lung consolidation and pulmonary infiltrates (infection, pulmonary disease, trauma, ventilator-induced injury, endotoxaemia).

Extrinsic restrictive pulmonary disorders: These disorders alter gas exchange by interfering with normal lung expansion. Causes include: pneumothorax, pleural effusion, mediastinal masses and increased intra-abdominal pressure due to ascites, pregnancy or gastrointestinal obstruction.

Drug	Indications	Dose	Possible side effects
Adrenaline (epinephrine)	CPA Hypotension Refractory bradycardia Anaphylaxis	0.01–0.2 mg/kg i.v., i.o., i.t. 0.01–0.03 µg/kg/min infusion 0.01 mg/kg i.v. slowly for anaphylactic reaction. Infusion may be required	Tachycardia Dysrhythmias
Albuterol	Bronchospasm Asthma Anaphylaxis	0.1–0.15 mg/kg inhaled	Tachycardia Dysrhythmias Hypotension
Aminophylline	Bronchospasm Asthma Anaphylaxis	Dogs: 2–6 mg/kg i.m., s.c. or slowly i.v. (over 15 minutes) Cats: 2–4 mg/kg i.m. or s.c. only	Tachycardia Dysrhythmias Hypotension
Amiodarone	Prolonged ventricular tachycardia or VF Non-physiological supraventricular tachycardia	5 mg/kg i.v.	Bradycardia Hypotension (due to risk of anaphylactoid reaction to be given with an antihistamine)
Antihistamines	Anaphylactic reaction	Diphenhydramine: 2.2 mg/kg slowly i.m. or i.v. Chlorphenamine 2.5–10 mg i.v. or i.m. total dose (depending on patient size) or 0.4 mg/kg i.v. or i.m.	Hypotension if given rapidly i.v.

31.1 Emergency drugs for use during general anaesthesia in cats and dogs. AV = atrioventricular; CNS = central nervous system; CPA = cardiopulmonary arrest; CPR = cardiopulmonary resuscitation; GI = gastrointestinal; i.o. = intraosseous; i.t. = intratracheal; i.v. = intravenous; VF = ventricular fibrillation. (continues)

Drug	Indications	Dose	Possible side effects
Atropine	Bradycardia AV block Sinus arrest Ventricular asystole	0.02–0.04 mg/kg i.m., i.v., i.t., i.o.	Tachycardia Central cholinergic syndrome Initial worsening of bradycardia and atrioventricular block possible
Calcium	Known hypocalcaemia Overdose of calcium channel blocker Hyperkalaemia	0.1–0.3 ml/kg 10% calcium chloride, slowly i.v. 0.5–1.0 ml/kg 10% calcium gluconate, slowly i.v.	Bradycardia Dysrhythmias
Corticosteroids	Anti-inflammatory Anaphylaxis Laryngeal oedema	Dexamethasone: 0.2–1 mg/kg i.v. (1–4 mg/kg for anaphylactic reaction) Methylprednisolone: 20 mg/kg i.v. (30 mg/kg for anaphylactic reaction) Prednisone sodium succinate: 10–25 mg/kg i.v. (for anaphylactic reaction)	Infection GI or renal ischaemia
Diltiazem	To slow conduction through AV node with non-physiological supraventricular tachycardia	0.05–0.15 mg/kg slowly i.v., repeat every 5 minutes to effect or until a total dose of 0.1–0.25 mg/kg	Bradycardia Hypotension
Dobutamine	Hypotension Myocardial dysfunction	2–10 µg/kg/min i.v. infusion	Tachycardia Dysrhythmias
Dopamine	Renal failure Hypotension Myocardial dysfunction Vasodilation	2–15 µg/kg/min i.v. infusion	Tachycardia Dysrhythmias
Ephedrine	Hypotension	0.02–0.05 mg/kg i.v. 1–5 µg/kg/min i.v. infusion	Tachycardia Dysrhythmias
Esmolol	Hypertension Tachycardia	0.05–0.5 mg/kg i.v. over 5 minutes 25–200 µg/kg/min i.v. infusion	Hypotension
Furosemide	Diuresis Pulmonary oedema Cerebral oedema Laryngeal oedema	1–2 mg/kg i.v.	Excessive diuresis Hypokalaemia
Glycopyrronium	Bradycardia	0.005–0.01 mg/kg i.v.	Tachycardia. Initial worsening of bradycardia and atrioventricular block possible
Isoproterenol	Refractory bradycardia Ventricular asystole	0.01–0.1 µg/kg/min i.v. infusion	Hypotension
Lidocaine	Ventricular premature contractions Ventricular tachycardia Ventricular fibrillation Acute vagally-mediated supraventricular tachycardia	Dogs: 1–2 mg/kg i.v. 25–100 µg/kg/min i.v. infusion Cats: 0.25–0.75 mg/kg slowly i.v.	Bradycardia Hypotension Seizures
Magnesium sulphate	Given with prolonged CPA or intractable ventricular fibrillation	30 mg/kg i.v. over 10 minutes	Hypotension CNS depression
Mannitol	Cerebral oedema	0.2–1.0 g/kg i.v. over 20 minutes	Volume overload
Noradrenaline (norepinephrine)	Hypotension Vasodilatory shock	0.1–1.0 µg/kg/min i.v. infusion	Increased myocardial work due to increased systemic vascular resistance (afterload)
Phenylephrine	Hypotension Vasodilatory shock	1.0–3.0 µg/kg/min i.v. infusion	Increased myocardial work due to increased systemic vascular resistance (afterload) Reflex bradycardia
Propranolol	Hypertension Tachycardia	0.02–0.1 mg/kg slowly i.v.	Hypotension
Sodium bicarbonate	Metabolic acidosis During CPR: • If pre-existing metabolic acidosis • If >10 minutes of CPR	0.5–1.0 mmol/kg i.v. over 20 minutes mEq of HCO_3^- to give = Base deficit x 0.3 x body weight (kg)	Metabolic alkalosis Respiratory arrest if given too quickly Hyperosmolality due to sodium overload
Terbutaline	Bronchospasm Asthma Anaphylaxis	0.01 mg/kg i.v., s.c. or i.m.	Tachycardia Hypotension Dysrhythmias
Vasopressin	CPA Vasodilatory shock (sepsis) Patients in VF unresponsive to defibrillation or adrenaline	0.2–0.8 IU/kg once i.v. 0.002–0.006 IU/kg/min i.v. infusion	Severe vasoconstriction Dysrhythmias

31.1 (continued) Emergency drugs for use during general anaesthesia in cats and dogs. AV = atrioventricular; CNS = central nervous system; CPA = cardiopulmonary arrest; CPR = cardiopulmonary resuscitation; GI = gastrointestinal; i.m. = intramuscular; i.o. = intraosseous; i.t. = intratracheal; i.v. = intravenous; s.c. = subcutaneous; VF = ventricular fibrillation.

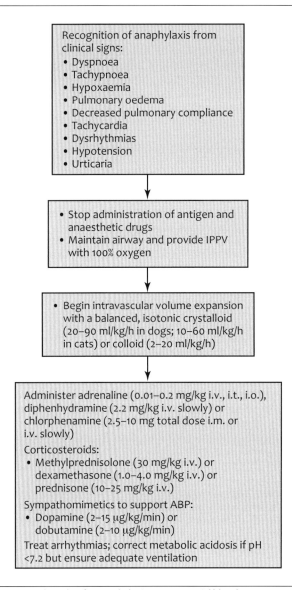

Recognition of anaphylaxis from clinical signs:
• Dyspnoea
• Tachypnoea
• Hypoxaemia
• Pulmonary oedema
• Decreased pulmonary compliance
• Tachycardia
• Dysrhythmias
• Hypotension
• Urticaria

↓

• Stop administration of antigen and anaesthetic drugs
• Maintain airway and provide IPPV with 100% oxygen

↓

• Begin intravascular volume expansion with a balanced, isotonic crystalloid (20–90 ml/kg/h in dogs; 10–60 ml/kg/h in cats) or colloid (2–20 ml/kg/h)

↓

Administer adrenaline (0.01–0.2 mg/kg i.v., i.t., i.o.), diphenhydramine (2.2 mg/kg i.v. slowly) or chlorphenamine (2.5–10 mg total dose i.m. or i.v. slowly)
Corticosteroids:
• Methylprednisolone (30 mg/kg i.v.) or dexamethasone (1.0–4.0 mg/kg i.v.) or prednisone (10–25 mg/kg i.v.)
Sympathomimetics to support ABP:
• Dopamine (2–15 µg/kg/min) or dobutamine (2–10 µg/kg/min)
Treat arrhythmias; correct metabolic acidosis if pH <7.2 but ensure adequate ventilation

31.2 Algorithm for anaphylaxis. ABP = arterial blood pressure; i.o. = intraosseous; IPPV = intermittent positive pressure ventilation; i.t. = intratracheal; i.v. = intravenous.

Treatment:

• Provide supplemental oxygen via nasal cannula, facemask or endotracheal intubation.
• Perform thoracocentesis to remove fluid or air and place chest drains if necessary (see Chapters 22 and 23).
• Correct atelectasis with an alveolar recruitment manoeuvre: use the reservoir bag to obtain a peak airway pressure of 30–40 cmH$_2$O for 20–30 seconds to reinflate atelectatic alveoli. Consider using PEEP to prevent recurrence of atelectasis.
• Treat underlying diseases (ARDS, endotoxaemia, pulmonary disease, infection). Details of treatments are beyond the scope of this book, but consider drugs such as furosemide, corticosteroids, antimicrobials, bronchodilators or surfactant therapy, depending on the underlying cause.
• Long-term ventilator therapy using specially designed critical care ventilators may be required for some conditions (e.g. ARDS). Details of patient management are found in books and articles on critical care, e.g. Silverstein and Hopper (2015).

Apnoea/respiratory arrest

Causes of apnoea include: rapid intravenous administration of induction agents, relative or absolute overdose of general anaesthetic agents, reflex apnoea secondary to endotracheal intubation or visceral traction, brainstem injury, cardiac arrest, or equipment failure (closed adjustable pressure-limiting (APL) valve (pop-off valve), ventilator malfunction).

Treatment:

• If the patient is not already intubated, immediate endotracheal intubation and provision of IPPV with oxygen supplementation are warranted.
• Rapid intubation and IPPV can help prevent cardiac arrest (which may quickly follow respiratory arrest).
• Rule out equipment failure (ventilator malfunction).
• If a closed APL valve is found to be the cause of apnoea, open the valve and immediately check for and treat possible tension pneumothorax and/or cardiac arrest.

Aspiration

Patients can aspirate regurgitated stomach contents, saliva, blood or mucus. Predisposing factors include: drugs that relax the lower oesophageal sphincter (anticholinergics, opioids, thiopental, volatile anaesthetics); factors that delay gastric emptying (fear, anxiety, pain, pregnancy, shock, use of opioids or anticholinergics); factors that increase intra-abdominal pressure (pregnancy, obesity, abdominal effusion, gastrointestinal obstruction, head-down positioning); and prolonged anaesthesia (>2 hours).

Preventive measures: Appropriate pre-anaesthetic fasting, rapid intravenous induction of anaesthesia and rapid control of the airway by endotracheal intubation will help to prevent aspiration. Use an ETT with a leak-tested cuff that can provide a seal at 20 cmH$_2$O airway pressure. Pretreatment with metoclopramide (increases lower oesophageal sphincter tone, speeds gastric emptying and lowers gastric fluid volume), H$_2$ receptor antagonists (e.g. cimetidine, famotidine and ranitidine, which decrease gastric volume and increase the pH of gastric contents) or proton pump inhibitors (e.g. omeprazole, raises gastric pH) may help to prevent aspiration or reduce morbidity if aspiration occurs. The use of maropitant, a neurokinin-1 receptor antagonist, reduces vomiting and reduces the risk of aspiration pneumonia.

Treatment once regurgitation has occurred:

• Ensure a secure airway by endotracheal intubation, confirm ETT cuff inflation and position the patient with the head down so that material flows out of the mouth.
• Use gentle suction to remove material from the oral cavity, oropharynx, nasopharynx and oesophagus.
• Check the pH of regurgitant material using indicator paper (e.g. litmus) or pH probe. Acidic contents can cause inflammation and possible oesophageal stricture formation.
• Lavage the oesophagus with saline or tap water and gently suction until suctioned fluids are clear. Be aware that lavage may increase the risk of aspiration.
• Instill 8.4% sodium bicarbonate diluted 1:1 with water (up to 0.6 ml/kg) or sodium citrate (0.6 ml/kg of a 10% solution) into the distal oesophagus using a urinary catheter if regurgitant fluid is proven to be acidic.

- Consider omeprazole to increase gastric pH (see Figure 10.5).
- Consider sucralfate to prevent oesophagitis and stricture formation (see Figure 10.5).
- If regurgitation has been triggered by accidental oesophageal intubation, leave the ETT in the oesophagus to facilitate drainage of materials away from pharyngeal and laryngeal areas; place another ETT into the trachea and inflate the cuff before removing the tube from the oesophagus.
- Suction the nasopharynx and oropharynx again just before extubation, and extubate with the ETT cuff slightly inflated.

Barotrauma or volutrauma

Trauma from pressure or shear stress may rupture alveolar walls and cause pneumomediastinum and pneumothorax, with possible subcutaneous emphysema. Hypoxaemia and cardiac arrest will follow if trauma is not recognized and treated immediately. Repetitive excessive peak airway pressure with IPPV will cause barotrauma in friable lung tissue, while repetitive collapse and re-expansion of normal or diseased lung during IPPV causes volutrauma (atelectrauma). A closed APL valve may result not only in volutrauma but also in a rapid reduction of venous return and cardiac arrest. Inappropriate and excessive use of the oxygen flush mechanism of the anaesthetic machine will rapidly cause barotrauma and volutrauma.

Prevention and treatment:

- Avoid high peak airway pressures: >30 cmH$_2$O in healthy lungs and >18 cmH$_2$O in diseased or compromised lungs.
- Use a smaller tidal volume (5–8 ml/kg), lower peak airway pressure (10–14 cmH$_2$O), faster rate (20–25 breaths/min) and mild PEEP (2–5 cmH$_2$O) to ventilate patients with compromised lungs.
- If lung damage is due to a closed APL valve, high peak airway pressure or incorrect use of oxygen flush, immediately correct the cause and treat possible tension pneumothorax and/or cardiac arrest.

Cardiovascular complications

Pathophysiology of cardiovascular complications

Many volatile and injectable anaesthetic agents produce a dose-related depression of myocardial contractility (negative inotropy) by altering intracellular calcium homeostasis. Most anaesthetics also cause a decrease in left ventricular diastolic function (negative lusitropy), a decrease in left ventricular afterload due to vasodilation, and depression of the baroreceptor reflex. These effects result in reduced venous return, bradycardia, hypotension and a decrease in CO, and are exacerbated in a failing heart. Isoflurane (mildly) and thiobarbiturates (moderately) can sensitize the myocardium to the arrhythmogenic effects of adrenaline and can facilitate the development of atrial or ventricular arrhythmias during myocardial ischaemia.

Cardiac arrhythmias

Bradyarrhythmias: Severe bradyarrhythmias can greatly reduce CO and tissue perfusion, particularly if there is limited ability to increase stroke volume through either increased myocardial contractility or increased venous return by venoconstriction. Severe bradyarrhythmias can

result in syncope in awake animals and severe hypotension in anaesthetized animals. Bradyarrhythmias observed during anaesthesia include sinus bradycardia, atrioventricular (AV) block (first and second degree), sinus arrest and atrial standstill. Causes include: drug effects (high dose mu opioid receptor agonists, alpha-2 adrenoceptor agonists), CNS disease (particularly if there is increased intracranial pressure (ICP)), high vagal tone, hypothermia, hyperkalaemia and sick sinus syndrome.

Prevention and treatment: See Figure 31.1 for drug doses.

- Consider including an anticholinergic agent in pre-anaesthetic medication for patients with high resting vagal tone (e.g. brachycephalic animals).
- Use an anticholinergic agent to treat bradyarrhythmias resulting from opioid administration.
- Use atipamezole to treat bradycardia and hypotension caused by alpha-2 adrenoceptor agonists before administering an anticholinergic agent.
- Use atropine rather than glycopyrronium if bradycardia is life-threatening, as it has a more rapid onset of action.
- Treat any other underlying causes of bradycardia (e.g. reduce ICP (see Chapter 28), correct hypothermia (see Chapter 3), correct hyperkalaemia (see Chapter 25)).

Supraventricular tachyarrhythmias: Severe tachyarrhythmias greatly reduce CO due to decreased diastolic filling, and reduce ejection and coronary perfusion times, resulting in myocardial ischaemia. Supraventricular tachyarrhythmias observed during anaesthesia include sinus tachycardia, atrial tachycardia and atrial fibrillation. Causes include: myocardial disease (see Chapter 21) and administration of certain drugs (anticholinergics, particularly atropine); tachyarrhythmias may also be secondary to SNS stimulation (e.g. due to pain, inadequate anaesthesia leading to awareness, hyperthermia, hypotension, hypovolaemia, hypoxaemia, hypercapnia, hypoglycaemia, hyperthyroidism, anaemia or phaeochromocytoma).

Treatment: See Figure 31.1 for drug doses.

- Physiological sinus tachycardia should be treated by correcting the underlying cause of SNS stimulation.
- If no underlying cause is identified, treat sinus tachycardia with beta blockers (propranolol or esmolol) if tachycardia is affecting blood pressure and CO.
- Non-physiological supraventricular tachycardia (e.g. atrial tachycardia, reciprocating tachycardia) can be treated with sodium channel blockers (lidocaine) or potassium channel blockers (amiodarone) to inhibit the arrhythmia, or with beta blockers (e.g. esmolol) or calcium channel blockers (diltiazem) to slow conduction through the AV node and the ventricular rate.
- Acute-onset vagally-mediated atrial fibrillation can be treated with lidocaine.

Ventricular tachyarrhythmias: The specialized conduction system of the heart is responsible for initiating cardiac depolarization, coordinating the electrical impulses throughout the atria and ventricles and coordinating ventricular contractions. It is critical that excitation and contraction be coordinated to maintain adequate CO and tissue perfusion. Ventricular arrhythmias observed during anaesthesia include VPCs, accelerated idioventricular rhythm, VT and VF. Causes include: gastric dilatation–volvulus; splenic trauma, torsion, tumour or splenomegaly; traumatic myocarditis; hypoxaemia; myocardial ischaemia (hypotension, severe anaemia); hypercapnia; acid–base imbalance; electrolyte imbalance (hypokalaemia, hypomagnesaemia); and the effects of certain drugs (thiobarbiturates, ketamine).

Treatment: See Figure 31.1 for drug doses.

- Always attempt to identify and treat the underlying problem (e.g. hypoxaemia, hypercapnia, electrolyte or acid–base imbalance).
- If the arrhythmia is related to administration of thiopental or ketamine, stop administration and alter the anaesthetic protocol.
- Accelerated idioventricular rhythm is usually benign and does not require treatment other than treating the underlying cause.
- Treat VPCs and VT with lidocaine (bolus ± constant rate infusion).
- CPR is required for VF.

Hypotension

See also Chapter 17 for information on hypotension.

Pathophysiology: Blood pressure is a measure of the force driving tissue perfusion. A mean arterial pressure (MAP) of at least 60 mmHg is necessary for perfusion of vital organs such as the brain, heart and kidneys. Hypotension is defined as a MAP <60 mmHg and/or a systolic arterial pressure <80 mmHg. Hypoperfusion of vital organs and the extremities results in inadequate delivery of oxygen to the tissues and inadequate removal of waste products, leading to clinical signs of shock and organ dysfunction. Causes of hypotension include:

- Hypovolaemia from haemorrhage, pre-existing fluid deficits, fluid loss due to evaporation and 'third spacing', or inadequate intraoperative fluid administration
- Vasodilation and reduced venous return due to anaesthetic drugs, severe metabolic or respiratory acidosis, hypoxaemia, endotoxaemia, septicaemia, or anaphylactic or anaphylactoid reactions
- Decreased myocardial contractility due to anaesthetic drugs, hypoxaemia or myocardial ischaemia, acid–base disturbances (respiratory or metabolic acidosis), endotoxaemia, electrolyte imbalances, cardiomyopathy or catecholamine depletion
- Cardiac arrhythmias that decrease CO, such as bradycardia, AV block, tachycardia, atrial fibrillation and VT
- Obstruction of venous return secondary to IPPV (increased intrathoracic pressure), pericardial effusion, tumours (especially mediastinal), tension pneumothorax, surgical packing or retraction of organs (cranial abdominal surgery)
- Reflex hypotension from bradycardia (oculo- or vago-vagal reflex) caused by excessive traction or pressure on the eye or viscera.

Treatment: See Figure 31.1 for drug doses; see also Chapters 17 and 18.
  The incidence of hypotension during anaesthesia can be reduced by appropriate pre-anaesthetic stabilization, administration of adjunct drugs with anaesthetic-sparing effects (balanced anaesthetic technique) and intravenous infusion of an isotonic balanced crystalloid solution. For treatment of hypotension:

- Rule out and correct hypoxaemia or hypercapnia
- Reduce depth of anaesthesia:
  - If the patient appears to be at too deep a plane, reduce rate of administration of anaesthetic agent
  - Administer anaesthetic-sparing adjunct drugs (opioids, ketamine) that permit use of decreased amounts of anaesthetic agents to maintain adequate anaesthesia.
- Treat bradyarrhythmias and tachyarrhythmias that may be affecting CO:
  - If an oculo- or vago-vagal reflex is suspected, stop surgical retraction of the eye or viscera and administer an anticholinergic.
- Administer a fluid bolus of 5–20 ml/kg of an isotonic balanced crystalloid solution or 2–5 ml/kg of a colloid solution to increase intravascular volume and improve venous return in patients without underlying cardiac disease (see Chapter 18):
  - With inhalant anaesthetic-induced hypotension in normovolaemic dogs, crystalloid boluses do not reliably increase ABP and may decrease oxygen delivery to the tissues as a consequence of haemodilution and tissue oedema formation; conservative use of crystalloid fluids is advised (see Chapter 18)
  - Colloids provide a more consistent increase in ABP but can also contribute to volume overload, so should be used conservatively in patients with cardiac disease.
- If the patient is receiving IPPV, reduce tidal volume (8–10 ml/kg) and peak airway pressure (<15 cmH$_2$O) and maintain an inspiration:expiration time ratio of 1:2 or 1:3 to minimize negative haemodynamic effects
- Provide sympathomimetic support (see Figure 31.1):
  - Dobutamine
    - Mainly beta-1 adrenoceptor agonist and a positive inotrope
    - Increases contractility, stroke volume and CO
    - Activation of beta-2 receptors may result in vasodilation and therefore a smaller than expected increase in ABP.
  - Dopamine
    - D$_1$, D$_2$, beta and alpha adrenoceptor agonist
    - Positive inotrope, chronotrope and vasoconstrictor, depending on infusion rate used
    - Beta-1 adrenergic agonist effects (increased contractility) predominate at 5–10 µg/kg/min
    - Mixed beta and alpha adrenergic agonist effects at 10–15 µg/kg/min (increased contractility and peripheral vasoconstriction to increase venous return)
    - Mostly alpha-1 (vasopressor) adrenergic effects at 10–15 µg/kg/min
    - Very high infusion rates can reduce splanchnic circulation
    - Results in increased venous return, perfusion pressure, cardiac contractility and CO, depending on infusion rate.
  - Ephedrine
    - Causes release of endogenous noradrenaline (norepinephrine) and is a direct alpha and beta adrenoceptor agonist
    - Provides positive inotropic and chronotropic effects as well as vasoconstriction to increase venous return, perfusion pressure and CO
    - Effects can be short lived; administration can be repeated but repeated boluses may not be as

effective due to depletion of noradrenaline stores
  – An infusion may be more effective (see Chapter 17).
- Noradrenaline
  – Mainly an alpha adrenergic agonist; provides vasoconstriction, increasing venous return and perfusion pressure
  – Minimal effects on myocardial contractility
  – Significantly increases left ventricular afterload and myocardial work. Decreased myocardial function may require concurrent administration of a positive inotrope such as dobutamine
  – Used for short-term treatment of refractory hypotension with endotoxaemia.
- Phenylephrine
  – Alpha adrenergic agonist; provides vasoconstriction, increasing venous return and perfusion pressure
  – Treatment for excessive alpha adrenergic blockade and vasodilation unresponsive to dopamine or ephedrine.
- Vasopressin
  – Provides vasoconstriction, increasing venous return and perfusion pressure
  – Used for CPR or vasodilatory shock in patients unresponsive to dopamine, ephedrine, noradrenaline or adrenaline (e.g. septic shock).
- Adrenaline
  – Mixed alpha and beta adrenergic agonist with potent vasopressor, positive inotropic and chronotropic effects
  – Excessive vasoconstriction can decrease splanchnic perfusion
  – Increases myocardial work and oxygen consumption; predisposes to myocardial ischaemia and arrhythmias at higher doses
  – Used for CPR or vasodilatory shock in patients unresponsive to dopamine, ephedrine, noradrenaline or vasopressin (e.g. septic shock, anaphylaxis).

Haemorrhage

Haemorrhage results in a decreased plasma volume and haemoglobin concentration, thus reducing the oxygen-carrying capacity of the blood. The body responds to these changes by increasing CO, minute volume and oxygen extraction by the peripheral tissues. Once maximal increases in CO, ventilation and oxygen extraction have occurred, oxygen delivery to the tissues becomes compromised with further haemorrhage. Arterial oxygen content must be increased or signs of inadequate tissue oxygen delivery (shock) will develop. The cardiovascular depressant effects of anaesthetic agents reduce the body's ability to compensate for blood loss. (See also Chapter 18.)

Treatment: Total blood volume can be estimated as 50–60 ml/kg in cats and 80–90 ml/kg in dogs.
Replace lost blood with blood products (whole blood, packed red blood cells or haemoglobin-based oxygen-carrying solutions (Oxyglobin®)) if loss is ≥20% of total blood volume in relatively healthy patients (i.e. animals that had a normal haemoglobin concentration before haemorrhage) or ≥10% of total blood volume in debilitated patients.
It is important to assess the individual patient (heart rate, blood pressure, end-tidal carbon dioxide, blood lactate, venous blood gases, co-existing disease).

Hypertension

ABP is the most important determinant of left ventricular afterload and cardiac work. Hypertension results in increased myocardial work and myocardial oxygen demand, potentially resulting in myocardial ischaemia and cardiac arrhythmias. Hypertension can also result in retinopathy, blindness and renal failure. Sudden hypertension during anaesthesia is an indication of SNS stimulation, and possible causes must be investigated and the cause identified.

Possible causes of hypertension include: pain and awareness, mild to moderate hypoxaemia, hypercapnia, metabolic acidosis, underlying renal or cardiac disease, phaeochromocytoma, stimulation of adrenal glands during surgery, or use of phenylephrine (e.g. during ophthalmic surgery). Note that the early stages of hypoxaemia, hypercapnia and metabolic acidosis result in SNS stimulation, tachycardia, peripheral vasoconstriction and hyper-tension. As the hypoxaemia, hypercapnia and acid–base disturbances become more severe, myocardial depression and vasodilation occur, resulting in hypotension and reduced CO.

Treatment: See Figure 31.1 for drug doses.

- Identify and treat the underlying cause where possible (awareness, pain, hypoxaemia).
- Increase the concentration of volatile agent and consider administering adjunct analgesics (opioids, ketamine) if hypertension is thought to be due to surgical stimulation.
- A temporary increase in isoflurane or sevoflurane concentration may be effective if hypertension is thought to be due to catecholamine release from a phaeochromocytoma or adrenal gland stimulation. Phentolamine and beta adrenergic blockers (esmolol, propranolol) may also be required. Alpha adrenergic blockade should be instigated before beta adrenergic blockade to avoid severe vasoconstriction (see Chapter 27).
- Acepromazine can be used to treat hypertension caused by phenylephrine used as a topical vasoconstrictor.

Miscellaneous complications
Hypoglycaemia

Because the CNS requires glucose as major energy source, hypoglycaemia during anaesthesia can result in: an unexplained increase in the depth of anaesthesia; tachycardia and hypertension; prolonged recovery or failure to recover from anaesthesia; and seizures or muscle tremors during recovery. Hypoglycaemia is common in neonatal and paediatric patients, but can also occur in patients with well controlled diabetes during fasting, and in patients with severe liver pathology, septicaemia or insulinoma.

Prevention and treatment:

- Monitor blood glucose every 30 minutes during anaesthesia and recovery in patients predisposed to hypoglycaemia and supplement glucose as necessary.
- Supplement glucose by administering 5% dextrose in sterile water (not a volume replacement fluid), or add 50 or 100 ml of 50% dextrose to 900-950 ml lactated Ringer's or Hartmann's solution to provide a 2.5% or 5% dextrose solution for volume replacement.

Myopathy or neuropathy

Pathophysiology: Hypoperfusion and ischaemic damage due to prolonged compression, inadequate padding and/or prolonged hypotension are the main causes of myopathy (myositis) during anaesthesia. Perioperative peripheral neuropathies occur as a result of nerve stretch or compression, generalized ischaemia, metabolic derangement (diabetes mellitus, severe anaemia), inadvertent injection of local anaesthetic agent into the nerve or surgical resection of the nerve. Axonal reactions to nerve injury include: transient ischaemic nerve block (no structural nerve damage), which lasts only minutes; neuropraxia (demyelination of peripheral fibres of the nerve trunk), where nerve function is recoverable in 4–6 weeks; axonotmesis (complete disruption of the axons within an intact nerve sheath), where recovery depends on regeneration of the distal nerve and complete recovery is unlikely; and neurotmesis (complete nerve disruption), where surgical repair, if possible, will return only partial function.

Prevention and treatment:

- Myopathy and neuropathy can be prevented by using adequate padding, careful positioning, short duration of anaesthesia and prevention of hypotension.
- Use of a nerve stimulator or ultrasound technique when performing locoregional nerve blocks to avoid inadvertent injection of local anesthetic into the nerve.
- Treatment includes intravenous fluids, anti-inflammatory drugs (corticosteroids or non-steroidal anti-inflammatory drugs (NSAIDs)), analgesics, sedatives and vasodilators (e.g. acepromazine).

Oliguria or anuria

Pathophysiology: The primary mechanism for oliguria or anuria during anaesthesia is reduced renal perfusion and a reduced glomerular filtration rate. In addition, volatile anaesthetic agents and full mu opioid receptor agonists increase secretion of antidiuretic hormone (vasopressin) and favour fluid retention. Urine production of <0.5 ml/kg/h is considered inadequate. Predisposing causes of oliguria or anuria in the perioperative period include: pre-existing renal disease; inadequate replacement of fluid deficits and ongoing losses; hypotension (particularly if severe or prolonged); and the use of NSAIDs when there is hypotension and renal hypoperfusion.

Prevention and treatment:

- Administer an isotonic balanced crystalloid fluid during anaesthesia and surgery, and maintain normotension to promote renal perfusion.
- If urine output is inadequate, administer a crystalloid fluid challenge of 5–20 ml/kg or colloid fluid challenge of 2–5 ml/kg, if no underlying cardiac disease is present.
- Administer diuretics: furosemide, dextrose or mannitol (osmotic diuresis).
- Administer dobutamine, dopamine or ephedrine to increase blood pressure and CO, and improve renal perfusion.

Anaesthetic mishaps and accidents

Anaesthetic mishaps can be categorized as preventable and unpreventable. Unpreventable mishaps include idiosyncratic drug reactions. The vast majority of accidents, however, are preventable. Accidents are commonly a result of human error, which can also contribute to equipment malfunctions. True equipment malfunctions are less common. Vigilance is important with all aspects of anaesthesia, and safety mechanisms should be put in place and used, for example check-lists and equipment alarms. An example of an anaesthesia check-list can be found on the Association of Veterinary Anaesthetists website (www.ava.eu.com).

Common human and equipment errors

- Lack of adequate training and familiarity with anaesthetic equipment:
  - Anaesthetic machine not set up properly
  - No machine check before induction of anaesthesia
  - Oxygen flowmeter turned off
  - Inadequate oxygen flowmeter setting
  - Unfilled or overfilled volatile anaesthetic vaporizers
  - Breathing system disconnected or not set up correctly
  - Unnoticed stuck or missing one-way valves
  - Exhausted absorbent granules
  - APL (pop-off) valve left closed.
- Monitoring device failure, or failure of personnel to observe the monitor.
- Ventilator failure, or failure to use ventilator correctly.
- Drug administration errors:
  - Drug interactions with concurrent medications
  - Wrong dose (underdose, relative or absolute overdose)
  - Wrong route of administration
  - Wrong syringe (always label syringes)
  - Wrong drug.
- Airway mismanagement:
  - Unrecognized oesophageal or endobronchial intubation
  - Premature extubation
  - Laryngeal injuries – vocal fold paralysis, granuloma, arytenoid dislocation
  - Tracheal perforation
  - Chemical tracheitis (due to inadequately rinsed tubes after using a chemical disinfectant)
  - Tracheal ischaemic necrosis or rupture from overinflated ETT cuff
  - Inadequate or excessive ventilation (wrong IPPV setting).
- Fluid mismanagement:
  - Fluid overload
  - Wrong type of fluid
  - Intravenous line disconnection, misplaced or migrated catheter, failure to check catheter placement
  - Failure to prime infusion set with fluids
  - Fluid bolus resulting in an accidental 'bolus' of drug(s) administered within the same fluid line.
- Burns:
  - Heating pads (never use electrical heating pads or push any heating blanket tightly against the body)
  - Radiant heat lamps
  - Airway burns (with some types of laser).
- Corneal abrasions or ulcers:
  - Failure to lubricate cornea with suitable eye lubricant
  - Warm air blowing on cornea
  - Damage from facemask.
- Post-anaesthetic blindness or renal failure secondary to:
  - Hypotension and inadequate perfusion of the optic nerve or kidneys during anaesthesia
  - Excessively wide opening of mouth with mouth gags in cats (blindness).

Anaesthetic emergencies

Anaphylactic reactions (type I – immediate)

For information on the treatment of anaphylaxis see Figure 31.2.

Hypersensitivity reactions are divided into four types:

- Type I (immediate)
- Type II (cytotoxic)
- Type III (immune complex)
- Type IV (delayed, cell-mediated).

Type I (immediate) hypersensitivity reactions are the most common and life-threatening hypersensitivity reactions that occur in the peri-anaesthetic period. An example of a type II hypersensitivity reaction is a haemolytic transfusion reaction.

Immunological anaphylactic (type I hypersensitivity) reaction (mediated by IgE)

Immunological anaphylactic reactions are an exaggerated response to an allergen. They appear within minutes of exposure to the allergen (antigen) in a sensitized patient. They are most commonly observed with antibiotic administration in the peri-anaesthetic period. Previous exposure to the allergen results in the production of allergen-specific IgE antibodies. On subsequent exposure to the allergen, these antibodies cause activation of mast cells and basophils and the release of chemical mediators. These mediators include leukotrienes, histamine, prostaglandins, kinins, cytokines, tumour necrosis factor-alpha and platelet-activating factor. There may also be a second, alternative pathway involving IgG antibodies and macrophages. Anaphylaxis may manifest as urticaria, angioedema, laryngeal and pulmonary oedema, bronchoconstriction, hypoxaemia, vasodilation, increased membrane permeability, hypotension, relative hypovolaemia, tachycardia, arrhythmias, shock and death.

Non-immunological anaphylactic (type I hypersensitivity) reaction (not mediated by IgE or other antigen–antibody interactions)

Non-immunological anaphylactic reactions (anaphylactoid reactions) manifest in a similar way to immunological anaphylactic reactions, but do not require previous exposure to an antigen to sensitize the patient. They are also more common during the peri-anaesthetic period. The triggering drug directly causes mast cell degranulation or activation of the complement system. Theoretically, this type of reaction could occur with any drug, but it has been reported to occur with administration of opioids, neuromuscular blocking agents, NSAIDs, dextrans, thiopental, propofol and radiocontrast agents.

Treatment of anaphylactic reactions

See Figure 31.2 for the anaphylaxis treatment algorithm and Figure 31.1 for details of drug doses.

Immunological and non-immunological anaphylactic reactions are clinically indistinguishable and both life-threatening, and treated in the same way:

- Discontinue drug administration and all anaesthetic agents
- Administer supplemental oxygen and use IPPV in order to maintain normal oxygen saturation
- Administer intravenous fluids up to shock rate (see Chapter 18)
- Administer adrenaline to treat bronchoconstriction and vasodilation
- Administer an antihistamine (diphenhydramine, chlorpheniramine) and a corticosteroid (methylprednisolone, prednisone or dexamethasone)
- Administer a bronchodilator (albuterol, aminophylline)
- Vasopressors (dopamine, ephedrine, vasopressin) may be required to treat hypotension
- Administer atropine if there is persistent bradycardia
- Treat severe metabolic acidosis (pH <7.2) with sodium bicarbonate.

Cardiopulmonary arrest

See Figure 31.1 for details of drug doses and Figure 31.3 for the cardiopulmonary arrest (CPA) algorithm.

CPA is the sudden cessation of functional ventilation and circulation. Cardiac arrest and respiratory arrest may occur simultaneously, but if respiratory arrest occurs first, cardiac arrest will swiftly follow unless there is rapid intervention to restore ventilation. CPA results in cessation of oxygen delivery to and removal of carbon dioxide from peripheral tissues. The anaerobic conditions result in increased production of lactate and hydrogen ions. A severe oxygen debt and mixed respiratory and metabolic acidosis quickly develop. Irreversible neurological damage will occur within minutes of cerebral oxygen deprivation.

Goals of CPR

The goals of CPR are to restore and optimize coronary and cerebral perfusion by restoring normal cardiac rhythm and effective respiratory gas exchange. CPR consists of basic life support (BLS), advanced life support (ALS), and post-resuscitation monitoring and support.

Causes and prevention of CPA

Common causes of CPA in the peri-anaesthetic period include: hypoxaemia, hypercapnia, electrolyte abnormalities (especially hyperkalaemia), acid–base abnormalities, hypotension, hypovolaemia, shock, significant hypothermia, autonomic nervous system imbalance (vagal stimulation), sensitization of the myocardium to catecholamines (xylazine, thiopental), anaesthetic agent overdose, severe trauma, systemic or metabolic disease, and significant underlying cardiac or respiratory disease.

Appropriate pre-anaesthetic assessment and stabilization, close monitoring, and prevention of hypoxaemia, hypercapnia, hypovolaemia, hypotension and hypothermia will help to prevent CPA. Comprehensive monitoring will also allow early detection of CPA.

Recognition of CPA

Signs of impending CPA: These include changes in respiratory rate, depth and pattern, such as bradypnoea or agonal gasping. Weak and irregular pulses, tachycardia or bradycardia, VPCs, hypotension that is poorly responsive to sympathomimetic agents, and cyanotic or grey mucous membranes are signs that may indicate impending CPA. Hypothermia that persists despite attempts to warm the patient, a sudden and unexplained increase in the depth of anaesthesia, or a decrease in level of consciousness in a non-anaesthetized patient are other signs of impending CPA.

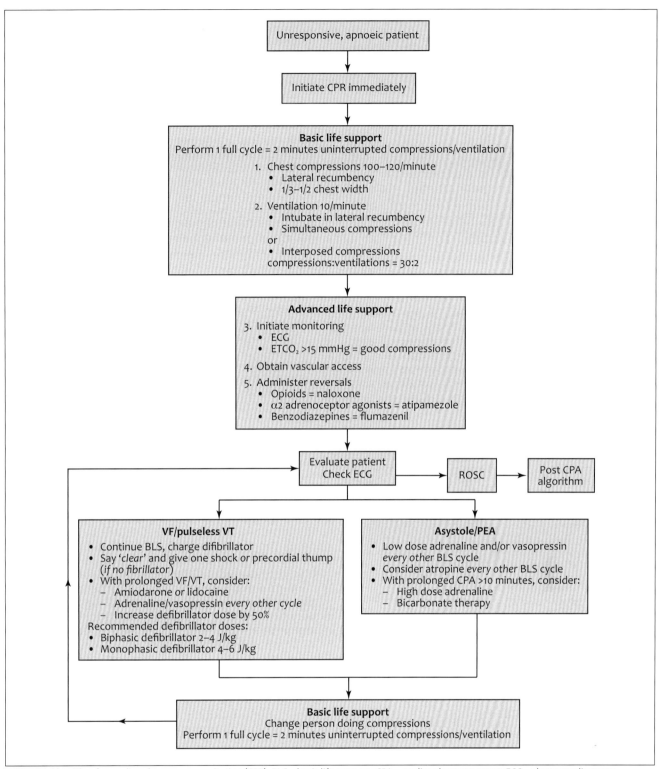

31.3 Algorithm for cardiopulmonary resuscitation (CPR). BLS = basic life support; CPA = cardiopulmonary arrest; ECG = electrocardiogram; ETCO₂ = end-tidal carbon dioxide; PEA = pulseless electrical activity; ROSC = return of spontaneous circulation; VF = ventricular fibrillation; VT = ventricular tachycardia.
(Modified from Fletcher *et al.*, 2012 with permission from the *Journal of Veterinary Emergency and Critical Care*)

Signs of CPA: These include loss of consciousness or an increase in the apparent depth of anaesthesia, loss of skeletal muscle tone, absence of heart sounds and agonal gasping or absent ventilation. Loss of palpable central pulses, such as the femoral pulse, can help to confirm CPA, but when used alone, this sign is unreliable as an indicator of CPA. Other signs of CPA include loss of pulse sounds on the Doppler monitor and a sudden decrease in end-tidal carbon dioxide (detectable by capnography). Pupils become

fixed and dilated, and mucous membranes may be cyanotic or pale. However, capillary refill time and mucous membrane colour can remain normal for several minutes after cardiac arrest, depending on the underlying cause. An abnormal rhythm may or may not be present on the electrocardiogram (ECG), as pulseless electrical activity (PEA) can appear 'normal' for several minutes after cardiac arrest has occurred.

CPR should be started if a femoral pulse cannot be palpated, especially if other signs of CPA are present.

Readiness

Readiness for CPA emergencies includes having a fully stocked emergency cart that is regularly audited for contents and is readily available in case of emergency. Contents of the cart should include emergency drugs and equipment to suction the airway, to ventilate the patient (ETT, ETT tie, cuff inflator, laryngoscope, tracheotomy kit), to ventilate the patient (artificial manual breathing unit ('Ambu bag'); Figure 31.4), oxygen source, breathing system), to place intravenous and intraosseous catheters for fluid/drug administration, to deliver drugs through the ETT (long, fairly stiff urinary catheters) and to perform thoracocentesis (butterfly catheters, needle, syringe, stopcock, chest tubes). A thoracotomy kit and electrical defibrillator should also be readily available. The cart should include printed copies of current CPR algorithms, checklists and dosage charts.

Having a trained resuscitation team with a designated leader and with specific roles assigned to each team member may improve the outcome of emergencies. It is recommended that personnel receive standardized resuscitation training at regular intervals (e.g. every 6 months) to refresh their skills. Training should include didactic components and opportunities to practice hands-on skills, assessment of performance and provision of constructive feedback. Post-resuscitation debriefing is also recommended after an emergency, with the aim of constructively improving the performance of the resuscitation team.

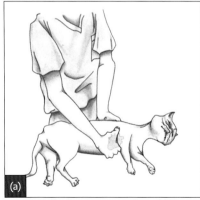

31.4 An artificial manual breathing unit ('Ambu bag') can be used to ventilate the lungs with either room air or air enriched with oxygen.

Basic life support

Basic life support (BLS) includes procedures to sustain artificial ventilation and coronary and cerebral perfusion. It consists of procedures for airway management, breathing and circulation.

It is critical that chest compressions be initiated as soon as possible in patients that are unresponsive, apnoeic or have agonal gasping, and not be delayed until after intubation. If there is any doubt whether the patient is in CPA, chest compressions should be initiated immediately while assessment continues.

Follow the mnemonic C, A, B.

Circulation (C): Two theories have been proposed for the mechanism by which external chest compressions during CPR create forward blood flow: the cardiac pump theory (Figure 31.5) and the thoracic pump theory (Figure 31.6).

According to the cardiac pump theory, compression of the chest wall directly over the heart compresses the heart chambers to create forward blood flow (Figure 31.5b). For cats and small dogs with high thoracic wall compliance, the cardiac pump can also be achieved by using a one-handed technique, with the operator's fingers wrapped around the sternum at the level of the heart (Figure 31.5a). The cardiac pump technique is most likely to be important in animals weighing <10 kg with compliant chest walls, but may also be used in dogs with narrow and deep chests, such as Greyhounds (Figure 31.5c).

The thoracic pump theory proposes that chest compressions increase overall intrathoracic pressure, which subsequently compresses the heart and the aorta and collapses the vena cava to produce forward blood flow. During elastic recoil of the chest, the subatmospheric intrathoracic pressure enhances venous return. This technique is more useful in medium to giant-breed dogs with rounded chests, in which direct compression of the heart is difficult. Chest compressions are delivered with the hands placed over the widest portion of the chest and with the patient in lateral recumbency (Figure 31.6a). Barrel-chested dogs (e.g. Bulldogs) can be placed in dorsal recumbency, with compressions performed over the sternum (Figure 31.6b). When using this technique, it is optimal to maximize high intrathoracic pressure by using simultaneous chest compressions and IPPV, and by keeping airway pressure low between chest compressions (i.e. no IPPV between compressions) to allow for venous return.

Regardless of the technique used, chest compressions must begin immediately in patients in CPA and should not be stopped during resuscitation, except when operators switch (see below). The goal of chest compressions is to maximize vital organ perfusion; this is achieved by maximizing the force and rate of compressions. Chest compressions are performed at a rate of 100–120/minute. Deep

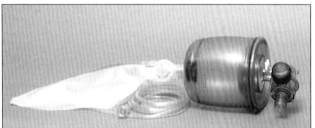

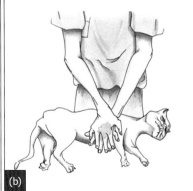

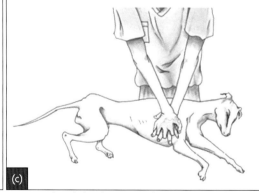

31.5 Cardiac pump technique. (a) For cats and small dogs (<10 kg) with compliant chests, use a one-handed technique to administer circumferential chest compressions with the hand wrapped around the sternum directly over the heart. (b) A two-handed technique applied directly over the heart may be used in larger cats and small dogs with low thoracic compliance. (c) Similarly, in deep, narrow-chested dogs like Greyhounds, perform chest compressions in either left or right lateral recumbency with the hands directly over the heart.

(Reproduced from Fletcher *et al.*, 2012 with permission from the *Journal of Veterinary Emergency and Critical Care*)

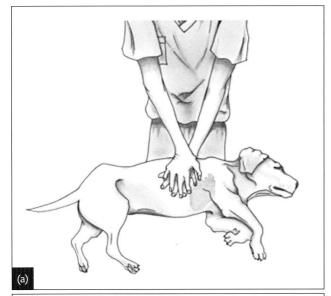

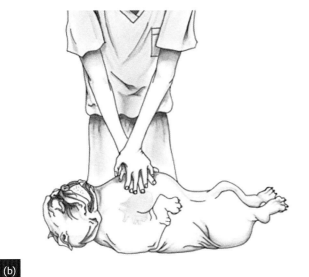

31.6 Thoracic pump technique. (a) For most dogs (>10 kg), perform chest compressions in either left or right lateral recumbency over the widest portion of the chest. (b) For barrel-chested dogs like Bulldogs, administer sternal compressions directly over the heart with the patient in dorsal recumbency.
(Reproduced from Fletcher *et al.*, 2012 with permission from the *Journal of Veterinary Emergency and Critical Care*)

compressions of 25–33% of the width of the thorax are recommended and full elastic recoil of the chest should be allowed (do not lean on the chest). Effective perfusion of the heart and brain is best achieved when chest compression consumes 50% of the duty cycle, with the other 50% devoted to the relaxation phase, allowing venous return. If possible, personnel performing chest compressions should alternate every 2 minutes to avoid fatigue, which increases the likelihood of an ineffective technique.

Airway management (A): Endotracheal intubation is recommended to secure the airway, facilitate administration of oxygen and allow IPPV. Use of a laryngoscope will facilitate visualization of the glottis and help to avoid oesophageal intubation. Suction may be required to remove blood, saliva, gastrointestinal contents, mucus, or pus from the airway. After visually confirming that the ETT is correctly placed, secure the tube in place and inflate the cuff to ensure an airtight seal between the tracheal mucosa and the ETT. If there is oral or pharyngeal swelling, manual

palpation and direction of the ETT into the trachea may be necessary. A tight-fitting facemask can be used in animals that are difficult or impossible to intubate orotracheally, or if the operator is awaiting help. Laryngeal mask airways or v-gel® devices (see Chapter 5) can aid in ventilation of animals that are difficult to intubate. Tracheotomy is sometimes necessary in patients that cannot be intubated due to anatomical difficulties or obstructions blocking the upper airway (e.g. bones, balls).

Breathing (B): Because hypoxia and hypercapnia both reduce the likelihood of return of spontaneous circulation (ROSC), securing the airway and providing IPPV with 100% oxygen is essential to maximize oxygen delivery to the tissues during CPR. Positive pressure ventilation is commonly provided using an anaesthetic breathing system and reservoir bag. Bag-valve devices (cat/small dog and larger sizes are available), also called 'Ambu bags', can be used for IPPV and to deliver up to 100% oxygen. High respiratory rates, longer inspiratory times and high tidal volumes will result in increased mean intrathoracic pressure, impairing venous return. Hyperventilation can also decrease cerebral and coronary perfusion by causing vasoconstriction. Currently, the recommended ventilation rate is 10 breaths/min using a tidal volume of 10 ml/kg and an inspiratory time of 1 second. Ventilation should be delivered in a way that achieves normal chest wall excursions while keeping the airway pressure low between breaths. Keep peak airway pressure during IPPV to <20 cmH$_2$O to avoid volutrauma and excessive decrease in venous return. However, a higher peak airway pressure may be needed in patients with poor pulmonary and thoracic compliance. If normal chest wall excursions are not observed and pulmonary/thoracic compliance seems to be reduced, recheck the ETT position and the tube cuff and rule out airway obstruction, pleural space disease (e.g. pneumothorax, pleural effusion) or severe lung parenchymal disease (e.g. pulmonary oedema).

Advanced life support

Advanced life support (ALS) comprises the procedures performed after BLS has begun. These procedures aim to achieve ROSC. ALS includes: therapy with drugs (vasopressors, positive inotropes and anticholinergics); fluid therapy to correct acid–base and electrolyte and volume abnormalities; and electrocardiography and electrical defibrillation, if required. It also includes treatments and strategies to reduce cerebral oedema.

The mnemonic D, E, F is used.

Drugs (D): See also Figure 31.1.

Adrenaline (epinephrine): Generation of adequate coronary and cerebral perfusion pressures requires vasoconstriction and an increase in venous return. Adrenaline is a non-specific adrenergic agonist used during CPR for its pressor effects via alpha-1 agonist activity. Adrenaline is also a beta-1 agonist, resulting in positive inotropic and chronotropic effects; these effects may actually be detrimental as they will increase myocardial oxygen demand during a period of reduced oxygen delivery, potentially worsening myocardial ischaemia. Currently, the recommendation is early administration of low-dose adrenaline (0.01 mg/kg i.v.) with subsequent re-administration every 3–5 minutes, or during every other 2-minute cycle of BLS. If CPR is prolonged (>10 minutes), high-dose adrenaline (0.1-0.2 mg/kg i.v.) may be considered.

Vasopressin: The pressor effects of vasopressin are mediated through peripheral V_1 receptors located on vascular smooth muscle. Unlike alpha-1 adrenoceptors, V_1 receptors remain responsive to stimulation even in acidic conditions. Vasopressin is a pressor that has no inotropic or chronotropic effects. Vasopressin (0.2-0.8 IU/kg i.v.) can be given as a substitute for (or alternating with) adrenaline every 3–5 minutes or during every other 2-minute cycle of BLS.

Atropine: Atropine is an anticholinergic that can be used to treat asystole or PEA that is associated with high vagal tone. A dose of 0.04 mg/kg i.v. is recommended.

Anaesthetics and reversal agents: Stop administration of general anaesthetics. Consider antagonism of opioids (with naloxone 0.04 mg/kg i.v.), alpha-2 adrenergic agonists (with atipamezole 100 μg/kg i.v.) and benzodiazepines (with flumazenil 0.01–0.03 mg/kg i.v.). Note that atipamezole is not licensed to be given via the intravenous route and should be used in this way only during CPR.

Antiarrhythmic drugs: With VF or pulseless VT that is refractory to defibrillation, amiodarone (5 mg/kg i.v.) or lidocaine (2 mg/kg i.v.) may be tried.

Calcium: Routine use of calcium is not recommended during CPR and it should be given only to patients with documented moderate to severe hypocalcaemia or severe hyperkalaemia.

Sodium bicarbonate: Sodium bicarbonate is not routinely used during CPR unless there is a pre-existing metabolic acidosis. It is also recommended that sodium bicarbonate (0.5–1 mmol/kg i.v.) be administered after >10 minutes of CPA, as the patient will almost certainly be acidotic at that point. Sodium bicarbonate therapy should be administered according to the base deficit if this has been calculated (see Chapter 18).

Corticosteroids: Routine use of corticosteroids during CPR is not recommended, although they may have a use during post-CPA supportive therapy (see later).

Prevention of cerebral oedema: Mannitol (0.2–1.0 g/kg i.v.) or hypertonic saline (2–4 ml/kg i.v.) should be given over 20 minutes once ROSC has been established, to prevent or reduce cerebral oedema.

Routes of administration: A cranial vena cava or jugular venous catheter is the best route for administration of drugs to patients in CPA, as this achieves drug delivery close to the heart. If a peripheral venous catheter is used for drug delivery it can take up to 2 minutes for drugs administered to reach the heart during CPR. If a peripheral catheter is used, a flush of 5–20 ml saline after the drug is administered may 'push' the drug into the central circulation; however, this technique may result in volume overload. It is imperative to pay close attention to the total volume of fluids administered. Administration of drugs via an intraosseous catheter (tibia, radius or ulna) can also be used. Administration via this route can be as fast as via a central venous catheter because the medullary cavity does not collapse during CPA. Certain drugs, such as adrenaline, atropine and vasopressin can be given via the ETT. When using this route, the dose should be administered into the distal trachea (just beyond the carina) using a sterile canine urinary catheter passed through the ETT; the drug will be rapidly absorbed into the pulmonary circulation from this site. The drug should be diluted in saline or sterile water before administration. It has been recommended anecdotally that the intravenous dose be doubled or even tripled when drugs are given by the tracheal route, but effective intratracheal doses have not been established empirically.

Electrocardiography (E): Placement of ECG leads is important for identification of the arrhythmia causing CPA, so that appropriate therapy can be given. Common CPA arrhythmias in veterinary patients include PEA (also known as electromechanical dissociation or pulseless idioventricular rhythm), ventricular asystole and VF. The underlying rhythm can change during CPR and these changes should be identified via the ECG and should guide treatment.

Pulseless electrical activity: This occurs when there is electrical activity without sufficient mechanical activity in the myocardium to produce adequate CO. Predisposing factors include hypovolaemia, hypoxaemia, acidosis, hypothermia, hyperkalaemia or hypokalaemia, tension pneumothorax and cardiac tamponade.

Treatment of PEA involves CPR and correction of the underlying problem, if possible.

Ventricular asystole: This is the absence of electrical and mechanical cardiac activity – apparent as the 'flatline' on the ECG. Causes of ventricular asystole include increased vagal tone, oculo- or vago-vagal response to manipulation of eyes or abdominal viscera, hyperkalaemia and severe hypoxaemia.

Treatment of ventricular asystole involves BLS, ALS and correction of the underlying problem, if possible.

Ventricular fibrillation: This is chaotic, disorganized, ectopic ventricular activity resulting in sustained systole. Because the activity is disorganized, there is no effective CO. Because there is no diastolic period during VF, no myocardial perfusion can occur and the ATP stores of the myocardium are very rapidly depleted. Predisposing factors include hypovolaemia, hypoxaemia, acidosis, hypothermia, hyperkalaemia or hypokalaemia, or severe multisystemic disease.

Treatment includes CPR and rapid defibrillation.

Technique for defibrillation: Immediate defibrillation is recommended when CPA is identified as being due to VF or pulseless VT of ≤4 minutes' duration or if VF is diagnosed during a rhythm check between cycles of CPR. If the patient has been in VF or pulseless VT for >4 minutes, myocardial energy substrates will be depleted and it is recommended that the patient receive a 2-minute cycle of BLS before defibrillation. In either case, BLS should begin while the defibrillator is activated.

To maximize current through the ventricles, the defibrillator paddles are placed on opposite sides of the thorax over the costochondral junction, directly over the heart. Defibrillator paste or gel (not alcohol) is applied to the paddles and they are held firmly against the chest wall to maintain the patient in dorsal recumbency. The operator must indicate the intent to defibrillate by announcing 'Clear', and ensure that no-one (including the operator) is touching the patient or table before defibrillation. Defibrillation should be followed by a rapid rhythm check and then immediate resumption of BLS for 2 minutes before applying the next countershock. Each subsequent countershock should be followed by 2 minutes of BLS.

For a biphasic defibrillator, the recommended dose is 2–4 J/kg. For a monophasic defibrillator, the recommended dose is 4–6 J/kg. In cats and dogs with VF or pulseless VT, the defibrillation energy should be increased by 50% if the first countershock is unsuccessful.

If the abdominal or thoracic cavity is open, internal defibrillation, using sterile defibrillation paddles, should be performed using a dose of 0.5–1 J/kg.

Automated external defibrillators (AEDs) designed for emergency use in humans should not be used for defibrillation in cats and dogs. Combined AED/defibrillator units should be used in the manual defibrillation mode not AED mode.

Fluid administration (F): Shock volumes of fluids are administered only if the CPA was preceded by severe absolute or relative volume depletion (haemorrhage, severe dehydration, anaphylactic or distributive shock). Euvolaemic or hypervolaemic patients should not be given supplemental intravenous fluids during CPR, other than to flush drugs into the central circulation (see earlier). If fluids are required, crystalloids, colloids or whole blood may be administered according to the patient's needs. Avoid fluids containing glucose, such as 5% dextrose in sterile water, as hyperglycaemia has been associated with poorer neurological recovery and outcome.

Open-chest *versus* closed-chest CPR

It is very important to establish a resuscitation code with the owner when the animal is admitted to the clinic. This should be indicated clearly on the patient records. Commonly used resuscitation codes include green (open-chest CPR if necessary), yellow (closed-chest CPR) and red (no CPR).

Closed-chest CPR will generate, at most, approximately 20–30% of the normal CO, while open-chest CPR may generate significantly more CO. Open-chest CPR should be performed when the abdominal or thoracic cavity is open at the time of CPA. Otherwise, the main indications for open-chest CPR are significant intrathoracic disease (tension pneumothorax, severe pleural effusion, pericardial effusion, or diaphragmatic hernia) and severe abdominal haemorrhage (ongoing blood loss occurring during CPR). A left lateral thoracotomy is performed at the 5th intercostal space to enable open-chest CPR.

Monitoring during CPR

ROSC will result in palpable pulses and a rapid increase in end-tidal carbon dioxide as pulmonary perfusion is re-established. Capnography is therefore helpful for assessment during CPR as it will help to identify ROSC; in addition, an end-tidal carbon dioxide of >15 mmHg (>2 kPa) indicates good CPR technique. Thoracic auscultation and the ECG should be checked during the pauses in chest compressions when the operators switch over. If a Doppler flow probe is in place, a return of spontaneous pulse sounds may be heard, but Doppler signals should be interpreted with caution as they may represent retrograde venous blood flow or motion artifact from chest compressions. Pulse oximeters may not function, due to peripheral vasoconstriction and poor-quality or absent pulses. Jugular venous blood samples will provide more accurate information than arterial blood samples on the acid–base status of the patient and the effectiveness of CPR.

Signs of successful resuscitation include return of the pupillary light reflex and palpebral reflex, spontaneous ventilation and airway protective reflexes.

Post-resuscitative monitoring and support

Post-resuscitative monitoring should include heart rate and rhythm, ABP, adequacy of oxygenation and ventilation, blood lactate and glucose, electrolyte and acid–base status, central venous pressure (if possible), body temperature, urine output and mentation.

Supportive measures to optimize CO and delivery of oxygen to the tissues should be implemented in order to help prevent a second arrest. Maximize tissue delivery of oxygen by maintaining normovolaemia, normotension, and adequate haemoglobin concentration and S_pO_2. Maintenance of adequate blood pressure (MAP 60–80 mmHg) may require vasopressors and positive inotropes (infusions of dobutamine, dopamine or adrenaline; see Figure 31.1). Supplemental oxygen should be titrated to maintain normal oxygenation (P_aO_2 80–100 mmHg (10.7–13.3 kPa); S_pO_2 94–98%). The successfully resuscitated patient may have rib fractures, pulmonary contusions, pulmonary oedema, pneumothorax, cerebral oedema and/or cardiac arrhythmias, and will benefit from oxygen therapy and analgesia. Both hypoxaemia and hyperoxaemia should be avoided.

Hypocapnia can lead to decreased cerebral blood flow, possibly resulting in cerebral ischaemia. Conversely, hypercapnia can lead to an increase in cerebral blood flow and increased ICP. Mechanical ventilation may be necessary to maintain normocapnia (30–32 mmHg (4.0–4.3 kPa in cats; 35–45 mmHg (4.7–6.0 kPa) in dogs). Serial monitoring of end-tidal carbon dioxide or arterial blood gases is ideal to ensure normocapnia and guide ventilatory support. Long-term ventilation may carry a poor prognosis (see references on critical care for more information). Patients that cannot maintain normal oxygenation with supplemental oxygen providing a F_iO_2 >60% may require endotracheal intubation and IPPV.

In humans, mild hypothermia leads to better cardiac and neurological outcomes after CPA. It is recommended that mild hypothermia (32–34°C) be established in cats and dogs that remain comatose after ROSC, and maintained for 24–48 hours; however, IPPV and careful monitoring will be required during this period. Patients that are hypothermic upon ROSC should be slowly rewarmed at a rate of 0.25–0.50°C/h. Rapid rewarming should be avoided.

Cerebral oedema and increased ICP commonly occur after resuscitation and are associated with a poor outcome (coma, cranial nerve deficits, decerebrate posture, abnormal mentation). Hypertonic saline or mannitol should be given to cats and dogs with neurological signs consistent with cerebral oedema as soon as ROSC occurs. Preventing hypoxaemia and inducing mild hypocapnia (32–35 mmHg (26–30 mmHg (3.5–4.0 kPa) in cats; 4.3–4.7 kPa) in dogs) with IPPV will help to reduce ICP by reducing cerebral blood flow. Maintaining normotension or slight hypertension (MAP 70–80 mmHg) will help to maintain cerebral perfusion if there is increased ICP. Patients should be closely monitored for seizures, and seizure prophylaxis may be required (see Chapter 28).

References and further reading

Aarnes TK, Bednarski RM, Lerche P, Hubbell JA and Muir WW 3rd (2009) Effect of intravenous administration of lactated Ringer's solution or hetastarch for the treatment of isoflurane-induced hypotension in dogs. *American Journal of Veterinary Research* **70**, 1345–1353

Beale RJ, Hollenberg SM, Vincent JL and Parrillo JE (2004) Vasopressor and inotropic support in septic shock: an evidence-based review. *Critical Care Medicine* **32**, S455–S465

Chen HC, Sinclair MD and Dyson DH (2007) Use of ephedrine and dopamine in dogs for the management of hypotension in routine clinical cases under isoflurane anesthesia. *Veterinary Anaesthesia and Analgesia* **34**, 301–311

Davis H, Jensen T, Johnson A *et al.* (2013) 2013 AAHA/AAFP fluid therapy guidelines for dogs and cats. *Journal of the American Animal Hospital Association* **49**, 149–159

DeFrancesco TC (2013) Management of cardiac emergencies in small animals. *Veterinary Clinics of North America: Small Animal Practice* **43**, 817–842

den Ouden DT and Meinders AE (2005) Vasopressin: physiology and clinical use in patients with vasodilatory shock: a review. *Netherlands Journal of Medicine* **63**, 4–13

Fletcher DJ, Boller M, Brainard BM *et al.* (2012) RECOVER evidence and knowledge gap analysis on veterinary CPR. Part 7: Clinical guidelines. *Journal of Veterinary Emergency and Critical Care* **22**, S102–S131

Jutkowitz LA (2004) Blood transfusion in the perioperative period. *Clinical Techniques in Small Animal Practice* **19**, 75–82

Long KM and Kirby R (2008) An update on cardiovascular adrenergic receptor physiology and potential pharmacological applications in veterinary critical care. *Journal of Veterinary Emergency and Critical Care* **18**, 2–25

Maton BL and Smarick SD (2012) Updates in the American Heart Association guidelines for cardiopulmonary resuscitation and potential applications to veterinary patients. *Journal of Veterinary Emergency and Critical Care* **22**, 148–159

Muir WW 3rd, Kijtawornrat A, Ueyama Y, Radecki SV and Hamlin RL (2011) Effects of intravenous administration of lactated Ringer's solution on hematologic, serum biochemical, rheological, hemodynamic, and renal measurements in healthy isoflurane-anesthetized dogs. *Journal of the American Veterinary Medical Association* **239**, 630–637

Pedro B, López-Alvarez J, Fonfara S, Stephenson H and Dukes-McEwan J (2012) Retrospective evaluation of the use of amiodarone in dogs with arrhythmias (2003–2010). *Journal of Small Animal Practice* **53**, 19–26

Plunkett SJ and McMichael M (2008) Cardiopulmonary resuscitation in small animal medicine: an update. *Journal of Veterinary Internal Medicine* **22**, 9–25

Rosati M, Dyson DH, Sinclair MD and Sears WC (2007) Response of hypotensive dogs to dopamine hydrochloride and dobutamine hydrochloride during deep isoflurane anesthesia. *American Journal of Veterinary Research* **68**, 483–494

Scroggin RD and Quandt J (2007) The use of vasopressin for treating vasodilatory shock and cardiopulmonary arrest. *Journal of Veterinary Emergency and Critical Care* **19**, 145–157

Shmuel DL and Cortes Y (2013) Anaphylaxis in dogs and cats. *Journal of Veterinary Emergency and Critical Care* **23**, 377–394

Silverstein DC and Hopper K (2015) *Small Animal Critical Care Medicine, 2nd edn.* Elsevier-Saunders, St. Louis, Missouri

Sinclair MD and Dyson DH (2012) The impact of acepromazine on the efficacy of crystalloid, dextran or ephedrine treatment in hypotensive dogs under isoflurane anesthesia. *Veterinary Anaesthesia and Analgesia* **39**, 563–573

Valverde A, Gianotti G, Rioja-Garcia and Hathway A (2012) Effects of high-volume, rapid-fluid therapy on cardiovascular function and hematological values during isoflurane-induced hypotension in healthy dogs. *Canadian Journal of Veterinary Research* **76**, 99–108

Wohl JS and Clark TP (2000) Pressor therapy in critically ill patients. *Journal of Veterinary Emergency and Critical Care* **10**, 21–34

Index

Page numbers in *italic* indicate figures